Diagnostic Medical Sonography

# ABDOMEN AND SUPERFICIAL STRUCTURES

## Diagnostic Medical Sonography

# ABDOMEN AND SUPERFICIAL STRUCTURES

### Third Edition

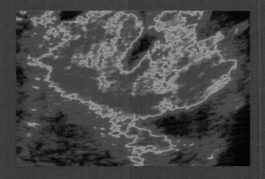

**Diane M. Kawamura, PhD, RT(R), RDMS**
Professor, Radiologic Sciences, Weber State University
Ogden, UT

**Bridgette M. Lunsford, MAEd, RVT, RDMS**
GE Healthcare - Ultrasound
Arlington, VA

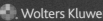 Wolters Kluwer | Lippincott Williams & Wilkins
Health
Philadelphia · Baltimore · New York · London
Buenos Aires · Hong Kong · Sydney · Tokyo

Publisher: Julie K. Stegman
Senior Product Manager: Heather Rybacki
Product Manager: Kristin Royer
Marketing Manager: Shauna Kelley
Design Coordinator: Joan Wendt
Art Director: Jennifer Clements
Manufacturing Coordinator: Margie Orzech
Production Services: Absolute Service, Inc.

351 West Camden Street
Baltimore, MD 21201

Two Commerce Square
2001 Market Street
Philadelphia, PA 19103

Third Edition

Printed in China.

**Library of Congress Cataloging-in-Publication Data**

Diagnostic medical sonography. Abdomen and superficial structures / edited by Diane M. Kawamura, Bridgette M. Lunsford. -- 3rd ed.
      p. ; cm.
   Abdomen and superficial structures
   Rev. ed. of: Abdomen and superficial structures / edited by Diane M. Kawamura. 2nd ed. c1997.
   Includes bibliographical references and index.
   ISBN 978-1-60547-995-8 (alk. paper)
   I. Kawamura, Diane M. II. Lunsford, Bridgette M. III. Title: Abdomen and superficial structures.
   [DNLM: 1. Abdomen--ultrasonography. 2. Digestive System--ultrasonography. 3. Ultrasonography--methods. 4. Urogenital System--ultrasonography. WI 900]

   617.5'5075--dc23

                      2011045980

Care has been taken to confirm the accuracy of the information presented and to describe generally accepted practices. However, the authors, editors, and publisher are not responsible for errors or omissions or for any consequences from application of the information in this book and make no warranty, express or implied, with respect to the contents of the publication. Application of the information in a particular situation remains the professional responsibility of the practitioner.

The authors, editors, and publisher have exerted every effort to ensure that drug selection and dosage set forth in this text are in accordance with current recommendations and practice at the time of publication. However, in view of ongoing research, changes in government regulations, and the constant flow of information relating to drug therapy and drug reactions, the reader is urged to check the package insert for each drug for any change in indications and dosage and for added warnings and precautions. This is particularly important when the recommended agent is a new or infrequently employed drug.

Some drugs and medical devices presented in this publication have Food and Drug Administration (FDA) clearance for limited use in restricted research settings. It is the responsibility of the health care providers to ascertain the FDA status of each drug or device planned for use in their clinical practice.

To purchase additional copies of this book, call our customer service department at (800) 638-3030 or fax orders to (301) 223-2320. International customers should call (301) 223-2300.
*Visit Lippincott Williams & Wilkins on the Internet* at **LWW.com**. Lippincott Williams & Wilkins customer service representatives are available from 8:30 AM to 6:00 PM, EST.

10   9   8   7   6

*To my husband, Bryan, for providing me with
confidence, for supporting my professional
endeavors, for giving of himself to help me, and
for being my favorite companion and best friend.
To our wonderful children, Stephanie and Nathan,
who continue to inspire me to appreciate
how important it is to learn new things.
To all my colleagues on campus and in the
profession who provide encouragement, support,
and stimulating new challenges.*

**Diane M. Kawamura**

*To my husband, James, with love and gratitude
for his constant support, encouragement, patience,
and understanding without which I would not
have had the courage to take on this task.
To my family for instilling a love of learning and
supporting me in all of my endeavors.
To my colleagues at GE from whom I have learned
so much and who continue to inspire me on a
daily basis to expand my knowledge and take on
new challenges.*

**Bridgette M. Lunsford**

*And to students and professionals
who will use this book:
"Any piece of knowledge I acquire today has a
value at this moment exactly proportioned to my
skill to deal with it. Tomorrow, when I know more,
I recall that piece of knowledge and use it better."*
—Mark Van Doren, *Liberal Education* (1960)

**DMK, BML**

# Contents

# Acknowledgments

Throughout the process, we appreciated the support and enthusiasm from Anne Marie Kupinski and Susan Stephenson as we collaborated on the three volumes of *Diagnostic Medical Sonography*. Their input and ideas were a significant contribution to the project.

Our thanks and gratitude goes to all the contributors of the third edition who gave of their expertise, time, and energy updating the content with current information to utilize in obtaining a more accurate imaging examination for our patients.

The image contributions became treasured moments. We thank the many sonographers and physicians for their assistance. A special thank you and recognition for ongoing support in image acquisition includes Taco Geertsma, MD, Ede, the Netherlands at Ultrasoundcases. info; Philips Medical Systems, Bothell, WA; GE Healthcare, Wauwatosa, WI; Joe Anton, MD, Cochin, India; Dr. Nakul Jerath, Falls Church, VA; and from Monica Bacani and Rechelle Nguyen at Nationwide Children's Hospital in Columbus, OH.

Many thanks to all of the production team at Lippincott Williams & Wilkins who helped edit, produce, promote, and deliver this textbook. We especially thank in the development of this edition Peter Sabatini, acquisitions editor, Kristin Royer, associate product manager, Jennifer Clements, art director, and Carol Gudanowski, illustrator, for their patience, follow-through, support, and encouragement.

To our colleagues, students, friends, and family, who provide continued sources of encouragement, enthusiasm, and inspiration, thank you.

**Diane M. Kawamura, PhD, RT(R), RDMS**
**Bridgette M. Lunsford, MAEd, RVT, RDMS**

# Preface

The third edition of *Diagnostic Medical Sonography: Abdomen and Superficial Structures* is a major revision. Educators and colleagues encouraged us to produce a third edition to incorporate new advances used to image, to refresh the foundational content, and to continue to provide information that recognizes readers have diverse backgrounds and experiences. The result is a textbook that can be used as either an introduction to the profession or as a reference for the profession. The content lays the foundation for a better understanding of anatomy, physiology, and pathophysiology to enhance the caregiving role of the sonographer practitioner, sonographer, sonologist, or student when securing the imaging information on a patient.

The first chapter introduces terminology on anatomy, scanning planes, and patient positions. Adopting universal terminology permits every sonographer to communicate consistent information on how he or she positioned the patient, how he or she scanned the patient, and how anatomy and pathology are sonographically represented.

The next four sections are divided into specific content areas. Doing this allowed the contributors to focus their attention on a specific organ or system. This simulates application in that while scanning, the sonographer investigates the organ or system, moves systematically to the next organ or system, and completes the examination by synthesizing all of the information to obtain the total picture.

We made every attempt to produce an up-to-date and factual textbook while presenting the material in an interesting and enjoyable format to capture the reader's attention. To do this, we provided detailed descriptions of anatomy, physiology, pathology, and the normal and abnormal sonographic representation of these anatomical and pathologic entities with illustrations, summary tables, and images, many of which include valuable case study information.

Our goal is to present as complete and up-to-date a text as possible, while recognizing that by tomorrow, the textbook must be supplemented with new information reflecting the dynamic sonography profession. With every technologic advance made in equipment, the sonographer's imagination must stretch to create new applications. With the comprehensive foundation available in this text, the sonographer can meet that challenge.

**Diane M. Kawamura, PhD, RT(R), RDMS**
**Bridgette M. Lunsford, MAEd, RVT, RDMS**

# Contributors

**Monica M. Bacani, RDMS**
Clinical Manager - Ultrasound
Nationwide Children's Hospital
Columbus, OH

**Heidi S. Barrett, RT(R), RDMS, RVT, RDCS**
Clinical Specialist – SF Bay Area
SonoSite, Inc.
San Francisco, CA

**Teresa M. Bieker, MBA-H, RT(R), RDMS, RDCS, RVT**
Department of Ultrasound
University of Colorado Hospital
Aurora, CO

**Kari E. Boyce, PhD, RDMS**
College of Allied Health
The University of Oklahoma
Oklahoma City, OK

**Joie Burns, MS, RT(R)(S), RDMS, RVT**
Sonography Program Director
Boise State University
Boise, ID

**Catherine Carr-Hoefer, BS, RT(R), RDMS, RDCS, RVT**
Assistant Manager, Diagnostic Imaging
Good Samaritan Regional Medical Center
Corvallis, OR

**Julia A. Drose, BA, RDMS, RDCS**
Department of Ultrasound
University of Colorado Hospital
Aurora, CO

**Kevin D. Evans, PhD, RT(R)(M)(BD), RDMS**
School of Allied Medical Professions
The Ohio State University
Columbus, OH

**Tim S. Gibbs, RT(R), RDMS, RVT, CTNM**
Ultrasound Supervisor
West Anaheim Medical Center
Anaheim, CA

**Joyce A. Grube, MS, RDMS**
Sonography Education Consultant
Jamestown, OH

**Kathleen Marie Hannon, RN, MS, RVT, RDMS**
Vascular Diagnostic Laboratory
Massachusetts General Hospital
Boston, MA

**Charlotte Henningsen, MS, RT(R), RDMS, RVT**
Chair and Professor, Sonography
    Department
Florida Hospital College
Orlando, FL

**Terri L. Jurkiewicz, MS, RT(R)(M), RDMS, RVT**
Assistant Professor, Radiologic Sciences
Weber State University
Ogden, UT

**Diane M. Kawamura, PhD, RT(R), RDMS**
Professor, Radiologic Sciences
Weber State University
Ogden, UT

**George M. Kennedy, AS, RT(R), RDMS, RDCS, RVT**
Department of Ultrasound
University of Colorado Hospital
Aurora, CO

**Zulfikarali H. Lalani, RDMS, RDCS**
Senior Staff Sonographer and
    Clinical Instructor
Alta Bates Summit Medical Center
Oakland, CA

**Wayne C. Leonhardt, BA, RDMS, RVT, APS**
Lead Sonographer, Technical Director, CE
    Coordinator
Alta Bates Summit Medical Center
Oakland, CA

**Bridgette M. Lunsford, MAEd, RVT, RDMS**
Clinical Applications Specialist
GE Healthcare - Ultrasound
Arlington, VA

**Janice L. McGinnis, RDMS**
Ultrasound Department
Bay Area Hospital
Coos Bay, OR

**Patrick R. Meyers, BS, RT(R), RDMS**
Owner
Musculoskeletal Ultrasound of SE WI LLC
Mequon, WI

**J.P. Moreland, RT(R)(CT), RDMS, RVS**
Director, Customer Education
GE Healthcare - Ultrasound
San Francisco, CA

**Rechelle A. Nguyen, RDMS**
Department of Ultrasound
Nationwide Children's Hospital
Columbus, OH

**Tanya D. Nolan, MAEd, RT(R), RDMS**
Assistant Professor, Radiologic Sciences
Weber State University
Ogden, UT

**Aubrey J. Rybyinski, BS, RDMS, RVT**
Ultrasound Section
The Hospital of the University of
 Pennsylvania
Philadelphia, PA

**Christine Schara, BS, RT(R)(N), RDMS**
Program Chair, Diagnostic Medical
 Sonography
Athens Technical College
Athens, GA

**Cathie Scholl, BS, RDMS, RVT**
Ohio Health Westerville Medical Campus
Westerville, OH

**Regina K. Swearengin, AAS, BS, RDMS**
Department Chair, Sonography
Austin Community College
Austin, TX

**John F. Trombly, MS, RT(R), RDMS, RVT**
Director, Medical Imaging Education
Red Rocks Community College
Arvada, CO

**Michelle Wilson, MS, RDMS, RDCS**
Instructional Designer
Sonography Sessions, L.L.C
Distance Education Specialists
Napa, CA

# Using This Series

The books in the *Diagnostic Medical Sonography* Series will help you develop an understanding of specialty sonography topics. Key learning resources and tools throughout the textbook aim to increase your understanding of the topics provided and better prepare you for your professional career. This User's Guide will help you familiarize yourself with these exciting features designed to enhance your learning experience.

## 18 Abnormalities of the Placenta and Umbilical Cord

Lisa M. Allen

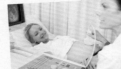

### OBJECTIVES

Recognize the sonographic appearance of placental and umbilical cord anomalies

Discuss developmental variations in placental size, shape, and configuration

Identify placenta previa classifications

Explain placental abruption and the associated risk factors

List placenta accreta classifications and known risk factors

Name the various abnormalities of umbilical cord insertion into the placenta

Describe cystic and solid masses of the umbilical cord

### KEY TERMS

succenturiate lobe | circummarginate placenta | circumvallate placenta | placenta previa | placental abruption | placenta accreta spectrum | chorioangioma | amniotic band syndrome | uterine synechiae | marginal insertion | battledore placenta | velamentous insertion | true knot | false knot | nuchal cord | cord prolapse | vasa previa | single umbilical artery | cord entanglement | umbilical cord hemangioma | umbilical cord coiling | umbilical coiling index

### GLOSSARY

**Aneurysm** Focal dilatation of an artery

**Bilobed placenta** Placenta where the lobes are nearly equal in size and the cord inserts into the chorionic bridge of tissue that connects the two lobes

**Body stalk anomaly** Fatal condition associated with multiple congenital anomalies and absence of the umbilical cord

**Breus' mole** Very rare condition where there is massive subchorionic thrombosis of the placenta secondary to extreme venous obstruction

**Extrachorial placenta** Attachment of the placental membranes to the fetal surface of the placenta rather than to the underlying villous placental margin

**False knot** Bending, twisting, and bulging of the umbilical cord vessels mimicking a knot in the umbilical cord

**Gastroschisis** Periumbilical abdominal wall defect, typically to the right of normal cord insertion, that allows for free-floating bowel in the amniotic fluid

**Limb–body wall complex** Condition characterized by multiple complex fetal anomalies and a short umbilical cord

**Marginal insertion (a.k.a. battledore placenta)** Occurs when the umbilical cord inserts at the placental margin instead of centrally

**Mickey Mouse sign** Term used to describe the cross-section of the three-vessel umbilical cord or the portal triad (portal vein, hepatic artery, common bile duct)

**Omphalocele** Central anterior abdominal wall defect of the umbilicus where abdominal organs are contained by a covering membrane consisting of peritoneum, Wharton's jelly, and amnion

**Placentomegaly** Term that refers to a thickened placenta

**Synechia (Asherman's syndrome)** Linear, extra amniotic tissue that projects into the amniotic cavity with no restriction of fetal movement

**Thrombosis** Intraplacental area of hemorrhage and clot

**True knot** Result of the fetus actually passing through a loop or loops of umbilical cord creating one or more knots in the cord

425

## CHAPTER OBJECTIVES

Measurable objectives listed at the beginning of each chapter help you understand the intended outcomes for the chapter, as well as recognize and study important concept within each chapter.

## GLOSSARY

Key terms are listed at the beginning of each chapter and clearly defined, then highlighted in bold type throughout the chapter to help you to learn and recall important terminology.

## PATHOLOGY BOXES

Each chapter includes tables of relevant pathologies, which you can use as a quick reference for reviewing the material.

## CRITICAL THINKING QUESTIONS

Throughout the chapter are critical thinking questions to test your knowledge and help you develop analytical skills that you will need in your profession.

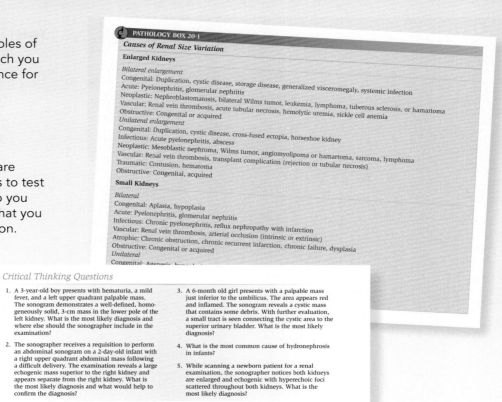

**PATHOLOGY BOX 20-1**

### Causes of Renal Size Variation

**Enlarged Kidneys**

*Bilateral enlargement*
Congenital: Duplication, cystic disease, storage disease, generalized visceromegaly, systemic infection
Acute: Pyelonephritis, glomerular nephritis
Neoplastic: Nephroblastomatosis, bilateral Wilms tumor, leukemia, lymphoma, tuberous sclerosis, or hamartoma
Vascular: Renal vein thrombosis, acute tubular necrosis, hemolytic uremia, sickle cell anemia
Obstructive: Congenital or acquired

*Unilateral enlargement*
Congenital: Duplication, cystic disease, cross-fused ectopia, horseshoe kidney
Infectious: Acute pyelonephritis, abscess
Neoplastic: Mesoblastic nephroma, Wilms tumor, angiomyolipoma or hamartoma, sarcoma, lymphoma
Vascular: Renal vein thrombosis, transplant complication (rejection or tubular necrosis)
Traumatic: Contusion, hematoma
Obstructive: Congenital, acquired

**Small Kidneys**

*Bilateral*
Congenital: Aplasia, hypoplasia
Acute: Pyelonephritis, glomerular nephritis
Infectious: Chronic pyelonephritis, reflux nephropathy with infarction
Vascular: Renal vein thrombosis, arterial occlusion (intrinsic or extrinsic)
Atrophic: Chronic obstruction, chronic recurrent infarction, chronic failure, dysplasia
Obstructive: Congenital or acquired

*Unilateral*
Congenital: Agenesis, hypoplasia

### Critical Thinking Questions

1. A 3-year-old boy presents with hematuria, a mild fever, and a left upper quadrant palpable mass. The sonogram demonstrates a well-defined, homogeneously solid, 3-cm mass in the lower pole of the left kidney. What is the most likely diagnosis and where else should the sonographer include in the examination?

2. The sonographer receives a requisition to perform an abdominal sonogram on a 2-day-old infant with a right upper quadrant abdominal mass following a difficult delivery. The examination reveals a large echogenic mass superior to the right kidney and appears separate from the right kidney. What is the most likely diagnosis and what would help to confirm the diagnosis?

3. A 6-month old girl presents with a palpable mass just inferior to the umbilicus. The area appears red and inflamed. The sonogram reveals a cystic mass that contains some debris. With further evaluation, a small tract is seen connecting the cystic area to the superior urinary bladder. What is the most likely diagnosis?

4. What is the most common cause of hydronephrosis in infants?

5. While scanning a newborn patient for a renal examination, the sonographer notices both kidneys are enlarged and echogenic with hyperechoic foci scattered throughout both kidneys. What is the most likely diagnosis?

## RESOURCES

You will also find additional resources and exercises online, including a glossary with pronunciations, quiz bank, sonographic video clips, and weblinks. Use these interactive resources to test your knowledge, assess your progress, and review for quizzes and tests.

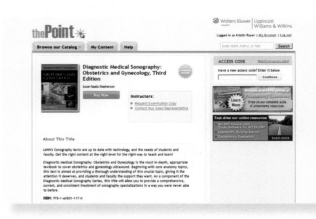

# 1 Introduction

Diane M. Kawamura

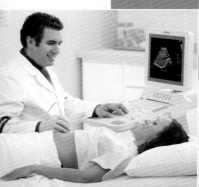

## OBJECTIVES

Identify anatomic definitions in regard to directional terms, anatomic position, and anatomic planes.

Demonstrate the sonographic examination to include patient position, transducer orientation, and image presentation and labeling.

Define the terms used to describe image quality.

Describe the sonographic echo patterns to demonstrate how normal and pathologic conditions can be defined using image quality definitions.

List and recognize the sonographic criteria for cystic, solid, and complex conditions.

Describe the appropriate patient preparation for a sonographic evaluation.

State what should and what should not be included in a preliminary report.

Calculate sensitivity, specificity, and accuracy using the four outcomes of true-positive, false-positive, true-negative, and/or false-negative.

## KEY TERMS

accuracy | anechoic | coronal plane | echogenic | echopenic | heterogeneous | homogeneous | hyperechoic | hypoechoic | isoechoic | sagittal plane | sensitivity | specificity | transverse plane

## GLOSSARY

**anechoic** describes the portion of an image that appears echo-free

**echogenic** describes an organ or tissue that is capable of producing echoes by reflecting the acoustic beam

**echopenic** describes a structure that is less echogenic or has few internal echoes

**heterogeneous** describes tissue or organ structures that have several different echo characteristics

**homogeneous** refers to imaged echoes of equal intensity

**hyperechoic** describes image echoes brighter than surrounding tissues or brighter than is normal for that tissue or organ

**hypoechoic** describes portions of an image that are not as bright as surrounding tissues or are less bright than normal

**isoechoic** describes structures of equal echo density

This chapter focuses on the sonography examination of the abdomen and superficial structures. It was written to assist sonographers in acquiring, using, and understanding the sonographic imaging terminology used in the remainder of this textbook. Accurate and precise terminology allows communication among professionals.

## ANATOMIC DEFINITIONS

The profession adopted standard nomenclature from the anatomists' terminology to communicate anatomic direction. Table 1-1 and Figure 1-1 illustrate how these simple terms help avoid confusion and convey specific information. A person in the conventional anatomic position is standing erect, feet together, with the arms by the sides and the palms and face directed forward, facing the observer. When sonographers use directional terms or describe regions or anatomic planes, it is assumed that the body is in the anatomic position.

There are three standard anatomic planes (sections) that are imaginary flat surfaces passing through a body in the standard anatomic position. The sagittal plane and coronal plane follow the long axis of the body and the transverse plane follows the short axis of the body[1] (Fig. 1-2).

**TABLE** **1-1**

Directional Terms

| Term | Definition | Example |
|---|---|---|
| Superior (cranial) | Toward the head, closer to the head, the upper portion of the body, the upper part of a structure, or a structure higher than another structure | The left adrenal gland is superior to the left kidney |
| Inferior (caudal) | Toward the feet, away from the head, the lower portion of the body, toward the lower part of a structure, or a structure lower than another structure | The lower pole of each kidney is inferior to the upper pole |
| Anterior (ventral) | Toward the front or at the front of the body or a structure in front of another structure | The main portal vein is anterior to the inferior vena cava |
| Posterior (dorsal) | Toward the back or the back of the body or a structure behind another structure | The main portal vein is posterior to the common hepatic artery |
| Medial | Toward the middle or midline of the body or the middle of a structure | The middle vein is medial to the right hepatic vein |
| Lateral | Away from the middle or the midline of the body or pertaining to the side | The right kidney is lateral to the inferior vena cava |
| Ipsilateral | Located on the same side of the body or affecting the same side of the body | The gallbladder and right kidney are ipsilateral |
| Contralateral | Located on the opposite side of the body or affecting the opposite side of the body | The pancreatic tail and pancreatic head are contralateral |
| Proximal | Closer to the attachment of an extremity to the trunk or the origin of a body part | The abdominal aorta is proximal to the bifurcation of the iliac arteries |
| Distal | Farther from the attachment of an extremity to the trunk or the origin of a body part | The iliac arteries are distal to the abdominal aorta |
| Superficial | Toward or on the body surface or external | The thyroid and breast are considered superficial structures |
| Deep | Away from the body surface or internal | The peritoneal organs and great vessels are deep structures |

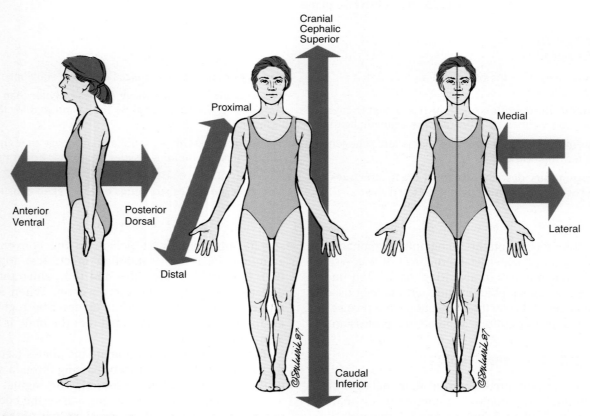

**Figure 1-1** Directional terms. The drawing depicts a body in the anatomic position (standing erect, arms by the side, face and palms directed forward) with the directional terms. The directional terms correlate with the terms in Table 1-1.

The word *sagittal* literally means "flight of an arrow" and refers to the plane that runs vertically through the body and separates it into right and left portions. The plane that divides the body into equal right and left halves is referred to as the median sagittal or midsagittal plane. Any vertical plane on either side of the midsagittal plane is a parasagittal plane (para means "alongside of"). In most sonography cases, the term sagittal usually implies a parasagittal plane unless the term is specified as median sagittal or midsagittal. The coronal plane runs vertically through the body from right to left or left to right, and divides the body into anterior and posterior portions. The transverse plane passes through the body from anterior to posterior and divides the body into superior and inferior portions and runs parallel to the surface of the ground.

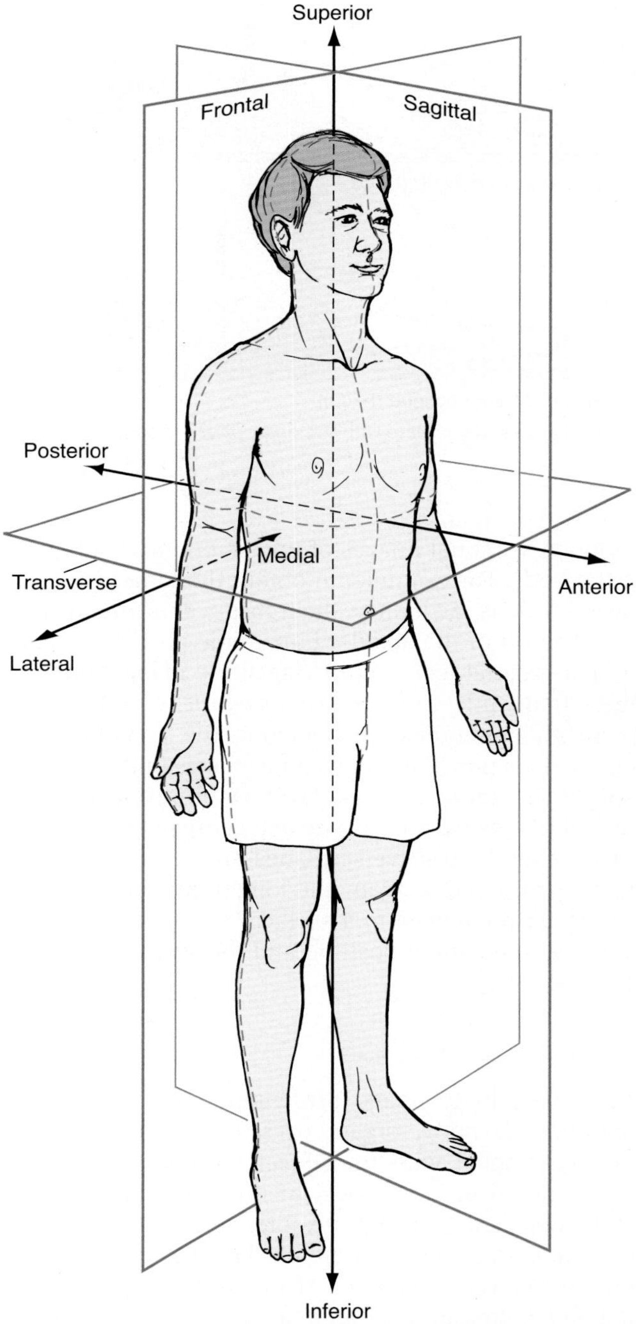

## SCANNING DEFINITIONS

### PATIENT POSITION

*Positional terms* refer to the patient's position relative to the surrounding space. For sonographic examinations, the patient position is described relative to the scanning table or bed (Table 1-2, Fig. 1-3). In clinical practice, patients are scanned in a recumbent, semierect (reverse Trendelenburg or Fowler), or sitting position. On occasion, patients may be placed in other positions, such as the Trendelenburg (head lowered) or standing position, to obtain unobscured images of the area of interest. Sonographers frequently convey information on patient position and transducer placement simultaneously. This terminology most likely was adopted from radiography, where it describes the path of the X-ray beam through the patient's body (*projection*), which results in a radiographic image (*view*). There is no evidence in the literature that this nomenclature has been adopted as a professional standard for sonographic imaging.

Figure 1-2 Anatomic planes. The standard anatomic position is used to depict the three imaginary anatomic flat surface planes. Both the sagittal and coronal planes pass through the long axis and the transverse plane passes through the short axis.

| TABLE 1-2 | |
|---|---|
| **Patient Positions** | |
| **Term** | **Description** |
| **Decubitus or Recumbent** | The act of lying down. The adjective before the word describes the most dependent body surface. |
| Supine or dorsal | Lying on the back |
| Prone or ventral | Lying face down |
| Right lateral decubitus (RLD) | Lying on the right side |
| Left lateral decubitus (LLD) | Lying on the left side |
| **Oblique** | Named for the body side closest to the scanning table. |
| Right posterior oblique (RPO) | Lying on the right posterior surface, the left posterior surface is elevated |
| Left posterior oblique (LPO) | Lying on the left posterior surface, the right posterior surface is elevated |
| Right anterior oblique (RAO) | Lying on the right anterior surface, the left anterior surface is elevated |
| Left anterior oblique (LAO) | Lying on the left anterior surface, the right anterior surface is elevated |

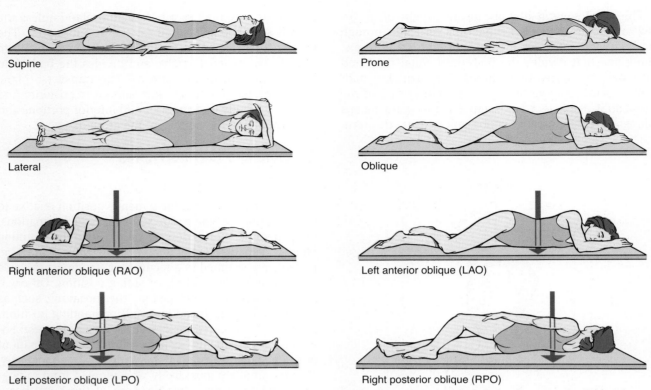

**Figure 1-3** Patient positions. The various patient positions depicted in the illustration correlate with the descriptions in Table 1-2.

Describing sonograms using the terms projection or view should be avoided. It is more accurate to describe the sonographic image stating the anatomic plane visualized, which is due to the transducer's orientation (i.e., transverse). A more specific description of the image would include both the anatomic plane and the patient position (i.e., transverse, oblique).

## TRANSDUCER ORIENTATION

The transducer's orientation is the path of the insonating sound and the path returning echoes are viewed on the monitor. Transducers are manufactured with an indicator (notch, groove, light) that is displayed on the monitor as a dot, arrow, letter of the manufacturer's insignia, and so forth. *Scanning plane* is the term used to describe the transducer's orientation to the anatomic plane or to the specific organ or structure. The *sonographic image* is a representation of sectional anatomy. The term *plane* combined with the adjectives sagittal, parasagittal, coronal, and transverse describes the section of anatomy represented on the image (e.g., transverse plane).

Because many organs and structures lie oblique to the imaginary body surface planes, sonographers must identify sectional anatomy accurately to utilize a specific organ and structure orientation for scanning surfaces. The sonography imaging equipment provides great flexibility to rock, slide, and angle the transducer to obtain sectional images of organs oriented obliquely in the body. For example, to obtain the long axis of an organ, such as the kidney, the transducer is oblique and is angled off of the standard anatomic positions: sagittal, parasagittal, coronal, or transverse plane. Sonographers frequently use the terms *sagittal* or *parasagittal* to mean longitudinal in depicting the anatomy in a long-axis section. Although some images in this text are labeled sagittal or parasagittal, they are, in fact, longitudinal planes because the image is organ specific. For organ imaging, transverse planes are perpendicular to the long axis of the organ, and longitudinal and coronal planes are referenced to a surface. All three planes are based on the patient position and the scanning surface (Fig. 1-4A–C).

## IMAGE PRESENTATION

When describing image presentation on the display monitor, the body, organ, or structure plane terminology, coupled with transducer placement, provides a very descriptive portrayal of the sectional anatomy being depicted. Current flexible, free-hand scanning techniques may lack automatic labeling of the scanning plane. With free-hand scanning technique, quantitative labeling may be limited, which means reduced image reproducibility from one sonographer to another sonographer. Sonographers usually can select from a wide array of protocols for image annotation or employ

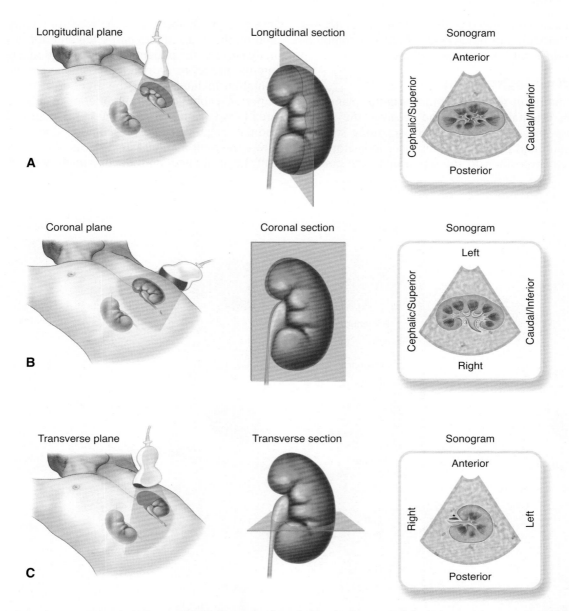

**Figure 1-4** Transducer orientation. **A.** A parasagittal plane provides a longitudinal section of the kidney on the sonogram. **B.** The coronal plane provides a coronal section on the sonogram. **C.** The transverse plane provides a transverse section on the sonogram. The sonogram is the image the sonographer observes on the monitor.

postprocessing annotation. This is extremely important when the image of an isolated area does not provide other anatomic structures for a reference location. To ensure consistent practice, sonographers must correctly label all sonograms. With today's equipment, standard presentation and labeling is easily achieved along with additional labeling of specific structures and added comment.

The anterior, posterior, right, or left body surface is usually scanned in the sagittal (parasagittal), coronal, and transverse scanning planes. For organ or structure imaging, these same body surfaces are scanned with different angulations and obliqueness of the transducer to obtain longitudinal, coronal, or transverse scanning planes. With few exceptions, the transducer at the scanning surface is presented at the top of the image.[1,2] Images obtained using an endovaginal probe are usually flipped so that they are presented in the more traditional transabdominal transducer orientation, whereas images obtained using an endorectal probe are presented in the transducer-organ orientation. With neurosonography (neurosonology), the superior scanning surface is presented at the top of the image when the transducer is placed on the head.

These six scanning surfaces, anterior or posterior, right or left, endocavitary (vaginal or rectal), and the cranial fontanelle coupled with three anatomic planes (sagittal, coronal, and transverse) produce a combination of 14 different image presentations.

### Longitudinal: Sagittal Planes

When scanning in the longitudinal, sagittal plane, the transducer orientation sends and receives the sound from either an anterior or posterior scanning surface. For a longitudinal plane, the transducer indicator is in the 12 o'clock position to the organ or to the area of interest. This always places the superior (cephalic) location on the image. From either the anterior or posterior body surface, the patient can be scanned in either erect, supine, prone, or an oblique position. The image presentation includes either the anterior or posterior, the superior (cephalic), and the inferior (caudal) anatomic area being examined[1,2] (Fig. 1-5A). Because the longitudinal, sagittal image presentation does not demonstrate the right and left lateral areas, the adjacent areas can be evaluated and documented with transducer

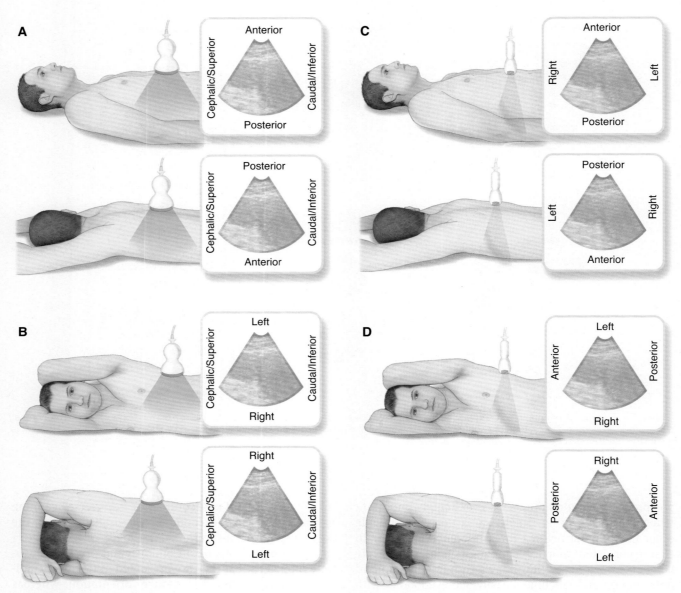

**Figure 1-5** Image presentations. **A.** Longitudinal, sagittal plane. With the patient being scanned from either the anterior or posterior surface with or without obliquity, the image seen on the monitor demonstrates the scanning surface (anterior or posterior) and the superior (cephalic) and inferior (caudal) area being examined. **B.** Longitudinal, coronal plane. With the patient being scanned from either the right or left surface with or without obliquity, the image seen on the monitor demonstrates the scanning surface (right or left) and the superior (cephalic) and inferior (caudal) area being examined. **C.** Transverse plane, anterior or posterior surface. With the patient being scanned from either the anterior or posterior surface with or without obliquity, the image seen on the monitor demonstrates the scanning surface (anterior or posterior) and the right and left area being examined. **D.** Transverse plane, right or left surface. With the patient being scanned from either the right or left surface with or without obliquity, the image seen on the monitor demonstrates the scanning surface (right or left) and the anterior and posterior area being examined. *(Continued)*

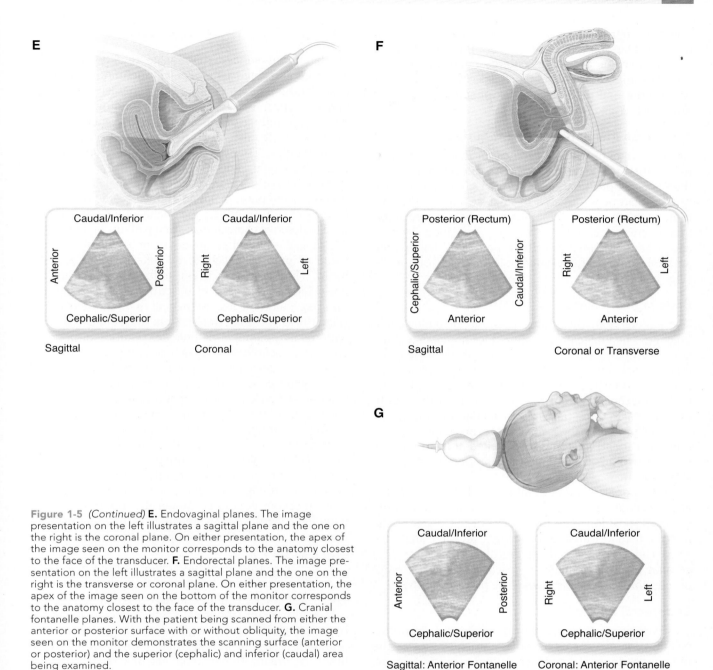

**E**

Caudal/Inferior

Anterior — Posterior

Cephalic/Superior

Sagittal

Caudal/Inferior

Right — Left

Cephalic/Superior

Coronal

**F**

Posterior (Rectum)

Cephalic/Superior — Caudal/Inferior

Anterior

Sagittal

Posterior (Rectum)

Right — Left

Anterior

Coronal or Transverse

**G**

Caudal/Inferior

Anterior — Posterior

Cephalic/Superior

Sagittal: Anterior Fontanelle

Caudal/Inferior

Right — Left

Cephalic/Superior

Coronal: Anterior Fontanelle

**Figure 1-5** *(Continued)* **E.** Endovaginal planes. The image presentation on the left illustrates a sagittal plane and the one on the right is the coronal plane. On either presentation, the apex of the image seen on the monitor corresponds to the anatomy closest to the face of the transducer. **F.** Endorectal planes. The image presentation on the left illustrates a sagittal plane and the one on the right is the transverse or coronal plane. On either presentation, the apex of the image seen on the bottom of the monitor corresponds to the anatomy closest to the face of the transducer. **G.** Cranial fontanelle planes. With the patient being scanned from either the anterior or posterior surface with or without obliquity, the image seen on the monitor demonstrates the scanning surface (anterior or posterior) and the superior (cephalic) and inferior (caudal) area being examined.

manipulation, changing the transducer orientation, or changing the patient position.[2]

## Longitudinal: Coronal Planes

When scanning in the longitudinal, coronal plane, the transducer orientation sends and receives the sound from either the right or left scanning surface. Because the transducer indicator is in the 12 o'clock position to the organ or to the area of interest, the superior (cephalic) location is always imaged. From either the right or left body surface, the patient can be scanned in either an erect, decubitus, or an oblique position and the image presentation includes either the left or right,

the superior (cephalic), and the inferior (caudal) anatomic area being examined[1,2] (Fig. 1-5B). Because the longitudinal, coronal image presentation does not demonstrate the anterior or posterior areas, the adjacent areas can be evaluated and documented with transducer manipulation, changing the transducer orientation, or changing the patient position.[2]

## Transverse Plane: Anterior or Posterior Surface

Using the anterior or posterior surface, the transducer orientation for a transverse plane places the transducer indicator in the 9 o'clock position on either the anterior or posterior surface to the organ or to the area of interest.

The right and left location is always imaged. From either the anterior or posterior surfaces, the patient can be scanned in either an erect, decubitus, or an oblique position. The image presentation includes either the anterior or posterior and the right and left anatomic area being examined[1,2] (Fig. 1-5C).

### Transverse Plane: Right or Left Surface

Using the right or left surface, the transducer orientation for a transverse plane places the transducer indicator in the 9 o'clock position on either the right or left surface to the organ or to the area of interest. From either the right or left surfaces, the patient can be scanned in either an erect, decubitus, or an oblique position. The image presentation includes either the right or left and the anterior and posterior anatomic area being examined[1,2] (Fig. 1-5D).

### Endovaginal Planes

The patient is in the supine position for endovaginal imaging. The image presentation does not change if the system employs either an end-firing or an angle-firing endovaginal transducer. For the sagittal (longitudinal) plane, the transducer is placed at the caudal end of the body with the indicator in the 12 o'clock position. Both the endovaginal sagittal and translabial transducer orientation produces the same image presentation. The inferior (caudal) anatomy is presented at the top of the monitor with visualization of the anterior and posterior anatomic areas.

The coronal plane is obtained with the transducer at the caudal end of the body and the indicator in the 9 o'clock position. The top (apex) of the image is the inferior (caudal) area and the right and left anatomic areas can be visualized on the display monitor. The coronal plane is sometimes described using an older description reference to transverse plane[1] (Fig. 1-5E).

### Endorectal Planes

The patient is most often in a left lateral decubitus position for placement of either the end-firing or the bi-plane endorectal transducer. When used for biopsy, both the end-firing and bi-plane endorectal transducer place the biopsy guide anterior toward the prostate. For either the sagittal plane or the transverse or coronal planes, the anterior rectal wall is the scanning surface and is assigned to the bottom of the display monitor (Fig. 1-5F).

### Cranial Fontanelle Planes

For neonatal brain examinations, the sagittal and coronal planes are most commonly accessed using the anterior fontanelle. For the sagittal plane, the transducer indicator is in the 6 o'clock position and indicates the anterior side of the brain. For the coronal plane, the transducer indicator is in the 9 o'clock position and indicates the right side of the brain (Fig. 1-5G).

## IMAGE QUALITY DEFINITIONS

Evaluation of sonographic image quality is learned and communicated using specific definitions. Normal tissue and organ structures have a characteristic echographic appearance relative to surrounding structures. An understanding of the normal appearance provides the baseline against which to recognize variations and abnormalities. These definitions describe and characterize the sonographic image.

An *echo* is the recorded acoustic signal. It is the reflection of the pulse of sound emitted by the transducer. Prefixes or suffixes modify the quality of the echo and are used to describe characteristics and patterns on the image.

*Echogenic* describes an organ or tissue that is capable of producing echoes by reflecting the acoustic beam. This term does not describe the quality of the image; it is often used to describe relative tissue texture (e.g., more or less echogenic than another tissue) (Fig. 1-6A,B). An aberration from normal echogenicity patterns may signify a pathologic condition or poor examination technique such as incorrect gain settings.

*Anechoic* describes the portion of an image that appears echo-free. A urine-filled bladder, a bile-filled gallbladder, and a clear cyst all appear anechoic (Fig. 1-6C). *Sonolucent* is the property of a medium allowing easy passage of sound (i.e., low attenuation). Sonolucent or transonic are misnomers that are often substituted for anechoic.[3] When the sonographic appearance is anechoic, sonographers frequently use the term *cystic*. When describing the appearance of the echo, the term anechoic is correct. When describing the histopathologic nature of an anechoic structure, cystic or cyst-like is correct (see "Interpretation of Sonographic Characteristics").

If the scattering amplitude changes from one tissue to another, it results in brightness changes on an image. These brightness changes require terminology to describe normal and abnormal sonographic appearances. *Hyperechoic* describes image echoes brighter than surrounding tissues or brighter than normal for a specific tissue or organ. Hyperechoic regions result from an increased amount of sound scatter relative to the surrounding tissue. *Hypoechoic* describes portions of an image that are not as bright as surrounding tissues or less bright than normal. The hypoechoic regions result from reduced sound scatter relative to the surrounding tissue. *Echopenic* describes a structure that is less echogenic than others or has few internal echoes. *Isoechoic* describes structures of equal echo density. These terms can be used to compare echo textures (Fig. 1-6D).

*Homogeneous* refers to imaged echoes of equal intensity. A homogeneous portion of the image may be anechoic, hypoechoic, hyperechoic, or echopenic. *Heterogeneous* describes tissue or organ structures that have several different echo characteristics. A normal liver, spleen, or testicle has a homogeneous echo texture,

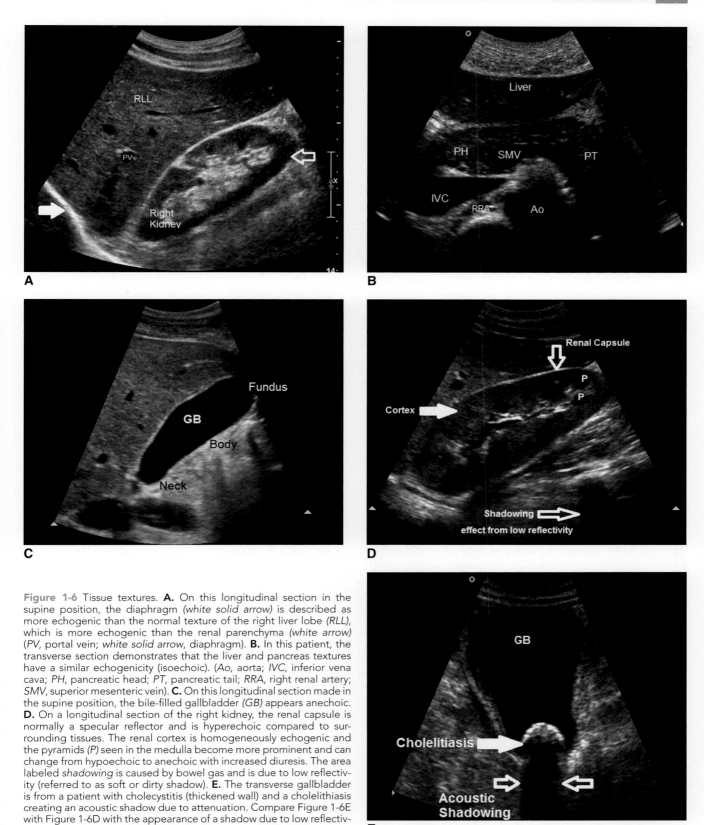

**Figure 1-6** Tissue textures. **A.** On this longitudinal section in the supine position, the diaphragm *(white solid arrow)* is described as more echogenic than the normal texture of the right liver lobe *(RLL)*, which is more echogenic than the renal parenchyma *(white arrow)* *(PV,* portal vein; *white solid arrow,* diaphragm). **B.** In this patient, the transverse section demonstrates that the liver and pancreas textures have a similar echogenicity (isoechoic). *(Ao,* aorta; *IVC,* inferior vena cava; *PH,* pancreatic head; *PT,* pancreatic tail; *RRA,* right renal artery; *SMV,* superior mesenteric vein). **C.** On this longitudinal section made in the supine position, the bile-filled gallbladder *(GB)* appears anechoic. **D.** On a longitudinal section of the right kidney, the renal capsule is normally a specular reflector and is hyperechoic compared to surrounding tissues. The renal cortex is homogeneously echogenic and the pyramids *(P)* seen in the medulla become more prominent and can change from hypoechoic to anechoic with increased diuresis. The area labeled *shadowing* is caused by bowel gas and is due to low reflectivity (referred to as soft or dirty shadow). **E.** The transverse gallbladder is from a patient with cholecystitis (thickened wall) and a cholelithiasis creating an acoustic shadow due to attenuation. Compare Figure 1-6E with Figure 1-6D with the appearance of a shadow due to low reflectivity. (Images courtesy of Philips Medical System, Bothell, WA.)

whereas a normal kidney is heterogeneous, with several different echo textures.

*Acoustic enhancement* is the increased acoustic signal amplitude that returns from regions lying beyond an object that causes little or no attenuation of the sound beam such as fluid-filled structures. The opposite of acoustic enhancement is acoustic shadowing and both are types of sonographic artifacts. *Acoustic shadowing* describes reduced echo amplitude from regions lying beyond an attenuating object. An example is cholelithiasis, which does not allow any sound to pass through (it is attenuated) causing a sharp, distinctive shadow (Fig. 1-6E). Air bubbles (bowel gas) do not allow transmission of the sound beam and most of the sound is reflected.[4] Often, sonographers refer to the shadowing caused by low reflectivity as soft or dirty shadowing.

## INTERPRETATION OF SONOGRAPHIC CHARACTERISTICS

Three other definitions are frequently used to describe internal echo patterns: cystic, solid, and complex.

The diagnosis of a cyst is made on many asymptomatic patients based on specific sonographic characteristic appearances and only in certain situations, with a correlation to the patient's history. The sonographic criteria for cystic structures or masses are as follows: (1) Cysts retain an anechoic center, which indicates the lack of internal echoes even at high instrument gain settings. (2) The mass is well defined, with a sharply defined posterior wall indicative of a strong interface between cyst fluid and tissue or parenchyma. (3) There is an increased echo amplitude in the tissue

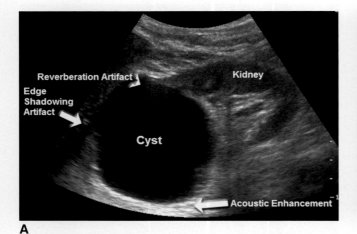

**A**

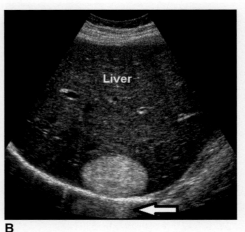

**B**

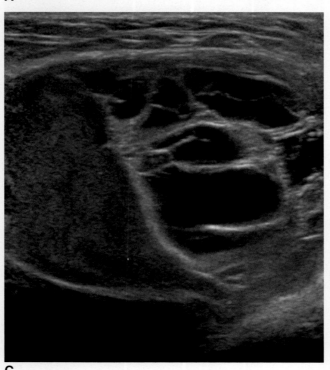

**C**

**Figure 1-7** Interpretation. **A.** Cystic. A longitudinal section of the right kidney demonstrates a renal cyst. The following sonographic criteria for a cyst are present: (1) anechoic center, (2) clear definition with a sharply defined posterior wall, (3) acoustic enhancement, (4) reverberation artifacts *(white arrowhead)*, and (5) edge shadowing artifact. **B.** Solid. A transverse section through the right lobe of the liver demonstrates a hemangioma. The benign solid mass presents with the following sonographic criteria for a solid mass: (1) internal echoes that increase with increased gain settings and (2) low-amplitude echoes *(arrow)* or shadowing posterior to the mass. Irregular walls may be present when the solid mass is a calculus or a malignant tumor. **C.** Complex. The encapsulated mass is a complex structure exhibiting septa between echogenic and anechoic areas. (Images courtesy of Philips Medical System, Bothell, WA.)

beginning at the far wall and proceeding distally compared to surrounding tissue. This increased amplitude is better known as *through-transmission* or the *acoustic enhancement artifact*. It occurs because tissue located on either side of the cystic structure attenuates more sound than does the cystic structure. (4) Reverberation artifacts can be identified at the near wall if the cyst is located close to the transducer. (5) Edge shadowing artifacts may appear, depending on the incident angle (refraction) and the thickness of the cystic wall at the periphery of the structure. The tadpole tail sign occurs with a combination of an edge shadow next to the echo enhancement (Fig. 1-7A).

A solid structure may have a hyperechoic, hypoechoic, echopenic, or anechoic homogeneous echo texture, or it may be heterogeneous because it contains many different types of interfaces. Usually, solid structure exhibit the following characteristics: (1) internal echoes that increase with an increase in instrument gain settings; (2) irregular, often poorly defined walls and margins; and (3) low-amplitude echoes or shadowing posterior to the mass due to increased acoustic attenuation by soft tissue or calculi (Fig. 1-7B).

A complex structure usually exhibits both anechoic and echogenic areas on the image, originating from both fluid and soft tissue components within the mass. The relative echogenicity of a soft tissue mass is related to a variety of constituents, including collagen content, interstitial components, vascularity, and the degree and type of tissue degeneration (Fig. 1-7C).

The amplitude of echoes distal to a mass, structure, or organ can be used to evaluate the attenuation properties of that mass. *Transonic* or *sonolucent* refers to masses, organs, or tissues that attenuate little of the acoustic beam and result in images with distal high-intensity echoes. An example is a cystic structure with the associated acoustic enhancement artifact. Masses that attenuate large amounts of sound show a marked decrease in the amplitude of distal echoes. An example is calculi, with the associated shadow artifact.

## PREPARATION

Before the patient is scanned, it is important for the sonographer to obtain as much information as possible. The sonographer should be aware of the indications for the study and of any additional clinical information such as laboratory values, results of previous examinations, and related imaging examinations. The sonographic examination should be tailored to answer the clinical questions posed by the overall clinical assessment.

Patient apprehension is reduced when the examination is explained. Apprehension may be lessened further by providing a clean, neat examination room, extending common courtesies and a smile, and letting the patient know that the sonographer enjoys providing this diagnostic service. It is important that patients know that they are the focus of the sonographer's attention.

The region of interest is visualized by planning the sonographic examination to image in multiple planes, two of which are perpendicular. Any abnormalities are imaged with differing degrees of transducer and patient obliquity to collect more information. The patient is released only after sufficient information is documented, because being called back for a repeat examination increases apprehension.

## THE PRELIMINARY REPORT

In many departments, sonographers provide a preliminary report. Legally, physicians can provide a diagnosis or an interpretive report, whereas sonographers cannot. To avoid litigation, the preliminary report is often referred to as the *technical impressions*. The preliminary report should give key sonographic findings. Ideally, the sonographer has an opportunity to discuss these findings with the sonologist. As a team, the sonographer and sonologist determine when the documentation is sufficient to complete the sonography examination. When immediate action is indicated by the sonographic findings and the sonologist is unavailable to provide the official interpretive report, the sonographer should provide the referring physician with as much information as possible immediately following the examination.

The report should describe the sonographic findings only on what is documented, without offering a conclusion regarding pathology. The terminology presented previously is very helpful. Include the scanning plane, normal tissue echogenicity, abnormal tissue texture (anechoic, hyperechoic, hypoechoic, isoechoic, cystic, solid or complex, focal or diffused, and shadowing or acoustic enhancement), measurements (vessels, ducts, organs, wall thickness, masses), location of measurements, and abnormal amounts of fluid collections. For example, describing an echogenic mass attached to the gallbladder wall that does not move as the patient changes position discusses the sonographic findings, whereas stating that the patient has a polyp located in the gallbladder is a diagnosis.

The department should have a policy regarding the preliminary report. Sonographers should be competent, through education and experience, to provide images of adequate quality and written documentation of the sonographic findings without legal obligation. Sonographers should not provide any verbal or written sonographic findings to the patient or the patient's family.

While demonstrating their sonographic evaluation expertise, sonographers should always adhere to the codes of medical ethics and/or professional conduct available from professional associations. These codes and clinical practice standards should also be included in the sonographer employment (job) description.

## SENSITIVITY, SPECIFICITY, AND ACCURACY

Sonographers should be aware of a few statistical parameters developed to judge the efficacy of sonographic examinations. These statistics are frequently reported in the literature. Knowing these statistics allows the sonographer to provide a sound rationale for why a diagnostic procedure should or should not be performed.

There are four possible results for each sonographic examination correlated to an independent determination of disease, such as a biopsy or a surgical procedure. (1) A *true-positive result* means that the sonographic findings were positive and the patient does have the disease or pathology. (2) A *true-negative result* means that the sonographic findings were negative and the patient does not have the disease or pathology. (3) A *false-positive result* means that the sonographic findings were positive but the patient does not have the disease or pathology. (4) A *false-negative result* means that the sonographic findings were negative but the patient does have the disease or pathology. Sonographers should strive to increase both the true-positive and true-negative results.

The examination's sensitivity describes how well the sonographic examination documents whatever disease or pathology is present. Mathematically, it is determined by the equation [true-positive ÷ (true-positive + false-negative) × 100]. If the number of false-negative examinations decreases, the sensitivity of the examination increases.

The examination's specificity describes how well the sonographic examination documents normal findings or excludes patients without disease or pathology. Mathematically, it is determined by the equation [true-negative ÷ (true-negative + false-positive) × 100]. If the number of false-positive examinations decreases, the specificity of the examination increases.

The accuracy of the sonographic examination is its ability to find disease or pathology if present and to not find disease or pathology if not present. Mathematically, it is determined by the equation [true-positive + true-negative ÷ (all patients receiving the sonographic examination) × 100].

There are two other statistics that sonographers should be aware of. The positive predictive value indicates the likelihood of disease or pathology if the test is positive. Mathematically, it is determined by the equation [true-positive ÷ (true-positives + false-positives) × 100]. The negative predictive value indicates the likelihood of the patient being free of disease or pathology if the test is negative. Mathematically, it is determined by the equation [true-negatives ÷ (true-negatives + false-positives) × 100].

The mathematical formulas presented provide a percentage. If sensitivity, specificity, accuracy, and positive and negative predictive values are expressed by fractions between 0 and 1 rather than by a percentage, the parameters were not multiplied by 100.

## SUMMARY

- Learning and understanding accurate and precise terminology allows communication among professionals.
- Developing standard protocols based on understanding patient positions, transducer orientations, and image presentations increases the accuracy of the sonography examinations.
- Sonographers describe sonographic findings with terminology that defines echo amplitude, echo texture, structural borders, characteristics of organs and anatomic relationships, sound transmission, and acoustic artifacts and identifies cystic, solid, and complex masses.
- The sonography examination relies on the skill, knowledge, and accuracy of the sonographer who must pay attention to the texture, outline, size, and shape of both normal and abnormal structures.
- The patient will benefit most when the sonographic appearance is correlated with patient history, clinical presentation, laboratory function tests, and other imaging modalities to compose a clinically helpful picture.

## *Critical Thinking Questions*

1. If the patient is lying on his or her right side and the transducer indicator is at the 12 o'clock position on the left lateral abdominal wall, what is the scanning plane and how is the image presented on the display monitor?

2. What anatomic areas are not visualized on a longitudinal, sagittal image presentation and how does the sonographer evaluate these areas?

3. Explain the mechanism and differentiate between acoustic shadowing and low reflectivity due to air bubbles.

## REFERENCES

1. American Institute of Ultrasound in Medicine Standard Presentation and Labeling of Ultrasound Images. A stage 2 standard. *J Clin Ultrasound*. 1976;4(6):393–398.
2. Tempkin BB. Scanning planes and scanning methods. In: Tempkin BB, ed. *Ultrasound Scanning: Principles and Protocols*. 3rd ed. St. Louis: Elsevier Saunders; 2009:11–24.
3. Laurel MD. *AIUM Recommended Ultrasound Terminology*. 3rd ed. Laurel, MD: American Institute of Ultrasound in Medicine; 2008.
4. Miner NS. Basic principles. In: Sanders RC, Winter T, eds. *Clinical Sonography: A Practical Guide*. 4th ed. Baltimore: Lippincott Williams & Wilkins; 2007:33–39.

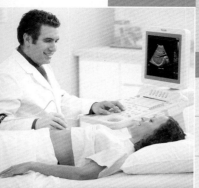

## 2

# The Abdominal Wall and Diaphragm

Terri L. Jurkiewicz

## OBJECTIVES

Locate the nine regions of the abdomen and the four quadrants of the abdominopelvic cavity.

Discuss the extent, the muscles, and the subcutaneous layers of the abdominal wall and diaphragm.

Describe the role of sonography, the sonographic technique, and the normal sonographic appearance of the abdominal wall and diaphragm.

Identify the etiology and sonographic appearance of acute and chronic abdominal wall inflammatory process to include resolution, organization, and abscess formation.

Describe the common etiologies and sonographic appearance of abdominal wall hematomas and trauma.

Identify the different types of abdominal hernias and their sonographic appearance.

List the neoplasms that affect the abdominal wall and describe their sonographic appearance.

Identify diaphragmatic pathologies that can be evaluated with sonography.

Identify technically satisfactory and unsatisfactory sonographic examinations of the abdominal wall and diaphragm.

## KEY TERMS

abdominopelvic cavity | abdominal hernia | abscess | aponeurosis | desmoid tumor | diaphragm | diaphragmatic hernia | diaphragmatic inversion | diaphragmatic paralysis | endometrioma | eventration | fascia | hematoma | inguinal canal | inguinal hernia | lipoma | neuroma | pleural effusion | rectus abdominis | rhabdomyolysis | sarcoma | seroma

## GLOSSARY

**abscess** a cavity containing dead tissue and pus that forms due to an infectious process

**ascites** an accumulation of serous fluid in the peritoneal cavity

**ecchymosis** skin discoloration caused by the leakage of blood into the subcutaneous tissues, which is often referred to as a bruise

**erythema** redness of the skin due to inflammation

**linea alba** fibrous structure that runs down the midline of the abdomen from the xyphoid process to the symphysis pubis separating the right and left rectus abdominis muscles

**omphalocele** a congenital defect in the midline abdominal wall that allows abdominal organs, such as the bowel and liver, to protrude through the wall into the base of the umbilical cord

**peristalsis** rhythmic wavelike contraction of the gastrointestinal tract that forces food through it

**pneumothorax** collapsed lung that occurs when air leaks into the space between the chest wall and lung

The human body contains two major cavities: the ventral (anterior) cavity and the dorsal (posterior) cavity. The dorsal cavity is divided into the cranial cavity and the spinal cavity. In the ventral cavity, the diaphragm muscle separates the thoracic cavity from the abdominopelvic cavity. The abdominopelvic cavity has an upper portion (the abdomen), a lower portion (the pelvis), and it is surrounded by the abdominal wall. This chapter focuses on the abdominal wall and diaphragm.

## REGIONS AND QUADRANTS

For clinical reasons used to describe the location of organs, pain, or pathology, the abdomen is divided into nine regions and the abdominopelvic cavity is divided into four quadrants. The nine regions are delineated by two horizontal (transverse) planes and two vertical (longitudinal) planes and the four quadrants are delineated by one horizontal (transverse) plane and one vertical (longitudinal, midsagittal, or sagittal) plane.[1,2] The nine regions are the (1) right hypochondrium, (2) epigastrium, (3) left hypochondrium, (4) right lumbar, (5) umbilical, (6) left lumbar, (7) right iliac fossa, (8) hypogastrium, and (9) left iliac fossa.[1,2] The four quadrants are the (1) right upper quadrant (RUQ), (2) left upper quadrant (LUQ), (3) right lower quadrant (RLQ), (4) and left lower quadrant (LLQ)[1,2] (Fig. 2-1A,B).

## ANATOMY

The abdominal wall is continuous but, for descriptive reasons, it is divided into the anterior wall, right and left lateral walls, and posterior wall. Because the anterior and lateral wall boundaries are indefinite, they will be combined in the presentation as they are combined in other references[1,2] (Fig. 2-2).

### ANTEROLATERAL ABDOMINAL WALL

The anterolateral wall extends from the thoracic cage to the pelvis. Superiorly, it is bounded by the cartilages of the 7th to 10th ribs and the xiphoid process. Inferiorly, it is bounded by the inguinal ligament and iliac crests, pubic crests, and pubic symphysis of the pelvic bones.

#### Layers

To better understand abdominal wall anatomy, it is important to distinguish between fascia and aponeurosis. A *fascia* is a fibrous tissue network located between the skin and the underlying structures. It is richly supplied with both blood vessels and nerves. The fascia is composed of two layers: a superficial layer and a deep layer. The superficial fascia is attached to the skin and is composed of connective tissue containing varying quantities of fat. The deep fascia underlies the superficial layers to which it is loosely joined by fibrous strands. It serves to cover the muscles and to partition them into groups. Although the deep fascia is thin, it is more densely

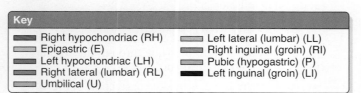

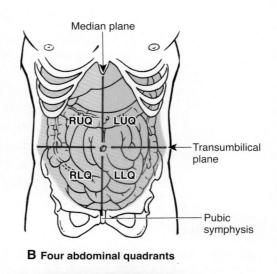

**Anterior views    A Nine abdominal regions**

| Key | |
| --- | --- |
| ▬ Right hypochondriac (RH) | ▬ Left lateral (lumbar) (LL) |
| ▭ Epigastric (E) | ▬ Right inguinal (groin) (RI) |
| ▬ Left hypochondriac (LH) | ▬ Pubic (hypogastric) (P) |
| ▬ Right lateral (lumbar) (RL) | ▬ Left inguinal (groin) (LI) |
| ▭ Umbilical (U) | |

**B Four abdominal quadrants**

| Key | |
| --- | --- |
| ▭ Right upper quadrant (RUQ) | |
| ▭ Left upper quadrant (LUQ) | |
| ▭ Right lower quadrant (RLQ) | |
| ▭ Left lower quadrant (LLQ) | |

**Figure 2-1** Abdominopelvic cavity subdivisions. **A.** The regions are formed by two sagittal (vertical) and two transverse (horizontal) planes. **B.** The quadrants are formed by the midsagittal plane and a transverse plane passing through the umbilicus at the iliac crest or the disk level between the L3-4 vertebrae. (Reprinted with permission from Moore KL, Agur AM. *Essential Clinical Anatomy*. 3rd ed. Baltimore, MD: Lippincott Williams & Wilkins; 2007:119.)

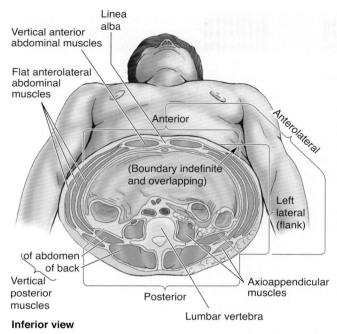

Linea
alba

Vertical anterior
abdominal muscles

Flat anterolateral
abdominal
muscles

Anterior

Anterolateral

(Boundary indefinite
and overlapping)

Left
lateral
(flank)

(of abdomen
of back)

Vertical
posterior
muscles

Posterior

Axioappendicular
muscles

Lumbar vertebra

**Inferior view**

**Figure 2-2** Abdominal wall subdivisions. The transverse section illustrates the structural relationships of the abdominal wall. (Reprinted with permission from Moore K, Dalley A, Agur A. *Clinically Oriented Anatomy.* 6th ed. Philadelphia, PA: Lippincott Williams & Wilkins; 2010:186.)

loosely to most of the subcutaneous tissue except it normally adheres firmly at the umbilicus.[1,2]

The subcutaneous tissue anterior to the muscle layers makes up the superficial fascia. Superior to the umbilicus, it is consistent with that found in most regions. Inferior to the umbilicus, the deepest part of the subcutaneous tissue is reinforced with elastic and collagen fibers and is divided into two layers. The first is a superficial fatty layer (Camper fascia) containing small vessels and nerves. Camper's fascia gives the body wall its rounded appearance. The second layer is a deep membranous layer (Scarpa fascia) and it consists of a combination of fat and fibrous tissue that blends with the deep fascia.[1,2] The membranous layer continues into the perineal region as the superficial perineal fascia (Colles fascia)[1] (Fig. 2-3).

The three anterolateral abdominal muscle layers and their aponeuroses (flat extended tendons) are covered by the superficial, intermediate, and deep layers of extremely thin investing fascia.[1] The investing layer of fascia is located on the external aspects of the three muscle layers and is not easily separated from the external muscle layer. Varying thicknesses of membranous and areolar sheets of endoabdominal fascia line the internal aspects of the wall. Although the endoabdominal fascia is continuous, different names account for the muscle or aponeurosis it is lining. For example, the portion lining the deep surface of the transversus abdominis muscle and its aponeurosis is the transversalis fascia. Internal to the transversalis fascia is the parietal peritoneum. The distance separating the parietal peritoneum from the transversalis fascia is determined by the variable amounts of extraperitoneal fat in the fascia.[1] The *parietal peritoneum* is a glistening lining of the abdominopelvic cavity formed by a single layer of epithelial cells and supporting connective tissue[1,2] (see Fig. 2-3).

## Muscles

There are five bilaterally paired muscles in the anterolateral abdominal wall and one unpaired muscle (Table 2-1). Located bilaterally on the anterior abdominal wall are the rectus abdominis muscles (see Fig. 2-2). The *rectus abdominis* is a long, broad, vertical, straplike muscle that is mostly enclosed in the rectus sheath. Also located on the anterior abdominal wall in the rectus sheath is the pyramidalis muscle. The *pyramidalis*, a

packed and is stronger than the superficial fascia; however, neither the superficial fascia nor the deep fascia possesses any notable internal strength since they are a condensation of connective tissue organized into definable homogeneous layers within the body.[3]

The *aponeuroses* are layers of flat fibrous sheets composed of strong connective tissue that serve as tendons to attach muscles to fixed points. An aponeurosis is minimally served by blood vessels and nerves. The aponeuroses are primarily located in the ventral abdominal regions with a primary function to join muscles to the body parts that the muscles act upon. An aponeurosis possesses good internal strength.[3]

The multilayered abdominal wall appears as a laminated structure when viewed from the superficial, outermost layer to the deep layer.[4] It consists of skin, subcutaneous tissue (superficial fascia), muscles and their aponeuroses, a deep fascia, extraperitoneal fat, and the parietal peritoneum.[1,2,4] The skin attaches

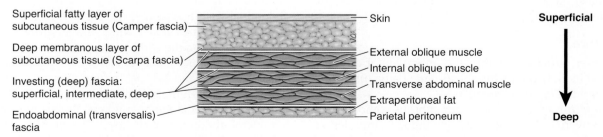

Superficial fatty layer of subcutaneous tissue (Camper fascia) — Skin — **Superficial**

Deep membranous layer of subcutaneous tissue (Scarpa fascia) — External oblique muscle / Internal oblique muscle

Investing (deep) fascia: superficial, intermediate, deep — Transverse abdominal muscle / Extraperitoneal fat

Endoabdominal (transversalis) fascia — Parietal peritoneum — **Deep**

**Figure 2-3** Anterolateral abdominal wall. The section of the anterolateral abdominal wall inferior to the umbilicus illustrates the multilayered, laminar-appearing tissue and muscles located anterior to the peritoneal cavity.

| **TABLE 2-1** | | |
|---|---|---|
| **Muscles of the Abdominolateral Wall**[1,2] | | |
| Rectus abdominis (Figs. 2-2 and 2-4A) | Bilaterally paired, vertical muscle<br>Origin: Arises from the front of the pubic bone and pubic symphysis<br>Insertion: Inserts into the fifth, sixth, and seventh costal cartilages and the xiphoid process<br>Action: Acts to flex the trunk, compress abdominal viscera, and stabilize and control pelvic tilt | |
| Pyramidalis (Fig. 2-4A) | Small, insignificant triangular muscle<br>Origin: Arises from the anterior surface of the pubis<br>Insertion: Inserts into the linea alba; lies anterior to the lower part of the rectus abdominis<br>Action: Acts to draw the linea alba inferiorly | |
| External oblique (Figs. 2-2 and 2-4B,C) | Bilaterally paired, flat muscle<br>Origin: Arises from the external surface of the lower eight ribs<br>Insertion: Inserts in linea alba via an aponeurosis and into the iliac crest and pubis via the inguinal ligament<br>Action: Acts to compress and support abdominal viscera, flexes and rotate trunk | |
| Internal oblique (Figs. 2-2 and 2-4B,C) | Bilaterally paired, flat muscle<br>Origin: Arises from the thoracolumbar fascia and the anterior two-thirds of the iliac crest<br>Insertion: Inserts into the inferior borders of the lower three ribs, linea alba, and pubis via a conjoint tendon<br>Action: Acts as a postural function of all abdominal muscles | |
| Transversus abdominis (transverse abdominal; Figs. 2-2 and 2-4B,C) | Bilaterally paired, flat muscle<br>Origin: Arises from the internal surfaces of the lower eight costal cartilages (7–12), the thoracolumbar fascia, the anterior two-thirds of the iliac crest, and the lateral third of the inguinal ligament<br>Insertion: Inserts into the xiphoid process, linea alba with aponeurosis of internal oblique, pubic crest, and pectin pubis via a conjoint tendon<br>Action: Same as external oblique; acts to compress and support abdominal viscera | |

small triangular muscle, is considered insignificant and is absent in approximately 20% of people[1,2] (Fig. 2-4A).

There are three flat, bilaterally paired muscles of the anterolateral group: (1) the external oblique (most superficial), (2) the internal oblique (middle layer), and (3) the transversus abdominis (also known as transverse abdominal)[1,2,4] (see Fig. 2-2 and Table 2-1). Coupled with the vertical orientation of the fibers of the rectus abdominis, the fibers in the three flat muscles are arranged to provide maximum strength by forming a supportive muscle girdle that covers and supports the abdominopelvic cavity. In the external oblique, the muscle fibers have a diagonal inferior and medial orientation. The fibers of the internal oblique, the middle muscle layer, have a perpendicular orientation at right angles to those of the external oblique. The fibers of the innermost muscle layer, the *transversus abdominis*, are oriented transversely[1,2] (Fig. 2-4B–D).

## Structures

The other structures within the anterolateral abdominal wall include the rectus sheath, linea alba, umbilical ring, and the inguinal canal.

The *rectus sheath* is the strong, fibrous compartment for the rectus abdominis and pyramidalis muscles as well as for some arteries, veins, lymphatic vessels, and nerves. The anterior layer and the posterior layer of the rectus sheath compartment are formed by the intercrossing and interweaving of the aponeuroses of the flat abdominal muscles. The posterior layer of the compartment has an area that is thin superior to the arcuate line (also known as linear semilunaris, semicircularis) and an area that is deficient superior to the costal margin.[4] The arcuate line is located approximately 8 cm superior to the pubis symphysis and refers to the transition terminating the posterior rectus sheath covering the proximal, superior three-quarters of the rectus abdominis.[4] The distal, inferior quarter is covered by the transversalis fascia, which serves as the only separation of the rectus muscles from the peritoneum[4] (Fig. 2-5A,B).

Throughout its length, the linea alba is formed as the fibers of the anterior and posterior layers of the sheath interlace in the anterior median line.[1,2] The linea alba is oriented vertically and courses the length of the anterior abdominal wall. It separates the bilateral rectus sheaths. Superiorly, the linea alba is wider and it narrows inferior to the umbilicus to the width of the pubic symphysis. The linea alba transmits small vessels and nerves to the skin. (Figs. 2-2, 2-4A, and 2-5A,B) In thin, muscular people, a groove is visible in the skin overlying the linea alba.

The *umbilicus* is the area where all layers of the anterolateral abdominal wall fuse.[1] The *umbilical ring* is a defect in the linea alba and is located underlying the umbilicus.[1,2] This is the area through which the fetal

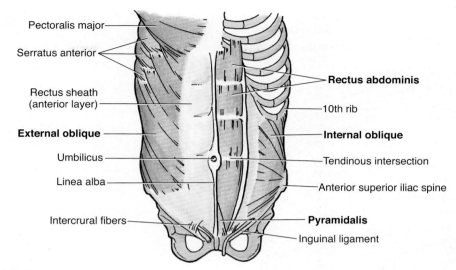

**A Anterior view**

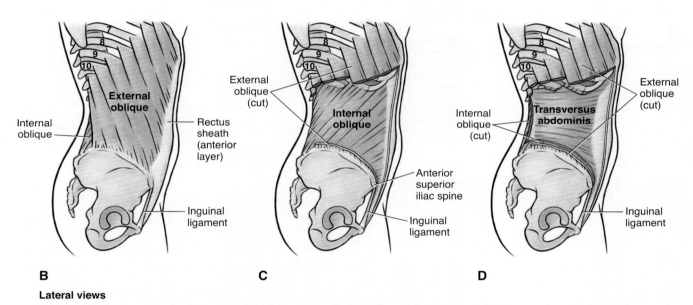

**B**

**C**

**D**

**Lateral views**

**Figure 2-4** Abdominolateral wall muscles. **A.** The bilaterally paired, vertically oriented rectus abdominis muscles and the small triangular pyramidalis muscle are located on the anterior wall. **B–D.** The three flat, bilaterally paired muscles comprising the anterolateral group include the external oblique, the internal oblique, and the transverse abdominal. The strength of the muscles can be contributed to the collaborative relationship of the orientation of the fiber of each muscle. (Reprinted with permission from Moore KL, Agur AM. *Essential Clinical Anatomy.* 3rd ed. Baltimore, MD: Lippincott Williams & Wilkins; 2007:122.)

umbilical vessels passed to and from the umbilical cord and placenta. After birth, fat accumulation in the subcutaneous tissue raises the umbilical ring and depresses the umbilicus.

The inguinal region extends between the anterior superior iliac spine and the pubic tubercle.[3] Located in the inguinal region is the inguinal canal, which is formed during fetal development. It is an important canal where structures exit and enter the abdominal cavity, and the exit and entry pathways are potential sites of herniation.[1,2] In adults, the *inguinal canal* is an oblique passage approximately 4 cm long. It has an inferior-to-medial orientation through the inferior part of the

anterolateral abdominal wall and lies parallel and superior to the median half of the inguinal ligament.[2] Functionally and developmentally distinct structures located within the canal are the spermatic cord in males and the round uterine ligament in females. Other structures included in the canal in both sexes are blood and lymphatic vessels and the ilioinguinal nerves. The inguinal canal has two openings. The deep (internal) inguinal ring serves as an entrance and the superficial (external) inguinal ring serves as the exit for the spermatic cord or the round ligament in females. Normally, the inguinal canal is collapsed anteroposteriorly against the spermatic cord or round ligament. Between the two openings,

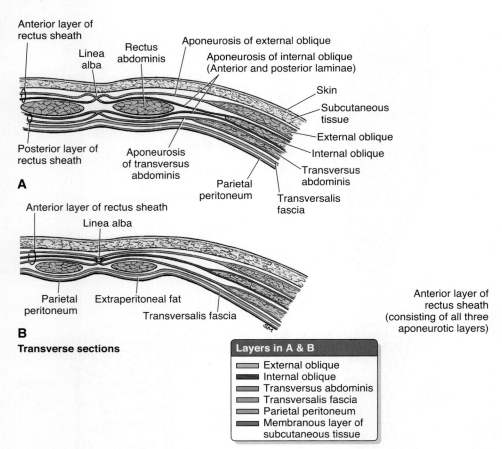

**Figure 2-5** Abdominal wall structures. Transverse sections of the anterior abdominal wall (**A**) superior to the umbilicus with the posterior layer of the rectus sheath. **B.** Inferior to the umbilicus, the rectus sheath is separated from the parietal peritoneum only by the transversalis fascia. (Reprinted with permission from Moore KL, Agur AM. *Essential Clinical Anatomy.* 3rd ed. Baltimore, MD: Lippincott Williams & Wilkins; 2007:123.)

(rings) the inguinal canal has two walls (anterior and posterior), a roof, and a floor[1,2] (Table 2-2, Fig. 2-6A,B).

## POSTERIOR ABDOMINAL WALL

The posterior abdominal wall is composed of the lumbar vertebra, posterior abdominal wall muscles, diaphragm, fascia, lumbar plexus, fat, nerves, blood vessels, and lymphatic vessels.

## Layers

The posterior abdominal wall is covered with a continuous layer of endoabdominal fascia, which is continuous with the transversalis fascia.[1,2] The posterior wall fascia is located between the parietal peritoneum and the muscles. The psoas fascia (sheath) is attached medially to the lumbar vertebrae and pelvic brim. Superiorly, the psoas fascia is thickened and forms the medial arcuate ligament. Laterally, the psoas fascia fuses with both

| TABLE 2-2 | | | |
|---|---|---|---|
| **Boundaries of the Inguinal Canal**[a] | | | |
| **Boundary** | **Deep Ring/Lateral Third** | **Middle Third** | **Lateral Third/Superficial Ring** |
| Posterior wall | Transversalis fascia | Transversalis fascia | Inguinal falx (conjoint tendon) plus reflected inguinal ligament |
| Anterior wall | Internal oblique plus lateral crus of aponeurosis of external oblique | Aponeurosis of external oblique (lateral crus and intercrural fibers) | Aponeurosis of external oblique (intercrural fibers), with fascia of external oblique continuing onto cord as external spermatic fascia |
| Roof | Transversalis fascia | Musculoaponeurotic arches of internal oblique and transverse abdominal | Medial crus of aponeurosis of external oblique |
| Floor | Iliopubic tract | Inguinal ligament | Lacunar ligament |

[a] See Figure 2-6.
Reprinted with permission from Moore K, Dalley A, Agur A. *Clinically Oriented Anatomy.* 6th ed. Philadelphia, PA: Lippincott Williams & Wilkins; 2010:204.

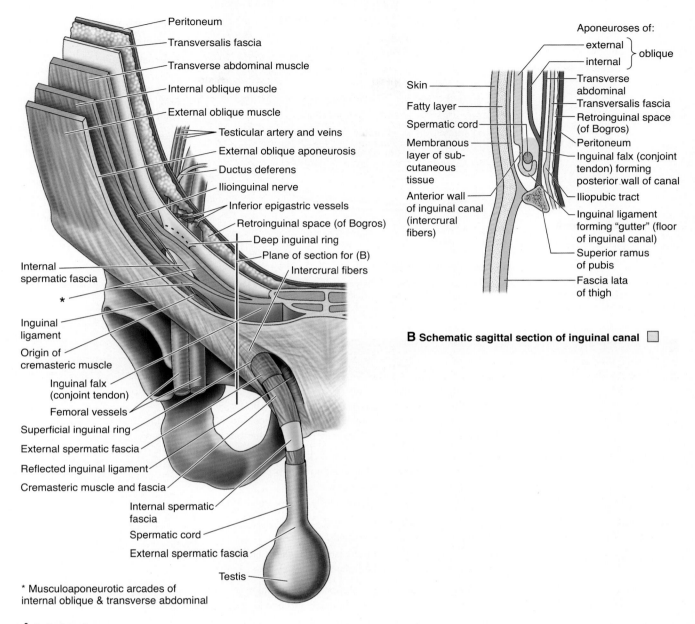

**A Anterior view**

**Peritoneum**
**Transversalis fascia**
**Transverse abdominal muscle**
**Internal oblique muscle**
**External oblique muscle**
**Testicular artery and veins**
**External oblique aponeurosis**
**Ductus deferens**
**Ilioinguinal nerve**
**Inferior epigastric vessels**
**Retroinguinal space (of Bogros)**
**Deep inguinal ring**
**Plane of section for (B)**
**Intercrural fibers**

Internal spermatic fascia
*
Inguinal ligament
Origin of cremasteric muscle
Inguinal falx (conjoint tendon)
Femoral vessels
Superficial inguinal ring
External spermatic fascia
Reflected inguinal ligament
Cremasteric muscle and fascia
Internal spermatic fascia
Spermatic cord
External spermatic fascia
Testis

* Musculoaponeurotic arcades of internal oblique & transverse abdominal

Aponeuroses of:
external
internal } oblique
Skin
Fatty layer
Spermatic cord
Membranous layer of subcutaneous tissue
Anterior wall of inguinal canal (intercrural fibers)
Transverse abdominal
Transversalis fascia
Retroinguinal space (of Bogros)
Peritoneum
Inguinal falx (conjoint tendon) forming posterior wall of canal
Iliopubic tract
Inguinal ligament forming "gutter" (floor of inguinal canal)
Superior ramus of pubis
Fascia lata of thigh

**B Schematic sagittal section of inguinal canal**

**Figure 2-6** Inguinal canal. The anterior and posterior wall, the roof, and the floor of the inguinal canal are illustrated. **A.** The abdominal wall layers and the coverings of the spermatic cord and testis are seen in the anterior view. In females, the canal serves as the passageway for the round ligament. **B.** At the plane shown in **(A)**, the sagittal section illustrates the composition of the canal. (Reprinted with permission from Moore K, Dalley A, Agur A. *Clinically Oriented Anatomy.* 6th ed. Philadelphia, PA: Lippincott Williams & Wilkins; 2010:204.)

the quadratus lumborum fascia and the thoracolumbar fascia. Inferior to the iliac crest, the psoas fascia is continuous with that part of the iliac fascia that covers the iliacus[1] (Fig. 2-7).

On the posterior abdominal wall, the thoracolumbar fascia is an extensive complex. Medially, it attaches to the vertebral column. In the lumbar region, the thoracolumbar fascia has posterior, middle, and anterior layers with enclosed muscles between them. The *fascia* is thin and transparent in the thoracic region it covers, whereas it is thick and strong in the lumbar region it covers. The posterior and middle layers of the thoracolumbar

fascia, which enclose the bilateral erector spinae muscles (vertical deep back muscles), are comparable to the enclosure of the rectus abdominis by the rectus sheath on the anterior wall.[2] When comparing the posterior sheath to the rectus sheath, the posterior sheath is stronger because it is thicker and has a central attachment to the lumbar vertebrae. The rectus sheath has no bony attachment and fuses with the linea alba. Like the rectus sheath, the lumbar part of the posterior sheath extending between the 12th rib and the iliac crest attaches laterally to the internal oblique and transversus abdominis muscles. The rectus sheath attaches to the

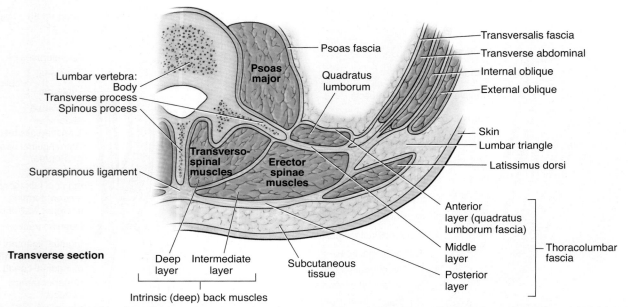

**Figure 2-7** Posterior abdominal wall fascia. The relationship of the psoas fascia, the three layers of the thoracolumbar fascia, and quadratus lumborum fascia with the muscles and vertebrae are illustrated on this transverse section of the posterior abdominal wall. (Reprinted with permission from Moore KL, Agur AM. *Essential Clinical Anatomy*. 3rd ed. Baltimore, MD: Lippincott Williams & Wilkins; 2007:300.)

**TABLE 2-3**

## Muscles of the Posterior Abdomen Wall[1,2]

| | |
|---|---|
| Psoas major (Figs. 2-6 and 2-7) | Bilaterally paired, long, thick, fusiform muscle<br>Origin: Arises from the bodies and transverse processes of lumbar vertebrae<br>Insertion: Inserts into the lesser trochanter of femur with iliacus via iliopsoas tendon<br>Action: Acts to flex the thigh; flexes and laterally bends the lumbar vertebral column |
| Iliacus (Fig. 2-7) | Bilaterally paired, triangular muscle<br>Origin: Arises from the iliac fossa and iliac crest and ala of the sacrum<br>Insertion: Inserts into the lesser trochanter of the femur<br>Action: Acts to flex the thigh; if thigh is fixed, it flexes the pelvis on the thigh |
| Quadratus lumborum (Figs. 2-6 and 2-7) | Bilaterally paired, thick muscular sheet<br>Origin: Arises from the iliolumbar ligament and iliac crest<br>Insertion: Inserts into the 12th rib and transverse process of first four lumbar vertebrae<br>Action: Acts to flex vertebral column laterally and depress the last rib |
| Psoas minor (Fig. 2-7) | Bilaterally paired, long, slender muscle anterior to psoas major<br>Origin: Arises from the bodies of the 12th thoracic and first lumbar vertebrae<br>Insertion: Inserts into the iliopubic eminence at the line of junction of the ilium and the superior pubic ramus<br>Action: Acts to flex and laterally bends the lumbar vertebral column |
| Iliopsoas | Formed by the psoas and iliacus muscles<br>Origin: Arises from the iliac fossa, bodies and transverse processes of lumbar vertebrae<br>Insertion: Inserts into the lesser trochanter of the femur<br>Action: Acts to flex the thigh, flexes and laterally bends the lumbar vertebral column |
| Latissimus dorsi (Fig. 2-6) | Bilaterally paired, broadest back muscle<br>Origin: Arises from the lower six thoracic vertebrae, lumbar vertebrae, iliac crest via thoracolumbar fascia, sacrum, lower three or four ribs, and inferior angle of scapula<br>Insertion: Inserts into the intertubercular (bicipital) groove on the medial side of the humerus<br>Action: Acts to abduct, medially rotate, and extend arm at shoulder |
| Erector spinae (Fig. 2-6) | Location: A group of three columns of muscle located on each side of the vertebral column<br>Action: Acts as the chief extensor of the vertebral column |
| Transversospinal (Fig. 2-6) | Location: An oblique group of three muscles deep to the erector spinae<br>Action: In the abdominal area, they act to stabilize vertebrae and assist with extension and rotation movements |

external oblique muscle, but the thoracolumbar fascia attaches to the latissimus dorsi[1] (see Fig. 2-7).

The anterior layer of the thoracolumbar fascia is the *quadratus lumborum fascia* and it covers the anterior surface of the quadratus lumborum muscle.[1,2] Compared to the middle and posterior layers of thoracolumbar fascia, it is a thinner and more transparent layer. The anterior layer attaches to the anterior surfaces of the lumbar transverse processes, to the iliac crest, and to the 12th rib. Laterally, the anterior layer is continuous with the aponeurotic origin of the transversus abdominis muscle. Superiorly, it thickens to form the lateral arcuate ligament and inferiorly, it is adherent to the iliolumbar ligaments[1] (see Fig. 2-7).

## Muscles

The muscles of the posterior abdomen are categorized as the superficial and intermediate extrinsic back muscles and the superficial layer, intermediate layer, and deep layer of intrinsic back muscles[1,2] (Table 2-3). The three main, bilaterally paired muscles comprising the posterior abdominal wall are the psoas major, iliacus, and quadratus lumborum (Fig. 2-8).

## DIAPHRAGM

The diaphragm is a double-domed, musculotendinous partition separating the thoracic cavity from the abdominal cavity.[1] The convex superior surface faces and forms the floor of the thoracic cavity and the concave inferior surface faces and forms the roof of the abdominal cavity. The concave surfaces form the right and left domes with the right dome slightly higher due to the

presence of the liver and the central part slightly depressed by the pericardium.[1] Its periphery is the fixed muscle origin, which attaches to the inferior margin of the thoracic cage and the superior lumbar vertebrae.[2,5] As the major muscle of inspiration, the central part descends during inspiration, ascends during expiration (to the fifth rib on the right and fifth intercostal space on the left), varies in postural position (supine or standing), and varies in height based on the size and degree of abdominal visceral distention.[1]

The muscular part of the diaphragm is located peripherally with fibers that converge radially on the trifoliate central aponeurotic part, the *central tendon*. The central tendon has no bony attachments and appears incompletely divided into what resembles the three leaves of a wide cloverleaf. Although it lies near the center of the diaphragm, the central tendon is closer to the anterior part of the thorax[1,2] (Fig. 2-9).

The area around the caval opening is surrounded by a muscular part that forms a continuous sheet. For descriptive purposes, the continuous sheet is divided into three parts based on its area of attachment: the sternal part, the costal part, and the lumbar part[1,2] (Table 2-4).

The diaphragmatic crura are musculotendinous bands that arise from the anterior surfaces of the bodies of the superior three lumbar vertebrae, the anterior longitudinal ligament, and the intervertebral discs. The right crus is larger and longer than the left crus and appears as a triangular mass anterior to the aorta.[5] It arises from the first three or four lumbar vertebrae and appears posterior to the caudate lobe of the liver.[1,5] The left crus arises from the first two or three lumbar vertebrae.[1]

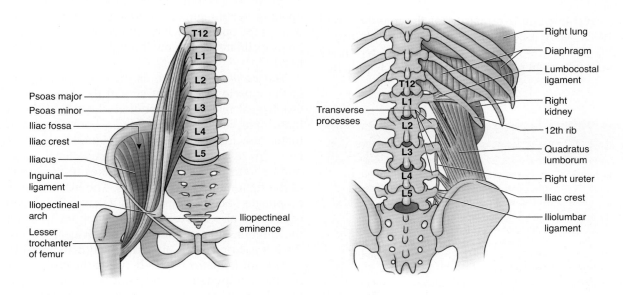

**Figure 2-8** Posterior abdominal wall muscles. The anterior and posterior sections illustrate the musculoskeletal relationship of the major posterior abdominal wall muscles. (Reprinted with permission from Moore K, Dalley A, Agur A. *Clinically Oriented Anatomy*. 6th ed. Philadelphia, PA: Lippincott Williams & Wilkins; 2010:311.)

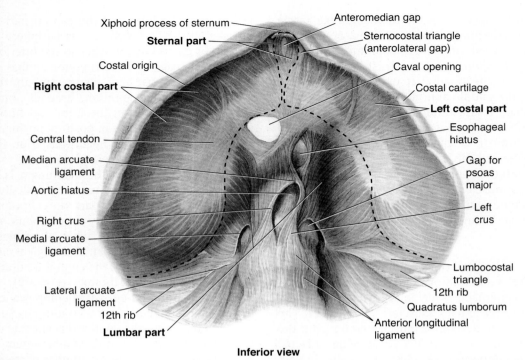

**Inferior view**

**Figure 2-9** Diaphragm. The view of the concave inner surface forming the roof of the abdominopelvic cavity illustrates the fleshy sternal, costal, and lumbar parts of the diaphragm (outlined with *broken lines*). Identify the relationship of how each part attaches centrally to the trefoil-shaped central tendon, the aponeurotic insertion of the diaphragmatic muscle fibers. (Reprinted with permission from Moore K, Dalley A, Agur A. *Clinically Oriented Anatomy.* 6th ed. Philadelphia, PA: Lippincott Williams & Wilkins; 2010:306.)

## Diaphragmatic Apertures

The diaphragmatic apertures (openings, hiatus) permit several structures (esophagus, blood vessels, nerves, and lymphatic vessels) to pass between the thorax and abdomen.[1,2] The three larger apertures are the caval, esophageal, and aortic, and there are a number of small openings.[1,5]

The caval opening is primarily for the inferior vena cava (IVC) as it ascends into the thoracic cavity.[1,5] The IVC shares the caval opening with the terminal branches of the right phrenic nerve and a few lymphatic

vessels passing from the liver to the middle phrenic and mediastinal lymph nodes.[1,5] Located to the right of the median plane, at the junction of the right and middle leaves of the central tendon, and at the level of the T8-9 intervertebral disk space, the *caval opening* is the most superior of the three large diaphragmatic apertures. Because the IVC is adherent in to the margin of the caval opening, diaphragmatic contraction during inspiration widens the opening, which allows the IVC to dilate and helps facilitate blood flow through this large vein to the heart.[1,2]

The *esophageal hiatus* is an oval opening located in the muscle of the right crus at the T10 level.[1,2] The esophageal hiatus is superior to the left of the aortic hiatus and, in 70% of individuals, both margins of the hiatus are formed by muscular bundles of the right crus. In 30% of individuals, a superficial muscular bundle from the left crus contributes to the formation of the right margin of the hiatus. The hiatus allows the esophagus to course from the thorax into the abdominal cavity and also serves as the opening for transmitting the anterior and posterior vagal esophageal branches of the left gastric vessels and a few lymphatic vessels.[1,5]

The aortic hiatus passes between the crura posterior the median arcuate ligaments at the inferior border of the T12 vertebra.[1,2] The hiatus is the opening posterior in the diaphragm for the aorta to course between the thoracic cavity to the abdominal cavity. The thoracic duct and sometimes the azygos and hemiazygos veins

| TABLE | 2-4 |
|---|---|
| **Diaphragmatic Peripheral Attachments[1,2]** | |
| Sternal part | Two muscular slips attach the diaphragm to the posterior aspect of xiphoid process. This part is not always present. |
| Costal part | Wide muscular slips bilaterally attach the diaphragm to the internal surfaces of the inferior six costal cartilages and their adjoining ribs. The costal parts form the right and left domes. |
| Lumbar part | The medial and lateral arcuate ligaments (two aponeurotic arches) and the three superior lumbar vertebrae form the right and left muscular crura that ascend and insert into the central tendon. |

are also transmitted through the aortic hiatus. The aorta does not pierce the diaphragm or adhere to the hiatus, which means diaphragmatic movements during respiration do not affect aortic blood flow.[1,2]

The *sternocostal triangle* (foramen) is a small opening between the sternal and costal attachments of the diaphragm. This triangle transmits lymphatic vessels from the hepatic diaphragmatic surface and the superior epigastric vessels. The sympathetic trunk passes deep to the medial arcuate ligament and is accompanied by the least splanchnic nerves. In each crus, there are two small apertures: one transmits the greater splanchnic nerve and the other the lesser splanchnic nerve.[1,2]

## VARIANTS

Anatomic variants are composed of individual variations in fat and muscle content. In more muscular individuals, each lateral muscle layer tends to be identifiable, whereas in less well-developed individuals, muscle groups tend to be indistinct. It is important to note that in obese patients, the fatty layer variation can be significant.

## SONOGRAPHIC APPEARANCES AND TECHNIQUES

### ABDOMINAL WALL

Sonography provides a valuable, inexpensive, and non-invasive method of imaging the normal abdomen wall and detecting pathologic processes such as inflammatory lesions, hemorrhage, hernia, or masses. Many clinical questions can be answered with the use of sonography in evaluating posttrauma or postsurgical patients. It is extremely important to understand the normal sonographic appearance of the abdominal wall and the appropriate instrumentation and scanning techniques necessary to achieve that appearance.

The superficial nature of the abdominal wall and its lesions demands excellent near-field imaging. Newer, high-frequency, short focal zone transducers (5–12 or 7–14 MHz linear array transducers) are the optimum tools for scanning this area.[6,7] Focal zone placement at the area of interest is especially important.

In some instances, a standoff device or other scanning technique may be indicated when scanning the superficial cutaneous layers to avoid a "main-bang" transducer artifact. Excellent standoff devices exist in the form of flotation pads constructed of liquid-filled microcell sponges, synthetic polymer blocks, and silicone elastomer blocks. Each of these substances is dense enough to stand alone and offers uniform consistency to minimize artifacts. When it is necessary to scan over a surgical wound, any protective dressings are removed and a commercially available adhesive plastic membrane can be applied directly to the wound to provide a smooth, safe scanning surface. The use of sterile gel and a sterile probe cover aids in protecting the patient from any bacterial contamination.[8] The sonographer should use light transducer pressure while scanning to eliminate distortion of the superficial layers.

Demonstration of the various layers of the normal abdominal wall and a contiguous diaphragm should not be limited to patients with superficial lesions. It should be an integral part of every high-quality sonographic abdominal study (Fig. 2-10A,B).

### DIAPHRAGM

The sonographic appearance of the diaphragm is of a thin, curvilinear, hyperechoic band on adults and hypoechoic structure on fetuses. The abdominal side of the diaphragm produces a thin, curved line representing the diaphragm–liver interface. An additional thin, echogenic line, an artifactual mirror image of the diaphragm–liver interface, may sometimes be seen on the thoracic side (Fig. 2-11). Another thick, echogenic line can be seen on the diaphragm–lung interface. Occasionally, reverberation artifacts from air in the lung originate from this area. The diaphragmatic crura lie anterior to the upper abdominal aorta and appear as thin, hypoechoic bands that thicken during deep inspiration. The crus of the right hemidiaphragm contain medium-density echoes. In some patients, diaphragmatic slips appear as round, focal, echogenic masses when seen in transverse section. They should not be mistaken for focal liver or peritoneal masses. They can be clarified by rotating the transducer from its transverse orientation and scanning along their long axis, noting their now elongated appearance.

## ABDOMINAL WALL PATHOLOGY

A thorough understanding of the anatomy and sonographic appearance of the superficial layers of the abdominal wall, and the tissues and organs directly beneath it, is essential before pathologic changes can be fully appreciated. Three major categories of disease affect the abdominal wall, the peritoneum, and the abdominal spaces. Both the tissues of the abdominal wall and the membranes lining its spaces are affected by inflammatory, traumatic, and neoplastic changes.

### INFLAMMATORY RESPONSE: ABSCESS

It is vitally important that sonographers understand the medical aspects of inflammation, as well as its sonographic appearance. Inflammation can be acute or chronic. Acute inflammation frequently results from cuts, scrapes, crushing injuries, or surgical trauma that produces tissue damage. Consequently, an inflammatory response can occur whenever bacterial infection damages the skin and underlying tissues. The four main indications of inflammatory response are heat, redness, pain, and swelling.[9]

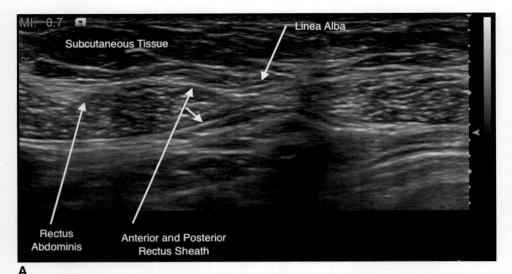

**A**

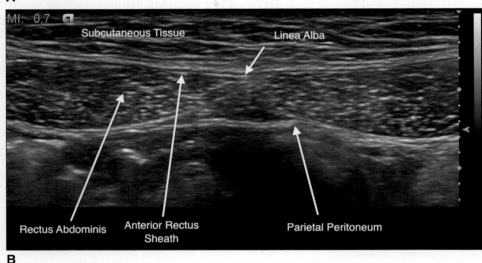

**B**

**Figure 2-10** Anterior abdominal wall. On transverse sections of the anterior abdominal wall, the subcutaneous tissue linea alba and rectus abdominis muscle can be visualized. On the sonogram **(A)** superior to the umbilicus, both the anterior and posterior rectus sheath are seen, but **(B)** inferior to the umbilicus, the rectus sheath is separated from the parietal peritoneum only by the transversalis fascia. Compare the sonographic anatomy with the illustrated anatomy in Figure 2-5A,B. (Images courtesy of Kacey R. Crandall, Tremonton, UT.)

In most patients with acute inflammations, the body will return to normal. This process of resolution can be hastened by the use of anti-inflammatory drugs. Such drugs block the body's natural inflammatory reactions, allowing removal of debris and fluid exudates associated with the inflammation via the circulatory and lymphatic systems.

If resolution occurs slowly, other consequences may result. Fibrous tissue growth invades areas of long-standing cellular and fluid exudates to form scar tissue. This process, called *organization*, is responsible for the development of adhesions following surgery. If sufficient necrosis of the involved tissues occurs, resolution does not take place and a cavity containing dead tissue and pus forms. The liquid pus in such a cavity consists of living and dead microorganisms, necrotic tissue, exudate, and granulocytes. The cavity itself is called an *abscess*.[9]

Abscesses are space-occupying lesions whose fluid content allows them to assume varied shapes (usually spherical or elliptical) (Fig. 2-12A,B). Because of their internal pressure, however, they can exert a mass effect on surrounding structures, causing compression, displacement, or both. Abdominal wall abscesses frequently occur as a result of postsurgical incisional infections or exist as extensions of a superficial intraperitoneal abscess. Less frequently, tuberculous paraspinal abscesses may also track along the musculofascial plane into the lateral and posterior abdominal walls.

Wherever abscesses occur, the usual treatment involves antibiotic therapy and sometimes drainage to facilitate resolution. Failure of an abscess to resolve can lead to thickening of its contents as a result of the reabsorption of water (inspissation), and eventually, calcifications develop. If the cause of the acute inflammation is not eliminated, the processes of tissue injury and repair will continue simultaneously, producing chronic inflammation.[9]

One variation is called *chronic suppurative inflammation* or *pyogenic inflammation*, in which an abscess is created as a result of persistent infection. Suppurative inflammation describes a condition in which a purulent

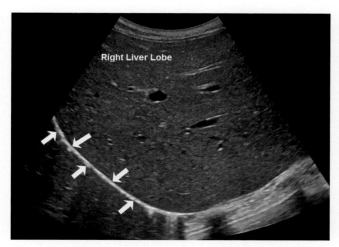

**Figure 2-11** Diaphragm. A longitudinal section through the right liver lobe shows the normal sonographic appearance of the thin, curvilinear, hyperechoic diaphragm *(arrows)*. On the chest side of the diaphragm, the mirror image artifact of the liver can be identified in the pleural cavity.

exudate is accompanied by significant liquefactive necrosis; it is the equivalent pus. The term *suppurative* refers to this formation of pus.[10] Body defenses may be poor because the blood supply to the area is limited. If so, chronic suppurative inflammation can easily occur, requiring surgical drainage and the use of specific antibiotics to affect a cure.[10]

Superficial abdominal wall abscesses can be caused by surgical or external trauma. In evaluating superficial abscesses, precise scanning is required to display the superficial layers of the skin, subcutaneous fat, muscle planes, and the peritoneum. The most clinically important aspect of treating abscesses is to determine whether the abscess is intraperitoneal or extraperitoneal. This is done by demonstrating the peritoneal line.

Superficial wound abscesses commonly result from intraoperative contamination. In such cases, sonography may have limited diagnostic value because the diagnosis can usually be made easily on physical examination.

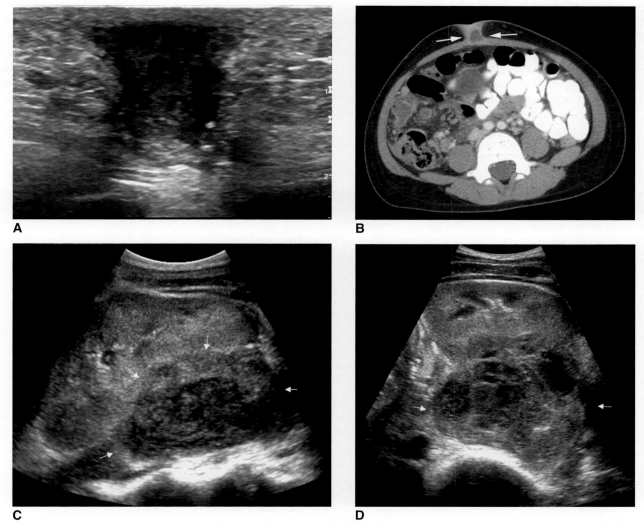

**Figure 2-12** A periumbilical abscess **(A)** presents with a mixed echo appearance with good acoustic transmission. **B.** The computed tomography examination demonstrates the size, shape, and periumbilical location *(arrows)*. (Images courtesy of Dr. Nakul Jerath, Falls Church, VA.) A left psoas muscle abscess *(arrows)* located near the left kidney and extending superiorly is visualized on **(C)** longitudinal and **(D)** transverse sections. The mixed echo appearance demonstrates good acoustic transmission. (Images courtesy of Philips Medical Systems, Bothell, WA.)

Most incisional abscesses are superficially located and display the clinical signs of erythema, tenderness, purulence, and crepitus around the wound.[11] However, if the abscess develops below the fascial plane, detection by physical examination alone can be difficult. Aspiration of the abscess under sonography guidance may be indicated so that the specimen can be sent to the laboratory for culture and sensitivity testing.[11]

The differential diagnosis of superficial abscesses includes rectus sheath hematomas and hernias, in addition to noninfected collections.[4,11,12]

Sonographically, most abscesses appear as homogeneous fluid masses. However, their internal patterns can range from uniformly echo-free to mildly or even highly echogenic. The presence of particulate debris or microbubbles floating within an abscess cavity is generally the cause of its increased echogenicity. If the particulate matter is uniformly distributed throughout the abscess, it may be difficult to recognize and differentiate the abscess from surrounding structures. Despite their variable internal textures, however, the majority of abscesses demonstrate posterior enhancement, revealing their fluid nature[13] (Fig. 2-12C,D).

Abscesses vary in contour from flat to oval or bonnet-shaped. Occasionally, large abscesses may compress adjacent structures and cause confusion in the differentiation of extraperitoneal versus intraperitoneal locations.[13]

Table 2-5 describes the common types of tissue changes associated with abscesses and their corresponding sonographic patterns. Because sonographic diagnosis is very technique- and operator-dependent, it is critical to understand how instrumentation and scan technique can alter the echo image from within an abscess.[14] Occasionally, septations may be seen within abscesses. Such findings require documentation because their presence contraindicates percutaneous drainage. Fortunately, septated abscesses occur infrequently within the peritoneal cavity.

To permit contact scanning, postoperative patients' surgical dressings must be removed. The face of the transducer should be cleansed with a sterilizing solution to avoid contamination. Caution must be used to avoid damaging the transducer's electrical connections when such a sterilizing process is used.[8]

The search for an abscess must be conducted in a systematic fashion, with special attention and care given to areas of swelling or tenderness. If there is any open wound, incision, drain site, or enterostomy, it is important to use sterile gel and a sterile transducer cover as a precaution against infectious contamination. Scan around such sites by angling the transducer to view the area beneath.

As the survey of such areas is made, special techniques may be necessary to enhance the appearance of any suspicious lesions. Because the gain setting may affect the overall appearance of lesions, it is important to vary the gain. When gain settings are excessively high, small fluid collections may be overlooked because of the "fill in." In contrast, when extremely low gain settings are used, there is a risk of making

| **TABLE 2-5** | | | |
|---|---|---|---|
| **Sonographic Appearances** | | | |
| **Collection** | **Location** | **Sonographic Characteristics** | **Acoustic Transmission** |
| Abscess | Near surgical site or painful area, subphrenic, subhepatic, paracolic gutters, and left perihepatic, perisplenic, and pelvis | Shape: Lenticular or shape of space. Anechoic, with irregular or smooth borders; may have internal echoes, septations, fluid-fluid level; abscesses that contain gas are echogenic and may shadow | Usually good |
| Hematoma | Near wound or surgical site | Shape: Lenticular or shape of space. Change with stage of resolution; fresh blood is hypoechoic, as is clotted blood; fragmentation of clot creates internal echoes and anechoic areas with some scattered echoes; fluid-fluid level may be caused by cholesterol in breakdown of red blood cells; long-standing hematoma may have thick contours | Coincides with stage; good to slow or decreased; may increase due to fluid portion |
| Ascites | Most dependent areas of body, cul-de-sac, Morrison pouch, paracolic gutter, pararenal areas, perihepatic, midabdominal | Anechoic if benign, ascites if exudative, internal echoes if malignant; bowel and implants in anechoic ascitic fluid | Increased |
| Urinoma | Adjacent to kidneys | Usually anechoic unless infected | Increased |
| Lymphocele | Adjacent to renal transplant | Usually anechoic but may have septations | Increased |

Courtesy Mimi Berman, PhD, RDMS.

a homogeneously solid mass appear cystic. Moderate gain settings are useful in demonstrating the far wall of an abscess, but low gain may also be required to avoid the strong reverberation artifacts frequently seen at, or obscuring, the near walls. By creating several images using different settings and scanning planes, it is possible to obtain maximum information about an abscess.

The shape of an abscess and its relationship to surrounding structures are valuable information if the clinician is planning percutaneous needle aspiration. Sonography aids in planning a safe aspiration route and monitoring the procedure, and it also provides a means of evaluating the effectiveness of therapy on follow-up examinations.

## TRAUMA

Abdominal muscles may be injured by penetrating wounds, by blows to the abdomen, or by hyperextension strain. Subcutaneous edema or muscle contusions are commonly seen with blunt trauma. A contused muscle will appear thicker and more anechoic if edema is present. In cases of extravasated blood and inflammatory reactions, a disorganized, coarse echo pattern is common. A similar appearance may be seen with rhabdomyolysis (the breakdown of muscle caused by injury).

With violent hyperextension strain, it is possible for the rectus muscle to rupture, causing tearing of the inferior epigastric artery. Such patients present with a tender mass, sonographically resembling the appearance of a superficial hematoma.

## HEMATOMAS

Hematomas are generally associated with muscular trauma that results in hemorrhage. They can also result from infection, debilitating disease, collagen disorders, pregnancy, and childbirth. Straining, coughing, anticoagulant therapy, and surgery can also be precipitating factors.[4,12]

Among the most common superficial abdominal wall hematomas are those occurring within the rectus sheath. Patients usually complain of pain and demonstrate a palpable abdominal mass that persists in both sitting and supine positions. Ecchymosis (discoloration) of the abdominal wall and a laboratory variance of a falling hematocrit value are often seen.

Rectus sheath hematomas may be unilateral or bilateral, small or large, and may extend along the entire length of the muscles or sheath. Although enclosed in the sheath, a hematoma may lie posterior to the muscles, surrounding them and conforming to the shape of the enclosed space. A hematoma usually enlarges caudally across the midline and over the lower abdomen. A large bleed may accumulate anterior to the bladder within the space of Retzius.[4] Such hematomas may produce asymmetry of the abdominal wall.

There is a higher incidence of complaints of pain and ecchymosis in patients whose bleeding is not confined to enclosed spaces.

Postsurgical hematomas are usually intimately related to an incisional site, frequently lying external to the anterior rectus fascia and presenting as a smooth-bordered, localized mass.

In all hematomas or thrombi, echogenicity will vary depending on the age and distribution of the hematoma and its cellular contents. During the acute phase, fluid–fluid levels may be seen within the hematoma, with clotted blood layering in the dependent part and unclotted blood or plasma floating on top. During active bleeding, it may even be possible to detect turbulent blood flow. If active arterial bleeding is identified or a hematoma is complicated by infection, surgery is indicated.[15]

The sonographic appearance will also depend where the bleed is located in relationship to the arcuate line. Above the arcuate line, the linea alba prevents the spread of hematoma across the midline and below the arcuate line, blood can spread to the pelvis or cross the midline. A hematoma above the arcuate line will appear ovoid transversely and biconcave in long axis; a hematoma below the arcuate line can form a large mass that indents on the dome of the urinary bladder (Fig. 2-13A,B).

Sonography is valuable during the conservative management of even large hematomas because of its ability to monitor their size and resolution as they resorb (hypoechoic phase) and liquefy (anechoic phase). An important reality is that hematomas are not limited to the anterior abdominal wall but can also involve the lateral or retroperitoneal muscles.

Sonographic patterns closely follow the pathologic evolution of the hematoma. Recent blood collections tend to appear echo-free, becoming more echogenic as they organize, although the reverse may also occur (see Table 2-5). Hematomas and thrombi behave differently, depending on their size and location. Generally, wound hematomas that occur within the body resolve. The borders of such masses differ in echo reflection from their centers. In contrast, abdominal wall hematomas or those surrounded by a capsule gradually change to an anechoic state.[15]

A *seroma* is a collection of serum in the tissue resulting from a surgical incision or from the liquefaction of a hematoma. The normal small seroma formation during the incisional healing process usually resolves. Without resolution, the seroma may require aspiration drainage to alleviate pain and/or visible swelling. The sonographic appearance of a seroma ranges from anechoic to hypoechoic (Fig. 2-13C,D).

When bleeding is secondary to anticoagulant therapy, a wide range of sonographic appearances is possible (Fig. 2-13E). Although it is uncommon to scan such patients during active bleeding, the relative lack of coagulation would likely produce an echo-free or

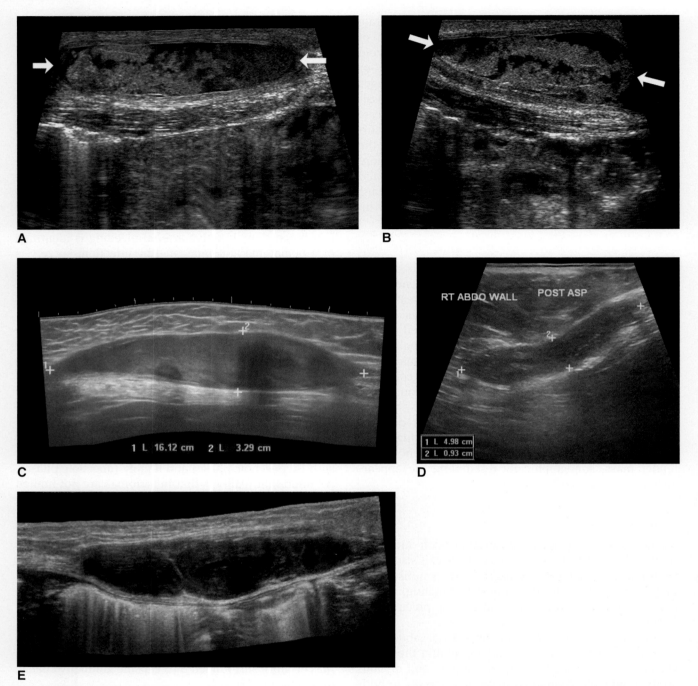

**Figure 2-13** Rectus sheath hematoma. A heterogeneous, lenticular-shaped hematoma (*arrows*) can be identified distal to the arcuate line on both **(A)** the longitudinal and **(B)** the transverse sonograms. (Images courtesy of Philips Medical Systems, Bothell, WA.) **C.** The transverse sonogram of the right abdominal wall slightly distal to the umbilicus visualizes a hypoechoic, homogeneous seroma measuring 16.12 cm × 3.29 cm. **D.** The longitudinal sonogram made postaspiration demonstrates the size change in the seroma that now measures 4.98 cm × 0.93 cm. (Images courtesy of Jill Hansen, Smithfield, UT.) **E.** The mixed echogenicity of the rectus sheath hematoma is from a 76-year-old woman. The patient presented with a clinical finding of a palpable mass, low hemoglobin, and uses anticoagulant therapy. The hematoma presents with a heterogeneous, complex pattern of anechoic, hypoechoic, and hyperechoic echo characteristics. (Image courtesy of Dr. Taco Geertsma, Gelderse Vallei, The Netherlands.)

an unusual layered appearance. The latter is due to the settling of moderately echogenic red blood cells to the bottom of the lesion. The fibrin content of the clot yields decreased echogenicity. Movement of blood can sometimes be produced in such patients by changing their positions. If turbulent blood flow is seen in a patient lying supinely in a fixed position, it indicates active bleeding.[12,15] The sequential use of modern high-resolution sonographic procedures, which clearly delineate the muscular layers of the abdominal wall, is a valuable way to study the response of such lesions to treatment.

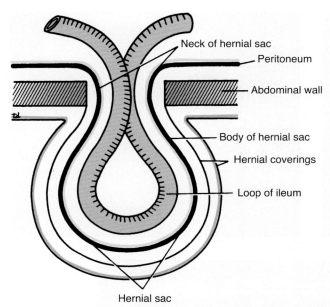

**Figure 2-14** Components of a hernia. Abdominal wall hernias consist of three parts: the sac, the contents of the sac, and the covering of the sac. (Reprinted with permission from Snell RS. *Clinical Anatomy.* 7th ed. Baltimore, MD: Lippincott Williams & Wilkins; 2003.)

## HERNIAS

There are two main categories of abdominal wall hernias: (1) ventral (anterior or anterolateral abdominal wall) and (2) groin (indirect inguinal, direct inguinal, and femoral).[16,17] Diaphragmatic hernias occur with less frequency and are presented later in this chapter. If the abdominal wall muscles are excessively weak through an acquired or congenital wall defect (omphalocele), the viscera lying beneath may protrude, resulting in a hernia. Natural weak areas include where vessels penetrate the abdominal wall; where fetal migration of testis, spermatic cord, or round ligament has occurred; and through aponeuroses.[18] Any condition that increases the pressure such as obesity, heavy lifting, coughing, or straining may contribute to either hernia formation or increased growth of an existing hernia.

Abdominal wall hernias consist of three parts: the sac, the contents of the sac, and the covering of the sac (Fig. 2-14). Hernia contents vary. Of the hernias diagnosed by sonography, most contain only fat, which may be intraperitoneal (mesenteric or omental) or peritoneal in orgin.[18] If a hernia does contain intraperitoneal fat, it may contain bowel later in its course.[18] When bowel is included in hernia contents, it increases the risk compared to those containing only intraperitoneal fat due to strangulation, which may result in ischemia caused by a compromised blood supply.[17,18] Some hernias contain free fluid of intraperitoneal origin.[16,18]

### Ventral Hernias

Ventral hernias are a category for all hernias occurring in the anterior and lateral abdominal wall. These include umbilical, paraumbilical, epigastric, and hypogastric hernias.[17] Other hernias and conditions to present with ventral hernia types, which also occur in the anterior and lateral abdominal wall, include spigelian, strangulation, incarcerated, incisional, and parastomal.[17]

Umbilical hernias are the most common type of ventral hernia. They are either congenital or acquired and are usually small. The umbilical hernia is particularly common in women. Infants and small children often acquire hernias in this area due to the weakness in the scar of the umbilicus in the linea alba (Fig. 2-15A). In most cases in children, these hernias decrease in size and disappear without event or treatment as the abdominal cavity enlarges. In adults, acquired hernias are more commonly termed *paraumbilical hernias* and are a large abdominal defect through the linea alba in the region of the umbilicus and are usually related to diastasis recti, which is a separation between the left and right side of the rectus abdominis muscle.[17] Adult paraumbilical hernias increase gradually in size and are the hernias that most often contain large intestine as well as omentum. Paraumbilical hernias occur with a higher incident in premature infants and in pregnant women (Fig. 2-15B).

Epigastric and hypogastric hernias occur in the linea alba above and below the umbilicus. Epigastric hernias occur through the widest part of the linea alba anywhere between the xyphoid process and the umbilicus. Usually, such hernias begin as a small defect of protruding extraperitoneal fat. Over a period of months or years, that fat is forced through the linea alba, pulling behind it a small peritoneal sac that often contains a small piece of the omentum.[17]

Although the clinical presentation of a spigelian hernia is rare, sonographically detected spigelian hernias are more common.[18] A spigelian hernia can occur anywhere along the course of the spigelian fascia, which is the complex aponeurotic tendon located between the flat anterolateral muscles.[17,18] Almost all spigelian hernias are located at the inferior end of the semicircular line, which is inferior to the arcuate line where the posterior rectus sheath is absent.[18] The spigelian hernia may be listed as an inguinal hernia since its location is within 2 cm of the internal inguinal rings and its symptoms are similar to indirect inguinal hernias[18] (Fig. 2-15C).

Two complications that may occur in midline hernias are strangulation (compromised blood supply causing ischemia) and incarceration or nonreducible (an irreducible sac where contents cannot be pushed back into the abdomen or through torn muscles).[16,17] Surgery is generally indicated because these two conditions are vulnerable to serious complications. With an incarcerated hernia, complicating factors may include edema of the protruding structure and constriction of the opening through which intra-abdominal contents have emerged. Strangulation of the bowel interrupts its blood flow, which progresses to necrosis and will require resection.[16]

An *incisional hernia* is a delayed complication caused by abdominal surgery, which leaves a weak abdominal wall. The hernias are more commonly encountered with

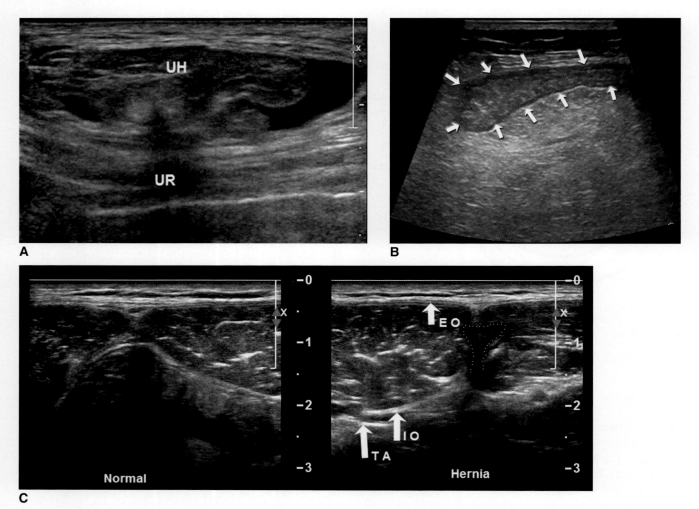

**Figure 2-15** Ventral and spigelian hernias. **A.** The longitudinal plane shows an umbilical hernia *(UH)* containing fat and bowel that passed through a dilated umbilical rings *(UR)*. **B.** On a different patient, the transverse plane shows a paraumbilical hernia *(arrows)* containing fat. **C.** The contiguous muscle can be seen on the normal abdominal wall on the left. On the left, the sonogram demonstrates a small spigelian hernia *(dotted outline)* as it herniated through both the torn transverse abdominis *(TA)* and the internal oblique *(IO)* muscles. The external oblique *(EO)* muscle is intact. On this obese patient, there is a large amount of fat seen between internal oblique and external oblique muscle. A mushroom-shaped or anvil-shaped hernia correlates with nonreducibility and the increased risk of strangulation. (Fig. 2-15A courtesy of Philips Medical Systems, Bothell, WA. Fig. 2-15B courtesy of Taryn Nichols, Providence, UT. Fig. 2-15C courtesy of Philips Medical Systems, Bothell, WA.)

vertical rather than with transverse incisions. Incisional hernias usually develop during the first few months after surgery. With most abdominal surgeries, their reported prevalence ranges from 0.5% to 13.9%, and for aortic surgery, it may be as high as 41%.[17] A subtype of an incisional hernia is a *parastomal hernia*. A parastomal hernia occurs adjacent to a stoma and is particularly difficult to detect at physical examination.[17] Elderly, obese, or malnourished patients are more prone to develop incisional hernias. Infection, which impairs wound healing, is also a predisposing factor.

### Groin Hernias

Groin hernias are a category for those occurring in the ilioinguinal crease at the junction of the abdomen and the thigh and the adjacent areas immediately above and below.[18] This definition limits it to inguinal hernias, but femoral hernias and, at times, spigelian hernias are also included in this category.[17,18]

Inguinal hernias, which make up 75% of all hernias, can be either direct or indirect, and can be either inguinal or femoral.[19] Indirect inguinal hernias are one of the most common forms of hernia and are 20 times more common in males than in females, and twice as common as direct hernias. Indirect hernias arise from the deep inguinal ring and extend superficially and interomedially down the inguinal canal (Fig. 2-16A,B). They can extend down into the scrotum in males, and the labium majorum in females. Nearly a third of inguinal hernias are bilateral, but unilateral hernias are located most often on the right side. Boys and young men are commonly seen with the indirect inguinal hernia in the inguinal canal area, where the testes descended during fetal development.

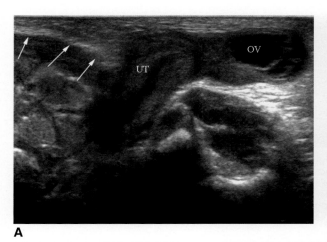 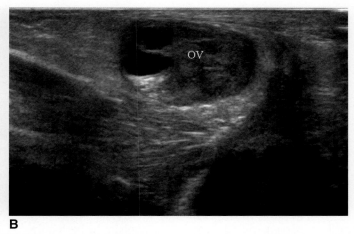

**A**  **B**

Figure 2-16 Inguinal hernia. **A.** The sonograms on this newborn female with a palpable right lower quadrant mass reveal the uterus *(UT)* and ovary *(OV)* herniated through the canal *(arrows)*. **B.** On another plane, the ovary *(OV)* is seen in the area of the mass. (Images courtesy of Dr. Nakul Jerath, Falls Church, VA.)

Direct inguinal hernias are caused by a weakness or tearing of the transversalis fascia, are usually found in elderly men with weak abdominal muscles, and are rarely found in women. Direct inguinal hernias are located medial and inferior to the internal inguinal ring and inferior epigastric arteries. Because the location is posterior to the spermatic cord, the hernia is prevented from extending down into the scrotum and labium majorum. A direct inguinal hernia will appear as nothing more than a generalized bulge.[19]

Femoral hernias occur less frequently than inguinal hernias and are located medial to the femoral vein and posterior to the inguinal ligament, usually on the right side. There is a higher incidence of femoral hernias occurring in females than in males.[17]

### Other Hernias

There are multiple other hernias that occur and these include sports hernia (groin and pubic area), lumbar hernia (defects in lumbar muscles or the posterior fascia below the 12th rib and above the iliac crest), pelvic hernias, traumatic hernias, recurring hernias, and multiple hernias.

### Sonographic Evaluation

Because groin hernias are generally palpable masses, the diagnosis is often made clinically and imaging may be used to evaluate the contralateral size. A diagnostic imaging referral is used because of the limitations of clinical assessment alone for a significant proportion of patients with symptoms suggestive of a hernia but without a lump or bump.[18,20] In one study, sonography was found to be accurate and have a higher sensitivity compared to herniography, which at one time was the imaging procedure of choice for hernia evaluation.[20] Patients are frequently referred for computed tomography (CT) or magnetic resonance (MR) imaging for hernia evaluation especially with nonspecific clinical findings.

The three major advantages of sonography over other imaging modalities are the ability to scan the patient in both upright and supine positions, the ability to include dynamic maneuvers such as Valsalva and compression, and the ability to document motion in real time.[16,18]

In many cases, employing the Valsalva maneuver demonstrates how the hernia content moves distally and the hernia widens. The hernia content moves back toward the abdomen and the sac narrows during the relaxation period following the Valsalva maneuver[16,18] (Fig. 2-17). Using the transducer for compression can reduce the hernia and push contents back toward the abdomen. When the compression is released, the hernia will return to the precompression position.[16,18] The third thing is to employ both supine and upright patient positions. In an upright position, most hernias enlarge or may only be present in the upright position.[16,18]

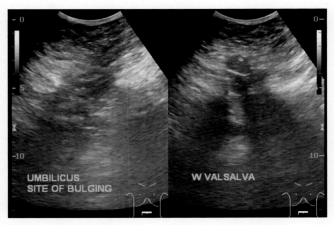

Figure 2-17 Valsalva maneuver. When the two transverse sonograms of an umbilical hernia without the Valsalva maneuver **(left)** and with the Valsalva maneuver **(right)** are compared, the image on the right demonstrates how the hernia widens as it moves distally. (Image courtesy of Taryn Nichols, Providence, UT.)

This scanning protocol allows for the documentation of a significant amount of information. The information includes (1) demonstrating an abdominal wall or groin defect; (2) determining the presence of bowel loops within a lesion; (3) exaggeration of the lesion on straining of the abdominal musculature; and (4) reducibility of the lesion with pressure.

Sonography can determine the location, size, and contents of a hernia. At the site of a hernia, interruption of the peritoneal line separating the muscles and abdominal contents is seen. Sonography can demonstrate the size of the defect and whether the hernia sac is fluid-filled or contains peristaltic bowel or mesenteric fat. Besides peristaltic motion, gas in the bowel produces the typical shadowing artifact. Mesenteric fat, which also appears to be highly reflective, lacks both peristalsis and shadowing. Ascites can complicate the appearance of hernia by producing a clearly fluid-filled sac. At times, the fluid can be evacuated out of the hernial sac and back into the peritoneal cavity when transducer pressure is applied to the area.

A high-frequency linear array transducer should be used to evaluate for a hernia, but a curved-array, lower frequency transducer may be required on obese patients. The larger field of view provides good visualization of landmarks. It is important to capture dynamic events and store these on video loops.

## NEOPLASMS

The primary abdominal wall tumors include (1) lipomas, (2) areas of calcification in old surgical scars, (3) desmoid tumors, (4) soft tissue sarcomas, (5) metastatic carcinoma, and (6) melanomas. Most lesions are readily diagnosed by the physical examination and clinical history. Sonography, CT, MR, and fine-needle biopsy, however, are all valuable tools when the distinction must be made between lipomas, hematomas, abscesses, hernias, and the more serious true neoplasms.

### Lipoma

Lipomas (fatty tumors) are among the most common benign masses of the abdominal wall and subcutaneous tissues. They can be found anywhere fat is present.[21] Lipomas are often surgically removed for cosmetic reasons, as they can grow to be very large. Surgical excision or liposuction can remove a lipoma depending on its size. A new injectable solution of deoxycholate can be injected subcutaneously causing the adipocyte to lyse.[22]

Lipomas are usually strongly echogenic to isoechoic and can be difficult to separate from adipose tissue if located superficially. Most lipomas unusually present with good through-transmission. They tend to be soft, compressible, and, in some cases, movable. The amount of transducer pressure applied must be moderate and consistent to prevent displacement of the mass during scanning (Fig. 2-18). If a suspected lipoma presents with an atypical sonographic appearance, its

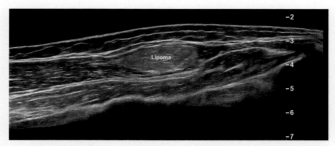

**Figure 2-18** Lipoma. A longitudinal image presents a superficially located, well-defined, and hyperechoic relative to the adjacent musculature lipoma. The intramuscular lipoma can be distinguished from the subcutaneous fat. (Image courtesy of Philips Medical Systems, Bothell, WA.)

recommended follow-up includes further diagnostic testing and MR imaging.

### Desmoid Tumors

Desmoid tumors may also be known as aggressive fibromatosis. They are generally benign fibrous tissue neoplasms commonly found in the anterior abdominal wall. The tumor is most frequently found in patients between the ages of 20 and 40 years. Although these tumors can occur in either sex, they are three times more frequent in women and the tumor is often related to pregnancy. Childbirth, trauma, or hormonal changes during pregnancy are thought to be predisposing factors. There is also a marked increase in desmoid tumors in patients with Gardner syndrome (familial polyposis syndrome). They are also often related to previous abdominal surgery.[23]

Desmoid tumors often present as nontender, benign masses, but can be infiltrating aggressive tumors that destroy adjacent structures.[23,24] Surgical excision is the treatment of choice whenever possible.[23] Follow-up is important because desmoid tumors tend to recur after local excision.[23,24] Recurrence treatment includes radiation therapy, nonsteroidal anti-inflammatory drugs (NSAIDs), hormones, interferon, and chemotherapy. Spontaneous regression of desmoid tumors has been recorded; the estimated recurrence rate is 50%.

Sonographically, desmoid tumors are relatively homogeneous, hypoechoic to isoechoic masses with only occasional internal echoes. Because they permit good through-transmission, the sonographer must use strict criteria for a cystic mass so as not to mistake the tumor for a cyst. The tumor should be evaluated with color Doppler as color flow may be seen within the tumor and is often noted with the more aggressive desmoid tumor.[23,24] Some desmoid tumors appear to be encapsulated sonographically, yet pathologic examination reveals no apparent capsule.

### Neuromas

Neuromas are most commonly found postinjury, normally after surgery when a nerve gets damaged and swelling occurs. Neuromas occur at the end of a severed nerve and are found in 37% posthernia repair patients.[25]

Sonographically, a neuroma is usually solitary, hypoechoic, and may or may not have enhancement. A neuroma does not demonstrate a specific blood flow pattern. It is important to assess patients with previous abdominal surgery for a neuroma when no other cause for pain can be found.[25]

## Endometrioma

An endometrioma of the abdominal wall is typically found postoperatively and usually occurs after cesarean sections or laparotomies. They are often mistaken for incisional hernias. The tumor is painful and the pain may or may not be related to the patient's menstrual cycle.[26]

The sonographic appearance of an endometrioma is nonspecific as it can present as a cystic, polycystic, mixed, and sometimes solid mass.[26]

## Sarcoma

Sarcomas arising from the abdominal wall include liposarcoma, rhabdomyosarcoma, and fibrosarcoma. These tumors can grow without evidence of clinical symptoms for a long time. As a result, they often attain a large size and are difficult to differentiate from large pancreatic tumors, renal tumors, or splenomegaly.[27,28] The sarcoma family of histiocytoma, osteosarcoma, angiosarcoma, fibrosarcoma, and a few rhabdomyosarcomas are seen postradiation in 0.03% to 8% of patients receiving radiation therapy.[28]

Sonographically, soft tissue sarcomas are hypoechoic or isoechoic in comparison to the surrounding muscle. Sonography can be used to locate and identify the mass, but MR imaging is usually performed to determine its size, shape, and if there is involvement with surrounding tissues (Fig. 2-19A–C).

## Metastatic Carcinoma

Metastatic carcinoma to the abdominal wall is frequently related to extension from a nearby primary carcinoma. For instance, in cases of primary ovarian carcinoma, there is a high incidence of clinically unsuspected metastases to the aortic and pelvic lymph nodes, diaphragm, peritoneum, and omentum. The abdominal wall may also be the site of distant metastases arising from laparoscopic port site surgery.[29,30] Note that superficial cutaneous melanomas (occult or recurrent) and pigmented nevi, which are clearly demarcated from normal skin, rarely occur in the anterior abdominal wall. Quite often, they are found subcutaneously. Metastasis may occur as an isolated finding, but more often it is seen in patients with widespread metastatic disease elsewhere.

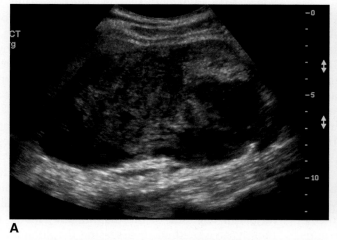

**A**

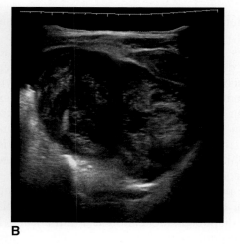

**B**

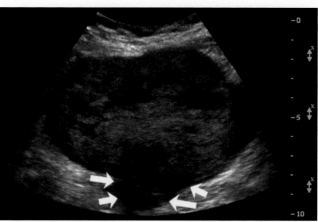

**C**

**Figure 2-19** Sarcoma in abdominal wall. The shape, size, and composition of a sarcoma are evaluated with sonography. **A,B.** This patient was diagnosed with a sarcoma, which is visualized as a heterogeneous mass located in the abdomen. Both images demonstrate good through-transmission, but do not demonstrate invasion of the mass. **C.** This patient was also diagnosed with a sarcoma. The heterogeneous mass shows the extent of involvement with surrounding tissues (arrows) and good through-transmission. Further evaluation on both patients should occur with magnetic resonance imaging and biopsy. (Images courtesy of Philips Medical Systems, Bothell, WA.)

The broad spectrum of sonographic patterns seen in both primary and metastatic carcinomas makes it imperative that sonographers take time to observe the boundaries of the mass and whether or not it encroaches into other areas. The sonographer can add color Doppler to evaluate an increase in vascularity. If at all possible, the sonographer should try to relate the abdominal wall mass to its primary source.

Some malignant masses are anechoic, with their deposits or extensions appearing very echogenic in contrast. Some are well circumscribed, whereas others are spiculated. When imaging a solid-appearing mass, the sonographer must use color Doppler, as malignant neoplasms will demonstrate vascularity.[27] Melanomas typically appear to be hypoechoic and may demonstrate enhanced through-transmission. Other masses, particularly rhabdomyosarcomas, are very echogenic. Tissue necrosis, of course, can produce echo-free areas within such masses. Varying the gain, and at times the transducer, during the studies and being alert to the subtlest changes that can be elicited are most desirable. Correlating what is seen on the sonogram with the physical appearance and clinical history of the patient is equally important.

## DIAPHRAGMATIC PATHOLOGY

The diaphragm is subject to pain, paralysis, herniation, eventration, and peridiaphragmatic abnormalities. Often, pleural effusions are seen adjacent to the diaphragm. Sonography is quickly replacing fluoroscopy as the method of choice for studying diaphragmatic motion because of its ability to examine children without the need for radiation and to easily perform bedside examinations of patients on respirators. In such settings, unassisted ventilation can be evaluated with the respirator disconnected for a few seconds.

The presence of fluid adjacent to the diaphragm (pleural effusion or ascites) prominently displays the central diaphragmatic tendon as a thin linear echo covering the dome of the liver. Peripheral muscle insertions may also be seen posteriorly (sagittal scan) and posterolaterally (transverse scan) as thick, triangle-shaped, hypoechoic bands. The presence of gas in the stomach and bowel makes the left hemidiaphragm more difficult to scan than the right.

### PLEURAL EFFUSION

Pleural effusion, also known as hydrothorax, is an accumulation of fluid within the pleural cavity. In newborns, a pleural effusion is most often caused by a malformed thoracic duct. They may also result from immune or nonimmune causes, such as Rh factors, congestive heart failure, lymphangiectasia, bronchopulmonary sequestration, hernia of the diaphragm,

metastatic diseases, and postsurgical and other unknown causes.[31] Occasionally, when there is a large amount of pleural effusion, or a tension pneumothorax, there is a slight possibility of a diaphragmatic inversion. Typically, the left side is affected, but it can involve the entire hemidiaphragm.[31]

Sonographic imaging for pleural effusions has increased detection by 40% and has decreased the pneumothorax rate to 3% as compared to 18% on clinical guidance alone. Sonography also has the advantage of being able to be performed at the bedside, with a preference for a patient in a seated position if possible.[32] There is an increase in visualizing actual pleural effusions because radiographically, pleural effusions are underestimated.[31] Sonographically, pleural effusion has the appearance of echo-free or anechoic areas on one or both sides of the chest superior to the diaphragm. Occasionally, septa can be seen within the fluid collection.[33,35] The lung does not change shape and the diaphragm appears as a hyperechoic band. Depending on how extensive the effusion is, often part of the lung can be seen floating on the effusion (Fig. 2-20A–C).

### PARALYSIS

Sonography is of particular investigative value when a chest radiograph demonstrates an elevated or obscured hemidiaphragm. Paralysis of one hemidiaphragm, caused by a damaged phrenic nerve, can be detected by showing absent or paradoxical motion on the affected side compared with a normal or exaggerated excursion on the opposite side.[32,35] Diaphragmatic paralysis can be demonstrated by minimal or no thickening of the hemidiaphragm during inspiration.[36] Unlike fluoroscopy, sonography can easily demonstrate the diaphragm even in the presence of peridiaphragmatic masses or fluid collections.[31,35,37,38]

The normal excursion of the diaphragm is easily visualized with sonography. Measuring the diaphragmatic thickness in the zone of apposition can show paralysis of one side of the diaphragm. This is an easy, noninvasive method of assessing diaphragmatic function.[32] Congenital eventration appears as an abnormal bulge or pouch in the diaphragmatic contour that moves normally with respiration. Normally, this pouch is filled with liver. When ascites is present, fluid may be seen filling the pouch separating the liver from the diaphragm.

### EVENTRATION

Eventration is the abnormal elevation of the diaphragm due to the failure of the muscle fibers to develop appropriately during gestation, and may be difficult to distinguish from other lesions or pathologies on a chest radiograph.[33,36] The diaphragm can give way abnormally, so that abdominal organs may protrude through

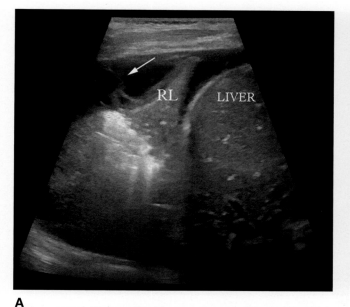

**A**

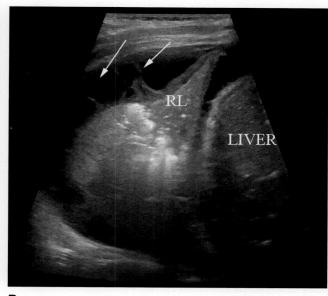

**B**

**C**

**Figure 2-20** Complex pleural effusion. **A,B.** The sonographic chest evaluation from the right posterior surface is performed on a pediatric patient with a history of pneumonia. The sonogram reveals a loculated pleural effusion with thick adhesions *(arrows)* seen superior to the right lobe of the liver. The right lung *(RL)* is seen as well. The adhesions can make thoracentesis more difficult, but sonography can help guide the procedure. **C.** Sonographic evaluation from the coronal right chest in a different pediatric patient demonstrates a complex pleural effusion *(PE)* superior to the right lobe of the liver. The right lung *(RL)* is also visualized.

a weakened section to form a diaphragmatic hernia. Elevation of the dome of the diaphragm was traditionally considered a developmental anomaly resulting from incomplete muscularization of the membranous diaphragm. Today, it is recognized that it may also be an acquired condition related to muscular weakness resulting from focal ischemia, infarct, or neuromuscular dysfunction. This condition accounts for 5% of all diaphragmatic defects.[33,36,39]

Diaphragmatic eventration may be partial (segmental) or complete (total), unilateral or bilateral. With segmental eventration, the anterior portion of the right hemidiaphragm is most often affected. Complete eventration occurs more often in men and on the left side.[33,39] Unilateral eventration is often associated with rib anomalies, whereas bilateral eventration is often associated with trisomy 13–15 and 18 and with Beckwith-Wiedemann syndrome.[39,41] It has the same effect as diaphragmatic

paralysis in that it limits movement of the diaphragm and inhibits ventilation.[33]

## HERNIA

Diaphragmatic defects may be either congenital or acquired. Congenital diaphragmatic hernia affects 1 in approximately 2,000 to 5,000 live births and results from diaphragmatic fusion failure, maldevelopment, or localized weakness. Approximately 56% of affected infants die from respiratory failure.[40] Diaphragmatic hernias may also develop following surgery, other trauma, or increased intrathoracic or intra-abdominal pressure.[33] Diaphragmatic hernias allow abdominal contents to enter into the thorax, and around 95% of hernias are through the left posterior lateral diaphragm. This allows stomach, small bowel, and even spleen to enter into the thorax, sometimes shifting the mediastinum and heart.[40,42]

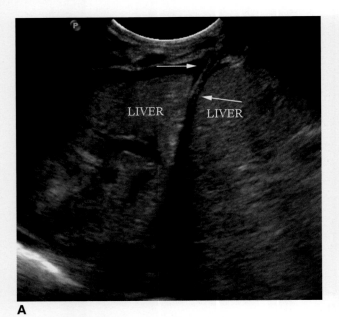

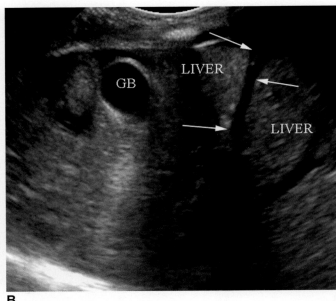

**A**    **B**

**Figure 2-21** Diaphragmatic hernia. **A.** The sonographic evaluation on a prenatal patient reveals a diaphragmatic hernia. The liver is seen on both sides of the diaphragm *(arrows)*. **B.** The gallbladder *(GB)* is also seen superior to the diaphragm. (Images courtesy of Dr. Nakul Jerath, Falls Church, VA.)

The normal fetal diaphragm appears as a thin, hypoechoic band separating the thorax from the abdomen. With congenital diaphragmatic hernia of the left side, sonography may show the presence of a fluid-filled stomach or bowel in the lower thorax, displacing the fetal heart.[40] On the right side, the liver, or bowel, will be seen within the chest cavity, the stomach will be below the diaphragm (Fig. 2-21A,B). In adults, usually the esophagus, and perhaps part of the stomach, can be seen within the chest cavity on the left.

## INVERSION

If a patient has inversion, a longitudinal section shows the hemidiaphragm bulging inferiorly in a convex fashion toward the abdomen. Respiratory distress, the result of air exchange between the two lungs in inspiration and expiration, causes the diaphragm to show little motion or to show asynchronous motion.

## RUPTURE

Penetrating injuries or blunt trauma may produce rupture of the diaphragm. With blunt thoracoabdominal trauma, 5% of patients have diaphragmatic rupture with the left side affected in 90% of the cases.[33,35,38,42,43] In rare instances, rupture may occur secondary to severe infection (e.g., amebiasis), or violent coughing.[38]

Posttraumatic diaphragmatic rupture requires surgical closure. The preoperative diagnosis of diaphragmatic rupture is difficult to make when multiple injuries and other life-threatening conditions exist simultaneously. Its presence may first be suggested by imaging studies such as chest radiography, peritoneal lavage,

sonography, scintigraphy, CT, and MR.[43] Any delay in making the diagnosis increases the chances of morbidity and mortality.[42-44]

The disruption of diaphragmatic echoes and visualization of herniated abdominal viscera are the sonographic signs of diaphragmatic rupture. Extensive (<10 cm long) ruptures have also been reported.[43]

## NEOPLASMS

The diaphragm is an uncommon site for neoplastic disease, either primary or secondary. The most common primary neoplasms are fibrous in nature or undifferentiated sarcomas. Secondary involvement usually occurs with local invasion by adjacent pleural, peritoneal, or thoracic and abdominal wall malignancies.[45-48]

Disruption or interruption of the diaphragm at the site of metastatic implants can be visualized sonographically, as well as partial or complete diaphragmatic inversion. The mass is usually heterogeneous with possible extension into contiguous organs.[46,48]

## SUMMARY

- The anterior abdominal wall extends from the xyphoid process to the symphysis pubis and is made up of the skin layer, the subcutaneous layer, and a musculofascial layer.

- The anterolateral abdominal wall is made up of the rectus abdominis, transverse, internal oblique, and external oblique muscles.

- Sonography provides a noninvasive method of imaging the abdominopelvic wall and detecting pathologic processes such as abscess, hematoma, hernia, or masses.

- Abdominal wall abscesses frequently occur as a result of postsurgical incisional infections, trauma, or as extensions of a superficial intraperitoneal abscess.

- Sonographically, an abscess can appear anechoic or have internal echoes, may be irregular or smooth bordered, and if the abscess contains gas, it may be echogenic with shadowing.

- Hematomas can be postsurgical or associated with trauma.

- The sonographic appearance of a hematoma varies with stage of resolution, but varies from hypoechoic to echogenic.

- A hernia occurs when the abdominal wall muscles are weak and the viscera lying beneath protrude.

- Hernias are normally classified ventral or groin and include umbilical, inguinal, femoral, epigastric, and spigelian.

- Sonographic criteria for abdominal wall hernia include demonstration of an abdominal wall defect, presence of bowel in the lesion, exaggeration of the lesion on straining of the abdominal muscles, and reducibility of the lesion with pressure.

- Neoplasms of the abdominal wall include lipomas, desmoid tumors, sarcomas, and metastatic tumors.

- Sonography can be used to visualize diaphragmatic paralysis, diaphragmatic hernia, inversion or rupture of the diaphragm, diaphragmatic neoplasms, and pleural effusion.

- The expanded and improved capabilities of diagnostic sonography available today demand a reassessment of the standard sonographic curriculum to include a fuller appreciation of the normal and abnormal appearances of the abdominopelvic wall and diaphragm. Only when these practices are utilized will patients receive the benefits of a complete abdominal sonography examination.

## Critical Thinking Questions

1. A 42-year-old patient presents with a recent history of abdominal surgery with pain and redness around the incision site. What type of transducer would you use to evaluate the area and what protocol would you follow? What do you expect to see?

2. A patient presents for an abdominal sonography to rule out an abdominal wall hernia. The patient complains of a palpable midline mass but, as you scan the patient supine, you are having a difficult time visualizing the mass. What technique should help you visualize the hernia and what do you expect to see?

3. You receive a request to evaluate a patient in the intensive care unit for diaphragmatic paralysis. Sonographically, how is diaphragmatic paralysis diagnosed?

## REFERENCES

1. Moore K, Dalley A, Agur A. *Clinically Oriented Anatomy.* 6th ed. Philadelphia, PA: Lippincott Williams & Wilkins; 2010.
2. Moore KL, Agur AM. *Essential Clinical Anatomy.* 3rd ed. Baltimore, MD: Lippincott Williams & Wilkins; 2007.
3. Fagan SP, Awad SS. Abdominal wall anatomy: the key to a successful inguinal hernia repair. *Am J Surg.* 2004; 188(6A Suppl):3S–8S.
4. Dempsey R. Rectus sheath hematoma. *JDMS.* 1997;13: 240–243.
5. Madden ME. *Introduction to Sectional Anatomy.* 2nd ed. Baltimore, MD: Lippincott Williams & Wilkins; 2008.
6. Gibbs TS. The use of sonography in identification, localization, and removal of soft tissue foreign bodies. *JDMS.* 2006;22:5–21.
7. Ahman H, Thompson L, Swarbrick A, et al. Understanding the advanced signal processing technique of real-time adaptive filters. *JDMS.* 2009;25:145–160.
8. Ridge C. Sonographers and the fight against nosocomial infections: how are we doing? *JDMS.* 2005;21:7–11.
9. Rote NS, Huether SE. Innate immunity: inflammation. In: MCanc3e, KL, Huether, SE, Brashers VL, et al. eds. *Pathophysiology: The Biologic Basis for Diseases in Adults and Children.* 6th ed. St. Louis, MO: Elsevier Mosby; 2010:183-216.
10. Murphy HS, Ward PA. Inflammation. In: Rubin, E, Gorstein F, Rubin R, et al., eds. *Rubin's Pathology: Clinicopathologic Foundations of Medicine.* 4th ed. Baltimore, MD: Lippincott Williams & Wilkins; 2005:41–83.
11. Hlava N, Niemann C, Gropper M, et al. Analytic reviews: postoperative infectious complications of abdominal solid organ transplantation. *J Intensive Care Med.* 2009; 24:3–17.
12. Osinbowale O, Bartholomew J. Rectus sheath hematoma. *Vasc Med.* 2008;13:275–279.
13. Schierloh H, Winter T. Fever of unknown origin. In: Sanders RC, Winter T, eds. *Clinical Sonography: A Practical Guide.* 4th ed. Baltimore, MD: Lippincott Williams & Wilkins; 2007:107–118.
14. Milburn DT. An overview: why we do the things we do (in ultrasound). *JDMS.* 2005;21:17–35.
15. Merton DA. Ultrasound examination of invasive procedure puncture site complications. *JDMS.* 1993;9: 297–305.
16. Rapp CL. Ultrasound of abdominal wall masses. In: Sanders RC, Winter T, eds. *Clinical Sonography: A Practical Guide.* 4th ed. Baltimore, MD: Lippincott Williams & Wilkins; 2007:125–132.
17. Aguierre DA, Santosa AC, Casola G, et al. Abdominal wall hernias: imaging features, complications, and diagnostic pitfalls at multi-detector row CT. *Radiographics.* 2005;25(6): 1501–1520.
18. Stavros AT, Rapp CT. Dynamic ultrasound of hernias of the groin and anterior abdominal wall. In: Rumack CM, Wilson SR, Charbonneau JW, et al., eds. *Diagnostic Ultrasound.* 4th ed., Vol. 1. Philadelphia, PA: Elsevier Mosby; 2011:486–523.
19. Guse JW. Ventral/incisional abdominal wall hernia with urinary bladder component. *JDMS.* 2003;19:107–109.
20. Robinson P, Henson E, Lansdown M, et al. Inguinofemoral hernia: accuracy of sonography in patients with indeterminate clinical features. *AJR Am J Roentgenol.* 2006;187(5):1168–1178.

21. Ahuja A, King A, Kew J, et al. Head and neck lipomas: sonographic appearance. *AJNR Am J Neuroradiol*. 1998; 19(3):505–508.

22. Rotunda A, Ablon G, Kolodney M. Lipomas treated with subcutaneous deoxycholate injections. *J Am Acad Dermatol*. 2005;53(6):973–978.

23. Stanek K. Intra-abdominal desmoid tumor. *JDMS*. 2007; 23:212–214.

24. Taggart R, Kavic T. Sonographic evaluation of fibromatosis (aggressive type) using color Doppler interrogation. *JDMS*. 2003;19:248–251.

25. Malpass S. Abdominal wall neuroma. *JDMS*. 2008;24: 225–227.

26. Blanco R, Parithivel V, Shah A, et al. Abdominal wall endometriomas. *Am J Surg*. 2003;185:596–598.

27. Stavros T. *Breast Ultrasound*. Philadelphia, PA: Lippincott Williams & Wilkins; 2004.

28. Rajaram V, Hill A, Doherty G, et al. Pleomorphic rhabdomyosarcoma of the anterior abdominal wall following multimodality treatment for carcinoma of the rectum. *Int J Surg Path*. 2004;12(2):161–165.

29. Wang P, Yen M, Yuan C, et al. Port site metastasis after laparoscopic-assisted vaginal hysterectomy for endometrial cancer: possible mechanisms and prevention. *Gynecol Oncol*. 1997;66(1):151–155.

30. Aoki Y, Shimura H, Li H, et al. A model of port-site metastases of gallbladder cancer: the influence of peritoneal injury and its repair on abdominal wall metastases. *Surgery*. 1999;125(5):553–559.

31. Piccoli M, Trambaiolo P, Salustri A, et al. Bedside diagnosis and follow-up of patients with pleural effusion by a hand-carried ultrasound device early after cardiac surgery. *Chest*. 2005;128(5):3413–3420.

32. Ledwidge M, Winter T. Rule out pleural effusion and chest mass. In: Sanders RC, Winter T, eds. *Clinical Sonography: A Practical Guide*. 4th ed. Baltimore, MD: Lippincott Williams & Wilkins; 2007:200–207.

33. Yang J. Left diaphragmatic eventration diagnosed as congenital diaphragmatic hernia by prenatal sonography. *J Clin Ultrasound*. 2003;31(4):214–217.

34. Tu CY, Hsu WH, Hsia TC, et al. Pleural effusions in febrile medical ICU patients. *Chest*. 2004;126(4):1274–1280.

35. Merino-Ramirez M, Juan G, Ramón M, et al. Electrophysiologic evaluation of phrenic nerve and diaphragm function after coronary bypass surgery: prospective study of diabetes and other risk factors. *J Thorac Cardiovasc Surg*. 2006;132(3):530–536.

36. Summerhill E, El-Sameed YA, Glidden TJ, et al. Monitoring recovery from diaphragm paralysis with ultrasound. *Chest*. 2008;133(3):737–743.

37. Mullinix AJ, Foley WD. Multidetector computed tomography and blunt thoracoabdominal trauma. *J Comput Assist Tomogr*. 2004;28(suppl 1):S20–S27.

38. Lerolle N, Guerot E, Dimassi S, et al. Ultrasonographic diagnostic criterion for severe diaphragmatic dysfunction after cardiac surgery. *Chest*. 2009;135(2):401–407.

39. Eren S, Ceviz N, Alper F. Congenital diaphragmatic eventration as a cause of anterior mediastinal mass in children: imaging modalities and literature review. *Eur J Radiol*. 2004;51(1):85–90.

40. Garne E, Haeusler M, Barisic I, et al. Congenital diaphragmatic hernia: evaluation of prenatal diagnosis in 20 European regions. *Ultrasound Obstet Gynecol*. 2002;19(4): 329–333.

41. Chen CP, Shu-Chin C. Prenatal sonographic features of Beckwith-Wiedemann syndrome. *J Ultrasound Med*. 2009; 17:98–106.

42. Daniel R, Naidu B, Marzouk J. Cough-induced rib fracture and diaphragmatic rupture resulting in simultaneous abdominal visceral herniation into the left hemithorax and subcutaneously. *Eur J Cardiothorac Surg*. 2008;34(4): 914–915.

43. Turham K, Makay O, Cakan A, et al. Traumatic diaphragmatic rupture: look to see. *Eur J Cardiothorac Surg*. 2008;33(6):1082–1085.

44. Al-Refaie R, Awad E, Mokbel E. Blunt traumatic diaphragmatic rupture: a retrospective observational study of 46 patients. *J Thorac Cardiovasc Surg*. 2009;9(1):45–49.

45. Eroglu A, Küçüoglu C, Karaoglanoglu N, et al. Extraskeletal Ewing sarcoma of the diaphragm presenting with hemothorax. *Ann Thorac Surg*. 2004;78(2):715–717.

46. Kumbasar U, Enon S, Osman A, et al. An uncommon tumor of the diaphragm malignant schwannoma. *J Thorac Cardiovasc Surg*. 2004;3:384–385.

47. Sem S, Discigil B, Badak I, et al. Lipoma of the diaphragm: a rare presentation. *Ann Thorac Surg*. 2007; 83(6):2203–2205.

48. Deniz P, Kalac N, Ucoluk G, et al. A rare tumor of the diaphragm: pleomorphic rhabdomyosarcoma. *Ann Thorac Surg*. 2008;85(5):1802–1805.

# 3 The Peritoneal Cavity

Joie Burns

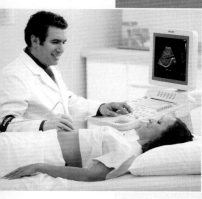

## OBJECTIVES

Identify the potential spaces of the peritoneum and the organs and/or ligaments that divide them on diagrams.

Identify the potential spaces of the peritoneum on sonograms.

State the organs located in the peritoneum.

Describe the scanning techniques used to image the potential spaces and diseases of the peritoneum.

Explain the role greater omentum and mesentery play in limiting the extent of pathology.

Recognize the sonographic appearance of benign and malignant changes seen in the peritoneum.

Analyze sonographic images of the peritoneum for pathology.

## KEY TERMS

abscess | ascites | biloma | FAST scan | hematoma | hemoperitoneum | lymphocele | mesothelioma | omental caking | peritoneal implants | pseudomyxoma peritonei | seroma | urinoma

## GLOSSARY

**abscess** a pocket of infection typically containing pus, blood, and degenerating tissue

**ascites** free fluid within the peritoneal cavity that may be associated with liver failure, abdominal trauma, or malignancy

**bare area** surface area of a peritoneal organ devoid of peritoneum

**biloma** a collection of extravasated bile that can occur with trauma or rupture of the biliary tract

**extraperitoneal organs** organs outside of the parietal peritoneum, but typically covered by parietal peritoneum on one side

**FAST scan** focused assessment with sonography in trauma scan. A triage sonography examination performed in the field or emergency department to detect free fluid within the chest and peritoneum that would indicate bleeding

**hematoma** an extravasated collection of blood localized within a potential space or tissue

**hemoperitoneum** extravasated blood within the peritoneal cavity

**hilum** area of the organ where blood vessels, lymph, and nerves enter and exit

**iatrogenic** treatment induced; may be intentional or unintentional

**lymphocele** an extravasated collection of lymph

**mesentery** two layers of fused peritoneum that conduct nerves, lymph, and blood vessels between the small bowel/colon and the posterior peritoneal cavity wall

**parietal peritoneum** peritoneum lining the walls of the peritoneal cavity

**peritoneal organs** solid organs within the peritoneal cavity that are covered by visceral peritoneum

**retroperitoneal organs** organs posterior to the parietal peritoneum that are typically covered on their anterior surface or fatty capsule by parietal peritoneum

**seroma** fluid collection composed of blood products located adjacent to or surrounding transplanted organs in the early transplantation period

**visceral peritoneum** peritoneum encasing peritoneal organs

Sonography can play a significant role in the identification of disease processes within the peritoneal cavity and, therefore, the peritoneal cavity is an important area of the body for sonographers to be familiar with. There are many disease processes of peritoneal organs that can result in pathology of the peritoneal cavity, including metastasis and a variety of fluid collections. Because of its ability to differentiate between cystic and solid lesions and collections, sonography excels at imaging the potential spaces within the abdominopelvic cavity. Sonography's real-time capabilities and use of sound waves instead of ionizing radiation make it an excellent technology for imaging as well as biopsy or aspiration guidance. A thorough understanding of the anatomy of the peritoneal cavity, especially its divisions, will assist sonographers in determining the presence and extent of disease processes.

## ABDOMINOPELVIC CAVITY

The abdominopelvic cavity can be described by two commonly accepted methods using superficial landmarks. The first, Addison lines, divides the abdominopelvic cavity into nine regions by drawing two sagittal (vertical) lines and two axial (horizontal) lines. The first of the axial lines is called the *transpyloric line* and is determined by drawing an imaginary line halfway between the manubrial notch and the superior pubic symphysis. Instead of using the transpyloric line, some choose to use the subcostal line, a line drawn at the inferior border of the last rib, for its ease of visualization. The second of the axial lines is called the *transtubercular line* and is determined by drawing an imaginary line halfway between the transpyloric line and the superior pubic symphysis. This line also intersects the anterior superior iliac spines (ASISs) of the pelvis. The sagittal lines are drawn halfway between the manubrial notch and the acromioclavicular joint called the *midclavicular line* or *mammary line*. These lines divide the abdomen into right and left hypochondriac; lumbar and iliac bilaterally; and epigastric, umbilical, and hypogastric centrally[1] (Fig. 3-1).

The abdominopelvic cavity may also be described in quadrants. One imaginary line is drawn vertically from the tip of the xiphoid process to the superior pubic symphysis along the sagittal midline plane, and a horizontal line is drawn at the level of the umbilicus. This divides the abdominopelvic cavity into the right upper quadrant (RUQ), right lower quadrant (RLQ), left upper quadrant (LUQ), and left lower quadrant (LLQ). This simpler method is the one most commonly employed in the clinical setting[1] (Fig. 3-2). The sonographer must be well versed in the anatomy that is found in each of these regions in order to correlate clinical findings with the sonographic examination.

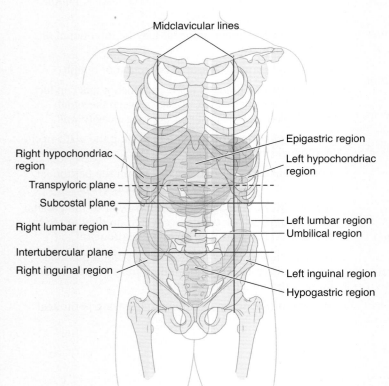

Midclavicular lines

Epigastric region

Right hypochondriac region

Left hypochondriac region

Transpyloric plane

Subcostal plane

Right lumbar region

Left lumbar region
Umbilical region

Intertubercular plane

Right inguinal region

Left inguinal region
Hypogastric region

**Figure 3-1** Addison lines. Nine regions of the abdominopelvic cavity based on Addison lines. The abdominal cavity is divided into nine regions by two sagittal midclavicular lines and two axial lines, the transpyloric line and the transtubercular line.

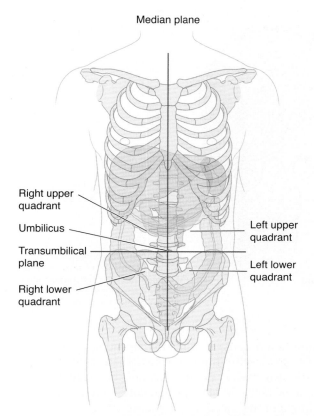

Figure 3-2 Quadrants of the abdominopelvic cavity. The abdominal cavity can be divided into four quadrants: right upper quadrant, right lower quadrant, left upper quadrant, and left lower quadrant.

## ANATOMY OF THE PERITONEAL CAVITY

A thin sheet of tissues called the *peritoneal membrane* divides the abdominal cavity into peritoneal and retroperitoneal compartments. The largest of the body cavities is the peritoneal cavity, encompassing the abdomen and pelvis.

The peritoneal cavity is formed by the fourth embryonic week and is derived from the mesoderm.[2] The abdominopelvic cavity is lined with a thin continuous layer of peritoneum. The cavity is completely sealed in males, but communicates with the external environment via the fallopian tubes in females. Peritoneum that envelopes the organs is referred to as *visceral peritoneum* and the peritoneal layer that lines the walls of the abdominopelvic cavity is referred to as *parietal peritoneum*. This thin layer coating all surfaces of the peritoneal cavity and its organs secretes a small amount of serous fluid, approximately 50 mL, which acts to lubricate visceral surfaces, allowing them to move without friction.[1]

As organs develop along the posterior abdominal wall and protrude into the peritoneal cavity, they are covered by visceral peritoneum except at their hilum where blood vessels, nerves, and lymph enter and exit the organ. The hila of peritoneal organs are considered

bare areas because they lack a peritoneal covering. These bare areas are part of the retroperitoneum.

## DIVISIONS OF THE PERITONEAL CAVITY

The peritoneal cavity is generally divided into two compartments: the greater sac and the lesser sac. The *greater sac* is the largest, housing the liver, spleen, stomach, first portion of the duodenum, jejunum, ileum, cecum, transverse colon, sigmoid colon, and the upper two-thirds of the rectum.[1] This large sac contains several potential spaces that must be evaluated for free fluid.

The *lesser sac* may be thought of as a diverticulum of the greater sac and is also referred to as the omental bursa by some. The lesser sac does not contain any organs. This potential space lies immediately posterior to the stomach, extending superiorly to the left suprahepatic recess between the posterior left lobe of the liver and the left hemidiaphragm. The lesser sac extends inferiorly into the fold of the greater omentum. This may also be referred to as the *inferior recess of the lesser sac* or *omental bursa*. Note that this fold is patent in infants and small children but generally fuses in adults, thereby significantly limiting the caudal extent of the lesser sac (Fig. 3-3A,B). The lesser sac's anterior wall is formed by the posterior stomach, whereas superiorly it is enclosed by the lesser omentum, also called *hepatogastric ligament*. The splenorenal and gastrosplenic ligaments create the left lateral wall of this pocket (Fig. 3-4). The omental foramen, also called the *foramen of Winslow*, is located at the right lateral aspect of the lesser sac and is the only opening communicating with the greater sac. This opening is found posterior to the *hepatoduodenal ligament*, the thickened right border of the lesser omentum that guides the portal triad into the liver (Fig. 3-4).

The lesser omentum—also called the *small omentum*, *gastrohepatic omentum*, and *gastrohepatic ligament*—is a fused double layer of peritoneum stretching between the lesser curvature of the stomach and the left sagittal fissure for the ligamentum venosum (transverse fissure). This ligament creates the anterior superior border of the lesser sac, separating it from the supracolic compartment of the greater sac (Fig. 3-5).

Within the greater sac is a large apron-like double-layered sheet of peritoneum called the *greater omentum* that extends inferiorly from the greater curvature of the stomach and transverse colon. The greater omentum extends inferiorly from the greater curve of the stomach, anterior to the bowel, folds inward, and travels superiorly to attach on the transverse colon. The anterior and posterior adjacent layers are separate in infants but typically fused in adults and contain a variable amount of fat[3] (Fig. 3-3). The greater omentum functions to prevent the parietal peritoneum of the anterior abdominal wall from adhering to the visceral peritoneum. This mesenteric drape is very mobile and moves to areas of inflammation, surrounding the inflamed area by creating adhesions to

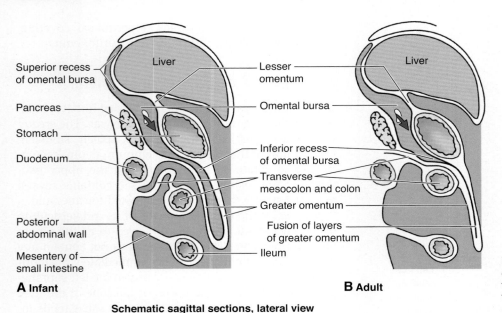

Superior recess of omental bursa

Liver

Lesser omentum

Pancreas

Omental bursa

Stomach

Duodenum

Inferior recess of omental bursa

Transverse mesocolon and colon

Greater omentum

Posterior abdominal wall

Fusion of layers of greater omentum

Mesentery of small intestine

Ileum

**A Infant**

**B Adult**

**Schematic sagittal sections, lateral view**

**Figure 3-3** Lesser sac. Note the patent inferior recess of the lesser sac in the infant **(A)** and the fused nature of the same space in the adult **(B)**. The *red arrow* indicates the omental foramen.

wall off infection (Fig. 3-6A,B). It also acts to cushion the abdominal organs to prevent trauma and acts to prevent the loss of body heat from abdominal organs.

The greater omentum subdivides the greater sac into a supracolic (above the colon) compartment and an infracolic (below the colon) compartment. The supracolic compartment is located anterior to the greater omentum and stomach and inferior to the liver. The infracolic compartment is posterior to the greater omentum, surrounding the small bowel and colon within the remainder of the greater sac (Fig. 3-7). This division is important because it limits the spread of infected materials, pus, ascitic fluid, and malignant cells within the peritoneal cavity. Communication between these two compartments is via the paracolic gutters, the lateral borders of the ascending and descending colon.

## POTENTIAL SPACES OF THE PERITONEUM

As organs grow into the peritoneal cavity, several pockets and recesses are formed by the organs, their vascular connections, and suspensory ligaments, thereby creating

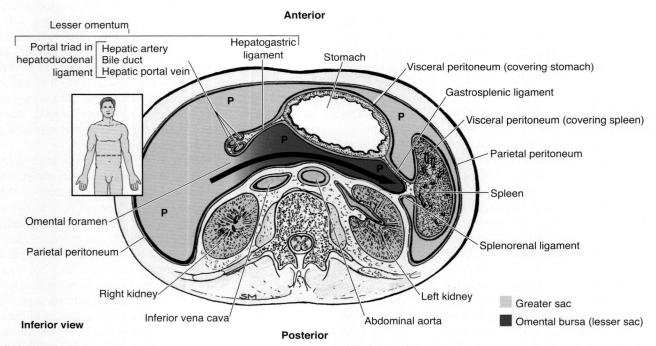

**Anterior**

Lesser omentum

Portal triad in hepatoduodenal ligament — Hepatic artery / Bile duct / Hepatic portal vein

Hepatogastric ligament

Stomach

Visceral peritoneum (covering stomach)

Gastrosplenic ligament

Visceral peritoneum (covering spleen)

Parietal peritoneum

Spleen

Omental foramen

Parietal peritoneum

Splenorenal ligament

Right kidney

Inferior vena cava

Left kidney

Abdominal aorta

**Inferior view**

**Posterior**

Greater sac

Omental bursa (lesser sac)

**Figure 3-4** Omental foramen. The *black arrow* extends through the omental foramen through the width of the lesser sac. The opening is posterior to the hepatoduodenal ligament. The lesser space is seen immediately posterior to the stomach.

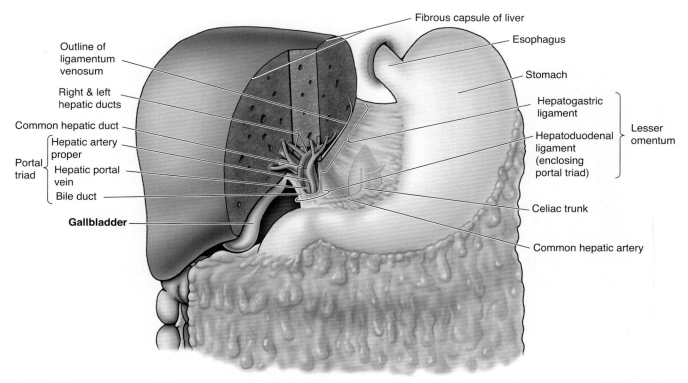

Fibrous capsule of liver

Outline of ligamentum venosum

Right & left hepatic ducts

Common hepatic duct

Portal triad {
Hepatic artery proper

Hepatic portal vein

Bile duct
}

**Gallbladder**

Esophagus

Stomach

Hepatogastric ligament

Hepatoduodenal ligament (enclosing portal triad)

} Lesser omentum

Celiac trunk

Common hepatic artery

**Figure 3-5** Lesser omentum. The lesser omentum is a double layer of peritoneum that stretches between the lesser curvature of the stomach to the left sagittal fissure for the ligamentum venosum.

a complex landscape for sonographers to examine when performing abdominal and pelvic examinations. Ligaments divide portions of the peritoneal cavity. Sonographers require a working knowledge of these ligaments in order to understand where to look for fluid within the peritoneal sac and how to image and describe its location. See Table 3-1 for a description of the ligaments of the peritoneal cavity.

Potential spaces are areas created by the peritoneal layer, reflecting between two organs or an organ and the peritoneal wall (typically posterior). A potential space is an empty fold; however, when disease is present, fluid or other materials may collect in this space. Because many pathologies present with excretions (ascitic fluid, blood, pus) into the peritoneal cavity, sonographers must examine these potential spaces and characterize

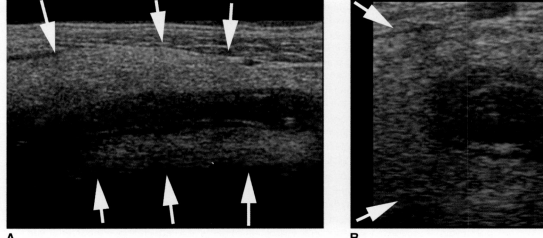

A

B

**Figure 3-6** Greater omentum. **A.** Longitudinal image in a patient with appendicitis demonstrates hyperechoic omental fat *(arrows)* surrounding the inflamed appendix. **B.** Transverse image again demonstrates the hyperechoic omental fat *(arrows)* seen surrounding the inflamed appendix. (Images courtesy of Dr. Taco Geertsma, Ede, The Netherlands.)

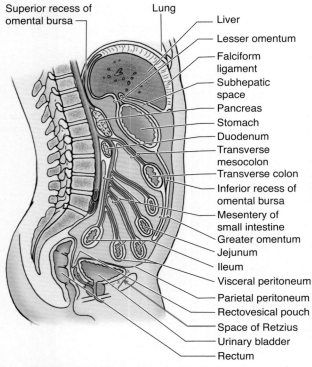

Superior recess of omental bursa
Lung
Liver
Lesser omentum
Falciform ligament
Subhepatic space
Pancreas
Stomach
Duodenum
Transverse mesocolon
Transverse colon
Inferior recess of omental bursa
Mesentery of small intestine
Greater omentum
Jejunum
Ileum
Visceral peritoneum
Parietal peritoneum
Rectovesical pouch
Space of Retzius
Urinary bladder
Rectum

**Figure 3-7** Divisions of the peritoneal cavity. *Green* represents the supracolic compartment of the greater sac; *pink* represents the infracolic compartment of the greater sac; and *blue* represents the lesser sac.

the fluid as part of the abdominal and pelvic examinations. The following text includes anatomic descriptions of each major potential space of the peritoneal cavity.

## Left Anterior Subphrenic Space

The left anterior subphrenic or suprahepatic space is an extension of the greater sac between the diaphragm and the anterior superior liver leftward of the falciform ligament.

## Left Posterior Suprahepatic Space

The left posterior suprahepatic space is also called the *superior recess of the lesser sac*; this space is an extension of the lesser sac between the diaphragm and the posterior superior liver. See Figures 3-3 and 3-7.

## Right Subphrenic Space

The right subphrenic or suprahepatic space is an extension of the greater sac between the right hemidiaphragm and the anterior superior liver rightward of the falciform ligament (Fig. 3-8).

## Hepatorenal Space

The hepatorenal space is also referred to as *Morrison pouch*. This peritoneal potential space is created by the peritoneum, reflecting from the liver over the right kidney and right posterior peritoneal wall. When the

| TABLE 3-1 | |
|---|---|
| **Ligaments of the Peritoneal Cavity** | |
| Gastrohepatic ligament | Also called the lesser omentum, smaller omentum, and gastrohepatic omentum. Connects the lesser curvature of the stomach and the left sagittal fissure for the ligamentum venosum (transverse fissure) of the liver. |
| Hepatoduodenal ligament | Thickened free edge of the lesser omentum through which courses the portal triad. Connects the liver to the duodenum. |
| Falciform ligament | Double-layered fold of peritoneum that ascends from the umbilicus to the liver. Contained within it is the ligamentum teres. The falciform ligament passes onto the anterior and then the superior surface of the liver before splitting into two layers. The right layer forms the upper layer of the coronary ligament; the left layer forms the upper layer of the left triangular ligament. |
| Coronary ligament | Bifurcation of the falciform ligament layers that fuse with the parietal peritoneum to form borders of the bare area of the liver, suspending the liver from the diaphragm. The right branch becomes the coronary ligament and the left branch becomes the left triangular ligament. Limiting the greater sac at its cephalad extent into anterior and posterior compartments in the right subphrenic area. |
| Left triangular ligament | Formed by the left branch of the falciform ligament and the parietal peritoneum. Forms the left extremity of the bare area of the liver. |
| Splenorenal ligament | Also called the lienorenal ligament, connects the splenic hilum to the posterior abdominal wall, through which the splenic vein and artery travel. |
| Gastrosplenic ligament | Connects the stomach to the spleen and inferior diaphragm. |
| Broad ligament | A suspensory ligament that extends from the lateral uterine sidewalls to the pelvic sidewalls dividing the pelvis into anterior and posterior compartments in the female. |
| Ligamentum teres | Remnant of the fetal umbilical vein, which is contained within the falciform ligament. It passes into a fissure on the visceral liver surface to join the left branch of the portal vein in the porta hepatis. |
| Ligamentum venosum | Exhibits as a fibrous band (remnant of the ductus venosus) attached to the left branch of the portal vein. It ascends in a fissure on the visceral liver surface to attach above the inferior vena cava. In fetal circulation, oxygenated blood flows to the liver via the umbilical vein (ligamentum teres). Most of the blood bypasses the liver via the ductus venosus (ligamentum venosum) and joins the inferior vena cava. |

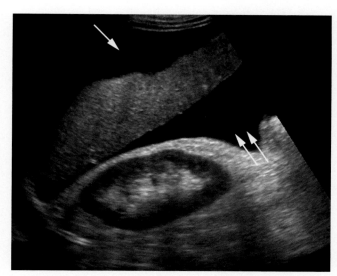

**Figure 3-8** Right anterior subphrenic space and hepatorenal space. Longitudinal image of the right upper quadrant demonstrates fluid within the right anterior subphrenic space *(single arrow)*; ascites is also seen within the hepatorenal space *(double arrows)*. (Image courtesy of Philips Medical Systems, Bothel, WA.)

patient is in a supine position, this space is the most gravity-dependent potential space of the abdominal cavity, collecting fluid from the supracolic area and the lesser sac. See Figure 3-8.

### Omental Bursa

The omental bursa, or lesser sac, is sandwiched between the posterior stomach and parietal peritoneum covering the anterior pancreas (front-to-back) and the splenorenal and gastrosplenic ligaments and epiploic foramen (side-to-side). In cases of posterior gastric wall perforation or inflammation or trauma to the pancreas, fluid or a pseudocyst may be identified in this space (Fig. 3-9).

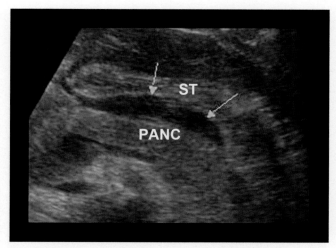

**Figure 3-9** Lesser sac. Transverse image of the epigastrium demonstrates a hematoma *(arrows)* within the lesser sac in a patient with acute pancreatitis. The posterior wall of the stomach *(ST)* borders the hematoma anteriorly. The pancreas forms the posterior border. (Image courtesy of Dr. Taco Geertsma, Ede, The Netherlands.)

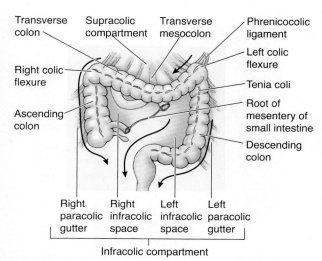

**Figure 3-10** Paracolic gutters. This diagram demonstrates the flow of fluid and other materials between the infracolic and supracolic compartments.

### Right and Left Paracolic Gutters

The right and left paracolic gutters are potential spaces or grooves found along the lateral ascending and descending colon that conduct fluids between the supracolic compartment of the abdomen and infracolic compartment of the inferior abdomen and pelvis. They are important in determining the extension of disease[1] (Fig. 3-10).

### Vesicorectal Space

The vesicorectal space or cul-de-sac in the male is the potential space created by the peritoneal reflection over the rectum and posterior bladder wall. When the male is in the supine position, this space is the most gravity-dependent potential space of the pelvic cavity draining fluid from the infracolic area. See Figures 3-7 and 3-11.

### Rectouterine Space

The rectouterine space is also called the *rectovaginal pouch*, *pouch of Douglas*, or *posterior cul-de-sac* in the female. This potential space is created by the parietal peritoneum draping over the anterior rectum, posterior vaginal wall, and posterior uterus. When the female is in a supine position, this space is the most gravity-dependent potential space of the pelvic cavity draining fluid from the infracolic area. See Figures 3-11B and 3-12.

### Uterovesicle Space

The uterovesicle space is also called the *uterovesicle pouch* or *anterior cul-de-sac* in the female, and is the potential space created by the peritoneal reflection over the uterine fundus, anterior uterus, broad ligament, and the posterior urinary bladder. See Figures 3-11B and 3-12.

### Space of Retzius

The space of Retzius is also called the *prevesicle* or *retropubic space* and is an extraperitoneal potential space located between the anterior wall of the urinary bladder and the pubic symphysis. See Figures 3-7 and 3-11A,B.

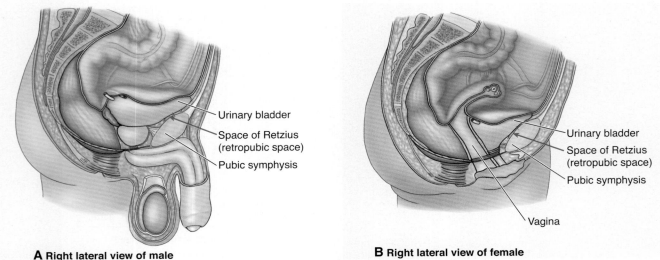

**A** Right lateral view of male

**B** Right lateral view of female

Figure 3-11 Male and female pelvic anatomy.

## SONOGRAPHIC EVALUATION OF THE PERITONEAL CAVITY

The parietal peritoneum lining the inner anterior abdominal wall may be visualized using a high-frequency 5- to 9-MHz linear transducer. The peritoneum appears as a thin hyperechoic continuous line posterior to the moderately hypoechoic internal oblique and rectus abdominis abdominal wall muscles. Bowel filled with gas, fluid, and fecal material will be identified deep to this anterior parietal peritoneum and can be observed to peristalsis. Sonographers may examine the anterior abdominal wall parietal peritoneum when evaluating for an abdominal wall hernia or delineating the position of an abscess or hematoma.

The visceral peritoneum and parietal peritoneum of the posterior peritoneal wall are typically not appreciated due to their depth. A lower frequency 2- to 5-MHz curvilinear or sector transducer is required to adequately visualize these deeper structures.

Generally, the peritoneal cavity is not evaluated as the primary focus of a diagnostic examination. Typically, the peritoneal organs are the focus of the examination, with the potential spaces of the peritoneal cavity viewed secondarily. A scanning technique that focuses specifically on the peritoneal cavity called *FAST* (focused assessment with sonography in trauma) has become more popular recently and may be used to assess the peritoneal potential spaces for free fluid in trauma situations.[4]

According to the *Ultrasound Guide for Emergency Physicians*, the FAST examination is performed by acquiring longitudinal and transverse images to include Morrison pouch (Fig. 3-13), the posterior right

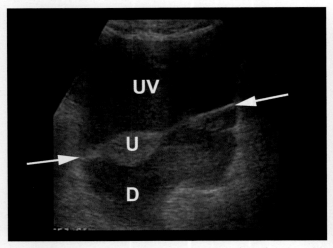

Figure 3-12 Female pelvis. Transverse image of the female pelvis demonstrates hemoperitoneum in the pouch of Douglas *(D)* and uterovesicle pouch *(UV)* outlining the uterus *(U)* and broad ligaments *(arrows)* bilaterally. (Image courtesy of Dr. Taco Geertsma, Ede, The Netherlands.)

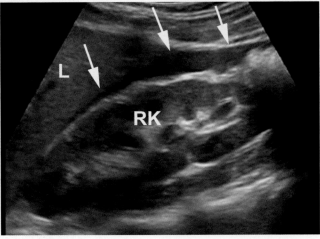

Figure 3-13 Morrison pouch. Longitudinal image of the right upper quadrant demonstrates a small amount of free fluid in Morrison pouch. (Image courtesy of Dr. Taco Geertsma, Ede, The Netherlands.)

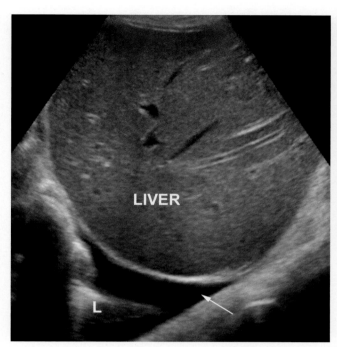

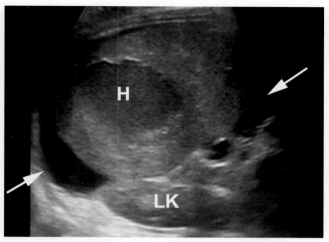

**Figure 3-15** Left upper quadrant. Transverse image of the left upper quadrant demonstrates free fluid *(arrows)* and a splenic hematoma *(H)* following abdominal trauma and splenic rupture. *LK*, left kidney. (Image courtesy of Dr. Taco Geertsma, Ede, The Netherlands.)

**Figure 3-14** Pleural effusion. Pleural effusion *(arrow)* is seen superior to the right hemidiaphragm within the chest cavity. Lung tissue *(L)* is seen suspended within the fluid. No fluid is seen inferior to the diaphragm in the subphrenic space. (Image courtesy of Philips Medical Systems, Bothel, WA.)

hemidiaphragm/liver interface (Fig. 3-14), the spleen/left kidney interface in the LUQ (Fig. 3-15), and the pouch of Douglas[4] (Fig. 3-16A,B). This triage scanning technique has proven to be sensitive in detecting as little as 200 mL of free fluid within the peritoneal cavity and 20 mL of pleural fluid. Additionally, the paracolic gutters and solid intraperitoneal organs may be imaged, depending on institutional protocol (Fig. 3-17). FAST

has proven to be very effective in hemodynamically unstable patients suffering blunt abdominal trauma. Computed tomography (CT) remains the gold standard for imaging hemodynamically stable patients with possible abdominal trauma whenever possible.[5,6]

When free fluid is observed within the peritoneal cavity, the sonographer should assess it for specific characteristics, taking images that demonstrate whether the fluid is simple or complex and to determine if it is loculated or freely mobile (Figs. 3-18 and 3-19). This may require using a higher frequency transducer, increasing the scanning gain above that optimally used during scanning, and imaging from multiple angles of incidence in order to detect fine septa or particles within the fluid. The patient's position may also be changed,

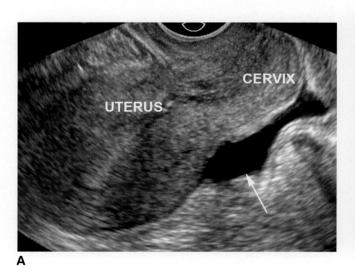

**A**

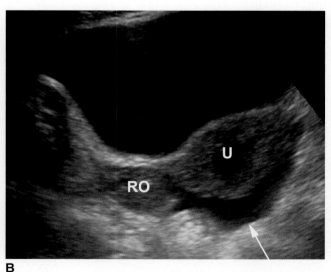

**B**

**Figure 3-16** Posterior cul-de-sac. (pouch of Douglas) **A.** Sagittal transvaginal image of the midline pelvis demonstrates free fluid in the posterior cul-de-sac *(arrow)*. **B.** Transverse transabdominal image of the female pelvis demonstrates free fluid in the posterior cul-de-sac *(arrow)*. *RO*, right ovary; *U*, uterus.

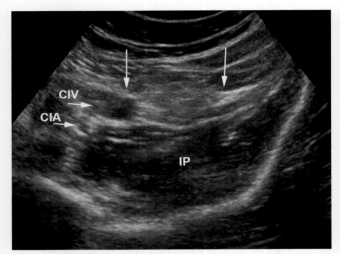

**Figure 3-17** Paracolic gutters. Transverse image of the left paracolic gutter demonstrates normal musculature and vasculature. The *arrows* demonstrate where free fluid could collect. *IP*, iliopsoas muscle; *CIV*, common iliac vein; *CIA*, common iliac artery.

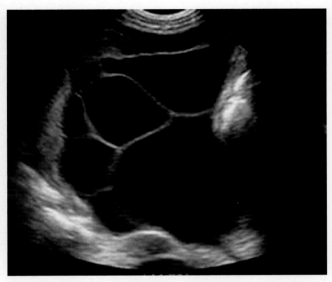

**Figure 3-19** Loculated ascites. Complex loculated ascites demonstrates multiple septa with apparent sequestered pockets of fluid. (Image courtesy of Philips Medical Systems, Bothel, WA.)

rolling the patient into a lateral decubitus or Trendelenburg position, to demonstrate fluid movement.

Free fluid must be differentiated from cystic masses of the peritoneum. Ascites will demonstrate bowel moving freely within it. Free fluid will follow the contour of peritoneal organs, filling sharp corners and interfaces of recesses and potential spaces. Cystic masses may demonstrate a mass effect on surrounding tissues, tending to have a circular or oval shape without sharp corners or angles (Figs. 3-20 and 3-21).

When assessing the paracolic gutters and posterior rectouterine/rectovesical space for fluid, it may be necessary to decrease the gain settings in order to identify small amounts of fluid adjacent to hyperechoic gas-filled bowel and to accommodate for enhancement posterior to a urine-filled bladder. Additionally, color and/or power Doppler

should be employed at the most sensitive settings possible to evaluate septa and other solid-appearing masses within the peritoneal cavity for blood flow. When blood flow is identified with color or power Doppler, it may be helpful to include spectral Doppler tracings with resistive indices.

## PATHOLOGIES OF THE PERITONEAL CAVITY

Although the peritoneum does normally secrete a small amount of serous fluid to lubricate the surfaces of the peritoneal organs, it is typically not appreciated during

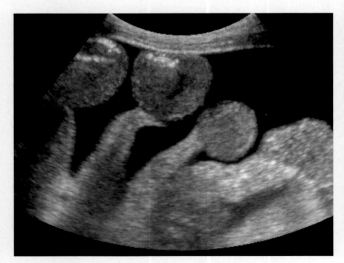

**Figure 3-18** Simple ascites. Sagittal view demonstrates simple ascites outlining the small bowel and mesentery floating freely within the fluid. (Image courtesy of Philips Medical Systems, Bothel, WA.)

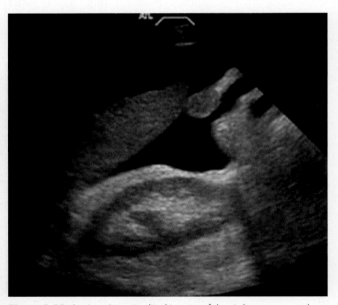

**Figure 3-20** Ascites. Longitudinal image of the right upper quadrant demonstrates simple ascites in Morrison pouch and the right subphrenic space. Note the sharp fluid-filled corners created at organ interfaces and how organs project into the fluid that fills the available spaces. (Image courtesy of Philips Medical Systems, Bothel, WA.)

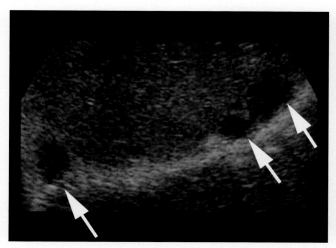

**Figure 3-21** Tuberculomas. Fluid-filled structures seen around the periphery of the liver represent tuberculomas. Note that these fluid collections are spherical and do not conform to the periphery of the organ or available space. (Image courtesy of Dr. Taco Geertsma, Ede, The Netherlands.)

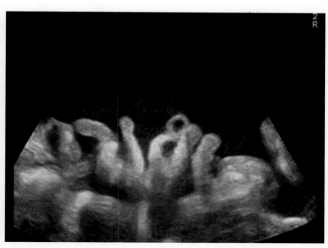

**Figure 3-22** Exudative ascites. Exudative ascites associated with peritoneal metastases is seen. Note the particulate appearance of the fluid and the bowel matted to the posterior wall. (Image courtesy of Dr. Taco Geertsma, Ede, The Netherlands.)

a sonographic examination. A small amount of fluid, up to 20 mL, is commonly seen in the pouch of Douglas following ovulation in menstruating females. Fluid and solid or semisolid materials identified in other potential spaces may indicate a pathologic process and should be investigated further. Common peritoneal abnormalities are discussed in this section.

## ASCITES

Ascites is ascitic or free fluid found within the peritoneal cavity that may be associated with a variety of causes including liver failure, abdominal trauma, or malignancy.[7,8] Ascitic fluid typically collects in Morrison pouch, the paracolic gutters, and the pouch of Douglas when the patient is in the supine position. There are two types of ascites: transudative and exudative. *Transudative ascites* is characterized by a lack of protein and cellular materials in the fluid.[5] Transudative ascites typically has a simple appearance and is often associated with portal hypertension and congestive cardiac disease[9] (Fig. 3-20). *Exudative ascites* is fluid that seeps out from blood vessels and contains a large amount of protein and cellular material.[10] Exudative ascites typically results in a more complex and echogenic appearance to the fluid and is associated with renal failure, inflammatory or ischemic bowel disease, peritonitis, and malignancy[9] (Fig. 3-22).

## PERITONEAL ABSCESS

A peritoneal abscess may be identified in a potential space or adjacent to an inflamed or perforated organ— the right subphrenic space being the most common due to the high frequency of appendicitis and duodenal ulcers.[1] Sonographically, the abscess typically appears as a thick-walled fluid collection that may contain ischemic tissue, pus, and blood components. The sonographic

appearance is variable and may be anechoic, solid appearing, multiseptated, or contain a debris or fluid–fluid level (Fig. 3-23). No blood flow should be visualized within the abscess pocket, but hyperemia may be demonstrated surrounding the thick, shaggy wall. Air may be present within the abscess demonstrating a hyperechoic anterior interface that is gravity dependent with a "dirty" shadow posterior. Scanning from a coronal horizontal approach to avoid bubbles may allow improved imaging of an air-containing abscess. Primary abscesses may occur adjacent to an inflamed organ such as the bowel with diverticulitis or appendicitis, or as a surgical complication. Additionally, parasitic abscesses may occur in peritoneal organs. These are often ingested and transported through the portal system into

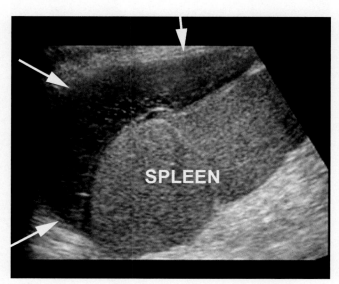

**Figure 3-23** Peritoneal abscess. Perisplenic abscess (*arrows*) is seen in the left upper quadrant. Note the complex echogenicity and the rounded edges that demonstrate this is not free fluid. (Image courtesy of Dr. Taco Geertsma, Ede, The Netherlands.)

the liver and spleen. The most common is *Echinococcus granulosus*. An existing fluid collection such as a hematoma or cyst may become an abscess when it becomes infected secondarily.

## HEMOPERITONEUM

Hemoperitoneum may be seen with blunt abdominal trauma resulting in abdominal viscera or vasculature bleeding into the peritoneum. The trauma may also be iatrogenically induced, such as following a biopsy, angioplasty, or other surgical intervention. Once the blood organizes, it is typically referred to as a *hematoma*.

## HEMATOMA

A hematoma is a blood clot or focal area of coagulated blood occurring as a postsurgical complication, following trauma such as an automobile accident, or occurring spontaneously in patients with hemophilia or other coagulation diseases, or those taking anticoagulant medications.[11] Large hematomas may be associated with a drop in hematocrit. Hematomas are typically found immediately adjacent to the tissue or vessel that has been disrupted, deep to a surgical incision, or in a dependent potential space of the peritoneum (Morrison pouch, the paracolic gutters, or the posterior cul-de-sac).

Hematomas have a variable appearance depending on their age (Fig. 3-24A,B). The evolution of clotting blood is relatively predictable when the patient is not taking blood thinning or thrombolytic medications. Initially, a hematoma is anechoic; however, within a few hours, the collection will become somewhat larger, more echogenic, and complex in appearance as fibrin is deposited. Over

a few days, the hematoma will become completely solid appearing with an echogenicity similar to the parenchyma of the normal spleen or liver. Color or power Doppler may assist the sonographer in identifying the hematoma as it will be devoid of blood flow and may demonstrate a mass effect on surrounding tissues. Eventually, the clot will progress into the lytic phase, retracting to become smaller in size with an increasingly complex appearance ending with complete or partial resorption by the body. Residual hematoma may be replaced by scar tissue resulting in a hyperechoic fibrotic retracted area. Longstanding hematomas may develop a thin eggshell calcification around the periphery. A thorough patient history will assist the sonographer in recognizing potential scar tissue in a patient with a history of trauma.

## PSEUDOMYXOMA PERITONEI

Pseudomyxoma peritonei (PMP) is a rare borderline malignant process that results when a benign appendiceal or ovarian adenoma ruptures, spilling epithelial cells into the peritoneum.[12–14] These cells develop into noninvasive peritoneal implants that secrete a gelatinous mucous into the peritoneal cavity.[13,14] The cells spread from the appendix in the right paracolic gutter into the right subdiaphragmatic space and into the intraperitoneal potential spaces of the pelvis. As the mucous accumulates within the abdominopelvic cavity, it takes up space around the bowel and causes fibrosis of the peritoneal membranes creating adhesions.[15] The 10-year survival rate of PMP patients is 30% because of the complications associated with recurrence and treatment.[15] Symptoms and imaging findings include abdominal pain and distention, omental caking, posterior fixation of bowel loops and mesentery,

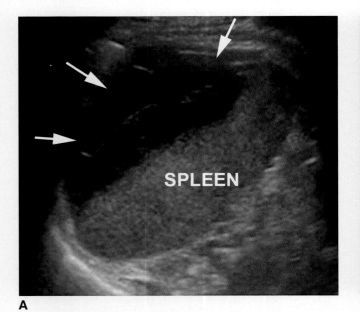

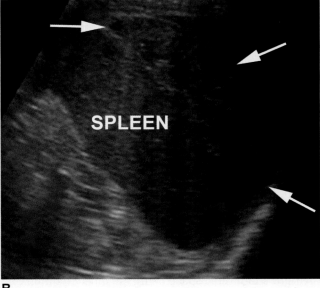

**A**    **B**

**Figure 3-24** Hematoma. **A.** Sagittal image demonstrates a hypoechoic fluid collection consistent with an acute splenic hematoma in a patient with recent abdominal trauma. **B.** Transverse image in the same patient a few weeks later demonstrates a nearly solid appearance. (Images courtesy of Dr. Taco Geertsma, Ede, The Netherlands.)

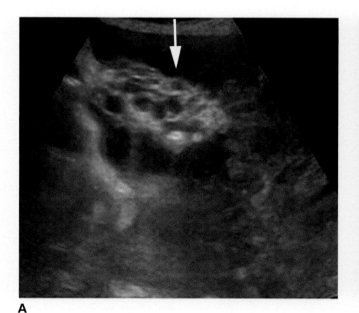

**A**

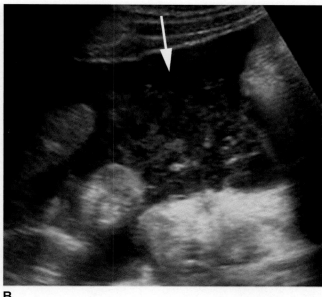

**B**

**Figure 3-25** Pseudomyxoma peritonei. **A.** A multicystic appearance of pseudomyxoma peritonei (PMP) *(arrow)* is seen within the peritoneal cavity secondary to a mucinous carcinoma of the appendix. **B.** Complex mucinous ascites *(arrow)* is seen in the same patient. (Images courtesy of Dr. Taco Geertsma, Ede, The Netherlands.)

bowel obstruction, and small bowel fistula.[16] Treatments include palliative surgical debulking to remove visible implants, chemotherapy, cytoreductive surgery, and perioperative/postoperative chemotherapy.[13,14] This final treatment is the most aggressive therapy that involves stripping parietal peritoneum from the abdominopelvic cavity and surgical removal of the right colon, greater and lesser omentum, spleen, gallbladder, and uterus and ovaries in females. Unfortunately, therapy is relatively ineffective in completely eradicating all of the cells, resulting in periodic recurrence over time.[16]

Sonographically, PMP most commonly appears as simple or multiloculated ascites. It may also present as several thin-walled cysts of varying sizes scattered throughout the peritoneum[16] (Fig. 3-25A,B). PMP may rarely appear as a hypoechoic solid mass.[16] Identifying the primary adenoma as well as the complexity of the concomitant ascites is important.

## FLUID COLLECTIONS

### Seroma

A seroma is a fluid collection composed of blood products located adjacent to or surrounding transplanted organs in the early postsurgical period. They are typically anechoic, but may contain septa.[5]

### Lymphocele

Lymphoceles are collections of lymphatic fluid outside of the lymph system due to disruption of the lymphatic vessels or lymph node resection. These collections are generally simple, but may contain septations. Lymphoceles are slower to develop following surgery and typically present

4 to 8 weeks after surgery.[17] The delayed onset can help establish the diagnosis of lymphocele. In the peritoneal cavity, a lymphocele may be seen following prostatectomy and lymph node dissection. The body may spontaneously resorb smaller collections, whereas larger collections may require more aggressive interventions ranging from percutaneous aspiration, surgery, or sclerosis.[5,17]

### Biloma

A biloma is an anechoic collection of bile located within the peritoneal cavity outside of the biliary tree.[11] It is typically associated with hepatic transplant due to a biliary leak or biliary tree ischemia, but it may also be the sequela of trauma, biopsy, or cholecystectomy (Fig. 3-26).

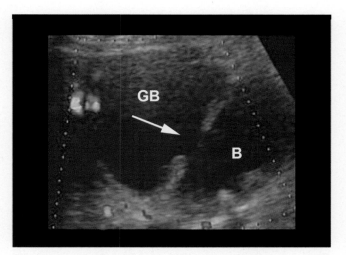

**Figure 3-26** Biloma. Gallbladder *(GB)* wall perforation *(arrow)* with adjacent biloma *(B)*. (Image courtesy of Dr. Taco Geertsma, Ede, The Netherlands.)

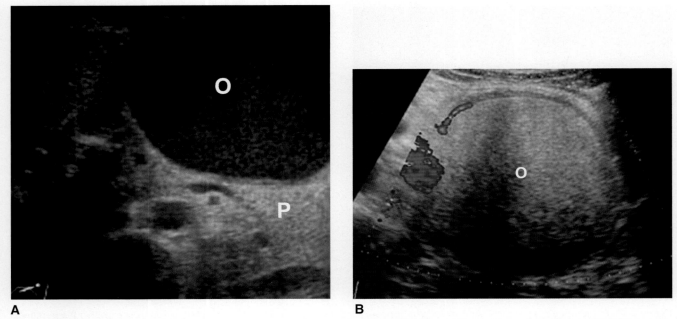

**A**    **B**

**Figure 3-27** Omental cyst. **A.** Transverse epigastric image demonstrates an omental cyst (O) anterior to the pancreas (P). **B.** Sonogram demonstrates an omental cyst nearly filled with clot. Color Doppler demonstrates flow around the periphery of the cyst. (Images courtesy of Dr. Taco Geertsma, Ede, The Netherlands.)

### Urinoma

A urinoma is associated with a rupture of the urinary tract. It is typically found adjacent to the kidney in the perirenal space of the retroperitoneum. When urine is free within the peritoneal cavity, it is more appropriately called *urine ascites*. Urine will appear as simple anechoic fluid. The bladder wall should be evaluated for discontinuity in cases of urine ascites.

## PERITONEAL MASSES

### Mesenteric Cysts

Mesenteric cysts may occur anywhere along the mesentery, but the majority originate from the small bowel mesentery.

Variable in size, these benign cysts grow slowly over time with peritoneal serous secretions. These unilocular cysts may be pedunculated and may torse, hemorrhage, or cause bowel obstruction due to a mass effect[16] (Fig. 3-27A,B).

### Mesenteric Adenopathy

Mesenteric adenopathy, also called lymphadenopathy, describes the enlargement of the lymph nodes along the mesentery or on the bowel. Adenopathy may be associated with inflammatory diseases of the bowel such as colitis and appendicitis and with viral infections. Adenopathy may also be associated with primary malignancy, such as lymphoma, or metastatic malignancy, such as colon cancer. Multiple lymph nodes become visible

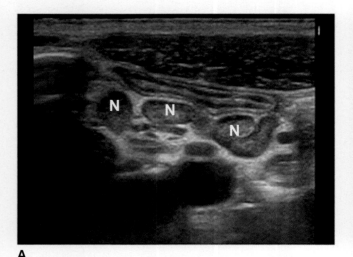
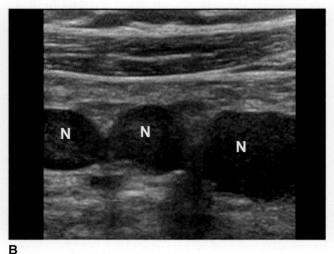

**A**    **B**

**Figure 3-28** Mesenteric lymphadenopathy. **A,B.** Mesenteric lymph node (N) enlargement in two patients with colitis. (Images courtesy of Dr. Taco Geertsma, Ede, The Netherlands.)

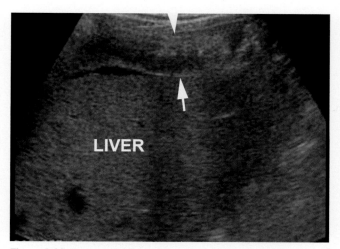

**Figure 3-29** Peritoneal mesothelioma. Peritoneal mesothelioma seen as a solid mass *(arrows)* of the peritoneum at the anterior aspect of the liver. (Image courtesy of Dr. Taco Geertsma, Ede, The Netherlands.)

along the mesentery adjacent to the inflamed bowel. The lymph nodes lose their oval shape and become more rounded as they increase in size (Fig. 3-28A,B).

### Peritoneal Mesothelioma

Peritoneal mesothelioma is a relatively rare primary malignant tumor of the peritoneum and is associated with asbestos exposure. Masses occur most frequently along the pleura and peritoneum, metastasizing by direct invasion into adjacent organs. The tumor may appear as a generalized thickening of the peritoneum, mesentery, omentum, and bowel, or as a discrete nodule (Fig. 3-29). It is frequently associated with a small amount of ascites and may demonstrate areas of calcification.[16]

### Peritoneal Implants and Omental Caking

Peritoneal implants are associated with peritoneal metastasis, appearing as multiple small polypoid masses projecting from the peritoneum. Concomitant findings of complex ascites and omental caking are commonly seen.[18] Peritoneal implants are most commonly associated with primary cancers of the ovary, stomach, and colon[12,16,18] (Fig. 3-30A,B).

Omental caking is a thickening of the greater omentum due to malignant infiltration.[3] Omental caking is indicative of peritoneal metastasis, also called peritoneal carcinomatosis, and is commonly associated with primary cancers of the ovary, stomach, and colon.[12,16,18] It is frequently associated with a significant amount of complex ascites and peritoneal implants of nodular metastatic masses along the parietal peritoneum.[18] Sonographically, an omental cake appears as a moderately echogenic homogeneous thick soft tissue layer deep to the anterior wall (Fig. 3-31A,B).

## INTERVENTIONAL APPLICATIONS

Because of its real-time capability and ability to demonstrate vasculature, sonography-guided biopsy and aspiration of the peritoneal cavity and its contents are frequently performed.

### PARACENTESIS

Paracentesis is the aspiration of ascitic fluid from the peritoneal cavity and may be done for diagnostic or therapeutic purposes.[7,8,17] This sterile procedure is typically performed by percutaneous placement of a Yueh catheter or other needle into the peritoneal cavity, typically in the area of the right paracolic gutter. In a diagnostic paracentesis, a small amount of fluid may be drawn into a syringe to be sent to the laboratory for testing. When greater amounts of ascitic fluid are present, a therapeutic paracentesis may be performed. Up to 6 L of fluid may be withdrawn for palliative purposes when the patient is experiencing respiratory difficulty and/or extreme abdominal pressure due to a large quantity of ascites. Large quantities of ascitic fluid are commonly associated with portal hypertension, requiring frequent drainage in the later stages of the disease.

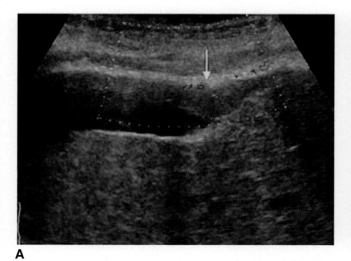

**A**

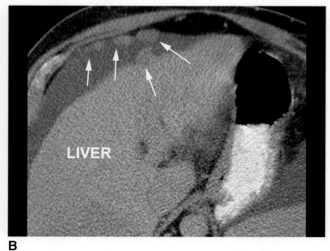

**B**

**Figure 3-30** Peritoneal implants. **A.** A lobulated solid mass *(arrow)* is seen projecting from the peritoneum anterior to the liver. A small amount of ascites is also seen. **B.** Computed tomography demonstrates solid polypoid masses *(arrows)* seen extending from the peritoneum consistent with peritoneal implants. (Images courtesy of Dr. Taco Geertsma, Ede, The Netherlands.)

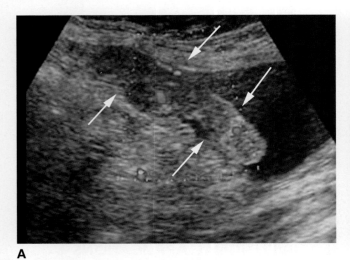

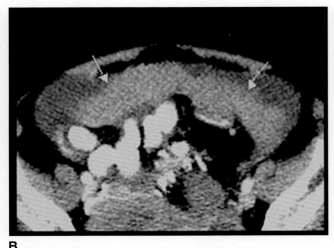

**A**    **B**

**Figure 3-31** Omental caking. **A,B.** Sonogram and computed tomography image demonstrate an omental cake *(arrows)* with some vascularity seen on color Doppler in a patient with ovarian cancer. (Images courtesy of Dr. Taco Geertsma, Ede, The Netherlands.)

## PERCUTANEOUS ABSCESS DRAINAGE

Percutaneous abscess drainage (PAD) is another sterile procedure that may be performed using sonographic guidance.[17] A small flexible catheter is inserted into the abscess pocket, and abscess contents are aspirated into a syringe to be sent to the laboratory for analysis.[19] The physician may choose to leave a drainage catheter in the abscess to allow for gravitational drainage and antibiotic instillation.

## SUMMARY

- Many disease processes and fluid collections can occur within the peritoneal cavity.
- The abdominopelvic cavity can be divided into nine regions: right and left hypochondriac, right and left lumbar, right and left iliac, epigastric, umbilical, and hypogastric regions.
- The abdominopelvic cavity can also be divided into four quadrants: right upper quadrant, right lower quadrant, left upper quadrant, and left lower quadrant.
- The quadrants and regions are used to describe the location of fluid collections and disease processes.
- The abdominopelvic cavity is lined with a thin continuous layer of peritoneum.
- The peritoneum that surrounds the organs is referred to as visceral peritoneum.
- The peritoneum that lines the walls of the abdominopelvic cavity is referred to as the parietal peritoneum.
- The peritoneum secretes a small amount of serous fluid that acts as a lubricant, allowing the organs to move without friction.
- The peritoneal cavity is divided into the larger greater sac, which contains the peritoneal organs, and the smaller lesser sac, which does not contain any organs.

- The greater omentum helps prevent the parietal peritoneum from adhering to the visceral peritoneum and also functions to move to areas of inflammation, surrounding the area and walling off infection.
- The greater omentum subdivides the greater sac into a supracolic and infracolic compartment; this separation helps limit the spread of infection and malignancy.
- Ligaments also divide the peritoneal cavity and form boundaries for potential spaces.
- A potential space is an empty fold except in the case of disease when fluid and other materials may collect.
- A FAST examination, or focused assessment with sonography in trauma, is used to evaluate for free fluid or blood in cases of abdominal trauma.
- When free fluid is visualized in the peritoneal cavity, it is important to determine if the fluid is simple or complex and freely mobile or loculated.
- Ascites is free fluid within the peritoneal cavity and may occur with liver disease, portal hypertension, cardiac disease, malignancy, or abdominal trauma.
- Morrison pouch, the paracolic gutters, and the pouch of Douglas are the most common locations for ascites to collect when the patient is supine.
- Transudative ascites is a simple ascites that lacks protein and cellular materials and is frequently associated with portal hypertension and congestive cardiac disease.
- Exudative ascites is fluid that seeps out of blood vessels, contains large amounts of protein and cellular material, and has a more echogenic or complex appearance. It is typically associated with renal failure, peritonitis, inflammatory bowel disease, and malignancy.
- A peritoneal abscess is a walled off collection of pus, ischemic tissue, and blood products. The sonographic appearance is variable.

- Hemoperitoneum refers to free blood within the peritoneal cavity.
- A hematoma is a blood clot or focal area of congested blood frequently occurring following trauma or surgical procedures, or occurring spontaneously in patients with clotting disorders.
- Pseudomyxoma peritonei occurs following the rupture of a benign appendiceal or ovarian adenoma. Epithelial cells are released into the peritoneum and secrete a gelatinous mucous into the peritoneal cavity.
- Sonographically, pseudomyxoma peritonei appears as a simple or multiloculated ascites or as several thin-walled cysts of various sizes.
- Seromas, lymphoceles, or bilomas may also occur in the peritoneal cavity following surgery or trauma.
- Mesenteric lymphadenopathy refers to enlargement of the lymph nodes along the mesentery or bowel and may be associated with inflammatory bowel disease.
- Peritoneal implants, complex ascites, and omental caking are commonly seen with metastatic cancers of the ovary, stomach, and colon.
- Paracentesis is a diagnostic or therapeutic procedure performed to remove ascites from the peritoneal cavity.
- Percutaneous abscess drainage may be performed under sonographic guidance.

## Critical Thinking Questions

1. Why is a FAST evaluation performed and what areas does this examination typically cover?

2. What are some of the common causes for accumulation of ascites?

3. A 45-year-old patient presents with a history of abdominal distention following surgery and chemotherapy for ovarian cancer. Your examination reveals multiple solid-appearing masses along the anterior abdominal wall, as well as a large amount of complex-appearing ascites. What is the most likely diagnosis?

4. A 62-year-old patient presents with fever, leukocytosis, and abdominal pain following an episode of colitis. Your examination reveals an irregular complex mass in the right lower quadrant. No blood flow is seen within the mass. What is the most likely diagnosis?

5. What is the difference between a therapeutic and a diagnostic paracentesis?

## REFERENCES

1. Moore KL, Dalley AF. *Clinically Oriented Anatomy*. 6th ed. Philadelphia, PA: Lippincott Williams and Wilkins; 2009:231–241.
2. Moore KL, Persaud TVN. *Before We Are Born: Essentials of Embryology and Birth Defects*. 7th ed. Philadelphia, PA: Saunders Elsevier; 2002.
3. Que Y, Wang X, Liu Y, et al. Ultrasound-guided biopsy of greater omentum: an effective method to trace the origin of unclear ascites. *Eur J Radiol*. 2009;70(2): 331–335.
4. Beck-Razi N, Gaitini D. Focused assessment with sonography for trauma. *Ultrasound Clin*. 2008;3:23–31.
5. Sanders RC, Winter TC. *Clinical Sonography: A Practical Guide*. 4th ed. Baltimore, MD: Lippincott Williams & Wilkins; 2006.
6. Reardon R, Hoffman B. Ultrasound guide for emergency physicians: an introduction. Ultrasound in Trauma—The FAST exam. Available at: http://www.sonoguide.com/FAST .html. Accessed July 17, 2011.
7. Hou W, Sanyal AJ. Ascites: diagnosis and management. *Med Clin North Am*. 2009;93:801–817.
8. Gines P, Cardenas A, Arroyo V, et al. Management of cirrhosis and ascites. *N Engl J Med*. 2004;350: 1646–1654.
9. Malde HM, Gandhi RD. Exudative v/s transudative ascites: differentiation based on fluid echogenicity on high resolution sonography. *J Postgrad Med*. 1993;39: 132–133.
10. Pick TP, Howden R, eds. *Gray's Anatomy: Anatomy, Descriptive and Surgical*. New York, NY: Random House; 1995.
11. Chen CJ, Chang WH, Shih SC, et al. Clinical presentation and outcome of hepatic subcapsular fluid collections. *J Formos Med Assoc*. 2009;108:61–68.
12. Joshi M. Sonography of adnexal masses. *Ultrasound Clin*. 2008;3:369–389.
13. Jarvinen P, Lepisto A. Clinical presentation of pseudomyxoma peritonei. *Scand J Surg*. 2010;99:213–216.
14. Teo M. Peritoneal-based malignancies and their treatment. *Ann Acad Med Singapore*. 2010;39:54–57.
15. Nagarajan P, Renehan A, Saunders MP, et al. Sugarbaker procedure for pseudomyxoma peritonei (Intervention Protocol). *Cochrane Database Syst Rev*. 2006;1:CD005659.
16. Dähnert W. *Radiology Review Manual*. 5th ed. Philadelphia, PA: Lippincott Williams & Wilkins; 2003.
17. Childs DD, Tchelepi H. Ultrasound and abdominal intervention: new luster on an old gem. *Ultrasound Clin*. 2009; 4:25–43.
18. Mironov S, Akin O, Pandit-Taskar N, et al. Ovarian cancer. *Radiol Clin North Am*. 2007;45:149–166.
19. Phillips CL, Williams PL, Watkinson AF. Pelvic drainage: image guidance and technique. *Ultrasound Clin*. 2009; 4:73–81.

# 4 Vascular Structures

Kathleen Marie Hannon

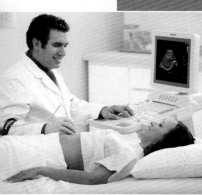

## OBJECTIVES

Identify the role of diagnostic medical sonography in the assessment of abdominal vascular structures.

Perform sonographic evaluation of the abdominal vascular system.

Describe the patient preparation, equipment considerations, and scanning techniques and Doppler protocols for normal and abnormal abdominal vascular structures.

Identify circulatory anatomy, name the layers of blood vessels, and distinguish the difference between arteries and veins.

Recognize the sonographic appearance and relational anatomy of the abdominal vascular system.

Describe the pathology, etiology, clinical signs and symptoms, and sonographic appearance or aortic pathology to include atherosclerosis, aneurysms, dissection, rupture, inflammatory aneurysms, stenosis, and vascular insufficiency.

Discuss the complications of an aortic graft, including pseudoaneurysms, graft aneurysms, hematomas, abscesses, and occlusions.

Describe the pathology, etiology, clinical signs and symptoms, and the sonographic appearance for each of the following venous abnormalities to include vena caval obstruction, tumors, venous enlargement, thrombosis, aneurysm, hepatic venous abnormalities (Budd-Chiari syndrome), and portal venous abnormalities (portal thrombosis and portal venous hypertension).

Formulate a list of differential diagnosis based on correlating the patient's clinical history, laboratory values, results of related diagnostic procedures, and the sonographic tissue characteristics.

Identify technically satisfactory and unsatisfactory sonographic examinations of the vascular system.

## KEY TERMS

anastomosis | aneurysm, pseudoaneurysm | Budd-Chiari syndrome | ectasia | Marfan syndrome | nutcracker phenomenon | postprandial, preprandial | parvus, pulsus tardus | splanchnic arteries | TIPS

## GLOSSARY

**anastomosis** a connection between two vessels

**arteriovenous fistula** connection allowing communication between an artery and vein

**ectasia** dilatation, expansion, or distention

**endograft** a metallic stent covered with fabric and placed inside an aneurysm to prevent rupture

**graft** any tissue or organ for implantation or transplantation

**prosthesis** an artificial substitute for a body part

**pseudoaneurysm** caused by a hematoma that forms as a result of a leaking hole in an artery; this pulsating, false (pseudo)aneurysm forms outside of the arterial wall

**thrombosis** the formation of a thrombus (clot) in a blood vessel

This chapter stresses the importance of learning how to identify normal and abnormal abdominal vessels and how to assess normal and abnormal blood flow. The many branches of arterial flow and the confluences of venous return provide a comprehensive road map for identifying normal and abnormal anatomy and anatomic relationships. Current sonography equipment makes it possible to accurately image smaller vessels and to detect intraluminal abnormalities such as thrombi and tumors.[1] Current instrumentation provides the ability to assess blood flow, to obtain hemodynamic information regarding the many factors that influence the dynamics of blood flow, and the hemodynamic consequences of vascular disease.

## SONOGRAPHY EXAMINATION

### PATIENT PREPARATION

It is recommended that all patients fast prior to vascular scanning. Fasting tends to reduce the amount of air in the abdomen, which has the potential to obscure the anatomy of interest. In emergency situations, however, scanning can be accomplished without any patient preparation.[2] If Doppler interrogation is desired, studies should be performed in a consistent manner to reduce result variability due to factors affecting blood flow hemodynamics such as ingestion of a meal, respiratory changes, and postural changes. In some instances, it may be helpful to perform preprandial and postprandial studies to aid in the diagnosis of abnormal blood flow states.

### EQUIPMENT CONSIDERATIONS

With an understanding of the relationship between resolution and beam penetration, the sonographer may select either a sector or linear transducer operating at the highest clinically appropriate frequency. For adults, the common gray scale scanning frequency is 5 MHz and lower. Doppler is essential for investigating blood flow hemodynamics. The Doppler frequency may vary from the imaging frequency. Color flow instrumentation provides rapid evaluation and visualization of blood flow and can reduce examination time.

### SCANNING TECHNIQUES

Most of the abdominal vasculature can be identified with the patient lying in the supine position. Standard scanning of the aorta and inferior vena cava (IVC) commences with the transducer placed in the subxiphoid position and oriented to the transverse plane. Because of their proximity, the aorta and the IVC can be demonstrated simultaneously and, once they are identified, gain settings should be adjusted to reveal their characteristic echo-free lumen. Some reverberation artifact may be present along the anterior aspect of each vessel. This is considered normal due to the strong reflective interface of each of the vessels' walls. Scanning continues inferiorly until the aortic bifurcation is reached. Images are recorded at 1- to 2-cm intervals along the course of the aorta and IVC and additional sections are recorded in any area of disease. Once transverse scanning is completed, the aorta and IVC should be imaged in longitudinal sections. Images are recorded in segments to demonstrate the entire length of each vessel.

If specific arterial branches or venous tributaries are being investigated, the examination should begin with the transducer positioned near the vessel's origin. Transducer manipulations are then carried out in an attempt to follow the course of the vessel. Images are recorded to demonstrate vessel length as clearly as possible and any disease that may be present.

A sonographer examining the many vascular branches and pathways in the abdomen must have a working knowledge of his or her general course throughout. Once each vessel's site of origin is known and the general course of the abdominal vasculature is learned, sonographic examination is made easier. Diligent Doppler sampling is the most reliable and accurate method for confirming arteries versus veins.

## VASCULAR ANATOMY

Blood is distributed throughout the body by a vast network of arteries and veins. In the systemic circulation, arteries transport blood from the heart to the muscles and organs, and veins transport blood from the muscles and organs back to the heart. Typically, blood vessels are composed of three distinct layers: (1) the tunica intima, (2) the tunica media, and (3) the tunica adventitia. The tunica intima, the innermost section of a vessel wall, consists of an endothelial lining and elastic tissue. Elastic fibers and smooth muscle constitute the second layer, the tunica media. The outer portion of the vessel wall, the tunica adventitia, is composed of elastic and collagen fibers.[3]

Although arteries and veins are histologically similar, there are differences in the distribution of each tissue within the walls that reflect pressure differences between the two systems. For example, arterial walls are thicker and contain more elastic and smooth muscle fibers than veins. This is true especially in the tunica media, which is the thickest layer of an artery and is largely responsible for its very elastic and contractile characteristics. Because of the thickness of arterial walls, they tend to maintain a constant shape and do not readily collapse in conjunction with low blood pressure.[3,4]

Because veins have less smooth muscle and elastic tissue, they are unable to contract to force through blood. Venous return to the heart is therefore accomplished through the pressure gradient difference between the arterial and venous network, breathing, and skeletal muscle contractions. Valves are also an important part of the veins located in the extremities.[5] The circulatory network of blood vessels, the vasa vasorum, is located within their walls.[5]

## ABDOMINAL AORTA AND AORTIC BRANCHES

### Anatomy

The aorta is the main artery of the chest and abdomen from which all other branch vessels are derived. For reference purposes, the aorta is divided into segments along its path (Fig. 4-1).

The aorta originates from the left ventricle. As it leaves the heart, systemic circulation begins. The aorta arises from the left ventricular outflow tract and then courses slightly posterior, a short distance medial, and then superior to form the ascending aorta. It then curves lateral and posterior to form the aortic arch. As the aorta completes its curve at the arch, it begins to descend inferiorly into the chest. This portion, the descending aorta, soon gives rise to the thoracic aorta. Once the aorta penetrates the diaphragm, it is termed the *abdominal aorta* until it bifurcates into the iliac arteries prior to entering the pelvic cavity. It is the abdominal aorta that is most accessible to sonographic examination (Fig. 4-2).

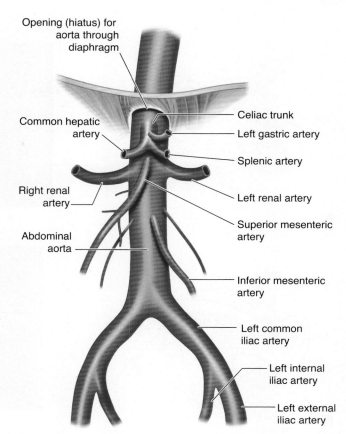

**Figure 4-2** Major branches. An anterior illustration of the abdominal aorta illustrates the anatomic location of its major branches.

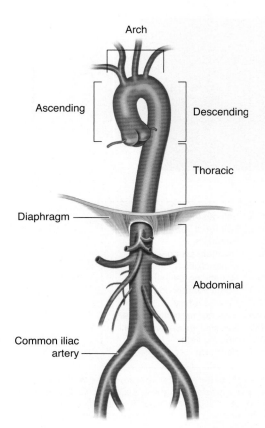

**Figure 4-1** Segments of the aorta. The common reference segments, ascending, arch, descending, thoracic, and abdominal aorta can be identified on the illustration.

As it courses through the abdomen, several major vessels branch off of the abdominal aorta. The first branch is the celiac axis (also known as the celiac trunk). It originates from the anterior aspect of the aorta and is usually found within the first 2 cm. The celiac axis is a short vessel, approximately 1 cm long. It divides into three branches: (1) the hepatic artery, (2) the left gastric artery, and (3) the splenic artery.[3,4] The vessel may present with anatomic variations on the number of branches (Fig. 4-3A–C).

The hepatic artery leaves the celiac axis at approximately a 90-degree angle and it crosses the midline and courses toward the right side of the abdomen, following the upper border of the pancreatic head. At the duodenum, the hepatic artery turns anteriorly to enter the liver hilum, following the course of the main portal vein. Intrahepatically, the artery then divides into left and right branches at the portal fissure to supply the left and right hepatic lobes, respectively.[3,4,6,7] The left gastric artery initially has an anterior and superior course from the celiac axis. It then turns lateral to the left side of the abdomen to supply the stomach and esophagus with blood.[3,4,6,7] The splenic artery takes a horizontal course from the celiac axis and follows the upper margin of the pancreatic body posteriorly. Along its route to the spleen, it generates arterial branches to the stomach and pancreas.[3,4,6,7]

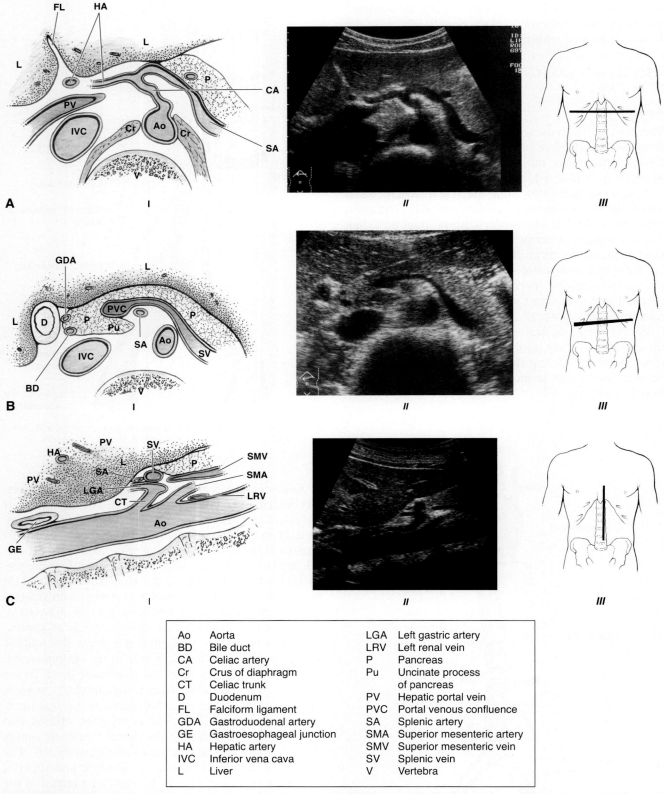

| Ao | Aorta | LGA | Left gastric artery |
| BD | Bile duct | LRV | Left renal vein |
| CA | Celiac artery | P | Pancreas |
| Cr | Crus of diaphragm | Pu | Uncinate process |
| CT | Celiac trunk | | of pancreas |
| D | Duodenum | PV | Hepatic portal vein |
| FL | Falciform ligament | PVC | Portal venous confluence |
| GDA | Gastroduodenal artery | SA | Splenic artery |
| GE | Gastroesophageal junction | SMA | Superior mesenteric artery |
| HA | Hepatic artery | SMV | Superior mesenteric vein |
| IVC | Inferior vena cava | SV | Splenic vein |
| L | Liver | V | Vertebra |

**Figure 4-3** Relationships. The abdominal aorta and its branches are illustrated along with representative sonograms. **A.** The level of the transverse section is made through the celiac trunk. **B.** The level of the transverse section is made through the pancreas. **C.** The level of a longitudinal section is made through the upper aorta. (Reprinted with permission from Moore K, Dalley A, Agur A. *Clinically Oriented Anatomy.* 6th ed. Philadelphia, PA: Lippincott Williams & Wilkins, 2010:322; Courtesy of Dr. A. M. Arenson, Assistant Professor of Medical Image, University of Toronto. See page 322 of resource book.)

The second major branch vessel, the superior mesenteric artery (SMA), also originates from the anterior surface of the aorta approximately 1 to 2.5 cm distal to the celiac axis (although this distance varies) and occasionally it may branch off of the celiac axis. As it begins to course inferiorly, it travels posterior to the pancreatic body and anterior to the uncinate process. It then continues inferiorly, paralleling the aorta. The left renal vein, duodenum, and uncinate process are located between the SMA anteriorly and the aorta posteriorly. The *nutcracker phenomenon* refers to the compression of the left renal vein between the aorta and the SMA (like a nut in a nutcracker). Several branches arise along the length of the SMA and are responsible for supplying the small and large bowel with blood (Fig. 4-3A–C).

The renal arteries are located just inferior to the SMA. The right renal artery tends to arise from the right lateral aspect of the aorta, whereas the left renal artery tends to arise from the left lateral or posterolateral aspect of the aorta. Both then course posterolaterally to enter the respective kidneys.[3,4,6,7]

The inferior mesenteric artery (IMA) is the last major branch to arise from the abdominal aorta before it bifurcates. It originates from the anterior aspect of the aorta and runs slightly inferiorly and to the left side of the abdomen. It is responsible for supplying the distal portion of the colon with blood.

At about the level of the umbilicus, the aorta bifurcates into the left and right common iliac arteries. These vessels course inferiorly and posteriorly, holding a position fairly deep in the pelvis. As a result, the iliac arteries can be very difficult to image. Full bladder techniques may be necessary to visualize them.[3,4,6,7]

## Sonographic Appearance

Sonographically, the lumen of the aorta and other vascular structures appear anechoic. It is important that the sonographer optimizes gain settings to demonstrate normal vessels as anechoic structures. In the longitudinal plane, slightly to the left of midline, the proximal aorta can be seen as an anechoic tubular structure following a somewhat anterior and inferior course within the abdomen. The spine lies immediately posterior to it, providing a highly reflective echo boundary. As the aorta courses inferiorly, it tapers and becomes smaller in caliber. In the proximal aspect of the aorta, both the celiac axis and the SMA can be seen as they arise anteriorly. A longitudinal section provides the best scanning plane to image the proximity of the celiac axis and SMA (see Fig. 4-3C; Fig. 4-4A–C).

In transverse scan planes, the aorta takes on a more rounded appearance and again can be seen to lie anterior to the spine. As the transducer is moved inferiorly from the xiphoid process, the first aortic branch to be encountered is the celiac axis. It appears as an anechoic tubular structure that divides into the hepatic artery and the splenic artery. If viewed in the appropriate plane, the image may resemble the spread wings of a seagull (see Fig. 4-3A). The hepatic artery branches off the right side of the celiac axis and can be followed transversely and superiorly as it travels to enter the liver hilum. The splenic artery branches off the left side of the celiac axis and courses to the left side of the abdomen to enter the splenic hilum (Fig. 4-5A). The splenic artery can be quite tortuous and is difficult to image in its entirety, especially in elderly patients.

The left gastric artery can occasionally be seen in its proximal aspect. This vessel, however, is usually smaller in caliber than the neighboring hepatic and splenic arteries and is more difficult to image consistently.

After moving the transducer inferiorly, the SMA can be seen. It appears rounded and is surrounded by an echodense collar consisting of mesentery and fat (see Fig. 4-3B).

Immediately inferior to the level of origin of the SMA are the origins of the renal arteries. They are best appreciated in the transverse plane because of their relationship to the acoustic beam. The renal arteries arise from the lateral aspect of the aorta and continue their course, respectively, to the right and left to enter the kidneys (Fig. 4-5B–D).

The IMA can be seen approximately midway between the renal arteries and the aortic bifurcation arising anterolaterally from the aorta. Soon after its origin, the IMA makes an abrupt turn in the posteroinferior direction. High-frequency probes and compression of overlying bowel loops greatly facilitate visualization of this artery, as does color flow Doppler.

At the level of the umbilicus, the right and left iliac arteries can be seen as they arise from the aortic terminus as rounded and anechoic vessels emerging from a common source (distal aorta). Further, more comprehensive imaging of the iliac arteries is accomplished by placing the transducer in the iliac fossa and angling medially with the scan plane oriented approximately 45 degrees from midline. Demonstration of the length of the iliac arteries is thus achieved. At times, successful imaging of the iliac arteries requires a distended urinary bladder. In this case, the transducer is placed in the midline of the pelvis and oriented 45 degrees from midline. Lateral angulation will result in visualization of the iliac vessels.

## ABDOMINAL VEINS

### Anatomy

The IVC is the large vessel that returns blood to the right atrium from the lower limbs, pelvis, and abdomen. It is formed by the junction of the paired common iliac veins slightly anterior and to the right of the fifth lumbar (L5) vertebral body. The IVC travels superiorly in the abdomen, enters the thoracic cavity, and enters the right atrium at the level of the eighth thoracic (T8) vertebral body. As the vena cava nears the heart, it courses somewhat anteriorly to form a hockey

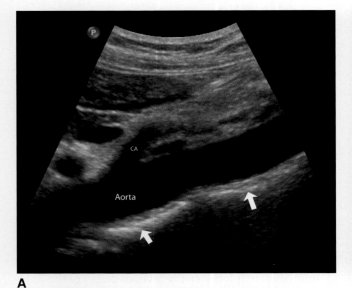

**A**

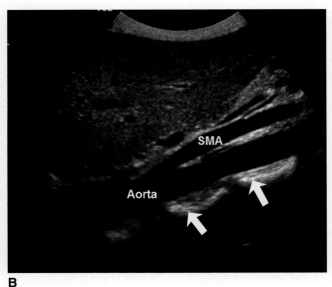

**B**

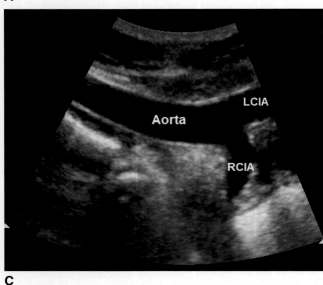

**C**

**Figure 4-4** Longitudinal aorta. **A.** A longitudinal sonogram through the proximal abdominal aorta demonstrates the origins of the celiac axis *(CA)*. **B.** The origin of the superior mesenteric artery *(SMA)* is seen on this longitudinal sonogram of the proximal aorta. On both sonograms, one can note the anterior aspect of the vertebral bodies *(arrows)*. **C.** At the level of the umbilicus, a longitudinal sonogram visualizes the bifurcation of the aorta into the right common iliac artery *(RCIA)* and left common iliac artery *(LCIA)*. (Images courtesy of Philips Medical System, Bothell, WA.)

stick–like configuration before it terminates in the right atrium (Fig. 4-6A,B).

There are many tributaries to the IVC, but most cannot be seen because of their small size. The veins most consistently seen entering the IVC are the common iliac veins at its formation, the renal veins, and the hepatic veins. The right renal vein is generally shorter than the left renal vein because of the right kidney's proximity to the IVC. The left renal vein traverses the abdomen, coursing anterior to the aorta and posterior to the SMA to finally enter the lateral aspect of the IVC.

The hepatic veins also drain directly into the IVC or right atrium. Normally, there are three hepatic veins: (1) the left, (2) the right, and (3) the middle (Fig. 4-7).

### Sonographic Appearance

Sonographically, the IVC is an anechoic structure slightly to the right of midline. Unlike the aorta, which has a relatively consistent diameter and a rounded appearance

in the transverse plane, the IVC tends to have a more oval shape. It also responds to respiratory variations. During inspiration, the IVC should collapse, owing to the decreased pressure within the thoracic cavity, allowing prompt blood flow from the IVC into the right atrium. The opposite is true for expiration, and the IVC expands during this maneuver. With suspended inspiration, the IVC expands due to increased intrathoracic pressure and decreased blood flow into the heart. During the Valsalva maneuver, the IVC collapses because of the increased abdominal pressure associated with this technique.[8,9]

The hepatic veins are best demonstrated in a transverse plane with the transducer just inferior to the xiphoid process and angled cephalic. Identification of the right, middle, and left hepatic veins is relatively easy because they converge to empty into the IVC (Fig. 4-8A). Partial imaging of the right hepatic vein with simultaneous imaging of the middle and left hepatic veins will result in a rabbit-ear appearance (Playboy bunny sign).

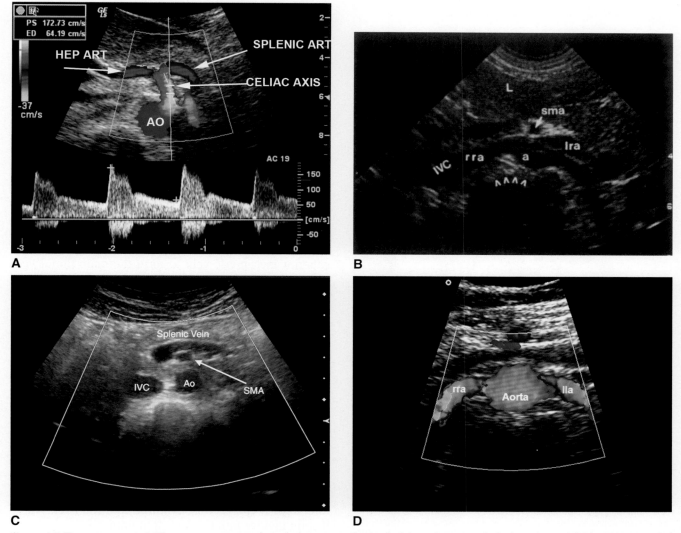

**Figure 4-5** Transverse aorta. **A.** Transverse sonogram through the aorta at the level of the celiac axis with the branching of the hepatic artery and splenic artery. **B.** The transverse sonogram at the level of the branching right renal artery *(rra)* and left renal artery *(lra)* off of the aorta *(a)* can be seen with its relationship to the superior mesenteric artery *(sma)* and inferior vena cava *(IVC)*. *L*, liver; *carets*, anterior aspect of a vertebral body. **C.** This transverse image displays the relationship of the splenic vein, superior mesenteric artery *(SMA)*, inferior vena cava *(IVC)*, and abdominal aorta *(Ao)*. **D.** A color Doppler image demonstrates the origins of the right renal artery *(rra)* and left renal artery *(lla)* branching off of the aorta. (Fig. 4-5A courtesy of GE Healthcare, Wauwatosa, WI; Fig. 4-5B courtesy of Kacey Crandall, Tremonton, UT; Fig. 4-5D courtesy of Philips Medical System, Bothell, WA.)

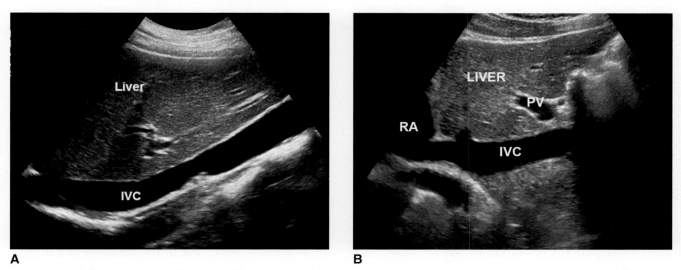

**Figure 4-6** Normal IVC. **A.** A longitudinal sonogram through the inferior vena cava *(IVC)* demonstrates the hockey stick configuration as the vessel as it nears the right atrium. **B.** This image displays the relationship of the inferior vena cava *(IVC)* draining into the right atrium *(RA)*. *PV*, portal vein. (Fig. 4-6A courtesy of Philips Medical System, Bothell, WA.)

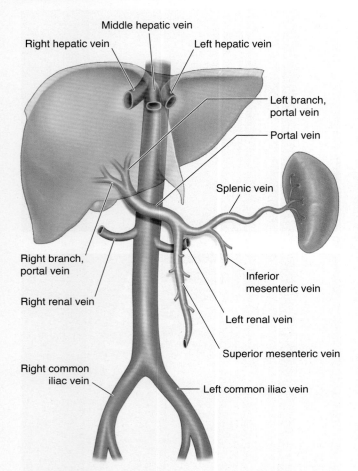

**Figure 4-7** Abdominal veins. The most often sonographically visualized veins and their relationships are depicted on the illustration of the inferior vena cava, its tributaries, and the formation of the portal venous system.

Optimal imaging of the renal veins is also accomplished using a transverse scanning approach. The renal veins should be visualized at about the same level as the renal arteries (just inferior to the origin of the SMA) (Fig. 4-8B). The right renal vein is best imaged with the transducer placed in the right lateral abdomen over the right kidney and angled medially. The renal vein is identified as an echo-free tube exiting the renal hilum. When attempting to visualize the left renal vein, the transducer is placed (in a transverse orientation) in the midline of the abdomen just inferior to the SMA origin (Fig. 4-8C). The left renal vein is seen as an anechoic tubular structure coursing between the SMA and the aorta to enter the lateral aspect of the IVC.

## PORTAL VENOUS SYSTEM ANATOMY

The portal venous system is composed of the veins that drain blood from the bowel and spleen and is separate from the IVC.

The main portal vein is formed at the junction of the splenic vein and the superior mesenteric vein, which

can be identified with sonography in most patients (see Fig. 4-7). To image the portal venous system, it is easiest to begin by placing the transducer in the midline of the abdomen substernally with a transverse orientation. The splenic vein can be used as an initial reference point, as it is easily seen in this plane. The splenic vein emerges from the splenic hilum and courses medial and superiorly within the abdomen, bordering the posterior surface of the pancreatic body and tail. It is identified sonographically as a tubular structure with a superomedial course within the abdomen coursing anterior to the SMA as it nears the midline. At its termination, the splenic vein can be seen to increase in diameter. This is the point at which the splenic vein merges with the superior mesenteric vein to form the main portal vein (Fig. 4-9A). The junction of the superior mesenteric vein and the splenic vein is known as the *portal confluence*, and this confluence is immediately posterior to the neck of the pancreas. Visualization of the superior mesenteric vein is accomplished by placing the transducer over the portal confluence (transverse orientation) and rotating the transducer 90 degrees. The length of the superior mesenteric vein will be displayed having a longitudinal course within the abdomen that parallels that of the SMA to its left (Fig. 4-9B).

The main portal vein travels somewhat obliquely and anteriorly within the abdomen before it enters the liver hilum (Fig. 4-9C). Placement of the transducer over the portal confluence and subsequent clockwise rotation eventually demonstrates the portal vein in its long axis. It can then be followed into the liver, where it soon divides into left and right branches.

Other vessels contributing to portal venous circulation include the inferior mesenteric vein, coronary vein, pyloric vein, cystic vein, and paraumbilical veins. These generally are not seen on routine abdominal examinations but may be identified in abnormal states and will be discussed later in this chapter.

## RELATIONAL ANATOMY OF THE ARTERIES AND VEINS

To perform sonography, it is clinically useful to know the relationship of abdominal arteries and veins to each other as well as to the ducts and organs.[10] Figure 4-10 illustrates the information summarized in Table 4-1.

## ARTERIAL ABNORMALITIES

### ATHEROSCLEROSIS

#### Description

Atherosclerosis is a form of arteriosclerosis in which the intimal lining of the arteries is altered by the presence of any combination of the following: focal accumulation of lipids, complex carbohydrates, blood and blood products, fibrous tissue, and/or calcium deposits. The media of the arterial wall is also changed.[11]

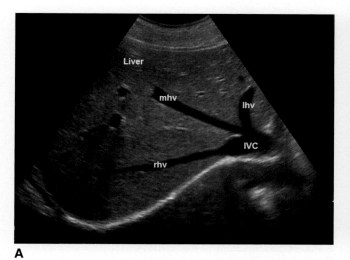

**A**

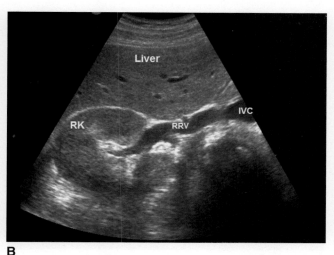

**B**

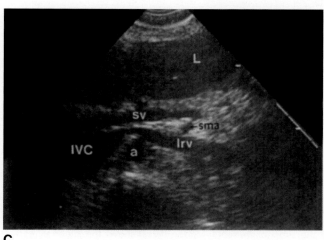

**C**

**Figure 4-8** Transverse sections. **A.** A transverse plane through the liver shows the right hepatic vein *(rhv)*, middle hepatic vein *(mhv)*, and left hepatic vein *(lhv)* draining into the inferior vena cava *(IVC)*. **B.** A transverse plane through the right kidney *(RK)* shows the right renal vein *(RRV)* as it courses to the inferior vena cava *(IVC)*. **C.** The transverse sonogram at the level of the left renal vein *(lrv)* shows its relationship to surrounding vessels. *a*, aorta; *IVC*, inferior vena cava; *sma*, superior mesentric artery; *sv*, splenic vein; *L*, liver. (Figs. 4-8A and 4-8B courtesy of Philips Medical System, Bothell, WA.)

### Etiology

The cause is not known, but several factors have been linked to the progression of atherosclerosis and they include hyperlipidemia, hypertension, cigarette smoking, and diabetes mellitus.[12]

### Clinical Signs and Symptoms

Generally, there are no symptoms of atherosclerosis until a significant stenosis develops. Then, symptoms vary and are related to the particular stenotic vessel. These are discussed later. Atherosclerotic disease also disposes to development of aneurysms. There are generally no symptoms unless complications arise.

### Sonographic Appearance

The sonographic findings of atherosclerosis include luminal irregularities (representative of the various changes of the intimal lining of the artery), tortuosity, and vessel wall calcification.

The wall irregularities detected by sonography can be seen as low-level echoes along the internal walls of the aorta with a propensity for development at the areas of bifurcation of the branch vessels.[1,13] In and of

themselves, these areas of plaque formation are not terribly important unless they produce hemodynamically significant stenosis of a particular branch artery. Detection of a hemodynamically significant stenosis is discussed in detail later in this chapter.

In elderly persons, tortuosity of the aorta is often seen leftward in the patient but occasionally can be right sided.[6] Imaging of the vessel is best carried out in the transverse plane, as this affords a clearer picture of the course of a tortuous aorta.

Aortic wall calcification is easily detected as an echogenic focus in the arterial wall, which at times may produce acoustic shadows (Fig. 4-11).

## ANEURYSMS OF THE ABDOMINAL AORTA

### Description

An aneurysm is a focal dilatation of an artery caused by a structural weakness in its wall. A fusiform aneurysm is a uniform dilatation. A saccular aneurysm is a saclike protrusion of the aorta toward one side or the other, is usually larger than a fusiform aneurysm, and is connected to the aorta by a channel or opening that varies

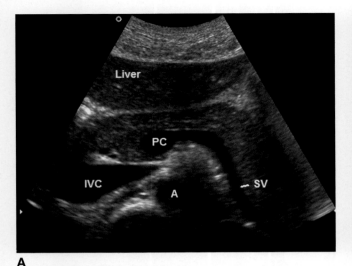

**A**

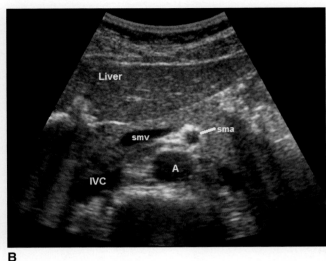

**B**

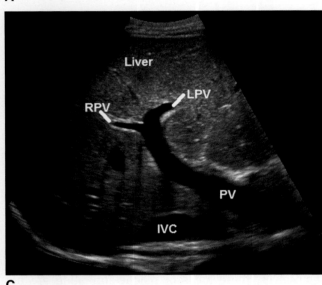

**C**

**Figure 4-9** Portal system. **A.** The vessels visualized on a transverse sonogram through the upper abdomen include the splenic vein *(SV)* as it merges with the superior mesenteric vein to form the portal confluence *(PC)*, which forms the beginning of the portal vein. *IVC*, inferior vena cava; *A*, aorta. **B.** Transverse plane made just below the origin of the superior mesenteric artery *(sma)* shows the superior mesenteric vein *(smv)*. *IVC*, inferior vena cava; *A*, aorta. **C.** An oblique plane through the right upper quadrant visualizes the portal vein *(PV)* as it enters the liver and branches into the right portal vein *(RPV)* and the left portal vein *(LPV)*. *IVC*, inferior vena cava. (Images courtesy of Philips Medical System, Bothell, WA.)

in size. A dissecting aneurysm is when a longitudinal tear in the arterial wall allows bleeding to occur into the wall. Fusiform and saccular aneurysm occur more often in the abdominal aorta, and dissecting aneurysms are less common and occur more often in the thoracic aorta (Fig. 4-12). Most abdominal aortic aneurysms occur below the level of the renal arteries.[12]

### Etiology

Atherosclerosis is the most common cause of aneurysms in the United States. Syphilis and other diseases can cause aneurysms, although these are not very common causes.[2,12]

### Clinical Signs and Symptoms

Generally, patients with aneurysms are asymptomatic, and the presence of an aneurysm is suspected during palpation of a pulsating mass in the region of the umbilicus, or by calcification seen on an abdomen

radiograph. Patients with an expanding aneurysm may have vague lower back or abdominal pain.[2]

### Sonographic Appearance

At the diaphragm, normal aortic diameters have been cited at approximately 2.5 cm.[6] During its course, inferiorly the aorta tapers, reaching a diameter of about 1.5 to 2.0 cm at the level of the iliac arteries.[6] Ectasia of the aorta, as seen with atherosclerosis, is manifested by a slight widening of the normal aortic diameter up to 3.0 cm. There are also aortic wall irregularities, owing to the atherosclerotic changes that take place in this disease process. A true aneurysm is identified sonographically as a dilatation of the aorta ≥3.0 cm near its bifurcation point, a focal dilatation along the course of the aorta, or lack of normal tapering of the aorta.[14–17]

Aneurysms vary in size and can range from 3 to 20 cm as a result of the abnormal blood flow patterns within an aneurysm. If thrombus is formed, it can usually be

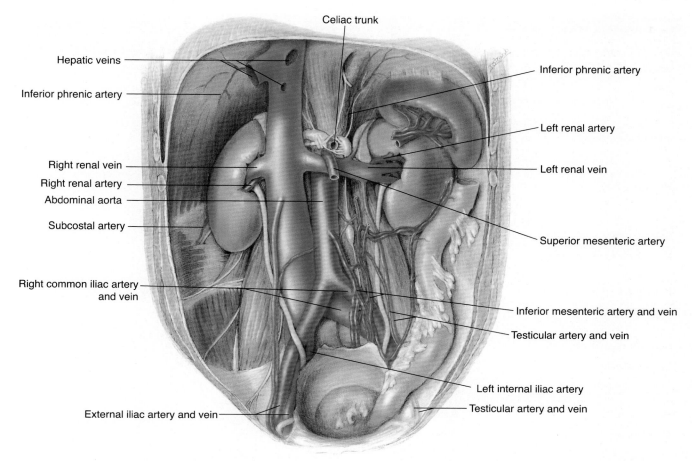

Celiac trunk

Hepatic veins

Inferior phrenic artery

Inferior phrenic artery

Left renal artery

Right renal vein

Left renal vein

Right renal artery

Abdominal aorta

Subcostal artery

Superior mesenteric artery

Right common iliac artery and vein

Inferior mesenteric artery and vein

Testicular artery and vein

Left internal iliac artery

External iliac artery and vein

Testicular artery and vein

**Figure 4-10** Relationships. Collective illustration of the major branches of the aorta, inferior vena cava, and the portal system helps visualize the abdominal vascular and organ relationships.

detected by sonographic techniques and is a common finding. Sonographically, thrombus typically produces a low-level echo pattern and tends to accumulate along the anterior and lateral walls of the aortic lumen[14,15] (Fig. 4-13A–E). Adequate demonstration of the thrombus may require that gain settings be increased from initial settings to display the low-level echoes associated with thrombus. It may also be necessary to scan coronally or obliquely through the aorta to demonstrate thrombus. These maneuvers may help reduce confusion between reverberation artifacts and actual thrombus. Occasionally, there may be calcification within the thrombus. An interesting phenomenon that has been reported in association with aortic aneurysm thrombus is that of an anechoic crescent sign (Fig. 4-13F). In these instances, the anechoic area within the lumen of the aneurysm was found at surgery to be serosanguineous fluid or liquefying clot. When evaluating the aorta for aneurysm formation, it is important to distinguish this finding from aortic dissection, as the surgical treatments are different.

Thrombus within the aorta may be difficult at times to visualize, especially in an obese or gassy patient. Anterior reverberation artifacts from a calcific anterior

aortic wall may obscure the clot as well. Instances have been reported in which an obstruction clot of the aorta was not detected sonographically.[18] If an obstructing clot is suspected on clinical grounds, Doppler examination of the aorta can confirm the presence or absence of flow within it, solving the problem (Fig. 4-13G).

If an aneurysm is detected during sonographic examination, it is prudent to attempt to identify the origins of the renal arteries as well as to extend the examination to the iliac arteries to look for aneurysmal involvement in these areas.

Associated renal artery aneurysm in conjunction with abdominal aortic aneurysm has been reported to be 1% or less.[19] Nonetheless, it is important for the surgeon to know of this coexistence because of the difference in treatment procedures. When the renal arteries are involved in an aneurysm, renal artery enlargement generally coexists with aortic dilatation. Demonstration of this complication, however, can be quite difficult because large aneurysms tend to displace surrounding bowel superiorly and subsequently cover the renal artery origins.[19] Consequently, diligent scanning techniques involving multiple patient positions and numerous transducer angulations may be necessary before

| TABLE 4-1 |  |
| --- | --- |
| **Relational Anatomy** |  |
| **Vessels** | **Relational Anatomy**[a] |
| Aorta | Anterior to the spine<br>Left of the inferior vena cava<br>More posterior proximally than distally |
| Inferior vena cava | Anterior to the spine<br>Right of the aorta<br>Courses anteriorly to enter right atrium |
| Hepatic artery | Anterior to the portal vein<br>Left of the common bile duct<br>Superior to the head of the pancreas |
| Splenic artery | Superior to the body and tail of the pancreas |
| Superior mesenteric artery | Posterior to the body of the pancreas and the splenic vein<br>Anterior to the aorta |
| Right renal artery | Posterior to the inferior vena cava |
| Splenic vein | Posterior to the body and tail of the pancreas<br>Inferior to the splenic artery |
| Superior mesenteric vein | Right of and parallel to the superior mesenteric artery |
| Left renal vein | Anterior to the aorta<br>Posterior to the superior mesenteric artery<br>Anterior to the right renal artery |
| Portal vein | Anterior to the inferior vena cava |
| Common bile duct | Anterior to the portal vein<br>Right of the hepatic artery |

[a]The left and right directional terms refer to the patient's anatomy.

adequate visualization of the renal artery origins is achieved. Color flow Doppler may also aid visualization of the renal arteries in such patients. If efforts to identify the renal arteries are unsuccessful, an attempt should be made to visualize the SMA. Because of the proximity of the renal arteries to the SMA, any aneurysm shown to involve the SMA also involves the renal arteries.

Abdominal aneurysms may also extend into the iliac arteries. When this occurs, the iliac arteries will be abnormally dilated and the thrombus may or may not be present in the dilated areas. Isolated iliac artery aneurysms are an occasional finding[2] (see Fig. 4-13D,E).

The accuracy rate for the sonographic detection of aortic aneurysms approaches 100% in most reports.[5,20–22] Because of this, sonography is a very good screening tool as the first step in evaluation of suspected aortic aneurysm and can be used to monitor the growth of

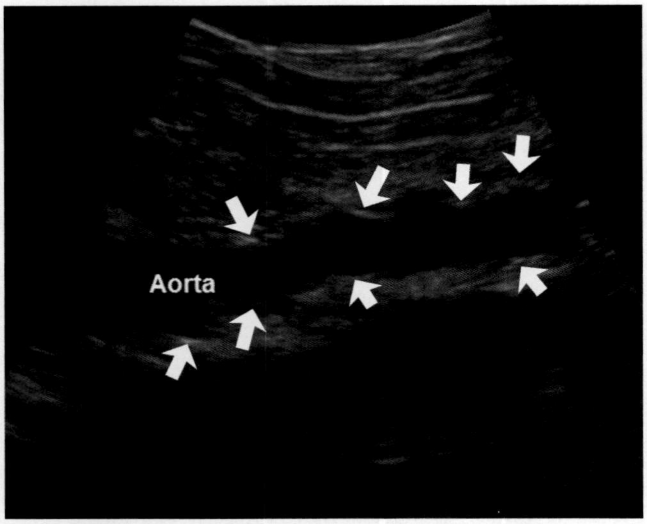

**Figure 4-11** Arteriosclerotic aorta. Diffuse plaque *(arrows)* with minimal acoustic shadowing can be seen in the longitudinal sonogram through the distal portion of an aorta. (Image courtesy of Philips Medical System, Bothell, WA.)

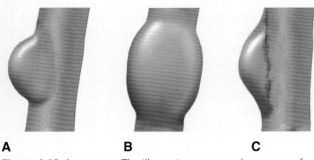

**A**    **B**    **C**

**Figure 4-12** Aneurysms. The illustration presents three types of aneurysms: **(A)** fusiform, **(B)** saccular, and **(C)** dissecting.

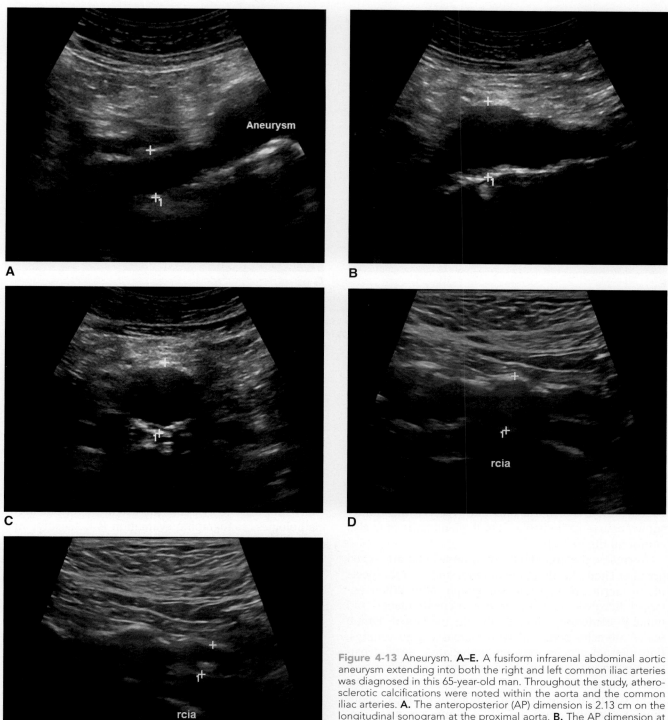

**Figure 4-13** Aneurysm. **A–E.** A fusiform infrarenal abdominal aortic aneurysm extending into both the right and left common iliac arteries was diagnosed in this 65-year-old man. Throughout the study, atherosclerotic calcifications were noted within the aorta and the common iliac arteries. **A.** The anteroposterior (AP) dimension is 2.13 cm on the longitudinal sonogram at the proximal aorta. **B.** The AP dimension at the infrarenal location is 3.58 cm and is seen on the longitudinal sonogram. **C.** On the transverse sonogram at the same infrarenal location, the measurement is 3.48 cm. **D.** The 1.6 cm diameter was measured in the right common iliac artery *(rcia)*. **E.** A large calcification is noted within the *rcia*. The sonographer should also note the size of the residual lumen compared to the total size of the aneurysm. *(continued)*

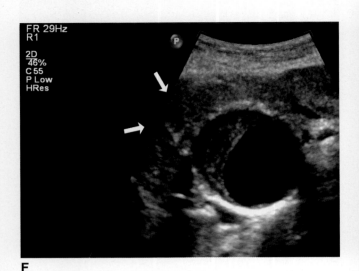

F

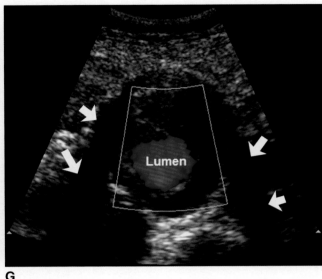

G

**Figure 4-13** *(continued)* **F,G.** These transverse sonograms display an abdominal aortic aneurysm. **F.** A transverse sonogram demonstrates the anechoic crescent sign *(arrows)* due to the area within the thrombus that has liquefied. **G.** A transverse sonogram with color Doppler provides evidence of blood flow as well as the residual lumen compared to the total size of the aneurysm. On both sides of the vessel, refraction creates shadowing artifacts *(arrows)*. (Figs. 4-13F and 4-13G courtesy of Philips Medical System, Bothell, WA.)

aneurysms over time.[23] However, there are some important considerations to keep in mind to avoid misdiagnosis of an aneurysm. Tortuosity may make the aortic diameter appear larger than it is. This occurs when the plane of imaging is not truly perpendicular to the aortic walls. Therefore, careful observations should be made of the aortic curvature in these instances to avoid misrepresentation of a tortuous aortic segment as an aortic aneurysm. Excessive air in the abdomen or obesity may obscure the distal aorta and iliac vessels and render some aneurysms invisible. Lymphadenopathy may also confound the picture.[21,22]

Normally, the abundant lymph nodes that are linked together chainlike along the anterior and lateral aspects of the aorta are invisible sonographically. When enlarged, however, their appearance can be dramatic—and initially confusing. Sonographically, enlarged lymph nodes are echo poor, but with increased gain settings, fine internal echoes may be appreciated. Several patterns of lymph node enlargement have been described: isolated large masses, which tend to develop along the aortic chain; mantlelike distributions of enlarged nodes draped atop the aorta and IVC; symmetric nodal enlargement along the aortic chain bilaterally; multiple spindle-shaped nodes dispersed in the mesentery; and large, confluent masses surrounding the aorta and IVC.[14] It is conceivable that the mantlelike configurations and the confluent mass effects may be confused with aortic aneurysm with thrombus. Close inspection of the area should reveal linear separations between lymph node masses. Also, the general appearance of extensive lymph node enlargement seems to be slightly more irregular, or "lumpy," than an aortic aneurysm. The most reliable and accurate tool to use to determine artery versus vein

versus lymph node is to Doppler sample for the presence or absence of arterial or venous flow patterns.

The rates with which sonography can accurately detect renal artery involvement and other abnormalities (ruptured aneurysm) are unfortunately not as high as those for aneurysm detection. Therefore, other diagnostic imaging tests are necessary to further evaluate these complications if they are suspected.[24]

Although other imaging procedures may be the primary tool used to evaluate the extent of various aortic pathologies, sonographic evaluation is a sensitive and specific imaging technique of choice for screening patients suspected of having aortic aneurysms. The sonographic measurements are accurate, repeatable, and noninvasive.[20,25]

## AORTIC DISSECTION

### Description

In aortic dissection, there is a separation of the layers of the arterial wall by blood or hemorrhage, which generally begins in the proximal portion of the aorta. According to the DeBakey model, there are three types of dissections (Fig. 4-14). Type I and type II involve the ascending aorta and the aortic arch; type III involves the descending aorta at a level below the left subclavian artery. There is a high incidence of mortality with type I and type II dissections because of the propensity of the dissection to extend into the pericardium. A lower mortality rate and a better prognosis are associated with type III dissections. Type I and type III dissections are more common than type II, which are often associated with Marfan syndrome. Once dissection has begun, it may extend for varying distances along the length of the aorta.[26,27]

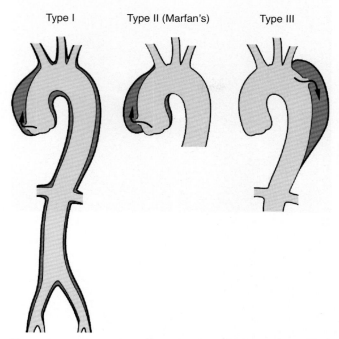

Type I          Type II (Marfan's)          Type III

**Figure 4-14** Aneurysm classifications. The three types of aortic dissections illustrated were categorized by DeBakey.

## Etiology

The etiology of aortic dissection is not clear. Presumably, the dissection results from a tear of the intimal lining of the aorta. It has been demonstrated, however, that this is not always the case, and postulation has been made that rupture of the vasa vasorum can initiate a dissection.[12,27] Hypertension is strongly associated with dissections, and cystic medial necrosis of the vessel is also well recognized as an underlying cause. Other entities that contribute to aortic dissection include Marfan syndrome, pregnancy, aortic valve disease, congenital cardiac anomalies (coarctation, aortic hypoplasia, bicuspid aortic valve, persistent patent ductus arteriosus, atrial septal defect, and tricuspid valve abnormalities), Cushing syndrome, pheochromocytoma, and catheter-induced needle wounds.[12,27-29]

## Clinical Signs and Symptoms

Intense chest pain is the most common symptom of aortic dissection. Abdominal, as well as lower back, arm, or leg, pain may also occur, depending on the extent of the dissection. There may also be vomiting, paralysis, transient blindness, coma, confusion, syncope, headache, and dyspnea, and extremity pulses may be absent.[26,27,29]

## Sonographic Appearance

Sonographically, aortic dissection appears as a thin, linear echo flap within the arterial lumen[30] (Fig. 4-15A). Because of the presence of blood flow along both sides of the dissection, there is usually motion of the flap with each cardiac cycle. Doppler interrogation is an additional diagnostic aid, providing demonstration

of arterial blood flow on both sides of the flap (Fig. 4-15B,C). When evaluating a patient for aortic dissection, it is important to utilize both longitudinal and transverse imaging planes to carefully examine the aorta, as an intimal flap can be overlooked if it is located laterally in the artery.[26]

## AORTIC RUPTURE

### Description

Abdominal aortic aneurysms of any size may rupture, but the risk increases with aneurysms larger than 7 cm in diameter.[21,31,32] Most aneurysms rupture into the peritoneal space, with no predilection for a specific site. They may also rupture into the duodenum, left renal vein, IVC, or urinary tract. An aortic rupture is a medical emergency as the mortality rate for untreated aortic rupture is virtually 100%; with surgery, the mortality rate ranges between 40% and 60%.[33]

### Clinical Signs and Symptoms

Typically, aortic rupture presents clinically as central back pain and hypotension.[6,12]

### Sonographic Appearance

Because of the leakage of blood outside of the vessel, aortic rupture may be diagnosed by identification of a hematoma in the abdomen in association with aneurysmal dilatation of the aorta. These hematomas may be located close to the aorta or may extend to varying degrees through the retroperitoneum. Aortic rupture may appear in a variety of stages, from a completely cystic mass to a complex mass. If large enough, the hematomas may also displace surrounding organs and structures.[12] Other findings suggestive of aortic aneurysm rupture include irregular intra-abdominal fluid collections in association with aortic aneurysm and diffuse irregular hypoechoic areas near an aortic aneurysm (Fig. 4-16A–F).

It is difficult to identify the actual rupture site by sonographic examination, although they may be inferred by hematoma "geography." Computed tomography (CT), on the other hand, is well suited for detection of aortic rupture and is the diagnostic test of choice because it allows for clear depiction of the extent and density of the hematoma as well as the site of rupture.[34] For high-risk patients, contrast-enhanced three-dimensional (3D) magnetic resonance angiography (MRA) is a preferred and accurate examination with iodinated contrast material or carbon dioxide contrast agents.[35]

## INFLAMMATORY ANEURYSMS

### Description

Inflammatory aneurysms are enveloped by a dense, fibrotic reaction, generally including many inflammatory cell infiltrates and fatty tissue. This fibrotic reaction is also vascular in nature and involves the retroperitoneum to different degrees. The inflammatory reaction

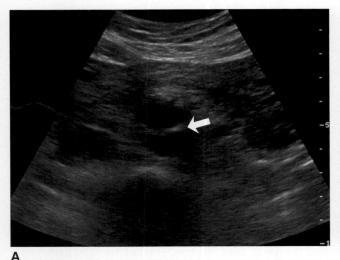

A

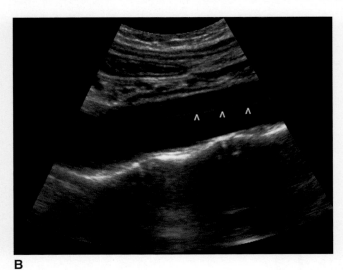

B

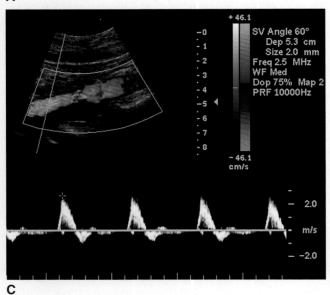

C

**Figure 4-15** Dissecting aneurysm. **A.** On a transverse plane, an aortic dissection appears as a linear echo flap *(arrow)* within the arterial lumen. **B.** On the longitudinal sonogram through the abdominal aorta, a thin linear echo flap *(carets)* is noted paralleling the anterior wall. **C.** The Doppler interrogation shows narrowing of an aorta flow with increased speed. (Images courtesy of Philips Medical System, Bothell, WA.)

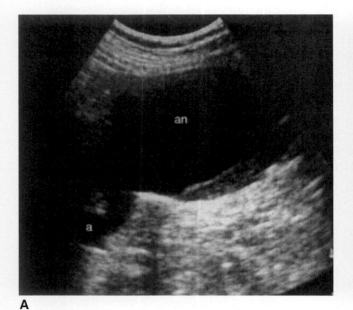

A

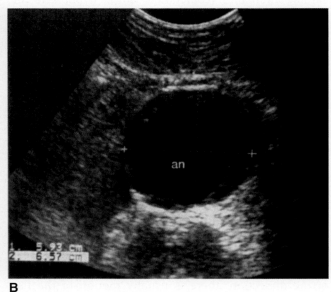

B

**Figure 4-16** Aortic rupture. **A,B.** The images are from the initial examination. The longitudinal **(A)** and transverse **(B)** sonograms show an aorta *(a)* with an intact, moderately large aneurysm *(an)*. *(continued)*

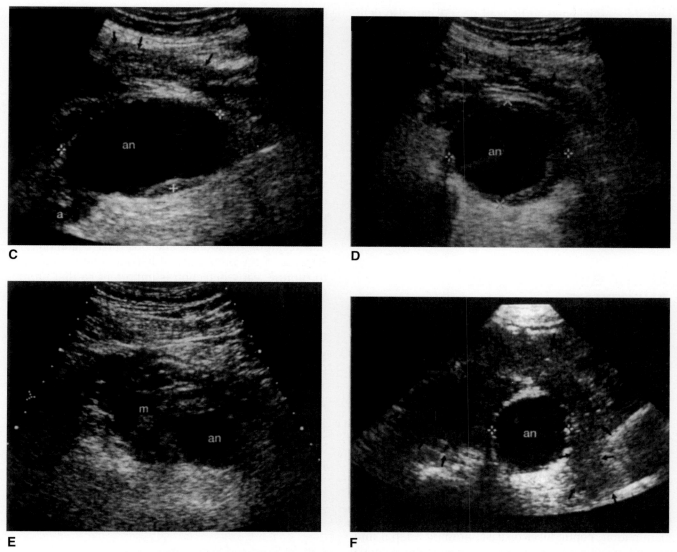

**Figure 4-16** *(continued)* **C,D.** Two days after the initial examination, the patient presented to the emergency department with acute abdominal/back pain and hypotension. The longitudinal **(C)** and transverse **(D)** sonograms were made through the aneurysm *(an)*. The adjacent, irregular hypoechoic mass *(arrows)* is representative of blood dissecting through the retroperitoneum. **E.** On a different patient, a collection of blood *(m)* is seen adjacent to the ruptured aneurysm *(an)* on this transverse sonogram. The aneurysm is almost lost in the collection of blood surrounding it. **F.** This patient has a diffuse dissection of an aneurysm *(an)* with blood leakage throughout the retroperitoneum *(arrows)*. This subtle example represents the difficulty sonography has in demonstrating aortic aneurysm rupture.

around the aneurysm may become adherent to the duodenum, sigmoid colon, small bowel, ureter, iliac vein, and inferior vena cava.[36–39]

Inflammatory aneurysms are an uncommon entity, reportedly between 5% and 20% of all aortic aneurysms.[37] They tend to occur in relatively younger persons than arteriosclerotic aneurysms. Even though the risk of rupture is less than that of a "normal" aneurysm, rupture is still a possible scenario.

### Etiology

The cause of inflammatory aneurysms is uncertain, but because they are always seen in the presence of aneurysm, it has been postulated that the aneurysm itself may be the cause of the inflammatory reaction.[36,38]

### Clinical Signs and Symptoms

Clinically, the symptoms of inflammatory aneurysms are similar to those of aortic aneurysm. Other symptoms may develop in accordance with the extent of inflammatory involvement to the neighboring areas. These may include leg edema, bothersome pulsations in the epigastrium, and constipation. Hydronephrosis with concomitant flank pain may develop in the presence of ureteral obstruction, and there may be anorexia, early satiety, and dyspnea if bowel adheres to the aneurysmal inflammation.[38,40]

### Sonographic Appearance

Typically, the sonographic features of an inflammatory aneurysm include aneurysmal dilatation of the aorta with a hypoechoic mantle, usually seen anterior and lateral to a thickened aortic wall.[36–38] CT can also demonstrate this phenomenon, and it is actually better able to depict the extension of the inflammatory process to the surrounding structures in the retroperitoneum.[37]

It is important to distinguish inflammatory aneurysms from a condition known as retroperitoneal fibrosis.[36] Whereas inflammatory aneurysms are always associated with an aortic aneurysm, retroperitoneal fibrosis is not. Also, the makeup of the two fibrotic reactions is somewhat different. Symptoms of retroperitoneal fibrosis generally do not occur until there is vascular or ureteral compromise. Sonographically, it appears as an echo-free area around the anterior and lateral aspects of the aorta, similar to that seen in association with inflammatory aneurysms, although no aneurysm is present.[41]

# AORTIC BRANCH VESSEL ANEURYSMS

## SPLANCHNIC ARTERY ANEURYSMS

### Splenic Artery Aneurysms

#### Description

Splenic artery aneurysms are the most common type of splanchnic artery aneurysm. These are usually multiple and occur in the main splenic arterial trunk. There is apparently a female preponderance. Splenic artery aneurysms, although not very common, are life threatening.[40,42]

#### Etiology

Causes of splenic artery aneurysm encompass fibromuscular disease of the renal arteries, pancreatic inflammation, peptic ulcer disease, primary arterial injury, and mycotic lesions. There is also a greater potential for patients with portal hypertension and multigravidas to develop splenic artery aneurysms.[32,40,42,43]

#### Clinical Signs and Symptoms

Symptoms vary and may range from none to nonspecific left side upper quadrant pain, nausea, vomiting, and a palpable mass if the aneurysm is large enough. There is about a 10% risk of rupture of a splenic artery aneurysm into the peritoneal cavity, with a lesser incidence of rupture into the gastrointestinal tract, spleen, or pancreas.[40]

### Hepatic Artery Aneurysms

#### Description

Hepatic artery aneurysms are the second most common type of splanchnic vessel aneurysms encountered. Seventy-five percent of all hepatic aneurysms are extrahepatic in origin. The remaining 25% occur intrahepatically, the right hepatic arterial branch being more often affected than the left.[44,45] Hepatic artery aneurysms are rare and tend to male preponderance.[40,42]

#### Etiology

The most common causes of reported hepatic arterial aneurysms are systemic infection, arteriosclerosis, and blunt abdominal trauma. Other, less common causes include iatrogenic trauma, vasculitis due to pancreatitis, chronic cholecystitis, polyarteritis, and congenital abnormalities.[45–49]

#### Clinical Signs and Symptoms

Generally, hepatic artery aneurysms are silent or asymptomatic until the aneurysm attains large size or tapers. When symptoms do occur, they are often vague and unclear and may include any of the following: epigastric pain (two-thirds of patients), gastrointestinal bleeding due to rupture of the aneurysm into the biliary tract and resulting hemobilia, and obstructive jaundice.[45,46] Because of the propensity of hepatic artery aneurysms to rupture, early detection is important so that prompt treatment can be obtained.

### Superior Mesenteric Artery Aneurysms

#### Description

SMA aneurysms are the rarest of the splanchnic arterial aneurysms (reported incidence approximately 1 in 12,000). Branch superior mesenteric arterial aneurysms are also quite rare.[40,42]

#### Etiology

The most common cause that has been cited in the pathogenesis of SMA aneurysms is cystic medial necrosis (mycotic aneurysm), which accounts for approximately 58% of the aneurysms detected. Arteriosclerosis, medial degeneration, and trauma have also been associated with SMA aneurysms.[42]

#### Clinical Signs and Symptoms

There may be intestinal angina and postprandial abdominal pain in association with an SMA aneurysm. General abdominal pain and fever (in association with the mycotic type aneurysms) may also be present.[40,42] Again, as with the other splanchnic vessel aneurysms, the symptoms are generally vague and nonspecific.

### Sonographic Appearance of Splanchnic Artery Aneurysms

Sonographically, splanchnic artery aneurysms appear similar to one another. The distinguishing feature is location in the abdomen. All splanchnic aneurysms may appear as an anechoic or a complex abdominal mass. Arterial pulsations or thrombus may or may not be discernable.[50] By demonstrating continuity of the mass with one of the splanchnic arteries, splanchnic artery aneurysms can be identified with a higher degree of confidence, but this is a difficult task to accomplish. Therefore, in order to confirm or refute the vascular nature of the lesion, Doppler sonography should always be used to further investigate an anechoic or complex mass in the upper abdomen. In the case of a splanchnic artery aneurysm, the Doppler signal demonstrates arterial pulsations. Color flow Doppler technology is also of benefit in this type of setting because the characteristic swirling blood flow patterns in these aneurysms are easily recognized.

## RENAL ARTERY ANEURYSMS

### Description

Renal artery aneurysms have been encountered with increasing frequency, although the overall incidence remains relatively low.[51] Most renal artery aneurysms tend to be extrarenal, but there are reports of intrarenal aneurysms. Generally, surgical intervention is required in the presence of aneurysms greater than 1.5 cm and there is associated pain, bleeding, or hypertension.[2] The prevalence of renal artery aneurysm rupture is about 20%.

### Etiology

Renal artery aneurysms are most commonly a result of atherosclerosis and polyarteritis, and represent true aneurysms; congenital abnormalities account for a relatively smaller portion of them. Aneurysms resulting from iatrogenic trauma, blunt trauma, or penetrating trauma are considered false aneurysms and tend to be among the least common types.[2]

### Clinical Signs and Symptoms

Symptoms encountered with renal artery aneurysm may include a palpable mass, hypertension, and blood in the urine along with flank pain.[2]

### Sonographic Appearance

A renal artery aneurysm appears as an anechoic mass along the extent of the renal artery, or occasionally intrarenally. Calcification of the wall may be present, and other findings may or may not include thrombus formation along the periphery of the mass and pulsations. Demonstrating continuity of the mass with the renal artery is a useful indicator of renal artery aneurysm. Doppler interrogations are an excellent method of distinguishing the vascular nature of a suspicious mass in this area because renal artery aneurysms will demonstrate arterial blood flow signals. Color flow Doppler can also rapidly demonstrate blood flow within an aneurysm.

Care must be taken in the evaluation of renal artery aneurysms because it is possible to mistake a normal left renal vein for a left renal artery aneurysm, especially in thin patients.[2] This is due to the fact that the left renal vein is prominent as it exits the renal hilum, but as it passes over the aorta to enter the IVC, it narrows. At this point, part of the aortic wall may not be visualized owing to the angle of incident sound beam and, subsequently, the renal vein may

appear to arise from the aorta. In order to clarify this situation, it may be helpful to study the area in question during suspended inspiration. If the structure is truly venous, the entire venous path should dilate, affording better visualization. If the vessel is arterial, inspiration techniques will not affect its size. Doppler investigation is probably the method of choice to determine the nature of the area in question. If the "mass" is found to have characteristic continuous low-velocity flow, it is most likely the renal vein. If arterial pulsations can be detected, the vessel is most likely the renal artery.

## ILIAC ARTERY ANEURYSMS

### Description

Iliac artery aneurysms are most often associated with (continuations of) abdominal aortic aneurysms. Isolated iliac aneurysms are possible, however, and when they occur, they tend to be bilateral. Isolated internal iliac aneurysms are rare. Half of all untreated iliac aneurysms rupture, making this the most common complication of iliac aneurysms.[2,52]

### Etiology

Most iliac aneurysms are arteriosclerotic in origin. Other less common causes include external or surgical trauma, pregnancy, congenital abnormality, syphilis, and bacterial infection.[2,52]

### Clinical Signs and Symptoms

Iliac artery aneurysms typically go unrecognized clinically and are often discovered unexpectedly. Because of compression on surrounding structures, large iliac aneurysms may produce urologic, gastrointestinal, or neurologic symptoms. Pain may also be present, and a mass may be palpable on physical examination.[2]

### Sonographic Appearance

An iliac artery aneurysm appears as a primarily anechoic mass in the pelvis. Smaller aneurysm may be difficult to identify in the presence of profuse bowel gas. Pulsations may be present. Thrombus may also be present along the periphery of the mass, and calcific changes may be visualized within the wall. Continuity with the iliac artery is a strong indicator for iliac artery aneurysm and Doppler interrogation reveals a turbulent arterial signal. Because of the strong tendency toward bilaterality, the contralateral iliac artery should also be examined carefully[2] (see Fig. 4-13D,E).

## AORTIC GRAFTS AND ASSOCIATED COMPLICATIONS

Diagnostic medical sonography is useful not only for the detection of arterial abnormalities such as aneurysms, but also for the assessment of aortic grafts and their related complications.

## Description

An aortic graft, endograft, or prosthesis is usually a man-made structure used to repair an aortic aneurysm. Grafts can be made of various materials including Teflon (DuPont, Wilmington, DE) and Dacron (INVISTA, Wichita, KS). The name of the graft is usually in reference to the vessel they are attached to, and the attachment may be anastomosed in an end-to-end anastomosis to the normal portion of the vessel after the aneurysm is removed.[53] In some instances, the original aneurysm may be retained and actually sewn around the prosthesis as a stabilizer.[13] In aortofemoral bypass surgery, the diseased segment of the aorta is left intact and end-to-side anastomotic technique is used, resulting in graft placement anterior and adjacent to the native vessel.[53] An endovascular repair of abdominal aortic aneurysms (EVAR) is a minimally invasive surgical procedure that involves deploying a stent graft into the aorta with subsequent exclusion of the aneurysm. In essence, an aortic stent graft is designed to prevent recurrent flow into the aneurysm sac by diverting the arterial flow through the graft material. Over time, due to the loss of dynamic arterial flow, the aneurysm sac is expected to contract and thereby is not likely to rupture.[54]

## Sonographic Appearance

Sonographically, graft replacements are easily detected by their characteristic wall brightness and, at times, it may also be possible to see their ribbing. The graft walls are also straighter than native vessel walls. At the level of the proximal anastomosis, the graft is usually seen to dive posteriorly and continue its course inferiorly with a slight angulation toward the anterior abdominal wall.[2] The graft then bifurcates, and a connection should be demonstrated at the iliac artery level or the common femoral artery level, depending on the extent of the prosthesis.

The sonographic appearance of EVAR grafts is characterized by wall brightness within the aneurysm sac and, like prosthetic grafts, endografts are straighter than the native vessel walls (Fig. 4-17A,B). Oftentimes, the endografts are of a bifurcated design where the bifurcated iliac limbs are visualized considerably more proximally in the aorta rather than at the aortoiliac bifurcation itself.

## Complications

### Pseudoaneurysms

Of all aortic graft complications, pseudoaneurysms are perhaps the most common.[2,53,55] They occur at the site of anastomosis and result from bleeding at this site or from trauma. In essence, there is a pulsating hematoma connected to the lumen of the graft-native vessel interface. The presence of a pulsating mass is usually the first clinical evidence that a pseudoaneurysm may be forming. It may be demonstrated as a graft ending abruptly in an anechoic mass, but is more often seen as a pulsating fluid collection near the site of anastomosis. Doppler interrogation of the mass reveals turbulent arterial signals, and color flow Doppler affords a dramatic representation of the swirling blood flow patterns within pseudoaneurysms as well as their leakage site.

### Graft Aneurysms

Graft aneurysms result from degeneration of the graft material and appear sonographically as focal dilatations of the actual graft material. These are not common complications of aortic grafts.

### Hematomas

Hematomas are a normal part of the healing process of graft replacement surgery. Sonographically, they may present as an anechoic or a complex mass in the area of the graft.

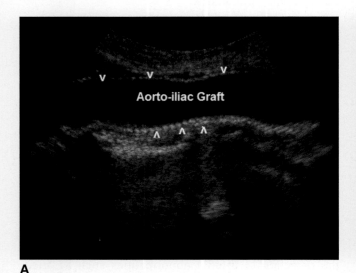

A

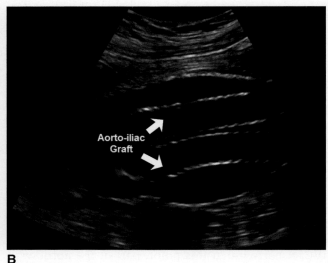

B

**Figure 4-17** Aortic graft. **A,B.** The longitudinal images made through end-to-end anastomoses of an aortoiliac graft can be seen with its characteristic ribbing *(carets)*.

## Abscess

Abscesses may also have a sonographic appearance consistent with an anechoic or complex mass in the area of a graft. Consequently, it may be impossible to differentiate between abscesses and hematomas by sonographic appearance alone. In these instances, clinical signs such as tenderness in the area, history of fever, leukocytosis, and local erythema may be useful in differentiating an infectious process from a hematoma. If there is any question, aspiration of the fluid under sonographic guidance will be diagnostic.

## Occlusion

Graft occlusion was an elusive complication for sonographers until the advent of Doppler technology. Now, it is relatively simple to verify flow through a graft. Once the graft is located by real-time scanning, the Doppler sample volume cursor is moved into the graft lumen. If flow is present, it registers as arterial pulsations. Absence of flow denotes occlusion of the graft. Often, even though there is a compete occlusion, real-time B-mode imaging cannot demonstrate the occluding clot.[53] Therefore, duplex Doppler is essential in this diagnosis. Color flow Doppler dramatically represents flow within a graft and can be used in conjunction with conventional Doppler to confirm graft patency.

## Endoleaks

Endografts have been associated with a device-related complications called *endoleaks*. Endoleaks occur as a result of an incomplete seal between the endograft and the native wall of the aorta or because the inferior mesenteric or lumbar arteries have not been excluded by the device and continue to provide a source of arterial flow into the aneurysm sac. There are also rare instances where an endoleak occurs as a result of endograft failure due to stump disconnection, fabric disruption, or graft porosity. A consequence of an endoleak is that there is continued blood flow around the graft within the aneurysm, which, in turn, may result in fatal consequences stemming from aneurysm expansion and eventual rupture.[56]

Endoleaks are identified on duplex by meticulous Doppler sampling and attention to the presence or absence of color outside of the endograft. Attention to the endograft in gray scale is critical to determine the presence of graft compression, luminal defects, and separation of modular junctions. Color flow Doppler is used to determine extra-stent flow. Use of the most sensitive color Doppler scale settings is required to determine low velocity leaks. Flow that is associated with an endoleak is relatively uniform, persists into diastole, and is reproducible in all scanning planes. Spectral Doppler should be used to determine the speed and flow direction for any suspected extra-stent flow. The endograft should be closely inspected at the proximal and distal fixation sites to document the presence or absence of endoleaks. The sonographer should also obtain velocity waveforms from each iliac limb extension to evaluate for any potential stenosis from graft compression.[57]

# VASCULAR STENOSIS

Discussion of arterial abnormalities would not be complete if the subject of stenosis was not mentioned. Until recently, angiography, and no other method of medical imaging, was very successful in the actual investigation of abdominal visceral artery stenosis. With continued improvement and refinements in duplex and color flow Doppler technology, much interest has been generated in developing criteria for evaluating suspected visceral artery stenoses.[58]

Several studies have shown that blood flow volumes through the visceral arteries can be assessed by Doppler techniques with a relative degree of accuracy when compared to more invasive methods.[59-65] Doppler blood flow volume studies are time consuming and their accuracy is limited by several inherent problems of the technique such as underestimation of vessel diameter and overestimation of average blood flow velocity. Even if Doppler techniques could precisely estimate flow volumes, its routine use in the clinical setting would seem to be limited, as evidenced by prior investigations of significant peripheral occlusive arterial disease. It has been established that volume flows are not particularly helpful in the assessment of stenotic lesions because collateral pathways "normalize" flow volume beyond areas of stenosis. Sonographers identify significant stenosis by recognizing the physiologic blood flow changes associated with significantly compromised arteries. Doppler findings in association with vascular stenosis are identified in Table 4-2. Because it may be difficult to visualize occlusive plaque in the visceral arteries with gray scale sonography, Doppler interrogation becomes very important in the assessment of visceral arteries. Before abnormal Doppler signals can be appreciated, it is essential to be familiar with normal Doppler waveform patterns of the major abdominal visceral arteries (Fig. 4-18A–F).

---

**TABLE** **4-2**

### Doppler Findings with Vascular Stenosis

1. Vessel lumen narrowed by atheromatous plaque or arteriosclerotic changes
2. Poststenotic dilatation
3. Increased velocities in the area of stenosis
4. Downstream changes: turbulence (increases as the percentage of stenosis increases), decreased velocities, slowed acceleration during systole, and relative elevation of diastolic velocities

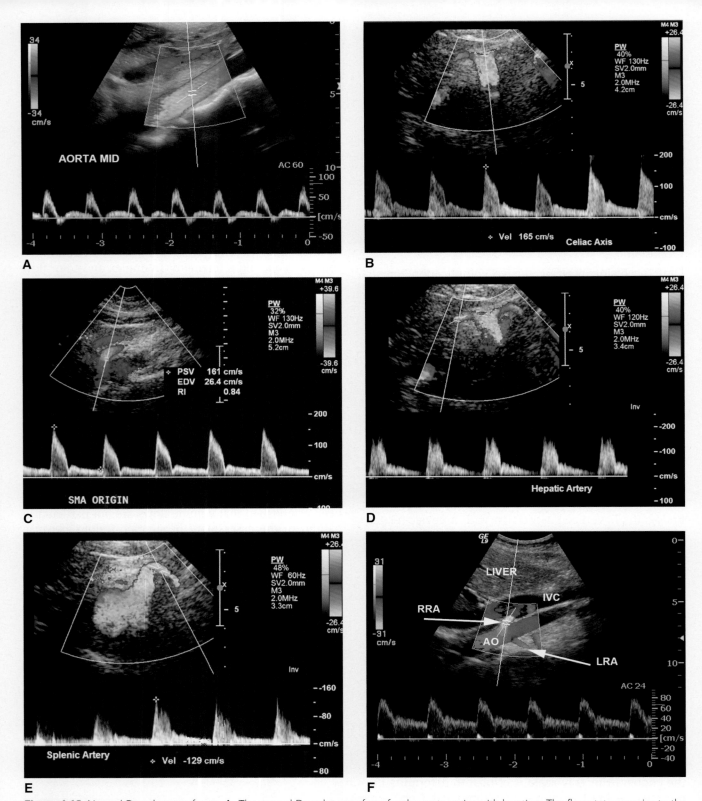

**Figure 4-18** Normal Doppler waveforms. **A.** The normal Doppler waveform for the aorta varies with location. The flow state superior to the renal arteries has a narrow, well-defined systolic complex with forward flow during diastole. The blood in diastole is represented as that part of the waveform closest to the zero baseline. **B.** The major branches of the celiac artery supply the liver and spleen organs that both have low-resistance arterial beds. The arterial waveform is affected by prandial states and caloric food composition. The normal peak systolic velocity (*PSV*) ranges from 98 to 105 cm/sec. If PSV is ≥200 cm/sec, it is considered abnormal and requires further evaluation.[66] **C.** The superior mesenteric artery (*SMA*) supplies the small bowel and proximal colon that also have low-resistance arterial beds. The arterial waveform is affected by prandial states, and the normal PSV ranges from 97 to 142 cm/sec. If PSV is ≥275 cm/sec, it is considered abnormal and requires further evaluation.[66] **D.** The hepatic arterial system has low-resistance flow characteristics with large amounts of continuous forward flow throughout diastole. When the hepatic artery and portal vein velocities are obtained in a fasting patient and compared, it is considered normal if the hepatic artery is equal to or slightly less than portal vein velocity. **E.** The splenic artery blood flow is normally a low-pulsatility Doppler signal but may have some turbulent flow due to its tortuous course from the splenic artery. With a PSV of 129 cm/sec and with an end-diastolic velocity of 45 cm/sec, the splenic artery may have turbulent flow due to its tortuous course. **F.** In this patient, the normal low-pulsatility right renal artery (*RRA*) Doppler spectrum is seen with a PSV of 80 cm/sec. The forward flow present in diastole is because of the low resistance in the renal vascular bed. *LRA*, left renal artery; *IVC*, inferior vena cava; *AO*, aorta. (Figs. 4-18A and 4-18F courtesy of GE Healthcare, Wauwatosa, WI.)

Although there is some variability between different investigators' data, there are accepted and established guidelines to follow when evaluating for potential renal artery and mesenteric artery stenosis.[66]

## RENAL ARTERY STENOSIS

### Description

Renal artery stenosis is a significant medical problem because of its association with uncontrollable hypertension. Other consequences of renal artery stenosis include decreased glomerular filtration rate and ischemic renal damage.[67,68] It is estimated that up to 6% of all hypertensive patients have significant renal artery stenosis as the underlying cause of their hypertension. Identification of these individuals allows corrective intervention that will reduce or minimize the progressive negative sequelae associated with renovascular hypertension.

### Etiology

Renal artery stenosis is caused by atherosclerotic plaque, generally located at its origin from the aorta or within its first 2 cm. It may also be caused by fibromuscular dysplasia. These lesions are usually located in the distal two-thirds of the renal artery.

### Patient Selection

Of all hypertensive individuals, it has been determined that those with a greater than 10% prevalence of having a significant renal artery stenosis include the following: children, onset age younger than 30 years (especially females), onset older than age 50 years (mostly male smokers), poorly controlled hypertension, rapidly worsening hypertension, severe hypertension (diastolic pressure >115 mm Hg), peripheral vascular disease, cerebrovascular disease, coronary artery disease, abdominal aortic aneurysm, aortic dissection, renal artery stenosis, renal insufficiency of unknown cause, renal function deterioration on angiotensin-converting enzyme, blood pressure that responds well to angiotensin-converting enzyme, elevated renin plasma, abdominal bruit, grade 3–4 hypertensive retinopathy, and unilateral small kidney.[69,70]

### Diagnostic Technique and Criteria

Sonography equipment provides color flow imaging to identify flow abnormalities and spectral Doppler measurements to provide the quantitative data to determine the severity of stenosis.[70] Two methods are used in sonography evaluation of renal artery stenosis, and a combination of the two methods will enhance the examination results. The direct method relies on detection of blood flow changes that occur at a hemodynamically significant stenosis, whereas the indirect method relies on identification of blood flow changes that occur distal to a significant stenosis. Both methods require attention to Doppler technique being crucial to the examination.

### Direct Method

The direct method involves direct visualization and Doppler interrogation of the aorta and renal arteries along their entire length. The examination begins with longitudinal images of the abdominal aorta. A central stream Doppler trace is obtained at or slightly above the renal artery origins, and an angle-corrected peak systolic velocity measurement is recorded. All velocity measurements should be made with a Doppler angle of less than 60 degrees. The renal arteries are then imaged, and the Doppler sample volume walked through their length. Doppler spectra and angle-corrected peak systolic velocities are recorded at the vessel origins and at their proximal, middle, and distal segments. The maximum peak systolic velocity from each side is noted and used to calculate the renal artery to aortic ratio (RAR).[71-76] Stenosis is diagnosed if there is a 50% to 60% reduction in the lumen diameter, which is considered hemodynamically significant (Table 4-3).[76-80]

Direct imaging and Doppler interrogation may be technically more difficult on obese individuals, as well as those with excessive bowel gas. Right lateral and left lateral decubitus patient positions may help in delineation of the renal arteries as well as multiple transducer positions and varying degrees of probe pressure. The major limitations of this method include incomplete visualization of the renal arteries, potential overestimation of blood flow velocities due to suboptimal

| TABLE 4-3 |
| --- |
| Criteria for Detection of at Least 50% to 60% Renal Artery Stenosis[70,78,81] |
| **Direct evaluation of the main renal artery** |
| PSV >180 to 200 cm/sec<br>RAR >3.3 to 3.5<br>Poststenotic turbulence |
| **Internal (intrarenal) evaluation of the segmental/interlobar arteries** |
| Absence of ESP<br>AT >0.07 sec (increasing the time to 0.10 increases specificity)<br>Tardus–parvus waveform<br>RI difference between kidneys exceeding −5 |
| **In stent stenosis** |
| PSV >250 cm/sec<br>Poststenotic turbulence |
| **Other hemodynamic parameters** |
| AI = measured from the slope of the initial acceleration point over the transmitted frequency<br>RRR = the ratio between PSV and the proximal or midsegment of the renal artery |

PSV, peak systolic velocity; RAR, renal-to-aorta ratio; ESP, end-systolic peak; AT, acceleration time; RI, resistive index; AI acceleration index; RRR, renal-to-renal ratio.

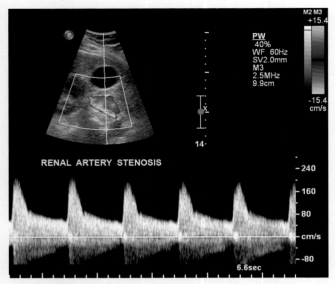

**Figure 4-19** Renal artery stenosis. Pulsed Doppler interrogation of the renal artery displays elevated peak systolic velocity of 200 cm/sec. (Image courtesy of Philips Medical System, Bothell, WA.)

Doppler angles (those >60%) and vessel tortuosity, and the inability to detect accessory renal arteries (Fig. 4-19).

There may be instances in which a Doppler angle of 60 degrees or less will not be obtainable despite the best efforts of the sonographer. Using a Doppler angle of greater than 60 degrees will lead to falsely elevated velocities. Abnormal velocities obtained with suboptimal Doppler angles should be viewed with suspicion. In these instances, poststenotic turbulence should be identified before significant stenosis is suggested.

A significant number of individuals have accessory renal arteries. Duplex Doppler and even color flow Doppler have not proven to be very helpful in identifying accessory renal arteries. A stenosis in an unrecognized accessory renal artery will result in a falsely negative examination.

### Indirect (Intrarenal) Method

The indirect method involves Doppler evaluation of the segmental or interlobar arteries in the upper, middle, and lower poles within the kidney. The rationale for evaluating each pole is to document if a stenotic accessory artery is feeding one of the renal poles. An abnormal waveform detected with Doppler in that segment compensates and adds information to the direct method where it is possible to miss accessory renal arteries.

Using color and/or power Doppler is essential and is helpful in identifying the intrarenal vessels and in determining an optimal angle of incidence. If a feeding artery has a high-grade stenosis, it can cause the pulsus tardus and parvus changes in intrarenal arterial flow

signals (*pulsus* is beat; *tardus* is slow; *parvus* is small). A tardus–parvus waveform demonstrates a delay in the time to maximum systole and an increase in the acceleration index. If the intrarenal segmental and interlobar arteries are normal, the waveform will display an early systolic peak (ESP) or notch at the beginning of systole. With renal artery stenosis greater than 60%, the ESP is absent.

The systolic acceleration time (AT) is measured from start of the systolic upstroke to the first peak or ESP. Systolic ATs greater than 0.07 seconds are consistent with a main renal artery stenosis exceeding 60%.[68,69,78,81] If 0.10 to 0.12 seconds is used as the cutoff for significant stenosis, it increases the specificity.[70] The resistive index (RI) is obtained from both kidneys. An RI difference more than –5 increases the probability of a stenosis in the kidney with the lower RI value (Fig. 4-20).[69]

It cannot be underestimated that either direct or indirect methods of obtaining accurate hemodynamic Doppler parameters require experience. The sonographer must pay attention to technique. With the patient in either a decubitus or oblique position, the scan plane through the posterior axillary line will result in a shorter Doppler distance and a better Doppler angle to interrogate the intrarenal vessels. Color Doppler should be used to visualize the vessel path to assist with the incident Doppler angle. Maintaining a Doppler incident angle between 0 to 30 degrees helps define the ESP. An angle greater than 30 degrees may not allow demonstration of the ESP.[83] To spread out the cardiac cycle to better visualize and measure each component, set the Doppler sweep speed to display only 2 to 3 seconds at a time. The pulse repetition frequency (PRF) is adjusted so the waveform fills the entire spectral window and the transducer frequency selected provides a large frequency shift and larger waveform. This enhances the definition of the ESP and improves caliper placement for measurements.

Limitations associated with indirect evaluation include obese body habitus, excessive bowel gas, inability to differentiate between severe stenosis and occlusion of the main renal artery, and inability to detect stenosis less than 60%.

### Postrenal Artery Stent Imaging

Postrenal artery duplex stent imaging is performed using the same protocol as nonstented renal arteries. The difference will be that the stent will be well visualized and brightly echogenic. After renal artery stents are placed, the diameter of the stented vessel may be slightly increased when compared to the diameter of the native artery distal to the stent. Because of this, a flow gradient may be present at the distal end of the stent due to diameter mismatch between the stented segment and the native renal artery. If so, the peak systolic velocity may increase slightly and disordered flow

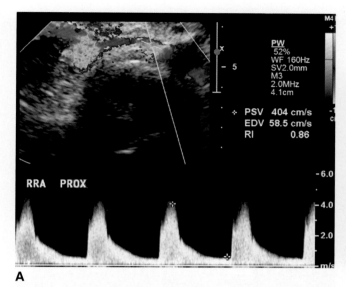
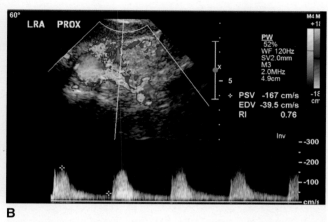

**A**

**B**

**Figure 4-20** Resistive index difference. A 76-year-old woman with history of uncontrolled hypertension, hyperlipidemia, coronary artery disease, and renovascular disease has had coronary artery bypass surgery and carotid endarterectomy presented for renal artery follow-up evaluation. **A.** The transverse image of the right renal artery displays peak systolic velocity *(PSV)* of 404 cm/sec, end-diastolic volume *(EDV)* of 58.5 cm/sec, and a resistive index *(RI)* of 0.86. **B.** The left renal artery displays *PSV* of 167 cm/sec, *EDV* of 39.5 cm/sec, and an RI of 0.76. There is a 0.10 cm/sec RI difference between the right renal arterial stenosis and the left renal artery.

will be apparent as the flow moves from the slightly larger diameter stented segment to the smaller diameter native arterial segment. Careful attention must be given to these flow patterns to make the distinction of whether the flow shift is due to size mismatch or the flow shift is due to a flow-reducing stenosis either in the stent or just distal to the stent docking site.[84] Velocity criteria for classification in stent stenosis of renal arteries include a peak systolic velocity of greater than 250 cm/sec and poststenotic turbulence must be present as well (Fig. 4-21).[84]

## MESENTERIC ARTERY STENOSIS (MESENTERIC INSUFFICIENCY)

### Description

Chronic mesenteric insufficiency is a complex problem that has been difficult to recognize clinically because presenting symptoms are vague and closely related to other abdominal disease processes. One vascular surgeon reports that the average time from initial patient complaint to actual diagnosis is 18 months.[85]

Mesenteric insufficiency results from lack of adequate blood supply to the intestinal tract due to underlying vascular compromise: either acute occlusion of the mesenteric vessels via embolic phenomenon, or atherosclerotic disease with associated significant stenosis and/or occlusion of the mesenteric vessels are implicated.

Individuals at increased risk of developing mesenteric arterial disease include those with a history of smoking, hypertension, coronary artery disease, peripheral

atherosclerotic disease, chronic renal insufficiency, and diabetes mellitus.

Classical symptoms of chronic mesenteric ischemia include progressive postprandial pain, weight loss, change in bowel habits, and an epigastric bruit.[86] Other symptoms that may be encountered include diarrhea, fear of eating, nausea/vomiting, and constipation.[87]

Acute mesenteric insufficiency is a catastrophic event necessitating immediate diagnosis and surgical intervention. Thus, angiography is still considered the primary diagnostic tool to demonstrate suspected acute mesenteric insufficiency.

Chronic mesenteric insufficiency results from hemodynamically significant stenosis and/or occlusion of two or the three arteries, which comprise the mesenteric circulation.[86,88] It is a much less ominous disease and can be corrected with minimally invasive methods or with bypass surgical techniques.[89] Because of the vague symptoms exhibited by a majority of patients and the reported uncommonness of chronic mesenteric insufficiency, physicians have been reluctant to pursue angiography, with its inherent risks, for many of these patients. Duplex and color flow Doppler sonography appears to be a more acceptable noninvasive technique to initially evaluate patients suspected of having chronic mesenteric ischemia.

### Examination

Because the diagnosis of chronic mesenteric ischemia depends on identifying significant stenosis and/or occlusion in two of the three mesenteric arteries, the examination

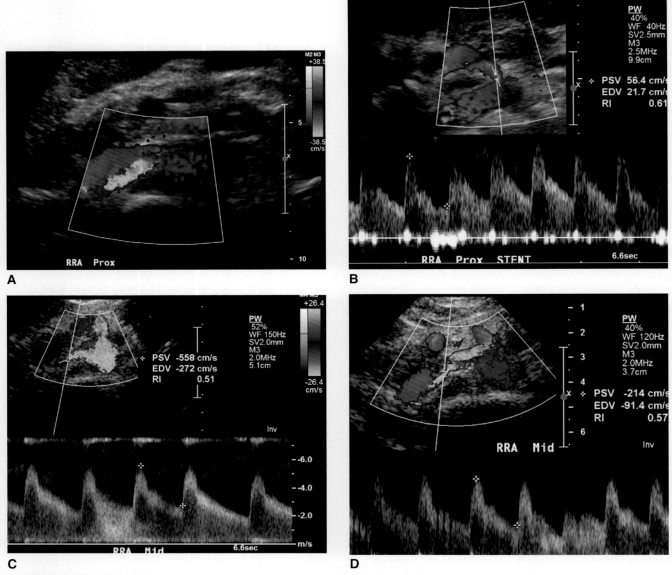

**Figure 4-21** Recurrent renal artery stenosis/stent imaging. This 19-year-old female college freshman noted sudden onset of headaches × 5 or more days. The college health center found her blood pressure to be 220/130 mm Hg. There were no associated neurologic symptoms with her headache. A computerized tomography angiography of the abdomen demonstrated a right renal artery (*RRA*) stenosis. Following a percutaneous balloon angioplasty and stenting of her RRA, this postintervention renal artery duplex was performed. **A.** The transverse color Doppler displays a wide, patent right renal artery. **B.** The longitudinal image displays a wide, patent RRA with normal velocity peak systolic velocity (*PSV*) of 56.4 cm/sec and end-diastolic volume of 21.7 cm/sec. **C.** Six months post-RRA stenting, the duplex RRA stent surveillance shows significantly elevated velocity of PSV of 558 cm/sec and EDV of 272 cm/sec. **D.** The patient had a repeat endovascular balloon dilatation and RRA stent. The postoperative RRA velocities returned to PSV of 214 cm/sec and EDV of 91.4 cm/sec. Note the resistive index (*RI*) on each image.

protocol should include sonography and Doppler evaluation of the CA, SMA, and IMA. The common hepatic artery (CHA) should also be evaluated because abnormal flow patterns in this location can confirm suspected CA occlusion.

Patients are evaluated after an overnight fast. Each vessel should be scanned throughout its length in search of focal velocity increases and associated poststenotic turbulence, paying particular attention to their proximal portions because this is where the majority of stenotic lesions are found. The SMA is usually best evaluated from a longitudinal imaging plane, whereas the CA should be evaluated from a variety of planes to best outline its course. Many times, axial scanning more clearly reveals the sometimes tortuous course of this artery. Velocity measurements are made with Doppler angles between 40 and 60 degrees. Color flow Doppler may be used as an aid in visualizing the mesenteric vessels in difficult patients and is also helpful in placing the Doppler sample volume and Doppler angle cursor.

Occasionally, a color bruit may be seen, and is a helpful finding in suggesting significant stenosis; however, duplex Doppler spectral tracings should always be used to confirm abnormal blood flow patterns demonstrated by color flow examination and common anomalies such as the SMA and CA sharing a common trunk.

Some institutions also perform postprandial scanning to help determine normal responses of SMA flow. Ensure has been used effectively as the "stress meal" for postprandial studies.

### Doppler Findings in Superior Mesenteric Artery

In a preprandial (fasting) state, Doppler spectral analysis of the normal SMA reveals a characteristic pattern that is associated with a highly resistant vascular bed. There is a sharp rise in flow during systole, and a rapid falloff during diastole with reversal of flow below the baseline (see Fig. 4-18C). In the postprandial state (after ingestion of a meal), the blood flow characteristics change and exhibit reduced or absent reversal of flow during the diastolic phase of the cardiac cycle concomitant with increased peak forward diastolic flow.[90] Velocity changes begin to occur within 15 minutes of meal ingestion, with near doubling of baseline peak systolic velocities occurring at about 45 minutes. After 90 minutes, blood flow velocity returns to baseline levels.[86] The diastolic flow goes through similar changes, with the maximum diastolic flow reaching approximately three times the baseline values at approximately 45 minutes postmeal.[86]

With a significant stenosis of the SMA, a loss of the reversed flow component, even in the preprandial state, occurs. Abnormally high velocities with associated poststenotic turbulence are also detected in the narrowed region of the vessel. Visually, poststenotic dilatation and arteriosclerotic plaque may be seen. A splanchnic peak velocity >275 cm/sec is considered highly indicative of a severely compromised blood flow, and CA peak systolic velocities >200 cm/sec have been associated with greater than 70% stenosis.[91] Because breathing may exert periodic effects on splanchnic arterial hemodynamics, which may affect an underestimation of arterial stenosis, it is recommended that mesenteric Doppler examinations be performed during expiration[91] (Fig. 4-22). Occlusion of the SMA is diagnosed when there is no Doppler signal detected in a reliably visualized vessel.

### Doppler Findings in the Celiac Artery

In a preprandial state, CA flow resembles that of other vessels supplying a low-resistant vascular bed with a rapid systolic upstroke followed by gradually decreasing velocities during diastole. Flow never reaches zero. During the postprandial state, some increase in CA velocities are noted, but not to the same extreme as those seen in the SMA.

Doppler findings suggesting significant celiac artery stenosis include a localized area of high velocity, a peak systolic velocity of >200 cm/sec, poststenotic

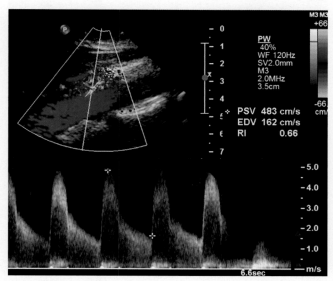

**Figure 4-22** Superior mesenteric artery (SMA) stenosis. Doppler evaluation of an SMA stenosis was made on this patient with a peak systolic velocity of approximately 483 cm/sec and end-diastolic volume of approximately 162 cm/sec.

turbulence, and blunted flow downstream from a high-grade stenosis. Visually, poststenotic dilatation may also be recognized (Fig. 4-23A,B).

### Doppler Findings in the Inferior Mesenteric Artery

Even though the IMA is a relatively important vessel, especially in regard to collateral flow in the presence of significant stenosis and/or occlusion of both the SMA and CA, it has not been studied much. Although sonographic examination is difficult due to its size and overlying small bowel, on a majority of patients referred for mesenteric arterial evaluation, it is feasible to demonstrate the IMA using high-frequency probes, bowel compression techniques, and color flow imaging.

Preprandial flow in the IMA resembles that of the SMA. There is, however, higher resistivity associated with the IMA. When the IMA provides collateral flow to the intestinal tract, it will enlarge, making it easier to identify.

### Postprandial Scanning

Postprandial scanning protocol begins with initial fasting evaluation of the mesenteric arteries for identification of stenosis. Afterward, the stress meal is given, and peak systolic velocities in the SMA are recorded at 5 to 10 minute intervals. A positive scan for chronic mesenteric ischemia consists of identification of significant stenosis of two of the three mesenteric arteries and no significant change in the SMA postprandial velocities.

### Pitfalls and Limitations

There are several pitfalls and limitations to be aware of when performing mesenteric insufficiency evaluation. Compression of the CA can occur from the median

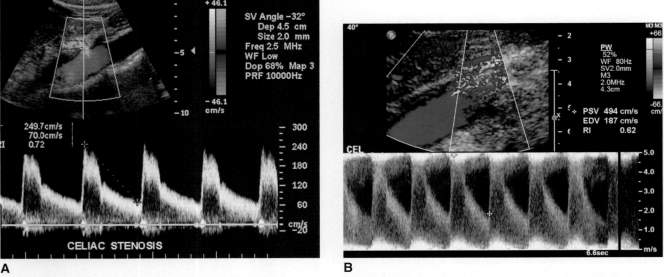

**Figure 4-23** Celiac artery stenosis. The Doppler evaluation was diagnosed as celiac artery stenosis on both of these patients. **A.** The first patient has a peak systolic velocity *(PSV)* of 249.7 cm/sec, end-diastolic volume *(EDV)* of 70.0, and resistive index *(RI)* of 0.72. **B.** The second patient has a PSV of 494 cm/sec, an EDV of 187, and an RI of 0.62. (Fig. 4-23A courtesy of Philips Medical Systems, Bothell, WA.)

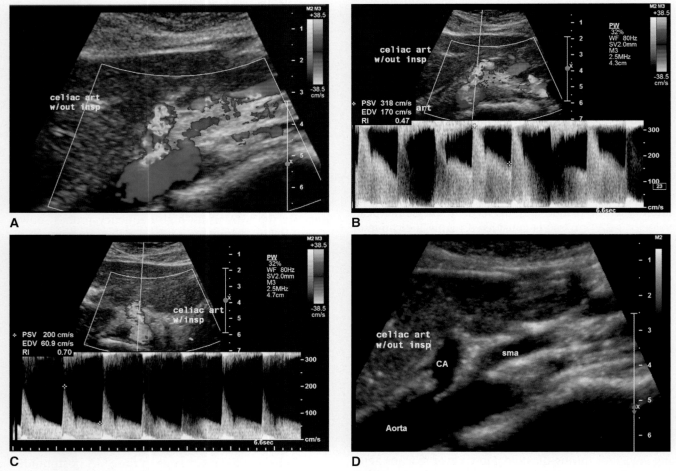

**Figure 4-24** Median arcuate ligament compression. This 32-year-old woman has an asymptomatic abdominal bruit during routine physical examination. Four months prior, her most recent pregnancy was complicated by a coronary artery dissection of the left anterior descending artery and myocardial infarction at approximately 3 weeks postdelivery. Initial treatment was an intra-aortic balloon pump and she did not require percutaneous coronary intervention. Postdischarge, the patient was managed medically and successfully completed cardiac rehabilitation. The aorta, celiac artery, and superior mesenteric artery *(SMA)* were obtained using Doppler angle correction with the cursors parallel to flow. **A.** A color bruit was present in the celiac artery on this longitudinal image. Using respiratory maneuvers, Doppler images were obtained of the celiac artery **(B)** with suspended respiration and **(C)** with deep inspiration. Gray scale images were also obtained of the CA **(D)** with suspended respiration and *(continued)*

arcuate ligament. This median arcuate ligament syndrome causes celiac artery compression by causing narrowing of the celiac artery at the end of deep expiration or at rest and in some patients at the end of inspiration. Median arcuate ligament compression syndrome can become the pathogenesis of hepatic and splenic artery disease (Table 4-4; Fig. 4-24).

Although much has been learned regarding mesenteric blood flow in normal and abnormal states, much still needs to be learned to help improve the accuracy and reliability of duplex and color flow Doppler in the evaluation of chronic mesenteric ischemia.

## HEPATIC ARTERY WITH A HEPATIC TRANSPLANT

### Description

The area of hepatic artery Doppler examination is important in the investigation of liver transplant recipients. The portable nature of the technique makes it a very good tool for the detection of postsurgical complications such as occlusion of the hepatic artery or occlusion of the portal system (which will be discussed in the following section, "Venous Abnormalities").

### Technique

Initially, the transducer is placed intercostally to identify the portal vein. After the portal vein is visualized, the transducer is maneuvered to identify the hepatic artery, usually located anterior to the portal vein. The Doppler sample volume is electronically moved into the area of interest to identify blood flow. Color flow Doppler instrumentation is very helpful for hepatic artery localization and subsequent placement of the sample volume. In a normal examination, the Doppler flow pattern is pulsatile and has a high diastolic flow component owing to the low resistance of the blood bed in the liver. Absent or very blunted flow is almost always indicative of hepatic arterial obstruction and is most critical in the immediate postoperative period.

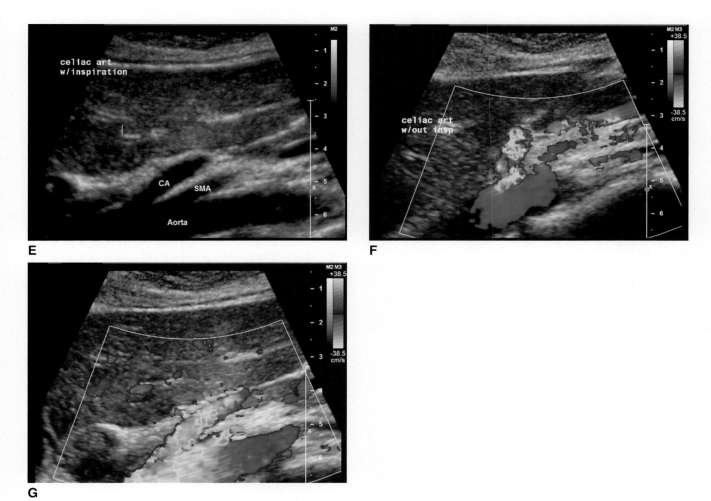

**E**

**F**

**G**

Figure 4-24 *(continued)* **(E)** with deep inspiration. The celiac artery peak systolic flow/diastolic flow at rest during suspended respiration was peak systolic velocity (PSV) of 318 cm/sec and end-diastolic volume (EDV) of 170 cm/sec. With deep inspiration, the celiac artery flow decreased significantly to PSV of 200 cm/sec and EDV of 70 cm/sec. **F.** Color flow changes of the celiac artery demonstrated the presence of significant mosaic turbulence at rest **(G)** that returned to laminar flow pattern with inspiration. Furthermore, on gray scale interrogation, the celiac artery trunk demonstrated evidence of luminal narrowing that resolved with deep inspiration.

**TABLE 4-4**

### Pitfalls and Limitations When Performing Mesenteric Insufficiency Evaluation

1. Due to body habitus, and overlying bowel gas, it may be impossible to interrogate the mesenteric arteries.
2. Incomplete interrogation of the vessel. Although most stenosis occurs at the vessel origins or within their first 2–3 cm, distal disease would be overlooked if the length of the vessel was not entirely examined.
3. Collateral flow may lessen the accuracy of Doppler parameters. There is speculation that adequate collateral perfusion through a normally patent mesenteric vessel may cause a decrease in the velocities detectable through a stenotic one. It has also been demonstrated that in isolated, single-vessel disease, compensatory flow increases occur in the nondiseased vessel, and this phenomenon, too, has the potential to negatively affect the accuracy of Doppler criteria.
4. Vessel tortuosity can cause confusing Doppler information. It may be difficult to differentiate between actual stenosis and vessel tortuosity.
5. The celiac compression syndrome may be mistaken for a celiac axis stenosis. Elevated celiac axis velocities and poststenotic turbulence can be detected in the celiac axis resulting from compression of the median arcuate ligament of the diaphragm. During inspiration, and subsequent Doppler evaluation, the high velocities and poststenotic turbulence disappear.

If hepatic arterial occlusion occurs in the later period of transplant recovery, its significance is not as profound because of the collateral circulation that has had a chance to develop.[92]

Although it is a less common complication of liver transplant, hepatic artery stenosis can be identified by Doppler and is recognized as a focal elevation of hepatic artery velocity with associated poststenotic turbulence.[93]

Originally, it was hoped that liver transplant rejection could be reliably detected using hepatic artery duplex scanning techniques as well. In these instances, the hepatic arterial Doppler signal was expected to show evidence of increased vascular resistance, depicted as a decreased diastolic flow component in the spectral tracing, but these findings turned out to be inconsistent.[92-94]

# VENOUS ABNORMALITIES

## VENA CAVAL OBSTRUCTION

In order to assess the IVC for the presence of obstruction, it is important to remember the effects of normal respiration on the IVC. These effects include (1) the IVC caliber decreases during initial inspiration; (2) after suspended respiration, the IVC enlarges to its maximum diameter; (3) the IVC caliber enlarges during expiration; and (4) during the Valsalva maneuver, the IVC caliber diminishes, nearly obliterating the lumen owing to the increased abdominal pressure created by this technique. Because of the variations in the caliber of the IVC during respiration, it is imperative that IVC examinations be done in a consistent manner. This is usually best accomplished by examining while the patient suspends inspiration.[8]

### Description

When blood flow in the IVC is obstructed, the normal response of the vessel is to increase in caliber below the point of obstruction. Because of the elastic capacity of the veins, the expansion of the IVC can be quite dramatic.

### Etiology

The most common cause of IVC obstruction is right-sided heart failure, which itself has many causes. IVC obstruction may also have its origins with an enlarged liver, para-aortic lymph node enlargement, retroperitoneal masses or tumors, and pancreatic tumors. A congenital IVC valve may also obstruct the lumen of the IVC.[12]

### Clinical Signs and Symptoms

Signs and symptoms may include abdominal pain, ascites, or tender hepatomegaly. Lower extremity edema may also be present in the more severe forms of IVC blockage.[12]

### Sonographic Appearance

In the presence of obstruction, the IVC tends to dilate below the level of obstruction. Respiratory changes are decreased or absent below the obstructed segment.[95]

In right-sided heart failure, the proximal IVC and hepatic veins become congested, resulting in a concurrent increase in diameter. Respiratory changes are markedly decreased or absent.

Solid, complex, or echo-poor tumors in the retroperitoneum or pancreas may be seen to impinge on the IVC. If large enough, they can obstruct the vessel and dilatation below the impingement would be recognized. Intravenous tumors, primary or metastatic, also obstruct flow within the IVC.[13,96] Again, dilatation of the vein below the tumor mass will be identified. Severe obstruction or compression of the IVC may result in enlargement of the ascending lumbar vein, which is recognized as an anechoic structure posterior to and midway between the aorta and IVC in transverse imaging planes.

In the superior vena cava obstruction syndrome, collateral vein formation and enlargement may develop involving the epigastric veins, the ligamentum teres, and the caudate lobe veins.[95]

## TUMORS OF THE INFERIOR VENA CAVA

Tumors of the IVC may be primary, metastatic, or an extension from a tumor.

### Primary Tumors

Primary tumors of the IVC, most of which are leiomyomas or leiomyosarcomas, tend to be uncommon (vascular incidence of only 2%). These types of tumors tend to develop in women, and the median age of detection is 61 years. With leiomyosarcomas, metastasis to the liver and lung has been reported in 40% to 50% of cases. A 36% recurrence rate is also reported, and prognosis is poor.[97,98]

### Metastasis or Extension of Tumors

Malignant invasion of the IVC may occur from renal carcinoma (the most commonly reported incidence at 9% to 33%), secreting and nonsecreting adrenal tumors, retroperitoneal sarcomas, hepatocellular carcinomas, teratomas, and lymphomas.[99]

### Clinical Signs and Symptoms

Symptoms are generally unremarkable, but this depends on tumor size and the degree of obstruction they present to the IVC. With tumors of large proportions, leg edema as well as ascites and abdominal pain may develop.[95] This is true for the primary tumors of the IVC as well as those that are metastatic.

### Sonographic Appearance

Tumors within the IVC tend to appear as echogenic foci. Occasionally, they may be isodense with the blood in the lumen, in which case they are more difficult to visualize. Tumors, especially the larger primary types, may be heterogeneous, with areas of necrosis.

Depending on tumor size and degree of obstruction, there may be normal or increased IVC caliber as well as loss of respiratory changes. Because of the similarity in echographic appearance of vascular tumor masses, the differential diagnosis is large and includes primary vascular neoplasm, malignant IVC mass, thrombus (chronic), and large primary tumors outside the vessel.[99] The latter differential is important because large tumors distort their surroundings, therefore making normal anatomy difficult to identify.

Doppler and color flow instrumentation can aid in the diagnosis of vena caval obstruction by tumors. Normally, blood flow in the mid and distal IVC is of low velocity and varies with respiration. Flow velocities decrease with inspiration and increase with exhalation. Near the heart, effects of right atrial hemodynamics become evident in the Doppler spectra, revealing complex triphasic waveforms. When the cava is partially obstructed, distinct blood flow patterns may be recognized, but these will depend on the degree of obstruction present. Milder forms of obstruction do not produce appreciable blood flow changes; however, with more severe forms of impingement and obstructive lesions, blood flow changes can be quite dramatic. Respiratory changes distal to a significant obstruction will be severely diminished or absent, whereas blood flow velocities within the narrowed segment caused by the obstruction lesion will elevate. With duplex Doppler technique, it is necessary to move the sample volume along the length of the IVC to look for increased flow velocity. Abnormal flow velocity findings may be useful in suggesting vena cava obstruction when the obstructing lesion is echopenic.

Color flow Doppler may be of greatest asset in these cases as the blood flow path is more easily seen than with conventional gray scale sonography (Fig. 4-25A–C). Complete occlusion of the IVC results in absence of detectable blood flow by Doppler interrogation.

When an IVC mass is identified during sonography, it is important to attempt to identify (1) the presence of a primary tumor and its site; (2) the cranial extent of the tumor mass (does it involve the hepatic veins or the right atrium?); and (3) possible tumor involvement or invasion of the wall of the vessel (CT is better able to show this type of involvement than sonography).[99] To localize a lesion in the IVC, it should be placed into one of the three (or a combination) designated segments because surgical management depends on its cranial extent. The upper IVC is that part of the vessel that is seen between the right atrium and the hepatic veins. The middle IVC includes the part between the hepatic veins and the renal veins, and the lower IVC is the portion that lies below the renal veins.[98]

## RENAL VEIN ENLARGEMENT

### Discussion and Etiology

There are several reasons why renal veins enlarge: increased flow due to a splenorenal or gastrorenal shunt in patients with portal hypertension or portal thrombosis, tumor involvement from a renal cell carcinoma, and increased flow from an arteriovenous malformation in the kidney are the most common.[100–102]

In portal hypertension, several collateral pathways are apt to develop as the pressure in the portal system increases. Consequently, blood flow is diverted to the collaterals, which may in turn fistulize to the left renal vein as a means of relieving the increased pressure.[103] The same mechanism can take place in a patient with portal venous thrombosis.

It has been determined that the prevalence of renal vein involvement in renal cell carcinoma is approximately 21% to 55%.[104] When invasion occurs, obstruction to the renal vein results in dilatation. Expansion may also be the direct result of tumor growth.

In arteriovenous malformation, there is an abnormal connection between the arterial and venous vessels. Because of the higher pressure in the arterial system, blood is routed directly from the artery into the vein, thus increasing blood flow through the veins. A natural response for the vein under increased blood volume is to dilate. Arteriovenous fistulas may occur for a number of reasons, including blunt or penetrating trauma, biopsy complications, tumor involvement, nephrectomy, and idiopathic causes.[102]

### Clinical Signs and Symptoms

Symptoms in the presence of an enlarged renal vein are generally associated with the underlying disease process and are not the result of the venous enlargement.

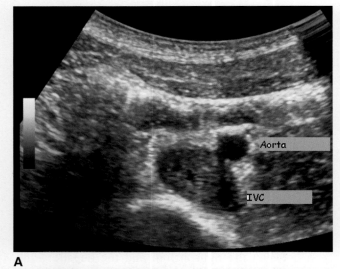

**A**

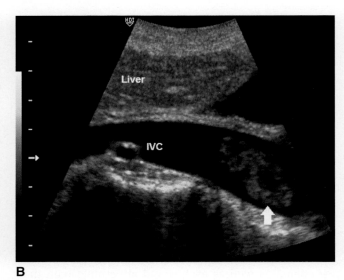

**B**

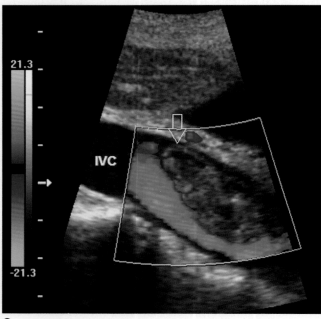

**C**

**Figure 4-25** Inferior vena cava thrombus. **A.** The thrombus seen in the IVC on this patient occludes a large section of the vessel diameter. In this patient, the **(B)** gray scale and **(C)** color Doppler images display a thrombus *(arrow)* in the inferior vena cava, diminishing much of the size of the vessel. During the sonography evaluation, respiratory influences or lack thereof should be noted. (Figs. 4-25B and 4-25C courtesy of Philips Medical Systems, Bothell, WA.)

With portal venous hypertension and gastrorenal or splenorenal shunting, there may be no obvious distinguishing clinical features.

Tumor involvement of the renal veins usually produces no specific symptoms that would lead to suspicion of tumor extension. Such findings are generally made during the routine workup of patients with known renal cell carcinoma.

In patients with small arteriovenous malformations, generally no clinically significant symptoms are recognized. With larger malformations, however, there may be hematuria, abdominal pain, abdominal bruit, congestive heart failure, and cardiomegaly with possible systolic hypertension, diastolic hypertension, and renal ischemia.[2,102]

## Sonographic Appearance

Evaluation of symmetry between the renal veins is useful in differentiating the types of disease processes that may cause venous enlargement.[101] If enlargement of the renal veins is bilateral or symmetric, the disease process most likely involves the IVC at a level above the insertion of the renal veins. Such may include congestive heart failure and tumor involvement or thrombosis of the IVC.

Unilateral renal vein enlargement may indicate tumor involvement, portal venous hypertension with renal vein collateral anastomosis, or arteriovenous fistula. In portal venous hypertension, there is isolated left renal vein involvement, whereas either the left or the right renal vein may be involved by tumor invasion or arteriovenous fistula.

Sonographically, an enlarged renal vein is defined as one with a diameter in excess of 1.5 cm. Another sonographic finding suggestive of increased flow volume into the renal vein is abrupt an IVC dilatation at the level of the renal insertion point.[101]

Blood flow patterns can be determined with Doppler techniques and may be useful in differentiating the various types of renal vein enlargement. For instance, in the presence of a gastrorenal or splenorenal shunt associated with portal hypertension or in the presence of an arteriovenous malformation, disturbed or turbulent venous flow signals are evident in the enlarged renal vein. Velocities may also be abnormally rapid.

With tumor involvement, an echogenic focus is usually present in the vessel lumen. If this is a finding during sonography examination, the IVC should be searched carefully to identify the extension of the tumor beyond the renal veins.

### Pitfalls

In a tumor-free vessel, reverberation artifact may mimic a tumor or possibly a thrombus. It is also possible that some metastatic tumors may appear isoechoic with the surrounding blood, making them very difficult to identify.

The left renal vein may appear enlarged at the point where it crosses over the aorta before entering the IVC. It should be noted that this is a normal finding in many persons. Dilatation should be suspected only if the entire length of the renal vein is enlarged, especially in conjunction with any of the other findings associated with renal vein enlargement.

Although duplication of the IVC is not common, it is possible that a duplicated IVC could be misinterpreted as left renal vein enlargement. To avoid this confusion, it is wise to follow the vessel in question to its origin if possible.[101]

## RENAL VEIN THROMBOSIS

### Etiology

Renal vein thrombosis may occur in any of the following disorders: nephrotic syndrome, renal tumors, renal transplantation, trauma, infant dehydration, and compression of the renal vein secondary to extrinsic tumor.[100]

### Clinical Signs and Symptoms

Symptoms of acute renal venous thrombosis may include loin or flank pain, leg swelling, proteinuria, and hematuria.[100]

### Sonographic Appearance

With renal vein thrombosis, the renal vein is dilated at a point proximal to the occlusion. In many cases, the thrombus is visible in the vessel lumen. Thrombus generally appears as an echogenic focus, especially in long-standing cases. In the more acute phase, however, thrombus may not appear echogenic, but isoechoic to the surrounding blood. In these instances, Doppler interrogation may be helpful (no venous signal is heard in the presence of renal vein occlusion). The acute phase of renal vein thrombosis causes enlargement of the kidney and loss of normal renal architecture.[100]

## VENOUS ANEURYSMS

### Description

Venous aneurysms are rare vascular abnormalities that may be incidentally discovered. They tend to occur principally in the neck or lower extremity veins. They have, however, been reported to occur in most major veins.[64] Portal vein aneurysm is the most common type of visceral venous aneurysm and have been reported in the main portal vein, the confluence of the splenic and superior mesenteric veins, and intrahepatic portal vein branches at bifurcation sites.[105] In recent years, there has been an increase in the number of venous aneurysm cases reported in the portal venous system.[106]

### Etiology

Several theories have been developed to explain the cause of venous aneurysms. They include weakening of the vessel wall by pancreatitis, portal hypertension, and embryonic malformations (congenital anomalies). There is a greater presence of aneurysms in patients who have chronic liver disease, portal hypertension, pancreatitis, trauma, and postsurgical complication.[105]

### Clinical Signs and Symptoms

Usually, no symptoms are associated with small aneurysms of the portal venous system. When an aneurysm enlarges, it may cause any of the following commonly reported symptoms: duodenal compression, common bile duct obstruction, chronic portal hypertension, jaundice, recurrent crampy abdominal pain, upper gastrointestinal bleeding, obstruction of the portal vein due to thrombus, and rupture of the aneurysm.[12]

### Sonographic Appearance

Sonographically, portal venous aneurysms can be recognized as anechoic, distended vessels that may or may not contain thrombus. Doppler techniques can be used to verify the venous nature of the echo-free structure by detecting a turbulent venous signal in the lesion. Included in the differential diagnosis (especially in the absence of Doppler data) are neoplastic cysts and visceral arterial aneurysms.

Once detected, pulsed and color Doppler examination can be used in follow-up of most patients. CT and MRA are more costly and invasive examinations that are used to determine location and relationship to adjacent organs, and angiography is used for surgical planning.[107] Employing Doppler helps define the pathology by being able to detect portal vein to hepatic vein fistulas by showing their connections and noting turbulent venous flow within the aneurysm. Doppler spectra in nonfistulated aneurysms do not show turbulent flow.

Other venous aneurysms are rare, but it stands to reason that they would resemble a portal vein aneurysm, except for their location within the abdomen. Doppler investigation should be used to help define the vascular nature of any suspicious anechoic lesion within the abdomen.

## HEPATIC VENOUS ABNORMALITIES

### Budd-Chiari Syndrome

#### Description and Etiology

Budd-Chiari syndrome is defined as the occlusion of some or all of the hepatic veins and/or occlusion of the IVC. Two types are recognized; primary Budd-Chiari syndrome is the resultant occlusion of the hepatic veins or IVC by a congenital web or fibrous cord. In secondary Budd-Chiari syndrome, occlusion of the hepatic veins and/or IVC occurs by tumor or thrombus formation.

#### Sonographic Appearance

Color flow Doppler is superior to gray scale sonography in the evaluation of suspected Budd-Chiari syndrome because of its ability to detect flow in otherwise unseen veins.[70,108,109] Recognized sonographic and Doppler findings of Budd-Chiari syndrome include absent or sluggish flow in the IVC (oftentimes, in the primary type), the obstructing membrane may be visualized, absent flow in some or all of the hepatic veins, reversed flow in portions of the obstructed hepatic veins, damped Doppler spectra with loss of normal triphasic flow pattern of obstructed hepatic veins, identification of intrahepatic venous-venous collaterals, and identification of extrahepatic collaterals. The intrahepatic collaterals appear as either a curved configuration resembling a hockey stick, or a spider web pattern.[108]

Evaluation of suspected Budd-Chiari should also include examination of the portal vein since a 20% incidence of portal venous occlusion has been reported in these patients.[70,110]

## PORTAL VENOUS ABNORMALITIES

### Portal Venous Thrombosis

#### Description and Etiology

Portal venous thrombosis can be caused by a variety of pathologic states: portal hypertension, inflammatory abdominal processes (appendicitis, peritonitis, pancreatitis, colon diverticulum), trauma, postsurgical complications, hypercoagulability states (oral contraceptives, pregnancy, migratory thrombophlebitis, antithrombin III deficiency, polycythemia vera, thrombocytosis), abdominal neoplasms (hepatocellular, colonic, pancreatic), renal transplant, and benign ulcer disease.[1,44,111-114] It can also be idiopathic. A potential complication of portal vein thrombosis is bowel ischemia and perforation.

### Clinical Signs and Symptoms

A patient with portal vein thrombosis may exhibit any of the following symptoms: abdominal pain, low-grade fever, leukocytosis, hypovolemia, and shock. Shock is unlikely unless there is an associated bowel infarction. Abdominal rigidity, elevated liver function test results, nausea, and vomiting may also be present. Changes in bowel habit, hematemesis, and melena can occur.[4,115]

### Sonographic Appearance

Portal venous thrombosis goes through several stages, and its sonographic appearance varies at different stages of the disease process.[112] In the first stage, there is echogenic thrombus in the vessel lumen; then thrombus and smaller collaterals are visible in the immediate area. Finally, larger collaterals (cavernomatous transformation of the portal vein) are observed in the absence of an identifiable portal vein. The latter two stages are usually seen in benign processes and are due to chronic disease.

Direct signs of portal venous thrombosis include visualization of a clot in the lumen of the portal vein (Fig. 4-26). Clot appears more echogenic than the surrounding blood, however, in the acute process—therefore, when thrombus is fresh, it may be very difficult to identify. A localized bulge of the vein at the clot level may also be recognized. Because improper gain settings and reverberation artifact may appear as clot within the lumen of the portal vein, careful attention to technique is critical to avoid misdiagnosis of portal vein thrombosis.

The normal caliber of the portal vein has been established to be smaller than 13 mm.[116] In the event of an acute thrombotic episode, the caliber is likely to exceed 13 mm, but in a more chronic process, it may indeed be less than 13 mm.[113]

Indirect evidence of portal vein thrombus includes lack of normal portal vein landmarks, collateral vessel formation in the area of the portal vein, and increased caliber of the superior mesenteric and splenic veins.[112] It has been demonstrated that in some cases of

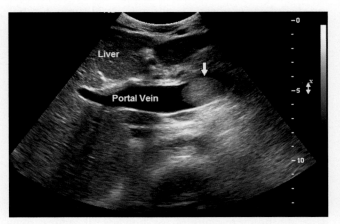

**Figure 4-26** Portal venous thrombosis. The transverse sonogram displays an echogenic clot in the portal vein lumen. (Image courtesy of Philips Medical Systems, Bothell, WA.)

complete obliteration of the portal vein by thrombus, the thrombus actually appeared isodense with the liver parenchyma. The only indication of portal involvement was echoic margins surrounding the clot, which were generated from the portal vein walls.[1]

In cavernous transformation of the portal vein, multiple wormlike, serpiginous vessels can be seen in the region of the portal vein. This particular process is the result of long-standing thrombus and subsequent collateral vessel formation.[117]

Duplex and color flow Doppler are proving more useful than conventional gray scale sonography in the detection of portal vein thrombosis.[104,118] With Doppler, the diagnosis of portal venous thrombosis is suggested by demonstration of absent flow within the vein. Several investigators have shown that the negative predictive value of portal vein thrombus is higher than its positive predictive value.[118] Reasons for false-positive Doppler scans include undetectable slow flow within the portal vein and technical factors. Some have proposed rescanning the portal vein in equivocal cases postprandially to confirm absence of flow.[93] Recently, it has been suggested that a hepatic artery RI of ≤0.50 may be useful in corroborating suspected portal venous thrombus.[118] This finding was determined more useful in acute portal vein thrombus as it was generally not seen in chronic portal venous thrombus with collateral formation.[118]

Sonography can also be used to detect rare superior mesenteric vein and splenic vein thrombosis.[111,112] Sonographically, signs of thrombosis appear similar to those seen in portal vein thrombosis. Echogenic material may be visualized directly inside the vessel lumen and the caliber of the superior mesenteric and splenic veins may be increased, especially in the acute phase. Absence of flow is detectable by Doppler techniques in the presence of total obstruction of the vein, whereas flow characteristics may be normal or diminished when thrombus is partially occlusive.

Color flow Doppler provides for easier demonstration of porta-hepatic collaterals associated with cavernous transformation of the portal vein. Color flow may also be better suited to detect partial portal vein thrombosis. In such instances, color flow voids within the portal vein may be apparent in areas of thrombus formation.[94]

It is difficult to differentiate between thrombus and tumor with sonography alone. Other findings, such as primary tumor or lymphadenopathy, may be useful in pinpointing the correct diagnosis. Some recent studies, however, have illustrated the potential utility of duplex and color flow Doppler in the differentiation of tumor thrombus from clot thrombus.[85,119,120] In all of the studies, the majority of tumor thrombi showed evidence of tumor vascularity. It was generally identified by color flow as a patchy or spotty pattern of color within the clot.[119,120] Doppler spectra revealed pulsatile arterial flow in two of the studies[85,119] and continuous venous flow with nearly constant amplitude in the other.[120]

## Portal Venous Hypertension

### Description

Portal hypertension is an increase in the portal venous pressure. Normally, pressure in the portal venous system is sustained between 0 and 5 mm Hg. In the pathologic state of portal hypertension, it increases to 10 to 12 mm Hg or more.[12]

### Etiology

Portal hypertension may be induced by an increase in the splanchnic blood flow or by increased hepatic vascular resistance.[12] Conditions associated with increased splanchnic blood flow include splenic, hepatic, and mesenteric arteriovenous fistulas resulting from either trauma or rupture of an aneurysm into the splanchnic vessel circulation. These particular mechanisms are not common causes in the United States.[12]

Conditions associated with increased resistance to hepatic vascular flow include extrahepatic obstruction of the portal vein, such as thrombosis and presinusoidal obstruction of portal vein radicles in which there is fibrosis of the portal triads. These can be idiopathic or associated with schistosomiasis, chronic arsenic or vinyl chloride toxicity, congenital hepatic fibrosis, granulomatous disease, or neoplastic infiltration. Perhaps the most common cause of portal hypertension in the United States is sinusoidal and postsinusoidal obstruction, as is seen with fatty infiltration and inflammation of the liver in patients with acute alcoholic hepatitis and cirrhosis. The Budd-Chiari syndrome or hepatic venous obstruction may also be a mechanism of portal hypertension. In these instances, hepatic venous occlusion results from congenital webs, thrombosis, or neoplasia.[12]

### Clinical Signs and Symptoms

In more advanced cases of portal hypertension, there may be ascites and gastrointestinal bleeding. Other complications include poor renal function and impaired coagulation,[67,101,121] but these symptoms are nonspecific, and the total clinical picture must be correlated with physical and sonographic findings to arrive at the correct diagnosis.

### Sonographic Appearance

In healthy persons, the portal vein diameter is usually less than 13 mm. It has been proposed that the presence of a larger portal vein is suggestive of portal venous hypertension, but this is not a consistent finding. Interestingly, in persons with known portal hypertension, portal vein caliber was frequently reported to be normal or small compared to that of normal persons. This is probably due to the development of collateral circulation pathways in patients with more severe portal hypertension. Increased portal vein caliber is not regarded as a reliable indicator of portal venous hypertension.[122] Measurements and diagnosis of portal venous hypertension should consider physiologic factors affecting portal vein measurements (meal, respiration, and posture). Goyal et al.[123] attempted to define discriminating measurement criteria of the portal veins keeping the physiologic factors constant. All measurements were taken in patients with an overnight fast, in a supine position, and at held deep inspiration. The largest diameters of the portal vein, splenic vein, and superior mesenteric vein were recorded and analyzed. Their results indicate that the upper limits of normal for the portal vein, splenic vein, and superior mesenteric vein are 16 mm, 12 mm, and 11 mm, respectively. Measurements above these discriminating values were 72% sensitive, 91% accurate, and 100% specific for the diagnosis of portal vein hypertension. It remains to be seen whether these criteria hold up in larger study populations.

In order to diagnose portal venous hypertension, it is important to look for the secondary effects of increased pressure within the portal system, which can include such things as collateral channel development and abnormal respiratory responses. More recently, Doppler techniques have been investigated in the hope they might allow the physician to more confidently diagnose portal venous hypertension, especially in the absence of visible collateral pathways or other changes associated with portal hypertension.

The collateral network associated with portal hypertension can be extensive and can involve many areas: coronary vein, gastroesophageal veins, umbilical vein, pancreatic duodenal veins, gastrorenal, and splenorenal veins.

It has been noted that a dilated coronary vein (vein of the stomach located in the midepigastric area and visualized as a tortuous anechoic structure measuring more than 5 mm and following the lesser omentum) was detected in a majority of patients with portal hypertension. This, along with the identification of esophageal varices, is a good indicator of portal hypertension. Because esophageal varices and coronary vein enlargement seem to be involved quite frequently in association with portal hypertension (80% to 90%),[124] it would be prudent to search the midepigastric region thoroughly to identify any of these collateral pathways. Of course, visualization of the collaterals depends on their size—larger ones being much more readily visible than smaller ones. Esophageal varices are also the most clinically significant of the collateral pathways because of their propensity to bleed, and a positive correlation between increasing size of the coronary vein and risk of variceal bleeding has been established.[125] Other collaterals are seen but not to the extent of the coronary vein and esophageal varices.

Ten percent to 20% of patients with portal hypertension may also have a patent umbilical vein. This structure is seen in the falciform ligament as a tubular area of 3 mm or greater.[126]

Pancreatic and duodenal collaterals may also be present. They would be located in the region of the descending duodenum, lateral to the pancreatic head. Depending on the amount of air in the duodenum at the time of study, as well as the size of the collateral vessels, they may be easy or difficult to identify.[121]

Splenorenal and gastrorenal venous involvement is detected in the area of the splenic hilum, renal hilum, and the greater curvature of the stomach, respectively. Their proximity may make it difficult to distinguish them from one another.[110] With this particular type of collateral, blood may also be spontaneously shunted to the left renal vein to relieve the high pressure in the system, in which case, the caliber of the left renal vein also increases. If unilateral left renal vein enlargement is present, portal venous hypertension with gastrorenal or splenorenal shunting may be a cause.[124] Other causes would include arteriovenous fistula of the kidney or tumor involvement.

Retroperitoneal and paravertebral collateral vessels as well as omental collaterals may be detected, although their position in the abdomen makes it difficult to do so.[124] Investigators have reported imaging dilated cystic veins of the gallbladder in patients with portal hypertension. The technique utilizes a high frequency transducer and pulsed-wave Doppler.[127]

Other related sonographic findings in the presence of portal hypertension may include a comma-shaped portal trunk, increased periportal echogenicity, increased caliber of the splenic and superior mesenteric veins, ascites, and an enlarged spleen.[28]

Respiratory effects on the portal system have been studied in an attempt to diagnose portal hypertension by abnormal findings. It has been stated that portal venous caliber does not change much with respiration[28]; therefore, respiratory dynamics of the superior mesenteric vein and the splenic vein have been investigated for usefulness in detecting portal venous hypertension.

In normal subjects, the caliber of both the superior mesenteric and splenic vein is less than 1 cm. During suspended inspiration, the diameters increased by 14% to 100% in the majority of normal subjects. In persons who developed portal hypertension as a result of cirrhosis, vessel diameters were usually 1 cm or greater and the inspiration-induced caliber changes were less than 10%.[128,129]

The role of Doppler sonography in the detection of portal venous hypertension is continually undergoing investigation.[130] One of the most useful aspects of color Doppler in the evaluation of portal venous hypertension is its superior ability to identify collateral vessels that are otherwise "invisible" with conventional gray scale sonography.[70,94]

Although current research has led to the conclusion that Doppler sonography can reliably measure portal flow, there is much variability between normal and abnormal flow and specific criteria has not been established to diagnose portal vein hypertension.[61,65,131,132] However, more recent studies indicate a more proactive role for duplex Doppler-derived flow estimates in determining the effectiveness of medical treatments by comparing individual patient baseline flows to postinterventional flows.[133]

Because of the inherent inaccuracies of Doppler-derived estimates and wider variability of portal flow, qualitative Doppler signs of portal vein hypertension are being sought to aid in its diagnosis.

The qualitative Doppler examination begins with visualization of the portal vein and its branches, by placing the transducer at the right intercostal spaces overlying the liver. This intercostal approach generally affords better detection of Doppler signals by virtue of better Doppler angles. Doppler interrogation is then carried out in the right, left, and main portal veins.[134] Once accomplished, flow is assessed in the superior mesenteric vein and along the splenic vein. Transducer positions for the latter examination are determined by the position of the vessels and the angle necessary to obtain Doppler data.

In normal subjects, portal vein blood flow velocity has been measured as 16.0 ± 0.5 cm/sec. In fasting adults, portal vein blood flow velocity ranged from 8 to 18 cm/sec. After ingestion of a meal, velocities increased by 50% to 100%. The flow characteristics in the majority of the normal subjects were a wavy continuous pattern (70%) and traveled toward the liver (hepatopetally). Flow in the superior mesenteric and splenic veins was also antegrade.[125]

Several blood flow abnormalities may be detected in patients with portal hypertension, including flow reversal (hepatofugal) in the portal veins—in some cases, this reversal of flow was detected only when the patient was asked to suspend inspiration. Reversed flow in the superior mesenteric vein suggested mesentericocaval shunting and prompted the examiner to look for collaterals in the pelvis. Reversed flow in the splenic vein and associated increase in left renal vein caliber along with high velocity, turbulent blood flow suggested splenorenal shunting. This prompted the examiner to look closely for collateral flow in the splenic and renal hilar areas. Hepatofugal flow was also detected in the left gastric (coronary), paraduodenal, and paraumbilical veins. The flow observed by Doppler techniques in collateral vessels tended to be fast and turbulent.[125]

It was also noted that the venous flow pattern in the portal system was continuous in approximately 72% of persons who had portal hypertension and associated cirrhosis. Blood flow velocity tended to be slower than in normal control subjects.[135] Because blood flow velocity in the portal vein is widely variable, consistent, useful criteria for the diagnosis of portal venous hypertension has not been forthcoming.[70]

There is still no clearly established role for Doppler sonography in the assessment of portal venous hypertension.[70,93] This is probably due in part to the complex nature of portal venous flow and resultant wide variations reported of normal and abnormal blood flow patterns.

# PORTOSYSTEMIC SHUNT EVALUATION

## Description

Major clinical complications of portal hypertension include variceal hemorrhage and ascites.[70] Sclerotherapy can be used to control variceal bleeding in some patients, but if it is not successful, other treatments are necessary to control the bleeding. The creation of surgical portosystemic shunts can be used to decompress the portal vein pressure, thus reducing the risk of variceal hemorrhage. Four types of shunts can be created, namely, portocaval, mesocaval, splenorenal, and, more recently, transjugular intrahepatic portosystemic.

## PORTOCAVAL SHUNTS

Portocaval shunts have been the most commonly used. These shunts are made by end-to-side or side-to-side anastomosis of the portal vein to the IVC. Portocaval shunts are generally amenable to sonography examination. Patency in these shunts can easily be confirmed with duplex and color flow Doppler by showing venous flow across the shunt from the portal vein into the IVC. Absence of flow would suggest shunt failure. Indirect signs of shunt patency in instances of nonvisualization of the shunt would include hepatopetal flow proximal to shunt anastomosis, and hepatofugal flow distal to shunt anastomosis. Persistent hepatopetal flow distal to shunt anastomosis would suggest shunt occlusion or severe stenosis.

## MESOCAVAL SHUNTS

Mesocaval shunts are created with an H configured synthetic graft connecting the midsuperior mesenteric vein with the IVC. These shunts are more difficult to evaluate because of their deep position within the abdomen and overlying bowel gas. Persistent scanning with the aid of color flow Doppler, however, generally results in adequate assessment of shunt patency. If the graft is visualized, duplex and color flow Doppler can be used to demonstrate flow across the shunt. If the graft cannot be visualized, graft patency can be inferred by demonstration of flow entering the IVC at a level below the renal veins.[70,93]

## SPLENORENAL SHUNTS

Splenorenal or Warren shunts are made by connecting the distal splenic vein to the renal vein, and these are the most difficult types of shunts to assess with sonography. Color flow Doppler seems essential for assessment of graft patency, which can be inferred by demonstration of well-defined splenic and renal limbs of the graft with appropriately directed flow.[70,93,94,136] The splenic limb of the shunt is usually best identified from an anterior approach, whereas the renal limb is best visualized from a coronal or flank approach. Graft occlusion or compromise is suggested by identification of collateral vessels in the left upper quadrant in lieu of well-defined limbs of the shunt, or occlusion of the distal splenic vein at the splenic hilum.[70,93]

## TRANSJUGULAR INTRAHEPATIC PORTOSYSTEMIC SHUNTS

Transjugular intrahepatic portosystemic shunts (TIPS) have been developed to avoid the surgical risks associated with the creation of portocaval, mesocaval, and splenorenal shunts. TIPS procedures involve placement of a metal stent between a hepatic vein and an intrahepatic portal vein via transcatheter route through the jugular vein. On sonography, the TIPS is usually easily seen as a bright tubular structure within the hepatic parenchyma connecting the portal vein with one of the hepatic veins (Fig. 4-27). Complications of these shunts include stenosis at either the portal or hepatic vein anastomosis, or occlusion of the shunt. Because identification of shunt dysfunction relies on the demonstration of relative changes in portal blood flow, it is important to perform both pre-TIPS and baseline post-TIPS examinations.[137]

Suggested protocol for evaluation of TIPS include that all scans be performed after the patient fasts and velocity measurements are taken with Doppler angles between 40 and 60 degrees (Table 4-5).[138–141]

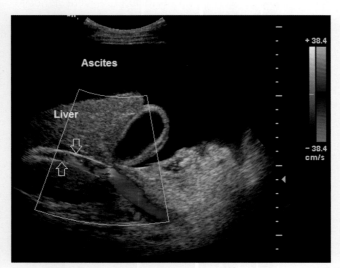

**Figure 4-27** Transjugular intrahepatic portosystemic shunts (TIPS). The image of a TIPS stent (*arrows*) can be identified with its echogenic walls in the portal vein. (Image courtesy of Philips Medical Systems, Bothell, WA.)

| TABLE 4-5 |
| --- |
| Protocol and Criteria for Evaluation of TIPS |

**Pre-TIPS examination includes:**

1. Measurement of maximum blood flow velocity and determination of blood flow direction within the extrahepatic portal vein, superior mesenteric vein, splenic vein at the confluence of the superior mesenteric vein, and the three hepatic veins
2. Identification of collaterals and blood flow direction within

**Post-TIPS examination includes:**

1. Repeat of pre-TIPS examination, PLUS
2. Evaluation of the shunt at three places: portal anastomosis, midportion, and hepatic vein anastomosis

**Reported signs of TIPS stenosis include:**

1. Drop in portal vein velocities to pre-TIPS levels
2. Focal, high-velocity blood flow within the shunt and associated poststenotic turbulence
3. Reversal of flow in the hepatic vein draining the TIPS (may also occur in TIPS occlusion)
4. More than 20% reduction of flow through the stent as measured at midstent from baseline studies
5. Detection of either an increase or decrease of midsegment shunt blood flow velocity in excess of 50 cm/sec

**Reported signs of TIPS occlusion include:**

1. Return of hepatopetal blood flow in the portal vein (may also occur in severe shunt stenosis)
2. Absence of blood flow within the TIPS stent

TIPS, transjugular intrahepatic portosystemic shunts.

## SUMMARY

- Current equipment provides the ability to assess blood flow, to obtain hemodynamic information regarding the many factors that influence the dynamics of blood flow, and the hemodynamic consequences of vascular disease.
- Blood vessels are composed of three distinct layers: (1) the tunica intima (innermost), (2) the tunica media (middle), and (3) the tunica adventitia (outermost).
- The aorta is the main artery of the chest and abdomen from which all other branch vessels are derived.
- The first branch is the celiac artery (also known as the celiac axis or trunk) and originates from the anterior aspect usually within the first 2 cm of the abdominal aorta.
- The celiac axis (CA) is approximately 1 cm long before it divides into the (1) hepatic artery, (2) left gastric artery, and (3) splenic artery.
- The second major abdominal aorta branch vessel is the superior mesenteric artery (SMA), which also originates from the anterior surface of the

aorta approximately 1 to 2.5 cm distal to the celiac artery.

- Inferior to the SMA, the right renal artery arises from the right lateral aspect of the aorta, whereas the left renal artery arises from the left lateral or posterolateral aspect of the aorta. Both then course posterolaterally to enter the respective kidneys.
- The inferior mesenteric artery (IMA) is the last major branch to arise from the abdominal aorta before it bifurcates.
- At the umbilicus, the aorta bifurcates into the left and right common iliac arteries that course inferiorly and posteriorly.
- The inferior vena cava (IVC) is the large vessel that returns blood to the right atrium from the lower limbs, pelvis, and abdomen.
- The IVC is formed by the junction of the paired common iliac veins slightly anterior and to the right of the fifth lumbar (L5) vertebral body and courses superiorly in the abdomen, enters the thoracic cavity, and enters the right atrium at the level of the eighth thoracic (T8) vertebral body.
- The veins most consistently seen entering the IVC are the common iliac veins at its formation, the renal veins, and the hepatic veins.
- The right renal vein is generally shorter than the left renal vein because of the right kidney's proximity to the IVC.
- The left renal vein traverses the abdomen, coursing anterior to the aorta and posterior to the superior mesenteric artery to finally enter the lateral aspect of the IVC.
- The three hepatic veins—(1) the left, (2) the right, and (3) the middle—drain directly into the IVC or right atrium.
- The effects of normal respiration on the IVC include: (1) IVC caliber decreases during initial inspiration; (2) IVC enlarges during expiration and is its maximum diameter after suspended respiration; and (3) during the Valsalva maneuver, the IVC caliber diminishes, nearly obliterating the lumen owing to the increased abdominal pressure created by this technique.
- The main portal vein is formed at the junction of the splenic vein and the superior mesenteric vein, which can be identified with sonography in most patients.
- The sonographic findings of atherosclerosis include luminal irregularities (representative of the various changes of the intimal lining of the artery), tortuosity, and vessel wall calcification.
- A true aneurysm is identified sonographically as a dilatation of the aorta ≥3.0 cm near its bifurcation

point, a focal dilatation along the course of the aorta, or lack of normal tapering of the aorta.

- Thrombus typically produces a low-level echo pattern and tends to accumulate along the anterior and lateral walls of the aortic lumen.
- Aortic dissection appears as a thin, linear echo flap within the arterial lumen.
- Aortic rupture with leakage of blood outside the vessels may be diagnosed by identification of a hematoma in the abdomen in association with aneurysmal dilatation of the aorta.
- Inflammatory aneurysms manifest with dilatation of the aorta with a hypoechoic mantle, usually seen anterior and lateral to a thickened aortic wall.
- The most common splanchnic artery aneurysms are splenic aneurysms followed by hepatic aneurysms with SMA aneurysms being the rarest.
- Renal artery aneurysms have been encountered with increasing frequency, although the overall incidence remains relatively low.
- Iliac artery aneurysms are most often associated with (continuations of) abdominal aortic aneurysms.
- An aortic graft, endograft, or prosthesis is usually a manmade structure used to repair an aortic aneurysm and is easily detected by their characteristic wall brightness, and at times their ribbing.
- Complications of aortic grafts include pseudoaneurysm, graft aneurysms, hematomas, abscesses, occlusions, and endoleaks.
- Renal artery stenosis, a significant medical problem associated with uncontrollable hypertension, can be evaluated using two methods that can be combined to enhance examination results.
- Both evaluation methods require attention to Doppler technique being crucial to the accuracy of the examination.
- The direct method involves direct visualization and Doppler interrogation of the aorta and renal arteries along their entire length relying on blood flow changes that occur at a hemodynamically significant stenosis.
- The indirect or intrarenal method involves Doppler evaluation of the segmental or interlobar arteries in the upper, middle, and lower renal poles and relies on identification of blood flow changes that occur distal to a significant stenosis.
- Postrenal artery duplex stent imaging is performed using the same protocol as nonstented renal arteries with the difference being the stent will be well visualized and brightly echogenic.
- Mesenteric insufficiency results from lack of adequate blood supply to the intestinal tract due to

underlying vascular compromise due to acute occlusion of the mesenteric vessels or atherosclerotic disease.

- In a preprandial (fasting) state, Doppler spectral analysis of the normal SMA reveals a characteristic pattern associated with a highly resistant vascular bed.

- In the postprandial state (after ingestion of a meal), the SMA blood flow characteristics change and exhibit reduced or absent reversal of flow during the diastolic phase of the cardiac cycle concomitant with increased peak forward diastolic flow.

- With obstruction, the IVC tends to dilate below the level of obstruction and respiratory changes are decreased or absent below obstructed segment.

- Tumors of the IVC may be primary, metastatic, or an extension from a tumor.

- Tumors within the IVC tend to appear as echogenic foci and occasionally isodense with the blood in the lumen.

- In arteriovenous malformation, there is an abnormal connection between the arterial and venous vessels.

- Doppler evaluation of symmetry and blood flow patterns between the renal veins is useful in differentiating the types of disease processes that may cause renal vein enlargement.

- An enlarged renal vein has a diameter in excess of 1.5 cm.

- With renal vein thrombosis, the renal vein is dilated at a point proximal to the occlusion.

- Venous aneurysms are rare vascular abnormalities that may be incidentally discovered.

- Portal venous aneurysms can be recognized as anechoic, distended vessels that may or may not contain thrombus.

- Doppler evaluation of portal venous aneurysms can be used to verify the venous nature of the echo-free structure by detecting a turbulent venous signal in the lesion.

- Primary Budd-Chiari syndrome is the occlusion of the hepatic veins or IVC by a congenital web or fibrous cord, and secondary Budd-Chiari syndrome is occlusion of the hepatic veins and/or IVC by tumor or thrombus formation.

- Portal venous thrombosis can be idiopathic or it can be caused by a variety of pathologic states and its sonographic appearance varies at different stages of the disease process.

- Direct signs of portal venous thrombosis include visualization of a clot in the lumen of the portal vein.

- Portal hypertension is an increase in the portal venous pressure.

- The collateral network associated with portal hypertension can be extensive and can involve many areas: coronary vein, gastroesophageal veins, umbilical vein, pancreatic duodenal veins, gastrorenal, and splenorenal veins.

- The creation of surgical portosystemic shunts can be used to decompress the portal vein pressure, which reduces the risk of variceal hemorrhage.

- Four types of shunts can be created, namely, portocaval, mesocaval, splenorenal, and, more recently, transjugular intrahepatic portosystemic.

- Optimize instrumentation settings to demonstrate normal arterial and venous lumen as anechoic structures.

- The sonography examination of the vascular system relies on the skill, knowledge, and accuracy of the sonographer who must pay attention to the texture, outline, size, and shape of both normal and abnormal structures.

- The patient will benefit most when the sonographic findings are correlated with patient history, clinical presentation, laboratory function tests, and other imaging modalities to compose a clinically helpful picture.

## Critical Thinking Questions

1. A Doppler spectral analysis of the normal superior mesenteric artery reveals a characteristic pattern associated with a highly resistant vascular bed. There is a sharp rise in flow during systole and a rapid falloff during diastole with reversal of the flow below the baseline. What does this characteristic pattern describe?

2. What is the most common location of aneurysm associated with the continuation of an abdominal aortic aneurysm?

3. Describe the calculation for the renal-to-aorta (RAR) velocity ratio.

4. What syndrome may occur because the left renal vein, duodenum, and uncinate process are located between the SMA anteriorly and the aorta posteriorly?

5. A 28-year old-man has abdominal pain, nausea, vomiting, and weight loss. The sonographer documents in the celiac artery significant variations in both the peak systolic flow and diastolic flow with normal respiratory cycles. What is the likely diagnosis based on the patient's history and the dynamic velocity changes associated with respiratory phases?

## REFERENCES

1. Boozari B, Bahr MJ, Kubicka S, et al. Ultrasonography in patients with Budd-Chiari syndrome: diagnostic signs and prognostic implications. *J Hepatol*. 2008;49(4):572–580.
2. Sutherland T. Demystifying abdominal ultrasound. *Aust Fam Physician*. 2009;38(10):797–800.
3. Moore K, Dalley A, Agur A. *Clinically Oriented Anatomy*. 6th ed. Philadelphia: Lippincott Williams & Wilkins; 2010.
4. Woolgar JD, Ray R, Maharaj K, et al. Colour Doppler and grey scale ultrasound features of HIV-related vascular aneurysms. *Br J Radiol*. 2002;75(899):919–929.
5. Schroedter WB, Holec SW. The definitive assessment of aneurysm by color flow Doppler. *J Diagn Med Sonogr*. 1991;7:201–204.
6. Hedayati N, Riha GM, Kougias P, et al. Prognostic factors and treatment outcome in mesenteric vein thrombosis. *Vasc Endovascular Surg*. 2008;42:217–224.
7. Hagen-Ansert SL. The vascular system. In: Hagen-Ansert SL, ed. *Textbook of Diagnostic Ultrasonography*. 6th ed. St. Louis, MO: Mosby; 2006:101–141.
8. Owen C, Meyers P. Sonographic evaluation of the portal and hepatic systems. *J Diagn Med Sonogr*. 2006;22(5):317–328.
9. Carter SA. Hemodynamic considerations in peripheral vascular and cerebrovascular disease. In: Zwiebel WJ, Pellerito JS, eds. *Introduction to Vascular Ultrasonography*. 5th ed. Philadelphia, PA: Elsevier Saunders; 2005:2–17.
10. Kim JM, Kim KW, Kim SY, et al. Technical essentials of hepatic Doppler sonography. *Curr Probl Diagn Radiol*. 2009;38(2):53–56.
11. Gotlieb AI. Blood vessels. In: Rubin E, Gorstein F, Rubin R, et al., eds. *Rubin's Pathology: Clinicopathologic Foundations of Medicine*. 4th ed. Baltimore, MD: Lippincott Williams & Wilkins; 2005:473–519.
12. Grisham A, Lohr J, Guenther JM, et al. Deciphering mesenteric venous thrombosis: imaging and treatment. *Vasc Endovascular Surg*. 2005;39:473–479.
13. Zwiebel WJ. Ultrasound assessment of the aorta, iliac arteries, and inferior vena cava. In: Zwiebel WJ, Pellerito JS, eds. *Introduction to Vascular Ultrasonography*. 5th ed. Philadelphia, PA: Elsevier Saunders; 2005:529–552.
14. Kunzli A, von Segesser LK, Vogt PR, et al. Inflammatory aneurysm of the ascending aorta. *Ann Thorac Surg*. 1998;65(4):1132–1133.
15. Davarn S, Reardon R, Joing S. Ultrasound use in the diagnosis of abdominal aortic aneurysm. *Acad Emerg Med*. 2007;14(4):323.
16. Gerhard-HM, Gardin JM, Jaff MR, et al. Guidelines for noninvasive vascular laboratory testing: a report from the American Society of Echocardiography and the Society for Vascular Medicine and Biology. *Vasc Med*. 2006;11:183–200.
17. American Institute of Ultrasound in Medicine. AIUM practice guidelines for the performance of diagnostic and screening ultrasound examinations of the abdominal aorta in adults, 2010. Available at: http://www.aium.org/publications/guidelines/abdominalAorta.pdf. Accessed January 31, 2011.
18. Mohler ER. Abdominal aorta imaging. In: Mohler ER, Gerhard-Herman M, Jaff MR, eds. *Essentials of Vascular Laboratory Diagnosis*. London, UK: Blackwell Publishing; 2005:68–71.
19. Di Candio G, Lencioni R, Ferrari M, et al. Abdominal aortic aneurysms: efficacy of sonography for preoperative assessment. *Eur J Ultrasound*. 1996;4(1):5–20.
20. Sprouse LR, Meier GH, Lesar CJ, et al. Comparison of abdominal aortic aneurysm diameter measurements obtained with ultrasound and computed tomography: is there a difference? *J Vasc Surg*. 2003;38(3):466–471.
21. Hudson P, Englund R, Hanel KC. What is the most important dimension of an abdominal aortic aneurysm? *J Vasc Tech*. 1996;20(4):213–216.
22. Devaraj S, Dodds SR. Ultrasound surveillance of ectatic abdominal aortas. *Ann R Coll Surg Engl*. 2008;90(6):477–482.
23. Lal B, Cerveira J, Seidman C, et al. Observer variability of iliac artery measurements in endovascular repair of abdominal aortic aneurysms. *Ann Vasc Surg*. 2004;18(6):644–652.
24. Pearce WH. Abdominal aortic aneurysm. *Medscape: eMedicine*. October 2009. Available at: http://emedicine.medscape.com/article/463354-overview. Accessed January 31, 2011.
25. Wilmink AB, Forshaw M, Quick CR, et al. Accuracy of serial screening for abdominal aortic aneurysm by ultrasound. *J Med Screen*. 2002;9:125–127.
26. Fojtik JP, Costantino TG, Dean AJ. The diagnosis of aortic dissection by emergency medicine ultrasound. *J Emerg Med*. 2007;32(2):191–196.
27. Catalano O, Siani A. Ruptured abdominal aortic aneurysm: categorization of sonographic findings and report of 3 new signs. *J Ultrasound Med*. 2005;24:1077–1083.
28. Rossi S, Rosa L, Ravetta V, et al. Contrast-enhanced versus conventional and color Doppler sonography for the detection of thrombosis of the portal and hepatic venous systems. *Am J Roentgenol*. 2006;186(3):763–773.
29. Clevert DA, Weckbach S, Kopp R, et al. Imaging of aortic lesions with color coded duplex sonography and contrast-enhanced ultrasound versus multislice computed tomography (MS-CT) angiography. *Clin Hemorheol Microcirc*. 2008;40(4):267–279.
30. Kaban J, Raio C. Emergency department diagnosis of aortic dissection by bedside transabdominal ultrasound. *Acad Emerg Med*. 2009;16(8):809–810.
31. Chaikof EL, Brewster DC, Dalman RL, et al. The care of patients with an abdominal aortic aneurysm: the Society for Vascular Surgery practice guidelines. *J Vasc Surg*. 2009;50(4 suppl):S2–S49.
32. Clevert DA, Schick K, Chen MH, et al. Role of contrast enhanced ultrasound in detection of abdominal aortic abnormalities in comparison with multislice computed tomography. *Chin Med J*. 2009;122(7):858–864.
33. Chaikof EL, Brewster DC, Dalman RL, et al. SVS practice guidelines for the care of patients with an abdominal aortic aneurysm: executive summary. *J Vasc Surg*. 2009;51(13):799–800.
34. Galesić K, Brkljacić B, Sabljar-Matovinović M, et al. Renal vascular resistance in essential hypertension: duplex-Doppler ultrasonographic evaluation. *Angiology*. 2000;51(8):667–675.
35. George H. Imaging of aortic aneurysm and dissection: CT and MRI. *J Thorac Imaging*. 2001;13(1):35–46.
36. Lee WK, Mossop PJ, Little AF, et al. Infected (mycotic) aneurysms: spectrum of imaging appearances and management. *Radiographics*. 2008;28(7):1853–1868.

37. Rogers S. Sonographic evaluation of arteritis. *J Diagn Med Sonogr*. 2005;21:128–134.

38. Paravastu S, Murray D, Ghosh J, et al. Inflammatory abdominal aortic aneurysms (IAAA): past and present. *Vasc Endovascular Surg*. 2009;43(4):360–363.

39. Willing SJ, Fanizza-Orphanos A, Thomas HA. Mycotic aneurysm of the abdominal aorta. Diagnosis by duplex sonography. *J Ultrasound Med*. 1989;8(9):527–529.

40. Vallina-Victorero Vazquez MJ, Vaquero Lorenzo F, Salgado AA, et al. Endovascular treatment of splenic and renal aneurysms. *Annals Vasc Surg*. 2008;23(2):258. e13– e17.

41. Chaubal N, Dighe M, Shah M. Sonographic and color Doppler findings in aortoarteritis (Takayasu arteritis). *J Ultrasound Med*. 2004;23(7):937–944.

42. Lorelli D, Cambria RA, Seabrook GA, et al. Diagnosis and management of aneurysms involving the superior mesenteric artery and its branches: a report of four cases. *Vasc Endovascular Surg*. 2003;37:59–66.

43. Kenningham R, Hershman MJ, Williams RG, et al. Incidental splenic artery aneurysm. *J R Soc Med*. 2002;95(9): 460–461.

44. Lee HK, Park SJ, Yi BH, et al. Portal vein thrombosis: CT features. *Abdom Imaging*. 2008;33(1):72–79.

45. Malkowski P, Pawlak J, Michalowicz B, et al. Thrombolytic treatment of portal thrombosis. *Hepatogastroenterology*. 2003;50(54):2098–2100.

46. Pasha FS, Gloviczki P, Stanson AW, et al. Splanchnic artery aneurysms. *May Clin Proc*. 2007;82:472–479.

47. Schweiger ML, Redick EL, Siegel LA, et al. Hepatic arterial pseudoaneurysm after placement of transjugular intrahepatic portosystemic shunt. *J Ultrasound Med*. 1997;16: 437–439.

48. Turkvatan A, Okten RS, Ersa K, et al. Hepatic artery aneurysm: imaging findings. *J Ankara University Faculty Med*. 2005;58:73–75.

49. Germanos S, Soonawalla Z, Stratopoulos C, et al. Pseudoaneurysm of the gastroduodenal artery in chronic pancreatitis. *J Am Coll Surg*. 2009;208(2):316.

50. Tulsyan N, Kashyap VS, Greenberg RK, et al. The endovascular management of visceral artery aneurysms and pseudoaneurysms. *J Vasc Surg*. 2007;45(2):276–283.

51. Zwiebel WJ, Mountford RA, Halliwell MJ, et al. Splanchnic blood flow in patients with cirrhosis and portal hypertension: investigation with duplex Doppler US. *Radiology*. 1995;194(3):807–812.

52. Richards T, Dharmadasa A, Davies R, et al. Natural history of the common iliac artery in the presence of an abdominal aortic aneurysm. *J Vasc Surg*. 2009;49(4):881–885.

53. Roth SM, Bandyk DF. Duplex imaging of lower extremity bypasses, angioplasties, and stents. *Semin Vasc Surg*. 1999;12(4):275–284.

54. Lee WA, Wolf YG, Fogarty TZ, et al. Does complete aneurysm exclusion ensure long term success following endovascular repair? *J Endovasc Ther*. 2000;7:494–500.

55. Bandyk DF. Surveillance after lower extremity arterial bypass. *Perspect Vasc Surg Endovasc Ther*. 2007;19: 376–383.

56. Nerlekar R, Warrier R, de Ryke R, et al. A comparative study of ultrasound and computed tomography for the follow up of abdominal aortic aneurysms after endovascular repair. *J Vasc Ultrasound*. 2006;30(2):81–85.

57. Johnson BL, Arko FR, Wolf Y, et al. Update: quantitative duplex ultrasound assessment of aortic aneurysms after endovascular repair. *J Vasc Surg*. 2003;27(3):165–170.

58. Taylor DC, Kettler MD, Moneta GL, et al. Duplex ultrasound scanning in the diagnosis of renal artery stenosis: a prospective evaluation. *J Vasc Surg*. 1988;7:363–369.

59. Radermacher J, Chavan A, Bleck J, et al. Use of Doppler ultrasonography to predict the outcome of therapy for renal artery stenosis. *N Engl J Med*. 2001;344:410–417.

60. Manoharan A, Gill RW, Griffiths KA. Splenic blood flow measurements by Doppler ultrasound: a preliminary report. *Cardiovasc Res*. 1987;21:779–782.

61. Gaitini D, Thaler I, Kaftori JK. Duplex sonography in the diagnosis of portal vein thrombosis. *Rofo*. 1990;153(6): 645–649.

62. Qamar MI, Read AE, Skidmore R, et al. Transcutaneous Doppler ultrasound measurement of celiac axis blood flow in man. *Br J Surg*. 1985;72:329–393.

63. Qamar MI, Read AE, Skidmore R, et al. Pulsatility index of superior mesenteric artery blood velocity waveforms. *Ultrasound Med Biol*. 1986;12:772–776.

64. Gillespie DL, Villavicencio JL, Gallagher C, et al. Presentation and management of venous aneurysms. *J Vasc Surg*. 1997;26(5):845–852.

65. Bombelli L, Genitoni V, Biasi S, et al. Liver hemodynamic flow balance by image-directed Doppler ultrasound evaluation in normal subjects. *J Clin Ultrasound*. 1991;19(5):257–262.

66. Mitchell EL, Moneta GL. Mesenteric duplex scanning. *Perspect Vasc Surg Endovasc Ther*. 2006;18(2):175–183.

67. Hoffman U, Edwards JM, Carter S, et al. Role of Duplex scanning for the detection of atherosclerotic renal artery disease. *Kidney Int*. 1991;39:1232–1239.

68. Poe PA. Color duplex ultrasound evaluation of renal and mesenteric arteries. *J Vasc Ultrasound*. 2003;27(3):177–183.

69. Lee H, Grant EG. Sonography in renovascular hypertension. *J Ultrasound Med*. 2002;21:431–441.

70. Pellerito JS, Zwiebel WJ. Ultrasound assessment of native renal vessels and renal allografts. In: Zwiebel WJ, Pellerito JS, eds. *Introduction to Vascular Ultrasonography*. 5th ed. Philadelphia, PA: Elsevier Saunders; 2005:612–636.

71. Dubbins PA. The kidney. In: Allan P, Dubbins P, McDicken WN, et al., eds. *Clinical Doppler Ultrasound*. 2nd ed. Philadelphia, PA: Churchill Livingstone Elsevier; 2006:185–213.

72. Taylor DC, Kettler M, Moneta G, et al. Duplex ultrasound scanning in the diagnosis of renal artery stenosis: a prospective evaluation. *J Vasc Surg*. 1988;7:363–369.

73. Hoffman U, Edwards J, Carter S, et al. Role of duplex scanning for the detection of atherosclerotic renal artery disease. *Kidney Int*. 1991;15:173–180.

74. Martin T, Nanra R, Wlodarczyk J, et al. Renal hilar Doppler analysis in the detection of renal artery stenosis. *J Vasc Tech*. 1991;15:173–180.

75. Moneta G, Lee R, Yeager R, et al. Mesenteric duplex scanning: a blinded prospective study. *J Vasc Surg*. 1993;17:79–86.

76. Rademacher J, Chavan A, Bleck J, et al. Use of Doppler ultrasonography to predict outcome of therapy for renal artery stenosis. *N Engl J Med*. 2001;344:410–417.

77. Zierler RE. Natural history of atherosclerotic renal artery stenosis. *Perspect Vasc Surg Endovasc Ther*. 1999;11:55–67.

78. Soares GM, Murphy TP, Singha MS, et al. Renal artery duplex ultrasonography as a screening and surveillance

tool to detect renal artery stenosis: a comparison with current reference standard imaging. *J Ultrasound Med.* 2006;25:293–298.

79. Coombs P. Color duplex of the renal arteries: diagnostic criteria and anatomical windows for visualization. *J Vasc Ultrasound.* 2004;28(2):89–95.

80. Raju S, Hollis K, Neglen P. Obstructive lesions of the inferior vena cava: clinical features and endovenous treatment. *J Vasc Surg.* 2006;44(4):820–827.

81. Motew SJ, Cherr GS, Craven TE, et al. Renal duplex sonography: main renal artery versus hilar analysis. *J Vasc Surg.* 2000;32(3):462–471.

82. Conkbayir I, Yucesoy C, Edguer T, et al. Doppler sonography in renal artery stenosis: an evaluation of intrarenal and extrarenal imaging parameters. *Clin Imaging.* 2003;27(4):256–260.

83. Crutchley TA, Pearce JD, Craven TE, et al. Clinical utility of resistive index in atherosclerotic renovascular disease. *J Vasc Sur.* 2009;49(1):148–155.

84. Rocha-Singh K, Jaff MR, Lynne K. Renal artery stenting with noninvasive duplex ultrasound follow up: 3 year results from the renaissance renal stent trial. *Catheter Cardiovasc Interv.* 2008;72(6):853–862.

85. Lencioni R, Caramella D, Sanguinetti F, et al. Portal vein thrombosis after percutaneous ethanol injection for hepatocellular carcinoma: value of color Doppler sonography in distinguishing chemical and tumor thrombi. *Am J Roentgenol.* 1995;164:1125–1130.

86. Zwolak RM, Fillinger MF, Walsh DB, et al. Mesenteric and celiac duplex scanning: a validation study. *J Vasc Surg.* 1998;27(6):1078–1087.

87. Armstrong PA. Visceral duplex scanning: evaluation before and after artery intervention for chronic mesenteric ischemia. *Perspect Vasc Surg Endovasc Ther.* 2007;19(4):386–392.

88. Bowie J, Bernstein JR. Retroperitoneal fibrosis: ultrasound findings and case report. *J Clin Ultrasound.* 2005;4(6):435–437.

89. Oderich G, Bower T, Sullivan T, et al. Open versus endovascular revascularization for chronic mesenteric ischemia: risk stratified outcomes. *J Vasc Surg.* 2009;49(6):1472–1479.

90. Bertino RE, Saucier NA, Barth DJ. The retroperitoneum. In: Rumack CM, Wilson SR, Charbonneau JW, et al., eds. *Diagnostic Ultrasound.* 4th ed., Vol. 1. Philadelphia, PA: Elsevier Mosby; 2011:447–485.

91. Seidl H, Tuerck J, Schepp W, et al. Splanchnic arterial blood flow is significantly influenced by breathing—assessment by duplex-Doppler ultrasound. *Ultrasound Med Biol.* 2010;36(10):1677–1681.

92. Radermacher J, Chavan J, Bleck J, et al. Use of Doppler ultrasonography to predict the outcome of therapy for renal artery stenosis. *N Engl J Med.* 2001;344:410–417.

93. Luong S, Miller J. Calcification and narrowing of the inferior vena cava. *J Diagn Med Sonogr.* 1991;7:154–156.

94. Williams C, Benson CB, Rhodes A, et al. American Registry of Diagnostic Medical Sonographers: survey of practice abdominal and in superficial sonography. *J Diagn Med Sonogr.* 1996;12(1):18–21.

95. Jia YP, Lu Q, Gong S, et al. Postoperative complications in patients with portal vein thrombosis after liver trans-

plantation: evaluation with Doppler ultrasonography. *World J Gastroenterol.* 2007;13(34):4636–4640.

96. England RA, Wells IP, Gutteridge CM. Benign external compression of the inferior vena cava associated with thrombus formation. *Br J Radiol.* 2005;78:553–557.

97. Singh-Panghaal S, Karcnik TJ, Wachsberg RH, et al. Inferior vena caval leiomyosarcoma: diagnosis and biopsy with color Doppler sonography. *J Clin Ultrasound.* 1997;25(5):275–278.

98. Sorrell K, Harris S, Hanna J, et al. Renal vein and inferior vena cava tumor thrombus: presentation and mapping of venous extension with color duplex ultrasound. *J Vasc Ultrasound.* 2006;30(1):9–15.

99. McGahan JP, Blake LC, deVere White R, et al. Color flow sonographic mapping of intravascular extension of malignant renal tumors. *J Ultrasound Med.* 1993;12:403–409.

100. Sidhu R, Lockhart ME. Imaging of renovascular disease. *Semin Ultrasound CT MR.* 2009;30(4):271–288.

101. Ferrante A, Di Stasi C, Pierconti F, et al. Incidental finding of right renal venous aneurysm in a patient with symptomatic ipsilateral renal carcinoma: a case report. *Cardiovasc Pathol.* 2005;14(6):327–330.

102. Yura T, Yuasa S, Ohkawa M, et al. Noninvasive detection and monitoring of renal arteriovenous fistula by color Doppler. *Am J Nephrol.* 1991;11(3):250–251.

103. Boozari B, Bahr MJ, Kubicka S, et al. Ultrasonography in patients with Budd-Chiari syndrome: diagnostic signs and prognostic implications. *J Hepatol.* 2008;49(4):572–580.

104. Valla DC. The diagnosis and management of the Budd-Chiari syndrome: consensus and controversies. *Hepatology.* 2003;38(4):793–803.

105. Gaba RC, Hardman JD, Bobra SJ. Extrahepatic portal vein aneurysm. *Radiology Case Reports* (Online). 2009;4:291. Available at: http://radiologycasereports.com/index.php/rcr/article/viewArticle/291/616. Accessed February 1, 2011.

106. Ozbek SS, Killi MR, Pourbagher MA, et al. Portal venous system aneurysms: report of five cases. *J Ultrasound Med.* 1999;18(6):417–422.

107. Jin B, Sun Y, LiY-Q, et al. Extrahepatic portal vein aneurysm: two case reports of surgical interventions. *World J Gastroenterol.* 2005;11(14):2206–2209.

108. Chaubal N, Dighe M, Hanchate V, et al. Sonography in Budd-Chiari syndrome. *J Ultrasound Med.* 2006;25(3):373–379.

109. Indeck M, Puyau F, Kerstein MD. Balloon septostomy for membranous obstruction of the vena cava in Budd-Chiari Syndrome. *Vasc Endovascular Surg.* 1984;18:399–402.

110. Andrew A. Portal hypertension: a review. *J Diagn Med Sonogr.* 2001;17:193–200.

111. Condat B, Pessione F, Denninger MH, et al. Recent portal or mesenteric venous thrombosis: increased recognition and frequent recanilization on anticoagulant therapy. *Hepatology.* 2000;32(3):466–470.

112. Bradbury MS, Kavanagh PV, Bechtold RE, et al. Mesenteric venous thrombosis: diagnosis and noninvasive imaging. *Radiographics.* 2002;22(3):527–541.

113. Miller VE, Berland LL. Pulsed-Doppler duplex sonography and CT of portal vein thrombosis. *Am J Roentgenol.* 1985;145(1):73–76.

114. Parmar HH, Shah JJ, Shah BB. Imaging findings in a giant hepatic artery aneurysm. *J Postgrad Med.* 2000;46:104–105.

115. Umpleby HC. Thrombosis of the superior mesenteric vein. *Br J Surg.* 1987;74(8):694–696.

116. Taourel P, Blanc P, Dauzat M, et al. Doppler study of mesenteric, hepatic, and portal circulation in alcoholic cirrhosis: relationship between quantitative Doppler measurements and the severity of portal hypertension and hepatic failure. *Hepatology.* 1998;28(4):932–936.

117. Gibson PR, Gibson RN, Donlan JD, et al. Duplex Doppler ultrasound of the ligamentum teres and portal vein: a clinically useful adjunct in the evaluation of patients with known or suspected chronic liver disease or portal hypertension. *J Gastroenterol Hepatol.* 1991;6(1):61–65.

118. Colli A, Cocciolo M, Mumoli N, et al. Hepatic artery resistance in alcoholic liver disease. *Hepatology.* 1998;28(5):1182–1186.

119. Evans K, Schneider J. Tumor masquerading as a portal vein thrombosis. *J Diagn Med Sonogr.* 2004;20(3):188–193.

120. Ciancio G, Vaidya A, Savoie M, et al. Management of renal cell carcinoma with level III thrombus in the inferior vena cava. *J Urol.* 2002;168(4 pt 1):1374–1377.

121. Iwao T, Toyonaga A, Oho K, et al. Value of Doppler ultrasound parameters of portal vein and hepatic artery in the diagnosis of cirrhosis and portal hypertension. *Am J Gastroenterol.* 1997;92(6):1012–1017.

122. Tchelepi H, Ralls PW, Randall R, et al. Sonography of diffuse liver disease. *J Ultrasound Med.* 2002;21(9):1023–1032.

123. Goyal AK, Pokharna DS, Sharma SK. Ultrasonic measurements of portal vasculature in diagnosis of portal hypertension, a controversial subject reviewed. *J Ultrasound Med.* 1990;9:45–48.

124. von Herbay A, Frieling T, Häussinger D. Color Doppler sonographic evaluation of spontaneous portosystemic shunts and inversion of portal venous flow in patients with cirrhosis. *J Clin Ultrasound.* 2000;28(7):332–339.

125. Goyal N, Jain N, Rachapalli V, et al. Non-invasive evaluation of liver cirrhosis using ultrasound. *Clin Radiol.* 2009;64(11):1056–1066.

126. Moneta GL, Taylor DC, Yeager RA, et al. Duplex ultrasound: applications to intra-abdominal vessels. *Perspect Vasc Surg.* 1989;2(2):133–148.

127. Taourel P, Blanc P, Dauzat M, et al. Doppler study of mesenteric, hepatic, and portal circulation in alcoholic cirrhosis: relationship between quantitative Doppler measurements and the severity of portal hypertension and hepatic failure. *Hepatology.* 1998;28(4):932–936.

128. Perisić MD, Culafić DjM, Kerkez M. Specificity of splenic blood flow in liver cirrhosis. *Rom J Intern Med.* 2005;43(1–2):141–151.

129. Bolognesi M, Sacerdoti D, Mescoli C, et al. Different hemodynamic patterns of alcoholic and viral endstage cirrhosis: analysis of explanted liver weight, degree of fibrosis and splanchnic Doppler parameters. *Scand J Gastroenterol.* 2007;42(2):256–262.

130. Kutlu R, Karaman I, Akbulut A, et al. Quantitative Doppler evaluation of the splenoportal venous system in various stages of cirrhosis: differences between right and left portal veins. *J Clin Ultrasound.* 2002;30(9):537–543.

131. Matveyenko AV, Donovan CM. Metabolic sensors mediate hypoglycemic detection at the portal vein. *Diabetes.* 2006;55(5):1276–1282.

132. Leen E, Goldberg JA, Anderson JR, et al. Hepatic perfusion changes in patients with liver metastases: comparison with those patients with cirrhosis. *Gut.* 1993;34(4):554–557.

133. Orban Schiopu AM, Balas BI, Diculescu M. The effect of a combined treatment with propranolol and isosorbide-5-mononitrate on Doppler ultrasound parameters in patients with cirrhosis and portal hypertension. *Rom J Gastroenterol.* 2005;14(2):123–127.

134. Segawa M, Sakaida I. Diagnosis and treatment of portal hypertension. *Hepatol Res.* 2009;39(10):1039–1043.

135. Cosar S, Oktar SO, Cosar B, et al. Doppler and gray-scale ultrasound evaluation of morphological and hemodynamic changes in liver vasculature in alcoholic patients. *Eur J Radiol.* 2005;54(3):393–399.

136. Culafic D, Perisic M, Vojinovic-Culafic V, et al. Spontaneous splenorenal shunt in a patient with liver cirrhosis and hypertrophic caudal lobe. *J Gastrointestin Liver Dis.* 2006;15(3):289–292.

137. Abbitt PL. Ultrasonography. Update on liver technique. *Radiol Clin North Am.* 1998;36(2):299–307.

138. Hirooka K, Hirooka M, Kisaka Y, et al. Doppler waveform pattern changes in a patient with primary Budd-Chiari syndrome before and after angioplasty. *Intern Med.* 2008;47(2):91–95.

139. Kruskal JB, Newman PA, Sammons LG, et al. Optimizing Doppler and color flow US: application to hepatic sonography. *Radiographics.* 2004;24(3):657–675.

140. Fung Y, Glajchen N, Shapiro RS, et al. Portal vein velocities measured by ultrasound: usefulness or evaluating shunt functioning following TIPS placement and TIPS revision. *Abdom Imaging.* 1998;23:511–514.

141. Abraldes JG, Gilabert R, Turnes J, et al. Utility of color Doppler ultrasonography predicting tips dysfunction. *Am J Gastroenterol.* 2005;100(12):2696–2701.

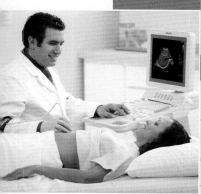

# 5 The Liver

Joyce A. Grube

## OBJECTIVES

Illustrate the normal anatomy of the liver including the liver lobes and segments, fissures, ligaments, and hepatic vasculature.

Describe the different methods used to classify lobar divisions of the liver including anatomical, segmental, and Couinaud's anatomical division.

List the functions of the liver and the laboratory values associated with liver function.

Explain the patient preparation, scan technique, and sonographic appearance of the normal liver.

Perform sonographic evaluations of the liver and hepatic system.

Discuss the pathophysiology and sonographic appearance of diffuse liver diseases including fatty infiltration, glycogen storage disease, hepatitis, and cirrhosis.

Describe the differential diagnoses, clinical signs and symptoms, and sonographic appearance of cystic and solid liver lesions.

Formulate a list of differential diagnosis based on correlating the patient's clinical history, laboratory values, results of related diagnostic procedures, and the sonographic tissue characteristics.

Identify technically satisfactory and unsatisfactory sonographic examinations of the vascular system.

## KEY TERMS

adenoma | Budd-Chiari syndrome | candidiasis | cavernous hemangioma | cirrhosis | diffuse hepatocellular disease | echinococcal cyst | epithelioid hemangioendothelioma | fatty infiltration | fibrolamellar hepatocellular carcinoma | focal nodular hyperplasia | glycogen storage disease | hepatic angiosarcoma | hepatitis | hepatocellular carcinoma | lipoma | liver abscess | liver hematoma | liver metastases | *Pneumocystis jiroveci* | polycystic liver disease | portosystemic shunt | schistosomiasis

## GLOSSARY

**AFP** $\alpha$-fetoprotein; a tumor marker frequently elevated in cases of hepatocellular carcinoma and certain testicular cancers

**ALP** alkaline phosphatase; an enzyme found in liver tissue that can be elevated with biliary obstruction

**ALT** alanine aminotransferase; a liver enzyme most specific to hepatocellular damage

**AST** aspartate aminotransferase; an enzyme found in all tissues, but in largest amounts in the liver, an increase can indicate hepatocellular damage

**falciform ligament** fold in the parietal peritoneum that extends from the umbilicus to the diaphragm and contains the ligamentum teres

**Glisson capsule** a fibroelastic, connective tissue layer that surrounds the liver

**hepatofugal** blood flow away from the liver; normal flow in the hepatic veins is hepatofugal

**hepatomegaly** enlarged liver

**hepatopetal** blood flow toward the liver; normal flow in the portal vein is hepatopetal

**jaundice** yellowish pigmentation of the skin and whites of the eyes caused by increased levels of bilirubin in the blood

**ligamentum teres** remnant of the obliterated left umbilical vein seen as a triangular echogenic foci dividing the medial and lateral segments of the left lobe of the liver in the transverse plane

**ligamentum venosum** remnant of the ductus venosus seen as an echogenic line separating the caudate lobe from the left lobe

**main lobar fissure** divides the right and left lobes of the liver; seen in the sagittal plane as an echogenic line between the gallbladder neck and the main portal vein

**porta hepatis** known as the gate to the liver, a fissure where the portal vein and hepatic artery enter the liver and the common hepatic duct exits

**Reidel lobe** anatomic variant in which the right lobe is enlarged and extends inferiorly as a tongue-like projection

The liver, often considered an accessory organ of digestion, is the largest solid organ in the body. The focus of this chapter is the liver. Its anatomy and physiologic function is so important to learn well because the liver is frequently involved with the disease, pathology, and pathophysiology affecting not only itself but many other systemic system disorders.

## ANATOMY

### EMBRYOLOGY

Early in the fourth week of fetal development, the liver, gallbladder, and bile duct system develop from an endodermal outgrowth, or hepatic diverticulum. During week 5, the diverticulum differentiates into the origin of the cystic duct and the gallbladder in the caudal portion; and, in the cephalic portion, two endodermal cellular buds begin forming the right and the left hepatic lobes.[1-3] These solid cell buds grow into columns or cylinders that branch and form networks and invade the vitelline and umbilical veins. The capillary-like vessels of the plexus eventually differentiate into the liver sinusoids. The endothelial cells of the plexus become the Kupffer cells. The columns of endodermal cells and the liver parenchyma grow into the surrounding mesoderm. The mesoderm provides the hemopoietic tissue and the connective tissue for the portal tracts and the fibrous liver capsule (Glisson capsule).[1,3] As the terminal branches of the right and left hepatic lobes canalize, the bile duct system is formed.

Both lobes are equal in size until the beginning of the sixth week, at which time the right lobe becomes larger, the caudate and quadrate lobes develop from the right lobe, and the left lobe actually undergoes some degeneration. At week 6, the liver fills most of the abdominal cavity and, relative to other organ development, the liver becomes less active.[1,2]

Hemopoiesis takes place in the liver at week 6, peaks at 12 to 24 weeks, and ceases at birth.[1,4] At week 10, lymphocyte formation occurs in the liver, which also ceases at birth. Coagulation factors are manufactured at 10 to 12 weeks and bile is produced by 13 to 16 weeks,[1] but the fetal liver does not function in digestion until after birth.[5]

Oxygenated blood and nutrients are delivered to the fetus through the umbilical vein, which ascends and divides into two branches.[6,7] The left branch joins the portal vein and enters the liver and the right branch, the ductus venosus, and flows directly into the inferior vena cava (IVC), bypassing the liver[5,8] (Fig. 5-1). Normally, both of these vessels deteriorate into fibrous cords sometime after birth. The left umbilical vein becomes the ligamentum teres, or round ligament, and the ductus venosus becomes the ligamentum venosum. In some individuals, the left umbilical vein may persist. Also, both the ligamentum teres and the ligamentum venosum can become recanalized as collateral vessels with certain disease processes such as portal hypertension.[8]

### LOCATION AND SIZE

The liver fills the right side and part of the left side of the upper abdomen, displaces gas-filled structures, and provides an acoustic window through which the upper abdomen and retroperitoneum may be imaged (Fig. 5-2A,B). Sonographically, it has a relatively homogeneous parenchymal background. The medium-level echo pattern is believed to be due primarily to nonspecular reflections, thought to be the lobules and their surrounding stroma. The homogeneous parenchymal background may be isoechoic or slightly more echogenic than the renal parenchyma and is isoechoic or slightly less echogenic than the pancreas. Interspersed within the parenchyma are tubular, fluid-filled structures representing branches of the portal and hepatic veins, and small, rounded, echogenic areas representing periportal, fibrofatty tissue, where the hepatic artery, bile duct, and portal vein lumina are too small to be imaged (Fig. 5-3A,B).

The largest internal organ of the body, the liver varies somewhat in shape and vascular disposition, depending on the patient's morphotype. It constitutes approximately 1/18th of an infant's total body weight and 1/36th of an adult's.[9] The exact weight varies but usually ranges from 1,200 g in adult women to 1,600 g in men.[3,7]

There is also a range of normal measurements. The greatest transverse portion ranges from 20 to 22.5 cm, the greatest anteroposterior measurement from 10 to 12.5 cm,[2] and the greatest length on the right surface from 15 to 17 cm.[10] Routinely taking liver measurements in the sagittal section will help detect hepatomegaly. Liver length and anteroposterior dimensions are obtained from sagittal and parasagittal sections obtained at the midclavicular line, which runs parallel to the spine halfway between midline and the right side of the body.[11]

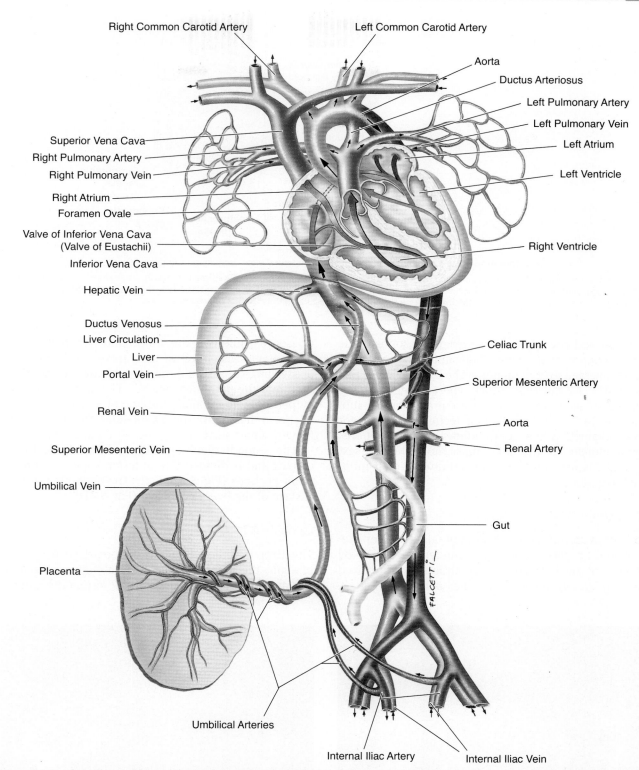

**Figure 5-1** Fetal circulation. The umbilical vein carries oxygenated blood from the placenta to the fetus, ascends the fetal abdomen, and courses toward the liver. A portion of blood flow is allowed to bypass the fetal liver via the ductus venosus. After birth, both veins close and exist as ligaments; the umbilical vein becomes the ligamentum teres and ductus venosus becomes the ligamentum venosum.

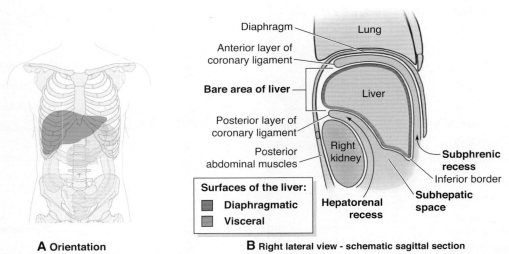

**Figure 5-2** Liver location. The liver occupies the right hypochondrium, the greater part of the epigastric region, and extends in varying degrees into the left hypochondrium as far as the mammary line.[3] The lateral segment of the left lobe and the length of the right lobe determine the contour and shape of the liver. Overall, the liver can be described as irregular, hemispheric,[2] or wedge shaped.[3]

Kratzer and coworkers did an extensive sonographic liver measurement study on 2,080 subjects. They found that the average liver diameter at the midclavicular line was 14.0 ± 1.7 cm (Fig. 5-2A). The average diameter for male subjects was 14.5 ± 1.6 cm and female subjects was 13.5 ± 1.7cm.[12] Their technique allows for easy assessment and accurate follow-up examinations. They demonstrated that body mass index, height, sex, age, and frequent alcohol consumption in men influenced liver size.[12]

## PERIHEPATIC RELATIONSHIPS

The liver is an intraperitoneal organ, almost completely covered by peritoneum and completely covered by a dense, fibroelastic connective tissue layer referred to as *Glisson capsule*.[5,13,14] A rather delicate structure,

Glisson capsule contains blood and lymphatic vessels and nerves. Distention of the capsule by liver disease or swelling causes pain, and the lymphatics may ooze fluid into the peritoneal space.[13] The areas not covered by peritoneum are along the line of attachment for the falciform ligament, the gallbladder fossa, the porta hepatis, areas surrounding the IVC, and a "bare area."[3]

The smooth diaphragmatic surface of the liver is convex and is divided into anterior, superior, and posterior portions (Fig. 5-4A–C).[2,3] The abdominal visceral surface of the liver is concave (Fig. 5-4D).

## LIGAMENTS

The liver is tethered to the undersurface of the diaphragm, the anterior wall of the abdomen, the lesser curvature of the stomach, and the retroperitoneum by

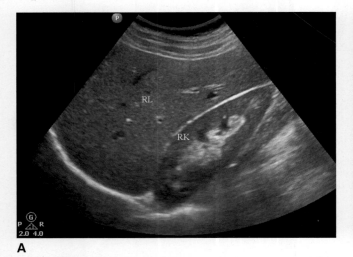

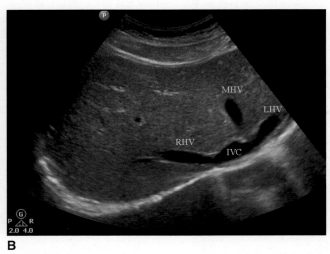

**Figure 5-3** Normal sonographic anatomy. **A.** A sagittal image of the right lobe *(RL)* of the liver demonstrates the homogeneous echo pattern of hepatic parenchyma as isoechoic or mildly hyperechoic in comparison to the renal parenchyma. *RK,* right kidney. **B.** A transverse image demonstrates the homogeneous echo pattern with hepatic veins *(RHV,* right hepatic vein; *MHV,* middle hepatic vein; *LHV,* left hepatic vein) and inferior vena cava *(IVC)* identified within normal hepatic parenchyma. (Courtesy of Katie Strayer, Kettering College, Kettering, OH.)

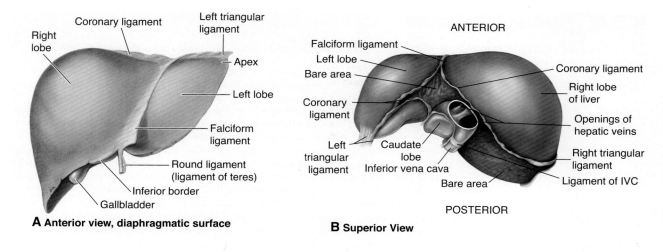

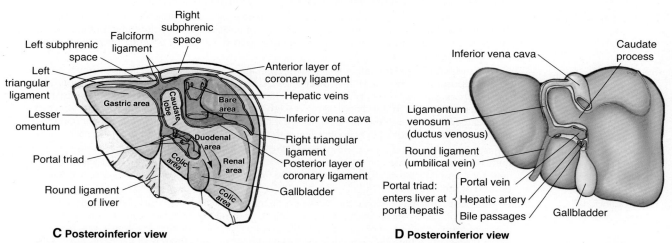

**Figure 5-4** Normal anatomy. **A.** Anterior surface. The border between the anterior surface and the visceral surface is the inferior margin.[3] Opposite the falciform ligament attachment, the anterior surface is marked by a deep notch, the umbilical notch, where the ligamentum teres extends from the umbilicus to the undersurface of the liver. Opposite the cartilage of the ninth rib is the notch for the gallbladder fundus.[3] **B.** Superior surface. The dome of the diaphragm separates the superior portion from the pleura and lungs on the right and the pericardium and heart on the left.[2] The surface is covered by peritoneum except along its posterior part, where it attaches to the diaphragm by the superior reflection of the coronary ligament. The coronary ligament separates the part covered with peritoneum from the bare area.[3] **C.** Posterior surface. The posterior portion is round and broad on the right but narrow on the left.[2] The central part presents a deep concavity as it is molded over the vertebral column and crus of the diaphragm. To the right of this concavity, the inferior vena cava *(IVC)* lies almost buried in its fossa and forms part of the posterior boundary of the porta hepatis.[2,3] Approximately 2 to 3 cm to the left of the IVC is the narrow fossa for the ligamentum venosus. The caudate lobe lies between these two fossae.[2,3] The posterior surface is in direct contact with the diaphragm and is attached by loose connective tissue. Most of the posterior surface is not covered by peritoneum, including the bare area, and is bounded by the superior and inferior reflections of the coronary ligament, which connect the liver to the diaphragm.[3] **D.** Visceral surface. The visceral surface is concave and faces posterior, caudal, and to the left. Peritoneum covers the visceral surface except at the gallbladder attachment and at the porta hepatis located in the left central part.[2,3] From lateral to medial, the right lobe has three impressions: the colic impression, a flattened or shallow area for the hepatic flexure; more posterior is the larger and deeper impression for the right kidney; and, lying along the neck of the gallbladder, the duodenal impression is a narrow, poorly marked area.[2] The quadrate lobe, located between the gallbladder and fossa for the umbilical vein, is in a relationship with the stomach's pyloric end, the duodenum's superior portion, and the transverse colon.[2] On the left, the gastric impression for the ventral surface of the stomach is a large hollow extending to the liver margin. The caudate process is just anterior to the IVC and connects the caudate lobe to the right lobe.[2]

eight ligaments—seven of which are either parietal or visceral peritoneal folds and one of which is a round, fibrous cord.[3] These are the coronary, falciform, ligamentum teres (round ligament), ligamentum venosum, right and left triangular, gastrohepatic, and hepatoduodenal ligaments. An understanding of the liver's ligamentous attachments and the caudate lobe's relational anatomy to the lesser sac is important for accurate localization of lobar structures and perihepatic fluid

collections. They are described in Table 5-1 and can be identified on Figures 5-4A–D and 5-5A,B.

## LOBES

Lobar divisions of the liver can be described as anatomic, based on external landmarks, or segmental, based on internal landmarks and hepatic function. Because some investigators may combine these methods

**TABLE 5-1**

## Ligament Attachments to the Liver

| Ligament | Description |
|---|---|
| Coronary | The coronary ligament connects the posterosuperior liver surface to the diaphragm and consists of an anterior and a posterior layer. The anterior layer is formed by the reflection of the parietal peritoneum, and the posterior layer is reflected from the caudal margin of the bare area onto the right adrenal gland and right kidney (hepatorenal ligament).[2,15] These two layers are continuous on each side with the right and left triangular ligaments and anteriorly with the falciform ligament.[15,16] |
| Falciform | The falciform ligament is a broad, thin anteroposterior fold of the parietal peritoneum.[15] It originates from the midportion of the coronary ligament; inserts itself in a parasagittal plane anteriorly and shifts obliquely to its posterior surface; separates the right and left liver lobes at the anterior surface; and extends from the liver to the abdominal wall between the diaphragm and umbilicus.[2,3,15,16] At its base or free edge, the ligamentum teres is released from between its layers.[15] |
| Ligamentum teres | The ligamentum teres (round ligament) is the fibrous cord resulting from the obliterated left umbilical vein.[3,15] It ascends from the umbilicus in the free margin of the falciform ligament to the notch in the anterior border of the liver. Here, it courses along a fissure on the visceral surface and continues as the ligamentum venosum as far back as the inferior vena cava.[3] |
| Ligamentum venosum | The ligamentum venosum, the obliterated ductus venosus, is usually attached to the left branch of the portal vein. It is a continuance of the ligamentum teres within the left intersegmental fissure on the superior, visceral surface of the liver. The upper part of the lesser omentum is also attached to the margins of the fissure. |
| Triangular | The right and left triangular ligaments are named because of their triangular shape. They are formed by the apposition of the upper and lower ends of the coronary ligament and extend from the diaphragm of the liver.[3] The right ligament is attached to the border at the right extremity of the bare area and passes to the diaphragm.[2] The left ligament is the larger of the two and attaches to the superior surface of the left lobe, where it lies anterior to the esophageal opening in the diaphragm.[3] Its anterior layer is continuous with the left layer of the falciform ligament.[2] |
| Gastrohepatic | The gastrohepatic ligament, also known as the *lesser omentum,* is composed of two folds of visceral peritoneum.[5] It originates on the undersurface of the liver, is continuous with the ligamentum venosum, and courses caudally to attach to the lesser curvature of the stomach and to the first portion of the duodenum.[16] |
| Hepatoduodenal | The hepatoduodenal ligament surrounds the portal triad (the portal vein, the hepatic artery, and the bile duct) prior to entering the porta hepatis. It is located on the right free edge of the gastrohepatic ligament forming the anterior boundary of the epiploic foramen (foramen of Winslow), a potential space representing the only communication of the lesser sac with the rest of the peritoneal cavity.[3] The inferior vena cava and caudate lobe form the posterior wall of the lesser sac.[3] The size of the caudate process, in part, determines the length of the hepatoduodenal ligament and its proximity to the inferior vena cava.[16] Below the caudate process, the portal vein, within the hepatoduodenal ligament, is contiguous with the posteriorly located inferior vena cava.[16] |

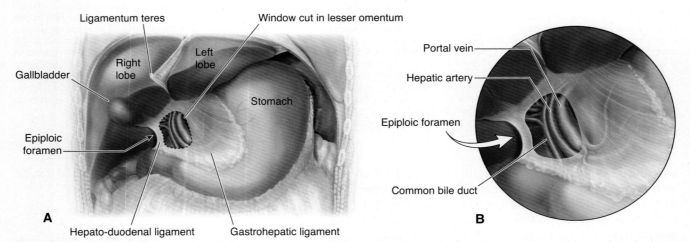

**Figure 5-5** Ligaments. **A.** The gastrohepatic ligament originates on the undersurface of the liver and courses caudal to attach to the lesser curvature of the stomach and the first portion of the duodenum. The hepatoduodenal ligament is located on the right free edge of the gastrohepatic ligament, surrounds the portal triad, and forms the anterior boundary of the epiploic foramen (of Winslow). **B.** Enlarged cutaway view of the hepatoduodenal ligament reveals the portal triad.

or may not specify which method is being used, the literature can be confusing and reports may appear to be contradictory. The next section presents each division separately. The sonographic images are presented in the segmental division because sonographers evaluate and document the liver using internal landmarks.

## Anatomic Division

The anatomic division of the liver is based on external markings. A broad division that uses the falciform ligament to divide the liver into the right and left hepatic lobes classifies the caudate and quadrate lobes as part of the right lobe. A more accurate anatomic approach is to divide the liver into right, left, caudate, and quadrate hepatic lobes. This system uses the falciform ligament and a simulated "H" configuration on the visceral surface (Fig. 5-6).

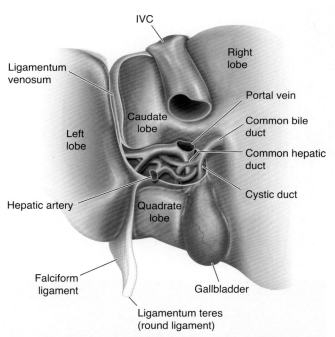

**Figure 5-6** Anatomic division. Viewing the "H" configuration on the visceral surface of the liver, the gallbladder fossa and inferior vena cava (IVC) fossa make the right vertical limb, the left intersegmental fissure (left sagittal fossa) makes the left vertical limb, and the porta fossa containing the porta hepatis and hepatoduodenal ligament forms the crossbar.[3,22] The gallbladder fossa, shallow and oblong, extends from the inferior margin to the right extremity of the porta hepatis.[2] The IVC fossa, a short, deep depression between the caudate lobe and the bare area, is separated from the porta hepatis by the caudate process.[2] The left intersegmental fissure is a deep groove extending from the notch on the inferior margin to the cranial border.[2] The porta hepatis joins it at right angles and divides it into cephalad and caudal parts.[2] The caudal part separates the quadrate lobe and the left lobe and is partially bridged by the pons hepatis, an extension of hepatic substance, which provides the ligamentum teres fissure.[2,3] The cephalad part lies between the left lobe and the caudate lobe and provides the fissure for the ligamentum venosum and the gastrohepatic ligament.[2,22] The porta fossa is short, about 5 cm, but deep.[2] It extends transversely across the left portion of the right lobe, joins the left intersegmental fissure at nearly a right angle, and separates the quadrate lobe from the caudate lobe.[2] It houses the portal triad, nerves, and lymphatics.[2]

### Right Lobe

The right lobe, six times larger than the left, occupies the right hypochondrium.[2] It is separated from the left lobe by the falciform ligament on its anterior surface and by the left intersegmental fissure on its visceral surface. It is somewhat quadrilateral. The anterior surface is marked by the falciform ligament, and its visceral and posterior surfaces are marked by three fossae: the porta hepatis, the gallbladder, and the IVC.[17]

### Caudate Lobe

The caudate lobe, anatomically distinct from the left and right liver lobes, is interposed between the IVC posteriorly, the left liver lobe anteriorly and superiorly, and the main portal vein (MPV) inferiorly.[18,19] The left margin forms the hepatic boundary of the superior recess of the lesser sac. The *caudate process* is a small elevation extending obliquely and laterally off the caudate lobe's right margin, as a tongue-like projection, coursing between the IVC and the portal vein and extending to the visceral surface of the right lobe.[19] Situated dorsal to the porta hepatis, it separates the gallbladder fossa from the commencement of the IVC fossa.[2] The shorter the caudate process, the longer the association between the IVC and portal vein.[20] The papillary process is an anteromedial extension of the caudate lobe.[2,21] It may appear separate from the caudate lobe and thus mimic lymph nodes or a pancreatic mass.

### Quadrate Lobe

The *quadrate lobe* is described by anatomists as a distinct lobe, but it is distinguished physiologically and sonographically as the medial segment of the left lobe. Situated on the visceral surface, it is bounded posteriorly by the porta hepatis, anteriorly by the inferior margin of the liver, and laterally by the gallbladder fossa on the right and the fissure for the ligamentum teres on the left.

### Left Lobe

The left lobe is situated in the epigastric and left hypochondriac regions. Anatomically, it is separated from the right hepatic lobe by the falciform ligament on its anterior surface. On the visceral surface, the fissure for the ligamentum teres separates it from the quadrate lobe, and the fissure for the ligamentum venosum separates it from the caudate lobe. The left lobe is flatter and smaller than the right but varies in size. Its superior surface is slightly convex, is molded to the diaphragm, and tapers off to the left at about the left mammary line.

### Segmental Division

Segmental division is based on two of the liver's most important functions, as a gland with bile ducts and as a vascular and storage organ supplied by blood from the portal veins and the hepatic arteries.[2] The internal lobar divisions do not coincide completely with those established by external markings. The functional lobar divisions are very important for sonographers to understand because they are clinically important in determining the segmental confinement of neoplasms, lesions, and other liver pathologies in preparation for possible surgical resection.

Using the *functional*, segmental method, the liver is divided into three lobes and four segments based on blood supply and biliary drainage: (1) the right lobe,

containing an anterior and a posterior segment; (2) the left lobe, containing a medial and a lateral segment; and (3) the caudate lobe. Using this nomenclature, the previously described quadrate lobe is now the medial segment of the left lobe. The *anatomic* left lobe is now the lateral segment of the left lobe. The caudate lobe is considered a separate, distinct lobe.

Sonographic landmarks are used to recognize the lobes and segments. These include the fissure planes, the hepatic veins, and the fissures for the ligamentum venosum and ligamentum teres (Fig. 5-7A). A combination of

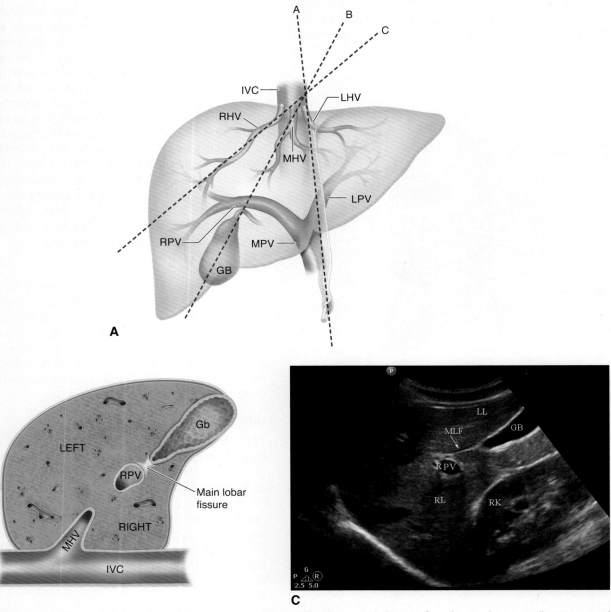

**Figure 5-7** Segmental division. **A.** A "see-through" anterior to posterior profile. The vertical planes, referred to in subsequent illustrations and sonograms, represent approximate scanning levels to document pertinent anatomy. (*GB*, gallbladder; *IVC*, inferior vena cava; *LHV*, left hepatic vein; *LPV*, left portal vein; *MHV*, middle hepatic vein; *MPV*, main portal vein; *RHV*, right hepatic vein; *RPV*, right portal vein. **B–P.** Segmental anatomy. **B.** A sectional illustration through vertical plane 1 (Fig. 5-5A), the main lobar fissure, located between the gallbladder neck and the RPV, divides the liver into the segmental right and left lobes. **C.** A parasagittal scan displays a portion of the main lobar fissure (*MLF*), seen as a linear band extending from the *RPV* to the *GB* separating the right lobe (*RL*) from the left lobe (*LL*). *RK*, right kidney. *(continued)*

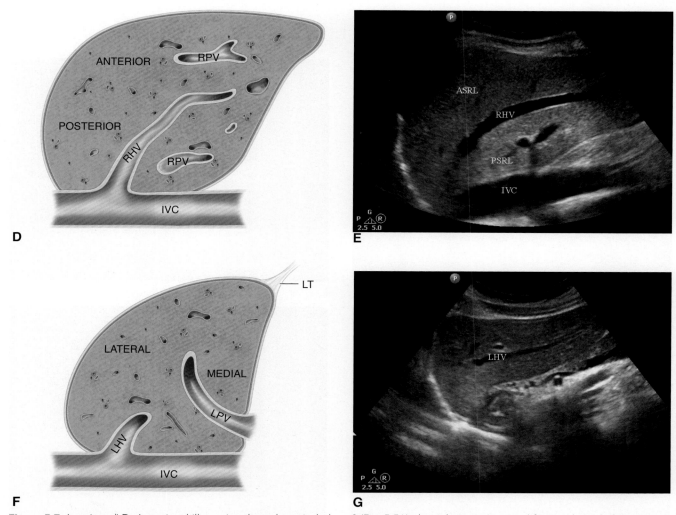

**Figure 5-7** *(continued)* **D.** A sectional illustration through vertical plane 2 (Fig. 5-5A), the right intersegmental fissure, the right hepatic vein (RHV) courses between the right anterior and right posterior branches of the portal vein, which supplies blood to the right lobe. **E.** A parasagittal scan through the *RHV* is the sonographic landmark dividing the right lobe of the liver into anterior and posterior segments. *ASRL,* anterior segment right lobe; *IVC,* inferior vena cava; *PSRL,* posterior segment right lobe. **F.** A sectional illustration through vertical plane 3 (Fig. 5-5A), the left intersegmental fissure, the left hepatic vein divides the left lobe into lateral and medial segments. **G.** A parasagittal scan through the left hepatic vein *(LHV)*. *(continued)*

scanning planes (transverse, oblique, sagittal, and para-sagittal) is needed to delineate all landmarks, which demarcate the lobes and segments.

### Right and Left Lobes

The right and left lobes are separated by the *main lobar fissure* (Fig. 5-7B). Sonographic landmarks that lie within the main lobar fissure are the middle hepatic vein (MHV), the gallbladder, and the IVC fossae. On sagittal or parasagittal scans, the incomplete main lobar fissure may be identified for a short distance between the gallbladder neck and the right portal vein (RPV), seen as an echogenic line (Fig. 5-7C).

The *right intersegmental fissure* divides the right lobe into an anterior segment and a posterior segment. The sonographic landmark for the right intersegmental fissure is the right hepatic vein RHV (Fig. 5-7D,E).

The *left intersegmental fissure* divides the left lobe into a medial and a lateral segment. The sonographic landmarks used to define this fissure are the left hepatic vein (LHV), the ascending branch of the left portal vein (LPV), and, more inferiorly, the hyperechoic ligamentum teres (Fig. 5-7F–I). In patients with ascites, the externally located falciform ligament may be a visible landmark for separation of the medial and lateral segments of the left lobe (Fig. 5-7J).

Hepatic veins run between segments (intersegmental) and lobes (interlobar), whereas portal veins, bile ducts, and hepatic arteries primarily travel within the segments (intrasegmental) (Fig. 5-7K). The RPV divides into the anterior segmental branch and the posterior segmental branch, taking blood to each respective segment (Fig. 5-7L). The LPV subdivides into the medial and lateral left segmental branches

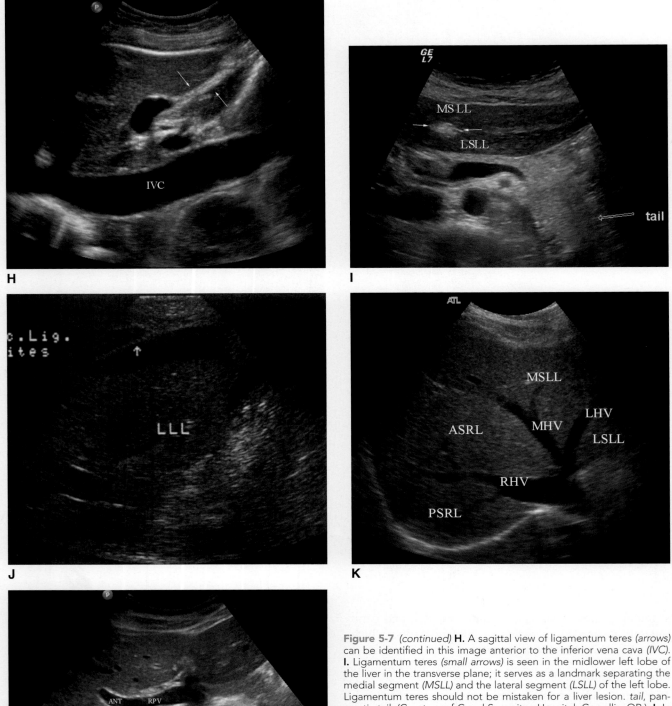

**Figure 5-7** *(continued)* **H.** A sagittal view of ligamentum teres *(arrows)* can be identified in this image anterior to the inferior vena cava *(IVC)*. **I.** Ligamentum teres *(small arrows)* is seen in the midlower left lobe of the liver in the transverse plane; it serves as a landmark separating the medial segment *(MSLL)* and the lateral segment *(LSLL)* of the left lobe. Ligamentum teres should not be mistaken for a liver lesion. *tail*, pancreatic tail. (Courtesy of Good Samaritan Hospital, Corvallis, OR.) **J.** In a patient with ascites, the falciform ligament *(arrow)* can be identified coursing between the anterior abdominal wall and the left lobe of the liver *(LLL)* on this sagittal scan. **K.** A transverse scan fully demonstrates the hepatic veins and liver segments. The middle hepatic vein *(MHV)* separates the right and left liver lobes. The left hepatic vein *(LHV)* separates the *MSLL* from the *LSLL*. The right hepatic vein *(RHV)* divides the anterior segment of the right lobe *(ASRL)* from the posterior segment *(PSRL)*. **L.** A transverse image demonstrates the division of the right portal vein *(RPV)* into anterior *(ANT)* and posterior *(POST)* branches. *(continued)*

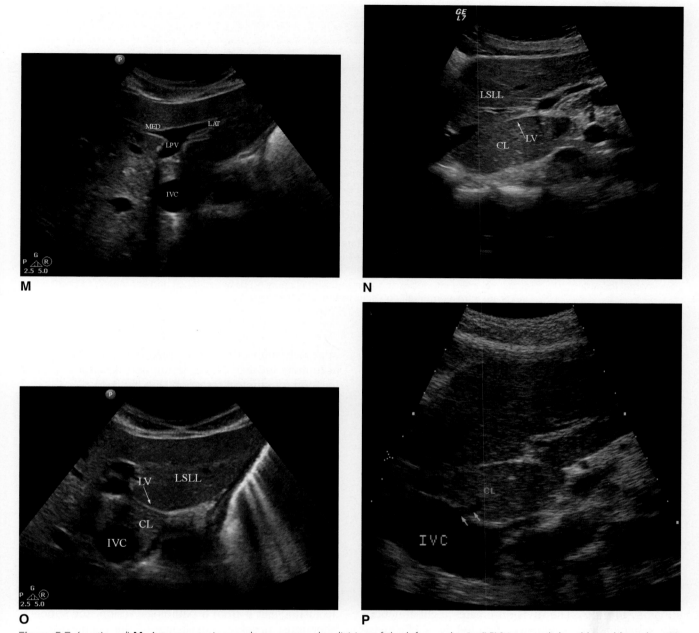

**Figure 5-7** *(continued)* **M.** A transverse image demonstrates the division of the left portal vein *(LPV)* into medial and lateral branches. **N.** A sagittal scan demonstrates the lateral segment *(LSLL)*, which is delineated from the caudate lobe *(CL)* by a linear band representing the ligamentum venosum *(LV)* *(arrow)*. (Image courtesy of Rey Aguila, Kettering Health Network, Kettering, OH.) **O.** The anatomy identified on the transverse scan includes the *LSLL*, which is delineated from the *CL* by the *LV* *(arrow)*. **P.** A parasagittal image demonstrates the small veins *(arrows)* draining directly from the *CL* into the *IVC*.

(Fig. 5-7M). Both portal veins and hepatic veins have distinguishing features on sonography examinations (Table 5-2).

## Caudate Lobe

The caudate lobe corresponds to the anatomic caudate lobe and is separated from the left lobe by the ligamentum venosum. Sonographically, three anatomic landmarks identify the caudate lobe: (1) the fissure for the ligament venosum sharply separates it from the left lobe and appears hyperechoic due to its fat content; (2)

the anechoic IVC appears on the right; and (3) the LPV courses over the anterior margin of the inferior caudate lobe, separating it from the more anterior left hepatic lobe (Fig. 5-7N,O).[19]

The caudate lobe is functionally distinct. It is not considered a right or a left lobe, as it receives its blood supply from both right and left portal radicles and from the hepatic arterial branches and has its own bile ducts.[19,20,22] It is drained by short venous channels that extend directly from the posterior aspect into the IVC (Fig. 5-7P).[19] This independent blood supply has

| TABLE | 5-2 |
| --- | --- |

## Sonographic Criteria for Differentiating the Portal Veins and Hepatic Veins

| | |
| --- | --- |
| Origin and drainage | Observe the point of origin and drainage of the vessels. Portal vein branches can be traced back to the main portal vein, distinguishing them from the hepatic veins draining into the inferior vena cava.[22] |
| Collagen content | Encased in a collagenous sheath and running in common with the hepatic artery and bile duct, the margins of portal veins are highly reflective, making them appear thicker and hyperechoic in contrast to the liver parenchyma.[22,49] By contrast, the hepatic veins are surrounded by parenchymal tissue and have rather imperceptible margins due to a minimal amount of collagen.[22] This is the simplest of the criteria, but it is also the least reliable.[23] A specular reflection may occur if the sound beam strikes the hepatic wall perpendicularly, resulting in a rather high-amplitude, echogenic margin,[23] similar in appearance to the portal vein branches.[22] |
| Branching patterns | An angle is formed by the limbs of a branched systemic venous structure and points in the direction of flow.[23] For the portal vein, branching is horizontal and the angle's apex is oriented toward the porta hepatis.[23,49] Hepatic vein branching is longitudinal, and the angle's apex formed at the communication points superiorly or supermedially toward the inferior vena cava.[23] |
| Caliber changes | The direction of blood flow also dictates the caliber of the venous radicles. The caliber of the hepatic veins becomes greater as it courses toward the inferior vena cava and diaphragm,[49] and the caliber of the portal veins decreases further from its point of origin, the porta hepatis. |
| Segmental location | Hepatic veins are interlobar and intersegmental, coursing between lobes and segments.[16] Portal veins are intrasegmental, coursing within lobar segments.[49] |

significant clinical implications that produce changes in cirrhosis as well as in Budd-Chiari syndrome.[24,25] The portal veins and hepatic arteries of the caudate lobe have a short intrahepatic course, which is not as readily affected by hepatic fibrosis. Caudate lobe enlargement and right lobe shrinkage seen in cirrhosis patients may be attributed to the discrepancy between blood perfusion in the two lobes.[20,25] Caudate lobe enlargement with associated compression of the underlying IVC is implicated in various cirrhotic complications such as IVC hypertension, ascites, portacaval shunt failure, and possibly hepatorenal syndrome (renal failure sometimes seen during the terminal stages of cirrhosis and ascites).

### Couinaud's Anatomy

A widely accepted and more detailed method of liver segmentation was described by C. Couinaud, a French surgeon, in 1957. The division creates eight functionally separate liver segments, counted in a clockwise fashion (Fig. 5-8A). The caudate and left lobes make up segments I through IV and the right lobe segments V through VIII (Table 5-3). The division is based on the hepatic veins and portal vein branches. Each of the eight segments has a central portal vein branch, hepatic artery, and bile duct. The hepatic veins provide the boundaries of each segment. Couinaud's nomenclature provides critical knowledge regarding hepatic surgery, with the potential to perform large resections while minimizing blood loss and morbidity. Major resections of up to 75% of liver tissue can be performed, provided two or three adjacent segments remain uncompromised.

In Couinaud's anatomy, the liver is divided vertically by the three planes of the hepatic veins (right, middle, and left). The liver is then also divided horizontally through the right and left portal veins.[21,26] This sonographic

approach allows the sonographer and the radiologist to accurately localize a liver lesion and describe a precise location for surgical resection (Fig. 5-8B–F).

### Anatomic Variations

Variations in anatomy include situs inversus (Fig. 5-9A,B), normal variations in shape, variations in lobe size, thinning of the left lobe, congenital absence of the left lobe, diaphragmatic indentations (pseudofissures), high posterior hepatodiaphragmatic interposition of the colon, and Reidel's lobe.[3,27,28] Reidel's lobe is an anatomic variant in which an unusually large right lobe gives the impression of hepatomegaly. It is more common in women than in men. Sonographically, Reidel's lobe is identified as a small handle, or a tongue-like projection, on the inferior right lobe that extends distally.[28] The caudal extension may reach as far as the iliac crest (Fig. 5-10A,B). To distinguish it from a pathologic lesion, the sonographer must observe consistency of the echotexture between Reidel's lobe and the right lobe of the liver.

| TABLE | 5-3 |
| --- | --- |

## Couinaud's Anatomy [21,26,27]

| | |
| --- | --- |
| Segment I | Caudate lobe |
| Segment II | Lateral segment of left lobe (superior) |
| Segment III | Lateral segment of left lobe (inferior) |
| Segment IV A | Medial segment of left lobe (superior) |
| Segment IV B | Medial segment of left lobe (inferior) |
| Segment V | Anterior segment of right lobe (inferior) |
| Segment VI | Posterior segment of right lobe (inferior) |
| Segment VII | Posterior segment of right lobe (superior) |
| Segment VIII | Anterior segment of right lobe (superior) |

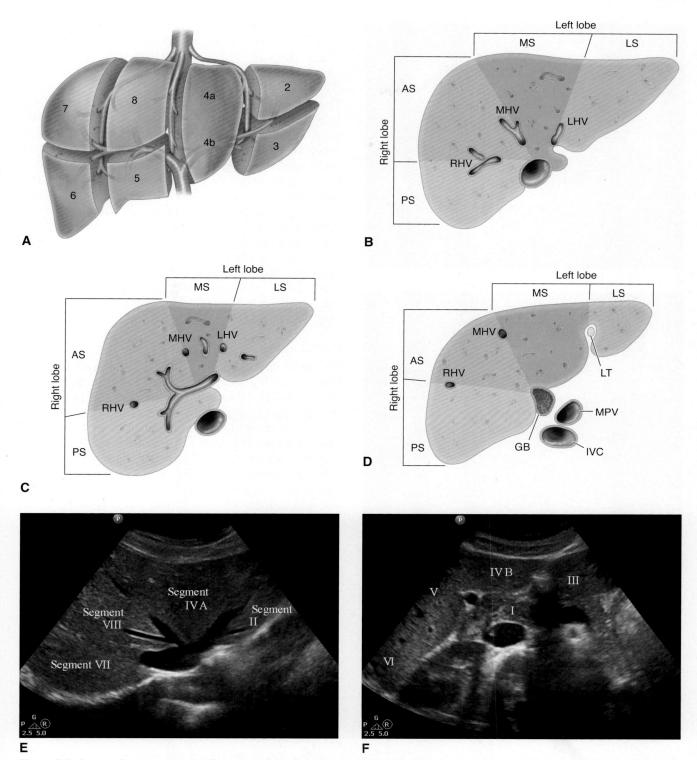

**Figure 5-8** Couinaud's anatomy. **A.** An illustration of the eight segments identified in a clockwise fashion. The hepatic veins divide the liver vertically into four segments and the portal veins divide the liver horizontally creating eight segments. **B.** A cross-sectional illustration high in the liver at the level of the hepatic veins identifies the four superior segments in Couinaud's anatomy (VII, VIII, IVa, and II) including the caudate lobe (I). **C.** A cross-sectional illustration at a midlevel through the liver identifies the right and left portal vein branches that correspond with the horizontal boundary. **D.** A cross-sectional illustration low in the liver at the level of the gallbladder and ligamentum teres identifies the four inferior segments in Couinaud's anatomy (VI, V, IVb, and III). **E.** A transverse scan at the level of the hepatic veins demonstrates the superior segments. **F.** A transverse scan through the gallbladder and ligamentum teres demonstrates the inferior segments.

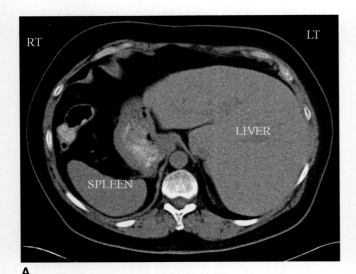

**A**

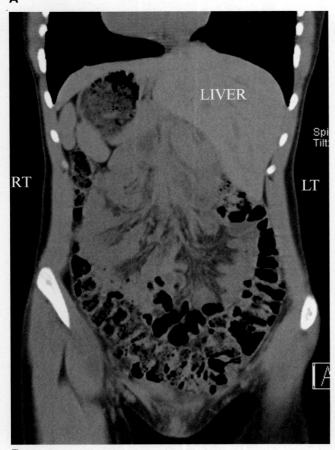

**B**

**Figure 5-9** Situs inversus. **A,B.** Axial and coronal computed tomography of a patient with situs inversus. Note the liver location in the left upper quadrant. (Images courtesy of Kettering Health Network, Kettering, OH.)

## VASCULAR SYSTEM

The liver is unique in that it receives a double blood supply. The hepatic arterial blood is oxygen rich, and the portal venous blood is nutrient rich after it traverses the walls of the gastrointestinal (GI) tract. The blood from the portal vein and hepatic arteries mix in the liver sinusoids and is drained by the hepatic veins (Fig. 5-11A–C).

### Hepatic Arteries

The common hepatic artery branches off the celiac axis and passes anterior and to the right to enter the right margin of the gastrohepatic ligament. Here it ascends, lying to the left of the common bile duct and anterior to the portal vein. As it turns cephalad, it gives origin to the gastroduodenal artery, the supraduodenal artery, and the right gastric artery. The proper hepatic artery is the continuation of the artery beyond the bifurcation of these vessels. It ascends and divides into several branches, most commonly into a right and a left ramus, which supply the right and left segmental lobes, respectively. The cystic artery arises off the right ramus, and the middle hepatic artery usually arises from the left ramus (Fig. 5-11D–H).

### Portal Veins

The MPV originates just to the right of midline at the junction of the splenic vein and superior mesenteric vein (SMV) and then courses cephalad and to the right into the porta hepatis.[22,29] At this point, the MPV normally measures 11 ± 2 mm (range, 6 to 15 mm), is anterior to the IVC, and is cephalad to the head of the pancreas (Fig. 5-11C,I). The MPV divides into a smaller LPV somewhat to the right of midline, more anterior and cranial, and into a larger RPV located more posterior and caudal.

The LPV courses cranially along the anterior surface of the caudate lobe, then arches, curving toward the left and anteriorly prior to its major bifurcation, giving a branch that courses back to the right to supply the medial segment of the left lobe (quadrate lobe)[22] and a branch for the lateral segment of the left lobe (Fig. 5-11J). Both are intrasegmental in their course.[29] Prior to the bifurcation is the umbilical portion, named because in utero, the umbilical vein is attached at this point.[22] The umbilical portion provides a blood supply to the caudate lobe through small branches that are not visualized sonographically.[22] The size of the LPV and its angle of bifurcation with the MPV vary, depending largely on the size and configuration of the left lobe.[17]

The main segment of the RPV is larger than the LPV, bifurcates from the MPV farther posterior, and has a long horizontal course.[20] It can be identified sonographically as a round or ovoid vessel positioned centrally in the right hepatic lobe. It bifurcates at various distances from the MPV to supply the right anterior and right posterior intrahepatic lobar segments (Fig. 5-11K–N).[3]

The common hepatic and intrahepatic ducts and the portal veins normally course parallel to each

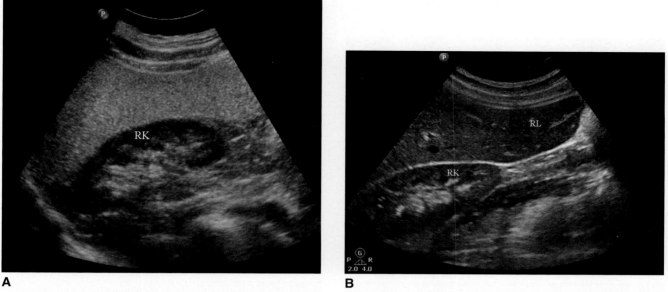

**Figure 5-10** Reidel's lobe. **A.** A Reidel's lobe can be seen on this image of a 36-year-old woman as an extension distal to the right kidney *(RK)*. **B.** This patient's Reidel's lobe *(RL)* extended well beyond the inferior margin of the right kidney *(RK)* into the right flank area. (Courtesy of Katie Strayer, Kettering College, Kettering, OH.)

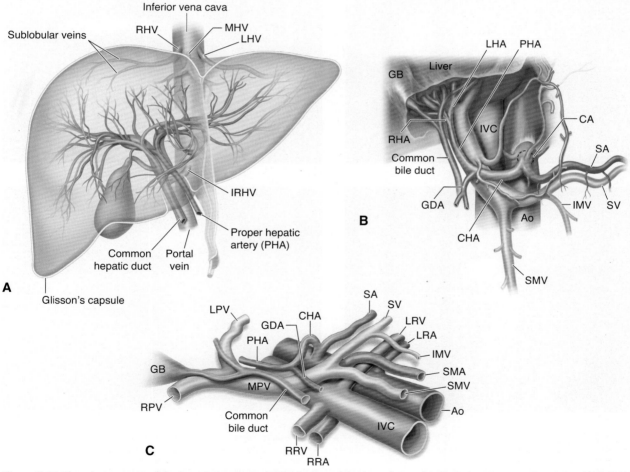

**Figure 5-11** Vascular anatomy of the liver. **A.** Intrahepatic distribution of the hepatic arteries, hepatic veins, portal veins, and biliary ducts. An accessory right hepatic vein draining directly into the inferior vena cava *(IVC)* is a variant identified in some patients. *IRHV*, inferior right hepatic vein; *LHV*, left hepatic vein; *MHV*, middle hepatic vein; *RHV*, right hepatic vein. **B.** The vessels and ducts of the upper abdomen. *Ao*, aorta; *CA*, celiac axis; *CHA*, common hepatic artery; *GB*, gallbladder; *GDA*, gastroduodenal artery; *IMV*, inferior mesenteric vein; *IVC*, inferior vena cava; *MPV*, main portal vein; *PHA*, proper hepatic artery; *SA*, splenic artery; *SMV*, superior mesenteric vein; *SV*, splenic vein. **C.** A recumbent view of the relationship between the vessels and ducts of the upper abdomen. *Ao*, aorta; *CHA*, common hepatic artery; *GB*, gallbladder; *GDA*, gastroduodenal artery; *IMV*, inferior mesenteric vein; *IVC*, inferior vena cava; *LPV*, left portal vein; *LRA*, left renal artery; *LRV*, left renal vein; *MPV*, main portal vein; *PHA*, proper hepatic artery; *RPV*, right portal vein; *RRA*, right renal artery; *RRV*, right renal vein; *SA*, splenic artery; *SMA*, superior mesenteric artery; *SMV*, superior mesenteric vein; *SV* , splenic vein. *(continued)*

115

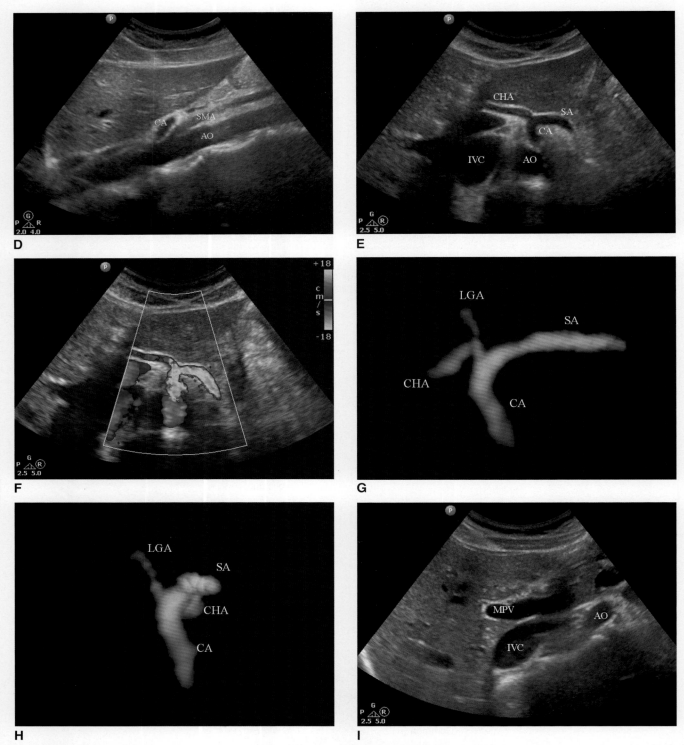

**Figure 5-11** *(continued)* **D.** A sagittal scan of the abdominal aorta *(AO)*, the celiac artery *(CA)*, and the superior mesenteric artery *(SMA)*. **E.** A transverse midline scan images the common hepatic artery *(CHA)*, splenic artery *(SA)*, celiac artery *(CA)*, aorta *(AO)*, and inferior vena cava *(IVC)*. **F.** Color Doppler image of the celiac artery and its branches. **G.** A three-dimensional (3D) power Doppler view with grayscale subtraction displays the *CA* branching into the *SA*, *CHA*, and the least often detected third branch, the left gastric artery *(LGA)*. **H.** A lateral view of the same 3D dataset offering superior visualization of the *LGA*. **I.** On an oblique section, the main portal vein *(MPV)* can be seen anterior to the *IVC*. *AO*, aorta. *(continued)*

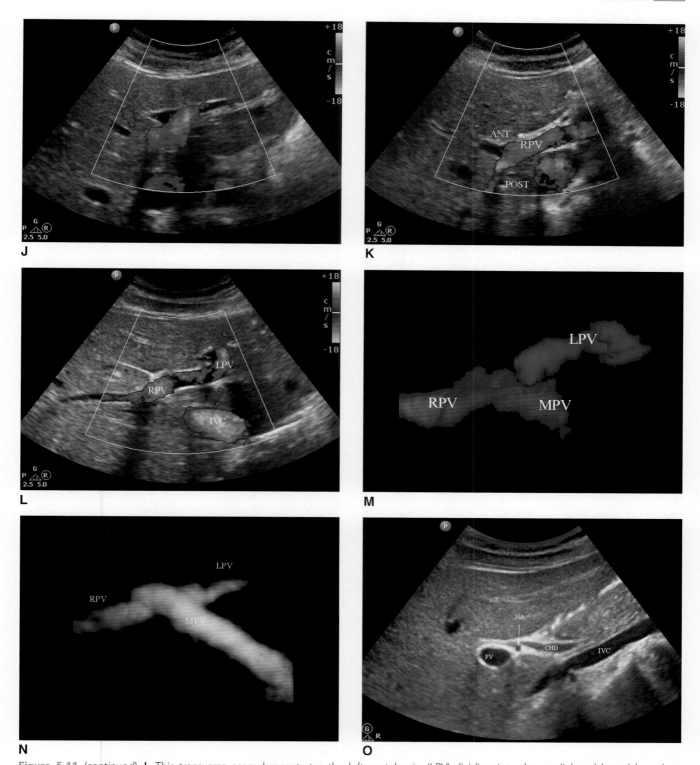

**Figure 5-11** *(continued)* **J.** This transverse scan demonstrates the left portal vein *(LPV)* dividing into the medial and lateral branches. **K.** A transverse scan shows the right portal vein *(RPV)* dividing into the anterior *(ANT)* and posterior *(POST)* segmental branches. **L.** An oblique color Doppler scan through the *RPV* and *LPV* demonstrates flow away from the transducer *(blue)* in the *RPV* branch and flow toward the transducer *(red)* in the *LPV* branch. *IVC,* inferior vena cava. **M.** A 3D reconstruction of the portal venous color Doppler signal with grayscale subtraction reveals the main portal vein *(MPV)*, *RPV*, and *LPV*. **N.** A 3D power Doppler grayscale subtraction image demonstrates the T-shaped bifurcation of the portal veins. **O.** Normal architecture of the relationship of the common bile duct *(CBD)* with the portal vein *(PV)* and hepatic artery *(HA)*. (Image courtesy of Stephanie Nieport, Kettering College, Kettering, OH.) *(continued)*

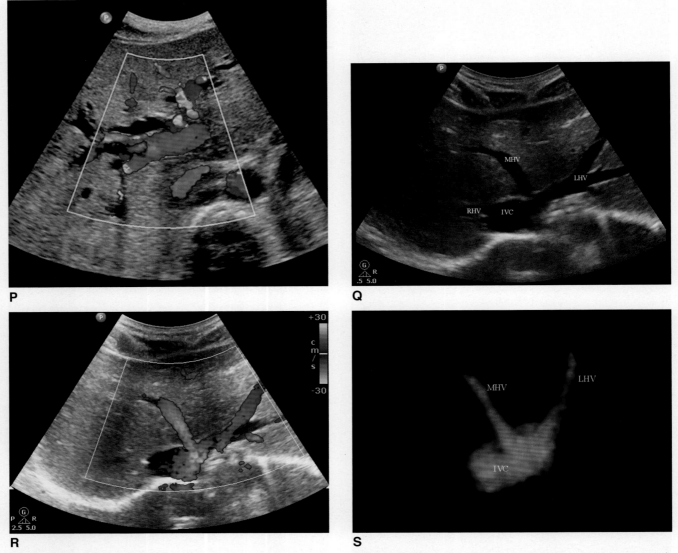

**Figure 5-11** *(continued)* **P.** The parallel-channel sign represents dilated bile ducts (structures void of color) and the portal veins (vessels with color). **Q.** The right hepatic vein *(RHV)*, middle hepatic vein *(MHV)*, and left hepatic vein *(LHV)* are seen in this transverse scan draining into the inferior vena cava *(IVC)*. Transducer placement is high in the liver. **R.** On the transverse color-flow image, the hepatic veins appear with hepatofugal flow representing flow exiting the liver. **S.** A 3D power Doppler grayscale subtraction image captures the "Playboy bunny" sign of the *IVC, MHV,* and *LHV.*

other; however, venous blood and bile flow in opposite directions (Fig. 5-11O). Intrahepatic ducts are not visualized routinely. If biliary radicles and portal venous radicles are imaged simultaneously side by side, the appearance, referred to as the *parallel-channel sign,* is used to diagnose biliary obstruction (Fig. 5-11P).

### Hepatic Veins

Hepatic veins are best visualized on transverse scans in the cephalad portion of the liver. They drain directly into the superior aspect of the IVC and all three should be demonstrated routinely: the RHV, the MHV, and the LHV (Fig. 5-11Q–S).

The RHV is the largest of the hepatic veins.[30] It courses between the anterior and posterior branches of the RPV,[31] is located in the right intersegmental fissure, and divides the cephalic aspect of the anterior and posterior segments of the right hepatic lobe.[29,30] The MHV is located in the main lobar fissure corresponding to the segmental division of the right and left lobes.[29] The smaller LHV is located in the cephalic portion of the left intersegmental fissure, dividing the left lobe into lateral and medial intrahepatic segments.[30]

The inferior right hepatic vein (IRHV) is a variant and can be difficult to visualize. It was identified in only 10% of the cases by Makuuchi and coworkers[32] but in 15.5% of liver examinations in a study by Sunder.[30]

When it can be identified, it is visualized on a transverse section at the level of the porta hepatis, on a longitudinal section situated behind the right portal venous branch,[30,32] or in a right intercostal coronal section; it measures 3 to 8 mm in diameter (Fig. 5-11A).[30] When identified, it may present as a *pseudo-parallel-channel sign* as it crosses the liver posteriorly and parallel to the right portal venous branch in the posteroinferior segment of the right lobe.[32] Attempting to identify an IRHV variant is clinically important for several reasons: (1) the entire main RHV is resected during hepatectomy because the right lobe can be preserved along with the hypertrophic IRHV; (2) thrombus has been identified in the IRHV in patients with hepatocellular carcinoma (HCC); (3) the right lobe's main drainage vein is the IRHV, as seen in primary Budd-Chiari syndrome; and (4) obstruction of the bile ducts presents a real parallel-channel sign, which needs to be differentiated from a false one.[32]

### Sonographic Distinction

The portal and hepatic vascular system is extremely important to identify sonographically. With ligaments, fissures, and fossae, it provides an important map for localizing specific abnormalities, affords the ability to distinguish dilated portions of the biliary tree, and can be used to perform follow-up examinations. The five criteria used to distinguish hepatic veins and portal veins are described in Table 5-2 and can be identified by comparing Figure 5-11I–S.

### PORTA HEPATIS

The porta (gate) hepatis (liver) is a fissure where the portal vein and hepatic artery enter the liver and the bile duct exits the liver.[2] In the normal relationship of these three structures within the hepatoduodenal ligament, the bile duct is ventral and lateral, the hepatic artery is ventral and medial, and the portal vein is dorsal (Fig. 5-11B,C).[2]

It is important to evaluate these structures and measure the bile duct in either a transverse or longitudinal section. To do this, locate the splenic vein on a transverse section and follow it to the right, where it is joined by the SMV and becomes the portal-splenic confluence (Fig. 5-12A). From the confluence, the MPV will course toward the liver and appear round. Oblique the transducer approximately 45 degrees (from right shoulder to left hip) until the long axis of the MPV, bile duct, and hepatic artery are identified (Fig. 5-12B). Make a measurement of the bile duct by placing the calipers along the inner wall to the opposing inner wall of the duct. Published values for the normal internal diameter of the bile duct vary from 4 to 8 mm. A transverse section through the portal triad has a Mickey Mouse appearance (Fig. 5-12C).

The bile duct and hepatic artery may be confused because of their proximity, their similar internal diameter (maximum internal diameter of the hepatic artery is reported to be 2 to 6 mm), and the common anatomic variations of the triad structures. Color Doppler can be particularly useful in distinguishing the bile duct from the hepatic artery due to the presence of flow in the artery and absence of flow in the bile duct (Fig. 5-12D,E). In addition, Berland and colleagues[33] found several reliable sonographic signs to differentiate the bile duct and hepatic artery, including evaluating the porta hepatis with Doppler techniques:

1. Only intrinsic pulsations should be exhibited by an artery or a vein.
2. A crossing artery can sharply indent a duct or a vein; the reverse is not true, probably owing to the lower venous and ductal pressures and a thicker, less easily deformed arterial wall.
3. The duct can occasionally decrease several millimeters in caliber during an examination and can have various calibers along its course, whereas arteries are uniform in caliber.
4. The artery may not parallel the vein or may do so only for a short distance, whereas the duct parallels the vein closely.
5. Arteries may be tortuous and loop in and out of the scanning plane.
6. Arteries produce pulsatile Doppler signals, veins produce continuous Doppler signals, and ducts produce no signal.

### MICROSCOPIC STRUCTURES

Hepatic lobes are made up of the basic functional unit: the liver lobule.[5,6] The liver parenchyma is made up of 50,000 to 100,000 individual lobules (Fig. 5-13A,B).[2,34] Within each lobule, small bile canaliculi lie adjacent to the cellular plates, receive the bile produced by the hepatocytes,[13,35] and carry it toward the bile duct branches in the triad regions (Fig. 5-13C).[6] These branches open into the interlobular bile ducts accompanying the hepatic artery and portal vein, except that bile flows in the direction opposite that of blood in these vessels.[2,6] Bile ducts join other bile ducts and form two main trunks, the right and left hepatic ducts, which eventually drain into the common hepatic duct.[6,7] The biliary duct walls consist of a connective tissue coat composed of muscle cells arranged both concentrically and longitudinally and an epithelial layer consisting of short columnar cells resting on a distinct basement membrane.[2,3]

## PHYSIOLOGY

The liver is an organ essential to life, as it performs more than 500 separate activities.[36] A single liver cell is so diversified in its activities that it is analogous to

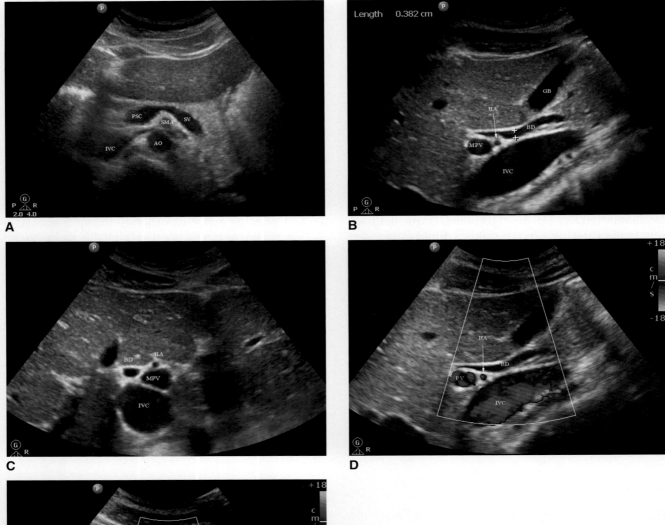

**Figure 5-12** Normal portal triad. **A.** A transverse section visualizes the splenic vein *(SV)* and portal-splenic confluence *(PSC)*. Locating the confluence at the level of the pancreas helps identify the formation of the main portal vein. **B.** An oblique section of the long axis of the portal triad demonstrates the dorsal main portal vein *(MPV)*, the ventral bile duct *(BD)*, and the hepatic artery *(HA)* coursing between the two structures. **C.** A scan through the cross-sectional portal triad has a Mickey Mouse silhouette: the *MPV* represents the face, the *BD* and *HA* represent the ears. **D.** A color Doppler scan of the long axis of the portal triad demonstrates flow within the portal vein *(PV)* and *HA* with absence of flow in the *BD*. **E.** A transverse, color-flow image confirms the same flow direction (hepatopetal) of the *PV* and toward the liver with no flow detected in the *BD*. *AO*, aorta; *GB*, gallbladder; *IVC*, inferior vena cava. (Courtesy of Angela Buehler, Kettering College, Kettering, OH.)

a factory for many chemical compounds; to a warehouse with short and long-term storage capabilities; to a power plant producing heat; to a waste disposal plant excreting waste; and to a chemist regenerating tissue that has not been too severely damaged. These functions are carried out by three types of cells in the parenchyma: the hepatocyte, which carries out most metabolic functions; the biliary epithelial cells, which line the biliary system, bile ducts, canaliculi, and gallbladder; and the Kupffer cells, which are phagocytic and belong to the reticuloendothelial system.[4]

It is not necessary to know all of these liver functions in great detail to obtain quality sonograms; however, because hepatic diseases alter these functions and produce identifiable clinical manifestations, it is important

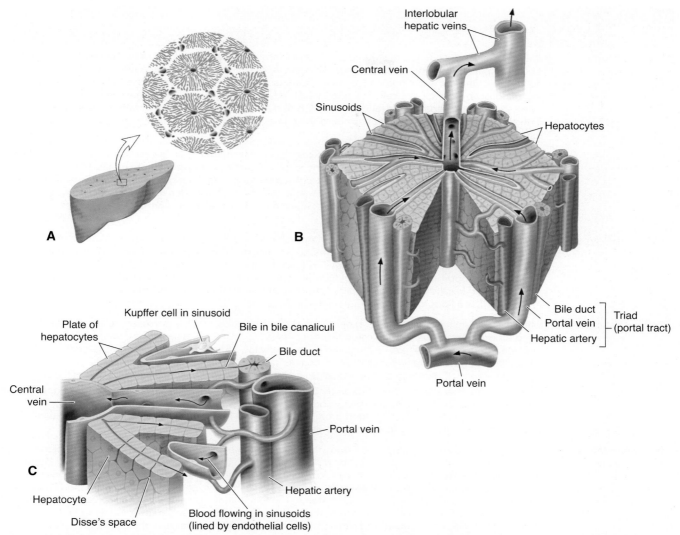

**Figure 5-13** Microscopic anatomy. **A.** An enlarged sectional cut of the liver shows the hexagonal or cylindrical shape of its lobules. Each lobule measures several millimeters in length and 0.8 to 2 mm in diameter.[2,4,35] **B.** The *arrows* indicate the direction of blood flow on this representation of one liver lobule. Constructed around a central hepatic vein, each lobule is composed principally of many cellular plates, or hepatocytes, the functional cells of the liver. The cellular plates radiate centrifugally from the central hepatic vein like wheel spokes.[4,35] Hepatocytes are capable of regenerating, which allows damaged or resected liver tissue to regrow.[13] A lobule has six corners. At each corner is a portal triad, so named because three basic structures are always present: a branch of the hepatic artery, a branch of the portal vein, and a bile duct.[6,7] **C.** An enlarged schematic view of a small portion of one liver lobule illustrates the sinusoids and portal triad. Sinusoids are small capillaries that have a highly permeable endothelial lining located between the cellular plates. They receive a mixture of portal venous and hepatic arterial blood.[4,13,35] The blood drains into the central hepatic vein in the middle of each lobule and flows into the interlobular hepatic veins.[13,35] Unlike other capillaries, sinusoids are also lined with phagocytic cells known as *Kupffer cells*.[5,6,13] Kupffer cells belong to the reticuloendothelial system and function to remove foreign substances from the blood, such as bacteria and depleted white and red blood cells.[5,6,36] Disse space, located between the endothelial lining and the hepatocyte, drains interstitial fluid into the hepatic lymph system.[13,35] Small bile canaliculi are adjacent to the cellular plates and receive the bile produced by the hepatocytes.[13,35]

to have a basic understanding of some normal functions (Table 5-4).

## LIVER FUNCTION TESTS

Liver enzyme names can generally be recognized because they normally end in *-ase*, but laboratory function tests are sometimes named with initials. Thus, ALP may not be immediately recognized as an enzyme test for alkaline phosphatase. Adding to the confusion, the transaminases often referred to in the literature have new names that are more chemically correct. Serum glutamic pyruvic transaminase (SGPT) is now called *alanine aminotransferase* (*ALT*), and serum glutamic oxaloacetic transaminase (SGOT) is now called *aspartate aminotransferase* (*AST*).

Alterations in any of the normal liver functions can produce a spectrum of disorders that can severely impair some liver functions and leave others entirely unaffected. Obstruction to the intrahepatic or extrahepatic biliary system or damage to the hepatocyte or Kupffer cells can alter the plasma chemistry. Understanding the

**TABLE 5-4**

## Hepatic Functions

| | |
|---|---|
| Bile formation and secretion | Bilirubin, or bile pigment, is a major end product resulting from the breakdown of hemoglobin by Kupffer cells[13] and other reticuloendothelial cells.[4] Bilirubin, bound to plasma protein, travels via the bloodstream to the liver, where it is conjugated (i.e., made water soluble) and excreted into bile. Bile is produced continuously by the hepatic cells at a rate of 700 to 1,200 mL a day.[13] Bile salts are formed from cholesterol in the hepatic cells, and emulsify fats and assist in the absorption of fatty acids from the intestinal tract.[4] Calculus formation occurs if the bile salt content is abnormally high due to cholesterol precipitation. |
| Carbohydrate metabolism | The liver acts as a glucose buffer. It removes excess glucose from the blood, stores it, and returns it to the blood when the glucose concentration begins to fall.[13] Functions of carbohydrate metabolism include (1) glycogenesis, the conversion of glucose to glycogen for storage[4]; (2) glycogenolysis, the reduction of glycogen to glucose[35]; and (3) gluconeogenesis, formation of glycogen from noncarbohydrates such as protein, amino acids, and fatty acids, which maintains a relatively normal blood glucose concentration.[4,13] |
| Fat metabolism | Fatty acids are a source of metabolic energy.[13] Approximately 60% of all preliminary breakdown of fatty acids occurs in the liver. Functions of fat metabolism include (1) $\beta$-oxidation of fatty acids and formation of acetoacetic acid, a soluble acid that passes from the liver cells into the extracellular fluid[4]; (2) formation of lipoprotein by synthesis of fat from glucose and amino acids[35]; (3) formation of cholesterol, which forms bile salts and phospholipids[4]; and (4) conversion of proteins and carbohydrates to fat to be transported as a lipoprotein for storage in the adipose tissue.[13] |
| Protein metabolism | Protein metabolism functions include (1) deamination of amino acids, which is necessary before they can be used for energy or converted into carbohydrates or fats[13]; (2) formation of urea by the liver, removing ammonia from the body fluid[4]; (3) formation of approximately 85% of the plasma proteins (except approximately 45% of the $\gamma$-globulins) at a maximum rate of 50 to 100 g per day[4,35]; and (4) interconversions or synthesizing of amino acids and other compounds vital to the metabolism of the body.[4]<br><br>The reticuloendothelial tissue performs an essential part in protein anabolism by synthesizing various blood proteins (prothrombin, bilinogen, albumins, accelerator globulin, factor VII) and other less important coagulation factors.[5,7] Blood proteins are essential for normal circulation, as they maintain water balance, contributing to the blood's viscosity.[6] |
| Reticuloendothelial tissue activity | The activity of the reticuloendothelial tissue in the liver starts before birth with the production of blood cells, a process called *hemopoiesis*.[1,7] By birth, this function is carried out by the bone marrow.[13] Plasma has three major types of protein: albumin, globulin, and fibrinogen.[4] All of the albumin and fibrinogen and 50% or more of the globulins are formed in the liver.[13] The rest of the globulins are formed by the lymphatic and other reticuloendothelial systems. The function of albumins is to provide colloid osmotic pressure, which prevents plasma loss from the capillaries. Fibrinogen polymerizes into long fibrin threads during blood coagulation, forming blood clots to help repair leaks in the circulatory system. Globulins perform a number of enzymatic functions in the plasma. The principal function of globulins is to provide natural and acquired immunity against invading organisms.[4,13]<br><br>After a circulation time of approximately 120 days, red blood cells die.[13,35] It is assumed that these cells simply wear out with age and rupture during passage through a tight spot in the circulatory system.[6] The reticuloendothelial tissue of the spleen and the liver digests the hemoglobin released from the ruptured red blood cells.[5] In this process, the iron from destroyed red cells is released back into the blood, bone marrow, or to other tissues.[4,35]<br><br>Large numbers of bacteria invade the body through the intestinal tract, passing through the mucosa into the portal blood. The sinuses of the liver where the blood passes are lined with Kupffer cells, which are tissue macrophages.[13] Kupffer cells form an effective particulate filtration system.[4,35] Almost all of the bacteria from the GI tract undergo phagocytosis.[49] |
| Storage depot | The liver has the capacity to store enough vitamin A to prevent a deficiency for as long as 1–2 years[4] and enough vitamin D and vitamin $B_{12}$ to prevent deficiency for 1–4 months.[4] The liver also stores glycogen, fats, and amino acids and can metabolize them into glucose or vice versa, depending on the body's needs.[13]<br><br>Aside from iron in the hemoglobin, by far the greatest proportion of iron is stored in the liver in the form of ferritin. When the body becomes iron deficient, the ferritin releases iron.[4] The liver is also the storage depot for copper and for some poisons that cannot be broken down or detoxified and excreted, such as dichlorodiphenyltrichloroethane. |
| Blood reservoir | Approximately 1,000–1,100 mL of blood flows from the portal vein through the liver sinusoids each minute, and another 350–400 mL flows through the hepatic artery.[4] As a blood reservoir, the liver has the capacity to enlarge and store 200–400 mL of blood with a rise of only 4–8 mm Hg in hepatic venous pressure. If there is hemorrhage and large amounts of blood are being lost in the circulatory system, the liver releases its blood from that stored in the sinusoids to help compensate for this loss in blood volume.[13] |

| TABLE 5-4 *(continued)* | |
|---|---|
| **Hepatic Functions** | |
| Heat production | The liver, a significant metabolizer, produces heat as a result of its chemical reactions. On average, 55% of the energy of food ingested becomes heat during adenosine triphosphate (ATP) formation. Even more heat is produced during the ATP cell formation process.[13] |
| Detoxification | To a great degree, the liver is a detoxifier, converting chemicals, foreign molecules, and hormones to compounds that are not as toxic or biologically active.[13] When amino acids are burned for energy, they leave behind toxic nitrogenous wastes that are converted to urea by the liver cells. These moderate amounts of urea are then easily removed by the kidney or sweat glands.[4] |
| Lymph formation | Under resting conditions, the liver produces between one-third and one-half of all the body's lymph. |

major tests performed to evaluate liver function helps in correlating the clinical history and presenting symptoms (especially in distinguishing obstructive from nonobstructive jaundice) with the sonographic visualization of hepatobiliary structures. The more common laboratory examinations are listed in Table 5-5. Because normal ranges vary by sex, age, and geographic region, they are not represented; usually they appear in parentheses on a laboratory report with an abnormal enzyme level clearly marked as high or low.

## SONOGRAPHIC EXAMINATION TECHNIQUE

### INDICATIONS FOR EXAMINATION

Indications for a sonographic examination of the liver may include the following: anorexia, fatigue and weakness, abdominal discomfort, fever, abnormal liver function tests (LFTs), jaundice, and hepatomegaly.[27] Other indications may include evaluating liver transplant patients, follow-up examination from positive findings on computed tomography (CT), serial evaluation of liver abscesses or tumors, evaluating the cancer patient for liver metastasis, and guidance for invasive procedures.

### PATIENT PREPARATION

Most of the liver can be visualized without special patient preparation, but because initial liver examinations should include a comprehensive study of all upper abdominal organs, the patient should fast (taking nothing by mouth) for 6 to 8 hours before the study. Patients who fast for longer periods may drink water to avoid dehydration. Patients should abstain from smoking, chewing gum, and excessive talking—activities that increase the amount of intestinal gas.

### PATIENT INSTRUCTIONS

#### Breathing Instructions

Normal and deep suspended inspiration techniques are generally used for optimizing sonographic liver assessment. A belly-out technique, which is accomplished

by pushing out the anterior abdomen by contracting the diaphragm, may occasionally be helpful. Both techniques allow the liver to descend below the ribs, displace bowel gas inferiorly, and provide better visualization. Suspended respiration often is best for intercostal imaging.

#### Patient Positioning

A subcostal and/or intercostal imaging approach is common while scanning the liver, with the patient in a variety of recumbent positions. Expansion of the rib spaces can be aided by having the patient raise the arms and place the hands near or under the head. The study begins with the patient in a supine position for initial documentation of liver size and anatomic evaluation. Additional planes may be imaged with the patient in the left posterior oblique and right posterior oblique positions. As the patient gradually shifts from the left posterior oblique position to the left lateral decubitus position, the right lobe of the liver typically descends inferiorly and rotates medially to expose more of the superior portion. With intercostal probe placement, the oblique or decubitus position may offer better visualization of the portal vein and common hepatic duct. The IVC also moves in position and can be identified anterior to the aorta. Patients with hepatomegaly should be examined in the oblique or decubitus position because, in the supine position, the large liver normally compresses the IVC. The lower liver segment may be better visualized with the patient in the right posterior oblique position. This allows the liver to displace the duodenum and transverse colon inferiorly.[17] Owing to the effects of gravity, an erect or semierect position may expose even more liver tissue.

### SCANNING TECHNIQUE

The liver is systematically evaluated in both the sagittal and transverse planes. Additional oblique scanning planes are utilized as necessary until the entire liver parenchyma, ligaments, fissures, vessels, bile ducts, and retroperitoneal spaces are adequately evaluated. Attention is paid to the size and echotexture of the liver, the

**TABLE  5-5**

## Liver Function Tests[37–41]

| Test | Explanation | Result | Clinical Indication |
|------|-------------|--------|---------------------|
| Bilirubin | Formed in large part from heme of destroyed erythrocytes or from breakdown of developing red blood cells in bone marrow or other hemoproteins. Heme is converted to biliverdin in the spleen, kidney, and liver. | Indirect increase | Diseases that cause hemolysis, such as hemolytic jaundice; diseases that affect the liver's ability to conjugate, such as Gilbert syndrome or Crigler-Najjar syndrome. |
|  | Unconjugated bilirubin, formed from biliverdin, is not water soluble and is not excreted in urine. Unconjugated, or direct, bilirubin is bound to albumin and transported to liver cells. Bilirubin is conjugated by liver enzymes, becomes water soluble, is not protein bound, and is excreted in urine. | Direct increase | Hepatocellular jaundice from hepatitis or cirrhosis; with decreased albumin and increased enzymes, parenchymal or obstructive liver disease; intrahepatic cholestasis from hepatic drug reactions, alcoholic hepatitis, primary biliary cirrhosis, or gram-negative septicemia; posthepatic jaundice from lower biliary tract obstruction. |
|  | Most laboratories report the total value and the direct (conjugated) value. The indirect (unconjugated) value is calculated by subtracting the direct value from the total. |  |  |
| Alanine aminotransferase (ALT), formerly serum glutamic pyruvic transaminase (SGPT) | Necessary enzyme in Krebs cycle for tissue energy production; largest amounts in the liver, smaller amounts in the kidney, heart, and skeletal muscle. When damage to these tissues occurs, ALT increases. ALT is a rather specific indicator of hepatocellular damage. It is used in conjunction with AST to help distinguish between cardiac and hepatic damage. AST levels are very high and ALT levels are only mildly elevated with cardiac damage. ALT can differentiate between hemolytic jaundice when there is no rise in ALT and jaundice due to liver disease with high ALT levels. Hepatitis, cirrhosis, Reye syndrome, and toxic drug treatment can be monitored with ALT. | Increase | Liver cell damage due to hepatitis, cirrhosis, or liver tumors. Reye syndrome, or biliary tract obstruction; other diseases involving the liver, heart failure, alcohol or drug abuse; elevated with some renal diseases, some musculoskeletal diseases, systemic lupus erythematosus, other conditions that cause trauma or hypoxia, and hemolysis. Ratio of AST to ALT can be meaningful. AST levels are higher in cirrhosis and metastatic carcinoma of the liver. ALT levels are usually higher in acute hepatitis and nonmalignant hepatic obstruction. |
| Aspartate aminotransferase (AST), formerly serum glutamic oxaloacetic transaminase (SGOT) | Enzyme found in all tissues, but largest amounts in cells that use the most energy, such as liver, heart, and skeletal muscles. AST is released with injury to cells. | Increase | In hepatitis, elevated before jaundice appears; cirrhosis, shock, or trauma may cause lesser elevation; other conditions include Reye syndrome and pulmonary infarction. Damaged cardiac cells have other correlating examinations. Ratio of AST to ALT is significant (see ALT). |
| Alkaline phosphatase (ALP) | Enzyme in the tissues of liver, bone, intestine, kidney, placenta; higher levels are normal with new bone formation in children and in pregnancy; normally excreted in bile. | Increase | Biliary obstruction from tumors or space-occupying lesions, hepatitis, metastatic liver carcinoma, pancreatic head carcinoma, cholelithiasis, or biliary atresia; elevation may also occur from bone or kidney origin and from congestive heart failure due to hepatic blood flow obstruction. |
| Lactic dehydrogenase (LDH) | An enzyme in all tissues, LDH normally is not used for liver evaluation because other enzyme values are more specific. LDH4 and LDH5 are found in liver, skeletal, kidney, placenta, and striated muscle tissue. | Increase $LDH_4$ and $LDH_5$ | Liver damage due to cirrhosis, chronic viral hepatitis, etc. |

| TABLE 5-5 | (continued) |
|---|---|

## Liver Function Tests[37-41]

| Test | Explanation | Result | Clinical Indication |
|---|---|---|---|
| γ-Glutamyl transpeptidase (GGTP or GGT) | Responsible for the transport of amino acid and peptide across cell membranes, it is found chiefly in liver, kidney, and pancreas, with smaller amounts in other tissues. The test is the most sensitive indicator of alcoholism and is also sensitive to other liver diseases. | Increase | Marked elevation in liver disease and posthepatic obstruction; moderate elevation with liver damage from alcohol, drugs, chemotherapy; elevation may also be due to pancreatic, kidney, prostate, heart, lung, or spleen disease. |
| Prothrombin time (PT) | Test used to determine pathologic deficiency of clotting factors due either to liver dysfunction or to absence of vitamin K. | Increase | Correlated with obstructive disease, PT can be corrected with parenteral vitamin K; when correlated with parenchymal disease, scarred nonfunctioning liver tissue does not produce prothrombin. |
| Albumin | The smallest protein molecule, it makes up the largest proportion of total serum protein. It is almost totally synthesized by the liver. Albumin plays an important role in total water distribution or osmotic pressure because of its high molecular weight. With dehydration, albumin levels increase. A lack of albumin in the serum allows fluid to leak out into the interstitial spaces and into the peritoneal cavity. | Decrease<br><br><br><br><br>Increase | Chronic liver disease, especially cirrhosis; ascites from cirrhosis, right-sided heart failure, cancer, or peritonitis; other conditions related to the GI tract, inflammation, pregnancy, and aging.<br>Hemolysis, other conditions related to dehydration, exercise, anxiety, depression. |
| Albumin/globulin (A/G) ratio | Albumin divided by globulins equals the ratio. When evaluating liver disease, serum globulin is produced by the Kupffer cells and albumin is synthesized in the liver. In chronic liver disease, the A/G ratio is reversed where albumin is decreased and globulin is elevated. | Decreased total protein with decreased albumin and elevated globulin (reversed A/G ratio) | Chronic liver disease, especially cirrhosis, ascites from cirrhosis; right-sided heart failure, cancers, or peritonitis and other conditions related to the GI tract; and inflammation, pregnancy, and aging. |
| α-Fetoprotein (AFP) | A globulin formed in yolk sac and fetal liver, it is normally present only in trace amounts after birth; produced with primary carcinoma of the liver and certain types of testicular cancer. | Increase | In nonpregnant adults, carcinoma of the liver, as in hepatocellular carcinoma. In the pediatric patient, hepatoblastoma. |

size of the intrahepatic and extrahepatic vessels and the IVC, the caliber of the bile ducts, and the pathology affecting the hepatobiliary structures.

## Sagittal Sections

Sagittal scanning typically begins in the midsagittal plane, just inferior to the sternum and xiphoid process, and proceeds to the left lobe and then the right lobe. The diaphragm and dome of the liver are best visualized by angling the transducer cephalad. The inferior margin of the right lobe of the liver may require a caudal transducer angle. In the average adult patient, the liver is typically larger than the imaging field of view. This presents a challenge to the sonographer and the radiologist regarding the inability to "fit" the entire liver in each sagittal imaging plane. Therefore, a complete sagittal assessment of all hepatic structures requires the sonographer to move the probe superiorly and inferiorly throughout the sagittal scanning process. Sonographers should be careful to image all aspects of the liver from the lateral margin of the left lobe to the lateral margin of the right lobe. Documented sagittal or parasagittal images should include the left lobe segments, the aorta, the IVC, the caudate lobe and ligamentum venosum, the porta hepatis, the gallbladder, the right lobe segments, the right kidney, and the right adrenal gland fossa (Fig. 5-14A–F). Specific sagittal protocols may vary, depending on liver size and shape; sonographic findings; and sonographer, radiologist, and referring physician preferences. A Reidel's lobe is best documented in the sagittal plane.

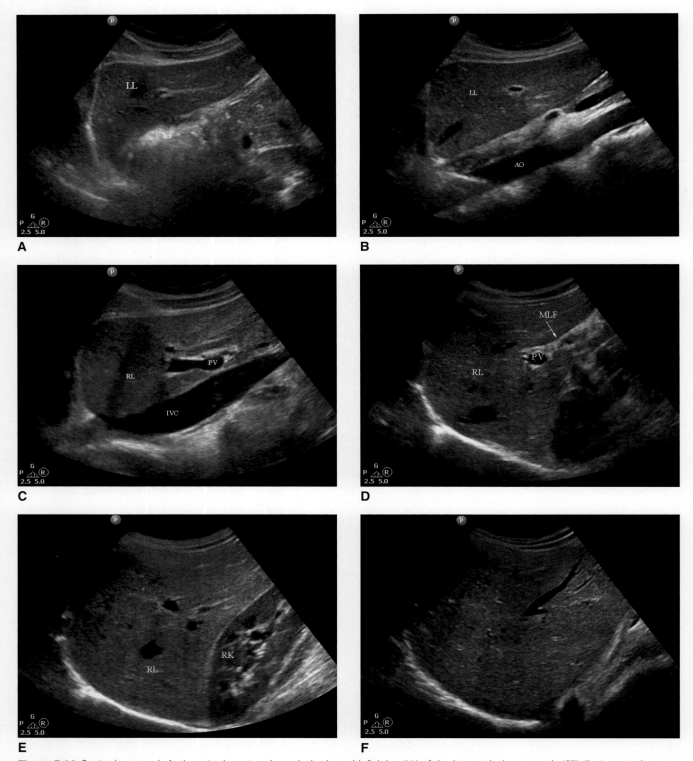

**Figure 5-14** Sagittal protocol. **A.** A sagittal section through the lateral left lobe *(LL)* of the liver with the stomach *(ST)*. **B.** A sagittal section through the *LL* with the aorta *(AO)*. **C.** A sagittal section through the right lobe *(RL)* of the liver with inferior vena cava *(IVC)*. **D.** A sagittal section through the *RL* near the main lobar fissure *(MLF)*. **E.** A sagittal section through the *RL* with liver/kidney *(RK)* interface. **F.** A sagittal section through the lateral *RL*. (Courtesy of Kara Tapalman, Kettering College, Kettering, OH.)

## Transverse Sections

In the transverse imaging plane, the transducer is swept cephalad from the dome to the inferior margin of the liver. Again, the size of the adult liver in the transverse dimension prohibits "fitting" the entire liver on each transverse image plane. Therefore, the sonographer usually begins the assessment at the midsagittal, subxiphoid location to image the left lobe in a transverse approach from superior to inferior then moves to a subcostal or intercostal probe position in order to image the right lobe from superior to inferior. The liver dome is best seen with cephalic transducer angulation. Portions of the heart may be seen just superior to the diaphragm. Documented transverse images should include the left lobe including the LHV and IVC, LPV, caudate lobe, ligamentum venosum, and aorta; and cross-sectional images of the right lobe including the dome, RHV, MHV, RPV, gallbladder, and right kidney (Fig. 5-15A–F). Specific transverse protocols may vary, depending on liver size and shape; sonographic findings; and sonographer, radiologist, and referring physician preferences.

## TECHNICAL CONSIDERATIONS

High-resolution two- and three-dimensional scanning with transducer frequencies ranging from 1 to 7 MHz are used in the sonographic evaluation of the adult liver. The highest frequency transducer should be selected in order to achieve the best possible resolution without compromising penetration. For optimal imaging, a multifocus transducer is ideal because it has a focus range for several depths. Curved array transducers with a wide sector image are more effective than linear array transducers for outlining the anatomic boundaries of the liver; however, a linear array transducer can be useful for evaluating the anterior liver capsule, especially in cases of cirrhosis.[25] Matrix array probes may offer superior resolution techniques, as well.

The time gain compensation (TGC) and the overall gain settings should be adjusted to give a uniform representation of the hepatic parenchyma from the anterior to posterior margins of the liver. The normal liver should display a relatively homogeneous texture of medium-level internal echoes that are isoechoic or slightly more echogenic than normal renal cortex. Careful attention to proper TGC settings is helpful in evaluating deep hepatic pathology or subdiaphragmatic fluid collections.

When using Doppler techniques, attention is paid to optimizing equipment settings for pulsed, color, and power-mode Doppler imaging. Improper selection of Doppler frequency, velocity scale, filter, gain, and incident angle may limit flow detection, cause errors in velocity readings, and cause Doppler artifacts.

## PITFALLS

Normal anatomy can sometimes have misleading sonographic characteristics. Anatomic variants and artifacts can simulate pathologic conditions. The normal ligamentum teres, fat anterior to the liver or between the liver and right kidney, acoustic shadowing from vascular and biliary structures, and air in the biliary tree have all been cited as causes of pseudolesions. The normal ligamentum teres can be well documented in the transverse plane close to the inferior margin of the left lobe of the liver. This fibrous structure surrounded by fat may appear as a hyperechoic lesion in the left lobe and may mimic a hemangioma or liver metastases (Fig. 5-16A).[42] On a transverse section or right costal margin view, perinephric fat may appear echopenic, rather than echogenic, and may mimic metastases. A sagittal section through the suspicious area that includes the kidney should clarify whether it is perirenal fat or a true metastatic lesion.[42]

The ribs can cause shadowing throughout the liver examination, especially when using the intercostal scanning approach. When shadowing is seen within the liver parenchyma, intraductal calculi should be considered. Other causes of shadows are calcified hematoma, infarct, granulomatous deposits, surgical metal clips, or air in the biliary ducts (Fig. 5-16B,C). A common scanning pitfall is stomach and bowel gas. Gas reflects sound and is always a problem, as it interferes with transmission. Thus, visualization of the liver parenchyma can be especially difficult if bowel loops are not located in the usual inferior and posterior positions.

It may be difficult to differentiate extrahepatic and intrahepatic masses, especially near the diaphragm. One area of confusion may be caused by the superimposition of a prominent left liver lobe between the spleen and diaphragm or chest wall. Careful scanning in the transverse plane should demonstrate the continuity of a prominent left hepatic lobe before a diagnosis of subcapsular hematoma or subdiaphragmatic abscess is rendered. The sonographic features most often observed in an extrahepatic mass include internal displacement of the liver capsule, capsule discontinuity, a triangular fat wedge anteromedially, shift of the IVC, and anterior displacement of the right kidney (Fig. 5-16D). The most often observed sonographic features of an intrahepatic mass are displaced hepatic vascular radicles, external bulging of the liver capsule, and posterior shifting of the IVC. The intrahepatic mass criteria can be noted on the sonograms in this chapter that demonstrate hepatic cysts, hepatic abscesses, benign neoplasms, and malignant neoplasms. These criteria should help define the anatomic origin and location of right upper quadrant (RUQ) masses.

## DIFFUSE HEPATOCELLULAR DISEASE

Hepatocellular disease (dysfunction of the hepatocytes) interferes with normal liver function.[20] The effect of the disease process on the whole liver ranges from simple fatty changes to more severe hepatitis or progressive cirrhosis. The parenchymal disease process produces changes that can decrease but more commonly increase

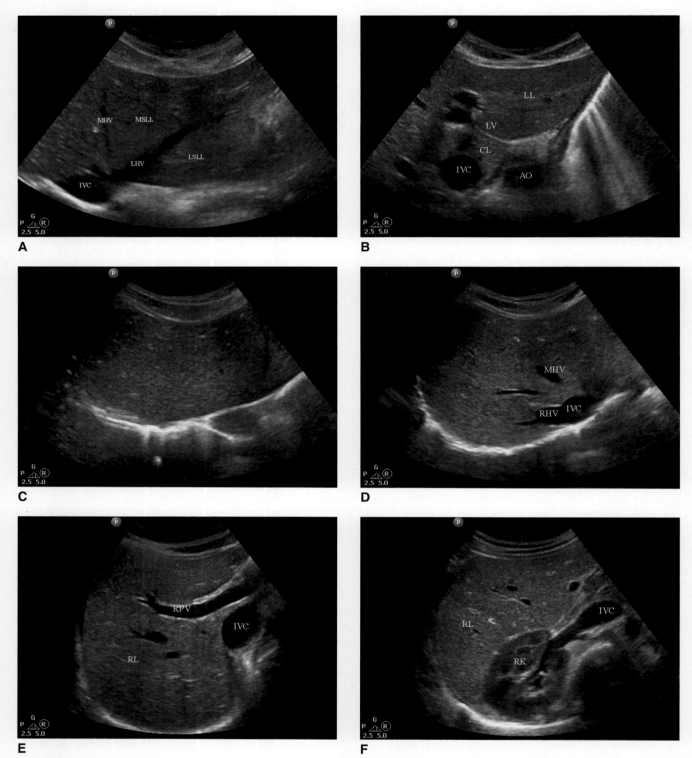

**Figure 5-15** Transverse protocol. **A.** A transverse section through the superior left lobe of the liver with the left hepatic vein. *AO,* aorta; *LHV,* left hepatic vein; *LSLL,* lateral segment left lobe; *MHV,* middle hepatic vein; *MSLL,* medial segment left lobe. **B.** A transverse section through the inferior left lobe *(LL)* with the caudate lobe *(CL)* and ligamentum venosum *(LV).* **C.** A transverse section through the superior right lobe of the liver at the dome. **D.** A transverse section through the right lobe with the middle *(MHV)* and right hepatic veins *(RHV).* **E.** A transverse section through the right lobe *(RL)* with the right portal vein *(RPV).* **F.** A transverse section through the inferior *RL* with the right kidney *(RK)* and inferior vena cava *(IVC).* (Courtesy of Kara Tapalman, Kettering College, Kettering, OH.)

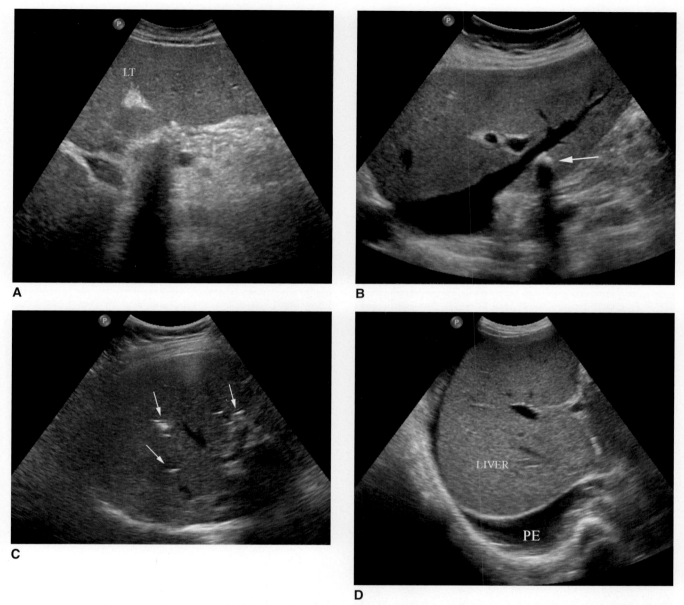

**Figure 5-16** Scanning pitfalls. **A.** In a transverse image of the inferior left lobe, the ligamentum teres (*LT*) serves as a landmark separating the medial and lateral segments of the left lobe. At times, the *LT*, a focal echogenic structure, may be mistaken for a liver lesion. (Courtesy of Rey Aquila, Kettering Health Network, Kettering, OH.) **B.** On a sagittal section of the right lobe of the liver, an isolated, echogenic structure (*arrow*) with distal acoustic shadowing is seen in the right lobe of an 80-year-old woman consistent with a granulomatous calcification. (Courtesy of Amy Stoudt, Kettering Health Network, Kettering, OH.) **C.** On a transverse scan, air within the intrahepatic bile ducts (pneumobilia; *arrows*) is displayed as echogenic linear bands in this postsurgical patient. Air can mimic periportal fibrosis. (Courtesy of Kettering Health Network, Kettering, OH.) **D.** On a transverse scan, an extrahepatic pleural effusion (*PE*) is identified by the fact that it displaces the liver anteriorly.

the normal echo density and often affect the liver's size. As the disease progresses, the liver is generally more difficult to penetrate owing to increased sound attenuation.[25] Sonography detects diffuse hepatocellular changes but cannot provide quantitative estimates of the severity of parenchymal damage.

## FATTY INFILTRATION

Fatty infiltration (steatosis) of the hepatocytes by itself usually does not significantly disrupt physiologic processes in the cells. Over time, however, the accumulation of fatty triglycerides within liver cells may cause the liver lobules to separate and increases the organ's weight.[43] Alcohol abuse and obesity are leading causes of the development of hepatic fatty infiltration.[28,44] Some other factors influencing fat deposition include diabetes, severe hepatitis, corticosteroid use or chemotherapy, parenteral hyperalimentation, protein malnutrition, metabolic disorders, pregnancy, cystic fibrosis, tuberculosis, some GI disorders, hyperlipidemia, Reye syndrome, and glycogen storage disease.[45] In the more advanced stages, liver function abnormalities occur. Elimination of the

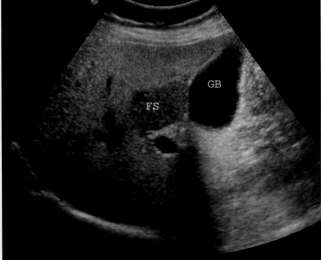

**Figure 5-17** Fatty infiltration. **A.** Hepatomegaly seen in this 48-year-old woman with classic heterogeneous appearance of the right lobe denoting fatty infiltration. **B.** A sagittal liver scan shows increased liver echogenicity, especially in the near field, and classic decreased sound penetration limiting visualization of the diaphragm (arrows). **C.** A 62-year-old woman with hepatomegaly and decreased penetration of the transverse right lobe. **D.** Focal fatty infiltration (arrows) noted in the right lobe of a 54-year-old man. *RK*, right kidney. **E.** Focal fatty sparing (FS) is seen as a hypoechoic, irregular-shaped area adjacent to the gallbladder (GB) in this patient.

process *causing* fatty metamorphosis may reverse the infiltration.

Sonographic features depend on the severity of fatty change and range from mild to severe. The key sonographic markers of fatty infiltration are diffuse increased echogenicity of the liver parenchyma and decreased acoustic penetration.[25] Hepatomegaly may be present. As the ratio of fat and fibrous tissue increases, the reflectivity and granularity of the liver parenchyma also increase.[10,28] Visualization of the normally bright intrahepatic vessel walls diminishes as the surrounding liver tissue becomes more hyperechoic. The cortex of the right kidney will appear unusually hypoechoic in contrast to the abnormally bright liver parenchyma. Increased sound attenuation makes penetration of the posterior liver and visualization of the diaphragm difficult (Fig. 5-17A–C).

Although the process is usually diffuse, fatty infiltration may be focal, resembling a hyperechoic mass. Although this focal fatty pattern may mimic "mass" formation, margins are typically more angular and vessels are not displaced (Fig. 5-17D).[10,46] Another sonographic appearance is that of focal fatty sparing making normal tissue appear as hypoechoic defects. Focal fatty sparing is usually detected in the medial segment of the left lobe near the porta hepatis, adjacent to the gallbladder, or in the caudate lobe (Fig. 5-17E).[46]

## GLYCOGEN STORAGE DISEASE

An autosomal recessive disorder that can have detectable features on sonography is glycogen storage disease. The most common type is classified as von Gierke disease (type 1). The disorder results from a defect in the enzyme glucose-6-phosphatase allowing excessive deposits of glycogen to be stored in the liver, intestinal tract, and kidneys.[47] Glycogen, normally broken down into glucose, is stored in the tissues, but the body is unable to synthesize it. This may cause severe hypoglycemia, abdominal distension, fatigue, and irritability.[48] Von Gierke disease begins in infancy, but with early therapy, survival can continue into adulthood.[47,48]

Sonographic features of type 1 glycogen storage disease are (1) a marked diffuse increase in parenchymal echogenicity and decreased penetration indicating a fatty liver, (2) hepatomegaly, and (3) the possible presence of solid liver masses. Typically, these masses are liver cell adenomas, which can occur in up to 40% of patients with von Gierke disease (Fig. 5-18).[49] Glycogen storage diseases types 3 and 4 are more often associated with cirrhosis and potentially with HCC.[50]

Of note in the literature is the opposite sonographic appearance of the liver in patients with decreased glycogen stores compared to those with steatosis (fatty infiltration). Cazier and Sponaugle[51] suggest there is a relationship between glycogen phosphate and the

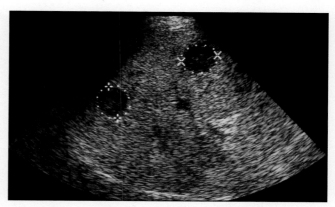

**Figure 5-18** Glycogen storage disease with liver cell adenoma. A transverse image in a man with known glycogen storage disease demonstrates fatty infiltration of the liver and hypoechoic liver lesions consistent with liver cell adenomas (*cursors*).

attenuation properties of the liver. Malnourished individuals or those fasting for several days have depleted glycogen stores. The sonographic result is a noticeable decrease in the attenuation of the liver and a resultant apparent increase in the echogenicity or delineation of the periportal vascular markings. The liver pattern resembles that of a "starry sky."[51] In some cases, the normal renal cortex may appear more echogenic than the liver. Normalization of the liver pattern relative to the kidney is achieved with adequate food intake if no other underlying process exists. Clinical correlation is necessary since decreased liver echogenicity can be seen with acute hepatitis, some diffuse infiltrative processes, necrosis, leukemia, and some lymphomas.

## HEPATITIS

Hepatitis means inflammation of the liver. Key causes are reactions to viruses or toxins such as drugs or alcohol.[28,43] Viral hepatitis may be mild or extensive. Types A, B, C, D, and E account for 95% of all acute hepatitis cases[52] (Table 5-6). Pathologic features of viral hepatitis are liver cell injury and swelling, varying cellular degeneration and possible necrosis, an immune system response, and regeneration.[49] Hepatitis A virus (HAV) is transmitted by a fecal–oral route, and symptoms typically resolve completely in less than 6 weeks.[49] Hepatitis B virus (HBV) occurs most frequently from blood transfusion or needle virus contamination and persists longer. *Non-A, non-B hepatitis* (NANB) is a term used for cases not due to HAV, HBV, Epstein-Barr virus, or cytomegalovirus (CMV). Most NANB cases are probably hepatitis C virus (HCV) infections. An estimated 90% of posttransfusion hepatitis is NANB.[43] Nearly half of all HCV cases develop into chronic hepatitis, and many chronic alcoholics with liver disease have antibodies to HCV.[43] Viral hepatitis accounts for 50% to 65% of all cases of fulminant hepatitis, although there are other causative agents such as viral infections.[43]

**TABLE 5-6**

Pathophysiology of Hepatitis[43,49,53]

| Hepatitis Type | Route of Transmission | Incubation Period (days) | Fulminant Hepatitis | Chronic/Carrier | Common Manifestations | Sonographic Appearance |
|---|---|---|---|---|---|---|
| Hepatitis A virus (HAV) | Parenteral (fecal–oral), contaminated water, milk, shellfish | 15–50 | Rare | No | *Incubation period:* Headache, nausea, vomiting<br>*Prodromal phase* (begins 2 weeks after exposure, lasts 3–12 days, ends with jaundice): Fatigue, anorexia, malaise, nausea with food odors; changes in taste suppress desire to smoke or drink alcohol; vomiting, headache, hyperalgia, cough, and low-grade fever; elevations of AST, ALT, LDH$_1$, LDH$_2$.<br>*Icteric phase* (jaundice, lasts 2–6 weeks): Abdominal pain and tenderness; elevated total bilirubin, dark urine, clay-colored stools; prothrombin time may be prolonged; may have pruritus if severe.<br>*Recovery phase* (resolution of jaundice 6–8 weeks after exposure): Symptoms diminish but hepatomegaly may persist; liver function tests return to normal within 2–12 weeks. | Normal at first<br>*Acute phase:* Hyperechoic portal vein walls; hypoechoic parenchyma due to swelling of liver.<br>*Chronic phase:* Increased amount of fibrous tissue and inflammatory cells surrounding hepatic lobules produces coarse echo pattern. |
| Hepatitis B virus (HBV) | Parenteral, sexual, mother to infant | 14–180 | Uncommon | Common (5%–10%) | | |
| Hepatitis C virus (HCV) | Parenteral | 60–180 | Uncommon | Common | | |
| Hepatitis delta (δ) virus | Parenteral, sexual | 28–180 | Common | Common | | |
| Hepatitis E | Parenteral (fecal–oral), contaminated water | 14–56 | Common in third trimester; uncommon otherwise | No | | |

With fulminant hepatitis, onset of symptoms is more sudden and severe, leading to shock, coma, and possibly, rapid death from marked liver necrosis. Liver transplantation may be lifesaving because massive hepatic necrosis is irreversible.[53]

The clinical features of the various viral hepatitides are difficult to distinguish, but those of clinical syndromes resulting from fulminating viral hepatitis, toxic reactions to drugs, and congenital metabolic disorders are fairly distinctive.[43,53] The degree of hepatitis symptoms varies. These symptoms include fever, chills, nausea and vomiting, RUQ pain, hepatomegaly, and jaundice. Hepatitis is a nonobstructive, hepatocellular cause of jaundice.

Laboratory values usually include elevated ALT and AST. During the icteric phase, both the conjugated and unconjugated fractions of serum bilirubin are elevated, and prothrombin time increases with the severity of disease (Table 5-6). Health care workers should avoid transmission of viral hepatitis by wearing gloves and washing their hands after examining patients with hepatitis A.[53] Direct contact with blood and body fluids must be avoided in cases of hepatitis B and C.[34,53]

The role of sonography in hepatitis is to (1) evaluate for parenchymal changes, (2) document hepatomegaly if present, and (3) exclude biliary obstruction as the source of jaundice. In the acute phase, the parenchymal pattern ranges from normal to hypoechoic secondary to diffuse swelling of the liver cells caused by inflammation.[28] The portal vein walls appear much more hyperechoic against the hypoechoic background of the edematous parenchyma. Periportal collagenous markings are easily seen extending peripherally in the liver.[28] Gallbladder wall thickening may be noted (Fig. 5-19A,B).[10,21,28] By contrast, fibrosis resulting from chronic hepatitis along with secondary fatty change produces a coarser and more hyperechoic texture. The portal vein walls are less discrete compared to the more reflective parenchyma. Chronic active hepatitis has more serious consequences than chronic persistent hepatitis, as more patients progress to develop cirrhosis or liver failure.[21]

## CIRRHOSIS

*Cirrhosis* is a general term for a diffuse process that destroys the normal architecture of the liver lobules. This process is the end result of chronic, severe damage to the liver cells, which leads to inflammation and subsequent necrosis.[10] Following inflammation, dense fibrous tissue septa form, which separate the liver lobules; parenchymal cells degenerate, followed by variable formation of regenerative nodules (regrowth).[10,43] Initial changes cause liver enlargement, but continued insult results in atrophy. The

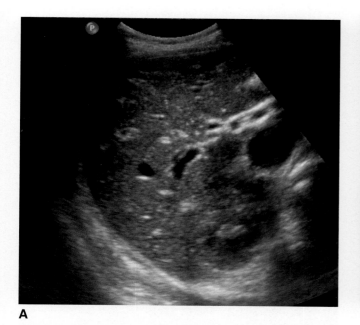
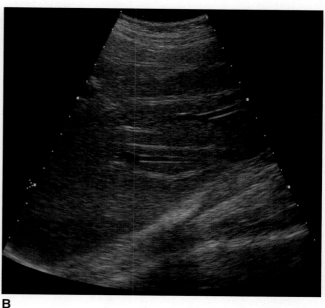

**A**    **B**

**Figure 5-19** Hepatitis. **A.** A right transverse scan demonstrates decreased liver echogenicity, and increased delineation of periportal and hepatic vessel tracts secondary to edematous changes from acute hepatitis. (Courtesy of Kettering Health Network, Kettering, OH.) **B.** A right sagittal image of a 44-year-old woman with acute hepatitis demonstrates mild markings. The vessels are seen as linear bands and could be delineated extending out to the periphery of the liver. (Courtesy of Good Samaritan Hospital, Corvallis, OR.)

parenchymal distortion may alter or compress biliary and vascular channels. Jaundice and portal hypertension develop.[8,24] The resulting jaundice develops more from impaired biliary excretion due to primary liver cell injury than from biliary obstruction.[3] New vascular channels can form collateral shunts, causing portal venous blood to bypass the liver (Fig. 5-20A).[24] Vascular changes compromise liver function, producing hypoxia, necrosis, and atrophy that ultimately lead to liver failure.[53]

Although precipitating factors vary, the leading cause of cirrhosis is alcohol abuse.[8] Seventy-five percent of deaths attributable to alcoholism are caused by cirrhosis.[34] However, the prevalence of cirrhosis among alcoholics is relatively low (approximately 25%).[53] Cirrhosis also develops in the course of other disorders, such as viral hepatitis, toxic drug and chemical reactions, biliary obstruction, and cardiac disease.[34] Cirrhosis is also associated with metabolic defects and storage diseases that cause minerals to be deposited in the liver: glycogen storage disease, hemochromatosis (iron deposition), Wilson disease (copper deposition), and galactosemia.[34,43] No matter what the cause, cirrhosis can take one of four forms: alcoholic (Laennec's, portal, or fatty), biliary (primary or secondary), postnecrotic, or metabolic[53] (Table 5-7).

LFT abnormalities depend on the stage and extent of disease. AST, ALT, lactic dehydrogenase (LDH4 and LDH5), and serum and urine conjugated bilirubin values are elevated. Serum ALP may also be elevated, whereas serum albumin is decreased and $\alpha$-globulin

proteins are increased. No symptoms may appear for a long time.

When clinical manifestations do occur, patients may present with fatigue, weight loss, diarrhea, hepatomegaly, jaundice, and possible ascites. Hepatomegaly causes stretching of Glisson capsule, and patients may complain of a dull, aching pain in the epigastric region or RUQ, with a feeling of fullness. As the disease progresses, the liver returns to normal size before the right lobe begins to atrophy; the caudate lobe is usually spared or hypertrophies, probably because of its unique blood supply.[20] The chronic effects of cirrhosis—alterations in normal liver function, portal hypertension, and liver failure—are detailed in Table 5-8.[43,49,53,54]

The sonographic features of cirrhosis vary during the disease progression. Early features include hepatomegaly and possible textural changes indicative of diffuse hepatocellular disease. These imaging features alone are nonspecific and unreliable in detecting the early histologic changes of cirrhosis. With superimposed fatty infiltration and fibrosis, the parenchymal pattern will display increased echogenicity compared to the normal renal cortex and decreased acoustic penetration. More specific sonographic features of cirrhosis are seen with late disease and can include (1) liver atrophy, especially the right lobe; (2) caudate lobe hypertrophy; (3) surface nodularity; (4) internal textural changes ranging from fine to coarse and from hypoechoic to hyperechoic; (5) loss of delineation of intrahepatic vasculature; and (6) possible findings related to portal hypertension (Fig. 5-20B–D). Parenchymal patterns can be inhomogeneous due

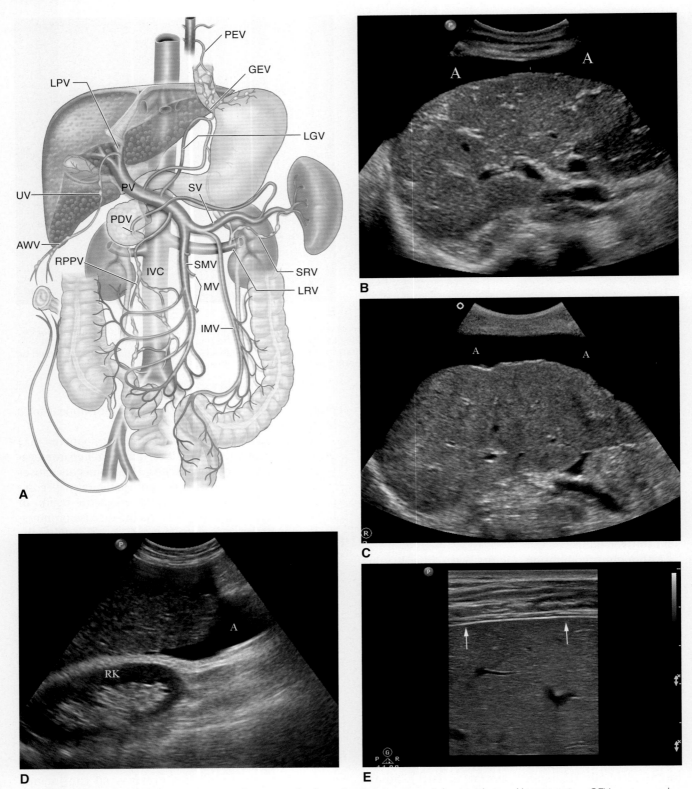

**Figure 5-20** Cirrhosis. **A.** A drawing illustrates the potential collateral vessels in severe cirrhosis with portal hypertension. *GEV*, gastroesophageal vein; *IMV*, inferior mesenteric vein; *IVC*, inferior vena cava; *LGV*, left gastric vein; *LPV*, left portal vein; *LRV*, left renal vein; *MV*, mesenteric vein; *PDV*, pancreaticoduodenal vein; *PEV*, paraesohpageal vein; *PV*, portal vein; *RPPV*, retroperitoneal-paravertebral vein; *SMV*, superior mesenteric vein; *SRV*, splenorenal vein; *SV*, splenci ven; *UV*, umbilical vein. **B.** A transverse scan demonstrates a cirrhotic liver with increased echogenicity and nodularity. Ascites *(A)* helps to delineate the irregular surface secondary to regenerating nodules. **C.** Another patient with cirrhosis and ascites *(A)*. Note the increased nodularity of the surface. **D.** A sagittal scan was obtained in a 59-year-old man with end-stage alcoholic liver disease. Ascites *(A)* outlines the liver margins of the inferior right lobe, which show considerable lobulation. (Courtesy of Melanie Willsey, Kettering Health Network, Kettering, OH.) **E.** Image of the liver capsule *(arrows)* in an asymptomatic patient demonstrates the normal smooth contour of the liver capsule. *(continued)*

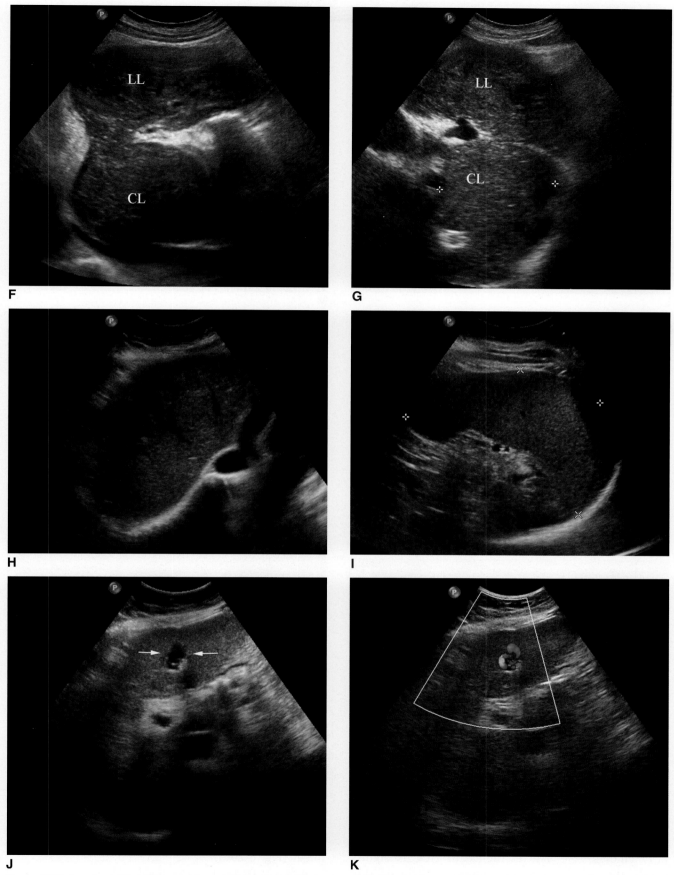

**Figure 5-20** *(continued)* **F.** A 53-year-old man with a history of cirrhosis now presents with considerable caudate lobe *(CL)* enlargement in the sagittal image. **G.** Same patient with *CL* enlargement on this transverse scan. **H–L.** A 48-year-old woman with a history of alcoholic cirrhosis presents for an annual serial examination. **H.** Sonographic assessment now reveals a coarse-appearing liver that was difficult to penetrate; **(I)** splenomegaly; **(J)** a complex cystic *(arrows)* structure in the transverse left lobe (LL) that **(K)** demonstrated flow. *(continued)*

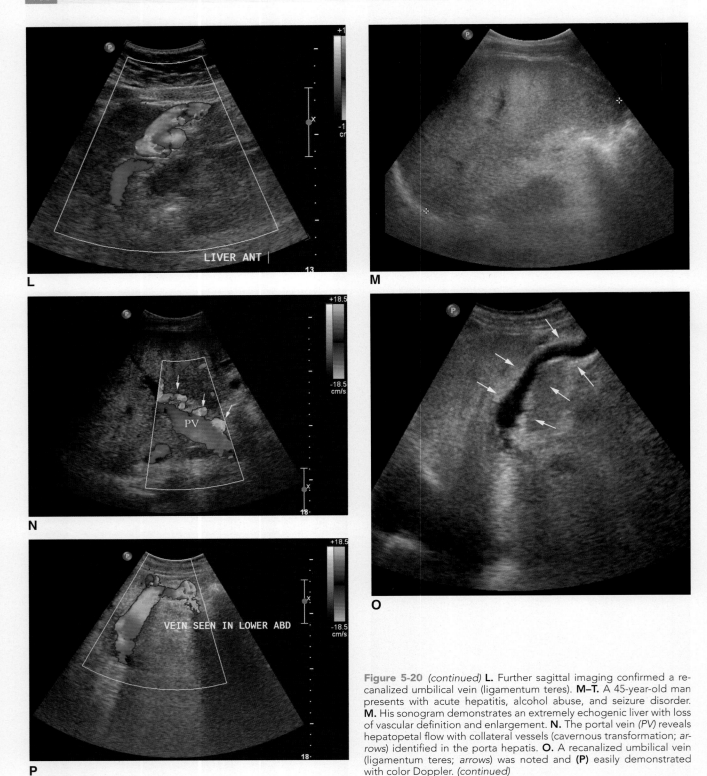

**Figure 5-20** *(continued)* **L.** Further sagittal imaging confirmed a recanalized umbilical vein (ligamentum teres). **M–T.** A 45-year-old man presents with acute hepatitis, alcohol abuse, and seizure disorder. **M.** His sonogram demonstrates an extremely echogenic liver with loss of vascular definition and enlargement. **N.** The portal vein *(PV)* reveals hepatopetal flow with collateral vessels (cavernous transformation; *arrows*) identified in the porta hepatis. **O.** A recanalized umbilical vein (ligamentum teres; *arrows*) was noted and **(P)** easily demonstrated with color Doppler. *(continued)*

to fibrosis, regenerative nodules, and superimposed fatty change.[25,28,55] The incidence of HCC is significantly increased with macronodular cirrhosis, but hepatomas may be difficult to differentiate from regenerating nodules.[55] Surface nodularity is diagnostic for cirrhosis and the anterior liver capsule can be

evaluated using a high-frequency linear array transducer (Fig. 5-20E).[25]

A lower frequency transducer may be necessary to compensate for areas of decreased sound penetration. It is useful to determine the caudate lobe/right lobe (C/RL) ratio to establish the presence of caudate hypertrophy

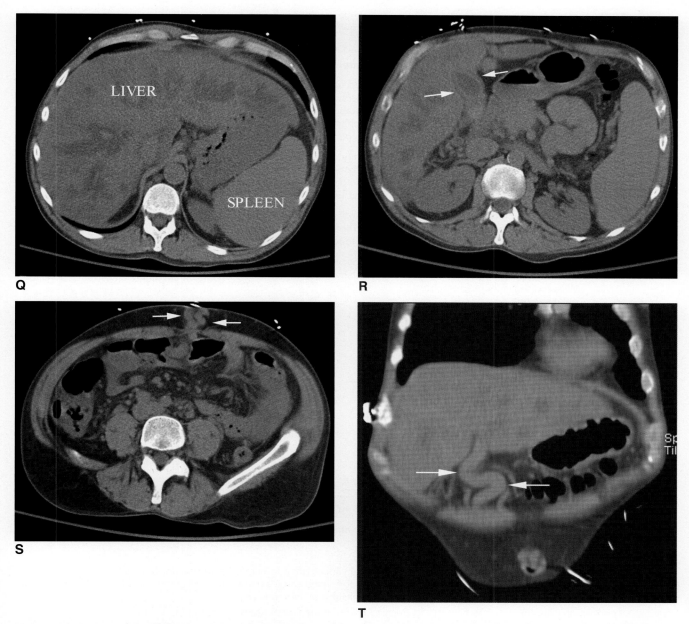

**Figure 5-20** *(continued)* **Q.** A follow-up computed tomography confirmed hepatomegaly and splenomegaly. **R.** The recanalized umbilical vein *(arrows)* was documented from the inferior margin of the left lobe **(S)** to the umbilicus. **T.** An anterior coronal view displayed the tortuosity of the umbilical vein *(arrows)*.

(Fig. 5-20F,G). This is accomplished by dividing the caudate lobe width by the right lobe width as measured on a transverse section using the MPV as a reference point.[49] A C/RL ratio above 0.65 has a 96% confidence level.[49]

Possible secondary findings of portal hypertension, splenomegaly, and ascites should be documented. Doppler scanning establishes patency and flow direction of the portal vein, hepatic artery, splenic vein, and collaterals. Organ resistance to inflow causes dilatation of the extrahepatic portal vein and splenic vein. Stasis can lead to thrombus with possible cavernous transformation. Reversed portal vein flow suggests collateral formation. Recanalization of the paraumbilical vein (ligamentum teres) with hepatofugal flow exceeding portal vein flow may limit the formation of GI varices, as it diverts blood away from the liver.[21,24] With cirrhosis, portal vein velocities are often reduced and hepatic artery flow velocities may be increased to maintain hepatic perfusion.[8] Doppler waveforms recorded from the hepatic veins show accelerated, continuous, turbulent flow, with loss of the normal multiphasic appearance secondary to noncompliance of the surrounding fibrous parenchyma (Fig. 5-20H–T).[8,24,25]

| TABLE 5-7 |
| --- |
| Cirrhosis[43,49,53] |

| Type | Etiology | Pathophysiology | Sonographic Appearance |
| --- | --- | --- | --- |
| Alcoholic | Toxic effects of chronic, excessive alcohol intake (alcohol is a hepatotoxin that induces metabolic changes that damage hepatocytes). | Fat accumulation, inflammation (alcoholic hepatitis), and derangement of the lobular architecture by necrosis and fibrosis (cirrhosis). | In early stages, hepatomegaly; liver may appear hyperechoic compared to normal renal parenchyma; diffuse parenchymal changes lead to a diagnosis of hepatocellular disease. As cirrhosis progresses, hepatic tissue begins to atrophy and attenuates more sound; fibrosis appears more coarse; vascular structures are not as readily visualized and may present an irregular contour due to nodular regeneration. With portal hypertension, splenomegaly and ascites may be seen. |
| Biliary | Primary: unknown, possible autoimmune mechanism; secondary: obstruction by cholelithiasis, stricture, or neoplasm. | Primary: lobular bile ducts become inflamed and scarred; secondary: bile ducts become inflamed and scarred proximal to obstruction. | |
| Postnecrotic | Viral hepatitis, drugs, toxins, autoimmune destruction. | Necrotic tissue is replaced with cirrhotic tissue, specifically fibrous, nodular scar tissue. | |
| Metabolic | Metabolic defects and storage disease (glycogen storage disease), Wilson disease; hemochromatosis, galactosemia. | Morphologic changes resulting in inflammation and scarring. | |

## VASCULAR ABNORMALITIES

A variety of conditions alter blood flow associated with the liver. Hemodynamic changes can range from simple vascular congestion to thrombosis and infarction with potential liver necrosis. Doppler scanning is a valuable tool for assessing changes within the hepatic artery and the portal-systemic and hepatic venous systems. Arterial inflow is characterized by a low-resistive Doppler waveform indicating forward flow throughout the cardiac cycle (Fig. 5-21A). Normal portal venous inflow is characterized by continuous monophasic flow with

| TABLE 5-8 |
| --- |
| Chronic Effects of Hepatic Cirrhosis[43,49,53,54] |

| Alteration in Function | Symptoms and Signs |
| --- | --- |
| **Portal Hypertension** | |
| Collateral vessel development | Esophageal varices often lead to GI bleeding and possible hemorrhage; hemorrhoids, caput medusa (a radiating plexus of dilated periumbilical subcutaneous veins) |
| Increased portal vein pressure | Recanalization of the ligamentum teres (umbilical vein) |
| Increased portal vein pressure and decreased serum albumin level | Ascites, peripheral edema |
| Splenomegaly | Hematopoietic disorders: anemia, leukopenia, thrombocytopenia |
| Hepatorenal syndrome | Elevated serum creatinine, azotemia, oliguria; precursor of hepatic coma |
| Postsystemic shunting of blood | Hepatic systemic encephalopathy (precursor of confusion, coma, and convulsions) |
| **Hepatocellular Dysfunction** | |
| Inability to remove conjugated bilirubin | Jaundice |
| Impaired bile synthesis | Malabsorption of fats and fat-soluble vitamins |
| Impaired plasma protein synthesis | Decreased level of albumin (precursor of edema and ascites) |
| Decreased synthesis of blood-clotting factors | Tendency to bleed |
| Impaired drug metabolism | Drug reactions and toxicity |
| Impaired gluconeogenesis | Glucose intolerance |
| Capillary congestion | Spider angiomas and palmar erythema |
| Decreased ability to convert ammonia to urea | Elevated blood ammonia level |
| Depressed metabolism of sex hormones | Women: menstrual disorders; men: testicular atrophy, gynecomastia, decrease in secondary sex characteristics |

little pulsatility.[8] Flow direction within the MPV is toward the liver (hepatopetal), with a flow velocity of 15 to 18 cm/sec.[56] Flow velocity can increase after eating (Fig. 5-21B).[8] Hepatic vein flow is away from the liver (hepatofugal) and toward the IVC.[24] In healthy individuals, pulsed spectral tracings of the hepatic veins show pulsatility relative to right atrial filling, contraction, and relaxation.[8,44] This triphasic hepatic venous pattern is sensitive to respiratory changes (Fig. 5-21C).[8]

A significant condition affecting liver hemodynamics is portal hypertension. The sonographic examination for portal venous hypertension and portal vein thrombosis is described in Chapter 4, and splenomegaly and splenic vein thrombosis are described in Chapter 8.

## HEPATIC VENOUS OUTFLOW OBSTRUCTION

Obstruction of the hepatic venous outflow tract by thrombus or tumor and the associated clinical features of abdominal pain, jaundice, hematemesis, ascites, hepatomegaly, and liver function abnormalities indicative of hepatocellular dysfunction are known collectively as *Budd-Chiari syndrome*. Distended superficial veins and lower extremity edema may be present if the IVC is also involved. The possible causes are varied. Although in a majority of cases the etiology is never determined,[20] thrombosis of the hepatic veins has been linked with several conditions such as oral contraceptive use; tumor invasion into the hepatic veins from HCC, renal carcinoma, or adrenal gland carcinoma; and radiation to the liver with obliteration of small hepatic veins.[24]

The sonographic findings of Budd-Chiari syndrome depend on the degree of venous obstruction and the underlying cause. The hepatic veins may not be visible or may appear thick-walled. In long-standing cases, the right lobe atrophies and there is hypertrophy of the lateral segment of the left lobe and of the caudate lobe,[57] the latter owing to its multiple small, direct connections to the patent portion of the IVC.[20]

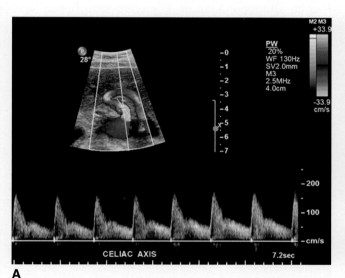

A

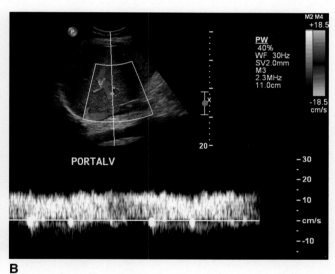

B

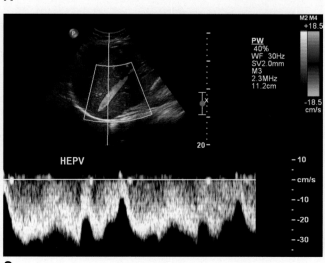

C

Figure 5-21 Normal hepatic vascular flow. **A.** Low resistive spectral tracing of the celiac artery. **B.** Continuous forward flow (hepatopetal) in the portal vein with spectral tracing. **C.** Triphasic, hepatofugal flow in the right hepatic vein.

As the disease progresses, sonographic appearances include hyperechoic areas from fibrosis and periportal regenerative nodules within infarcted areas, ascites, splenomegaly, pleural effusion, and an hourglass configuration of the IVC if there is coarctation.[57] Because blood flows to unobstructed vessels, flow may be to interlobular hepatic veins, to subcapsular arcades, or retrograde (hepatofugal), through branches of the portal veins. Vascular Doppler assessment is useful in demonstrating altered hemodynamics in the IVC, hepatic veins, and portal veins, as well as the level of obstruction.

## PASSIVE LIVER CONGESTION

Passive edema of the liver secondary to vascular congestion is a complication related to heart failure.[44] The large volume of blood exiting the liver must pass through the hepatic veins, to the IVC, and enter the right side of the heart. Resistance to flow into the right side of the heart from cardiac or pulmonary disorders will cause secondary dilatation of these vessels. In the more acute phase, the liver enlarges, causing RUQ discomfort. Sonographically, the liver is easily penetrated and dilated veins are readily visible. The IVC is dilated and does not change in caliber with respiratory maneuvers (Fig. 5-22A,B). Pulsed Doppler waveforms of the hepatic vein demonstrate a highly pulsatile W-type pattern,[44] showing flow reversal during systole secondary to tricuspid regurgitation.[8] Sample volume tracings in the portal vein are also more pulsatile than normal, with minimal or slight flow reversal during diastole. In chronic disorders, the liver shrinks and becomes more fibrotic, but hepatic veins remain distended.[3]

## HEREDITARY HEMORRHAGIC TELANGIECTASIS

Hereditary hemorrhagic telangiectasis, or *Osler-Weber-Rendu disease*, is an uncommon autosomal dominant disorder that leads to repeated incidents of hemorrhage.[21] This condition is characterized by thin-walled, dilated vascular channels forming arteriovenous malformations. Sites most affected are mucocutaneous tissues and the GI tract. Liver involvement occurs in approximately 30% of cases, with the lungs and brain affected less often. The condition can be found in some patients with hepatic fibrosis, cirrhosis, and HCC.[21,49]

Sonographic features noted in telangiectasis are (1) marked dilatation of the celiac artery, the hepatic artery, and its branches; (2) a tortuous intrahepatic tubular structure with turbulent arterial Doppler signals representing arteriovenous malformations; and (3) large draining hepatic veins showing biphasic or continuous flow.[21] The extrahepatic portal vein and spleen are usually normal in size, without collateral formation, unless an arterioportal shunt is present with hepatofugal flow. Liver enlargement is variable. In some patients, intrahepatic shunts lead to heart failure, pulmonary hypertension, and, to a lesser extent, portal hypertension. Doppler assessment is helpful in differentiating intrahepatic features from Caroli disease.

## PELIOSIS HEPATIS

Peliosis hepatis is a rare disorder that can occur in chronically debilitated patients with advanced tuberculosis, hematologic disorders, diabetes, carcinoma, and chronic renal disease, and from the use of anabolic

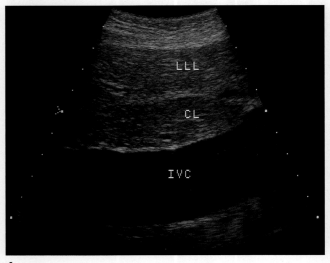

**A**

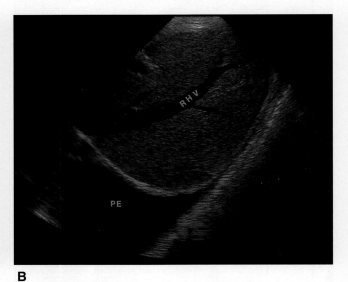

**B**

**Figure 5-22** Liver congestion. **A.** A sagittal scan of the inferior vena cava *(IVC)* shows dilatation with no respiratory change in a woman with right heart failure. *CL,* caudate lobe; *LLL,* left lobe liver. **B.** A sagittal scan of the right lobe of the liver demonstrates a dilated right hepatic vein *(RHV)* and pleural effusion *(PE).* Sonographically, the liver was easy to penetrate. The patient had heart failure, as well as pericardial fluid and ascites. (Courtesy of Good Samaritan Hospital, Corvallis, OR.)

steroids or oral contraceptives.[49,50,58] The condition is often asymptomatic and is discovered incidentally at autopsy. Classic parenchymal peliosis is characterized by the development of necrotic, blood-filled liver spaces that communicate with hepatic veins and adjacent sinusoids.[50,58] Periportal sinusoidal dilatation is more common with steroid use. Hepatomegaly is common. Sonographic findings include focal or diffuse, irregular-walled, cystic liver lesions representing ectatic vascular spaces. However, if the blood-filled spaces are small, the echo texture may be nonspecific, with a patchy hyperechoic and hypoechoic pattern. Correlation with the clinical history and histologic examination can confirm the diagnosis.[49]

# HEPATIC CYSTS

Liver cysts may be classified as congenital or acquired. True hepatic cysts are congenital and are further categorized as simple cysts or those related to hereditary disorders such as polycystic liver disease. Congenital cysts result from developmental anomalies in the formation of intrahepatic bile ductules, the proper involution of these ductules, or both.[49] The incidence increases with age.[28] Women are more frequently affected. Nonparasitic cysts are found during laparotomy in approximately 1/600 cases.[49] Acquired cystic lesions can result from trauma, parasites, or inflammatory reactions.[46]

## CONGENITAL CYSTS

Congenital cysts are better described as developmental since their prevalence increases with age.[36] The cysts are usually asymptomatic. They are discovered incidentally in fewer than 1% of patients less than 60 years of age but in 3% to 7% of older patients.[36] Solitary lesions are more common than multiple cysts, and the right lobe is affected twice as often as the left.[20,49] Cysts can be tiny or occupy large areas. In some patients, multiple or large cysts can cause hepatomegaly, palpable nodules, abdominal discomfort, and localized bile duct compression causing jaundice.[46] In these cases, LFTs may be mildly elevated.

The imaging modality of choice for hepatic cysts is sonography. Lesions are typically round or oval (Fig. 5-23A,B). Sonographically, the imaging criteria for diagnosing a simple liver cyst include demonstration of:
1. A well-defined, thin-walled, cystic mass with a sharp posterior wall
2. No internal echoes (anechoic)
3. Distal acoustic enhancement
4. Lateral wall refractive edge shadowing

Sonographic diagnosis of a hepatic cyst is 95% to 100% accurate. Correlation with the patient's history, including the patient's age, is necessary.

Sonographically, congenital cysts can be characterized, measured, and localized precisely for fine-needle aspiration. These cysts typically contain straw-colored or clear fluid. Cytologic evaluation may be needed if cyst walls are irregular or if internal debris or septations are present. Complex cysts may indicate superimposed hemorrhage or infection. Cysts with wall calcification can cause wall thickening and acoustic shadowing. Other differential diagnoses of complex cysts include bilomas, necrotic tumors, hepatic cystadenoma, parasitic masses, and intrahepatic hematoma or abscess (Fig. 5-23C).[20,46,49]

Polycystic liver disease is caused by an inherited developmental defect in the formation of bile ducts. Histologically, the cysts are lined with cuboidal epithelium and are scattered randomly throughout the liver, causing disruption of the normal echo appearance. Cysts are numerous, become detectable in the third or fourth decade, and more often affect women. One-quarter to one-half of all persons who have autosomal dominant polycystic kidney disease also have a polycystic liver; renal cysts are found in 60% of patients with polycystic liver disease. After the liver is evaluated, the kidneys, spleen, and pancreas should be scanned for associative cystic change. Hypertension is common in patients with renal involvement (Fig. 5-23D–G).

If a patient demonstrates multiple liver cysts but has no associated renal cysts or verifiable family history of polycystic disease, a diagnosis of multiple liver cysts is made. Other considerations include Caroli disease, multiple abscesses, hepatic cysts with tuberous sclerosis, degenerative metastasis, or multiple abscesses.

## ACQUIRED CYSTS

Acquired cystic masses can be categorized as traumatic (hematoma, biloma), parasitic (echinococcal), or inflammatory (abscess).[29] They are often suspected prior to scanning because patients are usually symptomatic. The sonographic appearance ranges from classic cystic features to complex masses. In addition to localizing and measuring these lesions, it is important to characterize the appearance of acquired cysts and to correlate the sonographic presentation with clinical findings.

### Hematoma

The liver's abundant vascular supply makes it highly susceptible to hemorrhage when blunt force trauma to the abdomen ruptures or tears hepatic tissue. In addition to trauma, hematomas can form secondary to interventional complications, from rupture of a vascular neoplasm or aneurysm, or can be associated with pregnancy-induced hypertension.[3,59] Symptomatically, the liver is tender. With a significant bleed, the patient may physically collapse and show signs of shock. The blood pressure and pulse rate decrease and the hematocrit level drops.

Liver trauma is categorized on the basis of severity and location. Classifications include contusion, subcapsular hematoma, central laceration, and transcapsular laceration with rupture through Glisson capsule.[60] Pregnancy-induced hypertension can cause spontaneous rupture of the liver capsule leading to massive intra-abdominal bleeding. With capsular disruption, both blood and bile can leak into the peritoneal cavity.

Although CT is the imaging modality of choice, high-resolution sonography is capable of detecting disruptions in the hepatic parenchyma associated with lacerations, localizing and measuring focal hematoma formation, and documenting hemoperitoneum. Doppler may be used to exclude pseudoaneurysm or arteriovenous malformation. Sonographically, the appearance of a hematoma depends on the age of the bleed. Intrahepatic hematomas are echogenic during the first day following injury as fibrin and erythrocytes are deposited.[49,60] Blood can be anechoic, but early in the evolution of a hematoma, acoustic enhancement may not be exhibited, as in a typical cyst. Margins may be less well defined. Gradually, as a hematoma becomes organized and develops a clot, it reveals internal echoes and septations, and presents a complex pattern that is both hyperechoic and hypoechoic. Eventually, it undergoes complete liquefaction and becomes a seroma, which again has an anechoic cystic pattern.

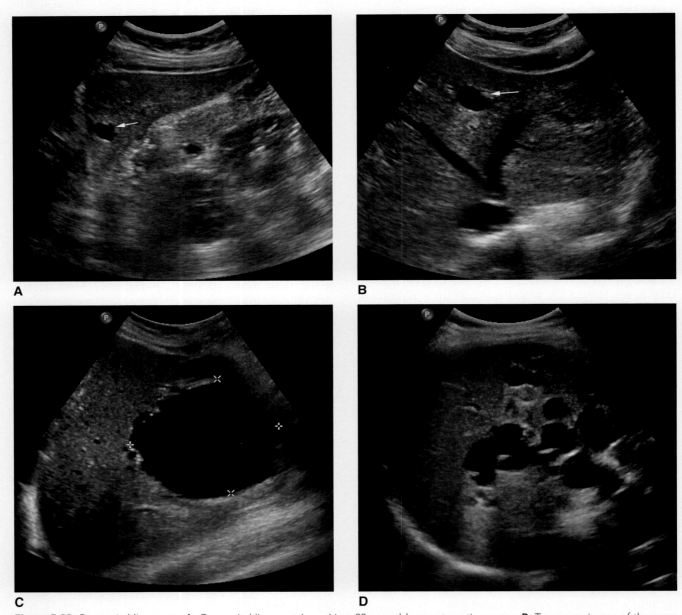

**Figure 5-23** Congenital liver cysts. **A.** Congenital liver cyst *(arrow)* in a 33-year-old asymptomatic woman. **B.** Transverse image of the same liver cyst *(arrow)*. Notice the posterior enhancement. **C.** This 80-year-old woman presented with a cystic liver lesion *(calipers)* following a laparoscopic cholecystectomy. The diagnosis was likely a biloma, rather than a congenital liver cyst. **D,E.** This 50-year-old woman presented with polycystic liver disease associated with polycystic kidney disease (PKD). *(continued)*

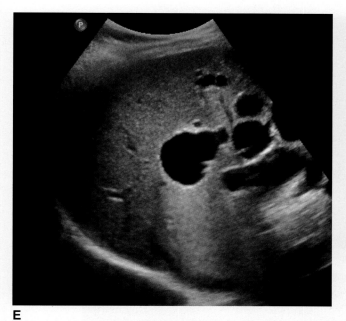

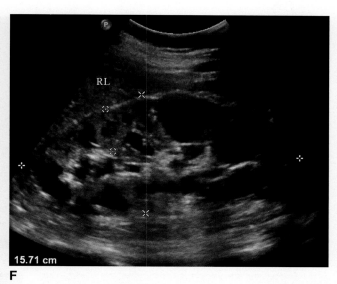

E

F

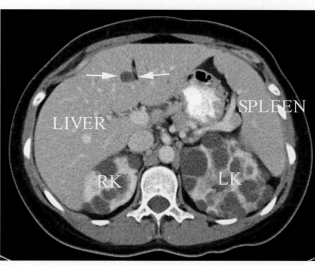

G

Figure 5-23 *(continued)* **F.** Note the cysts within the right kidney and significant enlargement of the kidney *(calipers)*. *RL,* right lobe of the liver. **G.** A computed tomographic scan demonstrates bilateral PKD with a liver cyst *(arrows)*. *LK,* left kidney, *RK,* right kidney.

Chronic hematomas may become calcified and produce characteristic acoustic shadows. Frequently, hepatic hematomas are contained by the liver capsule. A subcapsular hematoma produces a striking appearance as it displaces the liver medially. Subcapsular hematomas may have a crescent shape (Fig. 5-24A,B). Although posttraumatic intrahepatic biloma is a rare lesion, it may be suspected if there is acoustic enhancement (Fig. 5-24C).

### Echinococcal Cyst

The *Taenia echinococcus* or *Echinococcus granulosus* is a parasitic tapeworm.[3] When a dog eats infested animal organs, the tapeworms mature in the dog's intestine and the ova are passed in the feces. Cattle, sheep, hogs, and humans serve as intermediate hosts. The parasites were once confined to specific geographic areas, but world travel and world markets for food products (that have been fertilized with infected manure) have increased their transmission. Sanitary measures reduce the incidence of this cyst.[3] Larvae ingested by humans hatch in the intestine and migrate most often to the liver (and less frequently, to the lungs, the brain, or another organ).[3] The cysts may deform the organ, leading to unusual findings on palpation. Clinical symptoms range from anaphylactic shock, if the cyst ruptures and the hydatid fluid enters the circulatory system, to slight elevation of ALP and possible jaundice, if the daughter cysts obstruct bile ducts.[3]

If the larvae invaginate and develop, they become encysted and generations of daughter cysts develop.[27] The original unilocular-looking cyst is eventually filled in by

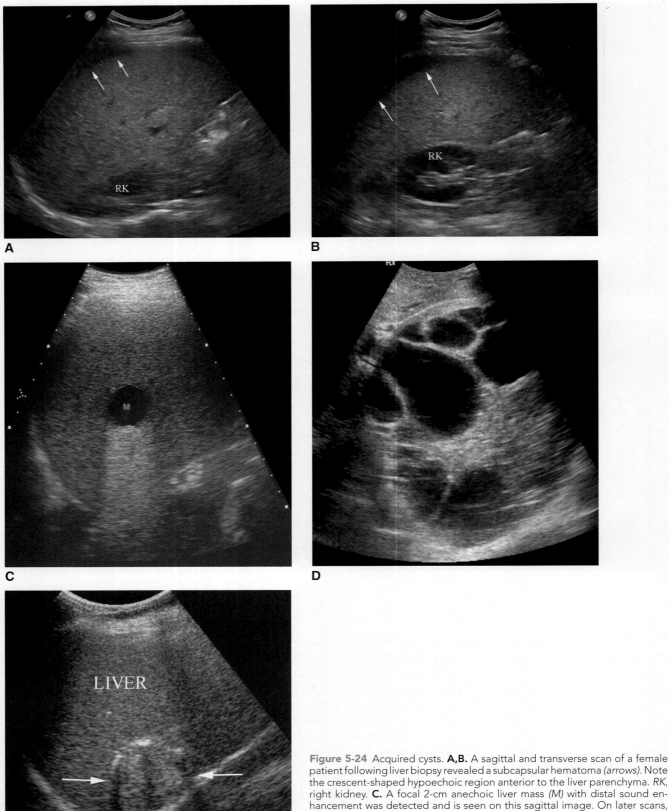

**Figure 5-24** Acquired cysts. **A,B.** A sagittal and transverse scan of a female patient following liver biopsy revealed a subcapsular hematoma *(arrows)*. Note the crescent-shaped hypoechoic region anterior to the liver parenchyma. *RK,* right kidney. **C.** A focal 2-cm anechoic liver mass *(M)* with distal sound enhancement was detected and is seen on this sagittal image. On later scans, the cystic mass enlarged and became thick-walled and complex. Aspiration revealed an infected biloma. **D,E.** These two sonograms from different patients display echinococcal cysts with **(D)** fluid collections with septa yielding a honeycomb appearance and **(E)** solid-looking cysts, presenting with calcification and shadowing. (Images **A–C** courtesy of Good Samaritan Hospital, Corvallis, OR. Images **D and E** courtesy of Robert DeJong, Baltimore, MD.)

multiple cysts of varying size. When it grows to approximately 20 cm, the patient experiences discomfort and pain. The daughter cysts float in a protein-free, highly irritating hydatid fluid, which also contains hydatid sand.[3]

The sonographic appearance of echinococcal cysts depends on the course of larval maturation. The possibilities include (1) a solitary cyst with possible mural (shell-like) calcification; (2) a mother cyst containing internal, peripherally placed daughter cysts; (3) fluid collections with septa yielding a honeycomb appearance; and (4) solid-looking cysts, presenting with or without calcification (Fig. 5-24D,E).[20,61] Larger cysts may rupture or compress adjacent vessels.[47] On occasion, a detached membrane may be seen undulating within the cyst's cavity.[47,61] During a stage of relative inactivity or parasite death, the germinal layer can fall away from the pericyst and infold within the cavity. This pattern has been referred to as the *congealed water-lily* sign.[61] Other descriptions of hydatid cysts include the *double-line,*[65] *ball of yarn, racemose,* and *whirl* sign.[61] As the lesion decreases in size, folds of the germinal layer become more tightly apposed and produce a more solid appearance.

## HEPATIC ABSCESSES

The cause of a hepatic abscess is usually a bacterial or parasitic (amebiasis) infection. Sonographic examination can noninvasively locate, measure, and characterize such hepatic masses. Hepatic abscesses have been located in the intrahepatic, subhepatic, and subphrenic areas.[17]

### PYOGENIC ABSCESS

A pyogenic abscess develops when the reticuloendothelial system is compromised by altered immune function or when there is severe sepsis. Bacterial infection reaches the liver from the biliary tree, portal vein, or hepatic artery by direct extension from a current infection or as a postoperative sequela.

Pyogenic abscesses produce varying symptoms, depending on the severity and extent of the process. Clinical symptoms may include fever, leukocytosis, elevated LFT values, RUQ pain, pleuritic pain, and hepatomegaly. An abscess in the subhepatic or subphrenic region is more likely the result of bacterial infection. A pyogenic abscess in the subhepatic region may result from cholecystectomy and is found in the gallbladder bed or Morrison pouch. In the subphrenic region, abscess formation results from bacteria spilling into the peritoneum at surgery, bowel rupture, perforated peptic ulcer, or trauma.[17] The mortality rate can be 100% in untreated cases.

Several sonographic features have been described: single or multiple masses measuring 1 cm or larger, 80% of which are located in the right lobe. The shape is variable but pyogenic abscesses may be round or ovoid, with walls that are usually irregular (90%) and poorly defined. The internal echo pattern is anechoic to hyperechoic (depending on the presence of debris, adhesions, or air microbubbles), but it is usually less echogenic than hepatic parenchyma. Distal acoustic enhancement occurs in 50% of cases (Fig. 5-25A–C). The clinical features and echo enhancement are important considerations in the differential diagnosis, which includes cyst, hematoma, biloma, necrotic tumor, echinococcal cyst, and primary or metastatic cystadenocarcinoma.[46]

### AMEBIC ABSCESS

An amebic abscess occurs when parasites (*Entamoeba histolytica*), usually from the colon, reach the liver through the portal vein. Once confined to specific geographic areas, amebic diseases are now transmitted to many developed countries. Humans serve as an intermediate host and are usually asymptomatic when the organism is confined to the GI tract.[20] With abscess development, patients may present with RUQ pain, hepatomegaly, diarrhea, fever, chills, anorexia, and black tarry stool.[20] Reactive hepatomegaly is common. Laboratory tests reveal moderate leukocytosis,[60] mild anemia, and elevated LFTs. Serologic tests are positive.[60] Fluid from the abscess can be aspirated and cultured. The fluid may be thick and chocolate colored; it becomes thinner with age.[3]

Sonographic features are variable. Before liquefaction, an echogenic mass may correlate with the presence of a new amebic abscess.[60] As the mass matures, it becomes more hypoechoic, contains fewer echoes, develops smoother walls, and demonstrates distal acoustic enhancement (Fig. 5-26). Amebic abscesses are typically located contiguous to the liver capsule, more often at the right liver dome or near the right hepatic flexure.[60] A serious complication of amebic abscess is its extension through the diaphragm to the chest or into the peritoneal cavity.[3] Most abscesses respond well to therapy. Sonography can monitor the involution and resolution of inflammatory processes. Incomplete resolution may result in a persistent cyst; residual calcification is possible.[60]

## OTHER PARASITIC AND INFECTIOUS PROCESSES

### SCHISTOSOMIASIS

Schistosomiasis is a common parasitic infection in certain parts of the world such as Africa, Asia, Indonesia, China, Japan, South America, and the Mediterranean.[3,47] In locations with contaminated water, immature worms can penetrate the skin and travel via the lymphatics and bloodstream to the mesenteric veins.[62] Eggs can travel to the intestine and urinary bladder or migrate up the

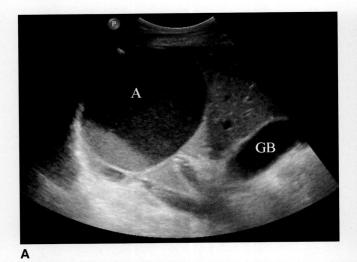

A

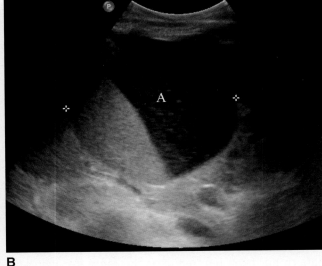

B

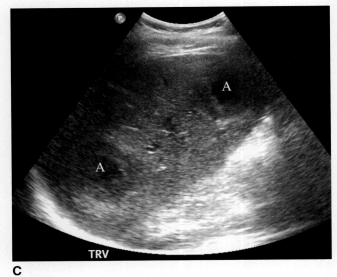

C

**Figure 5-25** Pyogenic abscesses. **A.** A sagittal scan of a middle-aged male with a debris-filled pyogenic liver abscess *(A)*. The gallbladder is identified *(GB)*. **B.** Transverse image from the same patient. The abscess measured 10 cm in diameter. **C.** A 49-year-old man presented with spiking fever and chills for 30 days. Sonogram revealed two liver masses consistent with abscesses *(A)*. During an open cholecystectomy procedure, the patient was also diagnosed with cholecystoduodenal and cholecystocolonic fistulas (the likely cause of bacterial liver invasion). (Courtesy of Margo Miller, Kettering Health Network, Kettering, OH.)

portal vein to the liver.[3,49,62] The ova penetrate the portal venous walls and lodge in the surrounding connective tissue. A granulomatous reaction occurs, inducing periportal fibrosis. Over a long period of time, portal hypertension may develop and cirrhosis is possible.[62]

Sonographic features include marked thickening and increased echogenicity of the periportal vein walls and radicles (Fig. 5-27A,B). Dilatation of the MPV and associated findings of portal hypertension are evident. Clinical correlation is needed. Initially, the liver may be enlarged and may have a normal parenchymal pattern; with time, the liver contracts as periportal fibrosis progresses and portal hypertension becomes more severe.

## HIV-AIDS

*Pneumocystis jiroveci* is the most common organism causing infection among patients with HIV and AIDS. The majority of people suffering from AIDS eventually develop *Pneumocystis* pneumonia. On occasion, *P. jiroveci* infection can spread outside the lungs to other

sites including the liver, spleen, pancreas, lymph nodes, and thyroid.[21] Extrapulmonary spread had increased with the use of aerosol pentamidine prophylaxis, which was believed to improve the survival of patients with HIV.[63] Yet, this treatment regimen is no longer in use yielding the decline of this infection. When liver involvement does occur, sonography often demonstrates a diffuse pattern of numerous tiny, brightly reflective parenchymal echoes presenting a "starry sky" pattern (Fig. 5-28A).[10,63] These hyperechoic foci may result from an inflammatory response to the offending organism.[49] They typically cast no acoustic shadows. However, as the disease progresses, acoustic shadowing may be noted from confluent areas of hepatic calcification. Multiorgan parenchymal calcification can indicate disseminated disease. Clinical correlation is needed since some other liver infections secondary to *cytomegalovirus* and *Mycobacterium avium-intracellulare* can display similar hepatic imaging patterns.[3] Visceral calcifications can also occur from histoplasmosis, granulomatous infection, tuberculosis, and as a sequela to traumatic and

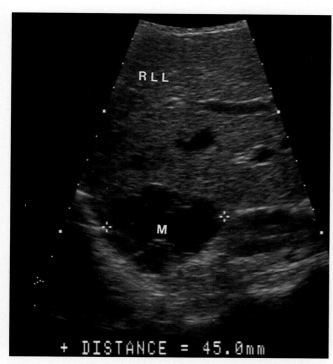

**Figure 5-26** Parasitic cyst. In the right lobe *(RLL)*, a 4.5-cm complex cystic mass *(M)* is detected in a woman who lived for a time in Indonesia.

other inflammatory processes (Fig. 5-28B). Differentiation between hepatic *P. jiroveci* and other opportunistic infections can be accomplished by core biopsy.

Some other hepatobiliary disorders affecting AIDS patients include fatty liver infiltration; hepatomegaly

(Fig. 5-28C); hepatitis; development of non-Hodgkin lymphoma,[44] candidiasis,[21] and cholangitis; cholecystitis; and biliary tract involvement from Kaposi sarcoma.[44] Kaposi sarcoma usually infiltrates the liver but generally produces no sonographic abnormality. If it is detected sonographically, Kaposi sarcoma can appear with increased periportal echogenicity, focal hypoechoic masses, or masses with mixed echogenicity (Fig. 5-28D).[64]

## CANDIDIASIS

A possible liver complication in patients with HIV or other immunocompromised conditions is hepatic candidiasis. Non-HIV conditions include hematopoietic malignancy, chronic granulomatous disease, chemotherapy, and organ transplantation.[17,47] Spread of this fungus (*Candida albicans*) is through the bloodstream. Patients may experience some RUQ pain and fever. This mycotic infection can cause hepatomegaly that is detectable by sonography. Fatty infiltration may be present, causing increased parenchymal reflectivity. Additionally, sonography may demonstrate the presence of focal liver masses (Fig. 5-29). The appearance of these lesions can change over the course of the disease process.[17,21,47,49] Initially, lesions may display a "wheel within a wheel" imaging pattern.[65] The center and outer portions are hypoechoic, with an intervening echogenic ring. The center eventually becomes more hypoechoic, yielding a "bull's-eye" appearance. Masses become progressively hypoechoic. A sequela of fibrosis and scar formation

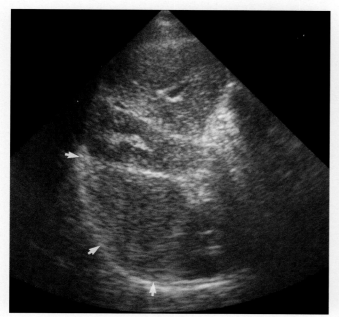

**A**

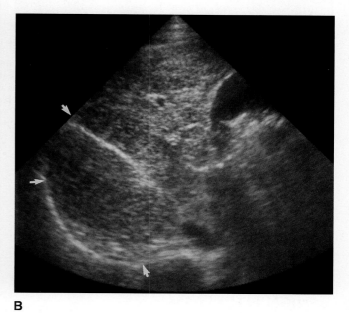

**B**

**Figure 5-27** Schistosomiasis. This 30-year-old woman presented with right back pain. A calcification was noted on a noncontrast abdominal radiograph, and the patient was referred for renal sonography evaluation. On both the sagittal **(A)** and transverse **(B)** sections of the liver, advanced periportal fibrosis provides the "turtle back" sonographic appearance *(arrows)*. (Courtesy of Charlotte Henningsen, Florida Hospital College of Health Sciences, Orlando, FL.)

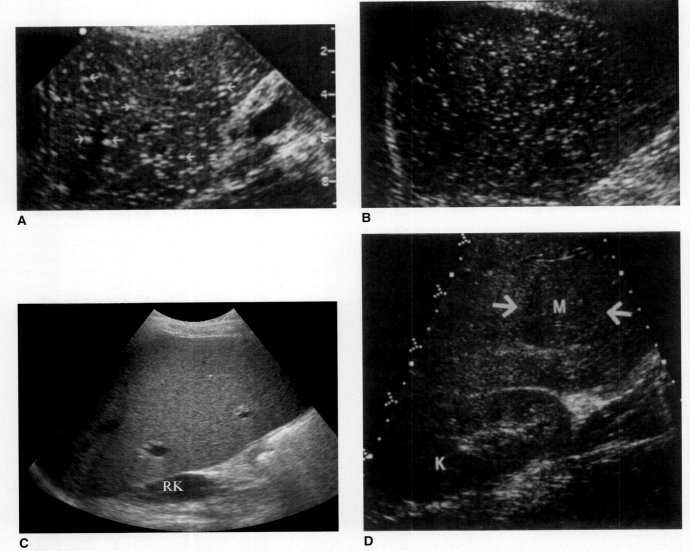

**Figure 5-28** HIV-AIDS–related liver disease. **A.** A sagittal scan of the left lobe of the liver reveals multiple tiny focal calcifications (starry sky) that are virtually invisible on computed tomography. This pattern is highly suggestive of, but not definitive for, disseminated *Pneumocystis* infection. **B.** An oblique longitudinal sonogram through the liver in this HIV-positive patient reveals a myriad of small focal calcifications. Although this pattern is most frequently seen in patients with disseminated *P. jiroveci* infection, other infectious processes in HIV patients may also produce this striking pattern. This patient had hepatic tuberculosis. Both mycobacterial and cytomegalovirus (CMV) infections occasionally produce findings similar to those illustrated here. (Images **A** and **B** reprinted with permission from Jeffrey RB, Ralls PW. *Sonography of the Abdomen.* New York, NY: Raven Press; 1995:142.) **C.** Hepatomegaly was documented on this scan of a 28-year-old male patient with AIDS. *RK*, right kidney. **D.** Kaposi sarcoma, focal mass. A subtle heterogeneous, mainly isoechoic mass (*M*) is noted on this longitudinal sonogram through the right lobe of the liver. Hepatomegaly, probably related to diffuse infiltration of the liver by Kaposi sarcoma, is present. *K*, right kidney. (Image **D** reprinted with permission from Jeffrey RB, Ralls PW. *Sonography of the Abdomen.* New York, NY: Raven Press; 1995:141.)

may result, offering a more coarse liver appearance with possible calcifications. Percutaneous aspiration of lesions can be performed for culture and histologic examination of affected liver tissue. Pathologic findings include the presence of yeast and mycelia contained in multiple microabscesses or small granulomas.[60]

## BENIGN NEOPLASM

In neonates and infants, benign hepatic tumors are more common than malignant ones[57]; in older children and adults, they are rarer than malignant ones,

whether primary or metastatic.[20] Primary liver tumors may originate from the parenchymal cells or bile duct epithelium or represent a mixture of the two. Sonography is an excellent imaging modality for liver tumors, although it lacks the necessary histologic specificity.

### CAVERNOUS HEMANGIOMA

Cavernous hemangioma is the most common benign liver tumor, occurring in up to 4% of the general population.[46,66,67] These lesions are not true neoplasms, as

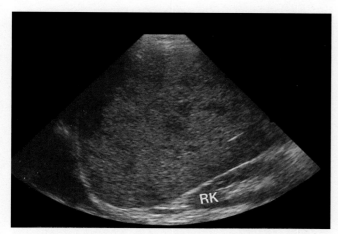

**Figure 5-29** Candidiasis: microabscesses. Multiple small, hypoechoic masses are seen in an immunocompromised patient receiving high-dose chemotherapy. Septic fever and hepatomegaly were present. A resolving right pelvic wall abscess was documented. Urinary tract infection and pulmonary infiltrates were part of the recent history. Although metastatic disease could represent some lesions, the rapid appearance of multiple masses between short-term imaging sessions was more indicative of septic emboli or fungal infection/candidiasis. *RK*, right kidney. (Courtesy of Good Samaritan Hospital, Corvallis, OR.)

histologically, they are composed of a large network of blood-filled vascular spaces lined with endothelium.[50,67] The spaces are separated by fibrous septa, which commonly proliferate centrally and extend peripherally. Hemangiomas are five times more common in women.[21] Lesions can occur at any age but increase in frequency with age.[67]

Most hemangiomas are found incidentally, as they cause no symptoms.[66,67] Most are solitary; 10% to 20% are multiple. Typical hemangiomas measure less than 3 cm, but larger lesions are possible.[21] They may grow slowly and enlarge during pregnancy, causing hepatomegaly and abdominal discomfort with degeneration and fibrosis. Occasionally calcifications are identified, but these phleboliths are rare.[50] Their location is typically in the posterior segment of the right lobe and in a subcapsular or marginal position (close to the periphery of the liver).[50]

Sonography is reported to be more reliable than CT in detecting cavernous hemangiomas, especially those smaller than 1 cm.[66] The classic sonographic appearance is a homogeneous (58% to 73%), hyperechoic (67% to 79%) mass with sharp, well-defined margins and possible posterior acoustic enhancement (Table 5-9, Fig. 5-30A–D).[21,67] When hemangiomas are smaller than 2.5 cm, acoustic enhancement may not be seen. Conventional color Doppler and power Doppler offer limited diagnostic information, because even though the tumor is a network of tightly woven blood vessels, the flow within them is too slow to be visualized with color Doppler.[28] Larger lesions present with more variable echo patterns—hypoechoic, isoechoic, heterogeneous[46]—as they become necrotic after depleting their internal blood supply. These atypical hemangiomas have the ability to mimic HCC (Fig. 5-30E–G).

If cavernous hemangioma is suspected after sonography, a short-term follow-up sonography examination is

| TABLE 5-9 | | | |
|---|---|---|---|
| **Benign Liver Neoplasms** | | | |
| **Neoplasm** | **Histologic Appearance** | **Clinical Signs** | **Sonographic Appearance** |
| Cavernous hemangioma | Large network of vascular endothelial-lined spaces with red blood cells. | No symptoms; 70% to 95% occur in women; frequency increases with age. | Usually homogeneous, hyperechoic mass with sharp, well-defined margins; may have posterior acoustic enhancement, usually in the posterior right segment. |
| Focal nodular hyperplasia | Hepatocytes, Kupffer cells, bile duct elements, and fibrous connective tissue; central fibrous band with radiating septa separates mass into nodules; no known malignant potential. | Usually asymptomatic, generally an incidental finding. | May be hypoechoic, hyperechoic, or isoechoic with normal tissue; 0.5-cm to 20-cm well-circumscribed mass. |
| Liver cell adenoma | Encapsulated, slightly atypical hepatocytes, often with areas of bile stasis, focal hemorrhage, and necrosis; malignant potential of a hepatoma; susceptible to hemorrhage. | Usually symptomatic; incidence increases in women of childbearing age and is associated with oral contraceptive use. | Usually hyperechoic relative to normal tissue; well-circumscribed mass; with hemorrhage, internal pattern ranges from anechoic to hyperechoic, depending on age of bleed. |

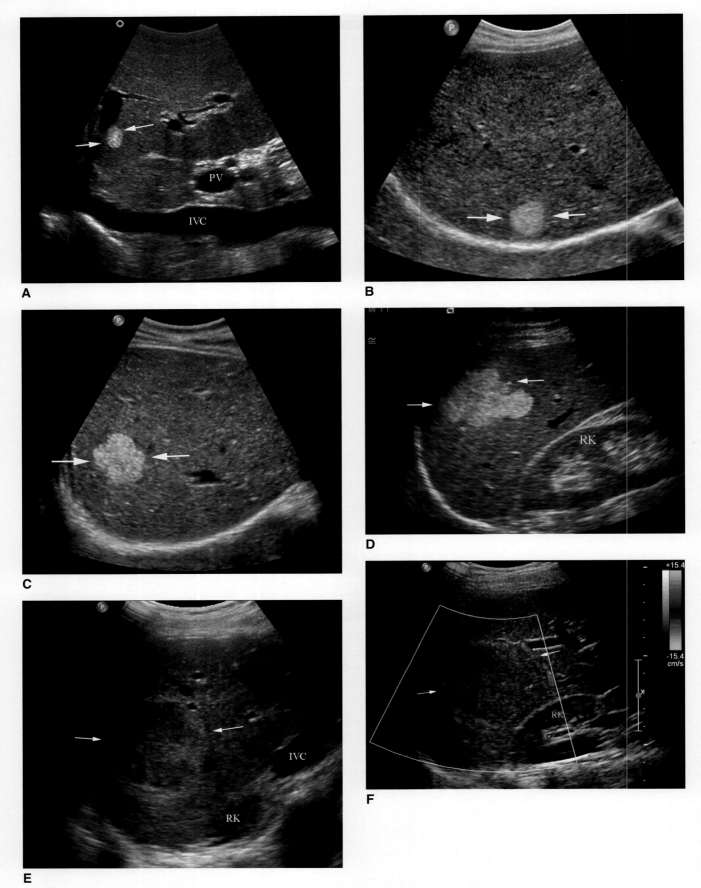

**Figure 5-30** Cavernous hemangioma. **A–D.** Four different patients are seen with classic sonographic appearances of cavernous hemangioma *(arrows)* ranging from small to large. *IVC,* inferior vena cava; *PV,* portal vein; *RK,* right kidney. **E–G.** A 37-year-old woman presented for a gallbladder examination. A 5.5-cm mass *(arrows)* was noted in the right lobe of the liver. Follow-up magnetic resonance imaging evaluation confirmed atypical liver hemangioma. *IVC,* inferior vena cava; *RK,* right kidney. *(continued)*

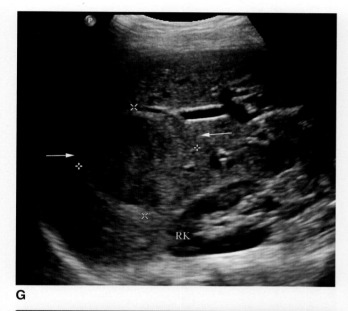

G

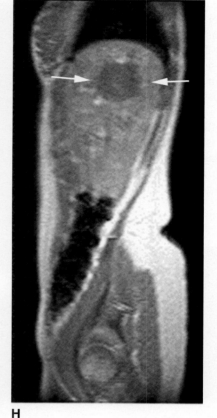

H

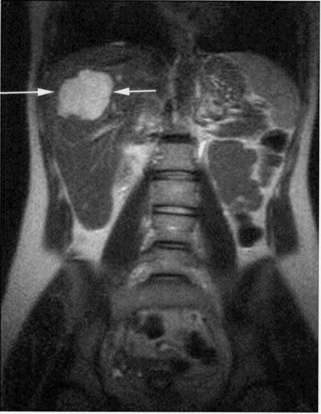

I

**Figure 5-30** *(continued)* **H.** A hypointense liver lesion *(arrows)* is noted on this T1-weighted magnetic resonance parasagittal image. **I.** The same lesion is demonstrated here on the T2-weighted coronal image as a hyperintense mass *(arrows)* confirming liver hemangioma.

accepted practice. If symptoms persist or characterization of a lesion with an atypical appearance is needed, another imaging modality may be useful. Clinicians regard magnetic resonance imaging (MRI) as the preferred modality in the confirmation of cavernous hemangiomas. On MRI, hemangiomas display low signal intensities on T1-weighted images with a markedly increased intensity on T2-weighted images (Fig. 5-30H,I). Hepatic

scintigraphy (nuclear medicine scan), using single photon emission computed tomography (SPECT) and technetium-99m–labeled red blood cells, is also sensitive and specific for diagnosing hepatic cavernous hemangiomas.[68] This procedure is preferable to CT and angiography if a hypoechoic or mixed echogenic hepatic lesion is found in a symptomatic patient who has abnormal LFT values or a known primary tumor. Dynamic CT can support the diagnosis of cavernous hemangioma if strict criteria are met.[21] After initial bolus injection of contrast material, vascular enhancement occurs along the periphery of the hypodense lesion and then completely fills in the lesion on delayed scans. Researchers are hopeful that contrast-enhanced sonography will offer definitive diagnosis of cavernous hemangiomas in the future.[21]

To establish stability, a 6-month follow-up sonography examination is recommended if a hyperechoic hepatic lesion is discovered incidentally in an asymptomatic patient with normal LFTs and no known primary disease. Large-gauge percutaneous needle biopsy should not be performed on these lesions because of the risk of potential hemorrhage.[50]

## FOCAL NODULAR HYPERPLASIA

Focal nodular hyperplasia (FNH) is a benign nodule that contains all the cellular elements of normal liver tissue (hepatocytes, Kupffer cells, bile duct elements, fibrous connective tissue) but lacks the normal hepatic architecture.[57] FNH is the second most common benign tumor of the liver.[21] This hyperplastic condition may occur at any age, although it is rare in children.[57] It is more common in women before the age of 21[69] and

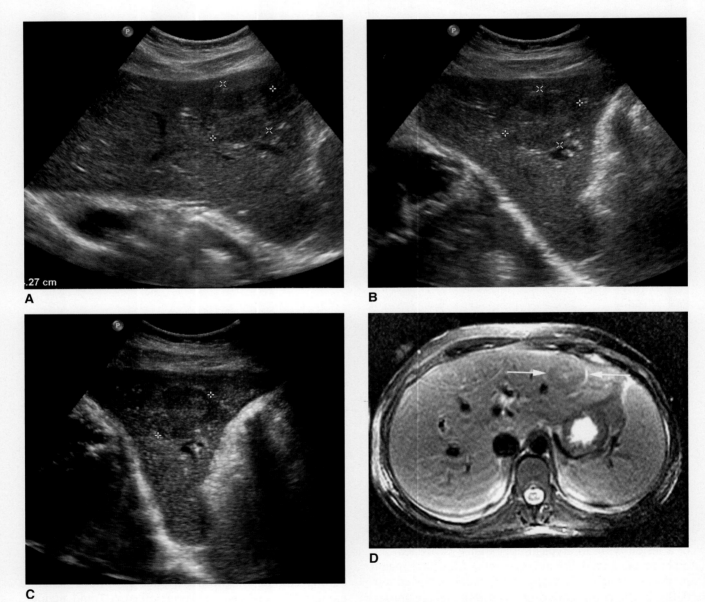

**Figure 5-31** Focal nodular hyperplasia. **A.** A 28-year-old female presented with abdomen and back pain, nausea and vomiting, and a history of gastric ulcers. A transverse scan shows a 4-cm subtle, isoechoic mass *(calipers)* detected in the left lobe. **B.** A sagittal image demonstrates the subtle mass *(calipers)* with **(C)** background color enhancement. **D.** A magnetic resonance image confirmed the lesion *(arrows)* as a focal nodular hyperplasia. (Courtesy of Jon Blaza, Kettering Health Network, Kettering, OH.)

there is controversial evidence of a relationship with long-term use of oral contraceptives. Individuals with FNH are usually asymptomatic unless lesions become large or hemorrhage.[50]

Sonographically, the classic appearance of FNH is a subtle, isoechoic lesion that is difficult to identify within the normal liver parenchyma (Fig. 5-31A–D).[67] FNH has also been described as a cirrhosis-like mass in normal tissue. The range of echotextures include hypoechoic, hyperechoic, or isoechoic.[46,66] Even though the mass is not encapsulated and multinodular, it is well circumscribed, with a characteristic depressed central or eccentric stellate scar composed of dense fibrous connective tissue, proliferating bile ducts, and thin-walled blood vessels, which may or may not appear on images.[46,66] Color Doppler imaging demonstrates impressive blood flow with rich vascularity in the center of the lesion (feeding vessel).

FNH lesions usually measure less than 8 cm[50] but can range in size from 0.5 to 20 cm. The mass is often located in the right lobe or lateral segment of the left lobe. In 13% of cases, lesions are multiple.[50,57] The reported sensitivity of various imaging modalities for FNH is as follows: ultrasonography with color Doppler, 100%; dynamic CT, 80%; enhanced MRI, 70%; and radionuclide scanning, 55%.[70] However, sonographic imaging features alone are not specific. Since these masses contain Kupffer cells that accumulate injected [99m]Tc-sulfur colloid and liver cell adenomas (LCA) do not, colloid uptake by a focal hepatic mass is virtually diagnostic of FNH.[68]

## LIVER CELL ADENOMA

LCA differ from FNH in that they contain no bile duct or Kupffer cells but are true hepatic encapsulated neoplasms, consisting of normal to slightly atypical hepatocytes, often with areas of bile stasis, focal hemorrhage, and necrosis. An LCA is usually solitary, with identifiable margins. When present, this uncommon mass occurs over 90% of the time in women, most often of childbearing age.[50] Its association with long-term oral contraceptive use in women is well documented.[21,59,67] Occasionally, LCA has been associated with androgen therapy in men[50] and is reported in patients with glycogen storage disease (type 1 von Gierke disease).[59,67] Lesions can shrink or disappear after the cessation of hormone administration.[50] In some cases, there is malignant potential related to adenomas.[67]

LCA produces no significant laboratory value changes and is sometimes an incidental finding. Usually adenomas cause symptoms ranging from a palpable mass and abdominal pressure to acute, severe RUQ pain due to rupture and sudden intraperitoneal hemorrhage.[59,67] Larger tumor size and hemorrhage are more common with LCAs than with FNH.

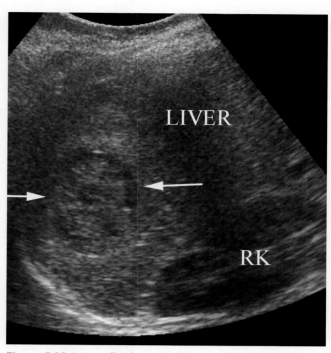

**Figure 5-32** Liver cell adenoma. The sonogram displays an encapsulated, well-circumscribed mass on a patient diagnosed with an adenoma. *RK*, right kidney. (Image courtesy of Robert DeJung, Baltimore, MD.)

The sonographic features are variable and may not be specific for LCA, FNH, metastatic disease, hepatoma, or even some hemangiomas (Table 5-9). Close correlation with clinical manifestations, radionuclide studies, CT, MRI, and, in some cases, angiography may be necessary to make a definitive diagnosis.[59] The usual appearance is of an encapsulated, well-circumscribed, hyperechoic mass, but it may appear hypoechoic or isoechoic relative to normal liver parenchyma (Fig. 5-32). As the tumor hemorrhages, the sonographic appearance varies with the age and extent of bleeding from anechoic to hyperechoic.

## LIPOMA

Intrahepatic lipomas are very rare and do not undergo malignant transformation.[47] Affected individuals are typically asymptomatic.[67] Masses may also be detected in children. Sonographic presentation of a lipoma is that of a highly echogenic lesion, which may not be distinguished from a hemangioma or hyperechoic metastases. Lipomas may result in speed error artifacts, a common acoustic misrepresentation. Because the speed of sound through fat is slower than through the normal liver, echoes distal to the mass will be displaced slightly deeper in the body.[47,49] Hepatic angiomyolipomas have been reported in patients with tuberous sclerosis.[49] Associated renal angiomyolipomas may also be present (Fig. 5-33). CT can confirm the fatty nature of these lesions.[21]

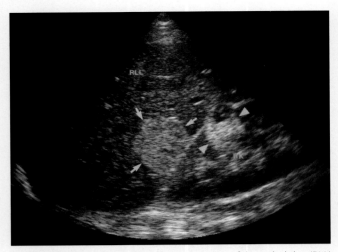

**Figure 5-33** Angiomyolipoma. A sagittal scan of the right lobe *(RLL)* reveals an echogenic mass *(arrows)* at the inferior edge. However, no significant sound distortion was noted posterior to this mass. The patient had known tuberous sclerosis. Bilateral echogenic cortical renal masses were also present. One of these is identified *(arrows)* on this scan displaying cystic degeneration *(arrowheads)* in the right kidney *(RK)*.

## MALIGNANT NEOPLASMS

### PRIMARY MALIGNANT TUMORS

Histologically, most primary malignant liver tumors are either HCC (80% to 90%), which develops in the hepatocytes, or cholangiocellular carcinoma (cholangiocarcinoma), which develops in the bile ducts (see Chapter 6). HCC, also known as hepatoma, is much less common in the United States than in densely populated parts of the Far East, southern Africa, China, Japan, and Greece.[53] It is the fifth most common cancer worldwide[71] and risk factors vary significantly. An epidemiologic study of primary liver carcinomas indicates that they may be related to exposure to carcinogens such as mycotoxins in the diet; chronic liver disease, especially cirrhosis; viral infections, especially HBV; and parasitic liver infections.[34,43] Individuals with hemochromatosis and some metabolic and glycogen storage diseases are at increased risk for developing cirrhosis and possible liver carcinoma.[47]

## HEPATOCELLULAR CARCINOMA

In the United States, the majority of HCCs develop in persons with preexisting cirrhosis.[21,28,60,67] It is unusual before age 40 and is most common in the sixth decade. Men are more often affected than women (5:1)[21] and blacks more often than whites. Morphologically, HCC may be: (1) focal, limited to one area; (2) multiple, occur in numerous nodules; or (3) diffuse, as infiltrates throughout the liver.[34,43,67] Physiologically, HCC interferes with normal hepatocyte function, causing biliary obstruction with jaundice, portal hypertension with ascites, portal vein thrombosis, and different metabolic disturbances. LFTs demonstrate increased levels of ALP, AST, and ALT. The most significant liver function anomaly is the presence of α-fetoprotein (AFP) in 70% of cases.[20,46] The pathophysiology may include invasion of the hepatic veins (producing Budd-Chiari syndrome)[24] and the portal veins,[67] resulting in metastasis to the heart and lungs and to other sites such as the brain, kidney, adrenal gland, spleen,[34] and bone.[47]

Patients usually present with RUQ pain, sudden deterioration of hepatic function in an already compromised liver, a palpable mass, rapid liver enlargement, fever of unknown origin, and ascites. By the time it is discovered, HCC is usually in an advanced stage and patients survive for only a few months. Greten et al.[71] published a retrospective study regarding survival rates in patients with HCC from 1998 to 2003. Of the 389 patients studied, the average survival rate was 11 months.[71] The diagnosis is based on clinical manifestations; laboratory function anomalies, especially the presence of AFP; imaging studies; and biopsy.

Sonographically, HCC has a range of appearances, evolving from progressively hypoechoic to isoechoic and as a lesion grows, it becomes unevenly hyperechoic (Fig. 5-34A–D). A few are diffusely hyperechoic initially and retain the same features throughout the disease process. Correlating sonographic and histologic findings reveal that hypoechoic lesions correspond to solid tumors without necrosis; complex masses are seen in tumors with some necrotic areas; and hyperechoic lesions are seen in two types of tumor: those with fatty metamorphosis and those with marked sinusoidal dilatation. Tumors usually do not calcify.[47] Because most patients with HCC have preexisting cirrhosis, differentiation of regenerating nodules from malignant tumors can be difficult.

The benefit of sonography is its ability to localize, measure, and characterize the presentation of HCC. Treatment and surgical resectability depend on the distribution and extent of liver involvement, the presence of vascular invasion, and the degree of metastatic spread. Detected tumors should be classified as focal, multiple, or diffuse, and affected liver segments should be recorded. Attention is paid to displacement or tumor invasion of intrahepatic vessels, the IVC, and the extrahepatic portal venous system. Portal vein thrombosis is reported in approximately 30% of HCC cases.[25] Tumors can compress bile ducts, causing localized dilatation. Sonography of the remaining abdomen can document ascites, regional lymphadenopathy, and other metastatic sites.

Doppler interrogation of larger HCCs tends to elicit increased vascularity and high-velocity signals.[21] More flow may be noted at the periphery and central part of

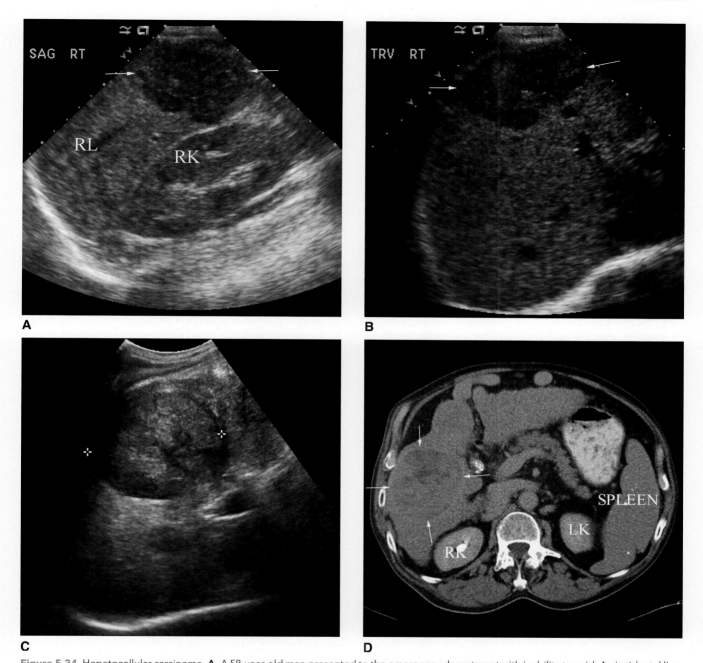

**Figure 5-34** Hepatocellular carcinoma. **A.** A 58-year-old man presented to the emergency department with inability to void. An incidental liver mass (arrows) was noted on his renal sonography evaluation. RK, right kidney; RL, right lobe. The mass has a hypoechoic, irregularly shaped appearance on this sagittal scan and **(B)** transverse image. Biopsy confirmed poorly differentiated hepatocellular carcinoma. It was later revealed that the patient was a polysubstance abuser with a history of hepatitis B and C. (Courtesy of Melanie Willsey, Kettering Health Network, Kettering, OH.) **C.** A 67-year-old man with a history of hepatitis C presents with an 8.5-cm liver mass consistent with hepatoma (calipers). **D.** A follow-up computed tomographic image confirmed the mass (arrows). LK, left kidney; RK, right kidney.

the mass compared to other liver tumors. However, the presentation is variable. Demonstration of tumor vascularity may be enhanced with the use of color and power-mode Doppler combined with sonography contrast agents.[67]

Oncologists continue to claim that the only potentially curative treatment for HCC is hepatic resection,[72] with survival rates between 30% and 50%. However, most patients have nonresectable tumors or are poor surgical candidates. Apart from traditional methods, nonresected hepatic neoplasms may be managed by transarterial chemoembolization[71,73] and percutaneous ethanol injection.[71,73] Other recently reported techniques for direct tumor treatment include percutaneous ablation therapy,[73] percutaneous microwave coagulation,[73] and interstitial therapies such as laser therapy, cryotherapy, and radiation therapy. In patients with a poor response to therapy, palliative transcatheter hepatic arterial embolization or, in some cases, hepatic transplantation is necessary. Unfortunately, donors are often scarce and tumor recurrence is possible. CT and sonography can be used as guidance techniques for an initial biopsy diagnosis and later for some percutaneous treatments of HCC.

## FIBROLAMELLAR HEPATOCELLULAR CARCINOMA

A subtype of HCC that typically manifests in adolescents and young adults is fibrolamellar HCC. This malignancy accounts for less than 11% of hepatomas.[47] Affected patients usually have no definable risk factors, and their long-term prognosis is better than that of patients with typical HCC. The average 5-year survival rate is 63%.[47] In this subtype, AFP values are normal.

Sonography reveals a solid-appearing liver lesion, typically solitary and often large, with variable echogenicity.[21,47] Lesions may be relatively homogeneous. Echogenic scarring and calcification are more common in fibrolamellar hepatomas than in typical HCC, leading to a heterogeneous appearance.[21,47]

## HEPATIC HEMANGIOSARCOMA

A rare but extremely aggressive malignant tumor is hepatic hemangiosarcoma (angiosarcoma). Hemangiosarcomas are malignant neoplasms that are composed of endothelial and fibroblastic tissue that surrounds the vessels of the liver.[27] It is the most common primary liver sarcoma.[50] There is a causative link with neoplastic development from exposure to arsenic, thorotrast, or polyvinyl chloride.[47,50] Development of symptoms may take decades. Presentation most often occurs between ages 60 and 80 years with rapid metastasis. Common metastatic sites include the lung, spleen, lymph nodes, bone marrow, thyroid, and peritoneal cavity. Thrombosis of the portal vein is possible.

Sonographic features depend on the time of presentation and may be nonspecific. Preceding tumor formation is a variable degree of portal and liver fibrosis with increased sound attenuation.[60] Sonographically, hepatic hemangiosarcomas appear as solid or mixed liver lesions. Small, diffuse lesions may be indistinguishable from fibrotic parenchymal changes.[60] Hemorrhage and necrosis yield lesions with mixed echo textures containing fluid-filled spaces.[47]

## EPITHELIOID HEMANGIOENDOTHELIOMA

Benign hemangioendotheliomas develop in infants. However, an uncommon malignant vascular tumor can occur in adults called *hepatic epithelioid hemangioendothelioma* (*EHE*).[21,50,60] In addition to the liver, concomitant lesions can develop within pulmonary and soft tissues.[67] On a sonography examination, liver lesions are typically hypoechoic and multiple in number, and may contain calcifications.[21,67] Lesions along the hepatic margins may lie close to each other and image as a larger mass.[67]

## METASTASES

The incidence of metastatic liver tumors is 18 to 20 times that of primary hepatic malignancies.[50] Primary cancers arising from the gallbladder, colon, stomach, pancreas, breast, and lung (decreasing order) are the most common forms contributing to metastatic liver disease.[21] Physiologically, the liver is vulnerable to metastatic carcinoma because of the large volume of blood it receives, the high nutrient level of the blood, and the large reserve of lymphatic drainage.[43] It is estimated that approximately 40% of patients with carcinoma have liver metastasis.[66] Clinically, metastases are frequently silent. The clinical course is related to the growth of the metastatic lesion and the site of the primary malignancy.[43] Symptoms may include hepatomegaly, jaundice, pain, nutritional wasting, and muscle wasting; other dysfunctions depend on the amount of hepatocellular involvement.[43] LFT values are frequently abnormal, especially ALP, AST, and ALT, and AFP is increased in many cases of liver metastasis. Multiple metastases give rise to multiple masses in the liver, suggesting that tumor seeding has occurred in episodes.[57] The prognosis is generally poor because of the poor response to treatment, the difficulty of resecting the tumor(s) surgically, and reseeding of the liver. Hepatectomy is the recommended treatment option for patients with resectable liver metastasis. The 5-year survival rate following surgery has been reported to be 20% to 30%.[23] Like HCC, however, most patients have nonresectable tumors or are poor surgical candidates.

Sonographically, metastases have a wide variety of appearances, reflecting the spectrum of tumor types: (1) hypoechoic, (2) hyperechoic, (3) isoechoic, (4) anechoic, (5) mixed (hyperechoic and hypoechoic), (6) bull's-eye or target appearance, or (7) complex (Fig. 5-35A–F).[20,57] Sonography examinations lack specificity for correlating the sonographic appearance of hepatic metastases with the organ or cell type of origin.[20,46] Some noted tendencies, however, are as follows: A majority of hyperechoic masses are from a primary colon tumor (54%)[66] and renal cell carcinomas[21]; cystic lesions may be associated with leiomyosarcomas and mucinous ovarian cancer[47]; and hypoechoic masses with lymphoma are seen.[57] Target-like metastases are frequently seen with lung cancer.[21] Additional findings include calcification within mucinous carcinomas[47] and in tumors that are partially involuting.[20] As with most tumors in the liver, an important finding is that hypervascular metastatic lesions are typically hyperechoic and hypovascular lesions are hypoechoic.[20]

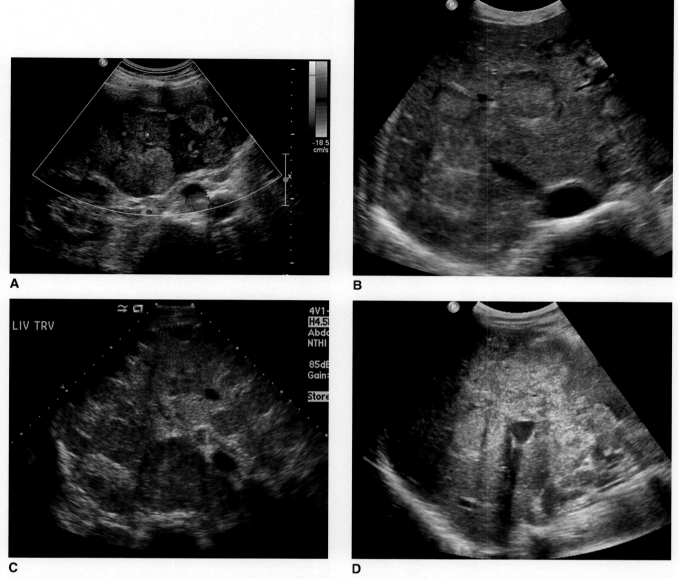

**Figure 5-35** Hepatic metastasis. **A.** A 48-year-old woman demonstrates multiple liver lesions with a 1-year history of colon cancer. **B.** A 73-year-old man now presents with stage IV squamous cell carcinoma of the mouth and jaw with metastasis to the liver, kidney, and adrenal gland. **C.** A 35-year-old man with a 7-year history of testicular cancer (teratoma and seminoma mix) now presents with chronic nausea and vomiting. Sonographic evaluation reveals multiple liver masses consistent with liver metastasis. **D.** These large hyperechoic liver masses were seen in a 55-year-old female patient with pancreatic cancer. *(continued)*

Sonography can be used to locate, measure, and characterize the initial lesion and as a noninvasive follow-up procedure to assess metastases for changes in size and appearance.[20] It is also valuable for distinguishing obstructive versus nonobstructive jaundice in patients suspected of having underlying malignant disease.[28]

Sonography can also aid in postsurgical hepatectomy assessment of liver regeneration and complications (Fig. 5-35G–I). Intrahepatic or perihepatic fluid collections, including hematoma, biloma, abscess, lymphoceles, and ascites, may be easily evaluated (Fig. 5-35J). Although sonography may not always be able to distinguish between the types of fluid collections, serial assessment can document progression or regression of findings.

## CONTRAST-ENHANCED ULTRASOUND

Contrast-enhanced ultrasound (CEUS) has proven useful in the evaluation of focal hepatic lesions. Although not yet approved by the U.S. Food and Drug Administration (FDA) for this use, CEUS of the liver is performed routinely in other parts of the world.[17,74] Similar to contrast-enhanced CT or MRI, CEUS allows for an evaluation of lesions based on their perfusion

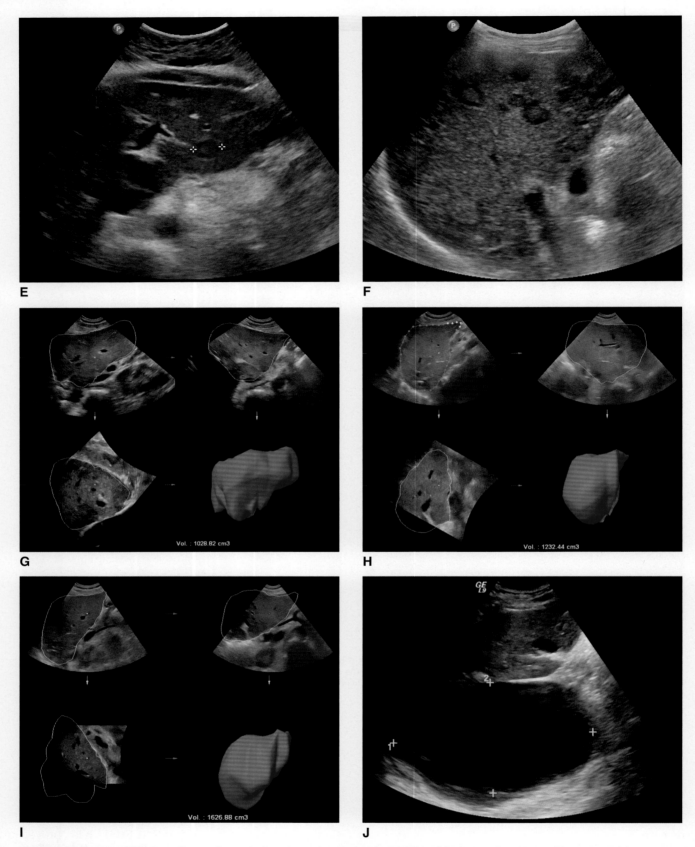

**Figure 5-35** *(continued)* **E.** A small target lesion *(calipers)* was identified in the left lobe of the liver in this 60-year-old woman with lung cancer. **F.** Multiple target lesions were easily identified on this sonogram of a 55-year-old woman with a history of breast cancer. **G–I.** A 59-year-old man with a history of colorectal cancer 1 year prior presents postsurgically following treatment of liver metastasis for sonographic evaluation of liver regeneration. Liver volume was calculated using a three-dimensional (3D) volume calculation. Presurgical liver volume measured 1,822 cm³. **G.** Twelve days following partial hepatectomy (extended right lobectomy), 3D sonography reveals a liver volume of 1,029 cm³. **H.** Twenty-four days after surgery, liver volume increased in size to 1,232 cm³. **I.** Thirty-six days postsurgery, the liver reached a volume of 1,627 cm. (Courtesy of John Walker, Jamestown, OH.) **J.** A large fluid collection *(calipers)* was noted in a partial hepatectomy patient prior to right lobe regeneration.

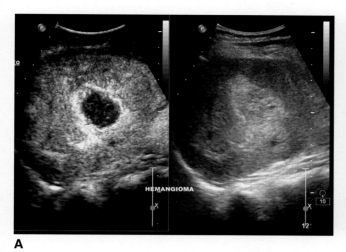

**A**

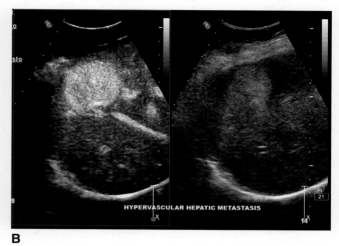

**B**

**Figure 5-36** Contrast-enhanced sonography. **A.** Contrast-enhanced ultrasound of the liver demonstrates a cavernous hemangioma. **B.** Contrast-enhanced ultrasound of the liver in another patient shows a hypervascular liver metastasis.

characteristics.[67,74] Grayscale sonography of focal liver lesions has limitations; the lesions may be difficult to see in the setting of a fatty or cirrhotic liver, and the sonographic appearances of many benign and malignant lesions overlap.[67,74] Studies have shown that without contrast, sonography is able to correctly characterize focal liver lesions 60% to 65% of the time; with contrast, the lesions are correctly characterized 86% to 95% of the time.[74] Conventional grayscale sonography was able to differentiate between benign and malignant lesions only 23% to 68% of the time, whereas CEUS was able to correctly make the distinction in 92% to 95% of patients.[74] CEUS is used to evaluate the vascularity and enhancement patterns of indeterminate lesions found on grayscale sonography or other imaging modalities. Benign and malignant liver lesions each have different enhancement patterns on CEUS, frequently allowing for a more definitive diagnosis without further testing (Fig. 5-36A,B).

## PORTOSYSTEMIC SHUNTS

Patients with portal hypertension, bleeding gastroesophageal varices, or Budd-Chiari syndrome may require shunt procedures for medical management.[24,44] Possible locations for shunts are between (1) the portal vein and IVC, (2) the SMV and IVC, (3) the splenic vein and left renal vein, and (4) intrahepatically between the MPV and hepatic vein.

Doppler sonography aids in the evaluation of shunts, allowing documentation of shunt patency and blood flow direction. Complications include thrombosis or stenosis of the shunt or stent, neointimal hyperplasia, and outflow obstruction.[24]

Percutaneous placement of intrahepatic shunts using expandable metal stents is an alternative to surgical shunts in some patients.[24,44] Transjugular intrahepatic portosystemic shunt (TIPS) is a temporary or palliative treatment option in patients with significant liver disease (Fig. 5-37A). TIPS dysfunction can be easily assessed with sonography. A baseline study should be obtained within 24 hours after insertion for serial evaluation. Color or power-mode Doppler and spectral analysis of the MPV, the stent, and the hepatic vein or IVC are optimized by attention to Doppler settings and insonation angle (Fig. 5-37B). Expected flow direction is from the portal vein to the hepatic vein or IVC. Reversed flow is normally detected in the RPV above the entrance to the shunt.[44] Spectral waveforms are obtained proximal and distal to the stent in the MPV and hepatic veins, as well as in the proximal, middle, and distal stent(s). Peak velocities are measured at each location. Attention is paid to focal increases in velocity at narrowed sections or to an increase or decrease in stent or prestent flow on serial exams. A decrease in flow velocity greater than 40 cm/sec or an increase greater than 60 cm/sec is indicative of stent dysfunction.[75] A flow velocity of less than 60 cm/sec or greater than 200 cm/sec within the stent is also suggestive of stenosis.[75] Absent flow suggests thrombosis. Patients with stenosis may demonstrate reverse flow in the hepatic vein, the intrahepatic portal vein, or both (Fig. 5-37C).

## SUMMARY

* The liver is an intraperitoneal organ and is the largest internal organ in the body, measuring 15 to 17 cm in a sagittal plane along the right lobe.

* The liver is divided into the right, left, and caudate lobes and is covered by a connective tissue layer referred to as *Glisson capsule.*

* Lobular divisions of the liver are described as anatomic, based on external landmarks, such as fissures and ligaments, or segmental, based on hepatic function.

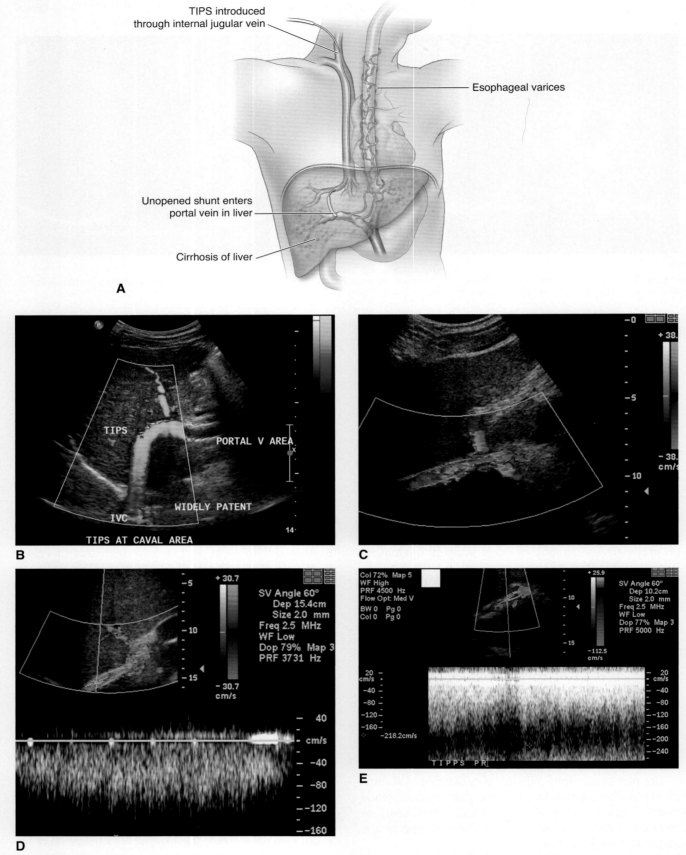

**Figure 5-37** Portosystemic shunt. **A.** An illustration shows TIPS. **B.** A liver sonogram of a 23-year-old woman with a history of autoimmune hepatitis and a single shunt placed between the main portal vein and inferior vena cava. Power Doppler assessment reveals a widely patent transjugular intrahepatic portosystemic shunt. **C–E.** On this patient with a stenosis, the images display the stenosis, poststenotic turbulence, and Doppler evaluation of the stenosis. (Images **C, D,** and **E** courtesy of Robert DeJong, Baltimore, MD.)

- The liver receives a unique double blood supply; the hepatic artery supplies oxygen-rich blood and the portal vein supplies nutrient-rich blood from the walls of the gastrointestinal tract. Both vessels can be seen entering the liver at the porta hepatis.

- The right, middle, and left hepatic veins drain directly into the IVC and are best visualized in a transverse plane with the transducer angled toward the cephalad portion of the liver.

- The liver performs over 500 functions including bile formation and secretion; the metabolism of carbohydrates, fats, and proteins; production of clotting factors; vitamin storage; blood reservoir; detoxification; and lymph formation.

- Liver function tests include ALT, which is most specific to hepatocellular disease, AST, ALP, lactic dehydrogenase, bilirubin, $\gamma$-glutamyl transpeptidase (GGT), prothrombin time, and albumin.

- Diffuse hepatocellular diseases, which affect the liver as a whole and interfere with normal liver function, include fatty infiltration, glycogen storage disease, hepatitis, and cirrhosis.

- Fatty infiltration of the liver can range from mild to severe and has many causes, but the most common are alcohol abuse and obesity. Sonographic features include a diffuse increase in the hepatic parenchymal echogenicity with a decrease in acoustic penetration.

- Hepatitis is an inflammation of the liver and can be caused by a virus or toxins such as drugs or alcohol. In the acute phase, the liver parenchyma may appear normal or hypoechoic due to diffuse swelling of the liver cells, whereas the portal vein walls appear more hyperechoic in contrast to the hypoechoic parenchyma. In the chronic phase, the parenchyma may appear hyperechoic, similar to that of fatty infiltration.

- Cirrhosis is a chronic, progressive disease that destroys the normal architecture of the liver lobules; caused most frequently by alcohol abuse, it can also be associated with biliary obstruction, metabolic disorders, and hepatitis.

- Sonographic features of cirrhosis vary with the stage of the disease and early on may include hepatomegaly and a diffuse increase in echogenicity; as the disease progresses, sonographic features can include a shrunken right lobe, hypertrophied caudate lobe, surface nodularity, hyperechoic parenchyma, loss of delineation of hepatic vasculature, possible portal hypertension, and ascites.

- Budd-Chiari syndrome is the obstruction of the hepatic venous outflow tract by tumor or thrombus in the hepatic veins or IVC.

- Hepatic cysts are more prevalent with increasing age, are usually asymptomatic, discovered incidentally, and should meet the diagnostic criteria for a simple cyst.

- Polycystic liver disease becomes detectable in the third or fourth decade and is an inherited disorder usually associated with autosomal dominant polycystic kidney disease.

- Acquired liver cysts can be categorized as traumatic (hematoma, biloma), parasitic (echinococcal), or inflammatory (abscess) and range in sonographic appearance from cystic to complex masses.

- Patients with AIDS may develop *Pneumocystis jiroveci* infection of the liver that presents sonographically as a diffuse pattern of numerous tiny brightly reflective echoes termed a "starry sky" pattern.

- Candidiasis is a fungal infection spread via the blood in patients with HIV and other immunocompromised conditions that causes hepatomegaly, fatty infiltration, and focal liver masses that may demonstrate a "wheel within a wheel" or "bull's-eye" appearance.

- Benign solid neoplasms of the liver include cavernous hemangiomas, focal nodular hyperplasia, lipomas, and liver cell adenomas.

- Hepatocellular carcinoma (HCC) is the most common primary malignant liver tumor and in the United States, the most common predisposing factor is cirrhosis.

- HCC or hepatoma interferes with normal hepatocyte function and may present as a focal nodule, multiple nodules, or may diffusely infiltrate the liver. LFTs are abnormal and AFP is elevated in 70% of cases.

- Hepatomas range in sonographic appearance from hypoechoic to hyperechoic, hepatic vein and portal vein invasion is common, and bile duct compression with subsequent dilatation is possible.

- Because of the large volume of blood the liver receives, metastatic liver tumors are 18 to 20 times more common than primary hepatic malignancies and may arise from many primary cancers including GI, breast, or pulmonary carcinoma.

- Sonographically, liver metastases may appear hypoechoic, hyperechoic, isoechoic, anechoic, complex, or have a bull's-eye or target appearance.

- Contrast-enhanced ultrasound is used to characterize focal liver lesions when the grayscale findings are indeterminant.

- Portosystemic shunts can be used to manage complications from portal hypertension, bleeding gastrointestinal varices, or Budd-Chiari syndrome. A transjugular intrahepatic portosystemic shunt (TIPS) typically connects the main portal vein to a hepatic vein and helps elevate symptoms of portal hypertension.

- CT, PET/CT, MRI, and radionuclide studies all play important roles in the diagnosis of liver disease.

- Radionuclide studies can be used to determine the cause and location of obstruction in patients with jaundice and can be used to confirm the diagnosis of a cavernous hemangioma.

## Critical Thinking Questions

1. How can portal veins be differentiated from hepatic veins sonographically?

2. A 38-year-old woman presents with a history of right upper quadrant pain and fullness. Your examination reveals simple cysts too numerous to count of varying sizes throughout an enlarged liver. What is the most likely diagnosis and which other organs should be evaluated to help confirm the diagnosis?

3. A 50-year-old diabetic man presents for an abdominal sonogram with slightly elevated LFTs. His liver is diffusely echogenic and is slightly enlarged. The posterior portion of the liver is difficult to visualize and the right kidney appears hypoechoic in comparison to the liver parenchyma. What is the likely diagnosis?

4. A 60-year-old man with a history of alcoholism presents with abdominal distention. Your examination reveals an echogenic liver with an irregular, nodular contour. Moderate ascites is present. What is the most likely diagnosis?

5. Which lab value is most diagnostic of hepatocellular carcinoma?

- CT is useful in evaluating trauma and jaundiced patients, demonstrating liver masses, evaluating for metastasis, and displaying the global relationship of abdominal anatomy.

- PET/CT displays both anatomical and functional information and is used to evaluate for distant metastases.[76]

- MRI has played a larger role in recent years in characterizing liver masses and evaluating for metastases.[76]

## REFERENCES

1. England MA. *Color Atlas of Life Before Birth: Normal Fetal Development.* 2nd ed. St. Louis, MO: Mosby; 1996.
2. Gray H. *Gray's Anatomy: Anatomy of the Human Body.* 29th ed. (American edition, Goss CM, ed). Philadelphia, PA: Lea & Febiger; 1973.
3. Netter FH. The CIBA collection of medical illustrations. In: Oppenheimer F, ed. *Digestive System.* 2nd ed. Vol. 3. Summit, NJ: CIBA Pharmaceutical Co; 1964.
4. Guyton AC, Hall JE. *Textbook of Medical Physiology.* 9th ed. Philadelphia, PA: WB Saunders; 1996.
5. Tortora GJ, Grabowski SR. *Principles of Anatomy and Physiology.* 10th ed. New York, NY: Wiley; 2003.
6. Marieb EN. *Human Anatomy and Physiology.* 6th ed. Redwood City, CA: Benjamin Cummings; 2003.
7. Seeley RR, Stephens TD, Tate P. *Anatomy and Physiology.* 8th ed. St. Louis, MO: McGraw-Hill; 2007.
8. Robinson KA, Middleton WD, AL-Sukaiti R, et al. Doppler sonography of portal hypertension. *Ultrasound Quarterly.* 2009;25:3–13.
9. Bonhof JA, Linhart P. A pseudolesion of the liver caused by rib cartilage in B-mode ultrasonography. *J Ultrasound Med.* 1985;4:135–137.
10. Tchelepi H, Ralls PW, Radin R, et al. Sonography of diffuse liver disease. *J Ultrasound Med.* 2002;21:1023–1032.
11. Wolson AH. Liver. In: Goldberg BB, McGahan JP, eds. *Atlas of Ultrasound Measurements.* 2nd ed. St. Louis, MO: Elsevier Health Sciences; 2006.
12. Kratzer W, Fritz V, Mason R, et al. Factors affecting liver size. *J Ultrasound Med.* 2003;22:1155–1161.
13. Huether SE. Structure and function of the digestive system. In: McCance KL, Huether SE, eds. *Pathophysiology: The Biologic Basis for Disease in Adults and Children.* St. Louis, MO: Elsevier Mosby; 2006.
14. Venes D, ed. *Taber's Cyclopedic Medical Dictionary.* 21st ed. Philadelphia, PA: FA Davis; 2009.
15. Spence AP, Mason EB. *Human Anatomy and Physiology.* Menlo Park, CA: Benjamin/Cummings; 1987.
16. Ralls PW. Hepatic section. In: Sarti DA, ed. *Diagnostic Ultrasound: Text and Cases.* 2nd ed. Chicago, IL: Year Book Medical; 1987.
17. Hagen-Ansert S, Zweibel W. Liver. In: Hagen-Ansert S, ed. *Textbook of Diagnostic Ultrasonography.* 6th ed. St. Louis, MO: Elsevier Mosby; 2006.
18. Abdel-Misih SRZ, Bloomston M. Liver anatomy. *Surg Clin N Am.* 2010;90:643–653.
19. Abdalla EK, Vauthey JN, Couinaud C. The caudate lobe of the liver: implications of embryology and anatomy for surgery. *Surg Oncol Clin N Am.* 2002;11:835–848.
20. Mittelstaedt CA. *Abdominal Ultrasound.* New York, NY: Churchill Livingstone; 1987.
21. Wilson SR, Withers CE. The liver. In: Rumack C, Wilson S, Charboneau J, eds. *Diagnostic Ultrasound.* 3rd ed. St. Louis, MO: Elsevier Mosby; 2005.
22. Kane RA. Sonographic anatomy of the liver. *Semin Ultrasound.* 1981;2:190–197.
23. Cervone A, Sardi A, Conaway GL. Intraoperative ultrasound (IOUS) is essential in the management of metastatic colorectal liver lesions. *Am Surg.* 2000;66:611–615.
24. Swart J, Sheth S. Role of vascular ultrasound in the evaluation of liver disease. *Ultrasound Clin.* 2007;2:355–375.
25. Shin DS, Jeffrey RB, Desser TS. Pearls and pitfalls in hepatic ultrasonography. *Ultrasound Quarterly.* 2010;26:17–25.
26. Ahuja AT, Griffith JF, Wong KT, et al. *Diagnostic Imaging Ultrasound.* Salt Lake City, UT: Amirsys; 2007.
27. National Education Curriculum (NEC) for Sonography. Joint Review Committee on Education in Diagnostic Medical Sonography (JRCEDMS). 2008.
28. Chong WK, Shah MS. Sonography of right upper quadrant pain. *Ultrasound Clin.* 2008;3:121–138.
29. Krebs CA, Odwin CS, Fleischer AC. *Appleton and Lange Review for the Ultrasonography Examination.* New York, NY: McGraw Hill; 2004.
30. Sunder T. Hepatic venous sonography: some variations and their implications on surgical anatomy. *JDMS.* 1988;4:185–188.
31. Smith NA, Sanders RC. Jaundice. In: Sanders RC, Winter TC, eds. *Clinical Sonography: A Practical Guide.* Philadelphia, PA: Lippincott Williams & Wilkins; 2006.

32. Makuuchi M, Hasegawa H, Yamazaki S, et al. The inferior right hepatic vein: ultrasonic demonstration. *Radiology*. 1983;148:213–217.

33. Berland LL, Lawson TL, Foley WD. Porta hepatis: sonographic discrimination of bile ducts from arteries with pulsed Doppler with new anatomic criteria. *Am J Roentgenol*. 1982;138:833–840.

34. Porth CM. Alterations in function of the hepatobiliary system and exocrine pancreas. In: Porth CM, ed. *Pathophysiology: Concepts of Altered Health States*. Philadelphia, PA: Lippincott Williams & Wilkins; 2008.

35. Guyton AC, Hall JE. *Human Physiology and Mechanisms of Disease*. 6th ed. Philadelphia, PA: WB Saunders; 1997.

36. Price SA, Wilson LM. *Pathophysiology: Clinical Concepts of Disease Processes*. 6th ed. St. Louis, MO: Mosby; 2003.

37. Chernecky CC, Berger BJ. *Laboratory Tests and Diagnostic Procedures*. Philadelphia, PA: WB Saunders; 2004.

38. Finley PR, Grady HJ, Olsowka ES, et al. Chemistry. In: Jacobs DS, DeMott WR, Finley PR, et al., eds. *Laboratory Test Handbook*. 3rd ed. Hudson, OH: Lexi-Comp; 1994.

39. Pagano KD, Pagano TJ. *Mosby's Diagnostic and Laboratory Test Reference*. 8th ed. St. Louis, MO: Elsevier; 2007.

40. Tilkian SO, Conover MB, Tilkian AG. *Clinical Implications of Laboratory Tests*. 3rd ed. St. Louis, MO: CV Mosby; 1983.

41. Wallach J. *Interpretation of Diagnostic Tests*. 8th ed. Philadelphia, PA: Lippincott Williams & Wilkins; 2007.

42. Smith NA, Sanders RC. Cold defects on liver scan: possible metastases to liver. In: Sanders RC, Winter TC, eds. *Clinical Sonography: A Practical Guide*. Philadelphia, PA: Lippincott Williams & Wilkins; 2006.

43. Bullock BL. *Pathophysiology: Adaptations and Alterations in Function*. 4th ed. Philadelphia, PA: JB Lippincott-Raven; 1996.

44. Kurtz AB, Middleton WD. Liver. In: Middleton, WD, Kurtz AB, Hertzberg BS, eds. *Ultrasound: The Requisites*. St. Louis, MO: Mosby; 2004.

45. Bayard M, Holt J, Boroughs E. Nonalcoholic fatty liver disease. *American Family Physician*. 2006;73:1961–1968.

46. Li D, Hann LE. A practical approach to analyzing focal lesions in the liver. *Ultrasound Quarterly*. 2005;21:187–200.

47. Dahnert W. *Radiology Review Manual*. Philadelphia, PA: Lippincott Williams & Wilkins; 2007.

48. Behrman RE. *Nelson Textbook of Pediatrics*. 17th ed. Philadelphia, PA: WB Saunders; 2004.

49. Grant EG. Liver. In: Mittlestaedt CA, ed.: *General Ultrasound*. New York, NY: Churchill Livingstone; 1992.

50. Phillips VM, Bernardino M. The liver and spleen. In: Putman C, Ravin C, eds. *Textbook of Diagnostic Imaging*. Philadelphia, PA: WB Saunders; 1994.

51. Cazier PR, Sponaugle DW. "Starry sky" liver with fasting. Variations in glycogen stores? *J Ultrasound Med*. 1996;15:405–407.

52. LaBreque DR. Acute and chronic hepatitis. In: Stein JH, Eisenberg JM, eds. *Internal Medicine*. 5th ed. St. Louis, MO: Mosby; 1998.

53. Huether SE, McCance KL, Tarmina MS. Alterations of digestive function. In: McCance KL, Huether SE, eds. *Pathophysiology: The Biologic Basis for Disease in Adults and Children*. St. Louis, MO: Elsevier Mosby; 2006.

54. Abbitt PL. *Ultrasound: A Pattern Approach*. New York, NY: McGraw-Hill; 1995.

55. Lefton HB, Rosa A, Cohen M. Diagnosis and epidemiology of cirrhosis. *Med Clin N Am*. 2009;93:787–799.

56. McGahan JP, Goldberg BB. *Diagnostic Ultrasound*. New York, NY: Informa Healthcare; 2008.

57. Bissett RAL, Khan AN. *Differential Diagnosis in Abdominal Ultrasound*. Philadelphia, PA: WB Saunders; 2002.

58. Choi SK, Jin JS, Cho SG, et al. Spontaneous liver rupture in a patient with peliosis hepatitis: a case report. *World J Gastroenterol*. 2009;15:5493–5497.

59. Casillas VJ, Amendola MA, Gascue A, et al. Imaging of nontraumatic hemorrhagic hepatic lesions. *Radiographics*. 2000;20:367–378.

60. Friedman AC. *Radiology of the Liver, Biliary Tract, Pancreas and Spleen*. Baltimore, MD: Williams & Wilkins; 1987.

61. Sabih DE, Sabih Z, Khan A. "Congealed waterlilly" sign: a new sonographic sign of hydatid cyst. *J Clin Ultrasound*. 1996;24:297–303.

62. Stone C. Schistosomiasis. *JDMS*. 2005;21:424–427.

63. Spouge AR, Wilson SR, Gopinath N, et al. Extrapulmonary pneumocystis carinii in a patient with AIDS: sonographic findings. *Am J Roentgenol*. 1990;155:76–78.

64. Luburich P, Bru C, Ayuso MC, et al. Hepatic kaposi sarcoma in AIDS: US and CT findings. *Radiology*. 1990;175:172–174.

65. Jeffrey RB, Ralls PW. *Sonography of the Abdomen*. New York, NY: Raven Press; 1995.

66. Tchelepi H, Ralls PW. Ultrasound of focal liver masses. *Ultrasound Quarterly*. 2004;20:155–169.

67. Kim TK, Jang HJ, Wilson SR. Hepatic neoplasms: features on grayscale and contrast enhanced ultrasound. *Ultrasound Clin*. 2007;2:333–354.

68. Weissleder R, Wittenberg J, Harisinghani MG. *Primer of Diagnostic Imaging*. 4th ed. St. Louis, MO: Mosby; 2007.

69. D'Agostino HB, Solinas A. Percutaneous ablation therapy for hepatocellular carcinomas. *Am J Roentgenol*. 1995;164:1165–1167.

70. Tao F, Heiden RA, Bieuei F. Focal nodular hyperplasia. *Applied Radiology*. 2000;29:30–33.

71. Greten TF, Papendorf F, Bleck JS, et al. Survival rate in patients with hepatocellular carcinoma: a retrospective analysis of 389 patients. *Br J Cancer*. 2005;23:1862–1868.

72. Zhou Y, Sui C, Li B, et al. Repeat hepatectomy for recurrent hepatocellular carcinoma: a local experience and a systematic review. *World J Surg Oncol*. 2010;8:55.

73. Minami Y, Kudo M. Radiofrequency ablation of hepatocellular carcinoma: current status. *World J Radiol*. 2010;28:417–424.

74. Bertolotto M, Catalano O. Contrast-enhanced ultrasound: past, present, and future. *Ultrasound Clin*. 2009;4:339–367.

75. Carr CE, Tuite CM, Soulen MC, et al. Role of ultrasound surveillance of transjugular intrahepatic portosystemic shunts in the covered stent era. *J Vasc Interv Radiol*. 2006;17:1297–1305.

76. Coenegrachts K. Magnetic resonance imaging of the liver: new imaging strategies for evaluating focal liver lesions. *World J Radiol*. 2009;1:72–85.

# 6 The Gallbladder and Biliary System

Teresa M. Bieker

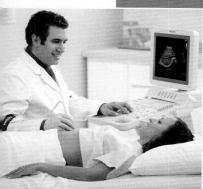

## OBJECTIVES

Illustrate surface, relational, and internal anatomy of the normal gallbladder and biliary system.

Discuss the embryologic development, common anatomic variants, and congenital anomalies of the gallbladder and biliary tree.

Describe the physiology of the gallbladder and biliary tree and include the laboratory values associated with normal and abnormal function.

Explain the sonographic evaluation of the gallbladder and biliary tree to include patient preparation, protocol, and demonstrate completing the examination procedure.

Describe the embryologic development, clinical signs and symptoms, and sonographic appearance for each of the following congenital anomalies: septate gallbladder, interposition of the gallbladder, biliary atresia, and choledochal cyst.

Identify gallbladder pathology in terms of etiology, clinical signs and symptoms, and sonographic appearance for acquired diseases to include biliary sludge, cholelithiasis, acute cholecystitis, acute acalculous cholecystitis, complicated cholecystitis, chronic cholecystitis, wall thickening, cholestasis, neoplasms, hyperplastic cholecystoses, and miscellaneous pathology.

Identify biliary system pathology in terms of etiology, clinical signs and symptoms, and sonographic appearance for acquired diseases to include postcholecystectomy, bile duct obstruction, cholangitis, other pathology, and AIDS cholecystopathy.

Differentiate between the advantages and disadvantages of utilizing other gallbladder and biliary system imaging procedures to include radiography, nuclear medicine, computed tomography, and magnetic resonance.

## KEY TERMS

acquired diseases | alanine aminotransferase (ALT) | aspartate aminotransferase (AST) | bilirubin | cholecystokinin (CCK) | congenital anomalies | extrahepatic biliary system | gallbladder

## GLOSSARY

**cholangitis** inflammation of the bile ducts

**cholecystectomy** surgical removal of the gallbladder

**cholecystitis** acute or chronic inflammation of the gallbladder

**cholecystokinin** a hormone secreted into the blood by the small intestine that stimulates gallbladder contraction

**choledocholithiasis** calculi within the bile duct

**cholelithiasis** the formation or presence of calculi or bile stones within the gallbladder

**common bile duct** duct that carries bile from the cystic and hepatic ducts to the duodenum

**cystic duct** the duct of the gallbladder that joins with hepatic duct to form the common bile duct

**gallbladder** a pear-shaped sac that lies on the undersurface of the liver; the gallbladder holds bile from the liver until released through the cystic duct

**junctional fold** a fold within the gallbladder neck or body

**phrygian cap** a fold within the gallbladder fundus

**pneumobilia** air within the bile ducts

**sludge** solid, semisolid, or thickened bile within the gallbladder or bile ducts

**sonographic Murphy's sign** pain over the gallbladder when the ultrasound transducer is used to compress the right upper quadrant

Sonography plays a key role in the evaluation of suspected gallbladder and biliary disease. Because the quality of sonographic examinations is strongly operator dependent, it is crucial to understand the anatomy, physiology, pathology, techniques, and pitfalls of scanning these structures. The quality of education and the experience of a sonographer are directly related to accuracy of findings.[1] This is especially true of the gallbladder and biliary tree because scanning may require patience, skill, and appropriate technique. Sonography is considered the modality of choice to evaluate gallbladder and ductal pathology.

## ANATOMY

The normal distended gallbladder is a pear- or teardrop-shaped sac measuring approximately 7 to 10 cm long and 3 cm in anteroposterior (AP) and transverse diameter. The wall measures less than 3 mm in thickness.[2,3] The gallbladder typically has a bile capacity of 30 to 60 mL.[4] The gallbladder is located in the main lobar fissure between the right and left hepatic lobes (Fig. 6-1). It lies under the visceral surface of the liver, lateral to the second part of the duodenum, and anterior to the right kidney and transverse colon[4] (Fig. 6-2A,B).

The gallbladder is divided into a neck, body, and fundus (Figs. 6-2B and 6-3A,B). The narrowest portion is the neck, which lies to the right of the porta hepatis. The body is the central or main portion. The fundus, varies considerably in position. Normally, the fundus is the most inferolateral portion of the gallbladder and it extends caudally and anteriorly below the inferior margin of the right hepatic lobe; however, it can extend as low as the right lower quadrant (RLQ) or as far left as the left anterior axillary line.[4,5]

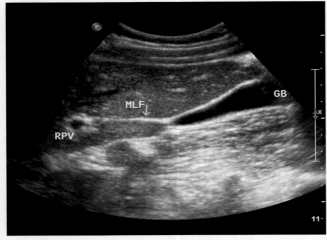

**Figure 6-1** Longitudinal image of the normal gallbladder (GB). Note the anatomic landmarks: the main lobar fissure (arrow, MLF) and the right portal vein (RPV).

Histologically, the gallbladder consists of an inner epithelial mucosa with folds, a muscular layer, a subserous layer, and an outer serosal surface. Mucous glands are found only in the gallbladder neck. Aberrant vestigial bile ducts of the liver may enter the adventitia (outermost covering) of the gallbladder and serve as a pathway for infection from the liver.[6]

The cystic duct arises from the superior aspect of the gallbladder neck and enters into the common bile duct (CBD)[3,4] (Fig. 6-4). It is 2 to 6 cm in length and its lumen contains a series of mucosal folds, the spiral valves of Heister, which prevent collapse or overdistention during sudden changes in position.[4]

The intrahepatic bile ducts run in juxtaposition to the portal veins and hepatic arteries. Together, these three structures form portal triads. The portal triads are surrounded by connective tissue and radiate through the lobes and segments of the liver. This fibrous connective tissue lines the portal vein walls, creating an echogenic appearance on sonography. The intrahepatic ducts join to form the right and left main hepatic ducts. The right and left main ducts unite at the porta hepatis to form the common hepatic duct (CHD). The cystic duct joins the CHD, forming the CBD. The CBD courses inferiorly within the hepatoduodenal ligament and anterior to the portal vein to the first portion of the duodenum and the head of the pancreas. In some cases, the CBD is surrounded by pancreatic tissue (Fig. 6-5A–D). The duct ends at the ampulla of Vater, which is difficult to visualize sonographically. Ducts can vary in their course, length, and site of anastomosis. For example, the CBD can be straight, curved, or angled.[3,4] There can also be accessory hepatic ducts.[4,6] Anatomically, the proximal duct is located at the liver, whereas the distal duct is located at the bowel. Central refers to the porta and peripheral is the branching within the liver.[3]

On sonography, the duct is measured inner wall to inner wall. A normal intraluminal measurement for the intrahepatic duct is 2 mm, or no more than 40% of the portal vein.[3] Measurements for the CBD and CHD are controversial; however, the CHD typically does not exceed 6 mm, and the CBD should measure less than 7 to 8 mm[7,8] (Fig. 6-6A–D). The bile duct diameter tends to remain constant throughout the day, as adequate relaxation of the sphincter of Oddi compensates for increased bile flow.[9] In elderly patients, the normal recoil of the elastic fibers of the duct may be lost, resulting in an ectatic "floppy duct."[10] There is debate in the literature over whether duct size increases with age. In the past, 1 mm was added for each decade of life after 50 years of age; however, this is no longer standard practice in all institutions.[3,8] Sonography can be performed repeatedly to assess dynamic physiologic or pathologic changes in duct size.[9]

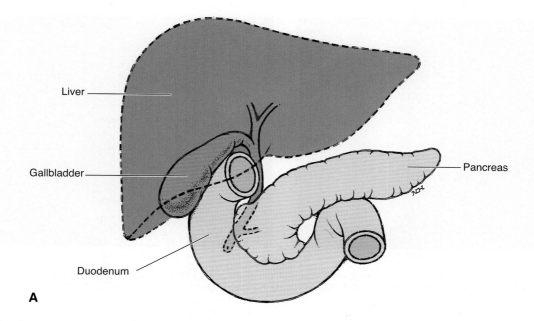

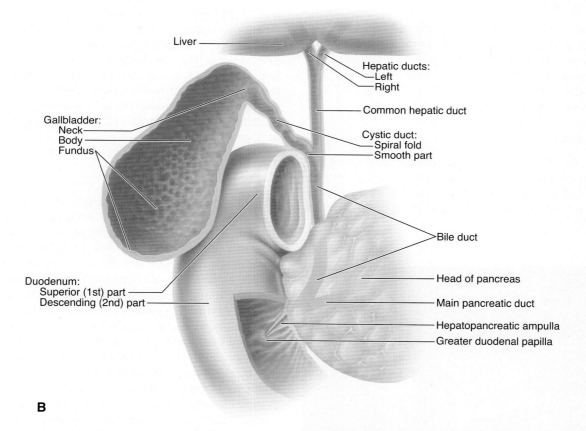

**Figure 6-2 A.** The illustration demonstrates the relationship of the normal gallbladder location to the liver, duodenum, and pancreas. **B.** The internal locations of the neck, body, and fundus and the ducts are labeled on this illustration. (**A**, Reprinted with permission: Lippincott Williams & Wilkins, The Neil Hardy Collection 2008-05; **B**, Reprinted with permission from Tank PW, Gest TR. *Atlas of Anatomy*. Baltimore, MD: Lippincott Williams & Wilkins; 2009:236C.)

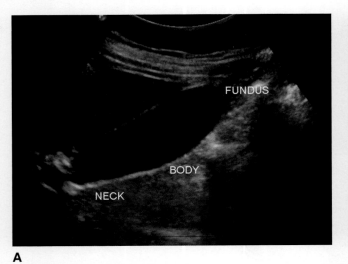

**A**

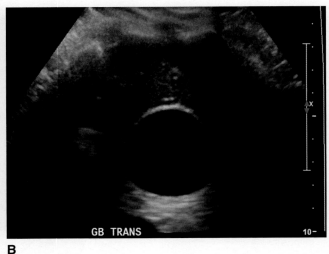

**B**

**Figure 6-3** Sonographic images of the normal gallbladder. **A.** Longitudinal gallbladder. The distal fundus is more bulbous, whereas the neck is the narrowest portion. **B.** Transverse mid-gallbladder at the body with a normal appearing wall.

## SECTIONAL VIEWS

Anatomic structures are sonographically identified by location and relationships with other structures. The schematic views with corresponding sonographic sectional images of the gallbladder and extrahepatic biliary tree demonstrate this relationship (Figs 6-7A–C, 6-8A,B, 6-9A–C, and 6-10A,B).

## VARIANTS

There are many common gallbladder variations, including different shapes (e.g., hourglass), positions, folds, and/or septations (Fig. 6-11A,B). The gallbladder may occasionally contain a small infundibulum

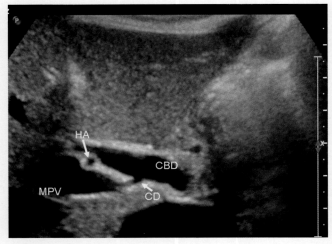

**Figure 6-4** Sonographic image of the porta hepatis. The cystic duct is seen entering the dilated common bile duct on the posterior margin. *CBD*, common bile duct; *CD*, cystic duct; *HA*, hepatic artery; *MPV*, main portal vein.

at the neck, Hartman pouch, where stones can collect. The phrygian cap is a common variant that forms when the fundus kinks or folds back on the body (Fig. 6-12). The gallbladder can be excessively mobile, ectopic (on the left, midline, transversely), or low in the RLQ. It can also be located partially or totally embedded in the liver parenchyma, completely surrounded by peritoneum, in the abdominal wall or falciform ligament, contained in the retroperitoneum, or above the liver.[4,6,11]

## PHYSIOLOGY

The biliary system transports bile, which is produced continually by hepatic parenchymal cells, to the duodenum, where it aids in digestion. Bile contains bile pigments (chiefly bilirubin), bile acids, cholesterol, lecithin, mucin, and other organic and inorganic substances. Bile helps to emulsify and promote the absorption of fats, and it also facilitates the actions of lipase, a pancreatic enzyme. The gallbladder concentrates and stores bile until needed and regulates biliary pressure.[4,6,11]

When food, especially fats, enters the small intestine, cholecystokinin (CCK) is secreted by the proximal small intestine, causing the gallbladder to contract and the sphincter of Oddi to relax. Bile is then released into the cystic duct, flows through the CBD, and enters the duodenum.[6] Gallbladder contraction can also be induced by commercially available "fatty meals" or by intravenous (IV) injections of CCK.[12] Gallbladder emptying may be diminished in some patients with gallstones. Residual gallbladder volume is known to increase during pregnancy. Sonography can monitor such gallbladder kinetics by measuring the gallbladder volume in various fasting and postprandial states. A complex sum-of-cylinders calculation can be used, but the ellipsoid method is

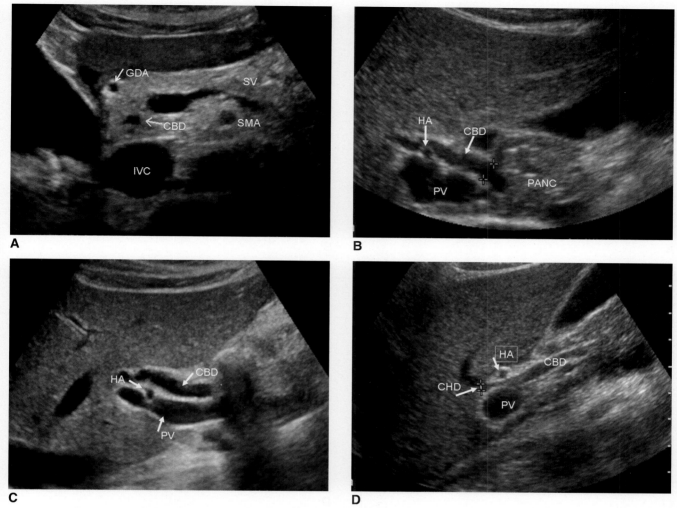

**Figure 6-5** Sonographic images of the extrahepatic biliary tree. **A.** Short axis of the common bile duct *(CBD)* at the level of the pancreatic head. **B.** Long-axis view of the CBD coursing from the liver to the pancreatic head. **C.** Portal triad at the porta hepatis. **D.** Occasionally, a re-placed hepatic artery is seen. The artery is located anterior to the duct, rather than between the duct and portal vein. *CBD,* common bile duct; *CHD,* common hepatic duct; *GDA,* gastroduodenal artery; *HA,* hepatic artery; *IVC,* inferior vena cava; *PANC,* pancreas; *PV,* portal vein; *SMA,* superior mesenteric artery; *SV,* splenic vein.

much simpler: V = 0.52 (length × width × height).[13,14] These two-dimensional volume measurements are less employed with the use of current equipment capable of producing three-dimensional sonography.

Several laboratory tests can be helpful in evaluating pathophysiology of the biliary tract. An increased WBC indicates infection. Aspartate aminotransferase (AST) and alanine aminotransferase (ALT) are enzymes produced by tissues of high metabolic activity, including the liver. Both values, but particularly the latter, can be mildly to moderately elevated in biliary obstruction. Lactic dehydrogenase (LDH), an enzyme, can be mildly elevated in obstructive jaundice. Alkaline phosphatase, another liver enzyme, markedly increases in obstructive jaundice. Bilirubin results from the breakdown of hemoglobin in red blood cells. Direct, or conjugated, bilirubin tends to elevate in obstructive (surgical) jaundice, whereas the indirect, or

unconjugated, bilirubin level rises in hepatocellular disease and hemolytic anemias.[4,15] Although helpful, the results of liver function tests can be nonspecific and must be considered with the clinical presentation and the findings of diagnostic imaging. Trends can be seen; therefore, it is important to evaluate the laboratory results over time to determine if function is improving or deteriorating.

## SONOGRAPHIC EXAMINATION, PREPARATION, PROTOCOL, AND PROCEDURE

Ideally, patients should not have anything by mouth for 6 to 8 hours prior to an examination of the gallbladder and biliary tree. Clear liquids are accepted. Fasting distends the gallbladder and reduces bowel gas for optimal visualization. The diagnosis of various gallbladder and

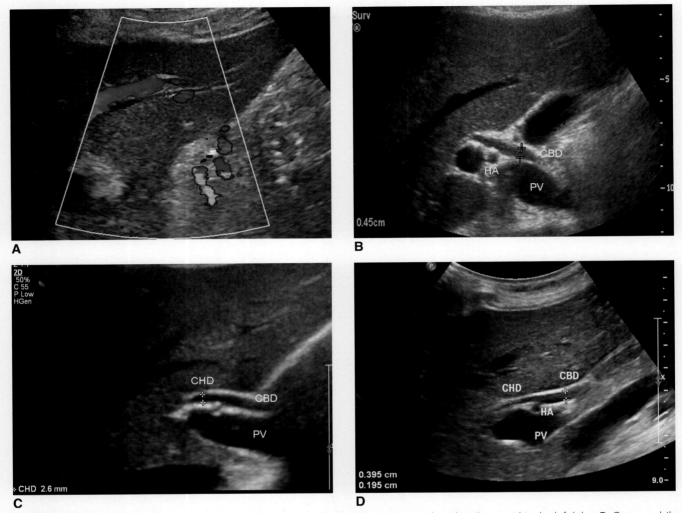

**Figure 6-6** Normal measurements of the ductal system. **A.** Intrahepatic duct measuring less than 2 mm within the left lobe. **B.** Common bile duct, less than 8 mm and **(C)** common hepatic duct, less than 6 mm at the porta hepatis. The ducts are measured inner wall to inner wall. **D.** Another example of normal duct measurements at the porta. *CBD,* common bile duct; *CHD,* common hepatic duct; *HA,* hepatic artery; *PV,* portal vein.

ductal pathologies can be made with a partially contracted, nonfasting gallbladder in emergent situations, when the patient is not fasting.

The chief complaint and pertinent medical or surgical history should be verified with the patient. This includes type, frequency, and duration of symptoms; location of pain; what aggravates or alleviates symptoms; prior similar episodes; and previous surgery or medical illnesses. Additional information, such as previous imaging studies, laboratory work, or clinic notes, is also helpful. The patient should also be evaluated physically. Note conditions such as jaundice and/or surgical scars.

The normal gallbladder has thin echogenic walls, an anechoic lumen, and posterior enhancement. The bile duct lumen should also appear anechoic; therefore, proper technique is important to avoid artifactual filling in of these structures. The gallbladder is located in

the main lobar fissure to the right of the ligamentum teres, anterior to the right kidney, and lateral to the pancreatic head. Although its position can vary, the neck has a constant relationship to the region of the porta hepatis[16] (Fig. 6-3A). The CBD is usually identified anterior to the portal vein and hepatic artery at the porta hepatis and should be followed throughout its course to the pancreatic head. The CHD and the right and left intraductal branches should also be evaluated. Dilated intrahepatic biliary ducts can be identified along the intrahepatic portal vein branches. The gallbladder and ducts are carefully evaluated for size, wall thickness, contents, course, and caliber. The presence or absence of pathology in the gallbladder, porta hepatis, and intrahepatic and extrahepatic biliary system should be documented.

Meticulous real-time examination of the gallbladder and bile ducts should be performed in all scan planes.

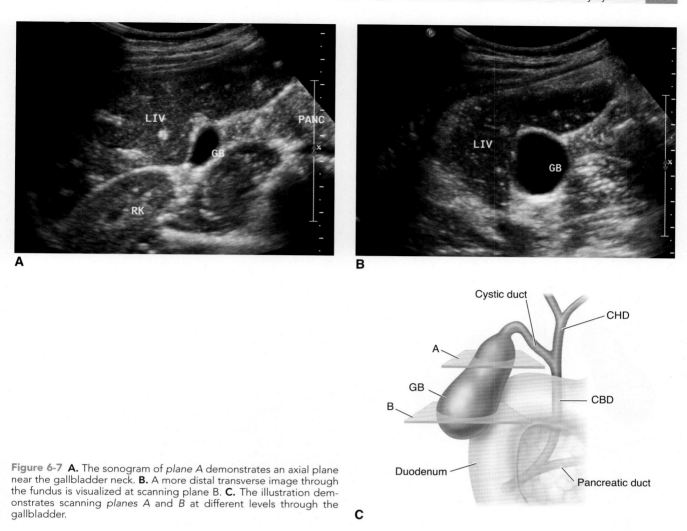

**Figure 6-7** **A.** The sonogram of *plane A* demonstrates an axial plane near the gallbladder neck. **B.** A more distal transverse image through the fundus is visualized at scanning plane B. **C.** The illustration demonstrates scanning *planes A* and *B* at different levels through the gallbladder.

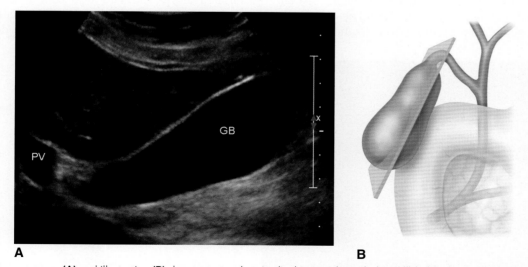

**Figure 6-8** The sonogram **(A)** and illustration **(B)** demonstrate a longitudinal image through the gallbladder body and fundus. *GB,* gallbladder; *PV,* portal vein.

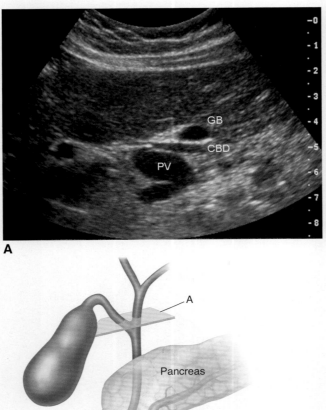

**A**

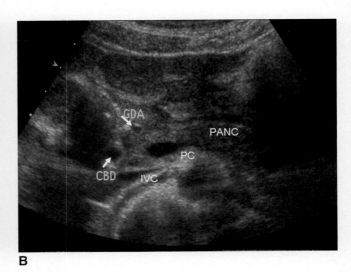

**B**

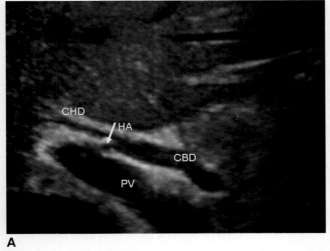

**C**

Pancreas

**Figure 6-9 A.** The transverse image at scanning plane A demonstrates the relationship of the gallbladder, proximal common bile duct, and portal vein. **B.** A transverse image at scanning plane B of the distal common bile duct demonstrates the ductal relationship with the pancreas and vessels. *CBD*, common bile duct; *GB*, gallbladder; *GDA*, gastroduodenal artery; *IVC*, inferior vena cava; *PANC*, pancreas; *PC*, portal vein. **C.** The illustration demonstrates transverse scanning plane at different levels.

A 3.5-MHz probe or higher should be utilized. In thinner patients, a 7.5-MHz probe can be used for optimal resolution. Proper setting of the overall gain, the time gain compensation (TGC), compression, spatial compounding, and dynamic range should be optimized to have adequate and accurate visualization of the gallbladder. Using harmonics is also helpful in reducing artifacts within the gallbladder as well as identifying small stones[7,17] (Fig. 6-13A,B). Adjust the focal zone for each area of interest. The focal zone is the narrowest segment of the beam, and suspected calculi (or other pathology) should lie within this zone to demonstrate

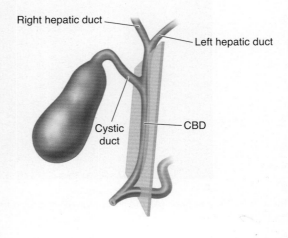

**A**

**B**

**Figure 6-10** The sonogram **(A)** and illustration **(B)** demonstrate a longitudinal scanning plane through the common bile duct. *CBD*, common bile duct; *CHD*, common hepatic duct; *HA*, hepatic artery; *PV*, portal vein.

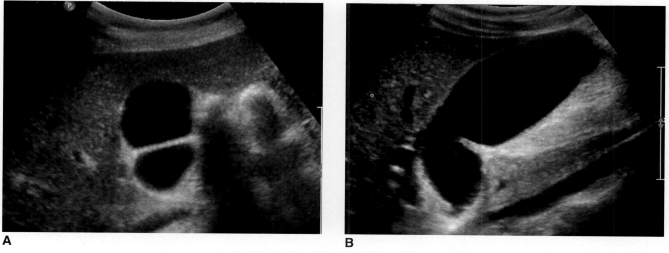

**Figure 6-11** Transverse **(A)** and longitudinal **(B)** images of a junctional fold.

shadowing. Even then, many small calculi may not shadow.[16] Changing the transducer frequency or angle may be necessary to bring the gallbladder into the focal zone.

The patient should be examined in two positions—typically supine and left lateral decubitus (LLD) or posterior oblique. A right lateral decubitus (RLD), erect (sitting or standing), or even prone positions may be necessary. While in the decubitus positions, small changes in the patient's angle, from 45 to 90 degrees, may improve visibility. The erect positions demonstrate gravity dependence. A prone position can show the mobility of stones and allows the liver to fall anteriorly, thereby providing an acoustic window and displacing bowel. Because the prone scanning position may be awkward, the technique may be varied by turning the patient prone for 10 to 15 seconds and then quickly

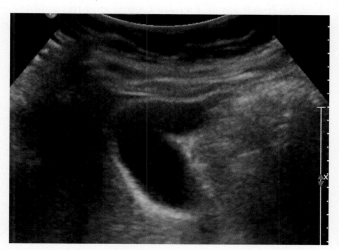

**Figure 6-12** Longitudinal sonogram of a phrygian cap, located at the fundus of the gallbladder.

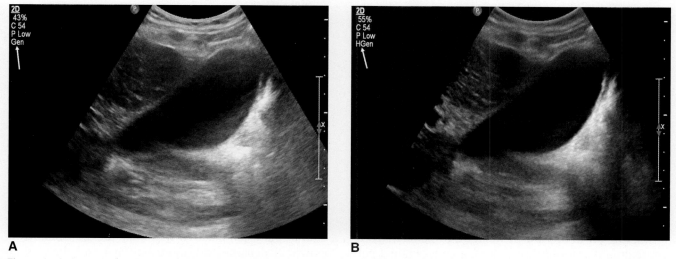

**Figure 6-13** Sonographic images of the gallbladder **(A)** without harmonics and **(B)** with harmonics on the same patient. Note the decrease in artifact within the gallbladder lumen. *Arrow* denotes settings.

returning the patient to an LLD position and rescanning the area.

Depending on the patient's body habitus and ability to cooperate, breathing techniques may also be beneficial. Suspended, full inspiration is often best, but sometimes, varying degrees of inspiration or expiration may also help. Breathing techniques are useful in moving organs inferiorly for improved subcostal access.

Another technique is to vary the scanning approaches. With the patient in an LLD position, scan subcostally with the transducer angled slightly toward the patient's right shoulder to elongate the portal vein and the bile duct at the porta hepatis. If this technique is not optimal, intercostally scanning may be necessary. Evaluate structures by scanning through many different windows to achieve the best angle and resolution. Gentle transducer pressure is useful for pushing bowel away from the field of view.

Due to absorption, gallstones should produce a clean shadow. If echogenic foci are seen within the gallbladder and does not shadow, several techniques should be attempted. First, reduce the gain distal to the foci. Second, increase the frequency of the transducer. Third, change the scanning angle to decrease the distance between the ultrasound beam and the stone. The focal zone should be at the stone.[18]

While scanning, it is also important to determine if there is a sonographic Murphy's sign. To evaluate, apply transducer pressure directly over the gallbladder. When positive, the patient will have focal pin-point tenderness. Care must be taken to ensure pressure is placed directly over the gallbladder and not the epigastrium or the liver. If the patient has received pain medication or is unresponsive, the sonographic Murphy's sign will not be accurate.[7]

It is also valuable to interrogate the gallbladder and biliary structures with color and/or pulsed Doppler. This may be helpful in evaluating hyperemia in inflammatory conditions, distinguishing solid masses from avascular pathology, and differentiating intrahepatic and extrahepatic bile ducts from blood vessels.[19]

A fatty meal may be needed to confirm an obstruction by observing changes in duct size or to evaluate gallbladder contractility and emptying. Patients with gallstones have exhibited higher resting gallbladder volumes, less fractional emptying after a fatty meal, and higher postprandial residual volumes.[20]

Meticulous scanning technique is crucial and can decrease or eliminate the need for other diagnostic tests.[21]

# CONGENITAL ANOMALIES

Embryonic development of the liver, gallbladder, and biliary duct system arises from the hepatic diverticulum of the foregut in the fourth week of gestation. This diverticulum divides into two parts: a larger cranial part, which gives rise to the liver, and a smaller caudal part, which develops into the gallbladder and cystic duct. At the beginning of the fifth week, the hepatic ducts, extrahepatic duct system, gallbladder, cystic duct, and pancreatic duct are demarcated as a solid cord of cells. Ductal lumina begin development during the sixth week in the common duct and slowly progress distally. The lumen extends into the cystic duct by the 7th week, but the gallbladder remains solid until the 12th week. Therefore, most gallbladder anomalies probably occur between the 4th and 12th week.[22,23]

Agenesis and duplication of the gallbladder are rare.[4] Anomalies of the gallbladder alone do not generally give rise to any characteristic symptoms. Although some of the defects predispose to bile stasis and attacks of cholecystitis, the attacks themselves have no unusual aspects. The symptoms only call attention to the anomaly.[22]

## SEPTATE GALLBLADDER

A gallbladder septum may result from a congenital mucosal diaphragm, adenomyomatosis, or a combination of the two. Because the gallbladder develops by cannulation of a blind sac, a septum will form if cannulation is incomplete. Although a gallbladder septum may be an incidental finding during an otherwise normal examination, stasis of bile in the distal segment predisposes to calculus formation.[24] A single septum appears as a thin linear echo separating the gallbladder into compartments. Simple junctional folds may mimic a septum.

The multiseptate gallbladder is one of the rarest congenital gallbladder malformations. There are two theories about its origin: incomplete vacuolization of the developing gallbladder bud or persistent wrinkling of the gallbladder wall. The septa consist of two epithelial layers with a muscular layer interposed. This anomaly may be associated with biliary colic or cholelithiasis or may be entirely asymptomatic without associated cholelithiasis.[25]

A multiseptate gallbladder can have variable sonographic appearances. There can be fine linear septa or a honeycomb pattern of clustered septations resulting in multiple communicating cyst-like compartments. Septa may cluster in the neck and body region of the gallbladder. Differential diagnoses include desquamated gallbladder mucosa (an unusual finding in acute cholecystitis) and hyperplastic cholecystoses (such as polypoid cholesterolosis or adenomyomatosis). Desquamated gallbladder mucosa appears as multiple, haphazardly arranged, linear, nonshadowing densities within the gallbladder lumen that do not consistently arise from the gallbladder wall as they do in multiseptate gallbladder. Polypoid cholesterolosis may more resemble multiseptate gallbladder, although the nonshadowing polypoid densities are more bulbous and there is no bridging of the lumen by septa as in the multiseptate gallbladder. In adenomyomatosis, Rokitansky-Aschoff sinuses could be confused with the honeycomb pattern, but cyst-like Rokitansky-Aschoff sinuses are smaller and are actually within the thickened gallbladder wall; there is no bridging of the lumen itself to form cyst-like compartments.[25,26]

## INTERPOSITION OF THE GALLBLADDER

Childhood jaundice is not unusual. Although interposition of the gallbladder (absence of the CHD and cystic duct) is a rare anomaly, its diagnosis is important because it is surgically correctable. Normally, the right and left main hepatic ducts join to form the CHD, which is entered by the cystic duct to form the CBD. In interposition, the main hepatic ducts drain, separately or together, directly into the gallbladder. The gallbladder then drains directly into the CBD, although variants can also occur (Fig. 6-14). The cause of interposition of the gallbladder is unknown.[23]

A patient with interposition of the gallbladder presents with jaundice, which may be intermittent, abdominal pain, and sometimes an enlarged gallbladder. Sonography may show enlarged intrahepatic ducts with a normal CBD, mimicking Caroli disease, or the ducts may appear to enter a cystic mass in the porta hepatis, mimicking a choledochal cyst. Although sonography may be difficult to interpret in this situation, it is still a good initial step, indicating that jaundice is due to an anatomic biliary abnormality.[23]

## BILIARY ATRESIA

Biliary atresia is the most common type of obstructive biliary disease in infants and young children.[27] Destruction of the extrahepatic biliary system occurs

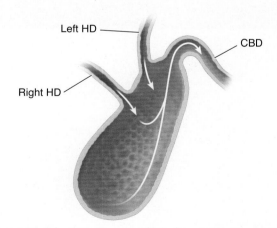

**Figure 6-14** Schematic diagram of bile flow pattern *(arrows)* in interposition of the gallbladder. The sonographic appearance reveals dilated intrahepatic ducts adjacent to a normal or enlarged gallbladder with no dilatation of the CBD. Differential diagnosis includes choledochal cyst, gallbladder hydrops, and Caroli disease.[27] *HD,* hepatic duct.

due to inflammation and sclerosing cholangiopathy.[28] Progressive obliteration of the extrahepatic ducts, and in many instances, the gallbladder takes place. This obliteration extends into the proximal intrahepatic duct system, which usually remains patent in the first few weeks of life. The severity varies with the duration of involvement. Fibrosis and obliteration of the biliary tree progress distal to proximal.[29]

More than 50% of neonates have transient jaundice characterized by mild elevation of serum bilirubin, which resolves spontaneously. Persistent or sudden onset jaundice after the first and second week of life may indicate a more serious abnormality, most commonly, biliary atresia or neonatal hepatitis. Less common causes include choledochal cysts, inspissated bile syndrome, enzyme deficiencies, metabolic abnormalities, hemolysis, hyperalimentation, and other congenital biliary anomalies.[23,29]

Biliary atresia is twice as common in males, whereas neonatal hepatitis is four times more common in females. It is important to distinguish biliary atresia from neonatal hepatitis because atresia may be treated surgically with a liver transplant or the Kasai procedure. The outcome is better with early surgical intervention. If surgical correction is not possible, death usually occurs within months; however, a few children survive several years.[6,29] Complications of untreated biliary atresia are cirrhosis, cholangitis, portal hypertension, malabsorption, and failure of biliary drainage.[28,29]

In normal neonates, the CHD is generally visible sonographically and measures no more than 1 mm. Intrahepatic duct dilatation combined with inability to visualize the CHD is suggestive of biliary atresia.[29] If only the cystic duct is obstructed, a hydropic gallbladder will develop.[6] Detection of both intrahepatic and extrahepatic dilatation excludes atresia and indicates obstruction (choledochal cyst, inspissated bile, biliary calculi). Also, if the gallbladder contracts within 30 minutes of feeding, biliary atresia is unlikely.[29] Large kidneys with increased echogenicity have been associated with some cases of biliary atresia. The mechanism for this is not known, and it should be recognized as a transitory phenomenon.[30]

## CHOLEDOCHAL CYSTS

There are five types of choledochal cysts, the most common being fusiform dilatation of the CBD. The right, left, and cystic ducts may be seen entering the choledochal cyst.[31] The less common type II is seen as one or more diverticula extending off of the CBD. Type III is a duodenal choledochocele and type IV is multiple cystic dilatations of the intrahepatic and extrahepatic ducts. Type V, Caroli disease (communicating cavernous ectasia), is a nonobstructive, saccular dilatation of communicating intrahepatic ducts.[3,31] Different causes of choledochal cysts have been cited, including congenital

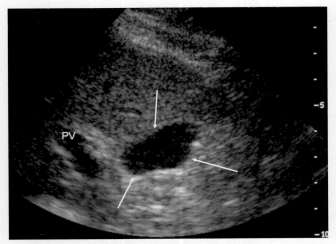

**Figure 6-15** Longitudinal image in post cholecystectomy patient. A choledochal cyst is seen at the porta hepatis *(arrows)*.

weakness of the duct wall, which results in the formation of a cystic structure, and angulation of the CBD, causing partial obstruction leading to dilatation and cyst formation.[6]

Clinically, the signs and symptoms include intermittent jaundice associated with colicky pain, failure to thrive, and sometimes a palpable subhepatic mass displacing the stomach and the duodenum.[6,31] Choledochal cysts are four times more common in females than males and often present early in life. Surgical management is recommended due to the increased incidence of malignant transformation that may occur later in life.[4,15]

Sonographically, choledochal cysts appear as a localized cystic mass separate from the gallbladder in the region of the porta hepatis or intrahepatically depending on the type (Fig. 6-15). To avoid mistaking a fluid-filled bowel loop for a choledochal cyst, the examiner should verify peristalsis.

## ACQUIRED DISEASES

### BILIARY SLUDGE

Sludge represents precipitates formed in the bile. It consists of a collection of calcium bilirubinate, mucus, and lesser amounts of cholesterol crystals within viscous

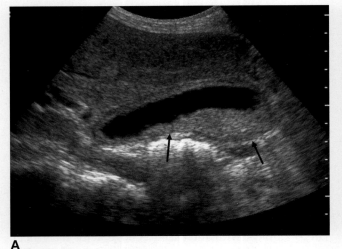

A

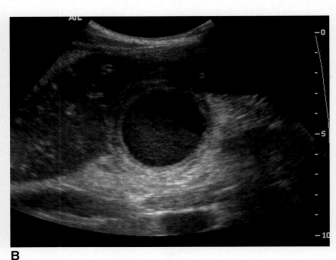

B

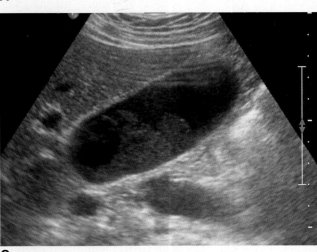

C

**Figure 6-16** Varying sonographic appearances of sludge. **A.** Layering sludge *(arrows)* that is isoechoic to the liver. **B.** Sludge that is more hypoechoic in appearance. **C.** Hypoechoic, more complex appearing sludge.

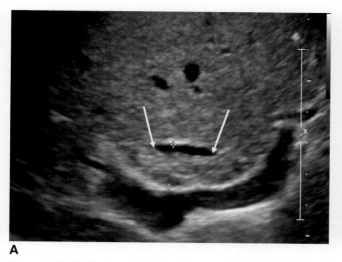
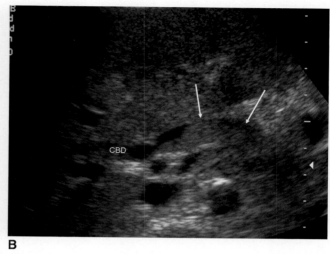

**A**    **B**

**Figure 6-17** Sludge has a similar appearance within the bile ducts. **A.** Homogeneous, layering sludge *(arrows)* within the bile duct. Calipers denote bile duct. **B.** Sludge *(arrows)* filling the proximal portion of the bile duct.

bile that contains high concentrations of mucus and other proteins.[18,32,33]

The pathogenesis, clinical significance, and ultimate prognosis of sludge remain uncertain. Sludge alone can produce biliary symptoms such as the classic pain of gallstones, and it can also be associated with other complications. Therefore, sludge associated with biliary pain can be a significant finding. The presence of sludge implies the formation of a precipitate and should not be regarded as normal. Sludge is sometimes a precursor to gallstone disease.[18,33]

Sludge may be caused by conditions such as prolonged fasting, total parenteral nutrition (TPN), bile stasis, pregnancy, rapid weight loss, or recent surgery.[3,18] Because gallbladder emptying is significantly reduced in patients fed parenterally, sequential CCK injections may help to induce gallbladder contraction.[34]

Sonographically, sludge produces a homogeneous, low-amplitude, nonshadowing echo pattern that tends to layer dependently (Figs. 6-16A–C and 6-17A,B). True sludge often forms a fluid–fluid level that remains constant in longitudinal and transverse images. Sludge slowly moves with changes in patient position. Sludge can disappear and reappear over time. Scattered brighter echoes within sludge may represent larger cholesterol crystals. If sludge completely fills the gallbladder (total bile sludging or hepatization of bile), it may be difficult to distinguish the echo-filled gallbladder from adjacent liver parenchyma (Fig. 6-18). Sludge may also lead to gallstones.[3,18]

Tumefactive sludge from long-standing biliary obstruction frequently does not layer but often resembles a polypoid mass that can mimic a gallbladder neoplasm (Fig. 6-19A,B). Color Doppler sonography can be useful in determining tumefactive sludge from a neoplasm.[35] Occasionally, mobile, round, echogenic, nonshadowing masses known as sludge balls are seen within the

gallbladder.[18] Also, sludge may be found in conjunction with gallstones (Fig. 6-20).

Using excessively high gain settings fills the gallbladder with artifactual echoes, giving a false appearance of sludge. This artifactual pattern has a snowflake appearance, whereas true sludge has a defined, low-level pattern. Increased echogenicity of surrounding organs is another clue of too much gain. It is also important to distinguish sludge from the "false debris" echo pattern of slice thickness artifacts.[32]

## CHOLELITHIASIS (GALLSTONES)

Gallstones can be large or small, single or multiple, symptomatic or silent. In the United States, approximately 25 million adults have gallstones.[18] The prevalence of gallstones is higher in females than in

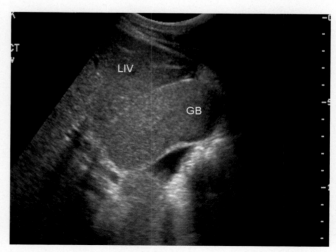

**Figure 6-18** Hepatization of bile. Sludge in the gallbladder *(GB)* has same echo texture as liver *(LIV)*.

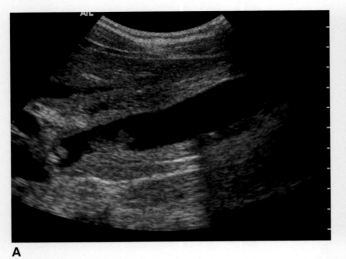

**A**

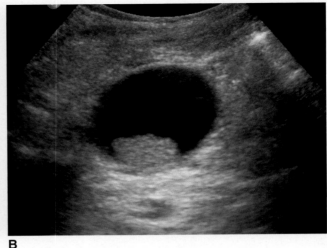

**B**

**Figure 6-19** Sonogram shows tumefactive sludge within the gallbladder. **A.** The sludge balls moved from the gallbladder neck to the body as the patient changed position. **B.** A larger collection of tumefactive sludge.

males. Gallstones are occasionally seen in fetuses and children[27,36] (Fig. 6-21A,B).

The majority of stones contain a mixture of cholesterol, bilirubin, and calcium. Approximately 75% of the gallstones in the United States are primarily cholesterol, with black or brown pigment stones accounting for 25% to 30% (Fig. 6-22). Many factors are associated with gallstone formation. Supersaturation of bile with cholesterol, abnormal gallbladder emptying, and altered absorption contribute to cholesterol stone formation.[37,38] Black pigment stones result from the presence of excessive deconjugated bilirubin and are associated with hemolytic diseases, cirrhosis, and TPN. Brown pigment stones are more common in Asian countries but are rare in the United States. They are associated with biliary tract infection and are usually located in the bile ducts rather than the gallbladder.[39]

The prime candidate for cholelithiasis is "female, fat, fair, forty, fertile, and flatulent."[27] Other associated risks include pregnancy, increasing age, fecundity, diabetes, rapid weight loss, and obesity.[3,18,40] Predisposing factors for cholelithiasis are short bowel syndrome, inflammatory bowel disease, hemolytic diseases (from hyperbilirubinemia), cirrhosis, TPN, cystic fibrosis, impaired release of CCK, and any condition that interferes with ileal absorption of bile acids.[27,34,37,38,41–44]

The majority (60% to 80%) of gallstones are asymptomatic, with most found during routine abdominal scanning. Patients with symptoms, however, generally present with right upper quadrant (RUQ) pain that is steady, occurs after meals, or radiates to the upper back, shoulder, or epigastric area. The patient may also have nausea or vomiting.[45] Because gallbladder disease can mimic the pain of ischemic heart disease, sonography of the biliary tree often plays a role in the workup of chest pain as well.[46] Pertinent laboratory values may include an elevated alkaline phosphatase and mildly elevated AST and ALT levels when the cystic duct or CBD is obstructed.[15]

Prognosis and treatment of cholelithiasis can vary depending on the frequency and severity of the attacks as well as the size of the stones. Small calculi tend to be more troublesome because they may exit the gallbladder and cause ductal obstruction.[45] Cholelithiasis may take a benign course and a low-fat diet may be sufficient treatment in some cases. Persistent symptoms may require surgical intervention, either laparoscopic or open cholecystectomy, to provide definitive treatment of gallstones.[47,48] Percutaneous cholecystostomy may assume a limited role in elderly patients and patients at high risk. Surgical cholecystostomy to remove stones is occasionally done but cholecystectomy is often necessary subsequently because of the

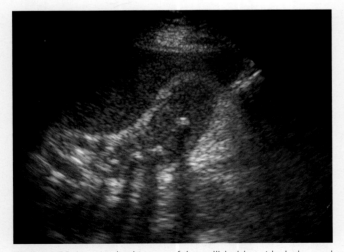

**Figure 6-20** Longitudinal image of the gallbladder with sludge and gallstones.

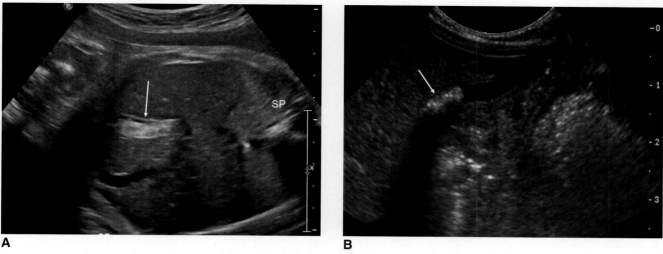

**Figure 6-21** Fetal and neonatal gallstones. **A.** Fetal gallstones in the third trimester. Gallstones within the fetal gallbladder *(arrow)* do not always create a shadow. *SP*, spine.) **B.** Stones with shadowing *(arrow)* within the neck of the gallbladder in this neonate.

high recurrence rate.[49] Sonography is the modality of choice for monitoring stones in these patients.[3]

The classic sonographic appearance of a gallstone is a mobile, gravity-dependent, echogenic foci within the gallbladder lumen that casts a posterior acoustic shadow[7] (Fig. 6-23A–F). If the proper technique and transducer are used, virtually all calculi over 5 mm can be accurately diagnosed. If less than 2 to 3 mm, stones can be more difficult to visualize. However, small stones are typically multiple and described as "gravel," thereby making detection easier[18] (Fig. 6-24A,B). Small gallstones that are located

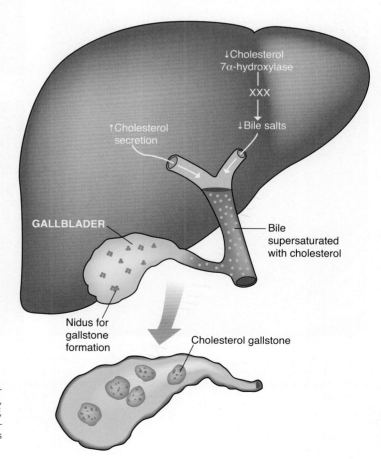

**Figure 6-22** Pathogenesis of cholesterol gallstones is a multifactorial process. (Reprinted with permission from Rubin E, Rubin R. The liver and biliary system. In: Rubin E, Gorstein F, Rubin R, et al, eds. *Rubin's Pathology: Clinicopathologic Foundations of Medicine.* 4th ed. Baltimore, MD: Lippincott Williams & Wilkins; 2005:804.)

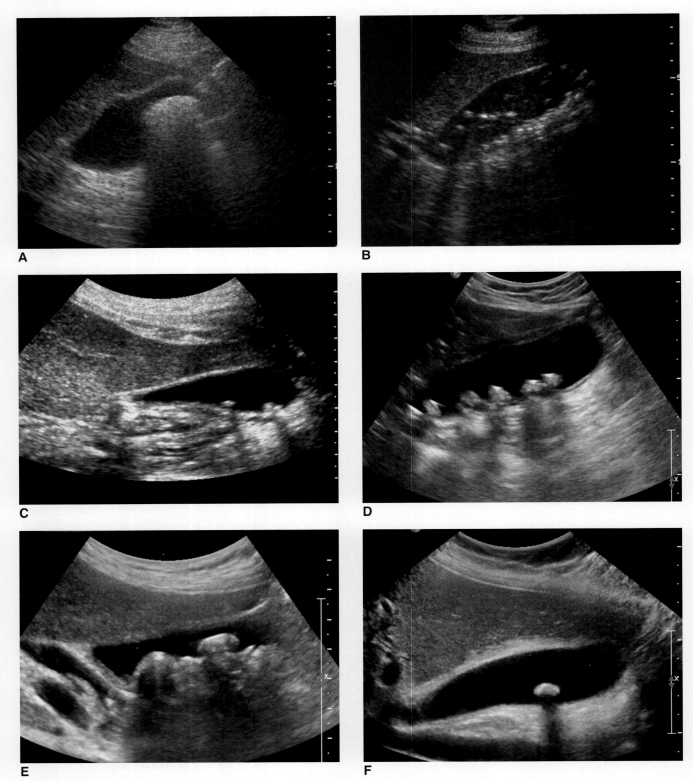

**Figure 6-23** Varying appearances of gallstones. **A.** Classic sonographic appearance of a gallstone within the fundus. **B.** Mixture of small shadowing stones along with sludge. **C.** Several, tiny stones that could exit into the duct. **D.** Multiple, shadowing, dependent stones within the gallbladder. **E.** Layering, irregular-shaped stones. **F.** Single, small, shadowing stone.

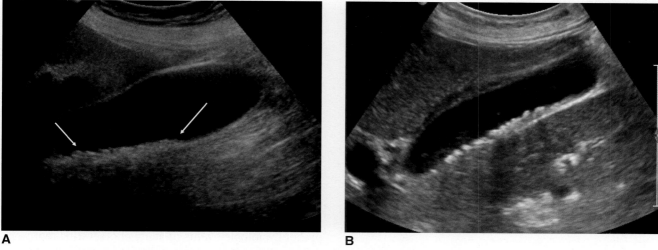

**A**    **B**

**Figure 6-24** Gravel. **A.** The thin layer of numerous small stones *(arrows)* in this longitudinal image of the gallbladder could be mistaken for bowel gas with shadowing just behind the gallbladder, but the small stones were observed to move within the gallbladder lumen. **B.** Longitudinal image showing gravel in another patient.

within the cystic duct or in the neck of the gallbladder can be more difficult to visualize.[7] The majority of gallstones produce "clean" shadows with distinct margins because only 20% to 30% of the incident beam is reflected. Calcified gallstones reflect a much larger percentage of the incident beam, but they produce reverberations within the shadow.[50] The visualization of reverberations and scattered echoes in the shadow are dependent on gain settings, transducer positioning, harmonics, and focusing.[17,50,51] Cholesterol stones or polyps can demonstrate reverberations and comet tail artifacts due to the rigidity and physical characteristics of cholesterol.[52] Other causes of echogenic foci with reverberation and comet tail artifacts within the RUQ include air in the biliary tree,

surgical clips in the gallbladder bed, gas in an intrahepatic abscess, drainage catheters, emphysematous cholecystitis, lead pellets, focal hepatic calcifications, and scars.[51,52]

As the patient changes position, gallstones should roll to the most dependent portion of the gallbladder (Fig. 6-25A,B). Stones that do not demonstrate mobility may be polyps, stones impacted in the gallbladder neck, or stones adherent to the gallbladder wall.[3,7]

There are many possible technical, anatomic, and diagnostic pitfalls of cholelithiasis (Table 6-1). Again, meticulous scanning in multiple planes using a variety of techniques, patient positions, and transducer frequencies is crucial for accurate diagnosis and proper patient management.

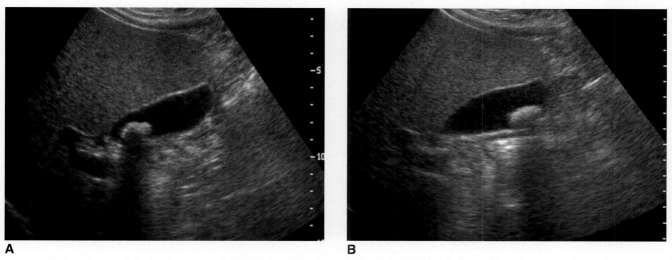

**A**    **B**

**Figure 6-25** **A.** With the patient supine, a distinct stone was seen along the posterior gallbladder wall. **B.** When the patient rolled into a left lateral decubitus position, the stone rolled to the fundus.

| TABLE | 6-1 |
|---|---|
| **Pitfalls in Identifying Cholelithiasis** | |

*False Positive*

- Bowel gas or ligamentum teres
- Junctional folds or valves of Heister
- Edge shadowing or other artifacts
- Scarring or surgical clips

*False Negative*

- Using inappropriate technique, transducer frequency, focal zone, or gain settings
- Stones within the phrygian cap or Hartman pouch
- Mistaking a thin layer of stones for bowel gas
- Small stones

## ACUTE CHOLECYSTITIS

In up to 95% of cases, acute cholecystitis or inflammation of the gallbladder, results from impacted stones within the neck of the gallbladder or the cystic duct.[7,18,35] Inflammation may result in necrosis, ulceration, swelling, and edema.[7] Various degrees of bacterial infection occur with acute cholecystitis leading to potential complications.[15]

Before 50 years of age, women are three times more likely to develop acute cholecystitis than men. After 50, the incidence is near equal.[18] Patients with acute cholecystitis may present with RUQ or epigastric pain, nausea and vomiting, and/or jaundice.[7] These acute attacks typically resolve after 4 to 6 hours or with passage of the stone. Another presentation is a longer attack of pain (greater than 24 hours) with a fever and laboratory values indicative of inflammation. These patients are more likely to have acute inflammation that is less likely to resolve.[18,53] Approximately 20% of patients with cholelithiasis will develop acute cholecystitis; however, only 20% to 35% of patients with RUQ pain will have acute cholecystitis.[7,35]

Clinically, the signs and symptoms of calculus are indistinguishable and somewhat nonspecific. Patients present with RUQ pain, positive Murphy sign, nausea, vomiting, distention, fever, a palpable RUQ mass, and/or jaundice.[15,35,54] These symptoms can be confused with acute pancreatitis, perforated peptic ulcer, liver abscess, or acute alcoholic hepatitis.[15] Laboratory results can also be nonspecific, possibly showing serum liver transaminase, leukocytosis, hyperbilirubinemia, or elevated alkaline phosphatase.[55]

On sonogram, a positive sonographic Murphy sign, wall thickening, and gallstones are strongly suggestive of acute cholecystitis. Pericholecystic fluid and, at times, a hydropic gallbladder are also seen.[7,35] Color or power Doppler may also be helpful in diagnosing acute cholecystitis by detecting hyperemia and an enlarged cystic artery. One of the aforementioned findings in isolation is not sufficient in making a diagnosis—a combination of several findings is needed[3] (Fig. 6-26A–E).

One thought is to manage the patient medically because 60% of acute cases resolve spontaneously and surgery should be saved until the acute attack has subsided. The preferred approach is to perform a cholecystectomy within the first several days of the onset of symptoms because early surgical intervention results in fewer complications and lower costs.[35,53] In patients with severe acute cholecystitis who are poor surgical candidates, are very ill, or are elderly, sonographically guided aspiration and percutaneous drainage of the gallbladder or antibiotic therapy is an alternative.[55] The pathophysiologic events of acute cholecystitis represent a dynamic process. Time is needed for these changes to occur. As a result, the clinical onset may precede the appearance of sonographic signs by as much as 12 to 24 hours.[56]

The major complications of acute cholecystitis include emphysematous cholecystitis, gangrenous cholecystitis, empyema, and perforation of the gallbladder.[18] The differential diagnosis of acute cholecystitis is broad and consists of pneumonia, pancreatitis, choledocholithiasis, hepatitis, liver abscess or neoplasm, peptic ulcer disease, and heart disease.[35]

## ACUTE ACALCULOUS CHOLECYSTITIS

In approximately 5% to 14% of acute cholecystitis cases, gallstones are not present. This is referred to as acute acalculous cholecystitis (AAC).[7] A combination of stagnant bile and direct vascular changes may be responsible for AAC. High concentrations of stagnant bile can be directly toxic and cause overdistension of the gallbladder leading to vascular compromise. Viscous stagnant bile can also act as a functional obstruction of gallbladder outflow, providing an excellent pathway for secondary bacterial invasion. Direct vascular changes, such as clotting, occur with severe burns and trauma. This leads to selective thrombosis of vessels supplying the gallbladder, followed by ischemia, necrosis, secondary bacterial involvement, infection, and possibly perforation through the gallbladder wall.[54,57,58]

The majority of acalculous cholecystitis cases occur in patients in the intensive care unit. There are multiple other causes of AAC, including trauma, surgery, severe burns, sepsis, long-term TPN, prolonged fasting, diabetes, and HIV.[3,7,18,35,55]

Clinically, the signs and symptoms of acalculous cholecystitis are indistinguishable and somewhat nonspecific. Patients often present with RUQ pain and a positive Murphy sign. Other symptoms include nausea, vomiting, distention, fever, and a palpable RUQ mass.[15,54] Symptoms of AAC can occur 24 hours

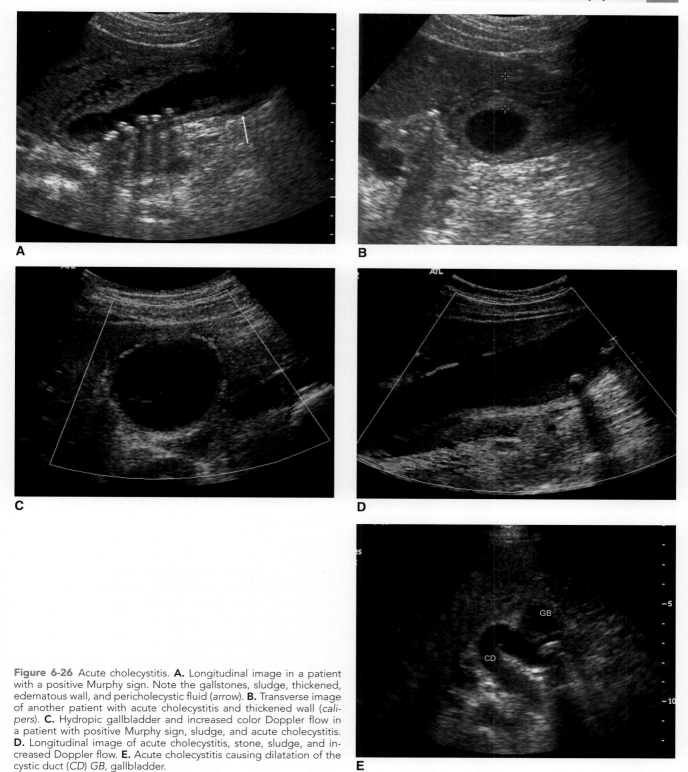

**Figure 6-26** Acute cholecystitis. **A.** Longitudinal image in a patient with a positive Murphy sign. Note the gallstones, sludge, thickened, edematous wall, and pericholecystic fluid (*arrow*). **B.** Transverse image of another patient with acute cholecystitis and thickened wall (*calipers*). **C.** Hydropic gallbladder and increased color Doppler flow in a patient with positive Murphy sign, sludge, and acute cholecystitis. **D.** Longitudinal image of acute cholecystitis, stone, sludge, and increased Doppler flow. **E.** Acute cholecystitis causing dilatation of the cystic duct (*CD*) *GB*, gallbladder.

to 50 days after the initial event but usually occur within 2 weeks.[57] Due to the difficultly in diagnosis, acalculous cholecystitis has a high morbidity and mortality rate.[35]

Sonographically, the gallbladder is often distended with a thickened wall and internal debris or sludge.[7]

Wall thickening with hypoechoic areas within the wall and pericholecystic fluid can also be seen.[18,55] Diagnosis, however, is often difficult due to the absence of gallstones. Also, the patient's mental status (i.e., patient is sedated) hinders the evaluation of a positive Murphy sign[7] (Fig. 6-27A–C).

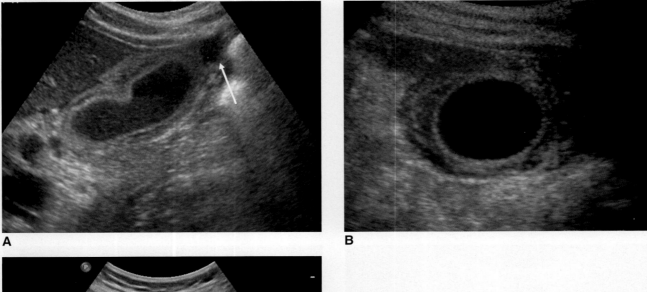

**Figure 6-27** Acute acalculous cholecystitis. **A.** Thickened gallbladder wall, sludge, and pericholecystic fluid *(arrow)* are seen in this longitudinal image. The patient had right upper quadrant pain, nausea, and vomiting. **B.** Transverse image showing a thickened gallbladder wall in this patient with acute acalculous cholecystitis. **C.** Longitudinal image in a patient with a positive Murphy sign and fever. The gallbladder wall is thickened and edematous.

There are two schools of thought regarding the treatment of acute cholecystitis. Mortality rates from AAC far exceed those from acute calculous cholecystitis. This could be due to several factors, such as the lack of clinical and laboratory specificity in the diagnosis of AAC.[54,59] Gangrene of the gallbladder can also occur in patients with AAC. Again, early diagnosis and treatment is the best way to avoid or minimize complications.[7]

## COMPLICATED CHOLECYSTITIS

Patients with acute cholecystitis are at risk for developing empyema, gallbladder perforation, gangrenous cholecystitis, or emphysematous cholecystitis.[7,18]

### Empyema

Empyema or suppurative cholecystitis, pus in the gallbladder, typically occurs in diabetic patients. The pus-filled gallbladder resembles sludge on a sonogram. Patients present with symptoms comparable to cholecystitis including fever, chills, and RUQ pain. Signs of sepsis can be present. A magnetic resonance image (MRI) or a percutaneous needle aspiration of the gallbladder is helpful to distinguish pus from sludge.[18,55] Patients with empyema are treated with cholecystectomy and IV antimicrobial therapy.[55]

### Gallbladder Perforation

Five to 10% of patients with acute cholecystitis will have a gallbladder perforation.[7,60] Typically, perforations occur in the fundus due to chronic inflammation and the low amount of blood flow to this area.[3,7] With an acute perforation, the bile leak will cause peritonitis; however, acute perforations are uncommon. Subacute perforations, which are more common, result in an abscess formation. The abscesses can occur in or around the gallbladder or liver or within the peritoneal cavity.[7] Gallbladder perforation is a life-threatening condition with a mortality rate of 19% to 24%.[35,61] An increased risk is reported with immunocompromised patients, such as diabetes or malignancy.[60]

Clinically, patients present with RUQ pain, nausea, vomiting, and fever. Laboratory work may reveal an

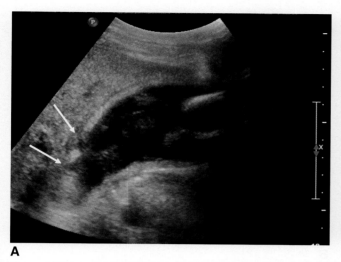

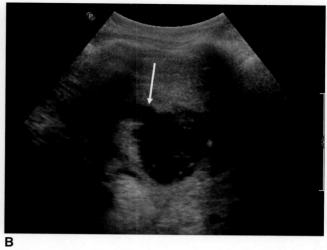

**Figure 6-28** Longitudinal **(A)** and transverse **(B)** images in a patient with gallbladder perforation. The defect seen on the anterior wall *(arrows)* is better demonstrated in the transverse section. Debris is also located within the gallbladder lumen.

increased WBC and abnormal liver function tests.[61] On sonogram, a complex fluid collection (abscess), irregular gallbladder wall, gallstones, inflammatory changes within the gallbladder fossa, and a focal defect of the gallbladder wall can also be seen.[7,18,60,61] Defects are typically focal and small; however, they can be large and involve a considerable portion of the wall (Fig. 6-28A,B). Computed tomography (CT) may be helpful in determining wall defects.[60] In order to avoid sepsis, an early cholecystectomy should be performed.[61]

## Gangrenous Cholecystitis

Gangrenous cholecystitis is due to absent blood supply or infection. The gallbladder wall becomes ischemic and eventually necrotic.[7,35] Approximately 2% to 38% of acute cholecystitis cases will develop into gangrenous cholecystitis.[35] Clinically, patients are acutely ill and a positive sonographic Murphy sign is present in one-third of patients; however, a positive sign may not be present due to nerve damage, therefore, the patient presents with diffuse versus localized pain.[7,55] Laboratory work may reveal an increased WBC.[55]

Sonography is often nonspecific in the diagnosis of gangrenous cholecystitis. A thickened, irregular gallbladder wall with both hyperechoic and hypoechoic striations is also suggestive of gangrenous cholecystitis.[7] Intraluminal membranes from sloughing off the walls and fibrous strands may be visualized on sonography. Gas within the gallbladder wall, or lumen, an absent gallbladder wall or an abscess may also be seen.[35] Gallbladder perforation occurs early or late in the course of acute cholecystitis and may take any of three forms: (1) localized with pericholecystic abscess, the most common form of perforation; (2) free perforation with generalized peritonitis; or (3) perforation into an adjacent hollow viscous such as in Bouveret syndrome.[14,62] The appearance of perforations varies

with the type, from free fluid in the peritoneal cavity to the diverse appearance of localized abscesses (Fig. 6-29A–D).

Due to the increased mortality and morbidity rates, early cholecystectomy and IV antimicrobial therapy is advised if gangrenous cholecystitis is suspected.[18,35,55]

## Emphysematous Cholecystitis

Emphysematous cholecystitis, a rare form of acute cholecystitis, is a condition in which gas-forming bacteria invade the gallbladder wall, lumen, pericholecystic spaces, and on occasion the bile ducts. This condition is more common in men and as many as 40% of cases are associated with diabetes. Many cases do not contain gallstones; however, they are more common in acute cases. Patients present with sudden progressive RUQ pain, fever, nausea, and vomiting. Patients with emphysematous cholecystitis are likely to develop a gangrenous gallbladder or abscess formation. Gallbladder perforation can also occur.[3,7,55,63] Emphysematous cholecystitis is fatal in about 15% of cases.[3]

Sonographically, gas bubbles appear as prominent non–gravity-dependent and changes with patient position. Air appears as echogenic foci within the gallbladder's wall or lumen, causing the gallbladder wall to appear echogenic. Ring down or comet tail artifacts are also seen.[3,35] This may make it difficult to visualize the gallbladder with emphysematous cholecystitis sonographically. To help differentiate gangrenous cholecystitis from a porcelain gallbladder, a porcelain gallbladder occurs in the wall, is smooth, and has a homogeneous shadow. With emphysematous cholecystitis, the near-field echoes tend to be dimpled and are not smooth as seen in the porcelain gallbladder (Fig. 6-30A–D). A CT or non-contrast radiography can be performed to distinguish air from calcification.[55,63]

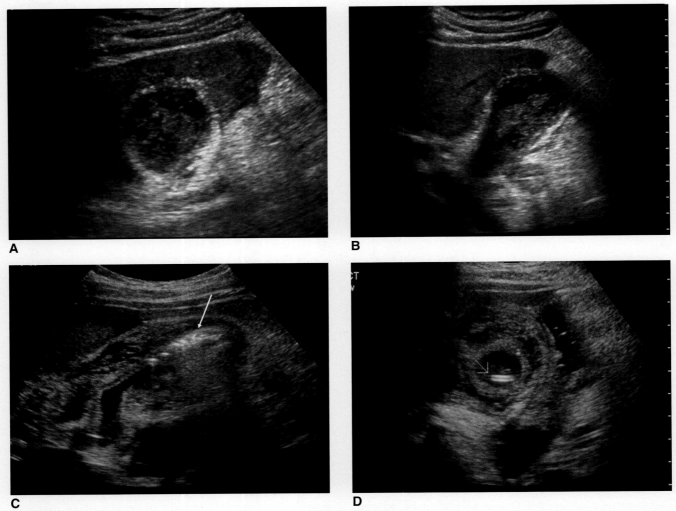

**Figure 6-29** Gangrenous cholecystitis. Transverse **(A)** and longitudinal **(B)** images in an acutely ill patient with right upper quadrant pain and fever. The wall is irregularly thickened and sludge was also seen. **C.** Longitudinal image in the latter stages of gangrenous cholecystitis. Air *(arrow)* is seen within the fundus of the contracted gallbladder. The wall is also thickened and edematous. **D.** A stent *(arrow)* was placed within the gallbladder in this patient with gangrenous cholecystitis. The patient was acutely ill and unable to have a cholecystectomy. Note the thick gallbladder wall and ascites.

In critical patients, percutaneous cholecystostomy and IV antimicrobial therapy can be used as a temporary treatment. Emphysematous cholecystitis is considered a surgical emergency and should be treated with cholecystectomy.[35,55]

## CHRONIC CHOLECYSTITIS AND ASSOCIATED CONDITIONS

Chronic cholecystitis, a common form of symptomatic gallbladder disease, is virtually always associated with stones.[55] By definition, there is chronic inflammation of the gallbladder wall and it is often incidentally found on sonography.[7,64] Repeated acute attacks produce a series of inflammatory changes that result in thickening and fibrosis of the gallbladder wall as well as contraction of the gallbladder.[7,55]

Chronic cholecystitis affects women more than men, and it occurs most often in the elderly.[64] The patient tends to have intolerance to fatty or fried foods, possibly associated with intermittent nausea and vomiting. There is often moderate RUQ and epigastric pain, which may radiate to the scapula. These attacks may be frequent or years apart. The patient, however, can also be asymptomatic.[3,4,15] Alkaline phosphates, AST, and ALT levels may be elevated. If jaundice is present, the direct bilirubin value is also elevated. It is possible for an attack of acute cholecystitis to be superimposed on underlying chronic disease, in which case some clinical and sonographic features of both entities could be present.[4,15]

Without cholecystectomy, complications sometimes arise from untreated chronic cholecystitis. *Bouveret syndrome,* or *gallstone ileus,* is a complication that

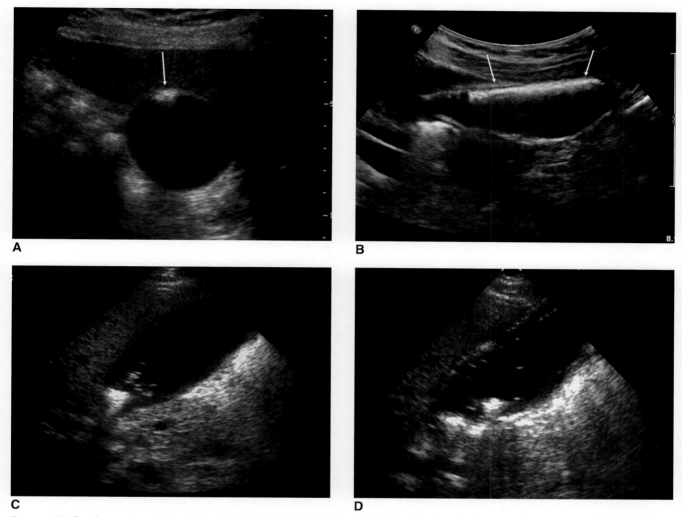

**Figure 6-30** Emphysematous cholecystitis. **A.** Transverse image of the gallbladder showing a small amount of air *(arrow)* within the gallbladder wall in a diabetic patient. **B.** Longitudinal image in a different patient with a larger amount of air *(arrows)* in the wall. With emphysematous cholecystitis, air can be seen within both the wall and gallbladder lumen. **C.** With the patient supine, air within the gallbladder is seen at the neck. **D.** When the patient rolls into a left decubitus position, the air moves out of the neck and swirls within the gallbladder lumen.

occurs when a biliary-enteric fistula forms between the gallbladder and duodenum. Large stones can erode through the gallbladder wall and into the duodenal bulb, where they become impacted in the duodenal lumen. There, the stone may cause gastric outlet obstruction (gastric dilatation) or distal bowel obstruction in the ileum, colon, or rectum, or it may be passed spontaneously. Although rare, this syndrome must be considered, especially in women older than 60 years with symptoms of upper intestinal obstruction as well as gallbladder disease.[65,66] Another possible complication of untreated cholecystitis is Mirizzi syndrome in which a gallstone becomes impacted in the gallbladder neck or cystic duct, exerting pressure on the adjacent common duct.[55]

The sonographic features of chronic cholecystitis are a small contracted gallbladder with stones and an evenly thickened, fibrous echogenic wall. A stone is often lodged within the neck[64] (Fig. 6-31A–D). With careful technique, the wall–echo–shadow (WES) triad or double-arc shadow sign may be seen (Fig. 6-32A,B). The first arc or curved echogenic line represents the thickened gallbladder wall. The second arc is from the surface of the stone followed by posterior acoustic shadowing.[2,5] With chronic disease, the gallbladder may be so contracted that it is difficult to visualize sonographically. The WES sign can be mimicked by residual barium, a porcelain gallbladder, or Bouveret syndrome.[4,65,66] Air-filled bowel loops in the RUQ may create shadowing, which can be mistaken for a contracted gallbladder with stones. The differential diagnosis for chronic cholecystitis is adenomyomatosis and gallbladder carcinoma.[64]

A porcelain gallbladder occurs when all or part of the gallbladder wall is calcified (Fig. 6-33A,B). It is a relatively rare manifestation of chronic cholecystitis and it is more common in men.[7,18] It is associated with a high

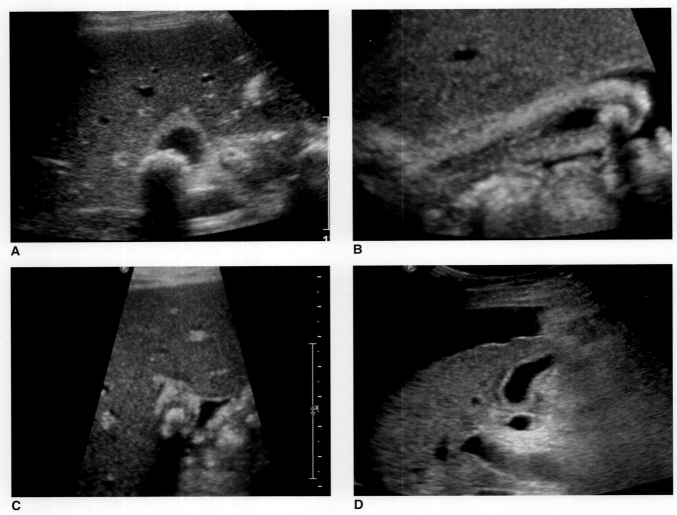

**Figure 6-31** Chronic cholecystitis. **A.** Longitudinal image in a patient with continued right upper quadrant pain. A stone is seen within the neck of a contracted gallbladder. The stone did not shift even though the patient moved into multiple positions. **B.** Longitudinal and **(C)** transverse images demonstrate thickened gallbladder wall, stone, and ascites. **D.** In a patient with chronic cholecystitis, cirrhosis, and ascites, a contracted gallbladder is seen on the sonogram.

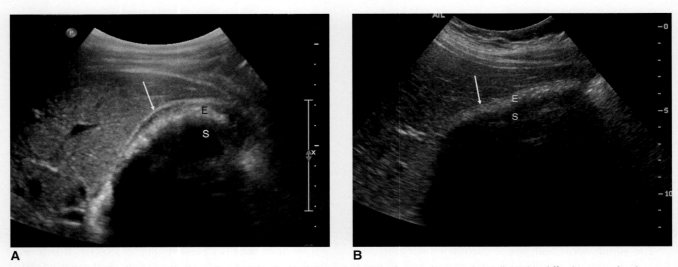

**Figure 6-32  A.** Longitudinal image of a wall–echo–shadow (WES) triad. **B.** With chronic disease, the wall can be difficult to visualize but was identified after careful evaluation. *Arrow*, gallbladder wall; *E*, echo from stone; *S*, shadow.

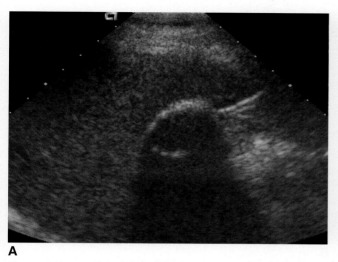

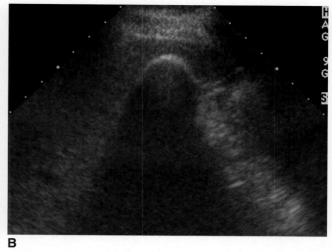

**A**

**B**

**Figure 6-33** Porcelain gallbladder. **A.** Transverse image showing a calcified anterior and posterior wall. **B.** At times, the anterior calcified wall is strongly calcified and the posterior wall cannot be seen.

incidence of gallbladder carcinoma.[3,18] Sonographically, a single echogenic line representing the calcified wall is seen. All or part of the wall may be calcified. If the wall is strongly calcified, a posterior shadow is also seen, which can obscure the gallbladder. Differential diagnosis consists of gallstones or emphysematous cholecystitis.[3,7] CT or non-contrast radiography may assist in the diagnosis of porcelain gallbladder.[18]

## GALLBLADDER WALL THICKENING

The gallbladder wall is thickened when it measures greater than 3 mm.[45] Approximately 50% of patients with acute cholecystitis will have gallbladder wall thickening. The nonfasting patient will also have a thickened gallbladder wall.[18] There are several other causes of gallbladder wall thickening including adenomyomatosis, gallbladder carcinoma, hepatic congestions, congestive heart failure, hypoalbuminemia, hypertension, and infections including hepatitis, pancreatitis, and HIV[7,18,35] (Pathology Box 6-1). Wall thickening alone is still a nonspecific finding, and further research is needed to determine whether analysis of specific morphologic features will help differentiate acute cholecystitis[67] (Fig. 6-34A–E).

## CHOLESTASIS AND PREGNANCY

Intrahepatic cholestasis occurs during the second and third trimesters of pregnancy and resolves shortly after delivery. The patient presents with pruritus. Laboratory values show elevated alkaline phosphatase, serum transaminase, and bile acids. Even though it is a benign condition for the mother, the fetus is at risk for prematurity, dysrhythmia, distress, or intrauterine death. By sonography, gallstones may be detected; however, there is no ductal dilatation.[28,68,69]

## GALLBLADDER NEOPLASMS

### Benign

Adenomas are pedunculated, well-circumscribed lesions within the gallbladder. Sonographically, they appear as a non–gravity-dependent echogenic mass

---

**PATHOLOGY BOX 6-1**

### *Causes of Gallbladder Wall Thickening*

**Intrinsic Causes**

Acute cholecystitis
Chronic cholecystitis
Gangrenous cholecystitis
Emphysematous cholecystitis
Adenomyomatosis
Polyp
Gallbladder carcinoma: primary or metastatic
Gallbladder torsion

**Extrinsic Causes**

Right-sided heart failure
Alcoholic liver disease
Hepatitis
AIDS
Sepsis
Hypoalbuminemia
Renal failure
Ascites (benign)
Multiple myeloma
Portal node lymphatic obstruction
Systemic venous hypertension
Gallbladder wall varices

**Physiologic Causes**

Contracted gallbladder after eating

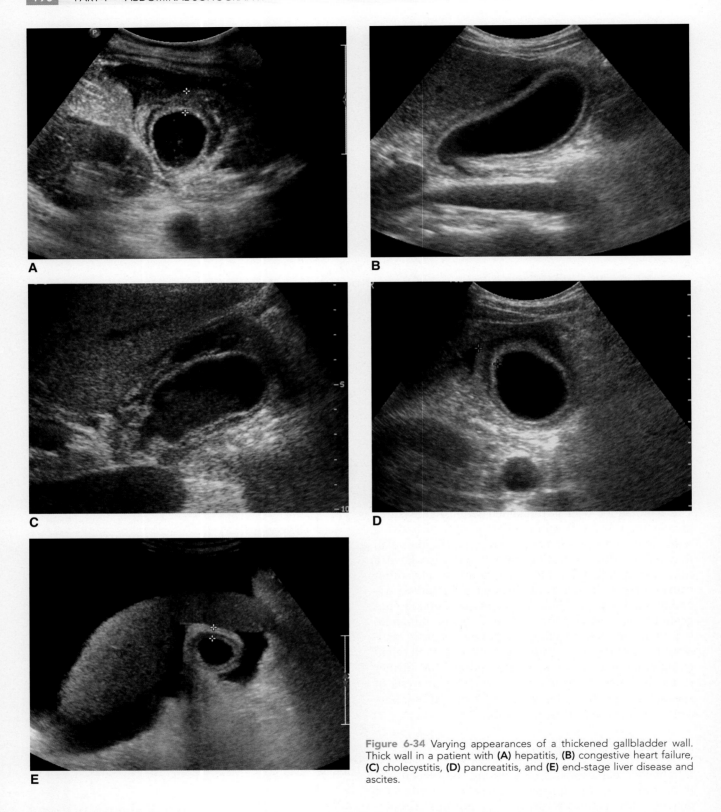

**Figure 6-34** Varying appearances of a thickened gallbladder wall. Thick wall in a patient with **(A)** hepatitis, **(B)** congestive heart failure, **(C)** cholecystitis, **(D)** pancreatitis, and **(E)** end-stage liver disease and ascites.

protruding into the gallbladder lumen. When large, adenomas may become more heterogeneous. Adenomas typically measure less than 2 cm. Malignant potential is considered low, although this is debatable.[7] Polyps greater than 1 cm, however, are suggestive of malignancy.[70]

Polyps are small, benign lesions that project into the gallbladder lumen on a stalk. Polyps may be adenomatous or, more frequently, cholesterol and therefore are not true neoplasms.[15] The majority of polyps are caused by chronic inflammation, hyperplasia of the gallbladder wall, or lipid deposits.[71] Polyps are fixed, nonmobile

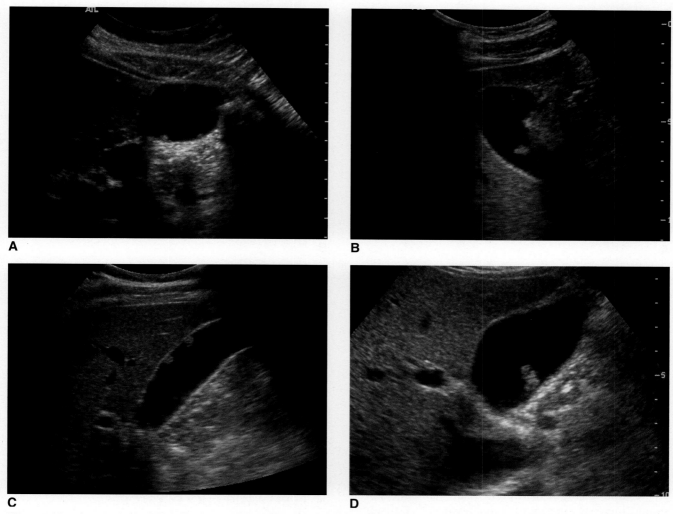

**Figure 6-35** Polyps can be small, large, single, or multiple **(A–D)**. Careful evaluation is needed to ensure polyps are not mistaken for gallbladder folds or sludge balls.

lesions that do not display a posterior shadow. They can be single or muliptle[70] (Fig. 6-35A–D). Care should be taken to not misdiagnose a polyp as sludge, gallstones, or a malignant lesion.[72] Treatment involves removal of polyps greater than 1 cm if the patient is over 50 years old. Any polyp that is growing, even when less than 1 cm, should be removed, due to the increased risk of malignancy.[7,71,73] Also, the gallbladder should be removed in the setting of polyps and primary sclerosing cholangitis (PSC).[73,74]

## Malignancies

The vast majority of gallbladder malignancies are adenocarcinomas.[74,75] The remaining small percentage is composed of wall tumors, metastases, or lymphoma. It predominantly affects women with an average age of 72. Even though gallbladder cancer is uncommon, it is the fifth most common malignancy of the digestive system. The primary risk factors are chronic cholecystitis and cholelithiasis; however, rapidly growing polyps and a porcelain gallbladder are also well-documented risks for developing gallbladder cancer.[7,45,76,77] Other risk factors include PSC, ductal anomalies, and choledochal cysts.[7] Gallstones are present in as many as 95% of cases and a porcelain gallbladder is seen in approximately 25% of gallbladder cancers.[75,78]

Gallbladder carcinoma can metastasize to the liver, lymph nodes, CHD, and other surrounding organs.[77] Intraductal spread occurs in at least 4% of cases and can clinically mimic pancreatic or bile duct tumors. Gallbladder cancer is often difficult to detect in its early stages, as patients may be asymptomatic or present with the signs and symptoms of cholelithiasis or cholecystitis. In addition, there are no laboratory alternatives to assist in early diagnosis. In the late stages of gallbladder carcinoma, patients will have jaundice, malaise, or weight loss.[75,77] The majority of gallbladder carcinomas are found incidentally during routine cholecystectomy. Fewer than 20% of gallbladder carcinomas are diagnosed preoperatively.[4] Cholecystectomy should be performed if metastasis has not yet occurred. The

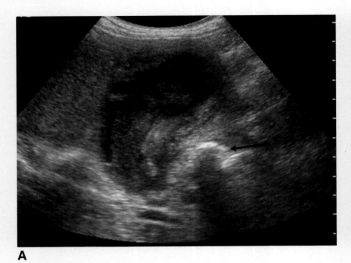

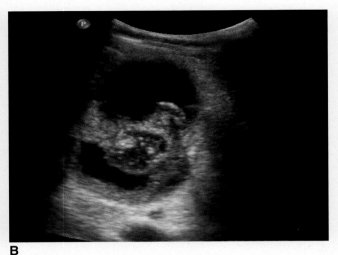

**Figure 6-36** Gallbladder carcinoma. **A.** Echoes completely fill the gallbladder lumen. A stone (arrow) was seen at the posterior portion of the gallbladder. Note the irregularly thickened, heterogeneous gallbladder wall. **B.** A heterogeneous mass extending from the gallbladder wall represents gallbladder carcinoma.

5-year survival rate for primary gallbladder carcinoma is less than 5%.[73]

If gallbladder carcinoma is diagnosed by sonography, it is typically in the advanced stage. At this point, a heterogeneous, irregular-shaped mass replaces the gallbladder. Tumefactive sludge or sludge balls can mimic a malignant gallbladder mass.[7,17,77] Direct invasion into the liver, irregular wall thickening, or a poorly defined polypoid mass may also be seen (Fig. 6-36A,B). In addition, a gallbladder mass greater than 1 cm, wall thickening greater than 1 cm, or disruption of the gallbladder wall should increase suspicion of malignancy.[7,77] Gallstones encased in tumor are also a sign of gallbladder carcinoma.[77] Color Doppler may be useful to establish the internal vascularity that is often present in malignancies.[79] Contrast-enhanced sonography may also be beneficial to differentiate benign from malignant masses.[17] Differential diagnosis for gallbladder cancer includes hepatocarcinoma, cholangiocarcinoma, or metastases. On the other hand, the benign differential diagnosis contains cholecystitis, polyps, and inflammatory and noninflammatory diseases. When a gallbladder malignancy is suspected, it is imperative to search the entire abdomen for other signs of malignancy such as liver metastases, vascular invasion, biliary dilatation, porta hepatis nodes, retroperitoneal adenopathy, or ascites.[77]

Melanoma is the most common tumor to metastasize to the gallbladder. Even with therapy, melanoma metastasis to the gallbladder carries a poor prognosis; however, long-term survival is occasionally seen.[80,81] Melanoma metastasis to the gallbladder is not associated with cholelithiasis, which differs from gallbladder cancer. Sonographic findings, however, are similar to asymmetric wall thickening and solitary or multiple masses within the gallbladder. Treatment of metastatic melanoma to the gallbladder is cholecystectomy.[82]

Other bloodborne metastases to the gallbladder can occur from the lungs, kidneys, and esophagus. Metastases from the stomach, pancreas, and bile ducts can reach the gallbladder by direct invasion. Malignancy of the liver, ovary, and colon can also metastasize to the gallbladder. Primary gallbladder cancer is strongly associated with stones and inflammatory gallbladder disease; however, metastatic disease is completely independent of cholelithiasis and cholecystitis.[83]

## HYPERPLASTIC CHOLECYSTOSES

Hyperplastic cholecystoses are a group of benign, noninflammatory conditions that are both degenerative and proliferative. They include adenomyomatosis, cholesterosis, neuromatosis, fibromatosis, and lipomatosis.[4,84]

Adenomyomatosis is a common condition characterized by excessive proliferation of the surface epithelium, with gland-like formations and outpouchings of the mucosa into or through a thickened muscle layer. These pouches, or diverticula, are called *Rokitansky-Aschoff sinuses*.[85,86] There are three forms of adenomyomatosis: (1) diffuse, involving the entire gallbladder; (2) segmental, in which the proximal, middle, or distal one-third is involved circumferentially; and (3) localized, the most common type, confined almost exclusively to the fundus.[18] It is more common in women, and patients generally present with RUQ pain. The sonographic appearance includes focal or diffuse wall thickening; small, round, anechoic spaces in the gallbladder wall represent Rokitansky-Aschoff sinuses and echogenic foci spaced at varying intervals in the gallbladder wall. These echogenic foci display acoustic shadowing or comet tail reverberation artifacts with a twinkle artifact on color Doppler.[18,85,86] Gallstones are also common[85] (Fig. 6-37A–D). Diagnosis is often made by sonography; however, adenomyomatosis

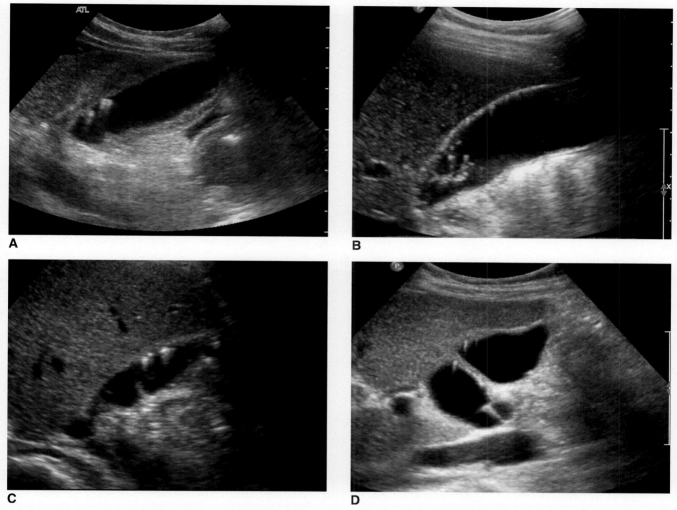

**Figure 6-37** Adenomyomatosis. **A.** Thickened wall with echogenic foci and comet tail artifact near the neck of the gallbladder. **B.** Adenomyomatosis throughout the majority of the anterior gallbladder wall. Sludge was also seen. **C,D.** Comet tail artifacts are seen at the body and fundus of the gallbladder representing adenomyomatosis.

can be misdiagnosed as gallbladder carcinoma, emphysematous cholecystitis, or chronic cholecystitis.[85,86]

Cholesterosis is characterized by lipid-laden macrophages that deposit within the gallbladder wall. Cholesterol polyps make up approximately 20% of these deposits; however, they represent 50% of all gallbladder polyps.[7] It occurs more frequently in women than in men.[6] The lesions may be diffuse, with no impairment of gallbladder function, or localized single or multiple polypoid lesions, which may be pedunculated and interfere with function.[4]

Neuromatosis and fibromatosis are rare proliferations of nerve and fibrous tissue, respectively. Lipomatosis is an excessive buildup of fat layers in the gallbladder wall. These three processes may or may not interfere with gallbladder function and are often not visualized sonographically.[4]

The hyperplastic cholecystoses are often asymptomatic, but when symptoms do occur, they often mimic those of cholelithiasis. Stones may or may not be present. Laboratory values are usually normal unless function is impaired. The risk of malignancy is low. Cholecystectomy should be considered in symptomatic patients.[4]

These lesions may not be detected sonographically, but when visible, the appearance can vary. Fixed polypoid lesions or a small misshapen gallbladder may be seen.[4]

## MISCELLANEOUS GALLBLADDER PATHOLOGY

An enlarged, distended, palpable, and nontender gallbladder in a jaundiced patient is referred to as a *Courvoisier gallbladder*. It occurs when there is obstruction of the CBD, typically due to a malignant neoplasm at the pancreatic head.[62] With any distal mass, dilation begins with the gallbladder, followed by the common duct, and finally the intrahepatic tree. Upon removal of the obstructing mass, the gallbladder decompresses

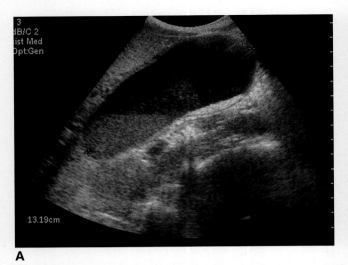

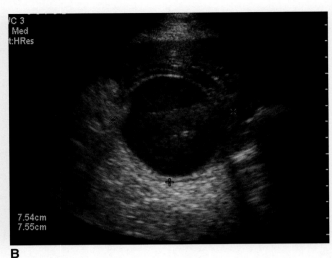

**A**  **B**

**Figure 6-38** Hydropic gallbladder. Longitudinal **(A)** and transverse **(B)** images in a patient with right upper quadrant pain, nausea, vomiting, and a palpable mass. The gallbladder measured greater than 4 cm in the anteroposterior diameter. Sludge and a thickened gallbladder wall were also noted.

actively (because of its contractile muscle), whereas the ducts passively return to normal in reverse order.[11]

A hydropic gallbladder is abnormally distended and filled with thick bile, mucus, or pus. The most common cause of hydropic gallbladder is a stone obstructing the gallbladder neck or cystic duct. There are numerous other causes including hyperalimentation, a variety of infections, and any obstruction of the CBD or cystic duct. The obstruction leads to gradual reabsorption of the bile despite continued accumulation of secretions from the gallbladder wall. The patient may be asymptomatic or present with RUQ pain, nausea, and vomiting; a palpable mass; and the symptoms of the underlying pathology. Sonographically, the gallbladder is rounded, distended, measures greater than 4 cm in AP diameter, and may have stones[87] (Fig. 6-38A,B).

Hydatid cysts of the gallbladder are rare. Parasitosis, caused by *Echinococcus granulosus*, enters the gallbladder through the cystic duct via the liver. The gallbladder can also become affected if there is an intrabiliary rupture of a cyst or a direct rupture of a cyst into the gallbladder. A primary hydatid cyst of the gallbladder is rare. On sonography, the appearance is described as a "cyst within a cyst."[88]

Torsion, or volvulus, of the gallbladder is rare, but its incidence may be increasing possibly due to the increase in life expectancy. It can occur at all ages but is more common in elderly patients. It is three times more frequent in women than men. The cause is uncertain but is thought to be lengthening of the gallbladder mesentery in old age that allows the gallbladder to be free floating on a pedicle. Vigorous bowel peristalsis, a mobile gallbladder fundus, gallstones, atherosclerosis of the cystic artery, and kyphosis have all been implicated as predisposing or contributing factors. Pathologically, the walls of the twisted gallbladder become thickened,

edematous, and hemorrhagic. Gangrene or a palpable mass may be present. The sonographic features include gross wall thickening and a distended tender gallbladder.[35,89,90] Color Doppler may be helpful to visualize the cystic artery. Gallstones are seldom present. The appearance and laboratory values are often nonspecific. Sonography is the modality of choice; however, CT, magnetic resonance cholangiopancreatography (MRCP), and hepato-iminodiacetic acid (HIDA) scan can be helpful. The diagnosis of torsion is seldom made preoperatively. The treatment is immediate cholecystectomy.[90]

Microabscesses in the gallbladder wall may be seen as hyperechoic foci in the wall, which may produce comet tail reverberations. Intramural diverticula filled with inspissated bile, small stones, or cholesterol crystals can have the same appearance.[91]

## THE POSTCHOLECYSTECTOMY PATIENT

In the postcholecystectomy patient, the gallbladder fossa is commonly filled with bowel loops, although closer examination may reveal echogenic foci with reverberations and/or shadows representing surgical clips. Occasionally, postoperative evaluation of the gallbladder fossa may demonstrate fluid collections. These range from asymptomatic simple anechoic collections to complex abscesses with the associated clinical presentation (Pathology Box 6-2).

Controversy exists over whether the size of the common duct should increase after the gallbladder is removed. Some indicate the duct may increase in caliber because it becomes a floppy, passive tube from previous episodes of inflammation, or as the result of surgical exploration of the duct at the time of cholecystectomy. Another theory is the duct may act as a reservoir for bile in the absence of the gallbladder.[92] Although some

*Causes of a Nonvisualized Gallbladder*

Patient is nonfasting
Postcholecystectomy
Contracted gallbladder with stones (chronic cholecystitis)
Congenitally absent gallbladder
Porcelain gallbladder
Hepatization of gallbladder
Mirizzi syndrome or gallstone ileus
Gallbladder neoplasms completely filling lumen
Ectopic gallbladder
Emphysematous gallbladder
Overlying bowel
Residual barium in nearby bowel

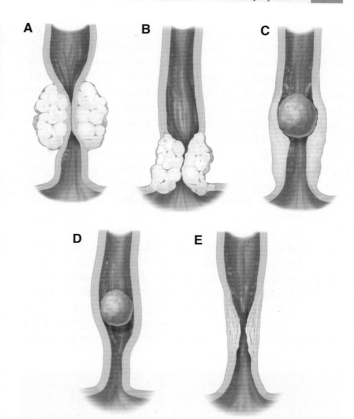

**Figure 6-39** Types of extrahepatic biliary obstruction. **A–C.** Complete common bile duct obstructions and **(D,E)** incomplete obstructions. **A.** Extrinsic cancer fixing and compressing duct, **(B)** intrinsic cancer, **(C)** impacted stone with edema of duct, **(D)** ball-in-valve stone causing intermittent obstruction, and **(E)** stricture of duct.

studies say that a normal postcholecystectomy common duct can measure up to 11 mm, others claim it should be considered dilated if it exceeds 6 mm in maximum intraluminal AP diameter.[21,93,94] Rescanning 30 to 45 minutes after a fatty meal may help determine whether obstruction truly exists. Fatty meals stimulate biliary flow and relax the sphincter of Oddi. If a normal or slightly dilated duct enlarges after a fatty meal or an abnormally large duct fails to shrink, CBD obstruction is strongly indicated. After a fatty meal, healthy, nondilated, patent ducts should decrease slightly in caliber if they change at all. A slight decrease in diameter virtually excludes obstruction.[92,94] Fatty meals are especially useful to confirm that an asymptomatic patient with equivocal or mildly prominent ducts has normal function.[94]

Postcholecystectomy syndrome is not a true syndrome; however, it refers to the recurrence of preoperative symptoms, particularly biliary colic. Incomplete relief may be due to an error in the original diagnosis of gallbladder disease. Retained common duct stones, biliary strictures, and chronic pancreatitis are the most frequent causes. Others include an excessive cystic duct stump, sphincter of Oddi spasms, biliary tract carcinomas, an amputation neuroma, and adhesions constricting the CBD.[62]

## BILE DUCT OBSTRUCTION

Bile duct obstruction, either intrahepatic or extrahepatic, causes a direct interference with the flow of bile (Fig. 6-39A–E). The obstruction can be from an intrinsic or extrinsic cause such as stones, benign or malignant tumors, and strictures.[7] Causes of biliary obstruction depend on the location. Intrahepatic biliary obstruction can be caused by PSC or any space-occupying mass within the liver. Obstruction at the porta hepatis can be due to cholangiocarcinoma, PSC, gallbladder cancer, or metastatic tumors. Biliary obstruction at the pancreas includes causes such as pancreatic cancer, pancreatitis, choledocholithiasis, or cholangiocarcinoma.[8] A previous episode of obstruction or inflammation with loss of elasticity or an ampullary dysfunction may also cause the duct to dilate.[92]

Clinically, the patient will present with RUQ pain, jaundice, and fever. In the obstructed patient, bilirubin or alkaline phosphatase can be elevated.[7] A duct can also appear normal despite abnormal laboratory values. This is more likely to occur in patients with fibrosed or infiltrated livers because the hardened, noncompliant liver prohibits the ducts from dilating. Conversely, a duct can be abnormal even though laboratory values are normal.[94] Significant sonographic biliary pathology can be present without clinical jaundice or an elevated serum bilirubin.[95] Duct size can also change sporadically because it is part of a dynamic system that responds as obstructions occur and resolve.[93]

By sonography, the bile ducts should be measured inner wall to inner wall[7] (Fig. 6-6). The CHD is considered dilated if the internal diameter measures greater than 6 mm or CBD measures greater than 8 mm.[3,79,95] Again, there is currently debate over whether the bile duct increases with age or after a cholecystectomy. The use of color Doppler is essential to distinguish bile ducts from small hepatic vessels.[77,96] Intrahepatic ducts measuring greater than 2 mm in diameter or more than 40% of the adjacent portal vein are considered dilated.[7] Additional sonographic criteria for intrahepatic dilatation include (1) the parallel channel sign (double-barreled shotgun sign), representing the dilated duct running anterior to its accompanying portal vein or hepatic artery; (2) irregular, jagged walls and branching patterns of the ducts (compared to smooth walls and smooth bifurcations of the portal venous system); and (3) stellate confluence of dilated ducts converging toward the porta hepatis[2,5,10,79] (Fig. 6-40A–D).

Sonography is also an important tool in locating the level and cause of obstruction (Fig. 6-41A,B). The findings depend on the type and location of the obstruction (dilatation may be intrahepatic, extrahepatic, or both).[2] With any type of blockage, the duct becomes dilated proximal to the obstruction.[8] For example, if the obstruction is at the porta hepatis, the intrahepatic ducts will become dilated, but the duct between the porta hepatis and pancreas will be normal.[3] With real-time scanning,

it is easier to trace the extent of ductal dilatation. It is also important to note whether obstruction is focal or diffuse. The entire course and caliber of the duct must be examined for dilatation (Table 6-2). It is also important to note the duct at the obstruction. If the duct tapers at the obstruction, it is typically a benign process. If, however, the duct ends abruptly, there is an increased association with malignancy. The ductal wall is also important to evaluate. Diffuse wall thickening is associated with cholangitis, whereas focal thickening is seen with stones, pancreatitis, and pancreatic carcinoma.[8]

Other conditions that can mimic dilated intrahepatic biliary radicles are Caroli disease (communicating cavernous ectasia of the intrahepatic ducts), enlarged hepatic arteries, cavernous transformation of the portal vein, and intrahepatic arteriovenous malformations.[5,10,79]

## Choledocholithiasis

Stones within the bile duct are the most common pathology of the biliary tract.[7,8] Common duct stones are usually formed in the gallbladder and then pass into the

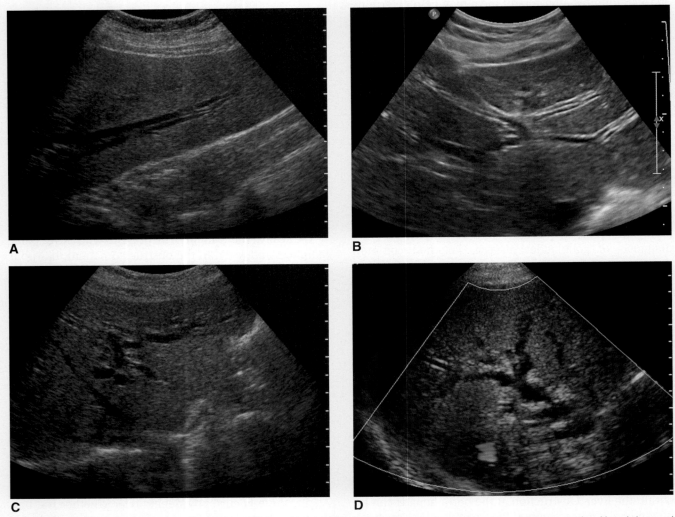

**Figure 6-40** Dilated intrahepatic ducts. **A,B.** Parallel channel sign of dilated intrahepatic ducts. One channel represents the dilated duct and the other its accompanying portal vein. **C,D.** Stellate confluence of irregular branching channels represents dilated intrahepatic ducts.

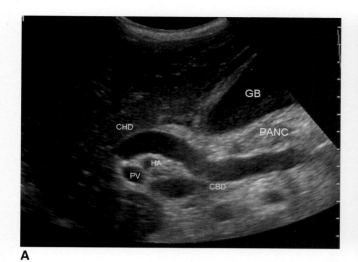

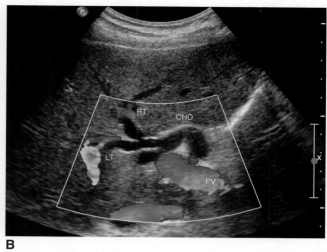

**Figure 6-41** Dilated common hepatic duct *(CHD)* and common bile duct *(CBD)*. **A.** Dilated CBD to the level of the pancreas. With an obstruction at the pancreas, the entire ductal system would be dilated. **B.** Dilated CHD at the porta hepatis. With an obstruction at the CHD, the intrahepatic ducts *(right* and *left)* would be dilated, but the CBD would remain normal. *GB*, gallbladder; *HA*, hepatic artery; *PANC*, pancreas; *PV*, portal vein.

CBD, where they may cause an obstruction (Fig. 6-42). After cholecystectomy, stones may be retained within the duct or they may form spontaneously. Choledocholithiasis may lead to cholangitis.[97]

Patients with choledocholithiasis may be asymptomatic unless obstruction occurs. Small stones may remain in the duct without obstructing or may pass silently out into the bowel. The clinical symptoms of ductal stones may include RUQ pain, intermittent or persistent obstructive jaundice, and cholangitis. With obstruction, bilirubin, alkaline phosphatase, and transaminase

values increase.[97] The patient may have temporary relief of symptoms if the stone passes into the duodenum or returns into the gallbladder.[45]

Common duct stones are found in 8% to 20% of patients undergoing cholecystectomy and 2% to 4% of patients following cholecystectomy.[8] Sonographically, stones can be visualized in dilated or nondilated ducts, although stones are typically easier to identify in the dilated duct. Bile duct stones can create a shadow, be single or multiple, large or small, mobile, or stationary[7,8] (Fig. 6-43A–C). Small stones may be difficult to detect due to their location and bowel gas.[45] The duct can also be packed with stones, producing a broad acoustic shadow, making it difficult to differentiate the duct from surrounding bowel. If visualization of the duct is not optimal, having the patient drink water may help displace the gas and improve visualization.[98,99] Other helpful

| TABLE | 6-2 |
| --- | --- |

**Defining the Level and Cause of Intrahepatic Biliary Dilatation**

**Causes of Intrahepatic Dilatation with a *Normal* CBD**

- Proximal bile duct tumors (benign and malignant)
- Klatskin tumor
- Cholangitis (primary sclerosing cholangitis)
- Tumors at the porta hepatis (adenopathy and metastases)
- Mirizzi syndrome
- Liver neoplasms compressing intrahepatic ducts
- Benign strictures

**Causes of Intrahepatic Dilatation with a *Dilated* CBD**

- Choledocholithiasis
- Carcinoma of pancreatic head
- Pseudocyst obstructing CBD
- Acute pancreatitis
- Chronic pancreatitis
- Choledochal cyst
- Lymphadenopathy
- Benign strictures
- Ampullary tumors

CBD, common bile duct.

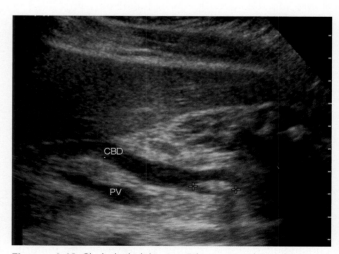

**Figure 6-42** Choledocholithiasis. Bile surrounding the stone *(calipers)* makes visualization easier. *CBD*, common bile duct; *PV*, portal vein.

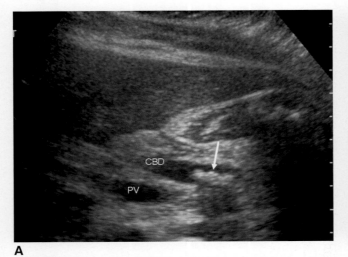

**A**

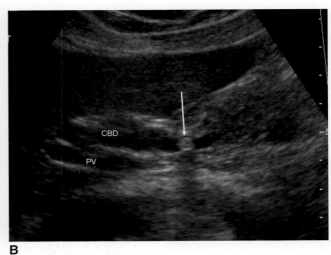

**B**

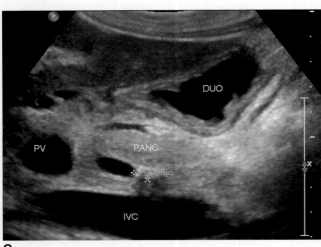

**C**

**Figure 6-43** Choledocholithiasis. **A.** Large stone *(arrow)* in distal portion of dilated common bile duct *(CBD)*. **B.** Small stone *(arrow)* in the distal common bile duct. **C.** Stone *(calipers)* at the distal common bile duct at the level of the pancreas. All of the stones have a distal shadow and cause dilatation proximal to the blockage. *DUO,* duodenum; *IVC,* inferior vena cava; *PANC,* pancreas; *PV,* portal vein.

techniques include harmonics, transducer pressure, and altering patient position.[7] If stones are visualized, an endoscopic retrograde cholangiopancreatography (ERCP) is used for removal and treatment.[35] If the obstruction or stones are not identified sonographically, an MRCP or ERCP could be helpful[7] (Figs. 6-44 and 6-45).

## Cholangiocarcinoma

Cholangiocarcinoma is a primary malignancy of the bile duct. The majority of these tumors are adenocarcinomas that grow slowly and may extend along the length of the CHD and CBD.[62] Cholangiocarcinomas may occur throughout the biliary tree; however, they are more common at the porta hepatis (Klatskin tumors).[7,8] Ampullary carcinomas may also include the distal portion of the CBD.[15,100]

Cholangiocarcinoma occurs equally in men and women, usually between 50 and 70 years of age.[15] Risk factors for developing cholangiocarcinoma include sclerosing cholangitis, choledochal cysts, and parasitic infections.[7] If detected early, the curative treatment for cholangiocarcinoma is surgery. However, the majority of patients present at the late stages. At this point, palliative treatment to prolong life is the goal.[101]

Signs and symptoms include marked icterus and a palpable gallbladder if the obstruction is distal to the cystic duct. Abdominal pain, anorexia, fatigue, weight loss, hepatomegaly, and ascites may be present.[92] A laboratory workup often reveals elevated serum bilirubin and alkaline phosphatase levels.[15,62]

By sonogram, ductal wall irregularity may be seen.[7,8] Tumors are typically small and are seldom seen by sonography; however, sonography is helpful in identifying the level of the ductal obstruction.[8] Cholangiocarcinomas vary in echogenicity from hypoechoic to hyperechoic. The portal vein should be evaluated for tumor involvement.[7] Other signs of malignancy such as liver metastases, ascites, and adenopathy should also be sought (Fig. 6-46A–D).

The list of differential diagnoses for cholangiocarcinoma is extensive. Other possible malignant intraductal tumors include hepatocellular carcinoma invading the bile duct, cystadenocarcinoma, metastases of melanoma to the bile ducts, lymphoma or other metastases in the porta hepatis simulating Klatskin tumors, and rhabdomyosarcomas.[100,102–104] Benign intraluminal tumors are very rare but include cystadenomas, papillomas, adenomas, granular cell myoblastomas, fibromas, neurinomas,

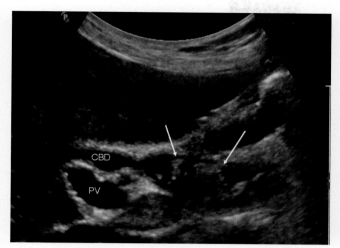

**Figure 6-44** More heterogeneous mass *(arrows)* within the duct was proven to be sludge by endoscopic retrograde cholangiopancreatography evaluation. *CBD,* common bile duct; *PV,* portal vein.

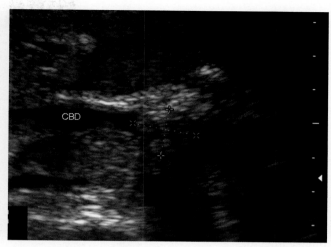

**Figure 6-45** A mass within the duct can also cause obstruction. This heterogeneous mass *(calipers)* within the common bile duct was an adenocarcinoma. *CBD,* common bile duct.

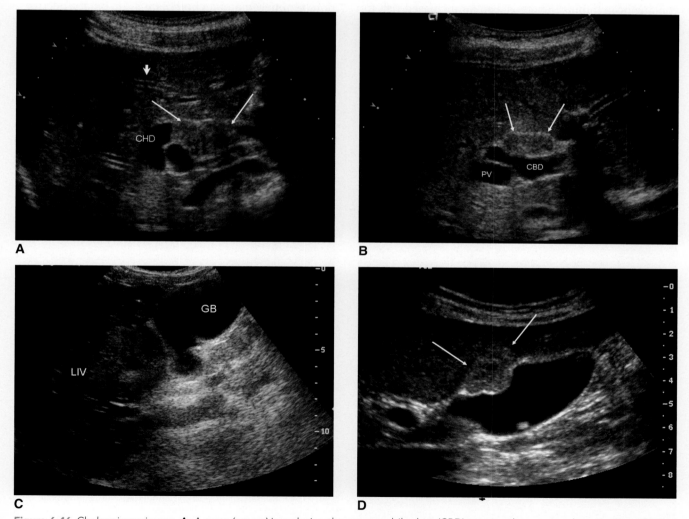

**Figure 6-46** Cholangiocarcinoma. **A.** A mass *(arrows)* is replacing the common bile duct *(CBD),* causing the common hepatic duct *(CHD)* to become dilated. The intrahepatic ducts are dilated as well *(arrowhead).* **B.** In a different patient, the cholangiocarcinoma *(arrows)* is compressing the duct at the porta hepatis. **C.** Metastasis to the liver from cholangiocarcinoma. The liver is heterogeneous, which represents multiple masses. The gallbladder is prominent as well. **D.** In this case, a mass *(arrows)* is compressing the gallbladder. A sludge ball is present as well. *GB,* gallbladder; *LIV,* liver; *PV,* portal vein.

leiomyomas, hamartomas, and lipomas.[100,103,104] Other causes of nonshadowing solid intraductal masses include material from a ruptured hydatid cyst, biliary sludge, blood clots, and nonshadowing calculi.[100,104] Extrinsic masses may also compress the duct externally and cause obstruction. Such masses include pseudocysts, adenopathy, lymphoma, or metastases in the porta hepatis region as well as pancreatic masses or inflammation.

## CHOLANGITIS

Cholangitis is a rare, chronic inflammatory and fibrosing disorder of the intrahepatic and extrahepatic biliary system. PSC is idiopathic, chronic, and sometimes familial, whereas secondary associated is due to a prior biliary infection.[7,74,105]

Patients with cholangitis may be asymptomatic or present with epigastric or RUQ pain, fatigue, pruritus, and jaundice. In the chronic stages, patient can progress to cirrhosis and liver failure. Patients are also at risk for cholangiocarcinoma.[7] There is also an increased risk for other carcinomas including hepatobiliary, hepatocellular, gallbladder, and pancreatic.[74] Laboratory tests may reveal an increased alkaline phosphatase value, elevated AST and ALT levels, increased WBC, and an increased direct bilirubin value (if jaundice is present).

The sonographic findings with cholangitis may include thickened and edematous duct walls that narrow the lumen, thus dilating the ducts proximally; however, diagnosis is difficult sonographically (Fig. 6-47A–C). The primary role of sonography in patients with cholangitis is to screen for cholangiocarcinoma. Cholangiography is typically the modality of choice to diagnose cholangitis while a biliary drain is placed to treat acute cholangitis[8,106] (Fig. 6-48). For PSC, liver transplant is currently the only treatment.[105]

## OTHER BILIARY TREE PATHOLOGY

Pneumobilia, air in the biliary tree, results from an extended communication of the bile duct to the gastrointestinal (GI) tract. This may occur following surgery, liver transplant, stent placement, fistula, ERCP, infection, emphysematous cholecystitis, or biliary necrosis. Sonographically, the air produces mobile bright echoes with dirty shadowing that follow the branching of the

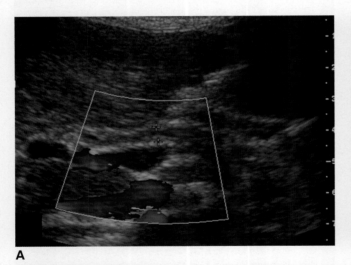

A

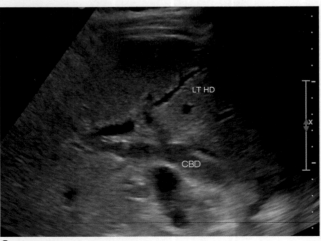

C

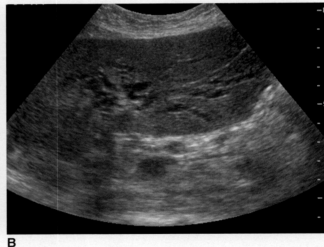

B

**Figure 6-47** Primary sclerosing cholangitis. **A.** The common bile duct walls (*calipers*) are thickened in this patient with primary sclerosing cholangitis. **B.** The thickened walls caused dilatation (*stellate pattern*) of the intrahepatic ducts. **C.** Dilated common bile and common hepatic ducts are seen in this patient with cholangitis. Note the echogenic, irregular walls of the bile ducts. *CBD*, common bile duct; *LT HD*, left intrahepatic duct.

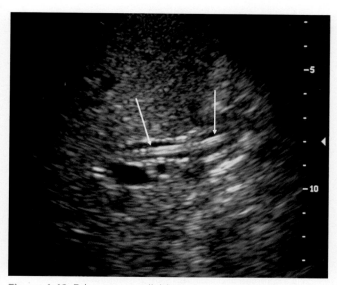

**Figure 6-48** Echogenic parallel lines *(arrows)* within the common bile duct represent a biliary stent.

portal venous tree[7] (Fig. 6-49A–D). It is important to determine whether the air is in the duct or the portal vein. Portal vein air is present with necrotic bowel.

Benign strictures of the extrahepatic bile ducts most often result from surgical trauma. The remaining cases are due to blunt abdominal trauma or erosion of the duct wall by a gallstone, which is known as *Mirizzi syndrome*. Mirizzi syndrome occurs when a stone obstructs the cystic duct, causing inflammation and obstruction of the common duct.[7] Depending on the degree of obstruction, the patient may be asymptomatic, icteric, or present with symptoms similar to cholangitis. Sonographically, strictures can mimic the appearance of cholangitis with dilated ducts if significant occlusion is present.[15]

Bilomas, collections of bile, can occur with laceration or rupture of the biliary tract and appear as upper abdominal fluid collections.[5] Following liver transplant, bilomas are cystic areas that can be seen along the falciform ligament or ligamentum venosum. They can be associated with hepatic artery thrombosis[3] (Fig. 6-50).

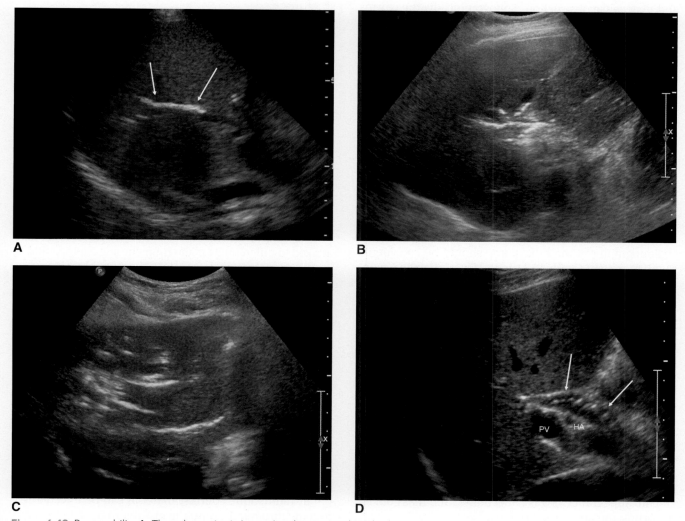

**Figure 6-49** Pneumobilia. **A.** The echogenic air *(arrows)* and posterior dirty shadowing are seen in the right hepatic lobe. **B,C.** Diffuse, extensive air within the intrahepatic ducts follows the branching pattern of the ducts and portal venous tree. The air moved under real-time observation. **D.** Air *(arrows)* was seen within the common bile duct after a liver transplant. *HA*, hepatic artery; *PV*, portal vein.

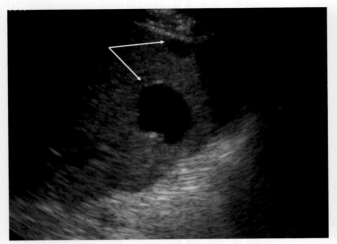

**Figure 6-50** Multiple bilomas (*arrows*) were seen in this post–liver transplant patient. Hepatic artery thrombosis was also seen.

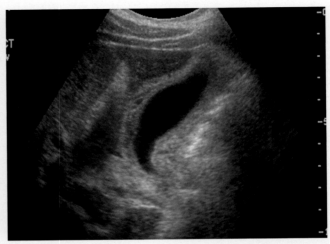

**Figure 6-51** Longitudinal image in a patient with elevated liver function tests demonstrates a markedly thickened gallbladder wall, which is a common finding in AIDS cholecystopathies.

In some areas of the world, roundworms (*Ascaris lumbricoides*) may infest the bile ducts and gallbladder and may cause obstruction. Sonographically, the worms appear as long, thin (20 to 30 cm in length and up to 6 mm thick), echogenic, linear structures within the bile ducts or gallbladder. Movement may also be seen.[3]

## AIDS CHOLECYSTOPATHY

The biliary system may become affected by HIV directly, opportunistic infections secondarily, or by AIDS. Cytomegalovirus (CMV), cryptosporidiosis, *Mycobacterium avium-intracellulare*, and other bacterial or fungal organisms have been responsible for biliary tract abnormalities and may lead to acalculous cholecystitis, sclerosing cholangitis, and gangrenous cholecystitis. AIDS-related neoplasms may lead to biliary tree obstruction and dilatation.[15,107,108]

Sonography of the biliary tree should be considered in AIDS patients with RUQ pain, fever, diarrhea, nausea and vomiting, jaundice, and abnormal liver function tests. Sonography may demonstrate a thickened gallbladder wall with possible striations, gallbladder dilatation, pericholecystic fluid collections, sludge, intrahepatic and extrahepatic biliary dilatation, and/or bile duct wall thickening[107–109] (Fig. 6-51).

## CORRELATION OF OTHER RELATED DIAGNOSTIC IMAGING PROCEDURES

Plain, non-contrast abdominal radiographs can reveal calcified gallstones (but only 15% contain sufficient calcium to be visualized), air in the biliary tree, porcelain gallbladder, gas-containing calculi (characteristic stellate appearance of gas collections), and mass effects distorting the abdominal organs.[15,16,59]

Oral cholecystography (OCG) is a rarely utilized radiography examination that requires the patient to ingest iodinated contrast medium. The examination was used to document gallbladder function, wall thickening, or strictures.[86]

Barium-contrast radiographic examinations such as a GI series may confirm the presence of biliary-enteric fistulas (i.e., gallstone ileus) because the barium refluxes into the biliary tree.[66]

Percutaneous transhepatic cholangiography (PTC) is an invasive procedure performed under X-ray guidance. A small needle is inserted through the liver into the biliary tree. Iodinated contrast medium is used to opacify the bile ducts, which allows an evaluation of the location and cause of obstructions. It may be used in patients whose bile ducts cannot be visualized by ERCP or to assess congenital biliary anomalies. Although it provides excellent detail, the morbidity and mortality rates are higher than with noninvasive tests.[15,23,110]

Scintigraphy examinations, such as the HIDA scan, are utilized to differentiate acute from chronic cholecystitis. It is a functional test to determine if the cystic duct is patent, thus ruling out acute cholecystitis. It will also demonstrate the major bile ducts and excretion of the tracer into the duodenum. Consequently, obstructive choledocholithiasis can also be diagnosed. Scintigraphy is used to evaluate acute gallbladder pathology; however, sonography has replaced scintigraphy in the majority of clinics.[35] For investigation of the gallbladder and biliary tree, nuclear medicine is approximately 85% accurate, but it can generate false-positive results. It does, however, only provide an isolated view in the workup of acute RUQ pain.[15,35,111,112] Also, it is a long exam, often taking up to 4 hours.[35]

ERCP is a standard test to evaluate biliary dilatation.[71] ERCP requires the insertion of an endoscope through the esophagus and stomach into the duodenum. At this point, radiopaque contrast material can be injected retrograde through the ampulla of Vater to opacify the pancreatic and biliary ducts for radiographic visualization. ERCP may be therapeutic as well as diagnostic because common duct stones can be effectively removed endoscopically via sphincterotomy or stent placement can be performed. Although it is an effective imaging procedure for biliary disorders, ERCP has definite risks, contraindications, and complications.[15,99,110,113]

MRCP is gaining an increased role in detecting choledocholithiasis and other acute biliary disease.[35,45,71] Gallstones and choledocholithiasis are best visualized on T2-weighted images, whereas gallbladder inflammation is seen on T1-weighted images.[18] Wall thickening, pericholecystic fluid, and inflammatory changes can also be seen.[55]

CT can provide information on the biliary system, if additional imaging is needed following a sonography examination.[35] Dilated bile ducts, intrahepatic and extrahepatic masses, choledocholithiasis, large gallstones, thickened gallbladder wall, pericholecystic fluid, and porcelain gallbladder may be detected by CT.[18,71,110] CT is also helpful in diagnosing gallbladder perforation and abscess.[18] CT can provide a global overview; however, it is inferior to sonography for diagnosing gallstones and other biliary pathology.[18,35,53]

Positron emission tomography (PET) is starting to have a role in diagnosing malignant conditions of the gallbladder and biliary tree, such as cholangiocarcinoma. More research is needed before PET becomes standard protocol.[101]

Intraductal ultrasound (IDUS) is also used to evaluate ductal pathology sonographically. IDUS uses a high-frequency probe that is inserted into the duct during an ERCP.[71] It can be used to evaluate malignant biliary structures and cholangiocarcinoma.[101]

Endoscopic ultrasound (EUS) is commonly used to evaluate ductal pathology sonographically. A small transducer is attached to an endoscope and is introduced into the duodenum. At this level, the bile duct can be visualized.[106] Small stones are more likely to be detected on EUS than conventional abdominal sonography.[45] EUS is safe and produces superior images of the bile duct. Because benign versus malignant biliary pathology is difficult to determine, a fine-needle aspiration can also be performed during EUS. Even though the majority of gallbladder masses are evaluated by conventional sonography or CT, EUS is a new resource that may be used more in the future.[71]

## SUMMARY

- The normal distended pear- or teardrop-shaped gallbladder is located in the main lobar fissure between the right and left hepatic lobes.

- Laboratory tests helpful in evaluating pathophysiology of the biliary tract include WBC, AST, ALT, LDH, alkaline phosphatase, and bilirubin.

- Sonography is the primary modality of choice to evaluate for RUQ pain or a positive sonographic Murphy sign indicating pain.

- Sonographic imaging of the gallbladder and biliary tree is accurate, quick, painless, noninvasive, inexpensive, and carries no risk of ionizing radiation.

- Sonography, along with clinical and laboratory values, is needed to perform an accurate diagnosis of RUQ pain.

- As new imaging technology develops, sonography will continue to play an important role in the diagnostic evaluation and management of gallbladder and biliary disease.

## *Critical Thinking Questions*

1. A 44-year-old woman presents with severe RUQ pain, nausea, vomiting, and leukocytosis. As the sonographer begins the examination, there is a positive sonographic Murphy sign. Both the longitudinal and transverse sonograms show diffuse gallbladder wall thickening measuring up to 6.5 mm. Based on this information, what is the most likely acquired gallbladder disease for this patient? What is the likelihood this patient will also have cholelithiasis? Identify two other complications for this acquired pathology.

2. While scanning the upper abdomen of a 62-year-old man with an elevated liver function test, the sonographer documents on both longitudinal and transverse gallbladder sonograms two echogenic, nonshadowing soft tissue masses. The masses appear to be on a short stalk on the posterior gallbladder wall and do not move to the most dependent portion of the gallbladder. What is the likely diagnosis for these two masses? What criteria suggest evaluating the mass as a malignant versus benign entity?

3. The sonograms show an enlarged, distended, palpable, and nontender gallbladder in a jaundiced patient being evaluated for adenocarcinoma of the head of the pancreas. What name is used to describe this sonographic appearance of the gallbladder?

4. A 66-year-old man with diabetes is being treated for acute cholecystitis and presents with progressive RUQ pain, fever, and nausea. Sonographically, the gallbladder wall is thickened, no calculi are identified, and air is seen in the neck with the patient in a supine position and in the lumen with the patient in a left decubitus position. What is the most likely diagnosis based on the patient's history and the sonographic findings?

5. The 72-year-old woman presented with RUQ pain, jaundice, and fever. Her laboratory values showed both an increase in bilirubin and alkaline phosphatase. The sonograms documented a normal gallbladder. The common bile duct measured 10 mm and appeared to end abruptly. What should the sonographer evaluate and document to complete the imaging examination?

## REFERENCES

1. Rickes S, Treiber G, Mönkemüller K, et al. Impact of the operator's experience on value of high-resolution transabdominal ultrasound in the diagnosis of choledocholithiasis: a prospective comparison using endoscopic retrograde cholangiography as the gold standard. *Scand J Gastroenterol*. 2006;41:838–843.

2. Weinberg KE. General abdominal sonography. In: Krebs CA, Odwin CS, Fleischer AC, eds. *Appleton & Lange Review for the Ultrasonography Examination*. 3rd ed. McGraw Hill Companies: Appleton & Lange; 2004:187–300.

3. Khalili K, Wilson SR. The biliary tree and gallbladder. In: Rumack CM, Wilson SR, Charboneau JW. *Diagnostic Ultrasound*. 3rd ed. Vol. 1. St. Louis, MO: Elsevier Mosby; 2005:171–212.

4. Anderhub B. *A Clinical Guide*. St. Louis, MO: Mosby; 1995.

5. Cooperberg PL. Gallbladder and bile ducts. In: Goldberg BB ed. *Abdominal Ultrasonography*. 2nd ed. New York, NY: John Wiley & Sons; 1984.

6. Netter FH. *The CIBA Collection of Medical Illustrations*. 2nd ed. Vol 3 (Digestive System), Part III (Liver, biliary tract, and pancreas). Summit, NJ: CIBA Pharmaceutical Company; 1964.

7. Rubens DJ. Ultrasound imaging of the biliary tract. *Ultrasound Clin*. 2007;391–413.

8. Baron RL, Tublin ME, Peterson MS. Imaging the spectrum of biliary tract disease. *Radiol Clin North Am*. 2002; 40:1325–1354.

9. Raptopoulos V, Smith EH, Karellas A, et al. Daytime constancy of bile duct diameter. *AJR Am J Roentgenol*. 1987;148:557–558.

10. Wing VW, Laing FC, Jeffrey RB, et al. Sonographic differentiation of enlarged hepatic arteries from dilated intrahepatic bile ducts. *AJR Am J Roentgenol*. 1985;145:57–61.

11. Van Gansbeke D, de Toeuf J, Cremer M, et al. Suprahepatic gallbladder: a rare congenital anomaly. *Gastrointest Radiol*. 1984;9:341–343.

12. Hopman WP, Rosenbusch G, Jansen JB, et al. Gallbladder contraction: effects of fatty meals and cholecystokinin. *Radiology*. 1985;157:37–39.

13. Dodds WJ, Groh WJ, Darweesh RM, et al. Sonographic measurement of gallbladder volume. *AJR Am J Roentgenol*. 1985;145:1009–1011.

14. Laing FC. The gallbladder and bile ducts. In: Rumack CM, Wilson SR, Charboneau JW, eds. *Diagnostic Ultrasound*. Vol. 1. St. Louis, MO: Mosby-Year Book; 1991:175–223.

15. Apstein MD, Hauser SC, Ostrow JD, et al. Liver biliary tree and pancreas. In: Stein JH, ed. *Internal Medicine*. 4th ed. St. Louis, MO: Mosby; 1994.

16. Cooperberg PL, Gibney RC. Imaging of the gallbladder. *Radiology*. 1987;163:605–613.

17. Inoue T, Kitano M, Kudo M, et al. Diagnosis of gallbladder diseases by contrast-enhanced phase-inversion harmonic ultrasonography. *Ultrasound Med Biol*. 2007;33:353–361.

18. Gore RM, Yaghmai V, Newmark GM, et al. Imaging benign and malignant disease of the gallbladder. *Radiol Clin North Am*. 2002;40:1307–1323.

19. Jeffrey RB Jr, Nini-Murcia M, Ralls PW, et al. Color Doppler sonography of the cystic artery: comparison of normal controls and patients with acute cholecystitis. *J Ultrasound Med*. 1995;14:33–36.

20. Kishk SM, Darweesh RM, Dodds WJ, et al. Sonographic evaluation of resting gallbladder volume and postprandial emptying in patients with gallstones. *AJR Am J Roentgenol*. 1987;148:875–879.

21. Laing FC, Jeffrey RB Jr, Wing VW, et al. Biliary dilatation: Defining the level and cause by real-time US. *Radiology*. 1986;160:39–42.

22. Hata K, Aoki S, Hata T, et al. Ultrasonographic identification of the human fetal gallbladder in utero. *Gynecol Obstet Invest*. 1987;23:79–83.

23. Stringer DA, Dobranowski J, Ein SH, et al. Interposition of the gallbladder—or the absent common hepatic duct and cystic duct. *Pediatr Radiol*. 1987;17:151–153.

24. Doyle TC. Flattened fundus sign of the septate gallbladder. *Gastrointest Radiol*. 1984;9:345–347.

25. Lev-Toaff AS, Friedman AC, Rindsberg SN, et al. Multiseptate gallbladder: incidental diagnosis on sonography. *AJR Am J Roentgenol*. 1987;148:1119–1120.

26. Kidney M, Goiney R, Cooperberg PL. Adenomyomatosis of the gallbladder: a pictorial exhibit. *J Ultrasound Med*. 1986;5:331–333.

27. Riddlesberger MM Jr. Diagnostic imaging of the hepatobiliary system in infants and children. *J Pediatr Gastroenterol Nutr*. 1984;3:653–664.

28. Rutherford AE, Pratt DS. Cholestasis and cholestatic syndromes. *Curr Opin Gastroenterol*. 2006;22:209–214.

29. Green D, Carrol BA. Ultrasonography in the jaundiced infant: a new approach. *J Ultrasound Med*. 1986;5:323–329.

30. Boechat MI, Querfeld U, Dietrich RB, et al. Large echogenic kidneys in biliary atresia. *Ann Radiol*. 1986;29:660–662.

31. Taylor LA, Ross AJ. Abdominal masses. In: Walker WA, Durie PR, Hamilton JR, et al, eds. *Pediatric Gastrointestinal Disease Pathophysiology, Diagnosis, Management*. Vol 1. Philadelphia, PA: BC Decker Inc.; 1991.

32. Fakhry J. Sonography of tumefactive biliary sludge. *AJR Am J Roentgenol*. 1982;139:717–719.

33. Lee SP, Maher K, Nicholls JF. Origin and fate of biliary sludge. *Gastroenterology*. 1988;94:170–176.

34. Cano N, Cicero F, Ranieri F, et al. Ultrasonographic study of gallbladder motility during total parenteral nutrition. *Gastroenterology*. 1986;91:313–317.

35. Hanbidge AE, Buckler PM, O'Malley ME, et al. From the RSNA refresher courses: imaging evaluation for acute pain in the right upper quadrant. *Radiographics*. 2004;24:1117–1135.

36. Sheiner E, Abramowicz JS, Hershkovitz R. Fetal gallstones detected by routine third trimester ultrasound. *Int J Gynecol Obstet*. 2006;92:255–256.

37. Bouchier IA. Gallstone: formation and epidemiology. In: Blumgart LH, ed. *Surgery of the Liver and Biliary Tract*. 2nd ed. Vol 1. New York, NY: Churchill Livingston E; 1994.

38. Jones RS, Jones BT. Cholecystitis and cholelithiasis. In: Rakel RE, ed. *Conn's Current Therapy 1994*. Philadelphia, PA: WB Saunders Company; 1994.

39. Everhart JE. Gallstones. In: Everhart JE, ed. *Digestive Diseases in the United States: Epidemiology and Impact*. US Department of Health and Human Services, Public Health Service, National Institutes of Health, National Institute of Diabetes and Digestive and Kidney Diseases. Washington, DC: US Government Printing Office; 1994: NIH Publication No. 94–1447.

40. Kaechele V, Wabitsch M, Thiere D, et al. Prevalence of gallbladder stone disease in obese children and adolescents: influence of the degree of obesity, sex, and pubertal development. *J Pediatr Gastroenterol Nutr*. 2006;42:66–70.

41. Chesson RR, Gallup DG, Gibbs RL, et al. Ultrasonographic diagnosis of asymptomatic cholelithiasis in pregnancy. *J Reprod Med*. 1985;30:920–922.

42. Connon J, Witt-Sullivan H. Gastrointestinal complications. In: Burrow GN, Ferris TF, eds. *Medical Complications during Pregnancy*. 4th ed. Philadelphia, PA: WB Saunders Company; 1995:21.

43. Graham N, Manhire AR, Stead RJ, et al. Cystic fibrosis: ultrasonographic findings in the pancreas and hepatobiliary system correlated with clinical data and pathology. *Clin Radiol*. 1985;36:199–203.

44. Williamson SL, Williamson MR. Cholecystosonography in pregnancy. *J Ultrasound Med*. 1984;3:329–331.

45. Portincasa P, Moschetta A, Petruzzelli M, et al. Gallstone disease: symptoms and diagnosis of gallbladder stones. *Best Pract Res Clin Gastroenterol*. 2006;20:1017–1029.

46. Fein AB, Rauch RF II, Bowie JD, et al. Value of sonographic screening in patients with chest pain and normal coronary arteries. *AJR Am J Roentgenol*. 1986;146:337–339.

47. Richter JM, Christensen MR, Simeone JF, et al. Chronic cholecystitis. An analysis of diagnostic strategies. *Invest Radiol*. 1987;22:111–117.

48. Vauthey JN. Cholecystolithiasis: which approach when? In: Blumbart LH, ed. *Surgery of the Liver and Biliary Tract*. 2nd ed. Vol 1. New York, NY: Churchill Livingstone; 1994.

49. Laffey KJ, Martin EC. Percutaneous removal of large gallstones. *Gastrointest Radiol*. 1986;11:165–168.

50. Parulekar SG. Ultrasonic detection of calcification in gallstones: "the reverberation shadow." *J Ultrasound Med*. 1984;3:123–129.

51. Suramo I, Päivänsalo M, Vuoria P. Shadowing and reverberation artifacts in abdominal ultrasonography. *Eur J Radiol*. 1985;5:147–151.

52. Cover KL, Slasky BS, Skolnick ML. Sonography of cholesterol in the biliary system. *J Ultrasound Med*. 1985;4:647–653.

53. Trowbridge RL, Rutkowski NK, Shojania KG. Does this patient have acute cholecystitis? *JAMA*. 2003;289(1):80–86.

54. Lin KY. Acute acalculous cholecystitis: a limited review of the literature. *Mt Sinai J Med*. 1986,53:305–309.

55. Smith EA, Dillman JR, Elsayes KM, et al. Cross-sectional imaging of acute and chronic gallbladder inflammatory disease. *AJR Am J Roentgenol*. 2009;192:188–196.

56. van Weelde BJ, Oudkerk M, Koch CW. Ultrasonography of acute cholecystitis: clinical and histological correlation. *Diagn Imaging Clin Med*. 1986;55:190–195.

57. Beckman I, Dash N, Sefczek RJ, et al. Ultrasonographic findings in acute acalculous cholecystitis. *Gastrointest Radiol*. 1985;10:387–389.

58. Munster AM, Goodwin MN, Pruitt BA Jr. Acalculous cholecystitis in burned patients. *Am J Surg*. 1971;122:591–593.

59. Becker CD, Vock P. Appearance of gas-containing gallstones on sonography and computed tomography. *Gastrointest Radiol*. 1984;9:323–328.

60. Sood BP, Kalra N, Gupta S, et al. Role of sonography in the diagnosis of gallbladder perforation. *J Clin Ultrasound*. 2002;30(5):270–274.

61. Konno K, Ishida H, Sato M, et al. Gallbladder perforation: color Doppler findings. *Abdom Imaging*. 2002;27:47–50.

62. Way LW. Biliary tract. In: Way LW, ed. *Current Surgical Diagnosis and Treatment*. 10th ed. Norwalk, CO: Appleton & Lange; 1994.

63. Bernstein D, Soeffing J, Daoud YJ., et al. The obscured gallbladder. *Am J Med*. 2007;120:675–677.

64. Sato M, Ishida H, Konno K, et al. Segmental chronic cholecystitis: sonographic findings and clinical manifestations. *Abdom Imaging*. 2002;27:43–46.

65. Fitzgerald EJ, Toi A. Pitfalls in the ultrasonographic diagnosis of gallbladder diseases. *Postgrad Med J*. 1987;63:525–532.

66. Maglinte DD, Lappas JC, Ng AC. Sonography of Bouveret's syndrome. *J Ultrasound Med*. 1987;6:675–677.

67. Cohan RH, Mahony BS, Bowie JD, et al. Striated intramural gallbladder lucencies on US studies: predictors of acute cholecystitis. *Radiology*. 1987;164:31–35.

68. Bacq Y. Intrahepatic cholestasis of pregnancy. *Clin Liver Dis*. 1999;3(1):1–13.

69. Rioseco AJ, Ivankovic MB, Manzur A, et al. Intrahepatic cholestasis of pregnancy: a retrospective case-control study of perinatal outcome. *Am J Obstet Gynecol*. 1994;170(3):890–895.

70. Park JY, Hong SP, Kim YJ, et al. Long-term follow up of gallbladder polyps. *J Gastroenterol Hepatol*. 2009;24:219–222.

71. Mishra G, Conway J. Endoscopic ultrasound in the evaluation of radiologic abnormalities of the liver and biliary tree. *Curr Gastroenterol Rep*. 2009;11:150–154.

72. Beck PL, Shaffer EA, Gall DG, et al. The natural history and significance of ultrasonographically defined polypoid lesions of the gallbladder in children. *J Pediatr Surg*. 2007;42:1907–1912.

73. Aldouri AQ, Malik HZ, Waytt J, et al. The risk of gallbladder cancer from polyps in a large multiethnic series. *Eur J Surg Oncol*. 2009;35:48–51.

74. Leung UC, Wong PY, Roberts RH, et al. Gall bladder polyps in sclerosing cholangitis: does the 1-cm rule apply? *ANZ J Surg*. 2007;77:355–357.

75. Miller G, Jarnagin WR. Gallbladder carcinoma. *Eur J Surg Oncol*. 2008;34:306–312.

76. Hsing AW, Gao YT, Han TQ, et al. Gallstones and the risk of biliary tract cancer: a population-based study in China. *Br J Cancer*. 2007;97:1577–1582.

77. Rodríguez-Fernández A, Gómez-Río M, Medina-Benítez A, et al. Application of modern imaging methods in diagnosis of gallbladder cancer. *J Surg Oncol*. 2006;93:650–664.

78. Weiner SN, Koenigsberg M, Morehouse H, et al. Sonography and computed tomography in the diagnosis of carcinoma of the gallbladder. *AJR Am J Roentgenol*. 1984;142:735–739.

79. Jeffrey RB, Ralls PW. Gallbladder and bile ducts. In: Jeffrey RB, Ralls PW, eds. *Sonography of the Abdomen*. New York, NY: Raven Press; 1995.

80. Katz SC, Bowne WB, Wolchok JD, et al. Surgical management of melanoma of the gallbladder: a report of 13 cases and review of the literature. *Am J Surg*. 2007;193:493–497.

81. Samplaski MK, Rosato EL, Witkiewicz AK, et al. Malignant melanoma of the gallbladder: a report of two

cases and review of the literature. *J Gastrointest Surg.* 2008;12:1123–1126.

82. Martel JPA, McLean CA, Rankin RN. Melanoma of the gallbladder. *Radiographics.* 2009;29:291–296.

83. Phillips G, Pochaczevsky R, Goodman J, et al. Ultrasound patterns of metastatic tumors in the gallbladder. *J Clin Ultrasound.* 1982;10:379–383.

84. Raghavendra BN, Subramanyam BR, Balthazar EJ, et al. Sonography of adenomyomatosis of the gallbladder: radiologic-pathologic correlation. *Radiology.* 1983;146:747–752.

85. Yoon JH, Cha SS, Han SS, et al. Gallbladder adenomyomatosis: imaging findings. *Abdom Imaging.* 2006;31:555–563.

86. Stunell H, Buckley O, Geoghegan T, et al. Imaging of adenomyomatosis of the gallbladder. *J Med Imaging Radiat Oncol.* 2008;52:109–117.

87. Krebs CA, Giyanani VL, Eisenberg RL. Biliary system. In: *Atlas of Disease Process.* Norwalk, CT: Appleton & Lange; 1993.

88. Yeola-Pate M, Banode PJ, Bhole AM, et al. Different locations of hydatid cysts. *Infect Dis Clin Pract.* 2008;16:379–384.

89. Quinn SF, Fazzio F, Jones E. Torsion of the gallbladder: findings on CT and sonography and role of percutaneous cholecystectomy. *AJR Am J Roentgenol.* 1987;148:881–882.

90. Lemonick DM, Garvin R, Semins H. Torsion of the gallbladder: a rare cause of acute cholecystitis. *J Emerg Med.* 2006;30(4):397–401.

91. Graif M, Horovitz A, Itzchak Y, et al. Hyperechoic foci in the gallbladder wall as a sign of microabscess formation or diverticula. *Radiology.* 1984;152:781–784.

92. Willson SA, Gosink BB, vanSonnenberg E. Unchanged size of dilated common bile duct after a fatty meal: results and significance. *Radiology.* 1986;160:29–31.

93. O'Connor HJ, Bartlett RJ, Hamilton I, et al. Bile duct caliber: the discrepancy between ultrasonic and retrograde cholangiographic measurement in the postcholecystectomy patient. *Clin Radiol.* 1985;36:507–510.

94. Simeone JF, Butch RJ, Mueller PR, et al. The bile ducts after a fatty meal: further sonographic observations. *Radiology.* 1985;154:763–768.

95. Gilbert F, Calder JF, Bayliss AP. Biliary tract dilatation without jaundice demonstrated by ultrasound. *Clin Radiol.* 1985;36:197–198.

96. Bressler EL, Rubin JM, McCracken S. Sonographic parallel channel sign: a reappraisal. *Radiology.* 1987;164:343–346.

97. Kondo S, Isayama H, Akahane M, et al. Detection of common bile duct stones: comparison between endoscopic ultrasonography, magnetic resonance cholangiography, and helical-computed-tomographic cholangiography. *Eur J Radiol.* 2005;54:271–275.

98. Cronan JJ. US diagnosis of choledocholithiasis: a reappraisal. *Radiology.* 1986;161:133–134.

99. O'Connor HJ, Hamilton I, Ellis WR, et al. Ultrasound detection of choledocholithiasis: prospective comparison with ERCP in the postcholecystectomy patient. *Gastrointest Radiol.* 1986;11:161–164.

100. Robledo R, Prieto ML, Perez M, et al. Carcinoma of the hepaticopancreatic ampullar region: role of US. *Radiology.* 1988;166:409–412.

101. Singh P, Patel T. Advances in the diagnosis, evaluation and management of cholangiocarcinoma. *Curr Opin Gastroenterol.* 2006;22:294–299.

102. Geoffray A, Couanet D, Montagne JP, et al. Ultrasonography and computed tomography for diagnosis and follow-up of biliary duct rhabdomyosarcomas in children. *Pediatr Radiol.* 1987;17:127–131.

103. Marchal GJ, VanHolsbeeck M, Tshibwabwa-Ntumba E, et al. Dilatation of the cystic veins in portal hypertension: sonographic demonstration. *Radiology.* 1985;154:187–189.

104. Subramanyam BR, Raghavendra BN, Balthazar EJ, et al. Ultrasonic features of cholangiocarcinoma. *J Ultrasound Med.* 1984;3:405–408.

105. MacFaul GR, Chapman RW. Sclerosing cholangitis. *Curr Opin Gastroenterol.* 2006;22:288–293.

106. Van Erpecum KJ. Complications of bile-duct stones: acute cholangitis and pancreatitis. *Best Pract Res Clin Gastroenterol.* 2006;20(6):1139–1152.

107. Rhodes M, Elerick C. Aids cholecystopathy: a comparison of ultrasound and computed tomography imaging. *J Diagn Med Sonogr.* 1995;11:234–239.

108. Teixidor HS, Godwin TA, Ramirez EA. Cryptosporidiosis of the biliary tract in AIDS. *Radiology.* 1991;180:51–56.

109. Romano AJ, vanSonnenberg E, Casola G, et al. Gallbladder and bile duct abnormalities in AIDS: sonographic findings in eight patients. *AJR Am J Roentgenol.* 1988;150:123–127.

110. Gibney RG, Cooperberg PL, Scudamore CH, et al. Segmental biliary obstruction: false negative diagnosis with direct cholangiography without US guidance. *Radiology.* 1987;164:27–30.

111. Coletti PM, Ralls PW, Lapin SA, et al. Hepatobiliary imaging in choledocholithiasis. A comparison with ultrasound. *Clin Nucl Med.* 1986;11:482–486.

112. Dykes EH, Wilson N, Gray HW, et al. The role of 99mTc HIDA cholescintigraphy in the diagnosis of acute gallbladder disease: comparison with oral cholecystography and ultrasonography. *Scott Med J.* 1986;31:170–173.

113. Chau EM, Leong LL, Chan FL. Recurrent pyogenic cholangitis: ultrasound evaluation compared with endoscopic retrograde cholangiopancreatography. *Clin Radiol.* 1987;38:79–85.

# 7 The Pancreas

Julia A. Drose

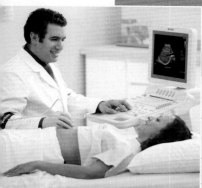

## OBJECTIVES

Describe pancreatic surface anatomy, vascular supply, and the common relational landmarks.

Discuss the most common pancreatic congenital anomalies to include pancreas divisum, annular pancreas, and ectopic pancreas.

Identify the endocrine and exocrine functions of the pancreas.

Correlate laboratory values and clinical indications associated with pancreatic abnormalities, disease, and pathology.

Explain the sonographic evaluation of the pancreas to include patient preparation, protocol, and demonstrate completing the examination procedure.

Differentiate normal from the varying sonographic appearances associated with pancreatic disease or pathology.

Describe the pathology, etiology, clinical signs and symptoms, and sonographic appearance for congenital diseases, inflammatory diseases, neoplastic diseases, and nonneoplastic cystic lesions.

## KEY TERMS

acute pancreatitis | chronic pancreatitis | pancreatic carcinoma | phlegmon | pseudocyst

## GLOSSARY

**acini cells** perform exocrine functions secreting digestive enzymes

**alpha cells** perform endocrine functions secreting glucagon

**amylase** enzyme that digests carbohydrates

**beta cells** perform endocrine functions secreting insulin

**delta cells** perform endocrine function secreting somatostatin

**endocrine** secreting into blood or tissue

**exocrine** secreting into a duct

**glucagon** hormone secreted by the alpha cells and functions to increase activity of phosphorylase

**insulin** hormone secreted by beta cells and functions to increase the uptake of glucose and amino acids by most body cells

**islets of Langerhans** endocrine portion of the pancreas made up of alpha cells and beta cells, which is the source of insulin and glucagon; also called pancreatic islet

**lipase** fat-digesting enzyme

**phlegmon** diffuse inflammatory reaction to infection spreading along fascial pathways, producing edema and swelling

**pseudocyst** an abnormal or dilated cavity resembling a true cyst but not lined with epithelium

**somatostatin** hormone secreted by delta cells and functions to regulate insulin and glucagon production

Sonographic imaging of the pancreas is often fraught with technical limitations, specifically overlying bowel gas. Although sonography may identify some pancreatic lesions, its primary use is often to identify abnormalities of other organs associated with pancreatic disease.

## ANATOMY

The pancreas is a nonencapsulated structure that lies obliquely in the anterior portion of the retroperitoneum. It consists of three main portions: the head, body, and tail. The head is located to the right and inferior to the body and tail. It has the largest anteroposterior

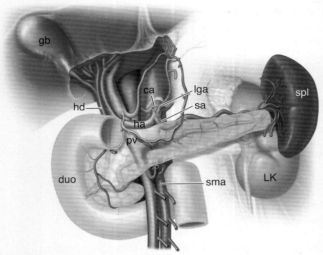

**Figure 7-1** Diagram showing the normal relationship of the pancreas to the prevertebral vessels and surrounding upper abdominal organs. *ca*, celiac axis; *duo*, duodenum; *gb*, gallbladder; *ha*, proper hepatic artery; *hd*, common hepatic duct; *lga*, left gastric artery; *LK*, left kidney; *pv*, main portal vein; *sa*, splenic artery; *sma*, superior mesenteric artery; *spl*, spleen.

dimension of the gland and is bordered by the C-loop of the duodenum[1] (Fig. 7-1).

Extending posterior and medial from the head is a curved projection of pancreatic tissue, the uncinate process. The uncinate process lies anterior to the inferior vena cava (IVC) and posterior to the superior mesenteric vein (SMV). The body and tail of the pancreas are bounded anteriorly and superiorly by portions of the stomach, duodenum, and left lobe of the liver.

The body of the pancreas lies anterior to the aorta, superior mesenteric artery (SMA), and left renal vein. Between these vessels and the body of the pancreas, the splenic vein may be identified as it courses from the spleen, toward its confluence with the SMV.

The neck of the pancreas lies just anterior to this confluence, where the vessels merge to form the portal vein. In many patients, the left lobe of the liver lies between the body and the anterior abdominal wall. Branches of the celiac axis—namely the hepatic, left gastric, and splenic arteries—course along the superior border of the body.

The tail of the pancreas extends from the body into the left anterior pararenal space. Bordered posteriorly by the splenic vein, it frequently extends to the splenic hilum. The tail is bordered anteriorly by the stomach and laterally by the left kidney. Because of its proximity to the stomach, the pancreatic tail is often obscured by gas on sonography.

The parenchyma of the pancreas consists of small groups of acini, which secrete digestive enzymes, clustered in multiple lobules, each surrounding a tributary duct. The smaller ducts merge into increasingly larger ducts, subsequently emptying into the main pancreatic duct, the duct of Wirsung. Enzymes secreted by the pancreas are carried by the main pancreatic duct into the alimentary tract via the ampulla of Vater. Near the ampulla, the main pancreatic duct merges with the distal common bile duct to form a single perforating channel into the duodenum (Fig. 7-2). A smaller accessory duct, the duct of Santorini, branches from the main pancreatic duct and perforates into the duodenum separately from the ampulla.[2]

Wedged within the acinar lobules are groups of endocrine cells known as the *islets of Langerhans*. These clusters contain various types of cells that release hormones directly into the bloodstream and lymph system. This allows them to be distributed throughout the body, where they stimulate other organs or functional tissues.

Blood supply to the pancreas is provided by branches of the splenic artery and the pancreaticoduodenal arteries. The superior pancreaticoduodenal artery arises from the gastroduodenal artery and perfuses the head of the pancreas. The gastroduodenal artery arises from the common hepatic artery and perforates the pancreatic parenchyma along the superior aspect of the head.[1] The body and tail sections of the pancreas are perfused by the inferior pancreaticoduodenal artery, which arises from the SMA. Branches of this and the splenic artery enter the pancreas at numerous points along the body and tail.[3]

## CONGENITAL ANOMALIES

Congenital anomalies of the pancreas are rare, but do exist. Pancreas divisum is the most common congenital anomaly, occurring in approximately 5% to 10% of the population.[4] It results from a failure of fusion of the dorsal and ventral pancreatic buds during embryologic development (Fig. 7-3). This variant results in anomalous drainage of the pancreatic ducts, but it usually is not associated with any significant sequelae.[5]

An annular pancreas is another congenital anomaly in which the head of the pancreas surrounds the second portion of the duodenum (Fig. 7-4). It occurs more frequently in males and has been associated with complete or partial atresia of the duodenum. Annular pancreas is associated with other congenital abnormalities in up to 70% of affected infants,[4] including duodenal stenosis or atresia (40%), Down syndrome (16%), tracheoesophageal fistula (9%), and congenital heart disease (7%).[6]

Ectopic pancreatic tissue may also occur. The reported incidence ranges from 1% to 13%.[7,8] In this setting, pancreatic tissue grows in other organs, usually the walls of the stomach, duodenum, or large or small intestine, or rarely the gallbladder, spleen, or liver. These formations of tissue comprised the acinar and ductal structures, similar to the pancreas. Because they are functional deposits of pancreatic tissue, they are susceptible to developing acute pancreatitis or tumor.

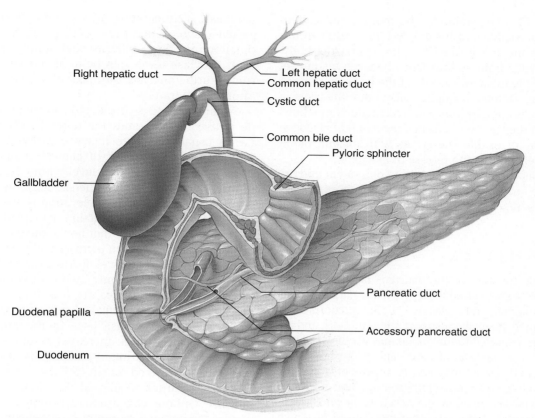

**Figure 7-2** Diagram showing the relationship of the common bile duct and main pancreatic duct as they merge and enter the ampulla of Vater. (Asset provided by Anatomical Chart Co.)

## PHYSIOLOGY

The pancreas is responsible for both endocrine and exocrine functions.

### ENDOCRINE FUNCTION

The endocrine function of the pancreas consists of hormone production, which occurs in the islets of Langerhans. Specialized cells, referred to as *alpha*, *beta*, and

*delta cells*, are contained within the islets of Langerhans. Each is responsible for the production of specific hormones. The majority of these cells are beta cells that produce insulin. Insulin aids in the metabolism of carbohydrates. By facilitating the transport of glucose across cell membranes, insulin increases the energy available for normal physiologic functions. It also influences the metabolism of proteins and fats. Insulin is released by the pancreas via a negative feedback mechanism. When the blood glucose level rises above a certain level, believed to be 100 mg/dL, the beta cells immediately secrete insulin.[9] When the blood glucose level falls, insulin secretion decreases. Other factors influencing insulin secretion include autonomic nervous system responses,

**Figure 7-3** Diagram showing pancreas divisum. The smaller ventral duct (*arrow*) drains the head and uncinate process of the pancreas, whereas the larger dorsal duct drains the rest of the pancreatic gland. (From Blackbourne LH. *Advanced Surgical Recall.* 2nd ed. Baltimore, MD: Lippincott Williams & Wilkins; 2004.)

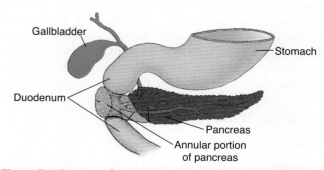

**Figure 7-4** Diagram of an annular pancreas. The head of the pancreas wraps around the duodenum and blocks or impairs the flow of food stuffs to the rest of the intestine.

the release of other endocrine hormones, and certain drugs.[2] Abnormalities of insulin secretion result in impairment of metabolic functions throughout the body. Diabetes results from an imbalance between insulin secretion and the metabolic needs of the body.

Glucagon, secreted by alpha cells within the islets of Langerhans, is another important hormone. It functions primarily in the liver and aids in conversion of glycogen into glucose, or usable energy. As with insulin, blood glucose levels initiate the release of glucagon.

Delta cells comprise the smallest component and are responsible for producing somatostatin, a hormone involved with regulating the production of insulin and glucagons.

## EXOCRINE FUNCTION

The exocrine function of the pancreas is to secrete enzymes, commonly referred to as *pancreatic juice*, that aids in food breakdown and digestion. These secretions accumulate in small intercellular spaces, the acini cells, and are eventually transported to the duodenum via the excretory ducts. Chemical analysis of pancreatic juice shows that in addition to digestive enzymes, it consists of water and inorganic salts such as potassium, sodium, and calcium.

The enzymes secreted by the pancreas are amylase, lipase, trypsinogen, and chymotrypsinogen—all of which are essential to the digestion and absorption of essential nutrients. *Amylase* breaks down complex carbohydrates into usable sugars; *lipase* is an enzyme that breaks down fats; and *trypsinogen* and *chymotrypsinogen* are preproteolytic enzymes that reduce proteins to their component amino acids. Additionally, some of these substances play an important role in the pathogenesis of pancreatic disease, especially in pancreatitis. The preproteolytic enzymes in the normal pancreas are inert. It is postulated that an inhibiting factor is secreted by the same cells that secrete exocrine enzymes. This inhibiting factor prevents trypsinogen and chymotrypsin from autodigesting the protein in the cell walls of the pancreas. With injury or disease, the inhibiting factor is unable to prevent the activation of proteolytic enzymes, which spill out into the surrounding parenchyma. Once the process begins, it can advance rapidly, each bursting cell releasing yet more digestive juice, reducing normal tissue to amorphous fluid.[10] Another component of pancreatic juice is the alkaline substance bicarbonate, which neutralizes the acidic gastric enzymes and triggers the action of the otherwise inert pancreatic enzymes in the duodenum. The pancreas is capable of secreting up to 4 L of exocrine fluid per day.[9]

# LABORATORY VALUES

## AMYLASE

Amylase, an enzyme essential in the digestion of carbohydrates, is one of the most useful laboratory values for the diagnosis of pancreatic disease. In a diseased pancreas, disintegrating acinar cells release their digestive enzymes into the organ's parenchyma, and ultimately into the capillaries that supply the diseased area. Amylase levels can be accessed with either serum or urine analysis. Normal values vary from laboratory to laboratory.

Serum amylase is considered elevated when the value is two to four times the normal reference range.[5] Levels usually begin to increase within 3 to 6 hours following the first onset of clinical symptoms. They usually reach a maximum level within 20 to 30 hours of disease onset, and often persist until the underlying cause is treated.[11] Amylase elevation is also associated with pancreatic duct obstruction, pancreatic malignancy, and biliary disease. Other non–pancreas-related processes may also cause an increased amylase level, such as perforated ulcers, bowel obstruction, and some cancers, but it is not commonly used to monitor these entities. With chronic pancreatitis, it is not uncommon for amylase levels to be normal or only slightly elevated.

An increased amylase level in the urine may lag behind the onset of an increased serum amylase. Additionally, in the setting of pancreatitis, urine amylase may remain elevated for up to 7 days after serum values have returned to normal. Elevation of the serum amylase without concurrent elevation of the urinary amylase value may represent a pathologic process not related to pancreatic disease such as decreased renal function.[12] Drugs such as aspirin, diuretics, alcohol, and oral contraceptives may also cause an increased amylase level.

A decreased amylase value has been associated with permanent damage to the pancreas, as well as hepatitis and cirrhosis of the liver.[13,14] The diagnosis of acute pancreatitis is often based on clinical symptoms rather than laboratory values.[15]

## LIPASE

Lipase is a fat-splitting enzyme excreted by the pancreas. It is released into the bloodstream in increased quantities in the setting of inflammatory, and occasionally neoplastic, pancreatic disease. With acute pancreatitis, lipase levels may be 5 to 10 times the normal reference range. Lipase rises within 24 to 48 hours of disease onset and can remain elevated for 5 to 7 days.[5] Lipase elevation also occurs in patients with obstruction of the pancreatic duct, pancreatic carcinoma, acute cholecystitis, cirrhosis, and severe renal disease.[16] Drugs associated with an increased lipase value include codeine, indomethacin, and morphine.

## FAT EXCRETION

Fecal fat excretion values reflect the amount of undigested fat molecules passing through the alimentary tract. Increased fecal fat (steatorrhea) is symptomatic of pancreatitis. Other abnormalities may also result in an increased discharge of fat into fecal matter, including celiac disease, inflammatory bowel disease, or short bowel syndrome. However, fat excretion is increased significantly in pancreatic disease.[5] Weight loss and leaking, oily stool are often associated with pancreatic steatorrhea.

## BILIRUBIN AND LIVER FUNCTION TESTS

An elevation of bilirubin and other liver function values may also occur with pancreatic disease.[5] This is due to the close anatomic relationships between the liver and biliary system with the pancreas. Pathologic processes in one structure may cause disease in the other. Neoplasia or inflammatory enlargement of the head of the pancreas frequently causes stenosis or complete obstruction of the distal common bile duct. In such cases, total serum bilirubin values are increased. Conversely, biliary duct disease, such as calculi and subsequent inflammation, may spread to the pancreas. Altered biliary and hepatic function values may suggest an underlying pancreatic process.

# SONOGRAPHIC EVALUATION

## INDICATIONS

The pancreas is usually sonographically evaluated as part of a complete abdominal sonography exam. Common indications include epigastric pain, abdominal pain or distension, or jaundice. Patients with abnormal laboratory values or a prior history of acute or chronic pancreatitis may also be referred for sonography. Sonography is not considered the best imaging test to evaluate for a pancreatic disease or neoplasm, but may be very useful in identifying secondary signs of a pancreatic process such as dilated biliary ducts, fluid collections, or gallstones.

## PREPARATION

Preparation for pancreatic sonography attempts to minimize the amount of gas in the stomach and duodenum by having the patient refrain from eating or drinking anything for 8 to 12 hours prior to the examination. Pancreatic sonography is contraindicated for patients who have undergone gastroscopic examination within 6 hours because large amounts of air are introduced into the stomach during this procedure. Because the head of the pancreas is intimately related to the duodenum, gas present here as well as in the transverse colon, which overlies the pancreas, may easily obscure visualization.

It is also recommended that the pancreas be the first organ evaluated when performing a complete sonographic evaluation of the abdomen. This is because patients are often asked to perform deep inspiration during the course of the exam. This often improves visualization of abdominal organs by displacing them

caudally. However, it also increases the amount of air within the bowel, which in turn obscures visualization of the pancreas.

### Transverse Imaging

In the transverse plane, the pancreas is identified as a crescent-shaped structure draping over the prevertebral vessels (Fig. 7-5). It has been described variously as horseshoe-, dumbbell-, or comma-shaped.[17] Normally, its echogenicity is equal to or greater than that of the liver, depending on the patient's age and body habitus.[18] Fat deposition in the interlobular areas accounts for the varying degrees of echogenicity and in some settings may cause contour alterations.[19] Children normally have less pancreatic fat than adults, so a hypoechoic pancreas in a pediatric patient is a normal finding.[20] In the adult population, a hypoechoic pancreas represents an abnormal finding.[18]

The main pancreatic duct, the duct of Wirsung, is frequently visualized sonographically in normal patients.[21,22] It appears as an echogenic lucency bordered by two parallel linear echoes traversing the body of the pancreas[23] (Fig. 7-6). The anteroposterior (AP) diameter of a normal pancreatic duct should not exceed 2 mm. The contour of the duct walls should be smooth without any areas of focal dilatation.[24] Color Doppler is useful in distinguishing the pancreatic duct from surrounding vascular structures.

The accessory pancreatic duct, the duct of Santorini, which drains the head of the pancreas, is not commonly seen.

The dimensions of the pancreas are best assessed using a true transverse plane of section. It is important to align the transducer so that the incident beam intersects the pancreas perpendicular to its transverse axis. This is usually a slight obliquity, with the head of the pancreas slightly lower than the tail.

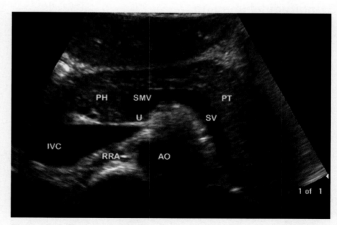

**Figure 7-5** Transverse image of the normal pancreas draping over the prevertebral vessels. *AO*, aorta; *IVC*, inferior vena cava; *PH*, pancreatic head; *PT*, pancreatic tail; *RRA*, right renal artery; *SMV*, superior mesenteric vein; *SV*, splenic vein. (Image courtesy of Philips Medical Systems, Bothell, WA.)

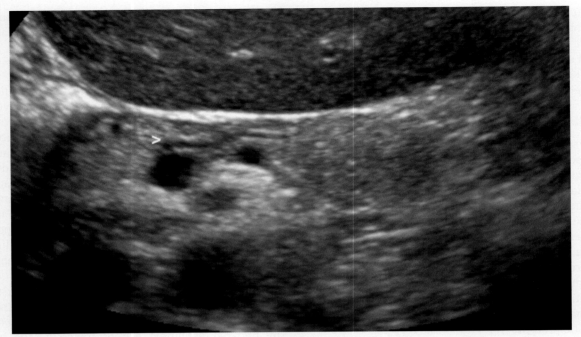

**Figure 7-6** Transverse image of the pancreas showing a normal main pancreatic duct (*arrowhead*). The duct of Wirsung.

The head of the pancreas is the widest portion of the gland, with the normal AP dimension measuring between 2 cm and 3.5 cm[1] (Fig. 7-7). The body of the pancreas is narrower and normally measures between 2 cm and 3 cm[17] (Fig. 7-8). The tail may be difficult to image from a projection that provides a true AP measurement, but in the normal gland, it measures 1 to 2 cm[25] (Fig. 7-9). A child's pancreas is smaller than an adult's but, relative to other upper abdominal organs such as the liver and kidneys, it may appear larger. Size, texture, and contour are all important considerations in identifying pancreatic disease.

In the transverse plane, the common bile duct should be seen in cross section entering the head of the pancreas.

### Longitudinal Imaging

On a longitudinal section, the pancreas is identified as an ovoid or circular structure lying anterior to the prevertebral vessels (Fig. 7-10). From a slightly oblique longitudinal section, the common bile duct may be seen entering the pancreatic head (Fig. 7-11). Anterior to the bile duct, the gastroduodenal artery is visualized. The neck of the pancreas appears as a narrow structure just anterior to the confluence of the SMV and the splenic vein. The body can be seen anterior to the SMA and posterior to the left lobe of the liver. In a true longitudinal section through the left anterior pararenal space, the tail appears thicker than the other portions because it is being transected as it dips posteriorly.

### EXAMINATION TECHNIQUE

The sonographic exam usually begins with the patient supine. Using the left lobe of the liver as a window, the transducer is aligned in a transverse position, just below the xiphoid process. A slight caudal angulation

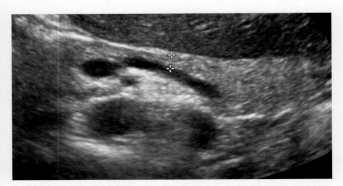

**Figure 7-7** Transverse image of the pancreas showing normal caliper placement for measuring the head of the pancreas.

**Figure 7-8** Transverse image of the pancreas showing normal caliper placement for measuring the body of the pancreas.

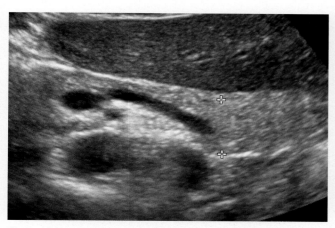

**Figure 7-9** Transverse image of the pancreas showing normal caliper placement for measuring the tail of the pancreas.

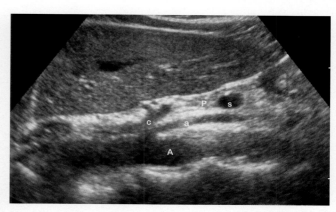

**Figure 7-10** Longitudinal image of the normal pancreas (P) lying anterior to the prevertebral vessels. *A,* aorta; *a,* superior mesenteric artery; *C,* celiac axis; *s,* splenic vein.

is applied, and the transducer position is adjusted so that the prevertebral vessels are identified. Instructing the patient to take a deep breath usually enhances the liver's usefulness as an acoustic window. During deep inspiration, the liver and diaphragm move inferiorly and over the pancreas. Because the head of the pancreas usually sits below the body and tail, rotating the probe counterclockwise a few degrees may permit visualization of the entire organ in a single image; however, additional acoustic windows may be necessary to image the various portions of the pancreas. In most patients with adequate preparation, the head and body of the pancreas are visualized 70% to 77% of the time.[2,26]

The pancreatic tail is often difficult to see. Bordered anteriorly by the stomach and splenic flexure of the colon, it is frequently obscured by air that has accumulated in the lumen of one or both of these organs. The tail of the pancreas is visualized in only 37% of patients on routine sonographic examination.[2] There are alternative approaches to imaging the tail using various acoustic windows. By rotating the patient into the right lateral decubitus or prone position, the examiner can attempt to image through the left lateral or posterior intercostal spaces. In using the lateral approach, it should be remembered that the plane of section is now coronal with the near field representing lateral and the far field representing medial.[27] With the patient prone,

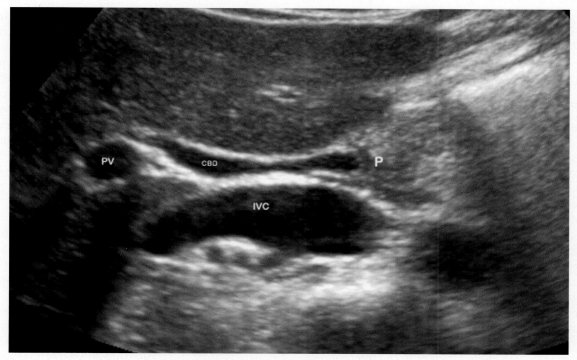

**Figure 7-11** Longitudinal image showing the common bile duct (CBD) entering the head of the pancreas (P). (IVC, inferior vena cava; PV, portal vein.

the tail of the pancreas may be seen anterior to the left kidney. Although this approach produces limited results, it may be useful when other approaches have failed.[28]

Another technique involves having the patient drink approximately 150 mL of water. The patient is then examined either upright or in the left lateral decubitus position, depending on which position provides the best acoustic window. Most examiners prefer to begin with the upright position, because air in the stomach rises above the water to lodge in the fundus.

# PATHOLOGY

## CONGENITAL DISEASES

### Cystic Fibrosis

Cystic fibrosis is the most common lethal genetic defect in the Caucasian population.[29] It is characterized by a dysfunction of epithelial chloride transport that affects multiple organs, including the lungs, liver, intestine, reproductive tract, and the pancreas. Cystic fibrosis is the major cause of pancreatic exocrine failure in children. This results in decreased enzyme production, which, in turn, leads to improper digestion of food and liquids. Approximately 85% to 90% of children with cystic fibrosis suffer from pancreatic insufficiency.[29,30] Recurrent acute and chronic pancreatitis can occur in this population and may even precede the diagnosis of cystic fibrosis by several years. Steatorrhea is also seen in affected patients.[31] On sonography, the affected pancreas will appear hyperechoic and small. Hypoechoic areas representing pancreatic fibrosis may be seen. Small cysts and calcifications may also be present. Gallstones and liver disease are also common.

## INFLAMMATORY DISEASES

### Acute Pancreatitis

In acute pancreatitis, all or part of the pancreas is inflamed. Biliary tract disease and excessive alcohol intake are the two most common causes. Gallstones are seen in approximately 60% of patients with acute pancreatitis.[1]

Acute pancreatitis is characterized by an edematous, enlarged gland; subsequently, there is a breakdown of the pancreatic architecture. It is believed that blockage of the pancreatic ductules leads to a release of digestive enzymes, which lyse cell walls.[2] Duct obstruction can be caused by biliary or duodenal reflux or hypersecretion of pancreatic enzymes. As the cell walls are destroyed by proteolytic digestive enzymes, more enzymes are released into the interstitial spaces, precipitating further destruction. Lipolytic enzymes, which break down fat, also effect changes in the internal morphology of the pancreas. Necrosis of blood vessel walls

may cause hemorrhage into or around the pancreas. An inflammatory reaction occurs and the gland becomes edematous.[32] Although alcohol and biliary tract pathology, especially gallstones, are the most common predisposing factors, abdominal trauma, drugs, viral infections, and many other causes exist.[33]

Although acute pancreatitis is frequently a self-limiting disease lasting about 5 days, a number of complications can occur. Pancreatic abscess may result from a localized suppurative process that results in pus collecting in or around the gland. Fluid collections in the pancreatic parenchyma break through the thin-walled connective tissue layer surrounding the organ and spill into surrounding areas. Most frequently, this fluid accumulates in the anterior pararenal space, although it may extend posteriorly to a potential space behind the renal fascia.[34,35] Pancreatic abscess is frequently associated with a left-side pleural effusion and splenomegaly resulting from splenic vein thrombosis.[36] In phlegmonous pancreatitis, the inflammatory reaction spreads to the soft tissues surrounding the pancreas. A phlegmon is an inflammatory process that spreads along fascial pathways, producing edema and swelling.[34] Other complications of acute pancreatitis include dehydration resulting from fluid loss, subsequent renal failure, pulmonary edema, and the development of chronic pancreatitis. Death may occur in a small percentage of patients from accompanying shock.[32] Complications of acute pancreatitis are varied. The course and prognosis of the disease depends on the severity of the complications and the underlying cause.

Clinically, the patient presents with sudden onset of severe abdominal pain, usually localized in the epigastrium or upper quadrants, often radiating to the back. The pain reaches a maximum within minutes or a few hours after onset of the disease and persists until the inflammation subsides. Characteristic of the pain associated with pancreatitis is the relief obtained by sitting up or bending at the waist. Nausea and vomiting are frequently present, and a mild fever may develop within the first few days. Serum amylase concentration increases to its maximum value within 24 hours after onset and gradually returns to normal over 3 to 10 days. An elevated white blood cell count (leukocytosis), proteinuria, and elevated bilirubin value may be present. Serum lipase concentration also increases and remains elevated longer than that of serum amylase.

Sonographically, an inflamed pancreas appears enlarged and hypoechoic, although in some cases, it may appear normal.[20] Additionally, the enlargement may be focal or diffuse. The pancreatic duct may appear enlarged secondary to obstruction.[37]

The echotexture of the pancreas may be hypoechoic due to edema, and the borders of the gland may appear irregular. Care must be taken in young patients whose pancreas may normally appear less echogenic to differentiate it from a diseased organ. In children, acute

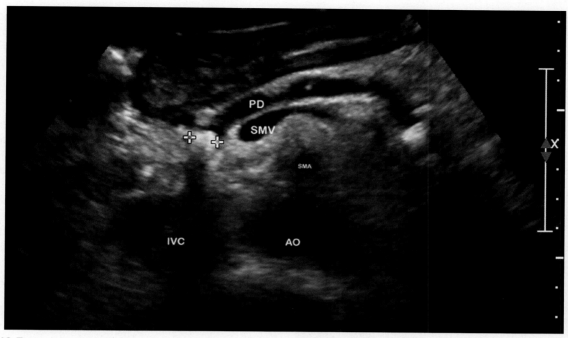

**Figure 7-12** Transverse image of the pancreas in a patient with acute pancreatitis resulting from a pancreatic duct stone *(calipers)*. The pancreatic duct *(PD)* is dilated secondary to obstruction. *AO*, aorta; *IVC*, inferior vena cava; *SMA*, superior mesenteric artery; *SMV*, superior mesenteric vein.

pancreatitis presents similar to an adult, with decreased echogenicity and increased AP diameter.[38] In children, diffuse or focal enlargement of the pancreas is generally a more reliable indicator of disease than altered echogenicity.[39]

Occasionally, when biliary calculi are the precipitating factor in acute pancreatitis, small stones may make their way through the ductal system and into the pancreatic duct. These may be seen sonographically as highly echogenic foci within a dilated duct (Fig. 7-12).

Pancreatic pseudocysts, encapsulated collections of the byproducts of tissue destruction, arise in about half of patients with severe disease.[40] Sonography may be used to follow pseudocyst maturation and, when necessary, to guide drainage. Although pseudocysts can occur anywhere in the abdominal cavity, they are most frequently found in or around the pancreas itself, especially in the area of the tail (Fig. 7-13). Hemorrhage of a pseudocyst may occur as a result of tissue necrosis (Fig. 7-14) and, if blood loss is significant, emergency surgical intervention may be indicated. Secondary infection of a pseudocyst may necessitate drainage.[41] Pseudocysts may contain pancreatic juice, blood, pus, and/or inflammatory byproducts.[34]

Because pseudocysts are a frequent complication of acute pancreatitis, any cystic-looking structures in the region of the pancreas should be carefully evaluated. They can have a varied sonographic appearances, from smooth-bordered and entirely cystic to poorly margin-ated, seemingly solid masses with no posterior acoustic

enhancement.[42] Septa or debris may be seen within and free fluid may be found in the retroperitoneal compartments.[35,43] The walls may be thin and smooth, or thick and irregular. Sonography is an excellent modality for detecting and following pseudocysts; its reported accuracy is 96%, owing to displacement of gas-containing bowel by the mass.[25]

Endoscopic sonography may be useful in the early diagnosis of acute pancreatitis. The procedure, which can be performed at the bedside noninvasively, often allows a more diagnostic evaluation of the pancreas because gas obscuration is not a factor. An enlarged pancreas with normal echogenicity is commonly visualized in patients with edematous pancreatitis. Focal hypoechoic

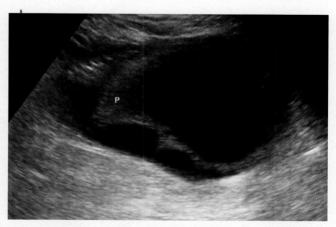

**Figure 7-13** Longitudinal image showing pancreatic pseudocysts arising from the tail of the pancreas *(P)*.

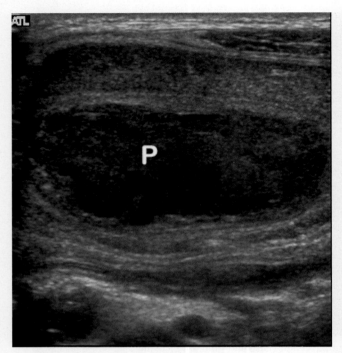

**Figure 7-14** Pancreatic pseudocyst *(P)* containing internal debris consistent with hemorrhage. (Image courtesy of Philips Medical Systems, Bothell, WA.)

areas representing intrapancreatic fluid collections may be seen if necrotizing pancreatitis is present. Computed tomography (CT) and magnetic resonance imaging (MRI) are also utilized to make a final diagnosis and delineate the extent of disease.

## Chronic Pancreatitis

Chronic pancreatitis results from repeated bouts of acute pancreatitis. Progressive interlobular fibrosis and destruction and atrophy of functioning tissue results. In the early stages, gross anatomic changes may be absent. As the disease progresses, the gland becomes small and atrophic. Interparenchymal fluid collections are frequently seen.[2] Calculi may be found within the pancreatic duct system, and cystic formations are common.

The prognosis for chronic pancreatitis is best when the causative agent can be removed, as in chronic cholecystitis, or alcohol-induced disease. Chronic pancreatitis may also occur in patients with hypercalcemia or hyperlipidemia.

In chronic pancreatitis, clinical symptoms include persistent epigastric pain radiating to the left lumbar region, nausea, vomiting, flatulence, and weight loss. Paralytic ileus is a common complication. Jaundice may also be present. During exacerbation of acute inflammatory disease, which frequently occurs in chronic relapsing pancreatitis, serum amylase and bilirubin levels may be elevated.

The sonographic findings in chronic pancreatitis are varied. Because gross anatomic changes may not occur in the course of this disease, sonography may not detect abnormalities. In cases where anatomic changes have occurred, however, sonographic evaluation most frequently reveals heterogeneous increased echogenicity secondary to fibrotic and fatty changes (Fig. 7-15). The pancreas may be enlarged with irregular borders, and the pancreatic duct may be dilated. A sonographic hallmark of chronic pancreatitis is the presence of calcifications within the parenchyma, which appear

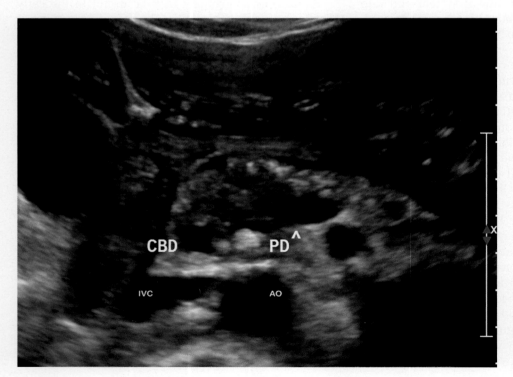

**Figure 7-15** Transverse image of the pancreas in a patient with chronic pancreatitis. The parenchyma of the pancreas is heterogeneous secondary to fibrotic and fatty changes. The common bile duct *(CBD)* and pancreatic duct *(PD)* are dilated. *AO,* aorta; *IVC,* inferior vena cava.

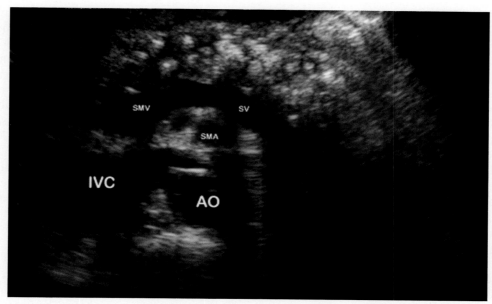

**Figure 7-16** Transverse image of the pancreas in a patient with chronic pancreatitis. Calcifications are seen throughout the parenchyma of the pancreas. *AO,* aorta; *IVC,* inferior vena cava; *SMA,* superior mesenteric artery; *SMV,* superior mesenteric vein; *SV,* splenic vein.

sonographically as bright reflections that may or may not cast a posterior acoustic shadow[25,44] (Figs. 7-16 and 7-17). Reported complications associated with chronic relapsing pancreatitis include a dilated biliary system resulting from common bile duct strictures,[45] pseudocyst formation, and venous thrombosis.[46]

## NEOPLASTIC DISEASE

Malignant tumors of the pancreas rank as the fifth leading cause of cancer-related deaths in the United States.[47] Early diagnosis is associated with a slightly better prognosis, but because many pancreatic malignancies do not produce symptoms until late in the disease,

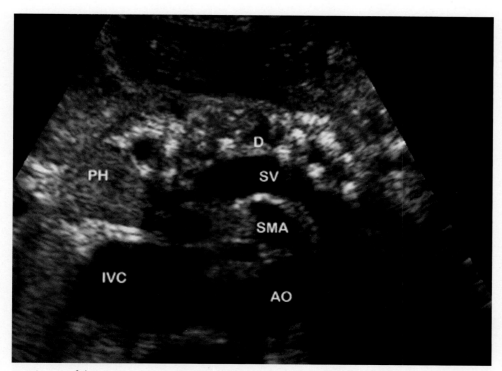

**Figure 7-17** Transverse image of the pancreas in a patient with chronic pancreatitis. Calcifications are seen throughout the body and tail of the pancreas. *AO,* aorta; *IVC,* inferior vena cava; *D,* pancreatic duct; *PH,* pancreatic head; *SMA,* superior mesenteric artery; *SV,* splenic vein. (Image courtesy of Philips Medical Systems, Bothell, WA.)

early detection is uncommon. Tumors most commonly occur in men older than 30 years of age and are approximately 50% more common in black men.[48] Risk factors include smoking, high-fat diet, chronic pancreatitis, diabetes, and cirrhosis of the liver.

Because of its dual role as an exocrine and endocrine gland, the pancreas is unique in cellular structure and physiologic function. Tumors may be classified according to the cell of origin.[49,50] Neoplasms of exocrine origin comprise the largest group of pancreatic tumors and include the single most common malignant lesion: acinar cell adenocarcinoma.[51–55] Adenocarcinomas account for 95% of all pancreatic malignancies.[1] Slightly more than 70% of these lesions occur in the head of the pancreas, with approximately 20% occurring in the body and 10% in the tail.[48] Adenocarcinoma is one of the most lethal of all malignancies with an overall 5-year survival rate of 2% or less. Anatomically, these lesions vary in size and gross appearance. Some are well-circumscribed, solid, ovoid masses, whereas others infiltrate surrounding pancreatic parenchyma so diffusely that the pancreas appears as a matted mass of tumor. Some small carcinomas that arise in the ampulla of Vater may be very difficult to detect sonographically. Tumors in the pancreatic head usually spread into the duodenum and compress the common bile duct and ampulla of Vater. Mechanical obstruction of the biliary tract causes dilatation of the ducts and frequently the gallbladder. A markedly distended and clinically palpable gallbladder, commonly referred to as a *Courvoisier gallbladder*, is easily visualized sonographically and is a reliable indicator of a lesion in the pancreatic head.[48]

Other exocrine lesions, benign solid adenoma and cystadenoma, cystadenocarcinoma, squamous cell carcinoma, and adenocanthoma are rare.[56] Benign solid adenomas and cystadenomas are more common in females.

Tumors of endocrine origin virtually always rise from islet cells and are, therefore, known as *islet cell tumors*. Islet cell tumors include insulinomas (70%), gastrinomas (20%), or glucagonomas (10%).[12] Most islet cell tumors are solid and are often very small, making them difficult to detect with sonography. These tumors can be singular or multiple and are more common in the body or tail of the pancreas.

## Solid Neoplastic Lesions

Sonographically, solid pancreatic tumors usually appear as echopenic or echogenic areas within the parenchyma.[57] Compared to the surrounding pancreatic tissue, these masses are hypoechoic. The borders may be well defined (Fig. 7-18), but more often they appear as poorly marginated, complex masses most commonly involving the pancreatic head[58–60] (Fig. 7-19). Color Doppler will often show increased vascularity to areas of tumor (Fig. 7-20). Because pancreatic carcinoma is rarely detected early in the disease process, by the time the patient is referred for diagnostic imaging procedures, the neoplasm has usually spread. Enlarged lymph nodes in the porta hepatis and in the para-aortic region indicate nodal metastasis. Inflammation of the pancreas is

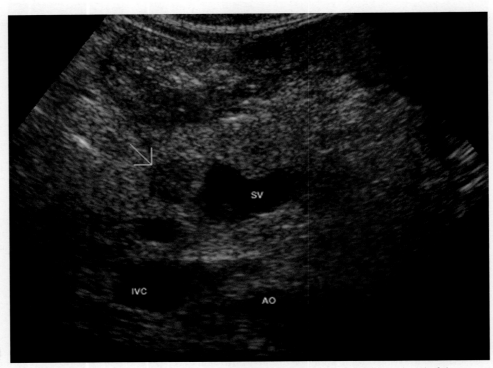

**Figure 7-18** Transverse image of the pancreas with a well-circumscribed neoplasm *(arrow)* within the head of the pancreas. *AO,* aorta; *IVC,* inferior vena cava; *SV,* splenic vein.

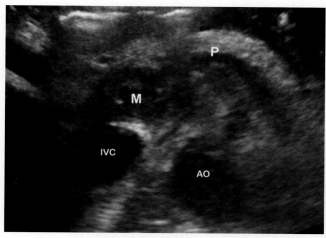

**Figure 7-19** Transverse image of the pancreas, showing a complex mass (*M*) within the pancreas (*P*) consistent with neoplasm. *AO*, aorta; *IVC*, inferior vena cava.

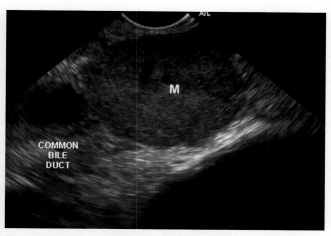

**Figure 7-21** Large malignant mass (*M*) within the head of the pancreas causing obstruction of the common bile duct. (Image courtesy of Philips Medical Systems, Bothell, WA.)

a common sequela in carcinomatosis, and the remainder of the organ may appear enlarged and hypoechoic.[61] Additionally, tumors in the head of the pancreas may cause obstructive jaundice, in which case, the common bile and intrahepatic ducts may appear dilated (Fig. 7-21). If the neoplasm is very small, the only sonographic indicator of an intrapancreatic abnormality may be the blunt termination of a dilated common bile duct in the head of the pancreas (Fig. 7-22).

Endoscopic sonography is more accurate in identifying small lesions (<2 cm) than transabdominal sonography, CT, or MRI. Endoscopic sonography is also the most sensitive means for detecting venous and gastric invasion.[44,62,63]

## Cystic Neoplastic Lesions

The majority of pancreatic tumors are solid, but cystic neoplasms do occur. When a fluid-filled structure is seen in or around the pancreas, the most likely diagnosis is

pseudocyst. Differentiation from a tumor can be made by analyzing laboratory results, which will most likely demonstrate inflammatory disease. In the absence of clinical suspicion of acute or chronic pancreatitis, cystic neoplastic disease must be considered.[64] Cystic neoplastic lesions are divided into two groups: benign microcystic adenomas and malignant mucinous cystic adenomas.[53,65,66] Microcystic adenomas are benign lesions composed of many cysts smaller than 2 cm. They occur more frequently in the head of the pancreas and may contain calcifications.[67] Morphologically, these tumors have thin, well-defined, fibrous capsules containing multiple cysts of varying size.[48] Mucinous cystic adenomas, also referred to as cystadenocarcinomas, are predominantly malignant lesions composed of larger cystic areas (greater than 2 cm) and may contain peripheral rim calcifications. They are usually large, unilocular, encapsulated masses, although some rare multilocular lesions have been reported.[68] About 60% occur in the tail of the pancreas, and are among the few pancreatic malignancies that have a good prognosis.[69]

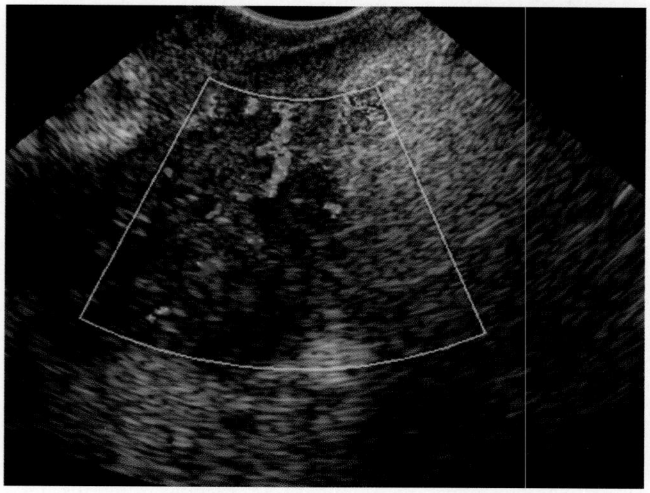

The patient with pancreatic carcinoma commonly presents with vague, diffuse pain located in the epigastrium that radiates to the back. As with acute pancreatitis, leaning forward or sitting upright may alleviate the pain. Jaundice occurs if the lesion produces biliary obstruction, and weight loss is common. Symptoms usually occur late in the disease. Laboratory results are generally nonspecific for pancreatic disease. Serum amylase and lipase values are occasionally elevated, steatorrhea does not occur in the absence of jaundice, and occult blood may be detected in stool when the tumor involves the ampulla of Vater.[69]

Primary cystic neoplasms have a variable sonographic appearance. Again, 85% to 90% of cystic masses in the pancreatic bed are related to inflammatory disease.[70] Microcystic adenomas appear sonographically as poorly marginated, mixed echogenic lesions.

**Figure 7-20** Color and spectral Doppler showing blood flow within a pancreatic neoplasm.

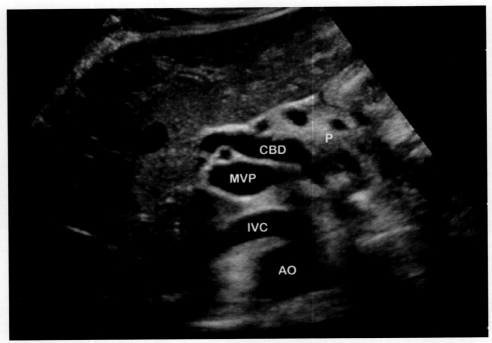

**Figure 7-22** Longitudinal image showing a dilated common bile duct *(CBD)* ending bluntly in the pancreatic head *(P)* of a patient with pancreatic cancer. The pancreatic parenchyma was heterogeneous although no discrete mass was identified. *AO*, aorta; *IVC*, inferior vena cava; *MVP*, main portal vein.

The cystic components are usually too small to be seen individually. Mucinous cystic neoplasms contain larger (greater than 5 cm) unilocular or multilocular areas, which may be seen sonographically. Mural excrescences may be seen projecting into the cystic area.[71-74] Other noninflammatory cystic lesions of the pancreas include polycystic disease and cystic fibrosis.

## NONNEOPLASTIC CYSTIC LESIONS

### Polycystic Disease

Polycystic disease is an autosomal dominant disease characterized by the presence of multiple small cysts in the kidney, liver, and, less commonly (10%), the pancreas.[75,76] Patients present with a family history of polycystic disease or are being worked up for hypertension, renal insufficiency, or pyelonephritis. The slowly multiplying and enlarging cystic masses eventually destroy the normal pancreatic tissue. The vast majority of patients with polycystic disease, however, succumb to renal failure well before the pancreas is physiologically affected. The finding of well-defined cystic lesions in the pancreas should alert the sonographer to the possibility of polycystic disease. In such cases, the liver and kidneys should be evaluated for the presence of multiple cysts. In the absence of renal or hepatic cysts, the diagnosis of polycystic disease cannot be made; instead, one of the above-mentioned inflammatory or neoplastic lesions should be considered.

### Von Hippel-Lindau Disease

Von Hippel-Lindau disease is an autosomal dominant disorder that involves the central nervous system. Pancreatic abnormalities associated with Von Hippel-Lindau include adenomas and islet cell tumors (Fig. 7-23). Pancreatic carcinoma has also been reported.[4] Seventy percent of individuals with Von Hippel-Lindau disease have pancreatic cysts at autopsy.[77] Peripheral calcifications may also occur in the pancreas.

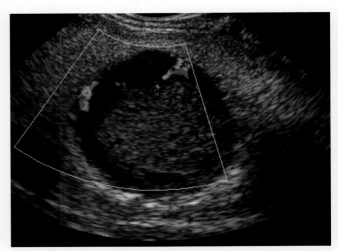

**Figure 7-23** Pancreatic islet cell tumor in a patient with Von Hippel-Lindau disease. Blood flow is appreciated within the mass with color Doppler. (Image courtesy of Philips Medical Systems, Bothell, WA.)

# Summary

- The pancreas is a nonencapsulated structure, with an oblique lie in the anterior portion of the retroperitoneum, and with three main portions (the head, body, and tail).
- Congenital anomalies of the pancreas are rare, with pancreas divisum being the most common.
- The pancreas is responsible for both endocrine (secreting into blood or tissue) and exocrine functions (secreting into a duct).
- Serum amylase is one of the most useful laboratory values for the diagnosis of pancreatic disease.
- Other values to monitor include lipase, fat excretion, bilirubin, and liver function tests.
- Patient preparation is an attempt to minimize the amount of gas in the stomach and duodenum by having the patient refrain from eating or drinking 8 to 12 hours prior to the exam.
- The pancreas exam includes evaluating the pancreas by making images and obtaining measurements in both the transverse and longitudinal sections.
- Cystic fibrosis is the most common lethal genetic defect resulting in multiple pancreatic pathologies.
- Inflammatory pancreatic diseases include both acute and chronic pancreatitis.
- Pancreatic pseudocysts are frequent complications of acute pancreatitis.
- Neoplastic pancreatic diseases include both solid and cystic neoplastic lesions.
- Polycystic disease and Von Hippel-Lindau diseases are autosomal dominant.
- Although sonography may not be considered as the primary imaging modality in evaluation of the pancreas, it is useful in detecting some lesions, particularly in an unsuspecting population.
- Sonography can aid in diagnosis-associated causes of pancreatic disease including biliary and hepatic abnormalities.

## Critical Thinking Questions

1. Sonographically, the pancreatic parenchyma is diffusely hyperechoic and small on a 13-year-old boy with cystic fibrosis. His symptoms include dyspnea and an abnormal glucose level. Why is the pancreas more hyperechoic and smaller than normal in a patient with cystic fibrosis?

2. A 37-year-old-man describes an acute and constant onset of epigastric and right upper quadrant pain radiating posteriorly for the past 20 hours. The laboratory findings include marked elevation of serum amylase, elevated lipase, and elevated bilirubin. Sonographically, there is cholelithiasis, all of the pancreas appears enlarged, and there is increased sound transmission posterior to the pancreas. Based on the clinical presentation, laboratory data, and sonographic findings, what is the most probable diagnosis?

3. The transverse and longitudinal sonograms shows a well-circumscribed, solid, ovoid mass in the pancreatic head; compression of adjacent structures; displacement of the vasculature normally surrounding the pancreas; Courvoisier gallbladder; and dilated extrahepatic and intrahepatic bile ducts. What is a reasonable explanation for the sonographic appearance?

4. A 43-year-old chronic alcoholic patient presents with a normal serum lipase, elevated serum amylase, and an enlarging mass in the epigastrium. The transverse and longitudinal sonograms at the tail of the pancreas show a well-defined, internally anechoic mass and posterior acoustic enhancement. What is the probable cause of the sonographic findings?

5. The sonographic examination on a patient with a history of chronic alcohol abuse and repeated episodes of acute pancreatitis document multiple calcifications throughout a diffusely hyperechoic, smaller-than-normal pancreas. For this patient, what is the most likely diagnosis?

## REFERENCES

1. Hagen-Ansert SL. The pancreas. In: Hagen-Ansert SL, ed. *Textbook of Diagnostic Ultrasonography. Vol 1. 6th ed.* St. Louis, MO: Mosby; 2006:235–270.
2. Nealon WH, Bhutani M, Riall TS, et al. A unifying concept: pancreatic ductal anatomy both predicts and determines the major complications resulting from pancreatitis. *J Am Coll Surg.* 2009;208(5):790–799.
3. Atri M, Finnegan PW. The pancreas. In: Rumack CM, Wilson SR, Charboneau JW, eds. *Diagnostic Ultrasound. Vol 1. 3rd ed.* St. Louis, MO: Elsevier Mosby; 2005:213–267.
4. Nijs ELF, Callahan MJ. Congenital and developmental pancreatic anomalies: ultrasound, computed tomography, and magnetic resonance features. *Semin Ultrasound CT MRI.* 2007;28:395–401.
5. Keller J, Aghdassi AA, Lerch MM, et al. Tests of pancreatic exocrine function—clinical significance in pancreatic and non-pancreatic disorders. *Best Pract Res Clin Gastroenterol.* 2009;23:425–439.
6. Skandalakis JE. The pancreas. In: Skandalakis J, Gray S, eds. *Embryology for Surgeons.* Baltimore, MD: Williams and Wilkins; 1994:336–404.

7. Prasad TR, Gupta SD, Bhatnagar V. Ectopic pancreas associated with a choledochal cyst and extrahepatic biliary atresia. *Pediatr Surg Int*. 2001;17:552–554.

8. Andronikou S, Sinclair-Smith C, Millar AJ. An enteric duplication cyst of the pancreas causing abdominal pain and pancreatitis in a child. *Pediatr Surg Int*. 2002;18:190–192.

9. Dietrich CF, Braden B. Sonographic assessments of gastrointestinal and biliary functions. *Best Prac Res Clin Gastroenterol*. 2009;23(3):353–367.

10. Uchida K, Yazumi S, Nishio A, et al. Long-term outcome of autoimmune pancreatitis. *J Gastroenterol*. 2009;44(7): 726–732.

11. Orebaugh SL. Normal amylase levels in the presentation of acute pancreatitis. *Am J Emerg Med*. 1994;12(1):21–24.

12. Beauregard JM, Lyon JA, Slovis C. Using the literature to evaluate diagnostic tests: amylase or lipase for diagnosing acute pancreatitis? *J Med Libr Assoc*. 2007;95(2):121–126.

13. Clark LR, Jaffe MH, Choyke PL, et al. Pancreatic imaging. *Radiol Clin North Am*. 1985;23(3):489–499.

14. Smotkin J, Tenner S. Laboratory diagnostic tests in acute pancreatitis. *J Clin Gastroenterol*. 2002;34(4):459–462.

15. Matull WR, Pereira SP, O'Donohue JW. Biochemical markers of acute pancreatitis. *J Clin Pathol*. 2006;59(4): 340–344.

16. Smith RC, Southwell-Keely J, Chesher D. Should serum pancreatic lipase replace serum amylase as a marker of acute pancreatitis? *ANZ J Surg*. 2005;75(6):399–404.

17. Mittlestaedt CA. *Abdominal Ultrasound*. New York: Churchill Livingstone; 1987.

18. Filly RA, London SS. The normal pancreas: Acoustic characteristics and frequency imaging. *J Clin Ultrasound*. 1979;7:121–124.

19. Marks WM, Filly RA, Callen PW. Ultrasonic evaluation of normal pancreatic echogenicity and its relationship to fat deposition. *Radiology*. 1980;137:475–479.

20. Berrocal T, Prieto C, Pastor I, et al. Sonography of pancreatic disease in infants and children. *Radiographics*. 1995; 15(2):301–313.

21. Didier D, Deschamps JP, Rohmer P, et al. Evaluation of the pancreatic duct: a reappraisal based on a retrospective correlative study by sonographic and pancreatography in 117 normal and pathologic subjects. *Ultrasound Med Biol*. 1983;9:509–518.

22. Weinstein DP, Weinstein BJ. Ultrasonic demonstration of the pancreatic duct: an analysis of 41 cases. *Radiology*. 1979;130:729–732.

23. Ohto M, Saotome N, Saisho HH, et al. Real-time sonography of the pancreatic duct: application to percutaneous pancreatic ductography. *AJR Am J Roentgenol*. 1980; 134:647–650.

24. Bryan PJ. Appearance of the normal pancreatic duct: a study using real-time ultrasound. *J Clin Ultrasound*. 1982;10:63–68.

25. Pochammer KF, Szekessy T, Frentzel-Beyme B, et al. Cranio-caudad dimension of the pancreatic head. *Radiology*. 1985;155:861–868.

26. de Graaf CS, Taylor KJ, Simonds BD, et al. Gray-scale echography of the pancreas: reevaluation of normal size. *Radiology*. 1978;129:157–165.

27. Lawson TL, Berland LL, Foley WD. Coronal upper abdominal anatomy: technique and gastrointestinal applications. *Gastrointest Radiol*. 1981;6:115–121.

28. Goldstein HM, Katragadda CS. Prone view ultrasonography for neoplasms of the pancreatic tail. *AJR Am J Roentgenol*. 1978;131:231–236.

29. Haber HP. Cystic fibrosis in children and young adults: findings on routine abdominal sonography. *AJR Am J Roentgenol*. 2007;189:89–99.

30. Walkowiak J, Lisowska A, Blaszczynski M. The changing face of the exocrine pancreas in cystic fibrosis: pancreatic sufficiency, pancreatitis and genotype. *Eur J Gastroenterol Hepatol*. 2008;20(3):157–160.

31. Taylor CJ, Aswani N. The pancreas in cystic fibrosis. *Paediatr Respir Rev*. 2002;3(1):77–81.

32. Crawford JM, Cotran RS. The pancreas. In: Cotran RS, Kumar V, Collins T, eds. *Robbins: Pathologic Basis of Disease*. 6th ed. Philadelphia, PA: Saunders; 1999: 902–929.

33. Goekas MC. Acute pancreatitis. *Ann Intern Med*. 1985; 103:86–91.

34. Donovan PJ, Sanders RC, Siegelman SS. Collections of fluid after pancreatitis: evaluation by computed tomography and ultrasonography. *Radiol Clin North Am*. 1982;20: 653–665.

35. Raptopoulos V, Kleinman PK, Marks S. Renal fascial pathway: posterior extension of pancreatic effusions within the anterior pararenal space. *Radiology*. 1986;158: 367–374.

36. Zaleman M, Van Gansbeke D, Matos C, et al. Sonographic demonstration of portal venous system thrombosis secondary to inflammatory disease of the pancreas. *Gastrointest Radiol*. 1987;12:114–121.

37. Doust B, Pearce JD. Grey-scale ultrasonic properties of the normal and inflamed pancreas. *Radiology*. 1976;120: 653–657.

38. Fleischer AC, Parker P, Kirchner SG, et al. Sonographic findings of pancreatitis in children. *Radiology*. 1983;146: 151–155.

39. Coleman BG, Arger PH, Rosenberg HK, et al. Gray-scale sonographic assessment of pancreatitis in children. *Radiology*. 1983;146:145–150.

40. Gonzales AC, Bradley EL, Clements JL. Pseudocyst formation in acute pancreatitis—ultrasonographic evaluation of 99 cases. *AJR Am J Roentgenol*. 1976;127:315–317.

41. Lawson TL. Acute pancreatitis and its complications. Computed tomography and sonography. *Radiol Clin North Am*. 1983;21:495–513.

42. Laing FC, Gooding GA, Brown T, et al. Atypical pseudocysts of the pancreas: an ultrasonographic evaluation. *J Clin Ultrasound*. 1979;7:27–32.

43. Jeffrey RB, Laing FC, Wing VW. Extrapancreatic spread of acute pancreatitis: new observations with real-time US. *Radiology*. 1986;159:707–714.

44. Tanaka K, Kida M. Role of endoscopy in screening of early pancreatic cancer and bile duct cancer. *Digestive Endoscopy*. 2008;21(1):S97–S100.

45. Lygidakis NJ. Biliary stricture as a complication of chronic relapsing pancreatitis. *Am J Surg*. 1983;145:804–806.

46. Lee SH, Bodensteiner D, Eisman S, et al. Chronic relapsing pancreatitis with pseudocyst erosion into the portal vein and disseminated fat necrosis. *Am J Gastroenterol*. 1985; 80(6):452–458.

47. American Cancer Society. *Cancer Facts and Figures*. Atlanta, GA: American Cancer Society; 2008:1–72.

48. Cadili A, Bazarrelli A, Garg S, et al. Survival in cystic neoplasms of the pancreas. *Can J Gastroenterol.* 2009;23(8): 537–542.

49. Cubilla AL, Fitzgerald PJ. Classification of pancreatic cancer (nonendocrine). *Mayo Clin Proc.* 1979;54:449–458.

50. Larsson L. Endocrine pancreatic tumors. *Human Pathol.* 1978;9:401–416.

51. Balthazar EJ, Subramanyam BR, Lefleur RS, et al. Solid and papillary epithethial neoplasms of the pancreas. *Radiology.* 1984;150:39–40.

52. Guillan RA, McMahon J. Pleomorphic adenocarcinoma of the pancreas. *Am J Gastroenterol.* 1973;60:379–386.

53. Herrera L, Glassman CI, Komins JI. Mucinous cystic neoplasm of the pancreas demonstrated by ultrasound and endoscopic retrograde pancreatography. *Am J Gastroenterol.* 1980;73:512–515.

54. Lack EE, Lavey R. Tumors of the exocrine pancreas in children and adolescents. A clinical and pathologic study of eight cases. *Am J Surg Pathol.* 1983;7:319–327.

55. Sommers SC, Meissner WA. Unusual carcinomas of the pancreas. *AMA Arch Pathol.* 1954;58:101–111.

56. Becker WF, Welsh RA, Pratt HS. Cystadenoma and cystadenocarcinoma of the pancreas. *Ann Surg.* 1965;161:845–859.

57. Wolson AH, Walls WJ. Ultrasonic characteristics of cystadenoma of the pancreas. *Radiology.* 1976;119:203–205.

58. Koenigsberg P. Focal lesions of the pancreas. *Semin Roentgenol.* 1985;20:3–21.

59. Shawker TH, Garra BS, Hill MC, et al. Spectrum of sonographic findings in pancreatic carcinoma. *J Ultrasound Med.* 1986;5:169–175.

60. Shawker TH, Linzer M, Hubbard VS. Chronic pancreatitis: the diagnostic significance of pancreatic size and echo amplitude. *Radiology.* 1985;154:568–574.

61. Niccoloni DG, Graham JH, Banks PA. Tumor-induced acute pancreatitis. *Gastroenterology.* 1976;71:142–145.

62. Helmstaedter L, Riemann JF. Pancreatic cancer-EUS and early diagnosis. *Langenbecks Arch Surg.* 2008;393:923–927.

63. Figueiredo FA, Giovannini M, Monges G, et al. Pancreatic endocrine tumors: a large single–center experience. *Pancreas.* 2009;38(8):936–940.

64. Freeny PC, Weinstein CJ, Taft DA, et al. Cystic neoplasms of the pancreas: new angiographic and sonographic findings. *AJR Am J Roentgenol.* 1978;131:795–802.

65. Hodgkinson DJ, Remine WH, Weiland LH. Pancreatic cystadenoma: a clinicopathologic study of 45 cases. *Arch Surg.* 1978;113:512–519.

66. Itai Y, Ohhashi K, Nagai H, et al. "Ductectatic" mucinous cystadenoma and cystadenocarcinoma of the pancreas. *Radiology.* 1986;161:697–700.

67. Logan SE, Voet RL, Tompkins RK. The malignant potential of mucinous cysts of the pancreas. *West J Med.* 1982; 136:157–162.

68. Compagno J, Oertel JE. Microcystic adenoma of the pancreas: a clinicopathologic study of 34 cases. *Am J Clin Pathol.* 1978;69:289–298.

69. Compagno J, Oertal JE. Mucinous cystic neoplasms of the pancreas with overt and latent malignancy. A clinicopathologic study of 41 cases. *Am J Clin Pathol.* 1978;69:573–580.

70. Wolfman NT, Ramquist NA, Karstaedt N, et al. Cystic neoplasms of the pancreas: CT and sonography. *AJR Am J Roentgenol.* 1982;138:37–40.

71. Carroll B, Sample WF. Pancreatic cystadenocarcinoma: CT body scan and gray-scale ultrasound appearance. *AJR Am J Roentgenol.* 1978;131:339–341.

72. Friedman AC, Lichtenstein JE, Dachman AH. Cystic neoplasms of the pancreas: radiological-pathological correlation. *Radiology.* 1983;149:45–50.

73. Lloyd TV, Antonmattei S, Freimanis AK. Gray-scale sonography of cystadenoma of the pancreas: report of two cases. *J Clin Ultrasound.* 1979;7:149–151.

74. Lo JW, Fung CH, Yonan TN, et al. Cystadenoma of the pancreas. An ultrastructural study. *Cancer.* 1977;39:2470–2474.

75. Mcgeoch JE, Darmady EM. Polycystic disease of kidney, liver and pancreas: a possible pathogenesis. *J Pathol.* 1976; 119:221–228.

76. Johnson PR, Spitz L. Cysts and tumors of the pancreas. *Semin Pediatr Surg.* 2000;9:209–215.

77. Levine E, Collins DL, Horton WA, et al. CT screening of the abdomen in von Hippel-Lindau disease. *AJR Am J Roentgenol.* 1982;139:505–510.

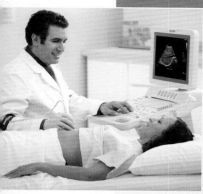

# 8 The Spleen

Tanya D. Nolan

## OBJECTIVES

Describe the normal anatomy and function of the spleen.

Describe the normal vasculature of the spleen.

List the common causes of splenomegaly.

Demonstrate the scanning techniques used to image the spleen.

Identify the sonographic appearance and etiology of benign focal lesions of the spleen including splenic cyst, abscess, infarct, hematoma, and hemangioma.

Discuss the sonographic findings of lymphoma, leukemia, and metastases of the spleen.

Identify technically satisfactory and unsatisfactory sonographic examinations of the spleen.

## KEY TERMS

AIDS | angiosarcoma | accessory spleen | asplenia | benign hemangioma | echinococcal cyst | Hodgkin lymphoma | leukemia | non-Hodgkin lymphoma | sickle cell disease | splenic ptosis | splenic trauma | splenomegaly

## GLOSSARY

**erythrocyte** red blood cell; contains hemoglobin and responsible for transporting oxygen

**erythropoiesis** process of red blood cell production; occurs in the fetal spleen from the fifth to sixth month of fetal life after which the bone marrow assumes the function

**hematocrit** laboratory value of the percentage of blood volume made up of red blood cells; can be low in cases of anemia, blood loss, and leukemia

**infarct** tissue death caused by an interruption of the blood supply

**leukocyte** white blood cell; main function is to protect against and fight infection in the body

**leukocytosis** elevated white blood cell count usually due to infection

**leukopenia** decreased white blood cell count; can be a result of many factors including viral infect and leukemia

**phagocytosis** process used by the red pulp to destroy old red blood cells

Every thorough sonographic examination of the upper abdomen includes images of the spleen. The location and shape of the normal spleen can present many challenges for the sonographer. Its variable and asymmetric shape makes it a challenge to orient the transducer to find its longest axis. Although radionuclide imaging and computed tomography (CT) are often the first studies conducted of the spleen, sonography is effective in characterizing masses, in evaluating the size and echotexture, in identifying the nature of palpated left-sided upper quadrant masses, in monitoring the course of trauma to the spleen, and in locating intraperitoneal blood collections. As always in sonography, one must appreciate the normal appearance and normal variations of the organ so that abnormalities can be easily recognized.

## EMBRYOLOGY AND NORMAL ANATOMY

The spleen develops from mesenchymal cells located between the layers of the dorsal mesentery of the stomach. These cells differentiate to form splenic pulp, supportive connecting tissues, and the splenic capsule.[1] The spleen is an intraperitoneal, ovoid organ entirely covered by peritoneum except at a small bare area at the hilum through which the splenic artery, splenic vein, and efferent lymphatic vessels pass. The spleen is a vulnerable organ located in the left hypochondrium, and its long axis parallels the ninth to eleventh ribs[2] (Fig. 8-1). The spleen is bordered anteriorly by the stomach; medially by the left kidney, splenic flexure

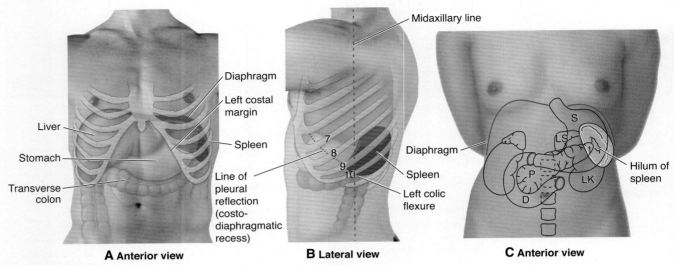

**Figure 8-1** The spleen in relationship to surrounding organs and structures.

of the colon, and pancreatic tail; and posteriorly by the diaphragm, pleura, left lung, and ribs[3] (Fig. 8-2). Although mobile, the spleen normally does not extend inferiorly beyond the left costal margin; therefore, clinically palpating the spleen through the anterior lateral wall is difficult without significant enlargement of the organ.[4,5] The neighboring organs and structures create indentations and impressions on the visceral surface of the spleen that may simulate masses; therefore,

knowledge of the normal variants is essential in preventing a misdiagnosis.[4]

At the hilus, the splenic arteries and veins are covered by the mesentery of the lienorenal ligament, which also houses the tail of the pancreas. The lienorenal and gastrosplenic ligaments attach the spleen to the left kidney and greater curvature of the stomach, respectively.[2,3] The phrenicocolic ligament is not directly attached to the spleen; however, it supports the inferior end of the

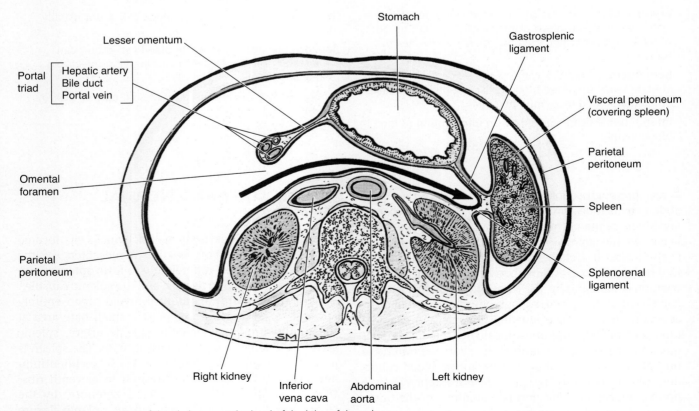

**Figure 8-2** Cross section of the abdomen at the level of the hilus of the spleen.

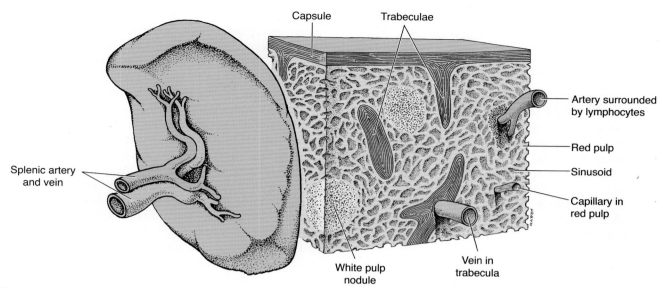

**Figure 8-3** Schematic of the cellular structure of the spleen.

organ. The lienorenal, gastrosplenic, and phrenicocolic ligaments work together to stabilize the spleen and hold it loosely in position. Laxity of peritoneal attachments allows for hypermobility and splenic enlargement up to 10 times its normal size.[5]

The average spleen measures 12 cm in length, 7 cm in width, and 3 to 4 cm in thickness.[2,6,7] In children, spleen length is highly correlated with age and body parameters (height, weight, and body surface area [BSA]).[6] The adult splenic size is commonly compared to that of a person's fist and weighs approximately 150 g.[8] Variations in the body's blood needs may affect its size. For example, the normal spleen may decrease in volume with advancing age or increase during digestion.[7]

A fibrous capsule composed of dense fibroelastic connective tissue surrounds the spleen and is thickened at the splenic hilum. Trabeculae (strands of connective tissue) project from the splenic capsule and divide the spleen into several compartments. These communicating compartments are filled of splenic lymphoid tissue termed *splenic pulp*, which filters the peripheral blood[2,4,8] (Fig. 8-3). The white and red splenic pulp make the spleen soft and friable, similar to a sponge. The white pulp is composed of lymphatic tissue consisting largely of lymphocytes and macrophages. The white pulp clusters around the splenic arterioles and is a major site for immunologic activity. Lymphatic follicles are responsible for the production of antibodies and therefore grow in number and size in response to antigens. The red pulp consists of a meshwork of blood-filled venous sinuses and reticular splenic cords, termed the *cords of Billroth*. The venous sinuses are capable of storing more than 300 mL of blood. Blood storage capacity increases with passive dilation of the venous sinuses. Reduction in systemic blood pressure results in

the constriction of the venous sinuses and the ejection of as much as 200 mL of blood into the venous circulation in order to restore blood volume and increase hematocrit.[4,8]

The highly vascular spleen receives its arterial blood from the splenic artery, a branch of the celiac axis (Fig. 8-4). The splenic artery initially divides into two major branches before separating into several minor arterioles within the spleen. These arterioles may be visible as small echogenic lines passing through the splenic parenchyma. It is important for the sonographer to remember that because there are no adequate anastomoses between arteries in the spleen, the organ is susceptible to infarction. Blood from the arterioles flows into the venous sinusoids and then exits through branches of the splenic vein. These branches leave the spleen through the splenic trabeculae and converge to form the splenic vein. The splenic vein is joined by the inferior mesenteric vein and traverses posterior to the tail and body of the pancreas. The splenic vein unites

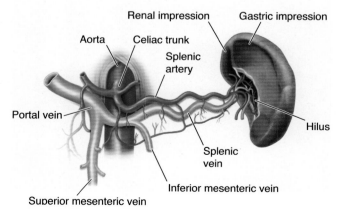

**Figure 8-4** Circulation of the spleen, including the splenic vein and splenic artery.

with the superior mesenteric vein posterior to the neck of the pancreas to form the hepatic portal vein.[2–4,8]

## NORMAL VARIATIONS

The spleen undergoes the same maturational changes as most body organs. Splenic maturation may be divided into at least four stages made distinctive by the distribution of lymphocytes.[9] Aplasia is a failure in normal embryogenesis that leads to the congenital absence of the spleen. This rare condition is commonly associated with other lethal malformations, and asplenic individuals are known to be at increased risk for infection with encapsulated bacteria.[10] Partial development may also occur and is associated with situs inversus and cardiovascular anomalies.

An accessory spleen is a relatively common anatomic variant seen in 10% to 30% of patients at autopsy and 16% of patients undergoing contrast enhanced CT of the abdomen. Most accessory spleens are small and measure between 1.5 and 2.0 cm. Approximately 75% of accessory spleens are found near to the normal spleen within the splenic hilum or gastrosplenic ligament omentum (Fig. 8-5). The other 20% are located within the tail of the pancreas where they may be mistaken for hypervascular pancreatic tumors. Differentiating accessory spleens from pancreatic masses or from hilar lymph nodes may be difficult, unless it is possible to trace their blood supply to the splenic artery. Rare locations for an accessory spleen include the pelvis or scrotum.[11,12] Following splenectomy, an accessory spleen may assume the function and size of the removed organ. In cases of hematologic disorders, residual splenic tissue and accessory spleens present after laparoscopic splenectomy may lead to a relapse.[13]

When a patient does not have a history of splenectomy and splenic tissue is not sonographically visualized in the normal anatomic location, the sonographer should extensively examine the entire left side of the patient from the thorax to the pelvis for an ectopic or wandering spleen. Splenic ptosis can occur if the supporting ligaments are dysfunctional or lax. Congenitally, incomplete fusion of the dorsal mesogastrium to the posterior abdominal wall during the second month of embryonic development may result in an unusually long splenic pedicle leading to the ectopia. Acquired mechanisms may exist in multiparous women secondary to hormone changes during pregnancy. Other factors associated with laxity of supporting structures include splenomegaly, trauma, extreme weight loss, weak abdominal muscles, and gastric distension; however, the precise etiology of wandering spleen is not completely understood.[5]

Because the wandering spleen lacks its normal peritoneal attachments, this variant is associated with a high incidence of splenic torsion and infarction. Clinically, patients may present as asymptomatic or demonstrate varying degrees of abdominal pain with an associated abdominal or pelvic mass. Contrast enhanced CT is the imaging modality of choice in diagnosing wandering spleen; however, variable echo patterns presented in sonography combined with duplex Doppler and color flow showing lack of flow in the splenic parenchyma secondary to torsion of the splenic artery is an excellent source of diagnostic information. The preferred treatment for wandering spleen is splenopexy in which a surgeon repositions the spleen in the left upper quadrant in order to prevent torsion of splenic vessels and preserve splenic function. Cavazos et al. found that laparoscopic splenopexy was more advantageous in returning function to the spleen, had minimal associated

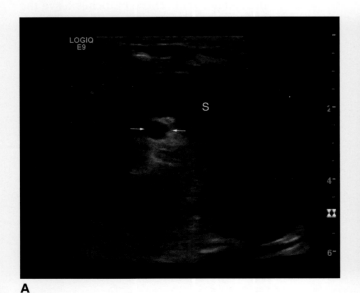

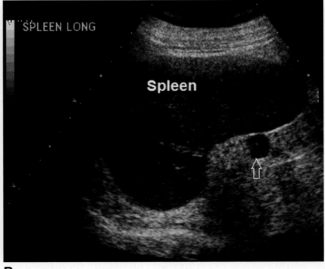

**A**  **B**

**Figure 8-5** Accessory spleen. **A:** Small accessory spleen *(arrows)* is seen in the splenic hilum *(S)*. **B:** On a different patient, an accessory spleen *(arrow)* is visualized in the splenic hilum. (Image **A** courtesy of GE Healthcare, Wauwatosa, WI; Image **B** courtesy of Natalee Braun, Ogden, UT.)

postoperative pain, allowed for early discharge from the hospital, and aided in a more rapid recovery when compared to open splenopexy or splenectomy.[14]

## PHYSIOLOGY

The spleen is an organ of mystery and perplexity for physiologists. Although the spleen is rarely the primary site of disease—as the largest secondary lymphoid organ of the reticuloendothelial system—it is often involved in inflammatory, hematopoietic, and metabolic disorders and is associated with immune and hematologic diseases. Functions of the spleen overlap those of other body organs making it possible for a person to live without the spleen; however, studies completed on individuals with splenic absence have given some indication to its important body functions. For example, patients who have undergone splenectomy often suffer from leukocytosis, decreased iron levels, greater volumes of circulating defective blood cells, and decreased immune function.[3,8] Currently, splenectomy may not be considered the first option of treatment because of the correlating risk of postsplenectomy sepsis.[15]

### FUNCTIONS OF THE SPLEEN

#### Reservoir and Filter

A small portion of the blood entering the terminal capillaries of the spleen will continue to microcirculate and enter highly distensible venous sinuses. This blood reservoir, crowded with red blood cells and platelets, may provide a transfusion type response to stresses imposed by hemorrhage.[2] The majority of circulating blood, however, will traverse through hyperpermeable capillary walls into the red pulp. The spleen's major function is to filter the peripheral blood. Red pulp is the principle site of filtration, and it performs three major functions related to blood cells. These include the removal of macrophages of ruptured, worn out, or defective blood cells; the storage of platelets; and the production of blood cells (hematopoiesis) during fetal life.[1]

#### Destruction of Red Blood Cells and Microorganisms

Within the red pulp, resident macrophages of the mononuclear phagocyte system phagocytose particles of debris, microorganisms, and old, damaged, or dead blood cells, particularly erythrocytes. Phagocytes come in contact with the blood in the reticulum cells. The blood is further exposed to phagocytes when it passes through the walls of the sinusoids on the way to the veins. The walls of the sinusoids also trap defective cells. The hemoglobin released from phagocytosed erythrocytes is catabolized, and the iron is stored in the cytoplasm of the macrophages or released back into the blood plasma.[4,8]

The removal of senescent, defective red blood cells occurs mainly in the cords of Billroth. This culling function of the spleen identifies and removes defective cells such as spherocytes, sickle cells, and thalassemic cells from circulation as they move through the walls of the sinuses because they lack the biconcave shape of normal red blood cells.

Red blood cells that are abnormal because they contain a granule, or even a parasite, are not culled. Rather, the nuclear fragments or membrane inclusions are milked from the erythrocytes, and the cleansed red blood cell returns to normal circulation. This process is referred to as *splenic pitting.*[16]

### Erythropoiesis

The spleen is responsible for erythropoiesis from approximately the fifth to the sixth months of fetal life. With age, the bone marrow assumes this function, but the spleen does retain its capacity to produce red blood cells throughout adult life.[4,8] The spleen's hematopoietic functions can be regained if chronic anemia develops or bone marrow parenchyma is lost.

### Defense Against Disease

All lymphoid organs are connected within the hematologic and immune systems because each organ is a site of residence, proliferation, differentiation, or function of lymphocytes and mononuclear phagocytes.[8] The white pulp plays a key role in lymphocyte circulation with memory of B-lymphocyte–producing and antibody-producing cells.[16] Bloodborne antigens encounter lymphocytes within the white pulp clumped around the splenic arterioles. These specialized cells initiate the immune response. There are many different types of lymphocytes, the most important of which are the T cells, B cells, and mature B cells or plasma cells.[8] The spleen is not merely a source of lymphocytes, macrophages, plasma cells, and antibodies, it can also phagocytose bacteria that have bypassed the lymph nodes.

### LABORATORY VALUES

Normally, there are approximately 5,000 to 10,000 white blood cells (WBCs) per microliter of blood. Leukocytosis occurs when the leukocyte count is higher than normal. When a physiologic stressor is present, leukocytosis is a normal response and commonly indicates the presence of inflammation or infection. In contrast, an abnormally low level of WBCs is referred to as *leukopenia.* Leukopenia is not a normal or beneficial finding. Leukocyte counts that decrease below 1,000/mm$^3$ open an individual to increased risk of infection. Patients with counts below 500/mm$^3$ are at jeopardy for serious life-threatening infection. Leukopenia may result from radiation therapy, chemotherapeutic agents, systemic lupus erythematosus, vitamin $B_{12}$ deficiency, cortisol treatment, and anaphylactic shock.

WBCs and platelets are affected by spleen sequestering but not to the same extent as the red blood cell concentration. Splenic pooling decreases circulating red blood cell concentrations, and sequestered red blood cells are exposed to splenic conditions that accelerate destruction and add to the reduced concentration. A laboratory hematocrit indicates the percentage of blood volume occupied by red blood cells. Abnormal findings in the level of hematocrit result from altered erythropoiesis, anemias, hemorrhage, Hodgkin disease, and/or leukemia.[4,8]

Abnormal laboratory tests, history of infectious disease, left upper quadrant pain, and a palpable enlarged spleen are all clinical manifestations and indications for a sonographic examination of the spleen.[2]

## NORMAL SONOGRAPHIC APPEARANCE AND TECHNIQUE

The normal echogenicity of the spleen is comparable with that of the liver and equal to or slightly hyperechoic to the kidney when the tissues are evaluated at the same distance from the transducer.[17] Splenic parenchyma is homogeneous with low-level to midlevel echoes, which are usually disrupted only by the arteries and veins in the area of the hilus[7,18] (Fig. 8-6). Within the splenic hilum, the splenic artery and its

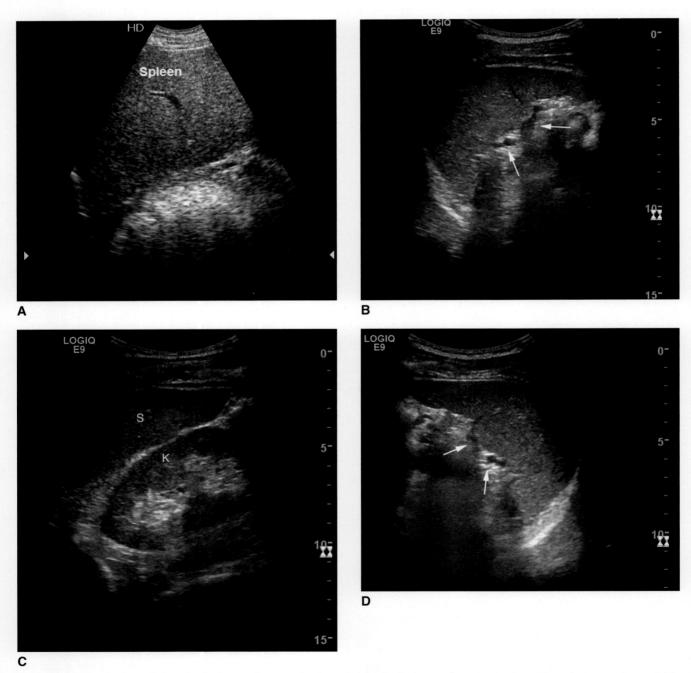

**Figure 8-6** Normal spleen. **A:** Longitudinal scan of a normal spleen. **B:** Longitudinal scan of a normal spleen. The splenic vessels are visible at the hilus (*arrows*). **C:** Longitudinal section lateral to the hilus of the spleen (*S*) outlines the splenic contour and shows its relationship to the left kidney (*K*). **D:** Transverse scan of a normal spleen. The vessels are visible at the hilus (*arrows*). (Image **A** courtesy of Philips Medical System, Bothell, WA; Image(s) **B**, **C**, and **D** courtesy of GE Healthcare, Wauwatosa, WI.)

bifurcations along with convergence of the splenic veins are visualized. Differentiation between these vessels is difficult without studying the Doppler signals (Fig. 8-7). Examining the spleen requires creative manipulation of the transducer and patient. When the patient is in the supine position, the transducer is placed between one of the left intercostals spaces posteriorly within the coronal plane.[7] The most common patient position is the right lateral decubitus position with the left arm raised over the head to separate the ribs and allow for better transducer access.[18] Additionally, the patient may vary respiration to optimize the image window. A large inspiration depresses the diaphragm and moves the spleen inferiorly away from bony thorax. A 2- to 5-MHz curvilinear transducer is commonly used to image the spleen. If necessary, a linear array transducer may be used to increase image detail; however, there is a slight disadvantage scanning in the intercostal space with a larger transducer footprint.[7] A smaller transducer head makes intercostal scanning more feasible.

Longitudinal imaging sections of the spleen should include the hilus with its blood vessels and several representational parenchymal images. Additionally, the left hemidiaphragm and the interface with the left kidney should be well demonstrated. The longest axis of the spleen and anteroposterior dimensions may be measured in this orientation. After completing evaluation and obtaining images of the spleen in longitudinal sections, the transducer should be rotated 90 degrees for transverse imaging. The organ should be measured in transverse orientation at its widest point when splenic volumetric index (SVI) is to be calculated. Fluids administered by mouth or through a nasogastric tube may help to define the stomach and the splenic margin.[18] When a mass is present in the left upper quadrant or the spleen is enlarged, visualization of the organ is often accomplished from an anterior approach. A spleen surrounded by free intraperitoneal fluid or associated with a pleural effusion is best visualized from an anterolateral approach.[7]

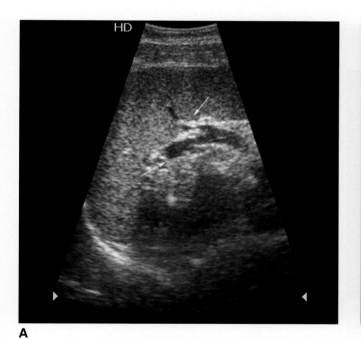

**A**

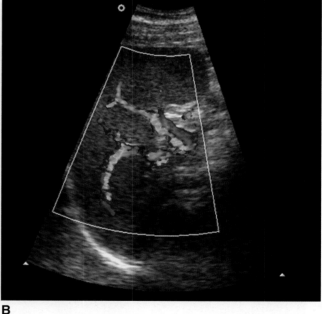

**B**

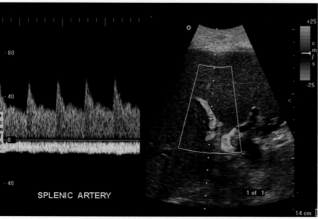

**C**

**Figure 8-7** Color and spectral Doppler. **A:** Longitudinal image of the normal spleen. Splenic vessels are visible at the splenic hilus *(arrows)*. **B:** Color Doppler imaging demonstrating splenic vessels at the splenic hilum. **C:** Pulsed Doppler waveform indicates the presence of the splenic arterial flow above the baseline and venous flow below the baseline. (Images courtesy of Philips Medical System, Bothell, WA.)

Due to the normal variations in splenic shape and size, in sonographic practice, length is the dimension primarily monitored for splenic enlargement. In 95% of adults, the normal spleen length is less than 12 cm, the breadth less than 7 cm, and the thickness less than 5 cm.[7,17,18] A long axis >12 cm is generally taken to indicate enlargement. Splenic enlargement may alter the echogenicity of the organ. For example, decreased echogenicity may be indicative of lymphoma whereas increased echogenicity may suggest the presence of myelofibrosis or infection.[18]

## DOPPLER AND COLOR DOPPLER

Spectral and color Doppler are invaluable in evaluating the splenic and perisplenic vasculature. Normal flow patterns in the splenic artery and vein are similar to those in all abdominal organs. Abnormalities in direction and flow dynamics characterize commonly seen pathology such as portal hypertension, with or without collateral vessels; splenic vein thrombosis; and aneurysms of the splenic artery. Absence of flow in areas of the splenic parenchyma is associated with avascular lesions, such as cysts or necrosis. Color Doppler is invaluable in illuminating hypoechoic vascular lesions that may be overlooked with gray scale imaging.

## DISEASES OF THE SPLEEN

Although attempts have been made to correlate alterations of splenic echogenicity and changes in blood flow with disease states, the most reliable sonographic criteria are those that affect the morphology of the organ.

## SPLENOMEGALY

The most common splenic abnormality observed sonographically is enlargement. Generally, if the lower splenic edge is palpated below the left costal margin at the end of inspiration, its enlargement is approximately three times its normal size.[2] Splenomegaly may induce symptoms of left upper quadrant fullness or pain from stretching of the capsule, stretching of the suspensory ligaments, or pressure on the adjacent organs, particularly the stomach and intestines. In addition, the patient often suffers from additional symptoms related to

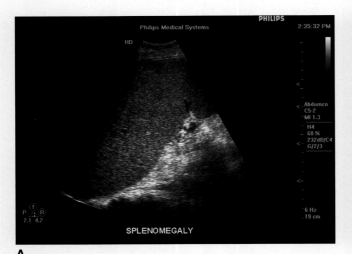

A

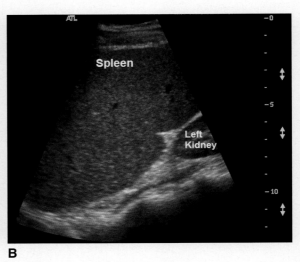

B

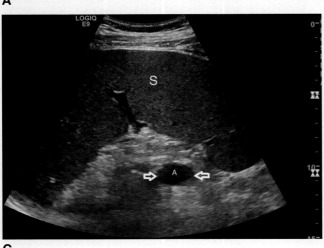

C

**Figure 8-8** Splenomegaly. **A:** The enlarged spleen fills the abdominal cavity and extends into the pelvis. **B:** Splenomegaly and associated left kidney. **C:** Enlarged spleen *(S)* is seen with an accessory spleen *(arrows)* near the splenic hilum. (Image(s) **A** and **B** courtesy of Philips Medical System, Bothell, WA; Image **C** courtesy of GE Healthcare, Wauwatosa, WI.)

underlying disease processes, such as jaundice, lymph-adenopathy, fever, or hemorrhage.

Historically, many criteria for splenomegaly have been developed. Serial section measurements of the spleen used to compute the volume are cumbersome and unpopular. Many sonographers use intuition and "eye-ball" the size of the spleen to determine enlargement, and visual inspection suffices when the enlarged spleen fills the abdominal cavity and extends into the pelvis. In cases of minimal or moderate splenomegaly, the spleen is considered enlarged when its length exceeds 13 cm[7,17–19] (Fig. 8-8).

A wide range of pathologic processes may produce splenomegaly. Diseases related to classification of splenomegaly may be broadly categorized as inflammation or infection, congestive, infiltrative, hematologic, metabolic, and traumatic[8] (Table 8-1). The single most common cause of splenomegaly is congestion secondary to portal hypertension, most often due to liver cirrhosis.[2] In cirrhosis, nodular parenchymal regeneration and fibrosis result in the reduction of blood flow and an elevation in portal venous pressure (portal hypertension). This increased pressure reverses normal flow through the portal and splenic veins toward the liver. The reversal of blood flow and damping of the normal respiratory variation in venous Doppler signals are characteristic of portal hypertension.[19] As pressure increases, the portal vein becomes enlarged and tortuous, and collateral vessels open between the portal veins and the systemic veins where pressure is considerably lower.[8] Collateral varices appear within the splenic hilus, retroperitoneum, and gastrohepatic ligament (Fig. 8-9). The most common varice is the splenorenal collateral where blood is directed from

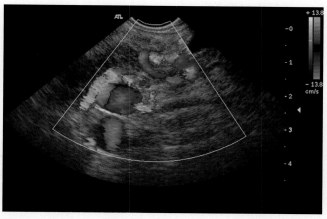

**Figure 8-9** Splenic varices. Dilated tortuous splenic varices secondary to portal hypertension. (Image courtesy of Philips Medical System, Bothell, WA.)

the splenic vein into the left renal vein then terminates at the inferior vena cava (IVC). Second, a recanalized umbilical vein in the ligamentum teres within the liver is pathognomonic for portal hypertention.[17–19] Sonographically, visualization of small, echogenic parallel lines, termed "reflective channels," within the splenic parenchyma has been shown to be a diagnostic criterion for differentiating among causes of splenomegaly due to acute systemic infections, hemolytic anemias, infiltrative processes, and portal hypertension. Color Doppler of these channels shows blood flow that proves them to be vascular. The echogenic walls are produced by dilated sinusoidal veins with collagen in their walls. The echogenic channels could be differentiated from splenic calcifications due to tuberculosis, histoplasmosis, and calcified infarcts of sickle cell disease by observing the parallel echoes and using color Doppler to detect blood flow.[19] The only other finding specific to portal hypertension includes occasional echogenic foci in an enlarged spleen caused by Gamna-Gandy bodies.

In abnormalities of red blood cell morphology, including hereditary spherocytosis, as well as in hemoglobin defects such as thalassemia, there is congestion of red blood cells with associated reticuloendothelial hyperplasia and splenomegaly.

Sickle cell disease has a variety of presentations dependent on the chronicity of the disease and whether it is homozygous or heterozygous. Acute splenic sequestration crisis occurs most frequently in children suffering from homozygous sickle cell disease. Large amounts of blood are acutely pooled within the liver and spleen; the spleen suddenly enlarges and is accompanied by a sharp decrease in hematocrit. Because the spleen can hold as much as one-fifth the body's blood supply at one time, mortality rates may increase up to 50% due to cardiovascular collapse.[8] Hypoechoic areas seen within the periphery of the spleen may represent subacute hemorrhage.

The most common malignant disease that affects the spleen is lymphoma (Hodgkin disease and non-Hodgkin

| TABLE | 8-1 |
| --- | --- |

**Disease Category or Pathologic Process Causing Splenomegaly**

| Disease Category | Pathologic Process |
| --- | --- |
| Congestive | Portal hypertension |
| Hematologic | Thalassemia, hereditary spherocytosis, autoimmune hemolytic anemia, sickle cell disease (in early stage) |
| Infiltrative | Leukemia, Hodgkin lymphoma, non-Hodgkin lymphoma |
| Metabolic | Gaucher disease, Niemann-Pick disease |
| Chronic inflammatory conditions | Sarcoid, tuberculosis, malaria |
| Hematopoietic malignancies | Acute lymphocytic leukemia, chronic myelogenous leukemia, chronic lymphocytic leukemia, agnogenic myeloid metaplasia |
| Trauma | Parenchymal hematoma, subcapsular hematoma |

lymphoma).[17] In leukemia and lymphoma, there may be diffuse infiltration of the spleen by malignant cell lines with associated enlargement. Diffuse infiltration of the bone marrow by these malignant cells may compromise its hematopoietic capability. As a consequence, the spleen may become the site of blood production, extramedullary hematopoiesis, enlarging the spleen.[8]

In metabolic diseases such as Gaucher and Niemann-Pick disease, the spleen is enlarged with macrophages distended with metabolic elements characteristic of each disease.[8]

Although the spleen parenchyma is very homogeneous, it may become more or less echogenic with enlargement. Unfortunately, one cannot differentiate

| TABLE 8-2 | |
|---|---|
| **Sonographic Characteristics of Disease Category or Process That Produces Focal or Diffuse Lesions** | |
| **Sonographic Appearance** | **Disease Category or Process** |
| **FOCAL LESIONS** | |
| *Splenic cysts* | |
| Anechoic, well-defined walls, enhanced sound transmission | Congenital |
| Sharply demarcated wall, multilocular internal structure representing daughter cyst, mural calcifications | Acquired echinococcal (hydatid) |
| Large cysts, dense, clearly defined walls | Epidermoid or epithelial |
| May not have well-defined wall, mural calcifications | Posttraumatic or postinflammatory pseudocysts |
| Single or multiple simple cysts | Polycystic kidney disease lymphangioma, extension of pancreatic pseudocyst |
| *Abscesses* | |
| Usually multiple, range from anechoic with well-defined borders to echo-filled and septate, gas creates dirty shadowing, air-fluid or fluid-fluid level might be visible | Bacterial endocarditis, diverticulitis, osteomyelitis, pelvic or other infection |
| *Infarcts* | |
| Well-demarcated, wedge-shaped or round, hypoechoic in acute phase; more echogenic in later stage; measure 1–2 cm and usually located in periphery with apex pointing medially | Bacterial endocarditis, tumor embolization, hemoglobinopathy, myeloproliferative disorders, leukemia, lymphoma, vasculitis (SLE, polyarteritis nodosa) |
| *Hematoma* | |
| Isoechoic to echogenic mass within parenchyma, which may become hypoechoic as hematoma resolves, may demonstrate fluid–fluid level, may produce splenomegaly | Trauma, coagulation disorder |
| Fractured spleen may appear only as enlarging spleen with normal echogenicity; blood might be found in pelvis, flanks, Morrison pouch, lesser and greater sacs; subcapsular hematoma may appear as normal spleen, or hypoechoic, or echogenic mass adjacent to clearly defined capsule; pericapsular hematoma may efface smooth contour of splenic capsule | Ruptured spleen secondary to trauma or enlargement |
| *Echogenic lesions* | |
| Sometimes with hypoechoic areas and accompanying splenomegaly | Primary benign and malignant neoplasms and metastases, abscesses, hematomas |
| **DIFFUSE CHANGES** | |
| *Calcifications* | |
| Echogenic foci with varying degrees of acoustic shadowing | Sequelae of granulomatous disease such as histoplasmosis or tuberculosis, from previous hematoma or infarction, cysts |
| *Hypoechoic nodules* | |
| Irregular, multiple hypoechoic parenchymal masses; occasionally hyperechoic lesions | Hodgkin and non-Hodgkin lymphoma, benign (i.e., hemangioma, hematoma, isolated lymphangioma) and malignant neoplasms (metastases) |

SLE, systemic lupus erythematosus.

between the degree of echogenicity and the pathological causes of enlargement.[7]

## FOCAL LESIONS

In addition to the diffuse involvement of the spleen described previously, a variety of processes involve the spleen focally. These include true or primary cysts, secondary or pseudocysts, infarctions, granulomas, abscesses, primary benign and malignant neoplasms, and metastases (Table 8-2).

### Cysts

Cysts in the spleen may be congenital or acquired. Within the acquired group, they may be postinflammatory, traumatic, or parasitic. Cysts arising from the epithelial or endothelial lining are considered primary cysts, and cysts resulting from trauma, infection, or degeneration are considered secondary cysts.[17] Worldwide, parasitic cysts are the most common benign cysts. These are overwhelmingly echinococcal (hydatid) in origin, attributable to *Echinococcus multilocularis* or *Echinococcus granulosus*. Sonographically, the appearance of the hydatid cysts varies from simple and centrally anechoic to complex, depending on the stage of the disease. All of these cysts should demonstrate well-defined posterior walls and acoustic enhancement (Fig. 8-10). Mural calcifications may also be identified.[7,20]

Although parasitic cysts are the most common benign splenic cysts wordwide,[20] pseudocysts are the most common in the United States. Typically, these pseudocysts are posttraumatic and are the sequelae of hematomas. In the case of trauma, a capsule of fibrous tissue develops around the resolved subcapsular or intraparenchymal hematoma, which ultimately liquefies to form the pseudocyst.[7] They lack the true epithelial lining of a primary cyst and are instead lined by debris and granulation tissue.[17] Clinically, posttraumatic pseudocysts present as

an abdominal mass with associated pain. Infection and rupture are potential complications.[21]

Primary congenital cysts, epidermoid, or epithelial cysts are epithelial in origin and have embryonic inclusion of epithelial cells from adjacent structures. These cysts originate from the splenic capsular mesothelium, which undergoes cystic dilation, and in some cases vascular metaplasia.[7,22] Epithelial cysts predominantly occur in children and young women and are usually asymptomatic unless they are very large in size and compress adjacent organs.[22]

A rare cystic mass that can involve the spleen focally or diffusely is the lymphangioma.[7] These are cystic, endothelial-lined spaces filled with proteinaceous material. Involvement of the spleen by this entity may be localized or may be part of a generalized lymphangiomatosis of the skin, lung, bone, and viscera. Differentiation from hemangioma is the most important diagnosis of lymphangioma.[23] Sonographically, they appear as multiseptated cystic masses.

### Abscesses

Single focal abscesses within the spleen are uncommon. Most often abscesses are multiple, the result of hematologic spread of infection, including bacterial endocarditis, diverticulitis, osteomyelitis, and pelvic infections.[17] Also, because of the proximity of the pancreatic tail to the splenic hilum, extension of pancreatic disease, such as pseudocysts, can occur.[24] Typically, these lesions are complex in appearance with mixed echogenic properties, and often they are indistinguishable from metastatic lesions or hematomas. When gas is present in the lesion, the characteristic high-level echoes and ring-down shadowing (dirty shadowing) will be observed.[7] Similarly, the demonstration of an air-fluid level when the transducer is held in a posterior or posterolateral position is helpful. Infected hematomas may present with identical sonographic properties. Immunocompromised patients are susceptible to fungal and microbacterial microabscesses, which present as target lesions or small hypoechoic nodules. Sonography-guided aspiration may be used in combination with antibiotic treatment or as a tool of diagnosis. Ruptured abscesses are associated with a high mortality rate.[7,17]

### Infarcts

Infarcts in the spleen are secondary to a wide range of pathologic causes, including hematologic disorders, atheromatous disease, diabetes, congenital abnormalities, or neoplasm.[17] Clinical features of splenic infarcts include left hypochondrial pain with fever and/or left pleural effusion. Laboratory values may indicate anemia, leukocytosis, and elevated lactate dehydrogenase (LDH).[25] Sonographically, splenic infarcts appear as well-demarcated hypoechoic wedge-shaped or round areas located at the periphery (Fig. 8-11). The echogenicity of the infarct is related to age. First, the acute

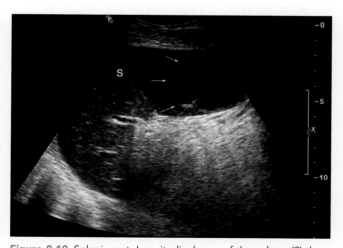

**Figure 8-10** Splenic cyst. Longitudinal scan of the spleen *(S)* demonstrating a simple, anechoic, intraparenchymal cyst *(arrows)*. (Image courtesy of Philips Medical System, Bothell, WA.)

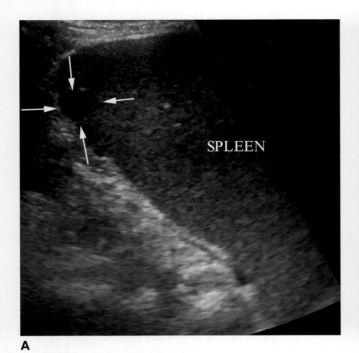

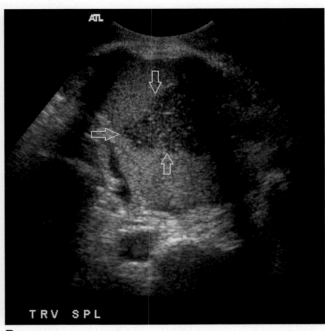

A

B

**Figure 8-11** Splenic infarct. **A:** A longitudinal plane displays a small wedge-shaped area located at the periphery representing a small infarct (*arrows*). **B:** In a different patient, this transverse plane visualizes a large, wedge-shaped splenic infarct (*open arrows*) in a pediatric patient with a history of left upper quadrant pain. After the examination, it was discovered she had leukemia. (Images courtesy of Robert DeJong, Baltimore, MD.)

inflammatory phase presents sonographically with hypoechoic features. These changes correspond to edema, inflammation, and necrosis. Later, as organization takes place, fibrosis and shrinkage supervene, giving rise to increased parenchymal echogencitiy.[7,17] Splenic infarcts are a rare cause of splenic rupture; however, the area should be monitored for increasing subcapsular hemorrhage, free peritoneal blood, and expanding liquefaction area within the infarct—all of which are risk factors for rupture.[25] Few, if any, features distinguish infarction from other sources of focal splenic disease, including small abscesses, metastatic disease, and lymphoma.[17]

## Trauma, Rupture, and Hematoma

The spleen is the organ most frequently damaged in blunt abdominal trauma. Blunt abdominal trauma is associated with a high mortality rate due to liver, spleen, and major blood vessel injury resulting in rapid exsanguination. In addition, injuries to the bowel or pancreas may lead to abdominal sepsis. The spectrum of injuries to the spleen include shattered spleen, fragmentation, disruption of hilar vessels, parenchymal lacerations, capsular tears, and contusions.[26] Because sonography is portable, highly sensitive to free peritoneal fluid, and may be performed quickly, the modality is well suited to a trauma setting. Sonography is not sensitive for the detection of parenchymal lesions and hemoperitoneum is not always present in patients with solid organ injuries; therefore, CT is often the modality of choice in cases

of trauma because it can image the entire body, depict the extension of lesions, and sensitively demonstrate vascular injury.[27]

When sonography is utilized, the spleen may appear normal if there is a small, fresh hematoma, or it may present as a heterogeneous mass if there are extensive parenchymal injuries. The appearance of a hematoma is variable based on the age of the bleed. Blood may initially appear isoechoic, making identification of acute trauma difficult. Assessment of the bleed may become more readily apparent on follow-up scans, as it evolves and becomes echogenic and then anechoic (possibly leading to pseudocyst formation)[17] (Fig. 8-12).

Subcapsular hematomas may also be isoechoic to the spleen. A double contour may be seen, produced by the collection between the capsule and splenic parenchyma, or the hematoma may compress the splenic parenchyma against the capsule. With time, the hematoma may become echogenic, complex, and then anechoic.[7,17]

An enlarging and sonographically heterogeneous spleen in the setting of acute trauma suggests the diagnosis of ruptured spleen (Fig. 8-13). The sonographer must examine the pelvis, Morrison pouch, and the flanks for free blood suggesting splenic rupture. Sonography may demonstrate pericapsular, subcapsular, or peritoneal blood collections.[7,17] Hemoperitoneum may be suggested by the sonographic demonstration of fluid in the lesser and greater sac on both sides of the gastrosplenic ligament. Early identification and regular follow up of patients with splenic trauma are important

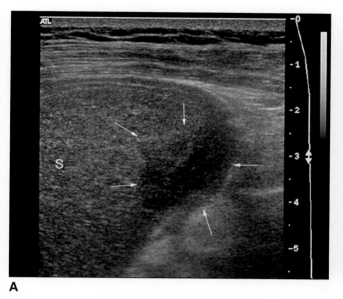
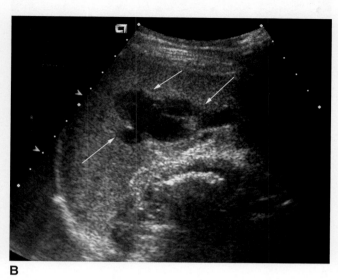

**Figure 8-12** Hematoma. **A:** Longitudinal scan of the spleen (S) demonstrating a resolving splenic hematoma (arrows). **B:** Longitudinal image of the spleen in a patient 6 months postblunt abdominal trauma demonstrating a resolving hematoma (arrows). (Image **A** courtesy of Philips Medical System, Bothell, WA.)

because delayed recognition may result in catastrophic splenic rupture days or weeks following the traumatic episode.[26,28] Currently, patients with splenic trauma are treated conservatively so as to reduce the risk of infection arising from splenectomy.[28]

An enlarged spleen may rupture spontaneously, whatever the cause of enlargement. Abnormalities that have been associated with rupture include Hodgkin disease, infectious mononucleosis, pneumonia, chickenpox, polycythemia rubra vera, and agnogenic myeloid metaplasia.

Splenosis occurs following splenic trauma or splenectomy. Splenic tissue may transplant in the peritoneal cavity in the small intestine, omentum, parietal peritoneum, colon, mesentery, and diaphragm. These implants cannot be differentiated from accessory spleens. Most of these masses do not produce symptoms and are located in areas not readily accessible with sonography.

## Splenic Calcification

Calcifications in the spleen appear echogenic and may demonstrate varying degrees of acoustic shadowing. They are usually the sequelae of granulomatous disease, most commonly histoplasmosis, tuberculosis, or extrapulmonary *Pneumocystis jiroveci*. Calcifications may also result from previous infarction or hematoma. Splenic artery calcification is common and should not be confused with calcification in a lesion[7] (Fig. 8-14).

## Malignant Neoplasms

Although Hodgkin disease usually begins in the lymph nodes, the spleen may be the primary site. In either case, eventually the spleen becomes involved.[29]

Irregular tumor-like nodules appear in the spleen. In both Hodgkin and non-Hodgkin lymphoma, involvement of the spleen may appear as focal hypoechoic or hyperechoic masses, diffuse splenomegaly, or normal splenic contour and size[17] (Fig. 8-15). Lymphoid neoplasms respond to a series of standard chemotherapeutic regimens; however, the majority of patients remain incurable.[29]

Vascular neoplasms of the spleen are rare, but they are the most common hematopoietic proliferation of the organ. These lesions include hemangiomas, lymphangiomas, hamartomas, littoral cell angiomas, hemangioendotheliomas, myoid angioendotheliomas, and angiosarcomas.[30] Angiosarcomas often present as a left upper quadrant mass and may be clinically associated with pain, malaise, fever, anemia, and weight loss. Spontaneous rupture with hemoperitoneum may be the initial presentation. They are equally distributed among men and women and the prognosis is very poor. Sonographically, angiosarcomas appear solid with nodular areas of mixed echogenicity[17] (Fig. 8-16).

## Metastatic Lesions

Despite its rich blood supply, metastases to the spleen seem relatively uncommon. Metastatic involvement of the spleen by carcinoma is usually seen in advanced cases of disease when the carcinoma has already metastasized or directly invaded other visceral organs.[31] Metastases spread from a variety of neoplasms, including those of the lung, breast, pancreas, and ovary. Overall, melanoma is the most frequent metastatic lesion of the spleen. Metastatic lesions usually present as hypoechoic masses,

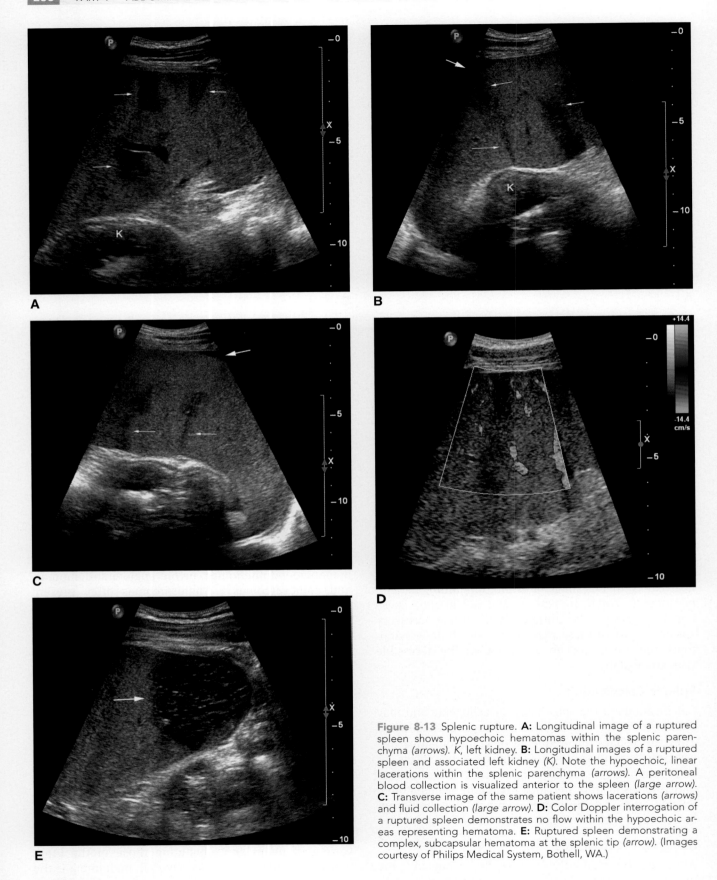

**Figure 8-13** Splenic rupture. **A:** Longitudinal image of a ruptured spleen shows hypoechoic hematomas within the splenic paren-chyma *(arrows)*. *K*, left kidney. **B:** Longitudinal images of a ruptured spleen and associated left kidney *(K)*. Note the hypoechoic, linear lacerations within the splenic parenchyma *(arrows)*. A peritoneal blood collection is visualized anterior to the spleen *(large arrow)*. **C:** Transverse image of the same patient shows lacerations *(arrows)* and fluid collection *(large arrow)*. **D:** Color Doppler interrogation of a ruptured spleen demonstrates no flow within the hypoechoic ar-eas representing hematoma. **E:** Ruptured spleen demonstrating a complex, subcapsular hematoma at the splenic tip *(arrow)*. (Images courtesy of Philips Medical System, Bothell, WA.)

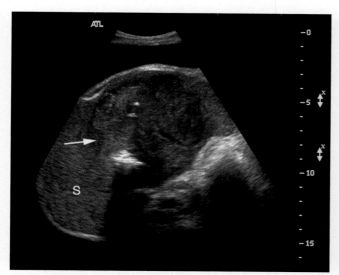

**Figure 8-14** Splenic mass. Longitudinal image of a complex splenic mass with calcifications *(arrow)*. (Image courtesy of Philips Medical System, Bothell, WA.)

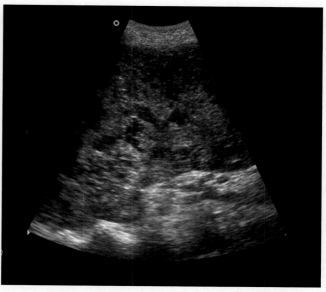

**Figure 8-16** Angiosarcoma. Diffusely abnormal spleen demonstrating mixed echogenicity consistent with angiosarcoma. (Image courtesy of Philips Medical System, Bothell, WA.)

although hyperechoic and complex lesions have been identified[7,17] (Fig. 8-17).There is no consistent correlation between the sonographic appearance of the lesions and the histologic type of primary tumor. Fine needle biopsy is a safe and efficient method of diagnosing splenic nodules and is necessary for definitive diagnosis. Needles with a caliber of 22- to 23-gauge should be used, and a bleeding diathesis should be excluded prior to the procedure to avoid unexpected hemorrhagic complications.[32]

## Acquired Aplasia and Hypoplasia

A small nonfunctional spleen is associated with repeated infarction, as occurs with sickle cell anemia. In such cases, the spleen is small, fibrotic, and calcified.

## Benign Hemangioma

Hemangiomas are the most common benign vascular neoplasm of the spleen and may be broadly described as congenital hamartomas.[7,17,33] They may be divided into capillary and cavernous types.[8] The sonographic appearance is variable, including well-defined, echopenic foci with enhanced through transmission, echogenic masses, and mixed complex masses, similar in appearance to hepatic hemangiomas. Rarely splenic hemangiomas may contain calcifications.[7,17] Differential diagnoses due to the complex appearance may include hydatid cyst, abscess, and metastases. Hemangiomas are generally isolated phenomena, but

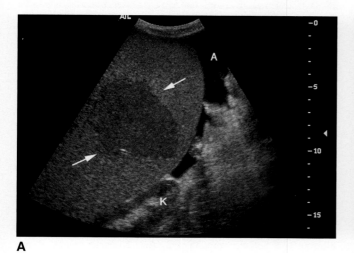

**A**

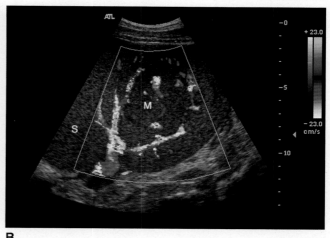

**B**

**Figure 8-15 A:** Hypoechoic intraparenchymal splenic mass *(arrows)* with associated ascites *(A)*. Left kidney *(K)* is compressed due to splenomegaly. **B:** Color Doppler of the splenic mass *(M)* demonstrating blood flow within the hypoechoic lesion. (Images courtesy of Philips Medical System, Bothell, WA.)

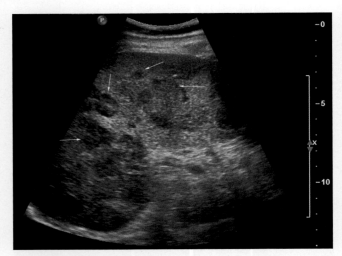

**Figure 8-17** Metastases. Longitudinal image of the spleen demonstrating multiple solid, hypoechoic masses characteristic of metastases. Many of the masses demonstrate a "bull's-eye" appearance with a hyperechoic center and a hypoechoic rim *(arrows)*. (Image courtesy of Philips Medical System, Bothell, WA.)

they may occur in association with Klippel-Trenaunay-Weber syndrome.[7,17] Duplex Doppler and color Doppler have demonstrated flow in the hypoechoic areas and may be useful in distinguishing between hemangiomas and infarctions, which are usually avascular. The introduction of microbubble contrast agents offers an option to improve the ability of sonography in characterizing splenic lesions[34] (Fig. 8-18). Symptoms are usually secondary to rupture or compression of adjoining structures. A pathologically involved spleen demonstrates enlargement, with nodular areas corresponding to cystic spaces containing serous fluid and coagulated blood. Other common lesions include lipomatous hamartomas and lymphangiomas.[30] These lesions cannot be differentiated sonographically.

## Acquired Immunodeficiency Syndrome (AIDS)

Human Immunodeficiency virus (HIV) is frequently accompanied by opportunistic infections and lymphoma, which affect the spleen as well as other abdominal

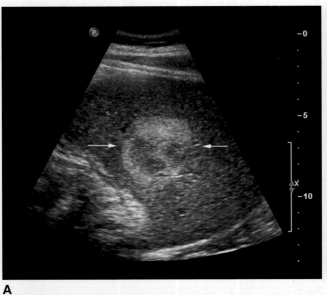

**A**

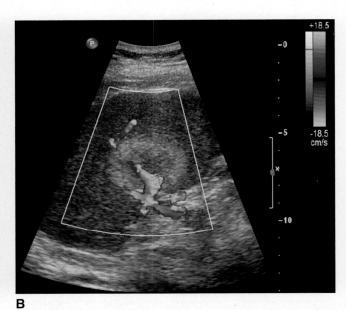

**B**

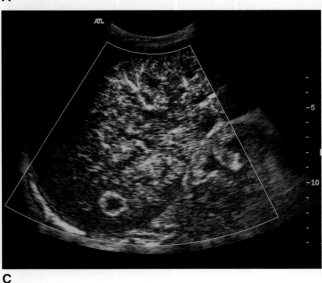

**C**

**Figure 8-18** Splenic hemangioma. **A:** Transverse image of the spleen demonstrates a focal, echogenic lesion consistent with a splenic hemangioma *(arrows)*. **B:** Color Doppler investigation of the splenic hemangioma. **C:** Splenic hemangioma imaged using contrast enhancement and power Doppler. (Images courtesy of Philips Medical System, Bothell, WA.)

## Critical Thinking Questions

1. A 22-year-old patient with a history of leukemia presents with left upper quadrant pain. The spleen is normal in size, but contains a hypoechoic wedge-shaped area. What does this likely represent?

2. A 45-year-old patient presents for an abdominal sonography examination to rule out gallstones. In taking a history, the sonographer learns that the patient had a splenectomy many years ago. While scanning the left side, the sonographer images an area that looks like the spleen. If the patient had a splenectomy, what could this area represent?

3. What are the most common causes of splenomegaly?

4. A patient with a history of Hodgkin lymphoma presents for an abdominal sonography examination to evaluate the spleen. What should the sonographer expect to find?

viscera and the retroperitoneum. Most commonly, an enlarged spleen, with or without associated adenopathy in the splenic hilus, is identified in HIV seropositive patients. Tuberculosis, lymphoma, and Kaposi sarcoma, associated with AIDS patients, appear as hypodense nodular implants within the splenic parenchyma. Patients with *Candida*, *P. jiroveci*, or *Mycobacterium avium* may demonstrate numerous punctuate nonshadowing calcifications typical of granulomatous disease within the spleen, liver, kidneys, and adrenal glands.[7,8]

## SUMMARY

- The spleen is an intraperitoneal organ located in the left upper quadrant of the abdomen.

- In the adult, the spleen measures approximately 12 cm in length and is surrounded by a fibrous capsule.

- The spleen serves a number of functions including acting as a reservoir for blood, destroying and removing red blood cells from circulation, and playing a role in the body's immune response.

- An accessory spleen, a normal variant in 10% to 30% of the population, usually measures 1.5 to 2 cm and is typically found in the splenic hilum or along the gastrosplenic ligament omentum.

- In cases of splenic ptosis, or wandering spleen, the supporting ligaments of the spleen are lax and allow the spleen to migrate along the left side from the thorax to the pelvis making it susceptible to torsion and infarction.

- Splenomegaly is the most common sonographically observed splenic abnormality and is diagnosed when the spleen measure greater than 13 cm in length.

- Splenomegaly can come from a number of causes, including portal hypertension, infection, metabolic and hematologic disorders, trauma, and infiltrative processes such as leukemia and lymphoma.

- Splenic cysts are either congenital or acquired. Acquired cysts can be parasitic (echinococcal), postinflammatory (final stage of an abscess), or traumatic (sequelae to hematoma or infarct).

- Splenic abscesses are typically multiple, complex lesions with mixed echogenicity and are often the result of infection spread through the bloodstream.

- Sonographically, acute splenic infarcts are well-defined, hypoechoic, wedge-shaped, or round areas seen along the periphery of the spleen.

- The spleen is frequently injured in cases of blunt abdominal trauma and fracture of the splenic capsule, parenchymal lacerations, and focal parenchymal or subcapsular hematomas may occur.

- In a trauma setting, an enlarging, heterogeneous spleen suggests a ruptured spleen.

- In Hodgkin and non-Hodgkin lymphoma, involvement of the spleen may appear normal, may have focal hypoechoic or hyperechoic masses, or may be diffusely enlarged.

- Although radionuclide imaging and CT are often the first studies conducted of the spleen, sonography is effective in characterizing masses, in identifying the nature of palpated left-sided upper quadrant masses, in monitoring the course of trauma to the spleen, and in locating intraperitoneal blood collections.

## ACKNOWLEDGMENT

The author would like to acknowledge Mimi Berman, Barbara Wajsbrot-Kandel, and Sherman S. Lipshitz for their work on the previous editions.

### REFERENCES

1. Tortora G, Grabowski S. *Principles of Anatomy and Physiology*. 9th ed. New York, NY: Biological Sciences Textbooks Inc; 2000.
2. Moore K, Dalley A, Agur A. *Clinically Oriented Anatomy*. 6th ed. Philadelphia, PA: Lippincott Williams & Wilkins; 2010.
3. Kelley L, Petersen C. *Sectional Anatomy for Imaging Professionals*. 2nd ed. St. Louis, MO: Elsevier Mosby; 2007.
4. Jenkins G, Kemnitz C, Tortora G. *Anatomy and Physiology: From Science to Life*. Hoboken, NJ: John Wiley & Sons, Inc; 2007.
5. Gomez D, Patel R, Rahman S, et al. Torsion of a wandering spleen associated with congenital malrotation of the gastrointestinal tract. *Internet J Radiol*. 2006;5:1.

6. Megremis SD, Vlachonikolis IG, Tsilimigaki AM. Spleen length in childhood with US: normal values based on age, sex, and somatometric parameters. *Radiology.* 2004;231(1):129–134.

7. Rumack C, Wilson S, Charboneau JW, et al. *Diagnostic Ultrasound.* St Louis, MO: Elsevier Mosby; 2004.

8. McCance K, Huether S. *Pathophysiology: The Biologic Basis for Disease in Adults and Children.* 5th ed. St. Louis, MO: Elsevier Mosby; 2006.

9. Steiniger B, Ulfig N, Risse M, et al. Fetal and early postnatal development of the human spleen: from primordial arterial B cell lobules to a non-segmented organ. *Histochem Cell Biol.* 2007;128(3):205–215.

10. Gilbert B, Menetrey C, Belin V, et al. Familial isolated congenital asplenia: a rare, frequently hereditary dominant condition, often detected too late as a cause of overwhelming pneumococcal sepsis. Report of a new case and review of 31 others. *Eur J Pediatr.* 2002;161(7):368–372.

11. Kim MK, Im CM, Oh SH, et al. Unusual presentation of right-side accessory spleen mimicking a retroperitoneal tumor. *Int J Urol.* 2008;15(8):739–740.

12. Jeanty C, Ismail L, Turner C. Incidental findings during routine antepartum obstetrical sonography. *JDMS.* 2008; 24(6):344–360.

13. Kirshtein B, Lantsberg S, Hatskelzon L, et al. Laparoscopic accessory splenectomy using intraoperative gamma probe guidance. *J Laparoendosc Adv Surg Tech.* 2007;17(2): 205–208.

14. Cavazos S, Ratzer ER, Fenoglio ME. Laparoscopic management of the wandering spleen. *J Laparoendosc Adv Surg Tech.* 2004;14(4):227–229.

15. Hedeshian MH, Hirsh MP, Danielson PD. Laparoscopic splenopexy of a pediatric wandering spleen by creation of a retroperitoneal pocket. *J Laparoendosc Adv Surg Tech.* 2005;15(6):670–672.

16. Stoehr GA, Stauffer UG, Eber SW. Near-total splenectomy: a new technique for the management of hereditary spherocytosis. *Br J Haematol.* 2005;241(1):40–47.

17. Henningsen C. *Clinical Guide to Ultrasonography.* St. Louis, MO: Mosby; 2004.

18. Sanders R, Winter T. *Clinical Sonography: A Practical Guide.* Baltimore, MD: Lippincott Williams & Wilkins; 2007.

19. Owen C, Meyers P. Sonographic evaluation of the portal and hepatic systems. *JDMS.* 2006;22:317–328.

20. Gerwe L, Haas, A. Echinococcal liver cyst. *JDMS.* 2003; 19(6):369–371.

21. Chandra S, NandaKishore M, Bhuvaneswari, V. Splenic pseudocyst with hypersplenism—Therapeutic implications of a rare association. *Internet J Surg.* 2007;9(2): 22–23.

22. Yigitbasi R, Karabicak I, Aydog, F, et al. Benign splenic epithelial cyst accompanied by elevated Ca 19–9 level: a case report. *Mt Sinai J Med.* 2006;73(6):871–873.

23. Takayama A, Nakashima O, Kobayashi K, et al. Splenic lymphangioma with papillary endothelial proliferation: a case report and review of the literature. *Pathol Int.* 2003;53:483–488.

24. Bieker T. Sonographic evaluation of a pancreatic pseudocyst in conjunction with portal vein thrombosis and cavernous transformation. *JDMS.* 2000;16:23–25.

25. Mahesh B, Muwanga CL. Splenic infarct: a rare cause of spontaneous rupture leading to massive haemoperitoneum. *ANZ J Surg.* 2004;74:1030–1032.

26. Mauritz W, Weninger P. Multislice computed tomography in blunt abdominal trauma. *Trauma.* 2007;9:195–212.

27. Valentino M, Serra C, Pavlica P, et al. Blunt abdominal trauma: diagnostic performance of contrast-enhanced US in children—Initial experience. *Radiology.* 2008;246(3): 903–909.

28. Whitfield C, Garner J. Beyond splenectomy options for the management of splenic trauma. *Trauma.* 2008;10: 247–257.

29. Musteata VG, Corcimaru IT, Iacovleva IA, et al. Treatment options for primary splenic low-grade non-Hodgkin's lymphomas. *Clin Lab Haem.* 2004;26:397–401.

30. Karim RZ, Ma-Wyatt J, Cox M, et al. Myoid angioendothelioma of the spleen. *Int J Surg Pathol.* 2004;12(1):51–56.

31. Kochar K, Vijayasekar C, Pandey U, et al. Primary carcinosarcoma of the spleen: case report of a rare tumor and review of the literature. *Int J Surg Pathol.* 2009;17(1): 72–77.

32. Kumar PV, Monabati A, Raseki AR, et al. Splenic lesions: FNA findings in 48 cases. *Cytopathology.* 2007;18: 151–156.

33. Ali TZ, Beyer G, Taylor M, et al. Splenic hamartoma: immunohistochemical and ultrastructural profile of two cases. *Int J Surg Pathol.* 2005;13(1):103–111.

34. Stang A, Keles H, Hentschke S, et al. Differentiation of benign from malignant focal splenic lesions using sulfur hexafluoride-filled microbubble contrast-enhances pulse-inversion sonography. *Am J Roentgenol.* 2009;193(3): 709–721.

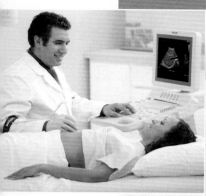

# 9 The Gastrointestinal Tract

John F. Trombly

## OBJECTIVES

Illustrate the anatomy of the gastrointestinal tract.

Define the process for sonographic evaluation of the gastrointestinal tract, including the transabdominal and endoluminal approaches.

List the five sonographic layers of the bowel wall.

Describe the normal sonographic appearance of the stomach, small bowel, appendix, and colon.

Discuss disorders of the stomach, small bowel, appendix, and colon that can be visualized sonographically.

## KEY TERMS

adenocarcinoma | appendiceal abscess | appendicitis | carcinoid tumor | Crohn disease | diverticulosis | duodenal ulcer | gastric carcinoma | gastric dilatation | gastric ulcer disease | gastritis | hematoma | intussusception | leiomyoma | leiomyosarcoma | lymphoma | mucocele | peptic ulcer | small bowel edema | small bowel obstruction | squamous cell carcinoma | ulcerative colitis | volvulus

## GLOSSARY

**appendicolith** a fecalith or calcification found in the appendiceal lumen

**dysphagia** difficulty swallowing

**ileus** failure of the intestine to propel its contents due to diminished motility

**peristalsis** rhythmic dilatation and contraction that propels the contents of the gastrointestinal tract

**ulcer** an erosion in the mucosal layer of the wall of the gastrointestinal tract; frequently located in the stomach or duodenum

**volvulus** abnormal twisting of the intestines that can lead to obstruction, gangrene, perforation, and peritonitis

The gastrointestinal (GI) tract is not often imaged by sonographers due to the difficulty in evaluating the structures. Gas in the GI tract can obscure details of the bowel wall and lumen as well as structures deep to the bowel such as the pancreas and the periaortic area of the retroperitoneum. Fluid or feces in the bowel lumen can be misinterpreted as non-GI disease. Development of specialized transrectal and endoscopic sonographic instruments now allow for successful and reliable sonographic evaluation of the GI tract.

## SONOGRAPHIC EXAMINATION TECHNIQUE

Real-time transducers provide the sonographic equivalent of fluoroscopy. The peristaltic activity visible on real-time examinations is nearly impossible to capture on still images but is invaluable to the sonographer who is identifying the GI tract and evaluating its function.

Two broad classes of sonographic examinations are performed on the GI tract: transabdominal and endoluminal. Transabdominal sonography is the traditional method, often used as a screening procedure to evaluate abdominal or pelvic pain or mass. Although the GI tract is not usually the primary focus of an abdominal sonogram, the clinician will find the examination more informative if the sonographer can identify GI lesions that may cause nonspecific abdominal symptoms.

Endoluminal sonographic examinations, however, are directed specifically at the bowel or the surrounding structures. Transrectal sonography, used to evaluate the prostate gland, is also suitable for evaluating the rectal wall and perirectal area and can be used to stage rectal tumors. The advantage of the endoluminal approach is that higher frequency transducers can be used and the layers of the bowel wall can be imaged.

Endosonography is not widely used by general sonographers but is performed by gastroenterologists using specialized endoscopes. Its chief advantage over optical endoscopy is its ability to "see" the layers of the bowel wall, making it useful for staging bowel malignancies and evaluating lesions of the deep layers of the wall that do not involve the superficial part of the mucosa.[1] Sonographically guided biopsy of such lesions enhances the diagnostic process.[1] Endosonography has been performed primarily on the upper GI tract: the esophagus, stomach, and duodenum. The method of examination is similar to conventional upper GI endoscopy. Following the usual premedication, the sonoendoscope is introduced into the esophagus with the patient in the left lateral decubitus position. When the lesion is identified visually, it can be examined with the attached sonographic transducer.

## PATIENT PREPARATION

Preparation of the patient for transabdominal sonography of the GI tract depends on the part of the tract that is of interest. Because examination of the upper abdomen looks at the gallbladder, pancreas, bile ducts, and upper GI tract, the patient should be advised to fast for about 4 hours before the examination to ensure distension of the gallbladder and to minimize stomach gas. If the stomach and duodenum are to be further evaluated, the patient can drink 10 to 40 oz of water through a straw to improve visualization. Having the patient drink fluid also helps in evaluating the mucosa and peristalsis of the jejunum and ileum. Oral fluid is, of course, contraindicated if the patient has GI obstruction or ileus or is scheduled for upper GI barium studies. For transabdominal examination of the colon, no special preparation is necessary, except for the rare occasion during pelvic sonography when a water enema is required to establish the position of the rectosigmoid colon. Before transrectal sonography, a cleansing enema may be helpful so that fecal material is not confused with mucosal lesions.

## ANATOMY OF THE BOWEL WALL

The GI tract is, essentially, a very long muscular tube, originating at the mouth and terminating at the anus (Fig. 9-1). The layers of the bowel wall are the same throughout the GI tract.[2] Described anatomically, the innermost layer is the epithelium, which in the esophagus is squamous and elsewhere a layer of cuboidal cells atop villi and glands. Deep to the epithelium lies the lamina propria, which in the esophagus is loose areolar tissue and elsewhere is glandular tissue. Immediately below the lamina propria is a very thin, smooth muscle layer called the *muscularis mucosa*. Just above and

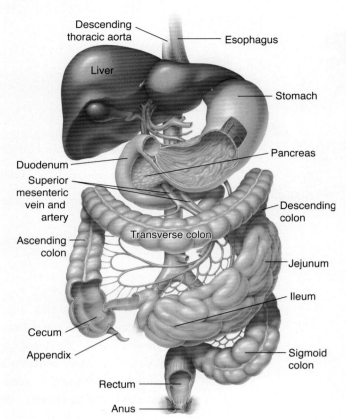

**Figure 9-1** Gastrointestinal tract. Anatomic drawing of the gastrointestinal tract.

below the muscularis mucosa are scattered patches of lymphoid tissue. Below the muscularis mucosa is more loose areolar tissue, called the *submucosa*. Deeper yet lies the muscularis propria, also known as the *muscularis externa*. This structure consists of an inner circumferential layer and an outer longitudinal layer of smooth muscle. The final layer of the wall is the serosa, a thin epithelial layer on the periphery of the bowel.

The structure of the bowel wall is sonographically visible using endoluminal transducers and is sometimes visible transabdominally, particularly in the stomach[1] (Fig. 9-2A). The innermost sonographic layer is an echogenic line that represents the fluid-mucosa interface.[2] Deep to that is a hypoechoic layer: the mucosa, lamina propria, and muscularis mucosa.[2] Deeper yet is the echogenic submucosa, followed by a hypoechoic layer, the muscularis propria, which in turn is followed by a thin echogenic layer, the serosa. Thus, the sonographic structure of the bowel is usually described as five layers: three echogenic layers separated by two hypoechoic ones[1,2] (Fig. 9-2B,C). Using high frequency transducers, the muscularis mucosa and the two layers of the muscularis propria can be resolved as well. Visualizing the layers of the bowel wall is useful in detecting certain pathologic conditions that will be discussed later.

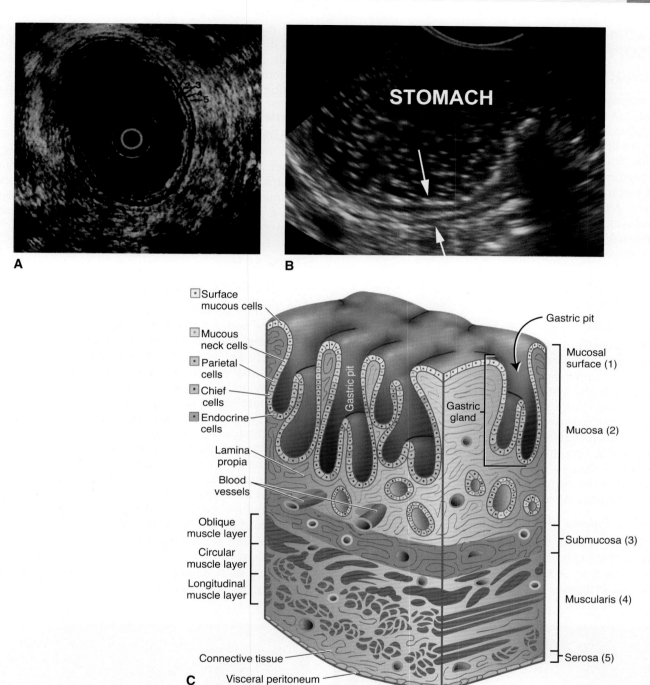

**Figure 9-2** Bowel wall. **A:** Endoscopic sonographic appearance of the normal gastric wall at the level of the body of the stomach. Five distinct layers of different echogenicity can be identified. (From Bolondi L, Casanova, P, Caletti GC, et al. Primary gastric lymphoma versus gastric carcinoma: endoscopic US evaluation. *Radiology*. 1987;165:821–826.) **B:** Sonographic image of the fluid-filled stomach demonstrates the five sonographically visible bowel wall layers (*arrows*): three echogenic and two hypoechoic layers. (Image courtesy of Philips Medical Systems, Bothell, WA.) **C:** Drawing of the gastric wall layers. The corresponding sonographic layers are numbered: mucosal surface (*1*), deeper part of the mucosa and the muscularis mucosa (*2*), submucosa (*3*), muscularis propria, which anatomically has a longitudinal muscle layer and a circular muscle layer (*4*), and serosa (*5*).

# ESOPHAGUS AND ESOPHAGOGASTRIC JUNCTION

## SONOGRAPHIC TECHNIQUE

Sonographic imaging of the esophagus is accomplished only via the sonoendoscope. With proper technique and equipment, the examiner can visualize fairly well the layers of the esophageal wall and surrounding mediastinal structures.[1] Sonographic endoscopy has demonstrated excellent sensitivity and specificity in the staging of esophageal cancer, particularly in the advanced stages.[1,3,4] Although esophageal varices are visible with sonoendoscopy, they can be assessed adequately with optical endoscopy. The esophagogastric junction can sometimes be viewed transabdominally (Fig. 9-3).

## DISORDERS OF THE ESOPHAGUS AND ESOPHAGOGASTRIC JUNCTION

### Carcinoma

Until recently, most carcinomas of the esophagus were squamous cell carcinomas.[4] These occur least commonly in the upper esophagus, and with about equal frequency in the middle and lower thirds. Squamous cell carcinoma of the esophagus affects older persons and more men than women. The lesions begin as longitudinal plaque-like areas, which quickly enlarge circumferentially; subsequently, strictures form and dysphagia develops. Because the esophagus lacks a serosa, extension into the surrounding mediastinum is unimpeded and few patients survive 5 years after diagnosis.

### Other Tumors of the Esophagus

Over the last 20 years, the incidence of adenocarcinoma of the esophagus has steadily increased, accounting for more than 50% of new cases of esophageal cancer. Adenocarcinoma of the esophagus primarily affects white males and is associated with gastroesophageal reflux disease. Rare malignant tumors of the esophagus include carcinosarcoma, lymphoma, mucoepidermoid carcinoma, and adenoid cystic carcinoma. The most common benign tumor of the esophagus is leiomyoma.

### Disorders of the Esophagogastric Junction

The esophagogastric junction can be evaluated with endosonography or, if the left lobe of the liver is large enough, with transabdominal sonography. The esophagogastric junction can be seen posterior to the left lobe and anterior to the abdominal aorta.[2] One can demonstrate a variety of abnormalities, including hiatal hernia, esophageal varices, and tumors.

# STOMACH

## SONOGRAPHIC TECHNIQUE

Of the entire GI tract, the stomach has the most potential for better sonographic diagnosis. The layers of the GI tract wall are thicker here than anywhere else and nearly always can be visualized transabdominally in the normal patient. A few special techniques are occasionally helpful. If uncertainty exists whether a cystic structure in the left upper quadrant represents the stomach, giving the patient a few sips of water through a straw produces a sparkling or swirling pattern in the stomach as the water flows. Usually, the stomach contains some air when the patient is supine. Turning the patient into the right lateral decubitus position moves fluid into the antrum, providing better visualization of that part of the stomach and confirming the identity of the stomach. Similarly, turning the patient into the left lateral decubitus position often improves visualization of the fundus.

When a solid-looking mass is suspected to be in the stomach, or when detailed evaluation of the gastric

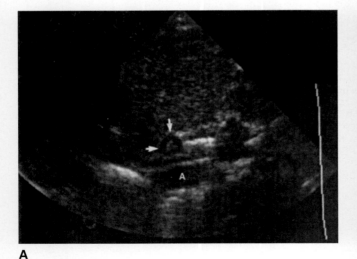
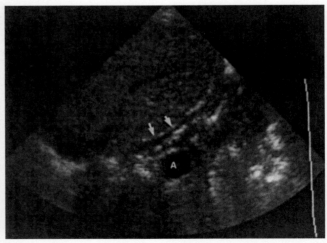

**A**    **B**

**Figure 9-3** Esophagogastric junction. Longitudinal **(A)** and transverse **(B)** normal esophagogastric junction (*arrows*) traversing between the aorta (*A*) and liver. Note the typical target appearance on the longitudinal view.

mucosa is required, the patient should sit up and slowly drink 40 to 50 oz of water and then be scanned in the upright, left lateral decubitus, supine, and right lateral decubitus positions, thus demonstrating most of the gastric mucosa. Some investigators recommend giving 1 mg of glucagon intravenously before the patient drinks the water to ensure retention of the fluid in the stomach—this should produce 30 to 60 minutes of gastric distention.

## NORMAL ANATOMY OF THE STOMACH

The stomach normally lies in the left upper quadrant of the abdomen. The fundus is medial to the spleen and anterior to the left kidney.[2] The body and antrum of the stomach lie posterior or inferior to the left lobe of the liver, anterior to the pancreas, and medial to the gallbladder and porta hepatis.[2] The antrum and body of the stomach often appear as a target-like structure inferior to the left lobe on longitudinal sonograms. If the left hepatic lobe is large enough, the esophagogastric junction can also be visualized as a target-like structure just below the diaphragm and just to the left of the spine. Gas, mucus, or fluid may fill the center of the stomach (Fig. 9-4). If the stomach is not distended, the bowel wall should measure 2- to 6-mm thick. When the stomach is distended to a diameter of ≥8 cm, the wall should measure 2 to 4 mm. Often, when fluid is present in the stomach, the rugal folds and posterior wall structure can be seen.

## DISORDERS OF THE STOMACH

### Gastric Dilatation

Many disorders can cause the stomach to dilate. Acute dilatation can occur after surgery or after placement of a body cast. It is not clear whether this dilatation is caused by reflex paralysis of gastric motility or obstruction of the duodenum by the superior mesenteric artery impinging on it. Tumor or ulcer disease may obstruct the gastric outlet. Pyloric muscle hypertrophy is rare in adults, but when it does occur, it is usually associated with gastritis or ulcer disease. Diabetes mellitus, scleroderma, or surgical vagotomy may bring about gastric dilatation as a complication of neuropathy. Observation of gastric peristalsis can be made to differentiate atonic from obstructive dilatation, but the distinction may be impossible in many cases because of rigidity of the stomach wall, often seen in tumor infiltration and gastric ulcer disease and the uncoordinated peristaltic waves seen in neuropathic conditions. Volvulus is another rare cause of gastric dilatation.

### Gastritis and Ulcer Disease

Chronic gastritis may present as enlarged rugal folds with generalized thickening of the mucosal layer of the wall (Fig. 9-5). This thickening may accompany either increased acid production, as in Zollinger-Ellison syndrome, or decreased acid production, as in Ménétrier disease. Chronic gastritis may also demonstrate hyperplastic and inflammatory polyps. Another variation is atrophic gastritis, in which the mucosa is thinned. This is difficult to see sonographically, but it is considered a precursor of gastric carcinoma.

Gastric peptic ulcers are one-third as common in the United States as duodenal ulcers. Benign peptic gastric ulcers can occur anywhere in the stomach but most often appear along the antral portion of the lesser curvature. Sonographically, there may be major wall

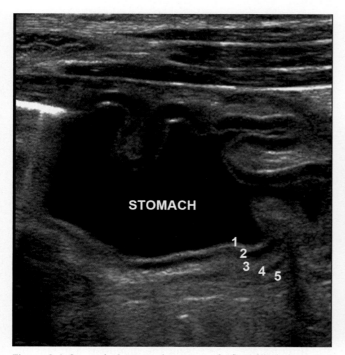

**Figure 9-4** Stomach. Sonographic image of a fluid-filled, distended stomach. Note the five sonographically visible layers of the stomach. (Image courtesy of Philips Medical Systems, Bothell, WA.)

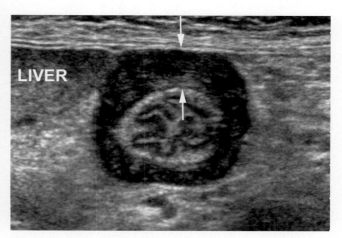

**Figure 9-5** Gastritis. Transverse image of an inflamed stomach demonstrates a thickened hypoechoic mucosal layer of the stomach wall (*arrows*). (Image courtesy of Philips Medical Systems, Bothell, WA.)

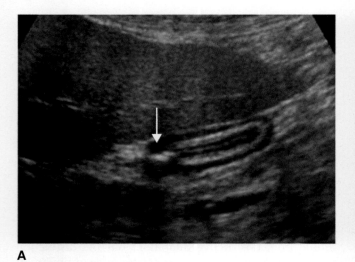

**A**

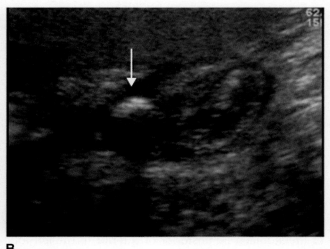

**B**

**Figure 9-6** Gastric ulcer. **A,B:** Longitudinal images demonstrate the gastric antrum in a patient with an air-filled benign gastric ulcer (*arrow*). (Images courtesy of Dr. Taco Geertsma, Hospital Gelderse Vallei, Ede, The Netherlands.)

thickening, usually caused by marked edema of the submucosa, with milder thickening of the gastric mucosa (Fig. 9-6A,B). Typically, the mucosa is undercut at the edge of the ulcer. A malignant ulcer, by contrast, should show more "heaping up" of the margin of the ulcer. The bowel layers adjacent to the ulcer may be obliterated in either benign or malignant ulcers. Ulcers can be detected sonographically, particularly if they are large, but often they are only suggested by focal or generalized edema of the wall. Peptic duodenal ulcers are even more difficult to identify, but mucosal edema can sometimes suggest their presence.

Complications of peptic ulcer disease, gastric or duodenal, include anterior or posterior perforation. Usually, anterior perforation results in free intraperitoneal air and, often, subsequent peritonitis, which may appear sonographically as ascites, loculated ascites, or dense debris in the peritoneal space. Thickening of the bowel serosa may be observed due to peritoneal irritation and reactive edema. Generalized peritoneal infection or localized abscess may also result. The chief complication of posterior duodenal perforation is bleeding, but posterior perforation of the stomach may result in pancreatitis.

### Gastroduodenal Crohn Disease

Crohn disease is an idiopathic inflammation that starts in the submucosa and spreads to all layers of the bowel wall. This disease usually occurs in young adults and affects the ileum primarily, and to a lesser extent the colon. Two percent to 8% of patients have stomach or duodenal involvement. Because the entire wall is involved at diagnosis, the sonographic appearance is that of a nonspecific hypoechoic target lesion if the lumen is viewed transversely. Advanced carcinoma, lymphoma, hematoma, and tuberculosis can appear similar.

### Other Inflammatory Conditions

Infection of the stomach can display marked thickening of the stomach wall and swelling of the gastric rugae, a condition called *phlegmonous gastritis*. Most cases are caused by α-hemolytic streptococci but *Staphylococcus, Escherichia coli, Clostridium welchii,* and *Proteus* species have also been found. Peritonitis occurs in 70% of cases. When gas-forming organisms such as *E. coli* or *C. welchii* are the cause, small gas bubbles may form in the gastric wall—this is a type of emphysematous gastritis. Swallowing a corrosive substance is a more common cause of emphysematous gastritis.

### Benign Gastric Tumors

Benign gastric tumors are rare and most are asymptomatic. Hyperplastic polyps and gastric adenomas are polypoid masses arising from the gastric mucosa; adenomas seem to have some malignant potential. Gastric cysts develop by cystic dilatation of gastric glandular tissue and enlarge into the submucosal space. Other types of tumors arise from the submucosal or muscle layer and spare the mucosa unless surface ulceration develops. Lipomas are generally echogenic. Smooth muscle tumors may show a typical swirled texture if they are large enough.

### Carcinoma

Gastric carcinoma is very common and is the second leading cause of cancer-related death in the world. Japan, Chile, Iceland, and Finland have gastric cancer rates up to seven times higher than that of the United States.

Survival rates range from 5% to 95% depending on the tumor stage. The earlier the diagnosis and staging, the better the prognosis.[3] Sonography is useful in the diagnosis and staging of gastrointestinal tumors.[5,6]

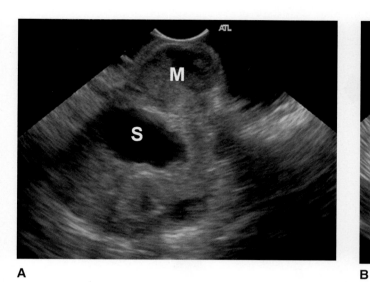

**A**

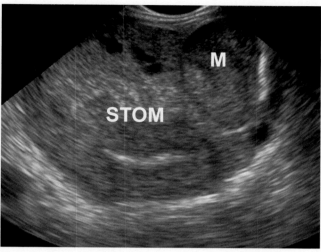

**B**

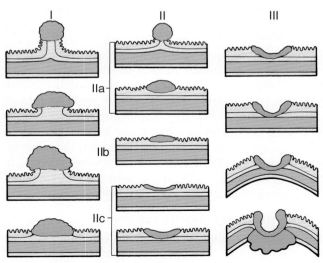

**C**

**Figure 9-7** Gastric carcinoma. **A,B:** Sonographic images of the stomach *(S, STOM)* demonstrate a thickened gastric wall and a well-defined hypoechoic mass *(M)*. Differential diagnosis of this mass includes leiomyoma and leiomyosarcoma. **C:** Sonographic image of a large heterogeneous gastric mass demonstrates color flow within the mass. (Images courtesy of Philips Medical Systems, Bothell, WA.)

Gastric carcinoma arises from the mucosa of the stomach, invading the submucosa and muscularis propria (Fig. 9-7A–C). Borrmann classification of gastric cancer divides lesions into four categories. In this system, a type 1 lesion is a focal polypoid mass. A type 2 lesion is a focal ulcerating tumor, and a type 3 lesion is also a tumor ulcer but has more extensive surrounding infiltration. A type 4 lesion demonstrates extensive infiltration of the stomach wall and may involve the entire stomach[7] (Fig. 9-8). Most gastric carcinomas spread primarily toward the serosa of the gastric wall. Some gastric tumors arise in the margin of a long-standing benign peptic ulcer.

## Lymphoma

Primary lymphoma of the stomach accounts for 3% to 8% of gastric malignancies. Reticulum cell sarcoma or lymphosarcoma are the most common, with Hodgkin

**Figure 9-8** Borrmann classification of gastric carcinoma.

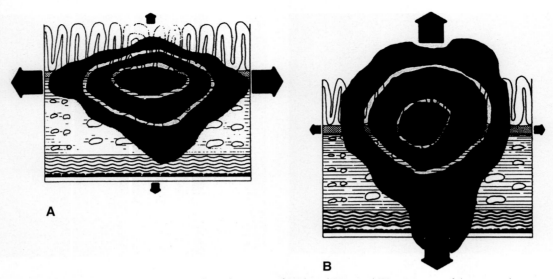

**Figure 9-9** Gastric tumor invasion. Growth pattern of **(A)** lymphoma and **(B)** carcinoma of the stomach.

lymphoma rarer.[8] The stomach is the most common site of primary lymphoma of the GI tract. The cells of origin are lymphocytes located just above and below the muscularis mucosa. Typically, lymphoma initially involves the outer part of the lamina propria and the inner part of the submucosa. Endosonography characteristically reveals this involvement as well as a tendency for the tumor to spread laterally following the muscularis mucosa rather than vertically through the layers of the wall as in gastric carcinoma (Fig. 9-9). The fact that the surface of the mucosa is not involved until quite late in the disease seems to be one of the primary reasons for interest in endosonography. Some lymphomatous lesions, however, do appear polypoid by endosonography and are difficult to differentiate from gastric carcinoma. By transabdominal sonography, the thickened, hypoechoic gastric wall and the marked rugal thickening may be revealed. Sonographically, gastric carcinoma is sometimes more echogenic than lymphoma, and in infiltrative lesions all layers are more equally involved than in lymphoma.

### Leiomyosarcoma

*Leiomyosarcoma* is a rare tumor accounting for 0.5% to 3% of all malignant tumors of the stomach.[9] This smooth muscle tumor arises from the muscularis propria and is, therefore, primarily exophytic. The appearance is similar to the sonographically familiar uterine fibroid. It is difficult to differentiate sonographically or histologically from its benign counterpart, the leiomyoma. Tumors smaller than 4 or 5 cm are considered unlikely to undergo malignant transformation; however, hemorrhage and cystic degeneration can occur.

### Other Malignant Gastric Lesions

Other gastric malignancies include carcinoid, hemangioendothelioma, hemangiopericytoma, Kaposi sarcoma, liposarcoma, myxosarcoma, fibrosarcoma, and

secondary tumors. The most common primary sources for metastasis to the stomach are malignant melanoma, breast carcinoma, and bronchogenic carcinoma.

## DUODENUM

### SONOGRAPHIC TECHNIQUE

The duodenum is best visualized by examining before and after ingestion of water. The valvulae conniventes, the folds in the inside bowel wall from which the microscopic villi protrude, can sometimes be demonstrated.

### NORMAL ANATOMY OF THE DUODENUM

The duodenal bulb, the first portion of the duodenum, normally lies to the right of the gastric antrum, anterosuperior to the pancreatic head, and medial to the gallbladder. Then the duodenum bends inferiorly to the right of the pancreatic head, this is the second portion. Next, it bends to the left, extending inferior to the pancreas and passing between the superior mesenteric artery anteriorly and the aorta posteriorly, forming the third portion. The fourth extends superiorly and to the left, posterior to the stomach, becoming the jejunum at the ligament of Treitz.

## SMALL BOWEL

### SONOGRAPHIC TECHNIQUE

Drinking fluid may enhance visualization of the mucosa of the jejunum and ileum and demonstrate peristalsis. The best time to view the small bowel depends on the transit time of the bowel. If ileus or obstruction is present, however, taking additional fluid by mouth is not helpful. If the small bowel is distended with fluid, the valvulae conniventes of the mucosa and other layers of the bowel wall are usually visible transabdominally.

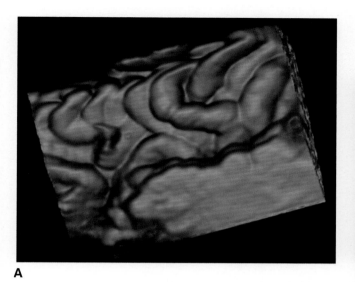
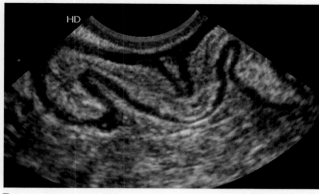

**A**    **B**

**Figure 9-10** Small bowel. **A:** Three-dimensional sonographic image of the small bowel. **B:** Longitudinal image of the normal, nondistended small bowel. (Image courtesy of Philips Medical Systems, Bothell, WA.)

## NORMAL ANATOMY OF THE SMALL BOWEL

The jejunum and ileum lie in the central portion of the abdomen, inferior to the liver and stomach and superior to the urinary bladder. With high resolution transabdominal transducers, loops in the small bowel can often be visualized even without distension by fluid or gas (Fig. 9-10A,B). These sections of bowel should be smaller than 3 cm in diameter and pliable on palpation and should demonstrate peristalsis. If fluid is present in the loops, the valvulae conniventes should be visible.

## DISORDERS OF THE SMALL BOWEL

### Ileus

*Ileus*, also called acute intestinal pseudo-obstruction, is characterized by failure of the intestine to propel its contents owing to diminished motility. The causes of ileus are numerous: peritonitis, spinal fracture, renal colic, acute pancreatitis, bowel ischemia, myocardial infarction, surgery, medications, hypokalemia, and infection, to name just a few. Sonographically, one sees small bowel distended with either air or fluid (Fig. 9-11A–C). Peristalsis is normal to somewhat increased. The bowel is less distended than when obstructed.

### Obstruction

Small bowel obstruction also has many causes, such as adhesions, inflammatory masses, neoplastic lesions, volvulus, intussusception, and luminal obstruction (such as fecal impaction).[10] Typically, the bowel loops are perfectly round in cross section, and peristalsis can

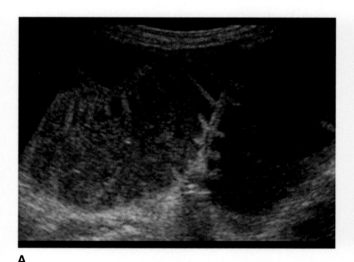
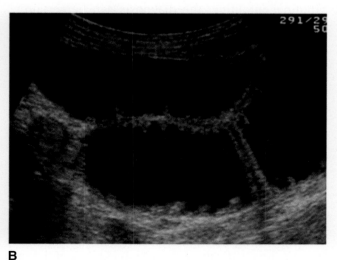

**A**    **B**

**Figure 9-11** Ileus. **A,B:** Longitudinal images demonstrate dilated fluid-filled bowel loops in a patient with ileus. *(continued)*

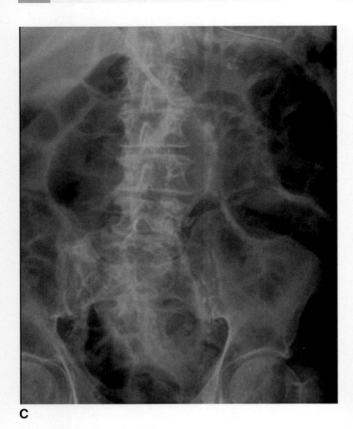

C

**Figure 9-11** *(continued)* **C:** Radiograph of the abdomen demonstrates dilated bowel loops consistent with ileus. (Images courtesy of Dr. Taco Geertsma, Hospital Gelderse Vallei, Ede, The Netherlands.)

vary from none to markedly increased. The valvulae conniventes are often visible (Fig. 9-12A–C).

In volvulus, the twisted, dilated loop appears C-shaped when viewed longitudinally, and often contains only fluid, no air. Intussusception, telescoping of the bowel into itself, is much rarer in adults than in children, and an identifiable bowel lesion is present in 75% to 80% of adults with this condition. The sonographic appearance of intussusception can be a nonspecific target lesion, but if one observes multiple concentric rings in the transverse view and longitudinal infolding, the diagnosis can be certain[10,11] (Fig. 9-13A,B).

### Hematoma

Hematoma of the bowel may result from trauma, ischemia, medication, or a hematologic abnormality such as hemophilia, Henoch-Schönlein purpura, anaphylactoid purpura, or thrombocytopenic purpura. Traumatic hematoma occurs most commonly in the duodenum because it is fixed in position and less able to move out of harm's way. In adults, a common cause of bowel hematoma is anticoagulant therapy. The most frequent cause of bowel ischemia is arterial obstruction. Sonographically, bowel hematoma is seen as nonspecific wall thickening of variable echogenicity. The thickening may be eccentric, and the mesentery may be involved. Often, there is thickening of the mucosal folds.

### Small Bowel Edema

Swelling of the valvulae conniventes can be caused by hypoproteinemia, which may be due to cirrhosis, kidney disease, or protein loss from the GI tract, as may occur in Ménétrier disease, Whipple disease, intestinal lymphangiomatosis, inflammatory bowel disease, and GI tumors. Blockage of mesenteric lymph channels, angioneurotic edema, and abetalipoproteinemia can also cause thickening of small bowel mucosal folds.

### Granulomatous Enteritis (Crohn Disease)

Crohn disease is the most common nonspecific inflammation of the small bowel. Its cause is unknown; the inflammation starts in the submucosa and becomes transmural, often with granulomatous features. The disease involves the ileum most often but may also affect the colon, jejunum, and stomach[12] (Fig. 9-14A–D). Ulcers, fistulae, and mucosal nodularity are frequently present.[13] Sonographically, the most obvious finding is hypoechoic thickening of the bowel wall and mesentery.[12] The resultant bull's-eye appearance is nonspecific and is often indistinguishable from tumor, hematoma, ulcerative colitis, pericecal abscess, or ruptured small bowel diverticulum.[14]

### Small Bowel Tumors

The most common primary neoplastic lesions of the small bowel, in order of occurrence, are smooth muscle tumors, carcinoid tumors, adenocarcinomas, and lymphoma. The bowel may also be involved as a part of multisystem

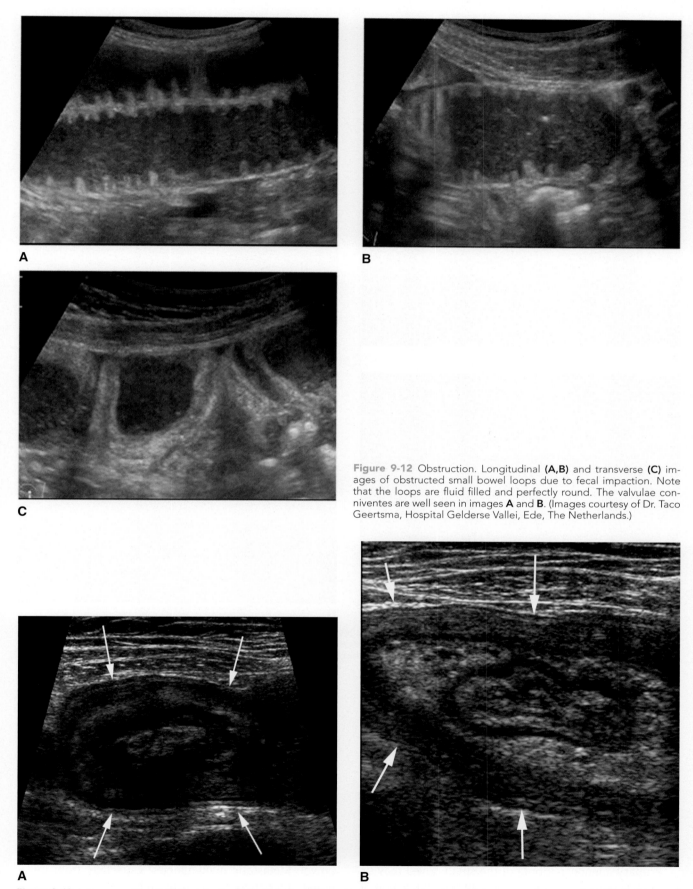

**Figure 9-12** Obstruction. Longitudinal **(A,B)** and transverse **(C)** images of obstructed small bowel loops due to fecal impaction. Note that the loops are fluid filled and perfectly round. The valvulae conniventes are well seen in images **A** and **B**. (Images courtesy of Dr. Taco Geertsma, Hospital Gelderse Vallei, Ede, The Netherlands.)

**Figure 9-13** Intussusception. **A,B:** Longitudinal images in two different patients demonstrate multiple concentric layers of small bowel (*arrows*) telescoping into the next segment consistent with intussusception. (Images courtesy of Philips Medical Systems, Bothell, WA.)

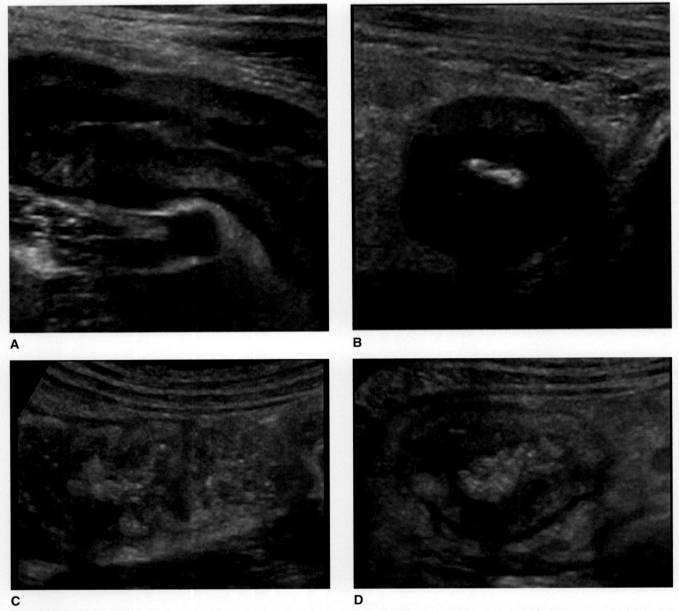

**A**

**B**

**C**

**D**

**Figure 9-14** Crohn disease. Longitudinal **(A)** and transverse **(B)** images demonstrate hypoechoic thickening of the submucosal layer in the terminal ileum in a patient with Crohn disease. Longitudinal **(C)** and transverse **(D)** images of the ascending colon in the same patient demonstrate mild wall thickening. (Images courtesy of Dr. Taco Geertsma, Hospital Gelderse Vallei, Ede, The Netherlands.)

lymphoma. When primary and multisystem lymphomatous involvements of the GI tract are combined, lymphoma is the most common neoplasia of the small bowel.

Lymphoma of the small bowel is usually part of a systemic involvement, most frequent by non-Hodgkin lymphoma (including Burkitt, undifferentiated, and histiocytic lymphoma). Fifty percent of patients with Hodgkin disease, however, also have involvement of the GI tract eventually. Sonographically, bowel wall involvement may appear as a target lesion. The mesenteric nodes may also be affected without involvement of the bowel wall.

Primary adenocarcinoma of the small bowel may be present as either a constricting circumferential lesion or

as a polypoid lesion. The lesions may range from 1 to 10 cm in diameter.

Leiomyoma is the most common benign tumor of the small bowel—it looks like leiomyomas elsewhere, including in the uterus. The tumor arises from the muscularis propria and is usually eccentrically located in the wall. Leiomyosarcomas can appear identical to larger leiomyomas, but larger tumors and tumors with central necrosis are more likely to be malignant.

Adenomas, lipomas, hemangiomas, and neurofibromas are other benign tumors that can arise in the small bowel. Metastatic malignancies, especially from melanoma and carcinomas of the lung, kidney, and breast, occur as either single or multiple intramural or intraluminal masses. These metastases may appear similar to smooth muscle tumors or lymphoma. Carcinoid tumors are discussed in the next section.

# VERMIFORM APPENDIX

## SONOGRAPHIC TECHNIQUE

The sonographic examination of the right lower quadrant begins with identifying the right colon, which is then followed downward to the cecum. By placing steady pressure on the transducer, one can displace gas-filled bowel loops to search for the appendix. The cecum and terminal ileum can often be seen. One can identify the normal appendix in some persons, but only inflamed, distended appendices can be visualized consistently.

## NORMAL ANATOMY OF THE APPENDIX

The normal appendix is not routinely visible transabdominally but can sometimes be visualized, especially when ascites is present. The normal appendix is a long tubular structure that is seen extending from the cecum and should measure no more than 6 mm in diameter, and the hypoechoic part of the wall should measure no more than 2-mm thick (Fig. 9-15). The appendix can be found under McBurney point, which is located by drawing an imaginary line from the right anterosuperior iliac spine to the umbilicus. The appendix is usually found at the midpoint of this line.

## DISORDERS OF THE APPENDIX

### Appendicitis

Appendicitis is usually associated with obstruction of the appendiceal lumen. Although it may occur in any age group, young adults are most often affected.

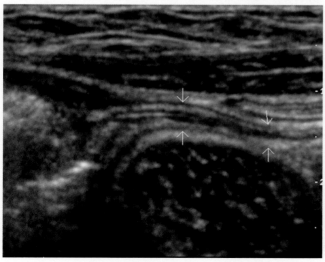

**Figure 9-15** Normal appendix. Longitudinal image demonstrates the normal thin walled appendix *(arrows)*. (Image courtesy of Philips Medical Systems, Bothell, WA.)

Appendicitis has generally been considered a clinical diagnosis, characterized initially by general periumbilical pain associated with leukocytosis, fever, and sometimes nausea. After a few hours, the pain localizes in the right lower quadrant, and there is point tenderness over the appendix and signs of peritoneal irritation such as rebound tenderness. Rebound tenderness and pain located over McBurney point is considered a positive McBurney sign and is clinical indicator of appendicitis.

Diagnostic studies have rarely been considered necessary traditionally; however, at appendectomy the appendix has been found to be normal in up to 40% of suspected appendicitis cases in young women, due to the numerous gynecologic causes of right lower quadrant pain in this population.[12,15] Also, there is much variation in the clinical presentation of appendicitis; many cases do not exhibit the classical symptoms. Sonography has a reported sensitivity and specificity of 78% and 83%, respectively, and compares with sensitivity and specificity of 91% and 90%, respectively, for computed tomography (CT).[16] Although CT is considered superior, sonography is highly effective in the evaluation of acute appendicitis and in patients for whom exposure to ionizing radiation is a concern, sonography provides a diagnostic alternative.[12,17,18]

The sonographic examination is performed with a 5- to 12-MHz transducer using the graded compression technique. Applying slow steady compression systematically to the right lower quadrant displaces or compresses normal gas- or fluid-filled bowel loops.[12,15] The graded compression technique also helps the sonographer to locate the area of maximum tenderness. Visualization of a noncompressible appendix >6 mm in diameter with mucus in the appendiceal lumen and with associated focal pain over the appendix is sufficient to establish the diagnosis of unruptured appendicitis (Fig. 9-16A,B). The appendiceal lumen is often distended and filled with mucus (Fig. 9-16C,D), but in some cases of appendicitis, the lumen is nondistended and appendiceal wall thickening is the primary finding. Retrocecal appendices, however, are particularly difficult to visualize sonographically. A calcified appendicolith is a strong indicator of appendicitis, even if a dilated appendiceal lumen is not seen (Fig. 9-16E).

Color flow and power Doppler imaging can add valuable information in the diagnosis of appendicitis. The increase in blood flow in the appendix may be patchy or may involve the entire appendix. Flow imaging is particularly helpful in equivocal cases in which the appendix is visualized but is normal or nearly normal; in this situation, a lack of flow on power Doppler suggests the appendix is normal, whereas increased flow suggests mild appendicitis (Fig. 9-16F). In appendicitis cases that are clearly abnormal on grayscale sonography, little or no power Doppler flow suggests wall ischemia and impending rupture. Retrocecal appendicitis may be easier to identify using flow imaging.

Although it was initially believed that any appendix visualized sonographically was abnormal, it is now clear that the normal appendix can frequently be identified.

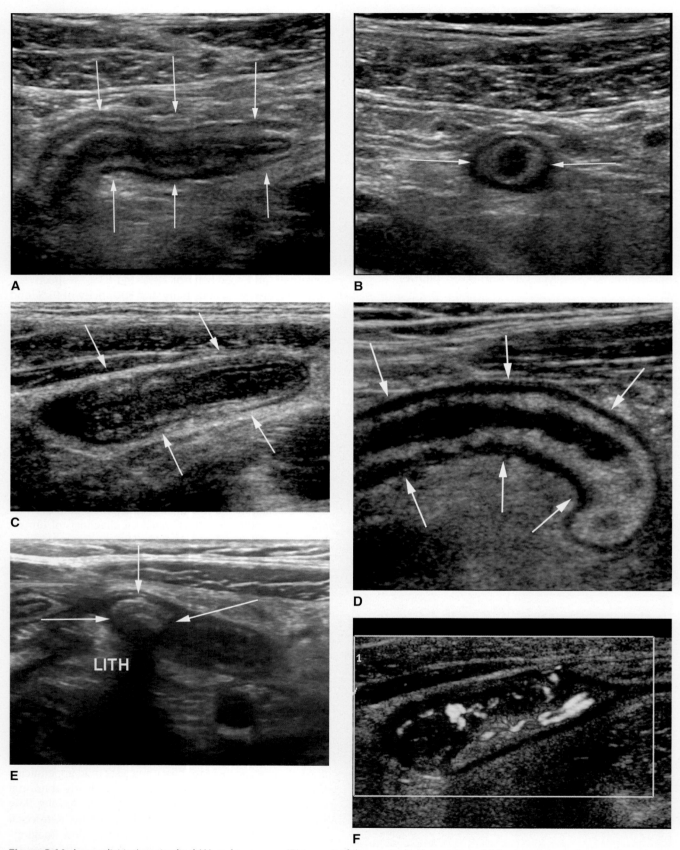

**Figure 9-16** Appendicitis. Longitudinal **(A)** and transverse **(B)** images of the appendix demonstrate thickening of the wall *(arrows)* consistent with appendicitis. **C,D:** Longitudinal images of two different patients with a dilated, inflamed appendix, with a thickened wall and dilatation of the appendiceal lumen. **E:** Longitudinal image of an inflamed appendix containing an echogenic appendicolith *(arrows)*. **F:** Longitudinal image demonstrates hyperemia within an inflamed appendix consistent with appendicitis. (Images A–D, F courtesy of Philips Medical Systems, Bothell, WA.)

It is also becoming clear that some cases of appendicitis can resolve without surgery, perhaps to recur later.

The chief complication of appendicitis is, of course, abscess formation or generalized peritonitis. Appendiceal rupture is not required for these complications to arise, as pathogens may travel through the intact wall. When the appendix has ruptured, it is much more difficult to visualize because the lumen is no longer distended and the anatomy is distorted by surrounding inflammation and adjacent abscess. Appendiceal abscesses may be echogenic because colon organisms may form gas within them. Gas in a tubo-ovarian abscess is less common. Characteristically, appendiceal abscesses are at the cecal tip or in the pericolic gutter, but sometimes they occur between small bowel loops medially, where they are much more difficult to find sonographically. The small bowel loops may be thickened due to inflammation from the adjacent abscess.

Power Doppler imaging can help differentiate between bowel wall thickening due to abscess and bacterial ileocolitis; in abscess cases, the increased blood flow will be greatest on the serosal surface of the bowel adjacent to the abscess, whereas blood flow will be greatest in the mucosa in cases of ileocolitis. Fluid collections near the appendix can be examined in a similar way; if increased blood flow is detected in omentum and peritoneum around the fluid, abscess must be suspected.

## Mucocele

Mucocele, distension of the appendix by mucus, is an uncommon lesion, found in 0.25% of appendectomies. It is slightly more common in men than in women and mean age at diagnosis is 52.7 years.[19] Right lower quadrant pain resembling appendicitis is the most common symptom, although patients may be asymptomatic. Mucoceles are classified into three groups: focal or diffuse hyperplasia, mucinous cystadenoma, and mucinous cystadenocarcinoma. Only the last is considered to have malignant potential. Mucocele rupture can cause massive accumulation of gelatinous ascites, called *pseudomyxoma peritonei*. If the mucocele is the mucinous cystadenocarcinoma variety, ascites is malignant and the patient has a poorer prognosis. An association has been noted between mucoceles and the presence of one or more other colon tumors.

Sonographically, the mucocele appears as a purely cystic or complex mass up to 7 cm in diameter, demonstrating through transmission posteriorly and located in the right lower quadrant. This lesion may be difficult to differentiate from ovarian cysts, mesenteric cysts, omental cysts, duplication cysts, renal cysts, or even abdominal abscess.

## Carcinoid Tumors

Carcinoids (argentaffinomas) arise from the argentaffin cells of the mucosa. In order of decreasing frequency, they arise in the appendix, small bowel, rectosigmoid colon, lung and bronchi, esophagus and stomach, pancreas, gallbladder, biliary tract, ovary and testis, and right colon.[20] Carcinoids have histologic features of malignancy, such as anaplasia and increased mitoses, but have relatively low metastatic potential. Local invasiveness is the best indicator of degree of malignancy. Appendiceal carcinoids rarely metastasize, whereas small bowel lesions are the most likely to do so.[21]

Sonographically, carcinoid tumors appear as sharply marginated hypoechoic masses without acoustic enhancement. The lesions are small: More than 95% are less than 2 cm in diameter. The larger the lesion, the more likely it is to metastasize. One-third of lesions greater than 2 cm in diameter will have nodal or distant metastasis.[22]

The tumors often produce hormones, principally serotonin and prostaglandin E, but because the liver inactivates serotonin received via the portal circulation, liver metastases are virtually always present if the patient experiences the carcinoid syndrome, which includes skin flushing, diarrhea, cyanosis, asthmatic attacks, and cardiac valve lesions.[20] If the primary site of the carcinoid is outside the GI tract (i.e., ovary, bronchus), metastasis is not required for the carcinoid syndrome.

### Other Disorders of the Appendix

Sonographic detection of adenocarcinoma of the appendix has been reported. The clinical presentation may be similar to that of acute appendicitis. Crohn disease of the appendix can occur as an isolated condition, or more commonly with Crohn disease of the colon or ileum. The sonographic appearance of these conditions is nonspecific.

### Bacterial Ileocolitis and Mesenteric Adenitis

When an abnormal appendix is not visualized sonographically, a search for other sonographic abnormalities in the right lower quadrant will sometimes show other GI findings. Enlarged lymph nodes adjacent to the cecum may be observed. Right lower quadrant lymphadenopathy without associated appendicitis is termed *mesenteric adenitis* and is the most common diagnosis at surgery if the appendix is normal. Abnormal lymph nodes are rounder in outline than normal nodes, and must be greater than 4 mm in anteroposterior diameter to be considered abnormal.

In some cases, the ileum, cecum, or both may show mild wall thickening as well as lymphadenopathy. *Yersinia, Campylobacter,* or *Salmonella* bacteria may be cultured from the stool in some of these patients. Bacterial ileocolitis is usually a self-limited disease that does not require surgery.

# COLON AND RECTUM

## SONOGRAPHIC TECHNIQUE

No special techniques are available for evaluating the colon. A normal person usually has more air in the colon than in the small bowel and the colon's larger diameter and prominent haustral indentations are often identifiable. A fluid-filled colon is unusual, generally indicating diarrhea or obstruction. The examiner may sometimes have difficulty differentiating a solid mass in the colon from a small bowel lesion. It is helpful to

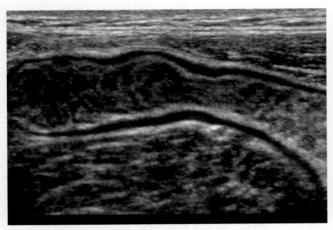

**Figure 9-17** Colon. Longitudinal image of the normal colon. (Image courtesy of Philips Medical Systems, Bothell, WA.)

know where the colon is usually located and to note the greater amount of air in the colon.

Endoluminal examination of the rectum should be performed in both the axial and longitudinal directions if possible because this allows better evaluation of the layers of the bowel wall involved, the extent of invasion of any tumor that may be present, and evidence of local lymphadenopathy.

## NORMAL ANATOMY OF THE COLON AND RECTUM

The colon usually lies in the periphery of the abdomen, laterally on the right and left, and superiorly along the liver margin in the upper abdomen. Because the colon hosts gas-producing bacteria, it is more often distended with gas than the rest of the bowel. Its customary position, its larger diameter, and its characteristic haustral folds, which are up to 3 to 5 cm apart,

can frequently help identify the colon (Fig. 9-17). The colon wall should measure 4- to 9-mm thick when not distended, and 2 to 4 mm when the colon is distended to a diameter of ≥5 cm.

## DISORDERS OF THE COLON

### Obstruction

The colon, usually, is at least partially filled with gas and, when colonic obstruction occurs, the obstructed loop is likely to be gas filled. This makes colon obstruction easy to diagnose radiographically and difficult to diagnose sonographically, although dilated loops of bowel may be identified. Although a specific diagnosis is not always possible, the location of the dilated loop may give some clues. Cecal volvulus is manifested by dilation of the right colon only. Sigmoid volvulus shows maximum dilatation in the central abdomen. Diverticulitis with obstruction usually causes dilatation of the left, and perhaps the entire colon, and an obstructing rectal carcinoma appears similar.

### Crohn Colitis (Granulomatous Colitis)

Crohn disease of the colon produces signs identical to Crohn disease of the small bowel. It tends to be a transmural inflammation, potentially developing fistulae and pericolonic abscesses. Multiple separate areas of the colon may be involved; the right colon is a frequent site, and associated ileal involvement is common. Typically, the bowel layers in the colon wall are not visible. Increased blood flow is usually present with color or power Doppler imaging.[23]

### Ulcerative Colitis

*Ulcerative colitis* is an inflammatory disease confined to the colonic mucosa and submucosa. The cause is not known, but a hypersensitivity or autoimmune

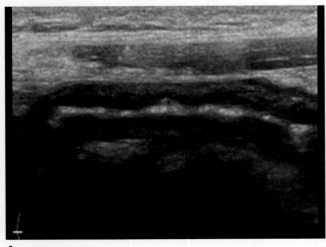

**A**

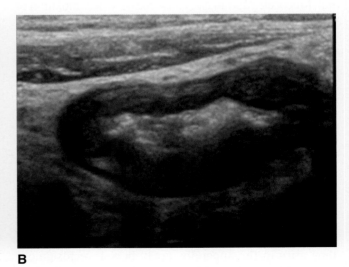

**B**

**Figure 9-18** Ulcerative colitis. Longitudinal **(A)** and transverse **(B)** views of the colon in a patient with ulcerative colitis. Note the absent haustration. (Images courtesy of Dr. Taco Geertsma, Hospital Gelderse Vallei, Ede, The Netherlands.)

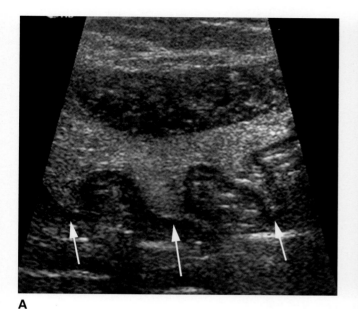

**A**

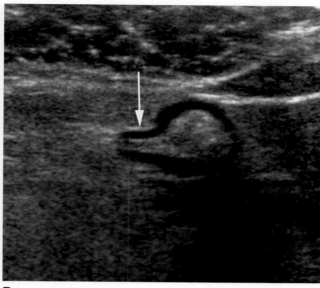

**B**

**Figure 9-19** Diverticulitis. Longitudinal **(A)** image of the colon in a patient with diverticulitis. Multiple diverticula are seen *(arrows)*. Note the thickened wall. **B:** Transverse image of the colon with a diverticulum *(arrow)*. (Images courtesy of Philips Medical Systems, Bothell, WA.)

mechanism is suspected. The inflammation starts in the rectal region and, as the disease progresses, extends up the left colon and may eventually involve the entire colon.[12] Unlike Crohn colitis, ulcerative colitis does not skip some areas, leaving them unaffected, but spreads in a continuous pattern. Patients with ulcerative colitis are at high risk of developing a particularly virulent form of colon carcinoma. The bowel wall appears thickened and is usually hypoechoic, although sometimes the layers of the bowel wall are visible sonographically (Fig. 9-18A,B).

## Diverticular Disease

*Diverticulosis* is an acquired condition in which small hernias of the mucosa (diverticula) form through the muscular layer of the colon. The rectosigmoid colon is most often affected. This condition, which is associated with a low bulk diet, affects >50% of people older than 50 years in Western countries. Diverticulosis is usually asymptomatic and is not sonographically detectable unless air or barium is present in the diverticula.

If one or more diverticula become filled with inspissated fecal material and then become inflamed, diverticulitis results. Often, there is also inflammatory thickening of the bowel wall. Pericolic abscesses may form because of diverticular rupture or transmural spread of infection. Sonographically, these abscesses appear as masses adjacent to the colon (Fig. 9-19A,B). They may be hypoechoic or may contain gas.

## Other Inflammatory Disorders

Other inflammatory colon conditions that may result in colon wall thickening include ischemia, amebiasis, shigellosis, tuberculosis, pseudomembranous colitis, radiation colitis, endometriosis, and pancreatitis. In

ischemic colitis, little or no flow is detectable with power Doppler imaging.

## Carcinoma

In Western countries, colon carcinoma is the third leading cause of death from cancer, after carcinoma of the lung and breast. Fifty percent of colon carcinomas arise in the rectum and rectosigmoid colon, 25% in the sigmoid, and 25% in the rest of the colon. Transabdominal sonography demonstrates a large colon cancer as a nonspecific hypoechoic target lesion (Fig. 9-20). Smaller polypoid lesions are much more difficult to identify because of gas or fecal material in the colon.

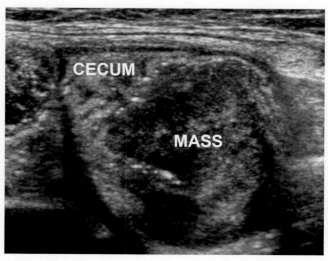

**Figure 9-20** Colon carcinoma. A large heterogeneous mass is seen in the cecum consistent with carcinoma of the colon. (Image courtesy of Philips Medical Systems, Bothell, WA.)

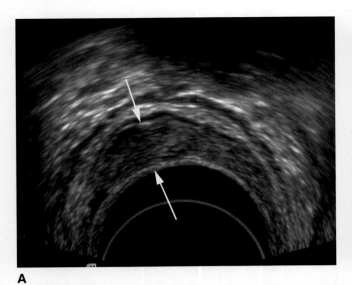

**A**

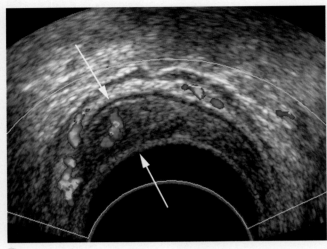

**B**

**Figure 9-21** Rectal mass. **A:** Transrectal sonogram demonstrates a hypoechoic ill-defined mass in the rectal wall. **B:** Color flow Doppler demonstrates flow within the mass. (Images courtesy of Philips Medical Systems, Bothell, WA.)

With high-frequency transrectal probes, the rectum can be imaged in transverse and longitudinal planes and can demonstrate the layers of the rectal wall. When rectal carcinoma is present, transrectal sonography can determine the degree of infiltration of the rectal wall and the perirectal area[24,25] (Fig. 9-21A,B). When staging local invasion, rectal sonography produced 96% sensitivity and 92% specificity.[26] Accurate presurgical staging of rectal tumors is vital for optimal planning of surgery and radiation therapy.[27]

## Lymphoma

Lymphoma of the colon appears similar to lymphoma of the small bowel. A hypoechoic lesion—annular, eccentric, or diffusely involving the bowel wall—may be observed.

## Benign Tumors

The same lesions seen elsewhere in the bowel can also involve the colon: leiomyomas, lipomas, fibromas, and hemangiomas.

| TABLE 9-1 | |
|---|---|
| **Sonographic Appearance of Gastrointestinal Lesion** | |

| Appearance | Lession |
|---|---|
| Target or pseudokidney sign (circumferential hypoechoic thickening of the bowel wall) | Lymphoma, intussusception, nonspecific inflammation, chronic ulcerative colitis, regional enteritis, hematoma, metastatic tumor |
| Focal hypoechoic lesions in the submucosa of the stomach | Neuroma, fibroma, gastric cysts, varices, ectopic pancreas |
| Focal hyperechoic lesions in the submucosa of the stomach | Ectopic pancreas, lipoma |
| Focal defect in the gastric mucosa with the mucosal layer preserved to the edge of the ulcer | Benign gastric ulcer |
| Defect in the gastric mucosa with indistinct mucosal layer at the ulcer edge | Benign or malignant ulcer |
| Focal hypoechoic lesions of the muscularis propria (exophytic) | Leiomyoma, leiomyosarcoma, metastatic tumor |
| Large cystic lesions | Obstruction, ileus, volvulus, mucocele |
| Thickening of the valvulae in the small bowel | Cirrhosis, renal disease, Ménétrier disease, Whipple disease, lymphangiomatosis, abetalipoproteinemia, inflammatory diseases |
| Mild thickening of the colon wall (<1 cm) | Chronic ulcerative colitis, regional enteritis, diverticulitis, pseudomembranous colitis, amebiasis, shigellosis, radiation colitis |
| Multiple concentric rings of bowel wall on transverse view, folded layers on longitudinal view | Intussusception |

## SONOGRAPHIC EVALUATION

Although sonography is not likely to replace barium studies of the GI tract as the principal method of visualizing GI anatomy and function, nor likely to replace CT in the overall staging of GI malignancies, its role in the evaluation of abdominal disorders is growing. The sonographic signs of GI lesions are summarized in Table 9-1. Sonography has the unique ability to visualize the layers of the bowel wall, either transabdominally or endoscopically, which is often useful in the diagnosis or staging of GI lesions. Additionally, the use sonographic endoscopy to direct biopsy and needle aspiration of GI lesions is developing as a valuable diagnostic tool.

## SUMMARY

- The GI tract is, essentially, a very long muscular tube, originating at the mouth and terminating at the anus.
- Sonography of the GI tract can either be performed transabdominally or endoluminally.
- Real-time sonography permits visualization of peristaltic activity that is helpful in identifying the GI tract and evaluating its function.
- When evaluating the abdomen, the patient should have nothing by mouth for 4 to 8 hours whenever possible; however, if the stomach and duodenum are to be further evaluated, the patient can drink 10 to 40 oz of water through a straw to improve visualization.
- Having the patient drink fluid also helps in evaluating the mucosa and peristalsis of the jejunum and ileum.
- Before transrectal sonography, a cleansing enema may be helpful so that fecal material is not confused with mucosal lesions.
- The layers of the bowel wall are the same throughout the GI tract. The innermost layer is the epithelium, followed by the lamina propria, muscularis mucosa, submucosa, muscularis externa, and the outermost serosa.
- The sonographic structure of the bowel is usually described as five layers: three echogenic layers separated by two hypoechoic ones.
- Sonographic endoscopy has demonstrated excellent sensitivity and specificity in the staging of esophageal cancer, particularly in the advanced stages.
- The stomach normally lies in the left upper quadrant of the abdomen with the fundus medial to the spleen and anterior to the left kidney and the body and antrum posterior or inferior to the left lobe of the liver, anterior to the pancreas, and medial to the gallbladder and porta hepatis.
- The antrum and body of the stomach often appear as a targetlike structure inferior to the left lobe on longitudinal sonograms.
- If the stomach is not distended, the bowel wall should measure 2- to 6-mm thick; however, when the stomach is distended to a diameter of ≥8 cm, the wall should measure 2 to 4 mm.
- Chronic gastritis may present as enlarged rugal folds with generalized thickening of the mucosal layer of the wall.
- Peptic ulcers most often occur in the antral portion of the lesser curvature and may demonstrate sonographically as a focal or generalized edema of the wall.
- Gastric carcinoma arises from the mucosa of the stomach, invading the submucosa and muscularis propria and is divided into four categories based on Borrmann classification.
- Ileus is characterized by failure of the intestine to propel its contents owing to diminished motility and may be caused by peritonitis, spinal fracture, renal colic, acute pancreatitis, bowel ischemia, myocardial infarction, surgery, medications, hypokalemia, and infection.
- Sonographically, ileus presents as small bowel distended with either air or fluid, although usually less distended than with obstruction, with normal to increased peristalsis.
- Small bowel obstruction also has many causes, such as adhesions, inflammatory masses, neoplastic lesions, volvulus, intussusception, and luminal obstruction (such as fecal impaction).
- Sonographically, with small bowel obstruction, the bowel loops are typically perfectly round in cross section, and peristalsis can vary from none to markedly increased.
- In volvulus, the twisted, dilated loop appears C-shaped when viewed longitudinally and often contains only fluid, no air.
- Intussusception is a telescoping of the bowel into itself and in adults is most commonly associated with an identifiable bowel lesion. Sonographically, intussusception appears as a nonspecific target lesion or as a mass with multiple concentric rings visible in transverse.
- Crohn disease is the most common nonspecific inflammation of the small bowel with inflammation starting in the submucosa and becoming transmural; the ileum is most often affected but may also affect the colon, jejunum, and stomach.
- Sonographically, the most obvious finding in Crohn disease is a hypoechoic thickening of the bowel wall and mesentery.
- The normal appendix is a long tubular structure that is seen extending from the cecum and should measure no more than 6 mm in diameter, and the hypoechoic part of the wall should measure no more than 2-mm thick.

## Critical Thinking Questions

1. While performing an abdominal sonogram, where would you expect to visualize the gastroesophageal junction?

2. Which of the following would not cause a target sign on sonography?
   A. Lymphoma of the small intestine
   B. Inflammation of the small intestine
   C. Intestinal ileus
   D. Intussusception

3. List the five sonographically visible bowel wall layers along with their normal echogenicity.

4. A 22-year-old man presents with right lower quadrant pain, nausea, and an elevated white cell count. Your examination reveals a noncompressible target-shaped lesion 7 mm in diameter at the point of maximum tenderness in the right lower quadrant. What is the most likely diagnosis?

5. A 27-year-old patient presents for an abdominal sonogram with a history of Crohn disease. What would expect to see on your examination?

- Appendicitis is usually associated with obstruction of the appendiceal lumen; although it may occur in any age group, young adults are most often affected.
- Appendicitis presents clinically as periumbilical pain that moves to the right lower quadrant with rebound tenderness, leukocytosis, fever, and sometimes nausea.
- Sonographically, appendicitis appears as a noncompressible appendix greater than 6 mm with mucus and possible appendicolith in the appendiceal lumen.
- Complications of appendicitis include perforation and abscess.
- Mucocele rupture can cause massive accumulation of gelatinous ascites, called pseudomyxoma peritonei.
- The colon usually lies in the periphery of the abdomen, laterally on the right and left, and superiorly along the liver margin.
- The colon wall should measure 4- to 9-mm thick when not distended, and 2 to 4 mm when the colon is distended to a diameter of ≥5 cm.
- Ulcerative colitis is an inflammatory disease confined to the colonic mucosa and submucosa that starts in the rectal region and, as the disease progresses, extends up the left colon and may eventually involve the entire colon. Unlike Crohn colitis, ulcerative colitis does not skip some areas, leaving them unaffected, but spreads in a continuous pattern.
- Colon carcinoma is the third leading cause of death from cancer, after carcinoma of the lung and breast and demonstrates sonographically as a hypoechoic target lesion.

### REFERENCES

1. Gutman JP, Ullah A. Advances in endoscopic ultrasound. *Ultrasound Clin.* 2009;4:369–384.
2. Sporea I, Popescu A. Ultrasound examination of the normal gastrointestinal tract. *Med Ultrason.* 2010;12: 349–352.
3. Puli SR, Reddy JB, Bechtold ML, et al. Staging accuracy of esophageal cancer by endoscopic ultrasound: a meta-analysis and systematic review. *World J Gastroentero.* 2008;14:1479–1490.
4. Brijbassie A, Shami VM. Esophageal cancer: ultrasonography. *Gastroenterol Clin North Am.* 2009;38:93–104.
5. Schwerk W, Braun B, Dombrowski H. Real-time ultrasound examination in the diagnosis of gastrointestinal tumors. *J Clin Ultrasound.* 2005;7:425–431.
6. Akahoshi K, Sumida Y, Matsui N, et al. Preoperative diagnosis of gastrointestinal stromal tumor by endoscopic ultrasound-guided fine needle aspiration. *World J Gastroenterol.* 2007;13:2077–2082.
7. Krstic AZ. Pathohistological findings in gastric cancer diagnosis. *Acta Medica Medianae.* 2009;48:15–19.
8. Ferreri AJ, Montalbán C. Primary diffuse large B-cell lymphoma of the stomach. *Crit Rev Oncol Hematol.* 2007; 63:65–71.
9. Saxena P, Nanda M. A rare presentation of a leiomyosarcoma of the stomach. *The Internet Journal of Surgery.* 2007;9. http://www.ispub.com/ostia/index.php?xmlFilePath = journals/ijs/vol9n2/stomach.xml.
10. Ilgen JS, Marr AL. Cancer emergencies: the acute abdomen. *Emerg Med Clin North Am.* 2009;27:381–399
11. Lehnert T, Sorge I, Till H, et al. Intussusception in children—clinical presentation, diagnosis and management. *Int J Colorectal Dis.* 2009;24:1187–1192.
12. Scott LM, Sawyers SR, Bokhari J, et al. Ultrasound evaluation of the acute abdomen. *Ultrasound Clin.* 2007;2: 493–523.
13. Gardiner KR, Dasari BV. Operative management of small bowel Crohn's disease. *Surg Clin North Am.* 2007;87: 587–610.
14. Válek V, Kysela P, Vavríková M. Crohn's disease at the small bowel imaging by the ultrasound-enteroclysis. *Eur J Radiol.* 2007;62:153–159.
15. Rybkin AV, Thoeni RF. Current concepts in imaging of appendicitis. *Radiol Clin North Am.* 2007;45:411–422.
16. van Randen AV, Bipat S, Zwinderman AH, et al. Acute appendicitis: meta-analysis of diagnostic performance of CT and graded compression US related to prevalence of disease. *Radiology.* 2008;249:97–106.

17. Terasawa T, Blackmore CC, Bent S, et al. Systematic review: computed tomography and ultrasonography to detect acute appendicitis in adults and adolescents. *Ann Inter Med*. 2004;141:537–546.

18. Gracey D, McClure MJ. The impact of ultrasound in suspected acute appendicitis. *Clin Radiol*. 2007;62:573–578.

19. Ruiz-Tovar J, Teruel DG, Castiñeiras VM, et al. Mucocele of the appendix. *World J Surg*. 2007;31:542–548.

20. Elsayes KM, Menias CO, Bowerson M, et al. Imaging of carcinoid tumors: Spectrum of findings with pathologic and clinical correlation. *J Comput Assist Tomogr*. 2011;35:72–80.

21. Pasieka JL. Carcinoid Tumors. *Surg Clin North Am*. 2009;89: 1123–1137.

22. Kulke MH. Clinical presentation and management of carcinoid tumors. *Hematol Oncol Clin North Am*. 2007;21: 433–455.

23. Maconi G, Sampietro GM, Sartani A, et al. Bowel ultrasound in Crohn's disease: surgical perspective. *Int J Colorectal Dis*. 2008;23:339–347.

24. Hinder JM, Chu J, Bokey EL, et al. Use of transrectal ultrasound to evaluate direct tumour spread and lymph node status in patients with rectal cancer. *Aust N Z J Surg*. 1990;60:19–23.

25. Puli SR, Reddy JBK, Bechtold ML, et al. Accuracy of endoscopic ultrasound to diagnose nodal invasion by rectal cancer: A meta-analysis and systematic review. *Ann Surg Oncol*. 2009;16:1255–1265.

26. Beynon J, Foy DM, Roe AM, et al. Endoluminal ultrasound in the assessment of local invasion in rectal cancer. *Brit J Surg*. 1986;73:474–477.

27. Giovannini M., Ardizzone S. Anorectal ultrasound for neoplastic and inflammatory lesions. *Best Pract Res Clin Gastroenterol*. 2006;20:113–135.

# 10 The Kidneys

Cathie Scholl

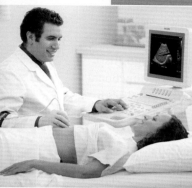

## OBJECTIVES

Discuss the normal anatomy of the kidneys from embryologic development to adulthood and include vasculature, location, size, and relational anatomy with other abdominal structures and organs.

Describe the microscopic internal renal anatomy to include the nephrons and juxtaglomerular apparatus.

Discuss the physiology of the upper urinary system.

State the common laboratory function tests and what a variance in each test indicates regarding renal function, disease, or pathology.

Demonstrate routine scanning procedure to include the patient preparation, patient instructions, patient positions, scanning techniques, technical considerations, and common scanning pitfalls.

Recognize sonographic anatomy to include the renal capsule, renal parenchyma (cortex, medulla, sinus, pelvis, and proximal ureter), anatomic variations and congenital anomalies (dromedary hump, junctional parenchymal defect, hypertrophied column of Bertin, renal sinus lipomatosis, and extrarenal pelvis), and vasculature.

Explain the pathology, etiology, clinical signs and symptoms, and sonographic appearance of urinary tract anomalies and abnormalities based on the amount of renal tissue (agenesis and hypoplasia), anomalies of number (collecting system duplications and supernumerary), and anomalies of position, form, and orientation (ectopic and horseshoe kidney).

Describe the pathology, etiologies, clinical signs and symptoms, and sonographic appearance of hereditary, developmental, and acquired cystic lesions of the kidneys.

Identify the systemic diseases that affect the kidneys.

Describe the sonographic appearance of common benign and malignant lesions of the kidneys.

Explain the intrinsic and extrinsic causes of hydronephrosis and the sonographic appearance of each grade.

Describe common causes and the sonographic appearance of urolithiasis.

Discuss the role of sonography in evaluating trauma to the kidneys.

List infections and inflammatory processes that affect the kidneys.

Describe the sonographic appearance of renal medical disease and list common causes of renal medical disease and renal failure.

Analyze sonographic images of the upper one-third of the urinary system for pathology.

Identify technically satisfactory and unsatisfactory sonographic examinations of the kidneys and proximal ureters.

## GLOSSARY

**azotemia** an overload of nitrogenous wastes such as blood urea nitrogen, uric acid, and creatinine in the blood that occurs with renal failure

**blood urea nitrogen (BUN)** blood test that evaluates the amount of nitrogenous waste in the blood and serves as a measure of kidney function

**creatinine** blood test along with BUN used to measure the kidneys' ability to remove waste products from the blood; creatinine elevates when the kidneys are not functioning properly

**diuresis** increased production of urine; can occur with diabetes mellitus, diabetes insipidus, acute renal failure, or increased fluid intake

**dysuria** painful urination

**Gerota fascia** also known as the renal fascia; dense connective tissue that surrounds and helps anchor the kidney, adipose capsule, and the adrenal gland

**hematuria** blood in the urine; referred to as gross hematuria (blood you can see in the urine) or microscopic hematuria (blood visible only under a microscope)

**hypernephroma** another term for renal cell carcinoma

**nephrectomy** surgical removal of a kidney

**nephropathy** kidney disease

**oliguria** low output of urine; many possible causes including dehydration, renal failure, or urinary obstruction

**proteinuria** protein in the urine; sign of chronic kidney disease

**pyuria** pus in the urine

**urosepsis** bacterial infection in the bloodstream as a result of a urinary tract infection

The urinary system consists of two kidneys, two ureters, the urinary bladder, and the urethra. Normally, the kidneys are located in the retroperitoneum on either side of the vertebrae and produce urine. The ureters convey the urine from the kidney to the urinary bladder, where it is stored in a temporary reservoir until it is discharged from the body through the urethra. This chapter discusses the upper third of the urinary system: the kidneys and proximal ureters. Chapter 11 presents the lower third of the urinary system (the distal ureters, urinary bladder, and urethra), Chapter 24 presents renal transplants, and Chapter 27 presents sonography-guided interventional procedures.

Sonography can be the first examination used to evaluate renal and juxtarenal tissue, as it is not dependent on renal function for real-time imaging. Current sonographic equipment provides morphologic information; permits identification and assessment of renal length, width, and thickness; demonstrates the appearance, size, and echogenicity of the renal capsule, cortex, medulla, and sinus; displays the distinctness of the corticomedullary junction produced by the interfaces of the arcuate vessels and the inward extensions of the cortex; and differentiates between solid and cystic lesions.

## ANATOMY

### EMBRYOLOGY[1-5]

As early as the third week of embryonic development, the kidneys begin to form from the columns of mesoderm (intermediate mesoderm). At successive intervals, three pairs of kidneys differentiate: the pronephros, the mesonephros, and the metanephros and paramesonephric ducts.

The pronephros (forekidney) is a transitory, nonfunctional structure that appears early in the fourth week of gestation. It degenerates rapidly, leaving nothing more than a duct to be utilized by the next kidney. Late in the fourth week, the mesonephros (midkidney) forms just caudad to the pronephros. This structure provides partial function while the permanent kidney continues to develop. By the end of the embryonic period and prior to degeneration, the mesonephros claims the pronephric duct and becomes known as the *mesonephric duct*. In the male, the mesonephric duct (wolffian) persists and develops into the male epididymis, the ductus deferens, and the ejaculatory duct. In the female, the mesonephric duct develops into the paramesonephric duct (müllerian), and eventually into the uterus and vagina.

During the fifth week of gestation, the metanephros (permanent kidney) appears as hollow ureteric buds that push upward from the mesonephric duct. The expanded distal ends form the renal pelvis, associated calyces, and collecting tubules; the mesonephric duct, the unexpanded proximal portion, forms the ureters. The nephrons, the functional units of the kidney, arise from the intermediate mesoderm around each ureteric bud. Nephron function begins at approximately 8 weeks.

With fetal growth, the kidneys appear to migrate from their pelvic location to the abdomen. This results from the rapid growth of the caudad part of the kidneys. As this so-called migration is not complete until 5 or 6 years of life, the kidneys in infants and young children are located more caudad.

## LOCATION AND SIZE[2,5,6–8]

The kidneys are about the size of a tightly clenched fist and are approximately 10- to 12-cm long, 5- to 7.5-cm wide, and 2- to 3-cm thick and weigh approximately 130 to 150 g.[2,5,6] The kidneys are typically within 2 cm of each other in length.[6,7] The paired kidneys are reddish brown organs with convex lateral borders and concave medial borders. On the medial border is an indentation or cleft, the renal hilus, which leads into a space called the *renal sinus*. Renal blood vessels, lymphatics, nerves, and the ureter enter or exit the kidney at the hilus and occupy the sinus (Fig. 10-1A).

Both kidneys are located in the retroperitoneum, lying along the posterior abdominal wall. Three layers of supportive tissues surround each kidney. The innermost layer is the fibrous renal capsule, which covers the surface, is continuous with the outer layer of the ureter at the hilus, and gives a fresh kidney a glistening appearance. The renal capsule serves as a barrier against physical trauma and infection. The middle layer is a mass of perirenal fat, the adipose capsule, which helps to hold the kidney in place against the posterior trunk muscles and cushions it against blows. The outermost layer, the renal fascia, is also referred to as Gerota fascia. (Chapter 14 differentiates the frequent reference to both the anterior and posterior as Gerota fascia, although it is more correct to reference the anterior renal fascia as Gerota fascia and the posterior

renal fascia as Zuckerkandl fascia.) The renal fascia is a dense, fibrous, connective tissue surrounding the kidney, the adipose capsule, and the adrenal gland, completely enclosing them and anchoring these organs to surrounding structures (Fig. 10-1B).

Renal vasculature and the fatty encasement are extremely important in holding the kidneys in their normal position; however, it is normal for both kidneys to demonstrate 3 to 4 cm of excursion when a patient changes from a supine to an erect position. *Ptosis*, an abnormal displacement to a lower position, occurs when the amount of fatty tissue dwindles (owing to rapid weight loss) and may precipitate a kinked ureter, resulting in hydronephrosis.

## RELATIONAL ANATOMY[3,4]

Understanding the location and relationship of the kidneys to surrounding structures is important, as displacement of those structures or an unusual renal position may suggest disease. The relational anatomy may be easier to understand when the kidney is viewed as having anterior and posterior surfaces, lateral and medial borders, and a superior and an inferior extremity.

### Anterior Surface

In most patients, the right kidney is 2 to 8 cm lower than the left owing to the presence of the liver. A narrow portion of the right anterior superior surface is in relation to the right adrenal gland. Inferior to this, approximately 75% of the anterior surface comes in contact with the renal impression on the visceral surface of the liver. The remaining right anterior surface is in contact with the descending portion of the duodenum. Laterally, the right superior anterior surface is in contact with the hepatic flexure and medially with the small intestine. The areas in contact with the liver and small intestine are covered by peritoneum; the adrenal, duodenal, and colic areas are devoid of peritoneum (Fig. 10-2).

The left anterior superior surface of the medial border is in proximity to the left adrenal gland. Close to the left anterior lateral border, a long strip is in contact with the renal impression on the spleen. At approximately the middle of the anterior surface lies a somewhat quadrilateral field marking the site of contact with the body of the pancreas. Superior to this is a small triangular portion, between the adrenal and splenic areas, marking the site of contact with the posterior surface of the stomach. Inferior to the pancreatic area, its lateral part is in relation to the colon's splenic flexure and its medial part lies in relation to the small intestine. The areas in contact with the stomach and spleen are covered by the omental bursa type of peritoneum, whereas the area in relation to the small intestine is covered by the peritoneum of the greater sac. The adrenal, pancreatic, and colic areas are devoid of

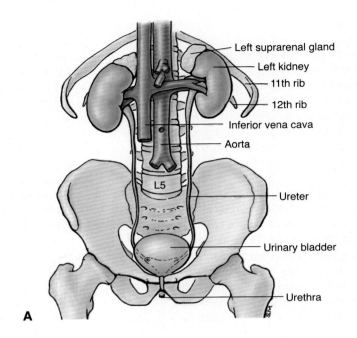

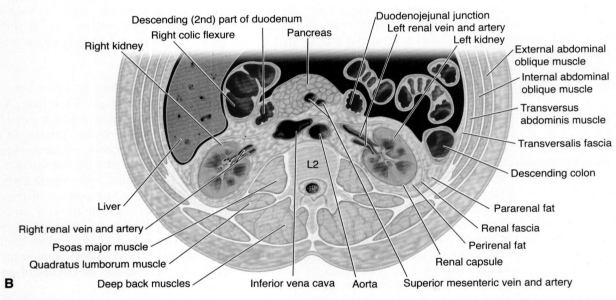

**Figure 10-1** Normal anatomy. **A:** The topographic anatomy relationship of the urinary system is seen in a female. **B:** A transverse section at the second lumbar vertebra level shows the retroperitoneal location and relational anatomy of the kidneys surrounded by the renal capsule, the perirenal fat (adipose capsule), and the renal fascia. Visualize the relational anatomy. (**A,** reprinted with permission from Agur AMR, Dalley AF. *Grant's Atlas of Anatomy.* 12th ed. Baltimore, MD: Lippincott Williams & Wilkins; 2009:165.**B,** reprinted with permission from Tank PW, Gest TR. *Atlas of Anatomy.* Baltimore, MD: Lippincott Williams & Wilkins; 2009:243.)

peritoneum (Fig. 10-2). Kidney surfaces in direct contact with other organs devoid of peritoneum are frequently referred to as *bare areas*.

## Posterior Surface

The posterior surface of both kidneys lies on the diaphragm, the medial and lateral lumbocostal arches, and the anterior surfaces of the psoas major, the quadratus lumborum, and the tendon of the transversus abdominis muscles (Fig. 10-2).

## Lateral and Medial Borders

The lateral convex border is directed toward the posterolateral wall of the abdomen. On the left side, it is in contact superiorly with the spleen. The median border is directed somewhat anteriorly and inferiorly. The superior and inferior extremities of the medial border are convex. The middle medial border is concave, presenting a deep longitudinal fissure, the renal hilus. Above the hilus, the medial border is in relation to the adrenal gland, below the hilus, with the ureter. The relative

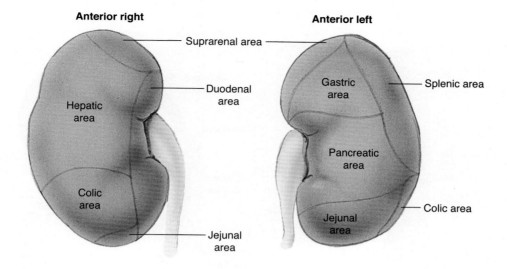

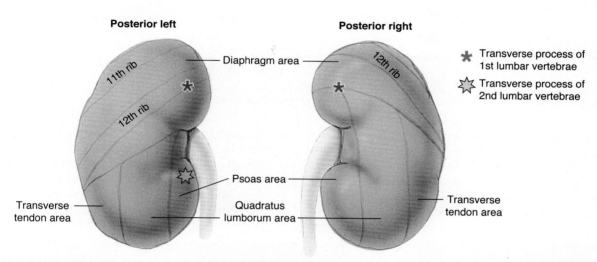

**Figure 10-2** Relationships. The topographic anatomy of the anterior, posterior, lateral, and medial renal surfaces illustrates anatomic relationships with other organs and structures.

position of the main structures in the hilus is as follows: the renal vein is anterior, the artery is in the middle, and the ureter is posterior and directed inferiorly[2] (Fig. 10-2).

### Superior and Inferior Extremities

The superior extremity of the kidney is thick and rounded, closer to the midline than the inferior extremity, and is topped by the adrenal gland, which also covers a small portion of the anterior surface. The inferior extremity is smaller, thinner, is farther lateral, and extends to within 5 cm of the iliac crest.

### VASCULAR ANATOMY[3–5]

Just inferior to the superior mesenteric artery (SMA), the renal arteries arise from the lateral aspects of the abdominal aorta. Because the aorta lies to the left of the midline, the right renal artery (RRA) is typically longer than the left. It courses transversely across the crus of the diaphragm posterior to the inferior vena cava (IVC), the right renal vein (RRV), the head of the pancreas, and the inferior portion of the duodenum. The left renal artery (LRA) courses posterior to the left renal vein (LRV), the splenic vein, and the body of the pancreas.

The RRV courses anterior to the RRA and enters the right lateral aspect of the IVC at a slightly lower transverse plane than the LRV. Because the IVC is situated to the right of the midline, the RRV is shorter than the left. The LRV courses from the left kidney hilus, passes anterior to the LRA, crosses over the aorta anteriorly, and passes posterior to the SMA before entering the medial aspect of the IVC (Fig. 10-1A, Fig. 10-2, Fig. 10-3A,B, and Table 10-1).

### NORMAL SONOGRAPHIC APPEARANCE

Although the position varies from patient to patient, the kidneys are normally located between the lower ribs and the iliac crest. For proper localization, surrounding

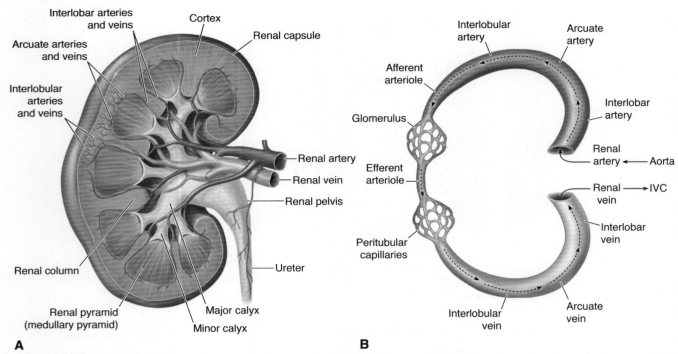

**A**

**B**

**Figure 10-3** Vascular anatomy. **A:** A coronal section shows the relationship of the vascular anatomy to the outer cortex, which surrounds the medulla (renal pyramids). **B:** A schematic depiction of the sequence of renal blood flow (see Table 10-1).

structures should be identified. In relative scanning planes, the liver, gallbladder, second portion of the duodenum, right adrenal gland, and IVC can be identified on the right. On the left, potentially identifiable structures include the spleen, pancreas, fourth portion of the duodenum, left adrenal gland, and aorta. The crus of the diaphragm, psoas muscle, and quadratus lumborum can be identified bilaterally.

Once the normal position and location of the kidneys have been established, the contour and internal architecture are observed. The shape and contour of a normal kidney appear smooth. Internally, the kidneys

| TABLE 10-1 | |
|---|---|
| **Renal Vasculature** | |
| Renal artery | Before or immediately after entering hilus, divides into five segmental (lobar) branches: (1) superior (apical) segmental artery, (2) anterior superior segmental artery, (3) posterior segmental artery, (4) anterior inferior segmental artery, and (5) posterior segmental artery |
| Segmental (lobar) arteries | Within renal sinus, each segmental artery branches to form interlobar arteries |
| Interlobar arteries | Pass between pyramids and branch into arcuate arteries at the base of pyramid |
| Arcuate arteries | Arching branches coursing between medulla and cortex parallel to kidney's surface |
| Interlobular arteries | Divisions of arcuate arteries produce a series of interlobular arteries, which travel through cortex toward kidney surface |
| Afferent arterioles | Interlobular arteries divide into several afferent arterioles, each of which supplies a renal corpuscle and forms a glomerulus, a tangled capillary network |
| Glomerulus | Blood comes in close contact with cells of glomerular capsule |
| Efferent arterioles | Reunited glomerular capillaries lead away from glomerular capsule, are smaller in diameter than afferent arterioles, and are unique, as blood usually flows out of capillaries into venules and not into other arterioles |
| Peritubular capillaries | Each efferent arteriole of a cortical nephron divides to form a network of capillaries around convoluted tubules called peritubular capillaries |
| Vasa recta | Efferent arterioles of a juxtamedullary nephron form straight, specialized portions from peritubular capillaries, called vasa recta, and course with loops of Henle into medulla |
| Interlobular veins | Peritubular capillaries unite to form interlobular veins, which unite to form arcuate veins |
| Arcuate veins | Follow same course as arcuate arteries and drain into interlobar veins |
| Interlobar veins | Course between pyramids and unite to form single renal vein |
| Renal veins | Exit kidney hilus |

have lobes without the lobular appearance seen in the lung. Each lobe is part of the collecting system and consists of a calyx, a conical medullary pyramid, cortical tissue, and vessels. In the adult there may be 8 to 18 minor calyces, but the average is 9. The minor calyces drain approximately 11 pyramids, and it is normal to have compound calyces draining more than one pyramid. This internal renal architecture presents specific echo amplitudes. Table 10-2 shows this normal echo amplitude and should assist in defining disease when alterations are encountered (Fig. 10-4A–E).

## Renal Capsule

The renal capsule is closely applied but not adherent to the renal parenchyma and appears sonographically as a strong, continuous, linear, specular reflector surrounding the cortex. Sparse perinephric fat, such as in infants, makes this line difficult to visualize. Fetal lobulation can persist into adulthood and give the kidney contour a scalloped appearance that should not be confused with scarring or cystic disease.[4]

## Renal Parenchyma[2]

A coronal section of a kidney reveals three distinct regions: the cortex, the medulla, and the pelvis. The granular-looking outer region, the renal cortex, extends from the renal capsule to the bases of the pyramids and into the spaces between them. The cortical extensions passing between the renal pyramids are called renal columns or columns of Bertin. Deep to the cortex, the renal medulla exhibits triangular or cone-shaped tissue masses called medullary (or renal) pyramids. The broader base of each pyramid faces the cortical area—its apex or papilla points are directed toward the center of the kidney. The striated (striped) appearance of the pyramids is due to the presence of straight tubules and blood vessels (Fig. 10-3A).

Surrounding the renal sinus, the two distinct areas of the kidney parenchyma, the cortex and medulla, can be separately distinguished sonographically (Fig. 10-4A). Differentiation between cortex and medulla is clearest in thin patients and in children. The corticomedullary junction is recognized by discrete, high-level, comma-shaped, specular echoes from the arcuate vessels and the inward extensions of the column of Bertin. The arcuate arteries are identified arching over the tops of the pyramids and serve as a marker for evaluation of cortical thickness.

## Renal Cortex

The normal adult renal cortex is homogeneously echogenic. In the traditional classification, echogenicity of the cortex is less than that of the liver, spleen, and renal sinus, although studies have shown that the cortex may appear isoechoic with the liver in adults with normal renal function. In neonates, the renal cortex is normally isoechoic or hyperechoic compared to the adjacent liver and spleen. In older children, the echo pattern of the cortex should be similar to that of adults. The echogenic comparison can only be made at the same depth and is valid only in the absence of hepatic or splenic disease. Scanning through a bile-filled gallbladder lying anterior to the kidney should be avoided, as it may artificially enhance the cortical echogenicity. A hyperechoic cortex is abnormal and should make the sonographer suspicious of renal medical disease.

## Renal Medulla

The inner portion of the renal parenchyma, called the medulla, contains the medullary pyramids separated by the columns of Bertin described previously. Sonographically, the medullary pyramids are cone-shaped or heart-shaped and are hypoechoic relative to the cortex.

| TABLE 10-2 | |
|---|---|
| **Sonographic Characteristics of the Normal Kidney and Related Structures** | |
| Echo amplitude of renal structures in ascending order | Renal medulla < renal cortex ≤ liver < spleen < pancreas < diaphragm < renal sinus = renal capsule |
| Renal capsule | Strong, continuous, linear specular reflector surrounds the cortex |
| Renal parenchyma | Resolves into more echogenic outer cortex from the hypoechoic inner medulla |
| Renal cortex | Homogeneously echogenic with closely spaced echoes of relatively low-level intensity; in adults, right kidney echogenicity ≤ that of normal liver; left kidney echogenicity ≤ that of spleen |
| Renal medulla | Rounded or blunted geometric, hypoechoic zones are best demonstrated on coronal sections, becoming more prominent with increased diuresis |
| Corticomedullary junction | Recognized by columns of Bertin extending inward and arcuate vessels |
| Arcuate vessels | Discrete, high-level, comma-like, specular echoes arching over the tops of the pyramids |
| Renal sinus | Intense, compact zone of central homogeneous echoes within the kidney sinus having an echo amplitude equal to that of the renal capsule |
| Vasculature | Linear, anechoic tubular structures entering and existing the renal hilus |
| Renal volume | V = length × width × thickening × 0.5 |

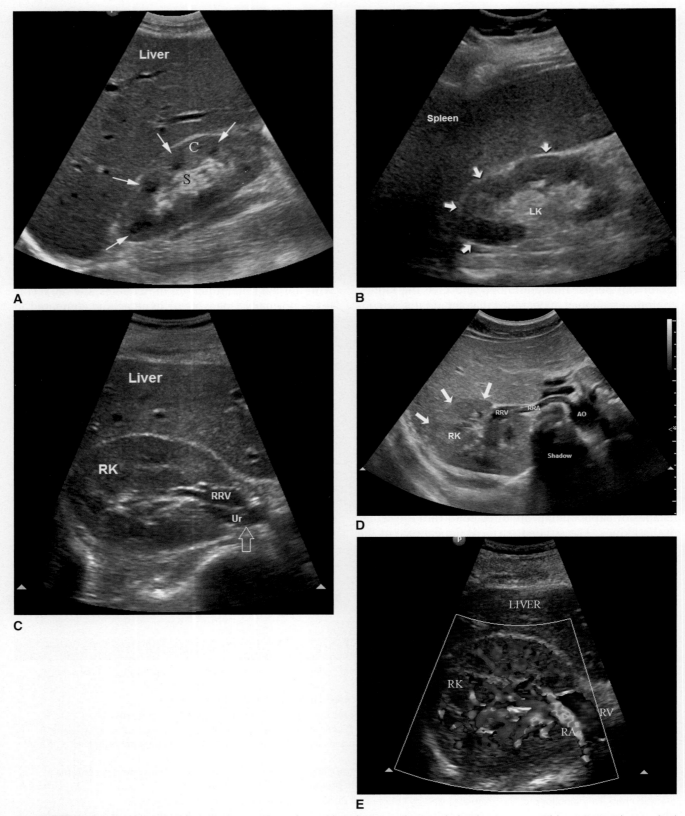

**Figure 10-4  A–E:** Normal sonographic anatomy (compare the sonographic appearance with the description in Table 10-2). **A:** A longitudinal section through the right kidney demonstrates the normal appearance of the renal cortex (C), hyperechoic renal sinus (S), and hypoechoic renal pyramids (arrows). **B:** A section through the left kidney (LK) on a technically difficult patient shows its relationship to the spleen. **C:** A transverse section made through the midportion of the right kidney displays the right renal vein (RRV) and proximal ureter (Ur) exiting (arrow) the renal pelvis. **D:** On a transverse section made through the midportion of the right kidney (RK, arrows), one can identify the right renal vein (RRV), the inferior vena cava (IVC) responding to inspiration, the right renal artery (RRA), the aorta (AO), and shadow caused by gas in the bowel. **E:** A transverse midsection through the right renal pelvis demonstrates the right renal artery (RRA) entering and the right renal vein (RRV) exiting the parenchymal vasculature. (continued)

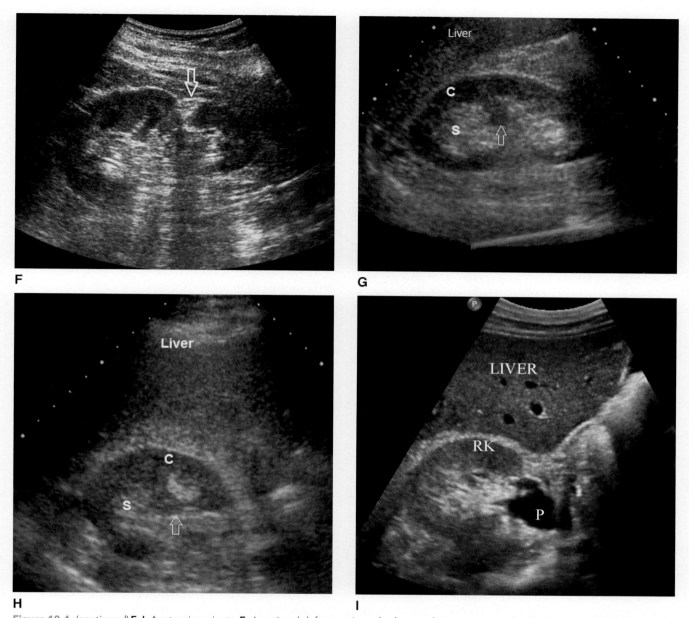

**Figure 10-4** *(continued)* **F–I:** Anatomic variants. **F:** Junctional defect: a triangular, hyperechoic area is noted midpole on this left kidney *(arrow)* consistent with a junctional defect. **G,H:** Hypertrophied column of Bertin. Longitudinal **(G)** and transverse **(H)** sections through the right kidney reveal the renal cortex *(C, arrow)* extending toward the center into the renal sinus *(S)*. **I:** Extrarenal pelvis. This transverse sonogram through the midpole of the right kidney demonstrates a central anechoic area outside of the renal pelvis, but communicating with the right kidney consistent with an extrarenal pelvis *(P)*. (**B–E, I**, Images courtesy of Philips Medical Systems, Bothell, WA; **F**, Image courtesy of Belinda Wilson, Columbus, OH.)

The medullary region is larger in children. The diuretic status of the kidney affects the detectability and sonographic characteristics of the medulla. With increased diuresis, the medullary pyramids become more prominent, anechoic, and more readily visible.

### Renal Sinus[9,10]

The renal sinus is imaged as an intense, compact zone of homogeneous central echoes within the kidney sinus. The echo intensity is caused primarily by hilar adipose tissue and secondarily by blood vessels and the collecting system. The echo amplitude results from the inherent scattering properties of fat cells and is not attributable to coexisting fibrous tissue septa. If renal sinus fat is minimal, as it is in infants, the central renal complex is less echogenic. In obese patients or patients with renal sinus lipomatosis, the central renal complex appears as an enlarged central echogenic complex, an anechoic to hypoechoic mass lesion, or a densely echogenic region with splaying of infundibular structures secondary to the increase in surrounding fat. When two lobulations of renal sinus fat are identified, a bifid renal pelvis or a double intrarenal collecting system should be suspected. The earliest renal sinus architectural change resulting from any infiltrative disease process, regardless of cause, is uneven widening of the interlobar septum.

### Renal Pelvis[2,5]

The renal pelvis is a large cavity medial to the hilus. Flat and funnel-shaped, it is continuous with the ureter, leaving the hilus (Fig. 10-4C–E). The papillae of the renal pyramid project into a cup-like chamber at the edge of the pelvis called the *minor calyces*. The 8 to 18 minor calyces join together to form two or three major calyces. The calyces collect urine, which drains continuously from the papillae and empties into the renal pelvis.

### Proximal Ureter[2,5]

From the renal pelvis, urine flows into the epithelium-lined, fibromuscular ureters, which are approximately 25- to 30-cm long and 6 mm in diameter. The smooth muscle wall of the calyces, pelvis, and ureters contracts rhythmically and propels urine by peristalsis to the bladder to be stored. Visualization of the collecting system and even the vessels in this area will depend on hydration and diuresis. When imaged in a transverse section, two echogenic interfaces are sonographically detectable. The proximal ureter is often sonographically identifiable as an anechoic structure emerging from the anteromedial renal pelvis posterior to the main renal vessels with a caudal course (Fig. 10-4C).

## Anatomic Variations

### Dromedary Hump[6,11–13]

A common renal variation, called a dromedary hump, is a local bulge of the lateral border of the kidney. The alteration in contour may mimic renal neoplasms. To distinguish bulges from an abnormal mass, document the location along the lateral renal border and demonstrate that the echogenicity of the focal widening is similar to that of the remaining cortex. Usually, a projection from the renal sinus can be identified pointing toward the dromedary hump.

### Junctional Parenchymal Defect[6,11,12,14,15]

The junctional cortical defect (junctional parenchymal defect or interpeduncular junction defect) is a common, normal variant that produces a wedge-shaped, hyperechoic defect in the anterior aspect near the junction of the upper and middle thirds of the kidney. It is frequently classified as a fetal lobulation anomaly but the term *lobation* is more correct, as the renal lobule is a microscopic unit. The anomaly is a remnant of the junction of reniculi, an incomplete embryologic fusion of the upper and lower poles, which occurs most often on the right kidney but can also occur on the left. A lobation appears as fine linear demarcations indenting the renal surface, separating normal lobes, and consists of a central pyramid and surrounding cortex. To distinguish it

from a scar or mass, its typical sonographic appearance is its location and triangular shape, whereas a scar is wider, less well defined, and associated with loss of renal cortex (Fig. 10-4F). Lobations typically overlie the space between the pyramids as compared with true renal scars, which are located overlying the medullary pyramids.

### Hypertrophied Column of Bertin[6,15,16]

A mass effect may be produced by hypertrophy of the renal column of Bertin. This common anatomic variant occurs when a double layer of renal cortex is folded toward the center of the kidney. They are usually located in the middle third of the kidney, more commonly on the left kidney than the right. If it is suspected, a coronal sonographic image of the renal column should be obtained. The image should have the following characteristics: (1) it indents the renal sinus laterally; (2) it is clearly defined from the renal sinus; (3) its largest dimension is less than 3 cm; (4) it is continuous or contiguous with the renal cortex; and (5) its echogenicity is close to that of the cortex (Fig. 10-4G,H).

### Renal Sinus Lipomatosis[10,16]

Renal sinus lipomatosis (fibrolipomatosis), excessive fatty infiltration of the renal pelvis, can be seen as an anatomic variant due to aging common in the sixth and seventh decades of life, associated with obesity, or a disease process associated with parenchymal atrophy or destruction. Often, it begins with renal calculi, which are found in 70% of cases. Nephrolithiasis is one of the predisposing factors for hydronephrosis, leading to associated infection that results in renal parenchymal atrophy. The void created by ongoing parenchymal atrophy may be filled by an abundant amount of fatty tissue. Thus, replacement lipomatosis can be seen as a sequela of atrophy, chronic calculous disease, and inflammation. Sonographically, lipomatosis may present as an enlarged, well-maintained reniform kidney that is outlined by the hypoechoic rim representing the residual parenchyma, renal capsule, and thick renal fascia. The sinus echo appearances are variable: (1) an enlarged central echogenic complex; (2) adipose tissue that may be relatively anechoic to hypoechoic, giving the impression of mass lesions; or (3) adipose tissue that may be densely echoic. The differential diagnosis includes infection, atrophy, and hydronephrosis.

### Extrarenal Pelvis[16,17]

Sonographically, the normal renal pelvis appears as a triangular structure lying within the renal sinus, and its axis is pointed inferiorly and medially. An intrarenal pelvis lies almost completely within the confines of the central renal sinus and is usually small and foreshortened. The extrarenal pelvis lies outside the renal sinus and tends to be larger, with long major calyces. On sonography, the extrarenal pelvis appears as a central cystic area located partially or entirely outside the kidney. Because it may mimic a pathologic condition, a transverse section should be made to document its continuity with the renal sinus (Fig. 10-4I).

## Renal Vasculature

The renal arteries are identified entering the hilus, posterior to the renal veins. They are not visualized as frequently as the veins, and care must be taken not to confuse them with the crus of the diaphragm. Longer than the LRA, the RRA courses posterior to the IVC. The renal veins are visualized at about the same level as the renal arteries. The RRV's size is altered by respiration and transmitted pulses from the IVC.[9] The LRV can be seen coursing between the SMA and the aorta to enter the lateral aspect of the IVC. The narrowing of the LRV between the aorta and the SMA is termed the nutcracker phenomenon (the vein is the nut between the two arteries, which represent the nutcracker) and should not be mistaken for pathologic change. The prominence of the LRV and the incompletely imaged normal aortic wall adjacent to it may give the false impression of a LRA aneurysm. In a patient with renal cell carcinoma (RCC), determining the patency of the renal veins is an important aspect of staging the disease. Venous tumor thrombus is diagnosed by the sonographic appearance of diffuse, low-intensity, intraluminal echoes or focal nodules, with or without luminal distention. Chapter 4 covers the renal hilar vasculature, and Doppler evaluation of intrarenal vasculature is discussed in the Scanning Technique section of this chapter.

## MICROSCOPIC ANATOMY

### Nephron[2,3,5]

The cortex and renal pyramids together constitute the renal parenchyma containing the kidney's basic histologic and functional unit, the nephron. Each kidney contains more than 1 million nephrons. Each nephron consists of (1) a renal corpuscle, an enlarged terminal end consisting of the glomerular capsule and its enclosed glomerulus; (2) a renal tubule divided into a proximal convoluted tubule, a perinephric loop (the loop of Henle), and a distal convoluted tubule; and (3) a vascular component. Table 10-3 describes the nephron's anatomy. Nephrons are frequently classified into two types. A cortical nephron's glomerulus is located in the outer cortical zone, and the remainder of the nephron rarely penetrates the medulla. A juxtamedullary nephron's glomerulus is usually closer to the corticomedullary junction, with longer loops of Henle extending farther into the medulla (Fig. 10-5A–C).

### Juxtaglomerular Apparatus[2,5]

The nuclei of the smooth muscle cells adjacent to the afferent (and sometimes efferent) arteriole are rounded instead of elongated. These modified cells are called

| TABLE 10-3 | |
|---|---|
| **Anatomy of the Nephron** | |
| **Renal Corpuscle** | |
| Glomerular capsule | Double-walled cup beginning in the cortex, composed of parietal and visceral layers separated by capsular space (often referred to as Bowman capsule) |
| Parietal layer | Outer wall composed of simple squamous epithelium |
| Visceral layer | Inner wall surrounding a capillary network called the glomerulus; consists of epithelial cells called podocytes (octopus-like branches terminating in foot processes or pedicles that intertwine with one another and cling to the basement membrane or glomerulus, forming part of filtration membrane) |
| Glomerulus | Tuft of capillaries associated with renal tubule; endothelium is fenestrated, so capillaries are exceptionally porous, allowing all substances except blood cells and most plasma proteins to pass from blood into glomerular capsule |
| **Renal Tubule** | |
| Proximal convoluted tubule | Wall consists of cuboidal epithelium with microvilli, cytoplasmic extensions, increasing surface area for reabsorption and secretion (convoluted means coiled and proximal signifies that the glomerular capsule is the origin) |
| Descending limb | Renal tubule straightens, becomes thinner, dips into medulla; consists of squamous epithelium |
| Loop of Henley | Diameter increases, bends into a U shape |
| Ascending limb | Ascends toward cortex and consists primarily of cuboidal epithelium |
| Distal convoluted tubule | Cuboidal epithelium with few microvilli (unlike proximal convoluted tubule); distal convoluted tubule of several nephrons empties into a common collecting tubule, which transports urine back into renal pyramids in medulla |

juxtaglomerular cells, and in response to lowered blood pressure, they are thought to secrete an enzyme called renin. Adjacent to the afferent and efferent arterioles, the cells of the distal convoluted tubule become narrower and taller. Collectively, these cells are called the *macula densa* and are thought to be chemoreceptors or osmoreceptors that respond to changes in the solute concentration of the filtrate. Each nephron's juxtaglomerular apparatus (JGA) is formed from these juxtaglomerular cells and the macula densa.

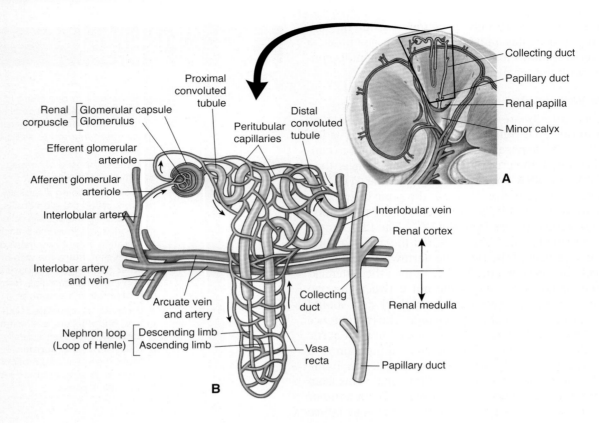

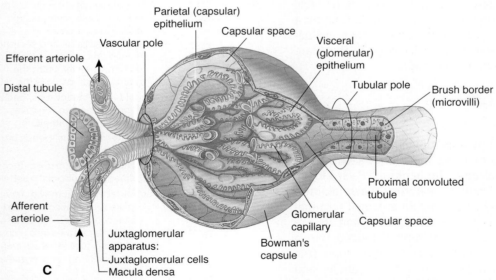

**Figure 10-5** Nephron anatomy. The illustrations show **(A)** the location and make-up of a nephron, **(B)** the distinction between a cortical and juxtamedullary nephron location, and **(C)** the structure of the cortical and juxtamedullary nephron (see Table 10-3). (**A**, reprinted with permission from Agur AMR, Dalley AF. *Grant's Atlas of Anatomy*. 12th ed. Baltimore, MD: Lippincott Williams & Wilkins; 2009:167.)

# PHYSIOLOGY[2,5,18]

To carry out the normal kidney functions of removing wastes from the blood and regulating its fluid and electrolyte content, approximately 1,100 to 1,200 mL of blood passes through the kidneys every minute. This represents 20% to 25% of the total cardiac output transported by the RRA and LRA. The enormous blood flow is related to the fact that, for the kidneys to maintain blood homeostasis, a considerable amount of blood must pass through the kidneys. More than 90% of the blood entering the kidney perfuses the cortex, containing the nephron, and only a small amount of the blood supplies the kidney's nutritive needs.

The kidneys, which process about 180 L (45 gal) of blood-derived fluid daily, are involved in both excretory and regulatory activities. Of the total amount of blood-derived fluid circulated through the kidneys, 99% is filtered and returned for circulation, whereas only about 1% is eliminated from the body as urine. The body depends on the efficient functioning of the glomeruli and the renal tubules (nephrons and collecting tubes) to filter the entire plasma volume approximately 60 times a day. As the smallest structural unit capable of producing urine, the nephron is so important that one-third of the nephrons must function simply to ensure survival. Three important nephron functions are (1) controlling blood concentration and volume by removing selected amounts of water and solutes, (2) helping to regulate blood pH, and (3) removing toxic wastes from the blood. The three processes involved in urine formation and the simultaneous adjustment of blood composition are described in Table 10-4.

Antidiuretic hormone (ADH), secreted by the posterior pituitary, increases the water permeability of the collecting tubule segments (facultative reabsorption) by enlarging the pores, so that water passes easily into the interstitial spaces.[19,20] Responsible for maintaining the body's fluid balance, ADH secretion increases in the event of increased water loss (sweating or diarrhea) or reduced blood volume or blood pressure (hemorrhage).

Aldosterone, secreted by the adrenal cortex, increases the rate of tubular resorption of sodium and produces a concurrent loss of potassium. Extracellular excess of potassium promotes aldosterone secretion, which in turn produces an increase in potassium excretion and sodium retention by the kidneys. Aldosterone secretion is also controlled by the renin-angiotensin system. Renin, secreted by the JGA, increases in response to decreased blood pressure in the afferent arteriole secondary to sodium depletion or to a change from the supine to the upright position. Renin acts as a catalyst on certain plasma proteins to produce angiotensin I, which is converted to angiotensin II by proteolytic enzymes. Angiotensin II increases systemic blood pressure. By acting as a potent vasoconstrictor,

it increases peripheral resistance and causes increased blood pressure, and by increasing the rate of aldosterone secretion and tubular reabsorption of sodium, it increases the kidney's ability to retain water and to produce a small volume of concentrated urine. In response to the increased volume of filtrate and increased sodium chloride passing through the JGA, renin secretion decreases.

## RENAL FUNCTION TESTS

Alterations in renal function produce a spectrum of disorders leading to severe impairment of some organ functions, whereas others remain entirely unaffected. Sonographers should have a basic understanding of normal and abnormal values to correlate the clinical history and presenting symptoms with the sonographic representation of anatomy, disease, or pathology. Table 10-5 presents several serum and urine laboratory tests related to renal function. Urea nitrogen, creatinine, and uric acid are used to evaluate renal function. Laboratory examination of urine specimens can detect the presence of red blood cells (RBCs), white blood cells (WBCs), and bacteria, which could indicate infection or tumor. Because normal values vary with sex, age, and geographic region, they are not presented in the table.

## SONOGRAPHIC SCANNING TECHNIQUE

### PATIENT PREPARATION

No patient preparation is required for sonographic examination of the kidneys but fasting augments visualization. If surrounding structures are of interest, such as the adrenal glands or the pancreas, it is recommended that the patient fast approximately 6 to 8 hours before the examination. If the examination's purpose includes assessment of associated ureteral and vessel pathology, the patient should drink 20 to 24 oz of liquid 30 to 45 minutes before the examination to ensure better visualization of the vessels and a urine-filled bladder. If possible,

| TABLE 10-4 | |
|---|---|
| **Urine Formation** | |
| Glomerular filtration | Nonselective process by which fluids and solutes are forced through membrane by pressure gradient; occurs in renal corpuscle across endothelial capsular membrane; portion of fluid entering nephron is called filtrate; filtrate consists of all raw materials in blood processed by renal tubules except formed elements and proteins too large to pass through the endothelial barrier |
| Tubular resorption | A discriminating process occurring as filtrate passes through renal tubules; depending on body needs, epithelial cells reabsorb water, glucose, amino acids, and electrolyte ions; the process allows the body to retain most of its nutrients; wastes such as urea are only partially reabsorbed |
| Tubular secretion | Active process that transports substances into nephron and adds material to filtrate from blood; secretion is for (1) disposing of substances not already in filtrate (penicillin and phenobarbital); (2) eliminating undesirable compounds reabsorbed by passive processes (urea and uric acid); (3) removing excessive potassium ions; and (4) regulating blood pH |

**TABLE 10-5**

Renal Functions Tests

| Test and Specimen | Explanation | Pathologic Variation | Clinical Indications |
|---|---|---|---|
| Blood urea nitrogen (BUN) Serum | Measures amount of urea nitrogen in blood; urea, an end product of protein metabolism is formed in liver and carried to kidney for excretion; BUN can be used to measure renal function | Increase | Acute or chronic disease of damaged kidneys: renal failure, congestive heart failure with decreased renal blood supply, obstructive uropathy, stress, dehydration, starvation, decreased blood volume (hemorrhage) |
|  |  | Decrease | Over hydration, liver failure, pregnancy, decreased protein intake, smoking |
| Creatinine clearance rate (Cr, CrCl) Serum or urine | Creatinine is a nonprotein, end product of breakdown of creatinine phosphate found in skeletal muscles; blood concentration is proportional to amount of active body muscle tissue and is normally maintained at a constant rate | Increase | Decrease in renal function (e.g., increase above 9.0 mg/dL may indicate 90% loss of nephron function); decreased glomerular filtration (uremia or azotemia if severe), glomerulonephritis, pyelonephritis, acute tubular necrosis, urinary tract obstruction, reduced renal blood flow, diabetes, nephritis, rhabdomyolysis, acromegaly, gigantism |
|  | Creatinine is removed by glomerular filtration, the rate of which is close to that of serum creatinine production; it is a very accurate test since creatinine production is not affected by protein intake, urine volume, hydration, or protein metabolism; if only one kidney is functioning, the opposite kidney, if normal, increases filtration rate | Decrease | Debilitation, muscle weakness or dystrophy, myasthenia, starvation, hyperthyroidism |
| Uric acid (UA) Serum or urine | Uric acid is an end product of purine metabolism; purine comes from dietary sources and from breakdown of proteins | Increase | Serum: gout, arthritis, uric acid renal stones, soft tissue deposits (tophi), lead poisoning, hypothyroidism, multiple myeloma, metastatic cancer, acidosis, toxemia, alcoholism, leukemias, hyperlipoproteinemia, diabetes mellitus, renal failure, stress, chemotherapy, shock, strenuous exercise, starvation |
|  |  |  | Urine: gout, chronic myelogenous leukemia, polycythemia vera, ulcerative colitis, febrile illness, liver disease, toxemia, high-purine diet |
|  |  | Decrease | Serum: Wilson disease, Fanconi syndrome, liver atrophy |
|  |  |  | Urine: renal disease (chronic glomerulonephritis, urinary obstruction, renal tubular degeneration), eclampsia, lead toxicity, chronic alcohol ingestion |
| Red blood cell (RBC) count Serum | Kidneys secrete erythropoietin, which stimulates production of RBCs in bone marrow; counted per milliliter of blood | Increase | Hypernephroma and renal cysts increase erythropoietin, causing erythrocytosis |
| Total white blood cell (WBC) count Serum | Counted per milliliter of blood | Increase | Infection or inflammation causes leukocytosis |
|  |  | Decrease | Toxic reactions, chemotherapy, or radiation therapy |

| Test | Description | Finding | Associated Conditions |
|---|---|---|---|
| Differential white cell count (Diff) Serum | Reports percentages of white blood cells (WBCs); granulocytes (neutrophils), eosinophils, basophils) and nongranulocytes (lymphocytes and monocytes) in blood; with elevation of WBC count, one or more cell types increase in number; the percentage increases per sample of 100, while the other cell percentages decrease, even though the absolute count does not; Diff provides specific information on stage and severity of disease or infection and host's ability to resist | Increase neutrophils (segs, or mature cells; band or stabs, young cells) | Bacterial infection, inflammation process, physical stress, tissue necrosis |
| Hematocrit (Hct) Serum | Percentage of red blood cells (RBCs) in plasma | Decrease | Acute hemorrhagic process secondary to disease or trauma |
| Lactic acid dehydrogenase (LDH) Serum | Enzyme found in cytoplasm of nearly all tissues | Increase | Acute renal infarction, chronic renal disorders |
| Urine pH Urine | Measures relative acidity (<7) or alkalinity (<7); normally, urine tends to be acidic due to diet (meat, eggs), whereas fruits and vegetables render it alkaline; alkaline urine promotes growth of certain organisms and calcium phosphate calculi in susceptible persons | Alkalinity | Renal tubular acidosis, diet, infection, respiratory alkalosis, metabolic alkalosis, drugs, bed rest |
| Specific gravity of urine Urine | Measures kidney's ability to concentrate urine; density of urine is compared to density of water (1,000); the higher the number, the more concentrated the urine unless it contains abnormal constituents | Increase | Dehydration, large number of solutes (iodinated contrast medium, glucose, intravenous albumin, protein), and increased secretion of antidiuretic hormone (trauma, stress, surgery) |
| | | Decrease | Hydration, presence of diuretic medication |
| Urine protein Urine | With proteinuria or albuminuria (excess of plasma proteins, principally albumin, in urine) blood concentration is lower | Increase | Acute or chronic glomerulonephritis, nephrotic syndrome, lupus nephritis, amyloidosis, severe renal venous congestion, nephrotoxic effect |
| Casts and cells Urine | Casts are formed in kidney as a result of agglutination of cells or cellular debris; casts in urine imply tubular or glomerular disorders; condition is associated with proteinuria or albuminuria since protein is necessary for cast formation | WBC casts | Pyelonephritis |
| | | RBC casts | Glomerulonephritis |
| | | Hyaline casts | Acute renal inflammatory disease, renal hypertension, heart failure, diabetic renal disease |
| | | Epithelial casts or cells | Renal tubular degeneration if seen in large quantities |
| | | Granular casts | Nephritis, acute tubular necrosis, advanced glomerulonephritis, pyelonephritis |
| | | Waxy casts | End-stage renal disease |
| | | Hematuria (blood cells) | Hemorrhagic cystitis or calculi in renal pelvis, tuberculosis, or tumors of renal collecting and tubule systems |
| Urinary glucose Urine | If blood glucose level is normal (no diabetes mellitus), the presence of sugar in urine indicates a low renal threshold for resorption | Glycosuria | Without diabetes mellitus, indicate renal tubule dysfunction (pregnancy, drugs, congenital metabolic disorders, Fanconi syndrome) |

schedule sonographic examinations first. Following a radionuclide renographic examination, residual radioactivity within the patient's urinary bladder is in proximity to the sonographer's hand.

## PATIENT POSITIONS AND SCANNING TECHNIQUES

The native kidneys can usually be accessed with the patient in a supine, posterior oblique, or lateral decubitus position and images can be obtained from anterior or lateral approaches. It is often advantageous to scan in more than one patient position and from more than one anatomic site.

Regardless of the approach selected, the kidney should be thoroughly imaged in at least two orthogonal planes and representative sectional planes should be studied. The sonographer should establish a protocol that includes evaluating the medial, lateral, superior, and inferior renal borders. The number of images made will vary. The minimum routine examination should include (1) longitudinal sections, coronal sections, or both in long axis for the renal length, sinus, and calyces, the lateral margin, and the medial margin pelvis and (2) transverse sections of the superior pole imaging the upper renal sinus, the midpole imaging the renal artery and vein and making measurements, and the inferior pole.

Using the liver as an acoustic window, the right kidney is best imaged with the patient in either a supine, left posterior oblique, or left lateral decubitus position, scanning through the anterior axillary line intercostally or subcostally. The left kidney is best imaged in the right posterior oblique or right lateral decubitus position, requiring transducer placement in an intercostal space along the posterior axillary line and using the spleen as an acoustic window.

The renal arteries and veins are best visualized in a transverse plane because of their perpendicular relationship to the ultrasound beam. The right renal vessels are best imaged with the transducer placed transversely over the right kidney and angled medially. To visualize the left renal vessels, the transducer should be placed in a transverse orientation in the midline of the abdomen, just inferior to the origination of the SMA. To appropriately evaluate vasculature, interrogation with pulsed wave Doppler and color Doppler should be performed.

A decubitus patient position will allow coronal sections to be obtained. Coronal sections provide better visualization of the renal parenchyma, the medial and lateral borders, and the proximal ureter. They also demonstrate the kidney's frontal plane so that lesions in the kidney, and in perirenal and pararenal spaces, can easily be located. A prone or supine position is better for demonstrating the posterior and anterior borders of the kidneys.

For patients who can be scanned only in a prone position, a pillow or rolled sheet placed under the abdomen at the kidney level compresses anterior soft tissue and stretches the posterior muscles. This reduces scattering and absorption of the sound beam and enlarges the acoustic window between the iliac crest and the ribs.

### Long Axis

With the upper pole more medial and posterior than the lower pole, the longitudinal renal axis is normally oriented in an oblique plane. The transducer is rotated from a transverse plane to a longitudinal position and manipulated until equal amounts of cortical tissue appear in both the upper and lower poles. If the imaging plane is skewed, the apparent renal length will be shorter.

## MEASUREMENTS[21–23]

Changes in renal mass accompanied by changes in renal architecture are easily detected by qualitative visual inspection while scanning. Alterations in renal mass without significant alterations in architecture require a quantitative method of detection. Accurate bilateral kidney length, width, and thickness measurements are normally obtained in the routine procedure. Renal measurements depend on a number of variables, including age, sex, body habitus, hydration, and the individual making the measurements. Compensatory renal hypertrophy occurs following removal of one kidney because of disease, injury, or transplantation. The best correlation of renal length is body height (Fig. 10-6A–D). The adult cortex is generally more than 1 cm in thickness over the pyramids. However, measurement of cortical thickness demonstrates greater interobserver and intraobserver variability as compared to other measurements of renal size.

From a physiologic standpoint, renal volume is more sensitive than any single linear kidney measurement and is the most useful and important variable in detecting disease and in evaluating renal allografts, monitoring children with urinary tract disease or assessing patients after unilateral nephrectomy. Using the formula length $\times$ width $\times$ thickness $\times$ 0.5, the renal volume averages 146 cm³ for the left kidney and 134 cm³ for the right kidney. Renal volume demonstrates the strongest correlation with height, weight, and total body area.

### Doppler Examination

For a discussion on Doppler evaluation of the hilar vessels, see Chapter 4.

Doppler examination requires education and experience to obtain useful information to contribute to the renal examination. The patient must be able to cooperate with instructions, remain immobile, and suspend respiration when required. With some pathologic conditions, it may be difficult to obtain this level of cooperation.

The patient can be positioned in either the posterior oblique or decubitus position for either the pulsed or color Doppler examination. The segmental, interlobar, and arcuate vessels can be examined with a 3- to 5-MHz

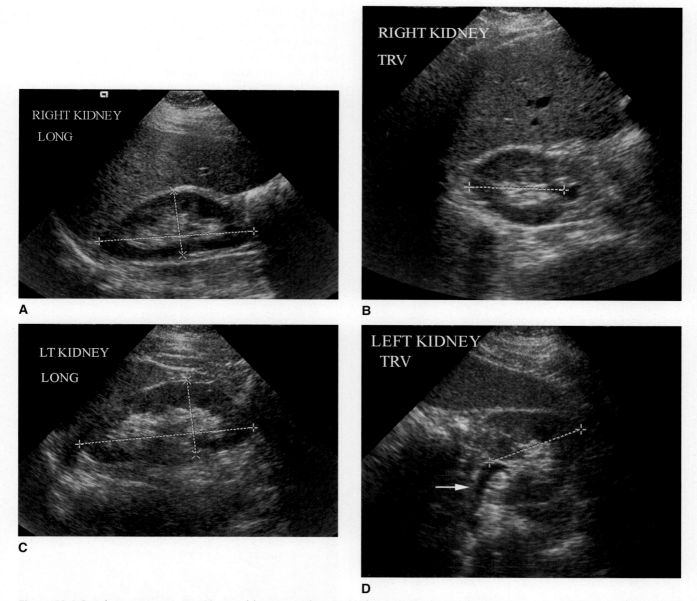

**Figure 10-6** Renal measurements in a 32-year-old woman with normal kidneys. **A:** The longitudinal section of the right kidney demonstrates correct locations *(calipers)* used to obtain the length and anteroposterior measurements. **B:** The correct width measurement *(cursors)* is obtained and is measured using a transverse section of the right kidney. **C:** The longitudinal section of the left demonstrates correct measurement locations *(cursors)* to obtain the length and anteroposterior measurements. **D:** The correct width measurement *(cursors)* is obtained using a transverse section of the left kidney. The proximal ureter is visualized exiting the renal hilum *(arrow)*.

transducer from a lateral intercostal approach. Transducer selection requires an adequate focal zone depth to interrogate the renal artery. The Doppler sample volume should be kept small (2 to 5 mm). All velocity measurements should be made with a Doppler angle of less than 60 degrees between the direction of flow and the Doppler beam. There may be instances in which a Doppler angle of less than 60 degrees will not be obtainable despite the sonographer's best efforts. This will lead to falsely elevated velocities, which should be viewed with suspicion. To offset problems related to inaccurate resistance measurements, the wall filter should be set as low as possible (≤50 Hz) so that important low-velocity information is not hidden. To minimize relative error and to maximize the Doppler tracings, use the smallest possible frequency range (pulse repetition frequency).

The Doppler sample volume is placed inside the renal hilum for the segmental arteries, along the border of the medullary pyramids for interlobar arteries, and at the corticomedullary junction for the arcuate arteries. The sonographer should obtain and analyze several consecutive identical waveforms and examine both kidneys. The resistive index (RI) is calculated to characterize intrarenal impedance. The RI is an index of pulsatility over a cardiac cycle determined by the following formula:

$$RI = peak\ systolic\ shift - minimum\ diastolic\ shift/\ peak\ systolic\ shift$$

To evaluate vascular or parenchymal disease, the segmental, interlobar, and arcuate intrarenal vessels are routinely examined. The normal pulse Doppler examination will show a low-impedance waveform with decreasing peak systolic velocities as the vessels are traced distally. The RI reported for the normal adult kidney ranges from 0.58 to 0.64 ± 0.05.[24] An RI of 0.70 is generally considered the upper limit of normal for the adult kidney. An RI value >0.70 shows excellent sensitivity and specificity in distinguishing renal obstruction from unobstructed dilatation. In cases of physiologic extremes of decreased heart rate and hypotension, the RI can be elevated even in the absence of renal pathology or a true change in renal vascular impedance.[24] Correlating the RI to heart rate and blood pressure is important (Fig. 10-7A,B).

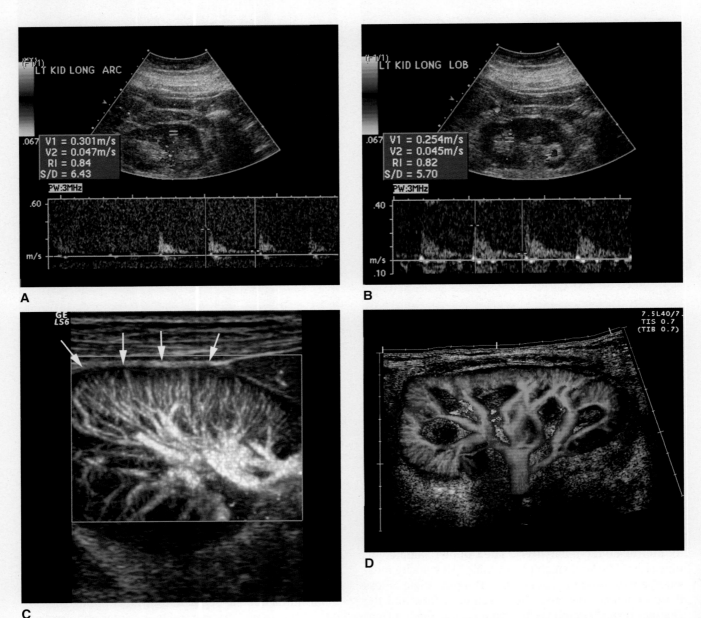

**Figure 10-7** Hypertension. **A,B:** The longitudinal sections of the left kidney were obtained on a woman with hypertension. The Doppler images presented are the **(A)** arcuate artery and the **(B)** interlobar artery. The data displayed include both peak systolic (V1) and end or minimum diastolic (V2) velocities, the systolic/diastolic (S/D) ratio, and resistive index, which are calculated by the equipment. **C:** Normal intrarenal flow. Transverse flow image of the kidney demonstrates flow into the periphery of the renal cortex. **D:** Power Doppler image of the kidney demonstrates the entire vasculature of the kidney from the renal artery to the intralobar arteries in the renal cortex. Flow is seen all the way to the renal capsule. Color and power Doppler delineates intrarenal vessels that are invisible on grayscale images and undetectable using other, noninvasive imaging techniques. The intensity of the color is related to the amplitude of the signal—that is, the number of red cells in each sample volume. (**A,B,** Images courtesy of Natalee Braun, Ogden, UT; **C,** Image courtesy of GE Healthcare, Wauwatosa, WI.)

When main renal veins or intrarenal parenchymal veins are examined, Doppler signals show continuous flow in the direction opposite arterial flow and variation due to both respiratory and cardiac activities.

Pulsed Doppler provides valuable physiologic information regarding intrarenal vascular flow, and spectral analysis is helpful to assess peripheral arterial resistance, hydronephrosis, and other diffuse renal diseases. Color Doppler is useful to evaluate renal artery occlusion and stenosis, aneurysm, pseudoaneurysm, arteriovenous (AV) fistula, AV malformation, and venous thrombosis. Power Doppler provides additional anatomic information by demonstrating the entire renovascular tree. The major advantage of power Doppler is that normal blood flow is demonstrated better, including renal cortical blood flow. Power Doppler is especially advantageous to evaluate renal perfusion in cases of flank pain or trauma, congenital and acquired renal vascular lesions, and hemorrhagic or tumor thrombus of the renal vein (Fig. 10-7C,D).

## TECHNICAL CONSIDERATIONS

For better kidney visualization, deep inspiration helps push the liver, spleen, and kidneys down below the ribs as much as 2.5 cm.[17] Visualizing some portions of the liver with the right kidney and the spleen with the left kidney is important, as their echo amplitude should always be compared to that of the renal parenchyma.

For adults, a 3.5- to 5-MHz transducer generally provides the highest frequency that affords adequate visualization of parenchymal detail in each scanning plane. Because acoustic energy attenuates exponentially as it penetrates tissue and because attenuation increases with frequency, optimal visualization of renal parenchyma requires varied gain, time gain compensation (TGC), and power output, making adjustments to optimize image quality while using the lowest exposure levels possible. To minimize the effect of TGC, it should be adjusted to achieve even uniform echo intensity throughout the depth of the homogeneous hepatic or splenic tissue and should be compared to the renal cortical echo amplitude at the same depth. The gain setting should be high enough to fill the cortex but low enough so as not to obliterate the medulla.

## PITFALLS

Although the kidneys are relatively easy to identify sonographically, there are pitfalls. The normal kidney is an anisotropic organ, which means that its appearance varies based on the angle of the ultrasound beam. On transverse sections, the kidney often appears more echogenic than on corresponding longitudinal images. This is due to the relative difference in the number of acoustic impedance mismatch interfaces encountered.

Respiratory motion or failure to visualize the true long axis of the kidney can lead to underestimation or overestimation of renal size.

Athletic patients and young men frequently have prominent hypertrophic psoas muscles that can simulate a renal or adrenal tumor and should not be mistaken for retroperitoneal fibrosis (Fig. 10-8A). A technique helpful in differentiating muscle from mass is to instruct the patient (lying in a supine position) to flex or pull up the legs while observing muscle contraction with real-time sonography.

Other anatomic structures—adrenal glands, liver, spleen, pancreatic head, and pancreatic tail—lie close to the kidney's upper pole and can simulate masses arising from this region. Congenital or developmental anomalies can make kidneys appear diseased or difficult to identify. Atrophic kidneys pose a significant challenge, as they are quite small and difficult to outline. Large or multiple cysts can be mistaken for hydronephrosis, and pseudohydronephrosis can appear secondary to overfilling of the bladder[10] or rapid hydration (Fig. 10-8B–G). An ectopic or transplanted kidney can be confused with a pelvic mass. Inappropriate TGC settings will not allow the determination of solid versus cystic masses.

Rib artifacts, especially at the upper poles of the kidneys, can cause shadowing and obscure pathologic processes. Duplication artifacts due to refraction of the sound beam can occur at liver–fat or spleen–fat interfaces, which can mimic an area of cortical thickening or a mass. The artifact occurs more commonly in the left kidney and occurs more frequently in obese patients. Changing the transducer position to entirely interpose the liver or spleen as an acoustic window in scanning renal tissue helps eliminate this artifact.

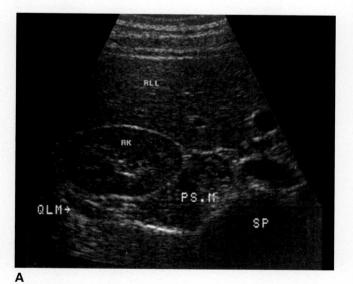

**A**

**Figure 10-8** Pitfalls. **A:** The anatomic locations of the psoas muscle (*PS.M*) and quadratus lumborum muscle (*QLM*) to the right kidney (*RK*) can be identified on this transverse section through the right upper quadrant. These muscles could be mistaken for either renal mass if the contiguous renal capsule is not observed or a retroperitoneal mass without an understanding of surrounding anatomy. Careful and complete scanning techniques must be employed on all patients to correctly identify normal versus abnormal anatomy. (*RLL*, right liver lobe; *SP*, spine.) (*continued*)

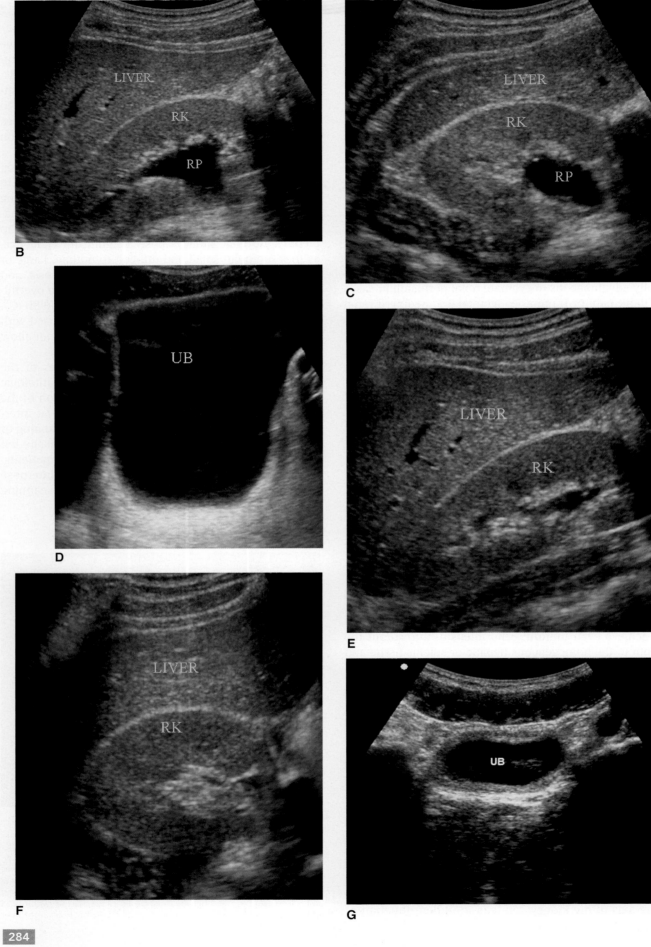

B

C

D

E

F

G

**Figure 10-8** *(continued)* **B:** Longitudinal and **(C)** transverse images of a right kidney with mild dilatation of the renal pelvis. **D:** Transverse image of the same patient's overly distended bladder. **E:** Longitudinal and **(F)** transverse images of the same right kidney taken after the patient voided. The dilatation resolved after voiding. **G:** Postvoid image of the patient's urinary bladder *(UB)*. The pseudohydronephrosis was due to an over-distended *UB* creating a false-positive diagnosis. (Images **B-G** courtesy of Taco Geertsma, MD, Hospital Gelderse Vallei, Ede, The Netherlands.)

A repertoire of scanning skills must be developed to help overcome these pitfalls. With careful scanning technique, the origin of any mass can be determined. In the evaluation of pelvic masses, visualizing the kidneys in their normal position rules out a pelvic kidney. Likewise, if one of the kidneys is not found in its proper location, checking the pelvic region is important. Post void images of the kidneys should be included within the exam protocol whenever any degree of hydronephrosis is encountered or when scanning a transplanted kidney. Obtaining the patient's clinical history and correlating it with the images is the most useful means of avoiding scanning pitfalls.

## CONGENITAL ANOMALIES

It has been estimated that 10% of infants have some form of urinary tract abnormality.[9] Congenital kidney anomalies can be classified according to (1) amount of renal tissue; (2) number; and (3) position, form, and orientation.

### AMOUNT OF RENAL TISSUE

#### Agenesis and Hypoplasia[16,25]

Renal agenesis is presumed to be due to unilateral absence of the nephrogenic primordium or failure of the wolffian duct to make contact with the mesodermal mass. The absence of function resulting from unilateral renal agenesis (absence of one kidney and ureter) or the diminished function caused by unilateral hypoplasia (reduced number of renal lobules and calyces) often produces hypertrophy of the contralateral kidney. Unilateral renal agenesis and hypoplasia are not considered life threatening, as the body can sustain life with one kidney. Sonographically, the two entities are difficult to distinguish. If no kidney or a small kidney is identifiable in the renal fossa along with hypertrophy of the contralateral kidney, agenesis or hypoplasia may be suspected, but an ectopic kidney should be included in the differential diagnosis.

Bilateral renal agenesis, complete absence of both kidneys, is not compatible with life. Bilateral renal agenesis can be detected in utero and is associated with oligohydramnios and absence of fetal urinary bladder filling. In a newborn, the adrenal glands enlarge and fill the renal fossae.

### ANOMALIES OF NUMBER

#### Collecting System Duplications[9,26]

Complete duplication of the ureter is the most common congenital anomaly of the genitourinary tract. More frequent in women than in men, it is associated with

early development of renal diseases. Two ureteral buds arise in the fourth gestational week from the wolffian duct, and initially the caudal ureter drains the lower pole, while the cephalic ureter drains the upper one. As the fetus develops, the cephalad ureter continues to migrate with the wolffian duct and enters the bladder at the trigone; however, it is usually associated with a short or absent submucosal tunnel and may become dilated due to vesicoureteral reflux or from an upper pole system obstruction. The upper pole ureter is malpositioned, enters the bladder below the trigone, and may be obstructed, leading to ectopic ureterocele (see Chapter 20).

Sonographically, identifying separation in the normal renal sinus echodensities contributes to the diagnosis (Fig. 10-9A). If dilatation is present, the sonographic characteristics simulate hydronephrosis or a large cyst. If an associated dilated ureter is present, its course should be followed in search of a ureterocele. When there is a question of possible collecting system duplication, sonography, which is independent of renal function, can be utilized to (1) determine the presence of kidneys, (2) exclude hydronephrosis, (3) exclude a duplication anomaly, (4) identify a ureterocele in the bladder, and (5) guide percutaneous puncture, if indicated. A major scanning pitfall is the inability to identify duplication sonographically when a nonfunctioning upper moiety is obscured by the lower moiety, which presents with marked lower pole hydroureteronephrosis due to reflux[27] (Fig. 10-9B). At times, a duplicated collecting system can be seen in the urinary bladder by observing the ureteral jets from the duplicated ureters (Fig. 10-9C).

#### Supernumerary Kidneys[4,16]

Complete duplication of the kidney, pelvis, and ureter is a rare condition believed to be due to splitting of the nephrogenic blastema before or at the time of union with the ureteric bud. This duplication occurs with equal frequency on the right and left sides and can be bilateral. A supernumerary kidney is an extra kidney with its own blood supply. The extra kidney usually is ectopic, and the ureter usually joins the upper kidney ureter, so that there is a common ureteral opening into the bladder trigone on the affected side.

If the condition is suspected, sonography can outline two separate kidneys; but if an extra kidney is not suspected and is ectopic, it may be overlooked during a routine examination. The hilar region should be carefully examined in a coronal longitudinal section to visualize the renal pelvis to verify the presence of a single ureter.

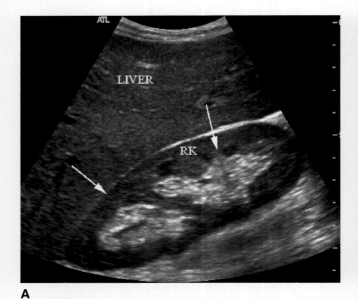

**A**

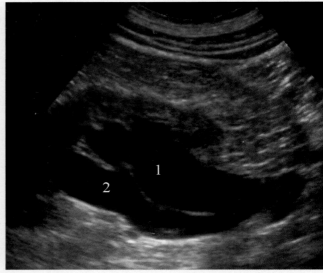

**B**

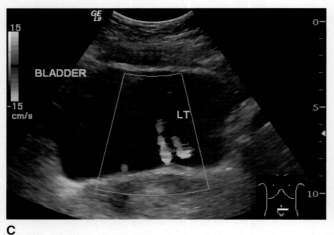

**C**

**Figure 10-9** Collecting system duplication. **A:** A right renal collecting duplication is recognized as the renal parenchyma extends anterior-posteriorly through the sinus. Two distinct renal sinuses are seen *(arrows)*. **B:** On a different patient, two dilated ureters are demonstrated exiting the renal hilum suggesting a duplicated system. **C:** This patient's left duplicated collecting system was imaged with the display of two left ureteral jets seen in the full urinary bladder. (**A**, Image courtesy of Philips Medical Systems, Bothell, WA; **B**, Image courtesy of Pam Thacker, Newark, OH; **C**, Image courtesy of Doug Amussen, Hyde Park, UT.)

## ANOMALIES OF POSITION, FORM, AND ORIENTATION

Fetal lobulations, the junctional cortical defect, junctional parenchymal defect, or the interpeduncular junction, and the renal column of Bertin are common anomalies and were discussed in the section on normal sonographic appearance.

### Ectopic Kidneys[1,4,5,16]

If early fetal vascular connections persist or if the metanephros develops in an abnormally low position, normal ascension of the kidney may not always occur. These kidneys are normal or slightly smaller than normal and lie just above the pelvic brim or sometimes even within the pelvis (Fig. 10-10A–C).

An intrathoracic kidney is a rare developmental anomaly that results when the kidney continues its craniad ascent. It is thought to be associated with delayed closure of the thoracic cavity. The pleuroperitoneal canal normally closes between the seventh and eighth weeks of fetal life. With an intrathoracic ectopic kidney, the diaphragm closes below or around the kidney. If kidney infection or obstruction develops, thoracic symptoms may occur.

In the third type of renal ectopy, both kidneys are located on one side of the body. This condition is relatively uncommon, and fusion to the contralateral kidney is more common than the unfused type. The upper pole of the crossed ectopic kidney is usually fused to the lower pole of the normally rotated ipsilateral kidney, and the ureter of the ectopic kidney crosses the midline to enter the bladder on the opposite side (Fig. 10-10D,E).

With all three types of ectopy, an associated rotational anomaly in which the kidney pelvis faces anteriorly is common. Vascular insertion into the aorta and IVC may be displaced, and the longer renal vessels have a more tortuous path, making kidney obstruction and infection more likely. Ipsilateral crossed ectopia and pelvic kidneys are associated with a higher incidence of bacterial infection and calculi because the ureter is kinked or tortuous, although it enters the bladder trigone in its

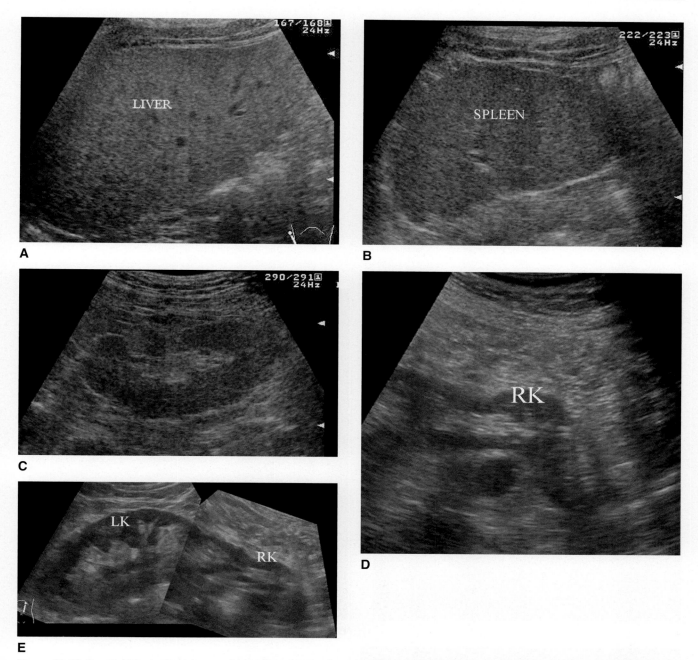

**Figure 10-10** Ectopic kidneys. **A:** An image of the right upper quadrant demonstrates an empty renal fossa. **B:** An image of the left upper quadrant reveals an empty renal fossa. **C:** A single pelvic kidney was found in the left lower quadrant. **D,E:** In this 53-year-old patient, a small right kidney **(D)** is fused to the inferior pole of the left kidney **(E)**. (Images courtesy of Taco Geertsma, MD, Hospital Gelderse Vallei, Ede, The Netherlands.)

normal position. Pelvic kidney can be confused with a palpable pelvic mass.

Sonography should be used to seek ectopic kidney or renal vasculature. Bowel gas may make a pelvic kidney more difficult to locate. Associated malrotation of the kidneys may require oblique scanning planes to image renal structures. The crossed, fused kidney may mimic a single kidney with a duplicated system or a kidney with a renal mass. Two separate sinuses should be demonstrated, as well as the absence of the contralateral kidney. Feces-filled colon or small bowel may occupy the normal

renal fossa and mimic a renal mass or a hydronephrotic kidney. Real-time sonography should be able to discern colon peristalsis or a change in configuration over time. Other imaging modalities such as computed tomography (CT), intravenous pyelogram (IVP), or radionuclide renal scanning can aid in confirming the diagnosis.

## Horseshoe Kidney[1,4,9,16]

Fusion of the upper or lower kidney poles during fetal development produces a horseshoe-shaped structure continuous across the midline and anterior to the great vessels. This is a common anomaly (occurring in 1 in 400 individuals). The majority are fused, with an isthmus composed of a simple cord or a fibrous band at the lower pole, although approximately 10% are fused at the upper pole. With lower pole fusion, the ureters usually pass anterior to the renal parenchyma. Generally asymptomatic and capable of normal function, horseshoe kidneys can be associated with hydronephrosis, infection, or calculus formation.

Patients with horseshoe kidney are often referred for evaluation of a pulsatile abdominal mass. Sonographically, when a mass is identified anterior to the abdominal aorta, a horseshoe kidney should be considered, along with an abdominal aortic aneurysm, lymphadenopathy, and pancreatic enlargement. Bowel gas may

obstruct visualization. After locating the long axis of the kidneys, follow the lower poles by angling and obliquing the scanning plane to determine if the lower poles fuse into the mass. Horseshoe kidneys are best identified by orienting the transducer in the plane of the isthmus and the adjoining renal poles. Lower fused poles are usually identified at the level of the iliac crest crossing the fourth or fifth lumbar vertebra with normal renal parenchyma or as a solid renal mass if the connection is fibrous tissue. Occasionally, a patient has very superficial renal tissue due to an exaggerated anteroposterior kidney axis (Fig. 10-11A–C). IVP and CT are two imaging modalities that will confirm the presence of a horseshoe kidney. To verify renal function in the connecting segment, a radionuclide scan can be performed.

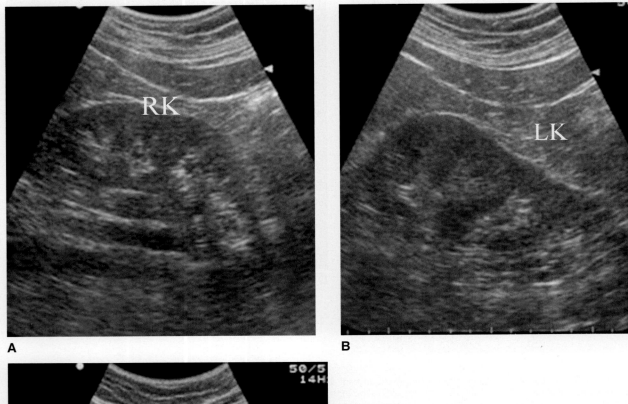

**Figure 10-11** Horseshoe kidney. On this patient, the sonographic examination demonstrated fusion of the lower poles. **A:** A longitudinal image on the right demonstrates a lack of definition of the inferior pole. **B:** A longitudinal image on the left also demonstrates an indiscernible inferior pole. **C:** A longitudinal image made over the midabdomen demonstrates the isthmus *(arrows)* anterior to the aorta, representing the inferior pole fusion of both the right and left kidney. (Images courtesy of Taco Geertsma, MD, Hospital Gelderse Vallei, Ede, The Netherlands.)

# CYSTIC RENAL MASSES

Cystic masses of the kidney may be hereditary alterations in differentiation, nonhereditary but developmental, or acquired disorders. For convenience and simplicity, they are discussed collectively here. As a group, renal cysts are important because they are reasonably common and often present diagnostic problems, some forms are major causes of renal failure, and occasionally they are confused with malignant tumors. Sonography is an excellent modality for defining the type of cystic disease because it is an anatomic examination, capable of distinguishing cystic from solid lesions, particularly suitable for renal imaging, and portable.

## POLYCYSTIC RENAL DISEASE

Cystic dysplastic kidneys, multicystic kidneys, and infantile polycystic kidneys (found in newborns and children) are discussed in Chapter 20.

### Autosomal Dominant Polycystic Kidney Disease[4,12,28–30]

Adult polycystic kidney disease is a relatively common disease (found in 1 in 1,000 to 1 in 2,000 persons worldwide) and accounts for 8% to 10% of the patients who require chronic dialysis or renal transplantation. The cause of this form of polycystic disease is unknown. In the majority of cases, it is inherited as an autosomal dominant trait. Approximately 10% of cases may be acquired through spontaneous mutation. The gene penetrance is such that morphologic evidence is seen in almost 100% of patients who survive to 70 to 80 years of age (1 in 1,000). Even though patients may remain asymptomatic throughout life,[30,31] autosomal dominant polycystic kidney disease (ADPKD) usually manifests clinically in the fourth decade and tends to cause kidney failure at the same age in members of an affected family. With this type of cystic disease, cystic dilatations form in the proximal convoluted tubules, Bowman's capsule, and the collecting tubules. With age, the cysts enlarge and renal function begins to decrease. The most frequent complications are infection and renal calculi, but cyst rupture, hemorrhage, and ureteric obstruction may also occur. The patient presents with abdominal and lumbar pain, hematuria, and hypertension. If calcifications are present and are associated with the cysts, they can appear thin, ring-like, curvilinear, or as small flecks and amorphous concretions. Death usually occurs about 10 years after the onset of symptoms. The most common causes of death are uremia (59%), cerebral hemorrhage (13%), and cardiac disease, usually associated with hypertension.[20] Concurrent with the disease, patients can also have cysts in the liver (25% to 50%), pancreas (9%), lungs, spleen, ovaries, seminal vesicles, testes, epididymis, thyroid, uterus, and bladder. Cerebral arterial (berry) aneurysms in the circle of Willis occur in 16% of patients, and 9% die from rupture.[12]

Sonographic examinations can safely be used to screen family members to diagnose polycystic disease that has not manifested clinically, to provide genetic counseling prior to procreation, and to learn more about the natural history of the disease. The examination protocol should include scanning both kidneys and making routine kidney measurements and measurements of major cysts. Because the disease may cause cyst formation in other organs, the liver, pancreas, spleen, and ovaries or testes should be imaged.

Sonographically, both kidneys are usually enlarged, with numerous discrete cysts in the cortical regions (Fig. 10-12A–D). If the cysts are too small to be resolved individually, innumerable abnormal, small echo complexes representing distorted renal cortex and medulla may be seen dotting the parenchyma.[11,16] There may be distortion of the central echo complex. A poorly demarcated renal contour is secondary to multiple peripheral cysts causing distortion and a decrease in specular reflections from the renal capsule. Once ADPKD is identified, the liver, pancreas, and spleen should be scanned carefully for evidence of cystic involvement (Pathology Box 10-1).

## MEDULLARY CYSTIC DISEASE

### Medullary Sponge Kidney[12,16,32]

The pathogenesis of medullary sponge kidney or tubular ectasia is a congenital autosomal recessive defect. It is a relatively common and usually innocuous structural change restricted to lesions of multiple cystic dilatation of the collecting ducts in the medulla. The condition occurs in adults, is usually bilateral, and is normally discovered as an incidental finding or sometimes in relation to secondary complications (calcifications in the dilated cysts, infection, urinary calculi). Renal function is usually normal, but calculi formation and infection may develop.

The bilateral characteristic ectatic collecting tubules are best seen on excretory urography. Sonographically, the medullary pyramids appear highly echogenic without shadowing, having an appearance similar to that of nephrocalcinosis (Fig. 10-13A,B). With discrete calcium deposits and stones seen in 10% to 15% of cases, discrete posterior acoustic shadowing may occur (Pathology Box 10-1). The differential diagnosis includes nephrocalcinosis and papillary necrosis.

### Nephronophthisis (Uremic Medullary Cystic Disease)[12,30]

Nephronophthisis, more commonly called uremic medullary cystic disease, is a rare, progressive, familial hereditary disorder that usually has its onset in young adults (autosomal dominant form) and children (autosomal recessive form). It is characterized by the presence of variable numbers of cysts in the medulla associated with significant cortical tubular atrophy and

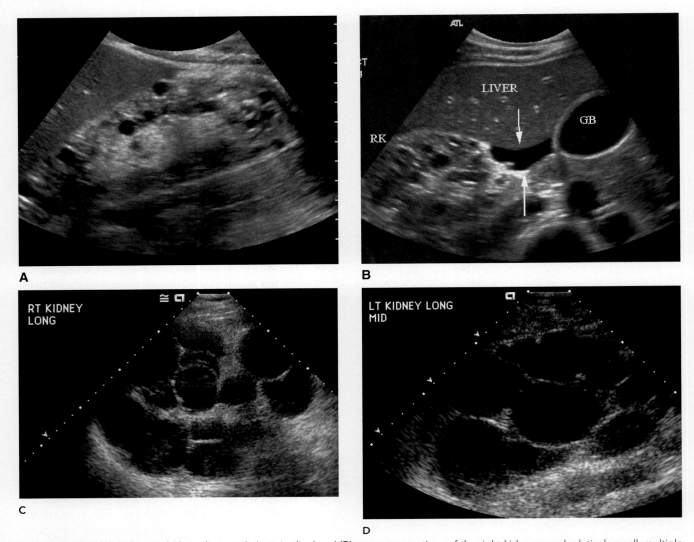

**Figure 10-12** Adult polycystic kidney disease. **A:** Longitudinal and **(B)** transverse sections of the right kidney reveal relatively small, multiple cysts seen throughout the kidney. Ascites is also seen *(arrows).* **C,D:** On a 70-year-old man, longitudinal views of the right kidney **(C)** and left kidney **(D)** demonstrate multiple cysts of various sizes, which replace the normal renal parenchyma. (**A,B,** Images courtesy of Philips Medical Systems, Bothell, WA; **C,D,** Images courtesy of Pam Endsley, Westerville, OH.)

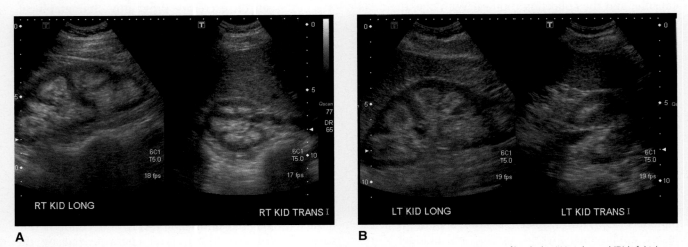

**Figure 10-13** Medullary sponge kidney. On this 27-year-old woman, the longitudinal and transverse sections of both the **(A)** right and **(B)** left kidneys reveal hyperechoic renal pyramids. This was an incidental finding, as the patient had no history of renal disease. Based on this, the diagnosis of medullary sponge kidney is favored although renal sinus lipomatosis could be considered as a differential. (Images courtesy of April Peters, Newark, OH.)

## PATHOLOGY BOX 10-1

### Congenital Cystic Renal Disease

| Entity | Cause | Clinical Features | Laboratory Values | Sonographic Features |
|---|---|---|---|---|
| Adult polycystic kidney disease | Autosomal dominant inheritance; multiple cyst formation on both kidneys leads to decreased function | Affects both sexes; onset usually in fourth decade; hypertension; abdominal, back, and flank pain | Proteinuria (50% of patients), azotemia, hematuria, uremia | Bilateral enlarged kidneys contain numerous cysts of various sizes; poorly demarcated renal capsule contour; may distort central echo complex; associated cysts in liver, pancreas, or spleen may be seen |
| Medullary sponge kidney | Congenital autosomal recessive defect; dilated tubules with calcium deposits | Usually asymptomatic; pain, hydronephrosis, infection may occur with associated calculi | Usually normal | Bilateral hyperechogenic areas with/without acoustic shadowing in regions of papillae |
| Uremic medullary cystic disease | Dominant and recessive hereditary disorder; multiple medullary and corticomedullary cysts 1–5 cm in diameter | Onset from age 3–5 years to early adulthood; renal failure, polyuria, thirst, renal salt wasting | Hyposthenuria, severe anemia, elevated serum alkaline phosphatase | Small cysts confined to the medullary portions of both kidneys; may have widening of central echoes with small cysts; normal sized or moderately small kidneys; loss of corticomedullary differentiation and increased parenchymal echogenicity |

interstitial fibrosis. The cortical tubulointerstitial damage is the cause of eventual renal insufficiency and progresses to terminal renal failure over a period of 5 to 10 years.

The most characteristic sonographic findings are multiple small cysts confined to the renal medulla. The presence of these cysts—associated loss of corticomedullary differentiation and increased parenchymal echogenicity along with anemia, salt wasting, progressive azotemia, and often polyuria—suggests the diagnosis of juvenile nephronophthisis (Pathology Box 10-1). The diagnosis is assisted by visualizing small kidneys with a sharply defined cortical surface; in contrast to polycystic disease which presents with cysts of variable size and location and enlarged kidneys with irregular cortical outlines. Furthermore, the capacity of ultrasound to identify cysts in the medullary region is limited.

## CORTICAL CYSTS

### Simple Cyst[12,30]

The most often encountered type of renal cyst is a simple serous fluid collection originating in the renal cortex. The origin of simple cysts is unknown. With the ability of the newer ultrasound equipment to resolve smaller structures, the simple cyst, once thought uncommon before age 40, is now being identified with increasing frequency in younger and even in pediatric patients. The prevalence of cysts increases markedly after age 40 and is identified in approximately 50% of all patients older than 50 years. Presumably to avoid confusing these cysts with polycystic disease, they are referred to in the singular (simple or solitary) renal cyst. Single cysts are more common, but simple cysts may be multiple, although they rarely number more than four per kidney. They have an epithelial lining and vary in size from 1 mm to giant cysts containing 5,000 mL of clear amber fluid. Simple cysts are usually unilocular, but may contain some septation or loculation. These cysts can be located anywhere in the kidney, including the adjacent tissues of the renal pelvis (peripelvic cyst) and the small divisions of the collecting system (Fig. 10-14A–D). Unless they obstruct portions of the collecting system, they remain asymptomatic and are most often discovered as an incidental finding. Simple cysts rarely cause other symptoms, although hypertension has been attributed to these lesions.

For a sonographic differential diagnosis, these lesions must meet the classic criteria for a cyst: (1) clear, smooth wall demarcation, especially a sharply defined far wall; (2) spheric or slightly ovoid shape; (3) absence of internal echoes; and (4) posterior enhancement (Pathology Box 10-2).

If all the criteria for a cyst are met, diagnosis of a simple renal cyst is 95% to 98% accurate; another 2% are due to hematomas, localized hydronephrosis, or septa in cysts.[25] Sonography cannot determine whether the cyst is benign or malignant. Most simple cysts are benign, but if mural growth is seen on follow-up examination, the cyst could be malignant. Five percent to 10% of complex renal cysts are proven to be tumors.[30] Diagnostic accuracy approaches 100% when the ultrasound examination is combined with cyst aspiration for cytologic and biochemical studies of the aspirate (Fig. 10-14B–E).

### Atypical Cysts

Atypical cysts are those that do not meet the criteria of simple cysts and require further investigation.

### Complex Cysts

#### Hemorrhagic Cyst[12,17,30]

Approximately 6% of simple renal cysts hemorrhage and the prevalence of hemorrhage increases in polycystic kidney disease. The reported incidence of neoplasm in these lesions approaches 30%. Depending on the age of the bleed, clot, and resorption, hemorrhagic cysts vary sonographically from anechoic to complex masses, with or without acoustic enhancement (Pathology Box 10-2 and Fig. 10-15A–C). These lesions, which do not always meet the classical criteria for a cyst on ultrasound, should be investigated by aspiration or CT. On CT, the presence of blood in any form increases attenuation, and hemorrhagic cysts appear hyperdense.

#### Infected Cyst[16,17,30,33]

Like hemorrhagic cysts, simple renal cysts can become infected by hematogenous dissemination of bacteria, by vesicoureteral reflux of infected urine, or as a complication of surgery. Infection is rare and accounts for only 2.5% of all complications. Patients present with fever and unilateral flank pain. An infected cyst is resistant to antibiotic therapy. The cysts usually contain cloudy fluid rather than the purulent contents of abscesses. Sonography is a useful diagnostic and treatment tool for guided aspiration and drainage. If the cyst content is sonographically clear and free of debris, it meets the classic sonographic criteria for a cyst, but a complex echo pattern is seen when particulate material floats in the fluid. This debris often shifts when the patient changes position. Necrotic exudate adherent to the cyst wall can sometimes be identified as discrete, hyperechoic, thickened mural masses with ill-defined borders (Pathology Box 10-2). The differential diagnosis includes hemorrhagic cysts, which can be confirmed with magnetic resonance imaging (MRI).

#### Septated or Multilocular Cysts[16,30]

The interior of a renal cyst is usually a single smooth cavity, although some cysts are trabeculated or divided by fibrous septa into two or more compartments. Usually there is free communication between loculi, as the

septa are usually incomplete. Septation has no pathologic significance unless papillary projections are demonstrated. Sonographically, septa appear as groups of linear internal echoes and should be evaluated to make sure they are thin, usually less than 1 cm in benign cysts. If the transducer is not perpendicular to the septum, the septal echoes may not appear linear and may suggest a solid mass within the cyst wall. Minimal cyst wall infoldings or small sacculations can also produce irregularity of the wall image. In such cases, cyst puncture becomes a vital diagnostic tool (Pathology Box 10-2 and Fig. 10-15D–G). The differential diagnosis includes nephroblastoma, cystic Wilms tumor, RCC, complicated renal cyst (hemorrhage, infection), abscess, cystic hypernephroma, obstructed upper pole moiety of a duplicated collecting system, large renal artery aneurysm, or calyceal diverticulum. Color Doppler is useful in helping to differentiate benign septated/multilocular cysts

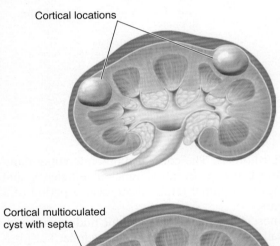

Cortical locations

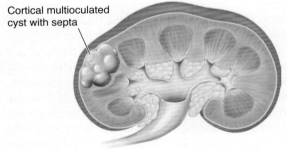

Cortical multioculated cyst with septa

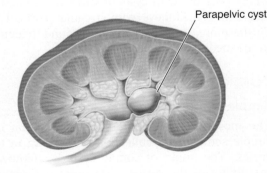

Parapelvic cyst

**A**

**Figure 10-14** Simple cysts. **A:** The illustration shows the common locations of simple and atypical renal cysts. *(continued)*

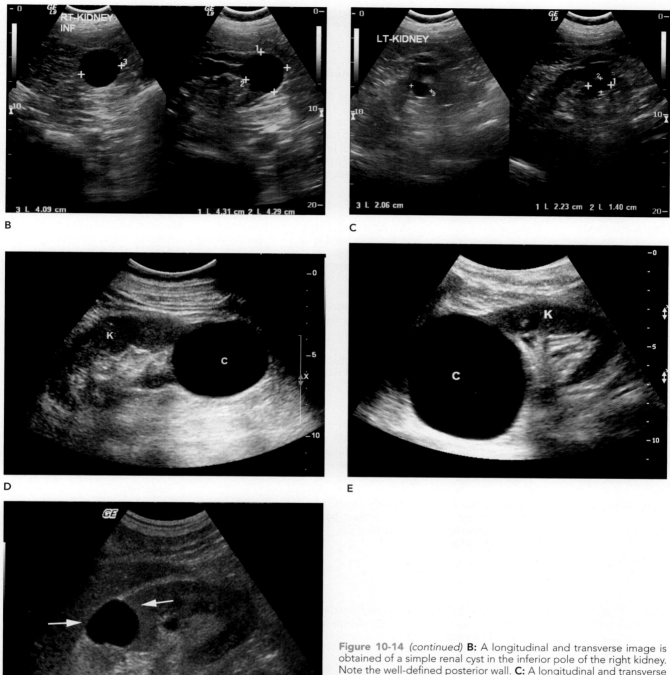

**Figure 10-14** *(continued)* **B:** A longitudinal and transverse image is obtained of a simple renal cyst in the inferior pole of the right kidney. Note the well-defined posterior wall. **C:** A longitudinal and transverse image displays a simple cyst in the medullary region of the left kidney. **D:** On a different patient, this longitudinal image demonstrates a renal cyst *(C)* arising from the inferior pole. **E:** This image from another patient demonstrates a large simple cyst located on the superior pole *(C)*. **F:** This longitudinal image demonstrates a simple cyst in the midpole of the kidney *(arrows)*. All of these cysts meet the criteria for simple cysts. **(B,C,** Images courtesy of Brian Johnson, North Logan, UT; **D,E,** Images courtesy of Philips Medical Systems, Bothell, WA; **F,** Image courtesy of GE Healthcare, Wauwatosa, WI.)

## PATHOLOGY BOX 10-2

### Developmental and Atypical Renal Cystic Masses

| Entity | Cause | Clinical Features | Laboratory Values | Sonographic Features |
|---|---|---|---|---|
| Simple cyst | Unknown | Discovered in 50% of patients after age 55 years; usually asymptomatic and discovered incidentally; rarely produces hypertension | Negative | Anechoic, clear, smooth wall demarcation, spherical or slightly ovoid, through-transmission; may be narrow band of acoustic shadowing edge artifact; single or multiple, but usually not more than four per kidney; usually 1–5 cm when unilocular, but may contain septations or loculations |
| Parapelvic and peripelvic cysts | Unknown | Asymptomatic; may be associated with hypertension or hydronephrosis | Hematuria, leukocytosis | Anechoic; parapelvic cysts are solitary, larger, with well-defined, sharp borders with through-transmission; peripelvic are smaller, multiple, or interconnecting network of cysts |
| Hemorrhagic cyst | Benign cysts can be transformed | Asymptomatic to abdomen, back, and flank pain | Hematuria | Anechoic to complex masses, with/without acoustic enhancement, with smooth to irregular walls |
| Infected or inflammatory cyst | Hematogenous bacterial spread, vesicoureteral reflux, infected urine, or surgical complication | If symptomatic, unilateral flank pain and fever | Leukocytosis | Anechoic mass meeting cyst criteria to complex mass, with/without particulate debris, smooth, thin to thick, irregular, ill-defined margins |
| Septate or multilocular cyst | Unknown; septation has no pathologic significance | Asymptomatic to abdomen, back, and flank pain | Negative | Anechoic, with one or more groups of linear, internal, thin echoes; wall infolding or sacculations can also produce irregularity |
| Calcified cyst | Can be acquired in benign cysts; many were hemorrhagic or infected previously | Asymptomatic to abdomen, back, and flank pain | Negative | Hyperechoic cyst wall with decreased sound transmission due to mural calcification; calcification may reflect enough sound, suggesting that the mass is solid; on a second scanning plane, there may be a calcium-free, anechoic portion |
| Milk of calcium in renal cyst | Formation is believed to be associated with low-grade inflammation and partial or complete obstruction in a calyceal diverticulum | Asymptomatic, incidental finding | Negative | Within calyx, an anechoic area containing hyperechoic foci with acoustic shadowing; foci may shadow movement with changing patient position |

from malignant RCC based on the neovascularity seen in malignant cysts.

## Calcification(s) in Cysts

### Calcified Wall

Mural calcification occurs in approximately 1% to 2% of all simple renal cysts, many of which were hemorrhagic or infected at one time. Sonographically, the layered, eggshell-thin cyst wall is hyperechoic, decreasing sound transmission and making an accurate diagnosis difficult. In certain areas, a densely calcified cyst can reflect enough sound to suggest falsely that it is solid. In these cases, it is important to obtain images from two scanning planes, as the cyst pattern can be identified in the calcium-free portions. Because mural calcifications are also associated with malignancy, correlation with other imaging procedures and

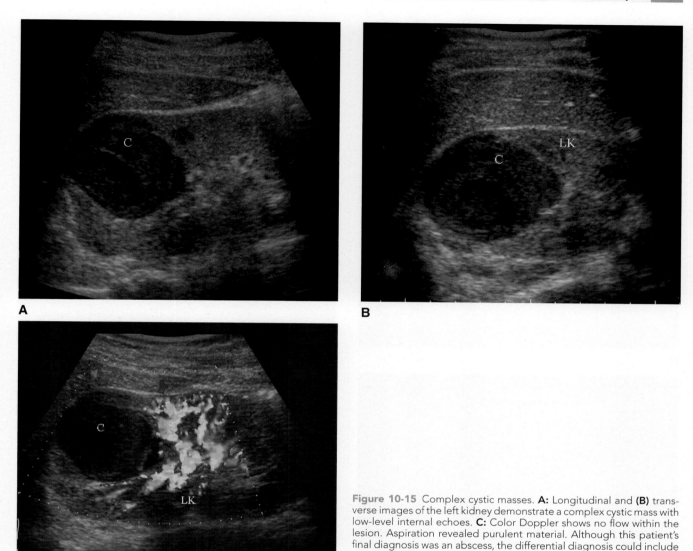

**Figure 10-15** Complex cystic masses. **A:** Longitudinal and **(B)** transverse images of the left kidney demonstrate a complex cystic mass with low-level internal echoes. **C:** Color Doppler shows no flow within the lesion. Aspiration revealed purulent material. Although this patient's final diagnosis was an abscess, the differential diagnosis could include a hemorrhagic renal cyst based solely on the sonographic appearance of this mass. *(continued)*

chemical analysis of the aspirate may be necessary to make a diagnosis (Pathology Box 10-2 and Fig. 10-16A–C).

*Milk of Calcium[17,30,34]*

Milk of calcium (MOC) in a renal cyst or calyceal diverticulum is quite common. It represents primarily small calcium carbonate crystals, although it can form from other substances. In most cases, MOC is deposited in calyceal diverticula, which may or may not have lost their communications with the calyceal system. When seen in a calyceal diverticulum, the formation usually occurs after a low-grade inflammation and partial or complete obstruction to urine flow with stasis. Unlike other lesions such as calculi or angiomyolipomas (AMLs), MOC is usually asymptomatic and requires no treatment. Sonographically, there is a layering, linear band of hyperechoic echoes with associated reverberation artifacts. Acoustic shadowing is possible if the

crystals are present in large amounts. The MOC may move within the cystic mass when the patient changes position (Pathology Box 10-2 and Fig. 10-16D,E). The differential diagnosis includes renal calculi, angiomyolipoma, calcified mural cyst, and prominent or calcified intralobar or arcuate artery.

## PARAPELVIC AND PERIPELVIC CYSTS[11,35]

Parapelvic cysts originate from renal parenchyma and protrude into the renal sinus, whereas peripelvic cysts are considered true sinus cysts. Neither of these two cysts communicates with the collecting system. Their cause is not known, but parapelvic cysts sometimes develop following urine extravasation into the renal sinus. Peripelvic cysts are believed to result from lymphatic ectasia or obstruction. Parapelvic cysts are generally solitary and large and meet the sonographic criteria for a cyst; peripelvic cysts are small, multiple,

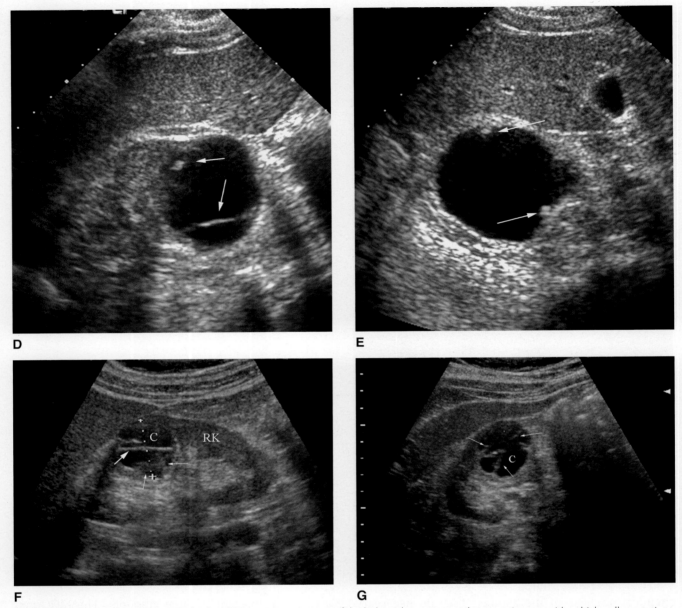

**Figure 10-15** *(continued)* **D:** Longitudinal and **(E)** transverse images of the kidney demonstrate a large cystic mass with a thick wall, septations, and mural calcifications. **F:** Longitudinal and **(G)** transverse images of a renal cyst containing multiple echogenic septations *(arrows)* and debris along the posterior wall *(small arrows)*. Cystic lesions that do not meet the requirements for a simple cyst can either be followed with sonography or computed tomography or undergo aspiration for a definitive diagnosis. **(A–C,F,G**, Image courtesy of Taco Geertsma, MD, Hospital Gelderse Vallei, Ede, The Netherlands.)

and often irregular in outline but are anechoic fluid collections.

Sonographically, a parapelvic cyst can resemble a dilated pelvis, but the remainder of the sinus echoes are normal (Fig. 10-17). Peripelvic cysts appear as pelvicaliceal dilatations sonographically and can be solitary, multiple, or a multilocular interconnecting network of small cysts appearing in the characteristic location in the normally compact central echo complex. Distributed along the calyceal infundibula or around the renal pelvis, they are usually not mistaken for the sonographic manifestations of hydronephrosis but are more often confused with sinus lipomatosis on excretory urography. Sonographically, neither parapelvic nor peripelvic renal cysts interconnect in the same way as a distended renal collecting system and there is no intrarenal system dilation as there is in hydronephrosis. In addition, both cysts are anechoic compared to the hypoechoic, ill-defined sinus fat deposits seen with lipomatosis (Pathology Box 10-2). If there is doubt, excretory urography or contrast-enhanced CT should provide a definitive diagnosis.

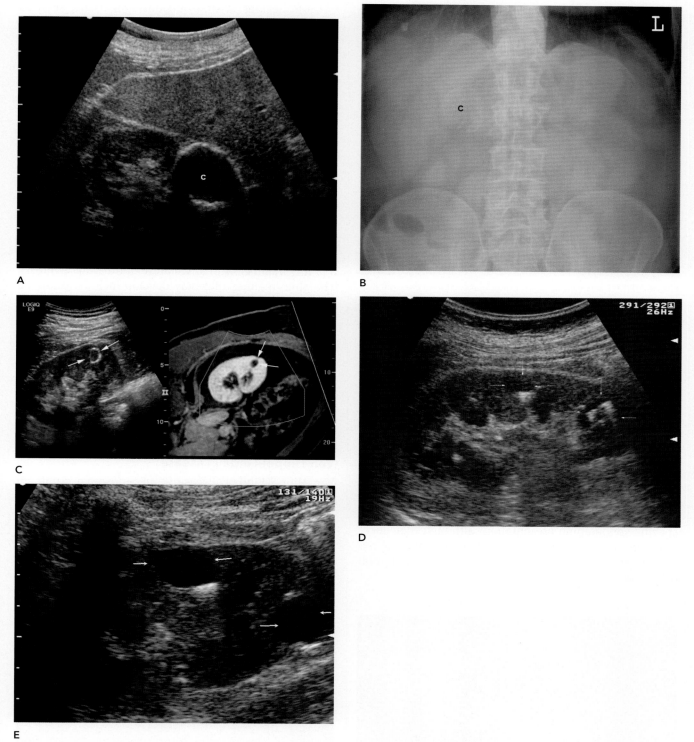

**Figure 10-16** Calcifications in cysts. **A:** Transverse image of the right kidney demonstrates a cyst **(C)** on the superior pole with a hyperechoic rim suggesting wall calcification. **B:** A radiograph from the same patient confirms the presence of a calcified right renal cyst. **C:** Volume navigation or fusion image of the kidney demonstrates a renal cyst with a calcified rim *(arrows)*. Fusion imaging allows the sonographer to fuse a previously acquired computed tomography (CT) or magnetic resonance imaging (MRI) dataset to the real-time ultrasound examination. This technology allows the sonographer to directly compare the findings of the CT or MRI examination while scanning in real time. **D,E:** In a different patient, longitudinal and transverse **(D)** images of the left kidney show cystic lesions *(arrows)* with linear hyperechoic areas suggestive of milk of calcium cysts **(E)**. (**A,B,D,E**, Images courtesy of Taco Geertsma, MD, Hospital Gelderse Vallei, Ede, The Netherlands; **C**, courtesy of GE Healthcare, Wauwatosa, WI.)

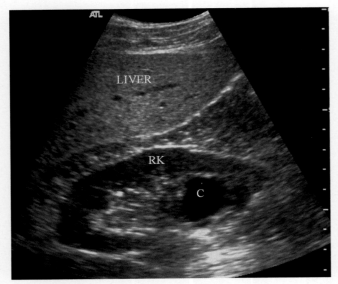

**Figure 10-17** Parapelvic cyst. A longitudinal section of the right kidney reveals a parapelvic cyst near the inferior pole. Parapelvic cysts should not be confused with dilatation of the renal pelvis. (Image courtesy of Philips Medical Systems, Bothell, WA.)

## ACQUIRED CYSTIC DISEASE

Most acquired cysts of the kidney occur when some process destroys renal tissue, leaving a lesion in the parenchyma that may or may not communicate with the collecting system. This category includes cavitating hematomas, inflammatory cysts (pyogenic and tuberculous abscess, parasitic cysts), necrotic neoplasm, calyceal diverticula, cystic diseases in patients receiving dialysis, and cystic diseases in native kidneys of renal transplant recipients. These acquired cysts have no specific sonographic presentation, although their location within the kidney, their configuration, and the patient's clinical history allow a more limited differential diagnosis.

Cystic lesions arising outside renal tissue, such as pancreatic pseudocysts, necrotic metastatic neoplasm, posttraumatic urinomas, renal artery aneurysms, and other less common lesions may occasionally be noted within the kidney on sonographic examination.

The section on Renal Failure discusses the complications of acquired cystic disease in the dialysis patient.

## CYSTS ASSOCIATED WITH SYSTEMIC DISEASE

### Tuberous Sclerosis[11,30,36–38]

Tuberous sclerosis is a multisystemic disorder associated with renal cyst formation and neoplasms. Patients present with the classic clinical triad of mental retardation, seizures, and cutaneous lesions (adenoma sebaceum). The disorder can be sporadic or inherited as an autosomal dominant trait, although only 50% of patients have a family member with any feature of tuberous sclerosis. The abnormalities that may develop include lesions in the kidneys, central nervous system (CNS), cardiovascular system, pulmonary system, and skeletal system.

The kidneys are affected in approximately 95% of adult patients, with 50% to 80% having multiple, bilateral AMLs. Renal cysts occur in 20% to 40% of patients and occur more often in infancy and childhood. The cysts may be the initial or occasionally the only manifestation of tuberous sclerosis in early childhood. The etiology of the cysts is unclear. They do not usually cause severe renal impairment (Fig. 10-18A,B).

### Von Hippel-Lindau Disease[11,30,38–41]

Von Hippel-Lindau disease is an autosomal dominant disorder with variable penetrance predisposed to form a variety of visceral cysts and neoplasms. It is usually not clinically evident until the third to fifth decade of life. Patients most often present with signs and symptoms related to cerebellar or spinal cord hemangioblastomas or retinal angiomas. Patients may also develop pancreatic

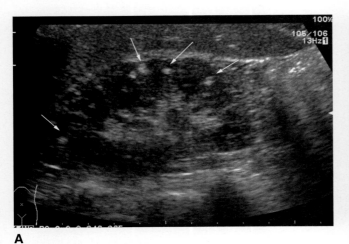

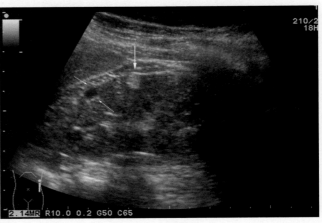

**Figure 10-18** Tuberous sclerosis. **A:** In this 15-year-old man with tuberous sclerosis, multiple hyperechoic angiomyolipomas (*arrows*) were identified in the right kidney. **B:** The left kidney also demonstrated multiple angiomyolipomas (*arrow*) and a small anechoic cyst (*small arrows*). (Images courtesy of Taco Geertsma, MD, Hospital Gelderse Vallei, Ede, The Netherlands.)

islet cell tumors, pheochromocytomas, and epididymal cystadenomas. Occasionally, abdominal cancers are diagnosed prior to the CNS and orbital symptoms. The kidneys are involved in approximately 59% to 63% of patients with von Hippel-Lindau disease. Renal cysts may be the first manifestation of the disease and usually precede solid tumors by 3 to 7 years. Although usually multiple, they generally do not cause hypertension, renal insufficiency, or an overall enlargement in renal size, as is seen in patients with ADPKD. Over time, approximately 70% of renal cysts are stable; however, approximately 20% enlarge on follow-up studies, and 10% become smaller or involute completely. Because the cysts can contain neoplastic elements in their walls and can evolve into RCC, benign-appearing cysts should be monitored.

In patients with renal involvement, RCC occurs in 24% to 45% of patients; the tumors are bilateral in up to 75% of cases and multifocal in 80% to 90% of cases. Unlike the sporadic form of RCC, the tumors develop at an earlier age and the typical male predominance is not present in patients with von Hippel-Lindau disease.

Approximately half of the siblings and half of the children of affected individuals will develop the disease. At-risk individuals should be evaluated in late adolescence with diagnostic tests directed at detecting the major manifestations of the disease. In addition to the brain, spinal cord, and orbit, the possible involvement of the kidneys, pancreas, and adrenal glands means that CT is probably the preferred mode of screening. Sonographic evaluation is valuable in diagnosing indeterminate renal and pancreatic masses. Treatment includes surgical resection, preserving as much normal renal parenchyma as possible. Intraoperative sonography helps localize the suspicious lesion(s) and can minimize the amount of renal parenchyma resected.

# SOLID RENAL MASSES/ NEOPLASMS[42,43]

A neoplasm (tumor) represents any new abnormal growth and is usually classified as benign or malignant (primary neoplasm). In contrast to benign neoplasms, malignant neoplasms show a greater degree of anaplasia and have the properties of invasion and metastasis. Metastasis (secondary neoplasms) is the dissemination of cancer cells from the location of origin to other areas in the body. Staging of neoplasms is based on the size of the primary tumor and the spread of the tumor to regional lymph nodes or other distant areas.

With sonography and CT, the detection of small renal parenchymal tumors has increased dramatically, especially in the kidneys. Differentiating between benign and malignant neoplasms and nonneoplastic masses (cysts) is more problematic. The sonographer plays a very important role in providing an examination to help

differentiate various conditions, which include (1) simple and atypical cysts; (2) pseudotumors, represented by anomalies or hypertrophied renal parenchyma (i.e., column of Bertin); (3) renal infarction or focus of infection; (4) angiomyolipoma (hamartoma); (5) lymphoma; (6) metastatic neoplasm to the kidney; (7) benign mesenchymal tumors such as fibroma or leiomyoma; and (8) RCC, adenoma, and oncocytoma. In addition to the imaging findings, whether on sonography or CT, clinical information is extremely important. Sonography may not be as sensitive as contrast-enhanced CT in depicting small masses, but many of these masses are detected incidentally during an ultrasound examination. The sonographer's role in patient assessment includes obtaining as complete a medical history as possible and performing a sonographic examination that will (1) identify the exact location of any mass; (2) distinguish between cystic, complex, and solid tissue by demonstrating the echo pattern (i.e., homogeneous or heterogeneous) and echotexture (i.e., anechoic, hypoechoic, hyperechoic, or isoechoic) to help distinguish the tissue composition (e.g., fat seen in an angiomyolipoma is echogenic); (3) manipulate gain, TGC, and focal ranges to provide an accurate representation of the tissue and its attenuating properties; (4) document the number of masses and evaluate the contralateral kidney (lymphoma and metastatic disease to the kidney is usually multiple and is seen in other areas, and the patient's history indicates its presence); (5) make precise linear and volume measurements; (6) document the growth rate of a mass on any follow-up examination; and (7) assess the vascularity of solid masses (e.g., RCCs are hypervascular and contain numerous AV shunts). All tumors are capable of distorting renal architecture and hindering renal function. With renal masses, symptoms are late in developing and may include dull pain in the flank area or hematuria.

## BENIGN NEOPLASMS

Sonography is extremely valuable in detecting some benign tumors and in determining their composition. In rare cases, the sonographic appearance alone determines the tumor type. Pathology Box 10-3 presents the most known benign renal tumors.

### Adenoma[6,20,44]

Often an incidental finding at surgery or autopsy, cortical adenomas are the most prevalent benign kidney tumors. Usually measuring 1 cm or less and rarely larger than 3 cm in diameter, they are asymptomatic unless they enlarge. Originating from renal tubular epithelium, these vascular benign masses are believed to be the counterpart of malignant RCCs. One theory is that adenomas smaller than 3 cm rarely metastasize, but adenomas and adenocarcinomas usually occur in the sixth or seventh decade of life and have the same male

## PATHOLOGY BOX 10-3

### Benign Renal Tumors

| Tumor | Characteristics/Treatment | Sonographic Features |
|---|---|---|
| Adenomas | Distinguished histologically; treated as malignant | Echogenic cortical mass usually <3 cm; vascular; attenuates sound |
| Oncocytoma | Distinguished histologically; treated as malignant | Generally nonspecific; can have stellate, hypoechoic central scar characteristic of oncocytoma; renal cell carcinoma can have central scar |
| Angiomyolipoma-hamartoma | If asymptomatic and thin computed tomography sections detect fat, no treatment; if symptomatic, <4 cm, embolization; if >4 cm or if recurrence, partial nephrectomy; if <1 cm, follow up with sonography | Homogeneous, hyperechoic cortical mass; 80% are comparable to renal fat; 20%–30% have some degree of acoustic shadowing; 12% are heterogeneous; 8% are isoechoic or hypoechoic |
| Lipoma | Composed of fatty tissue; combines with angiolipoma, angiomyolipoma, and fibroma; most common mesenchymal-type tumor, female:male ratio 6:1 | Sharply circumscribed; <5 mm diameter; if seen, hyperechoic mass |
| Leiomyoma | Retroperitoneal tumors formed from renal capsule or vessels | Hyperechoic mass found in retroperitoneum |
| Juxtaglomerular tumor (reninoma) | Rare, secretes renin; young female preponderance (mean age, 31 years); signs and symptoms relate to hypertension; associated with elevated plasma renin and secondary aldosteronism with severe diastolic hypertension; treatment is nephrectomy | Hypovascular, solid renal mass; well circumscribed or encapsulated: arising near corticomedullary junction |
| Hemangioma | Rare; no sex preference; occurs in third and fourth decades; patients may have hematuria with no other explanation; capillary type more common than cavernous type, and both types are intermixed with fibrous stroma | Hyperechoic; <1 cm in diameter |
| Fibroma | Fibrous mass in medulla; female preponderance; finding in 26%–42% of autopsies | Hyperechoic mass(es) in medulla, rarely in cortex; 2–3 mm in diameter |
| Multilocular cystic nephroma | Encapsulated cystic region; preponderance in young men and older women; distinguished histologically; treated as malignant; partial or radical nephrectomy | Large, anechoic space (up to 10 cm); similar in appearance to cystic renal cell carcinoma or cystic Wilms tumors |

to female ratio of 3:1. Adenomas may be responsible for painless hematuria.

Sonographically, renal adenomas have a pattern similar to that of RCC. The highly vascular tumor has many internal echoes and associated sound attenuation (Fig. 10-19A).

## Oncocytoma[6,11]

Oncocytomas, or oxyphilic adenomas, are a class of very large vascular adenomas that usually occur in middle to old age, with a male to female ratio of 1.7:1. Patients are usually asymptomatic but may have pain or hematuria. An enlarging mass may outstrip its blood supply with concurrent infarction, hemorrhage, and necrosis, which produces a central stellate fibrotic scar resulting from the organization and healing of the hemorrhage.

Sonographically, oncocytomas usually cannot be distinguished from typical RCCs, which may explain why oncocytomas account for 2% to 14% of renal tumors preoperatively thought to be cancer and 5% of all renal neoplasms. Typically, they range from 0.3 to 26 cm in diameter and are well defined, smooth, and homogeneous, similar to RCC. If a central stellate scar is imaged

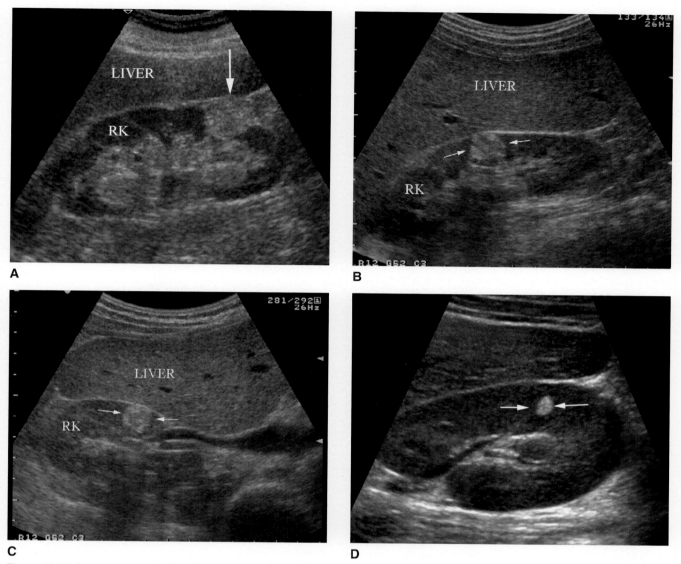

**Figure 10-19** Benign masses. **A:** On a longitudinal section of the right kidney, an echogenic lesion *(arrow)* is identified arising from the cortex, which could represent a benign adenoma, although angiomyolipoma and renal cell carcinoma are also part of the differential diagnosis. The remainder of the kidney appears normal and the patient has no symptoms relating to renal dysfunction. Longitudinal **(B)** and transverse **(C)** images from another patient reveal a hyperechoic mass within the midpole of the right kidney. The diagnosis of angiomyolipoma (AML) was made. **D:** A small hyperechoic lesion within the renal parenchyma demonstrates the classic sonographic appearance of an angiomyolipoma. The mass is very echogenic, homogeneous, and well circumscribed. (**A-C**, Images courtesy of Taco Geertsma, MD, Hospital Gelderse Vallei, Ede, The Netherlands; **D**, image courtesy of Philips Medical Systems, Bothell, WA.)

an oncocytoma should be suspected, but RCCs may also have a central scar.

## Angiomyolipoma [6,11,16,30,36,38]

AMLs are benign hamartomatous, mesenchymal mixed tumors composed of fat cells intermixed with smooth muscle cells and aggregates of thick-walled blood vessels in varying proportions. They occur in two distinct clinicopathologic forms: (1) a unilateral solitary mass, three times more common in women than in men, usually developing in the fourth to sixth decades and not associated with tuberous sclerosis; and (2) multiple bilateral masses, occurring in 80% of patients with tuberous sclerosis complex.

Most AMLs are asymptomatic; however, the walls of the tumor vessels lack normal elastic tissue, and they can bleed internally or into the renal parenchyma, collecting system, or retroperitoneum. Patients can present with flank pain, hematuria, or life-threatening hemorrhage and hypertension, and renal failure may occur. Focal hemorrhage with evidence of necrosis, cystic degeneration, and calcification within the lesion is common. Malignant transformation is thought to be extremely rare, if indeed it ever occurs.

The striking sonographic appearance of AMLs alone often leads to the diagnosis. Approximately 80% are homogeneous and are markedly hyperechoic (like renal fat) compared to renal cortex. Because of their cortical location, this comparison is easy to visualize. AMLs are among the most acoustically reflective of all renal masses. Their strong echogenicity, even at low gain settings, is due to their high-fat content and heterogeneous cellular architecture, as well as their hypervascularity. Approximately 20% to 30% have some degree of acoustic shadowing, but most display good sound transmission despite their numerous interfaces and solid nature (Fig. 10-19B–D). Small RCC tumors (<3 cm) may mimic the sonographic appearance of an AML, whereas larger RCCs are less likely to have similar appearance.[45] With hemorrhage, necrosis, and a predominance of nonfatty elements, 12% of AMLs are hyperechoic but heterogeneous, and 8% are either isoechoic or hypoechoic.

## MALIGNANT NEOPLASMS

### Renal Cell Carcinoma[6,11,12,20,30,37,41,44–48]

RCC, also referred to as *hypernephroma* or *adenocarcinoma,* represents 1% to 3% of all visceral cancers. RCCs are the most common malignant tumor of the kidney, accounting for approximately 80% to 90% of all renal malignancies in adults. The lesion occurs most often after age 50 and has a 2:1 male to female ratio. There is 10% to 25% incidence of bilateral or multifocal RCC in patients with von Hippel-Lindau disease and in patients with ADPKD undergoing dialysis, and there is an increased incidence in ADPKD, tuberous sclerosis, and other diseases and syndromes associated with multiple renal cysts. Another characteristic of RCC is that the abnormal cells frequently produce hormones or hormone-like substances (i.e., erythropoietin, parathyroid-like hormone, renin, gonadotropins, or glucocorticosteroids), which produce paraneoplastic syndromes, which may be the first manifestation of the disease. The classic symptoms include costovertebral angle pain, a palpable mass, and hematuria. Only 15% of patients present with all three symptoms, and hematuria is the most significant of the three. Other symptoms include fever, weight loss, hypertension, and possible masculinization or feminization if the tumor produces gonadotropin.

Histologically, RCCs are described by cell type (clear cell or granular cytoplasm) and cellular morphology (well differentiated, poorly differentiated, or undifferentiated). Tumor size varies greatly and sometimes is enormous. The tumors may infiltrate throughout the kidney, even though they often appear to have a capsule or pseudocapsule sharply delimiting them from the adjacent normal parenchyma (which may be compressed). By local extension, RCC spreads into the perinephric fat and renal vein. Lymphogenous and

| TABLE 10-6 |
| --- |
| **Staging of Renal Carcinoma** |

| Disease Entity | Stage | Five-Year Survival Rate |
| --- | --- | --- |
| Tumor within kidney (small or large) | I | ≈ 80% – 100% |
| Tumor in perinephric fat but confined to Gerota fascia | II | ≈ 65% – 75% |
| Tumor in renal vein, regional lymph nodes, or vena cava | III | ≈ 25% – 50% |
| Adjacent organ invasion, distant metastases, tumor in juxtaregional lymph nodes | IV | ≈ 0% – 20% |

hematogenous spread often allow metastases to develop before there are any local symptoms of the primary lesion. Approximately 30% of patients have metastases at the time of diagnosis, with 75% of these belong to the lung. The pattern of the disease is spread to regional nodes, lungs (50%), bone (33%), the opposite kidney (10% to 15%), liver, adrenal, and brain. The survival rate is based on the stage of the disease. The average survival time after surgical removal for lesions at each stage is presented in Table 10-6 and Figure 10-20A.

Often highly vascular, RCCs contain numerous areas of hemorrhage, necrosis, or cystic degeneration. Approximately 10% are hypovascular, and many of these represent a microscopic subclassification referred to as *papillary cystadenocarcinoma.* Compared to renal parenchymal malignancy, papillary cystadenocarcinoma is characterized by slower growth, less extensive involvement at the time of diagnosis, and a better prognosis.

The RCC mass is seen with varied sonographic appearances. Compared to normal adjacent renal parenchyma, 50% appear hyperechoic, 40% appear more echogenic, and 12% appear markedly hyperechoic, similar to the echogenicity of the renal sinus or an AML. Isoechoic masses are detected when they are exophytic or distort the renal contour (Fig. 10-20B). Hypoechoic appearances and irregular wall contours have also been reported. It was once believed that neovascularity correlated with echogenicity, but no correlation exists between tumor vascularity and tumor echogenicity (Fig. 10-20C–E). The degree of hemorrhage and necrosis does determine the degree of echogenicity. In 20% to 30% of RCC cases, calcification is identifiable and may appear punctate, amorphous, or mottled. The extent of sound attenuation is ascertained by comparing the intensity of the echoes at the far wall of the mass with those at the near wall and with those transmitted through the normal kidney, liver, and spleen. The RCC mass that does not attenuate sound is one that has undergone complete cystic or hemorrhagic transformation.

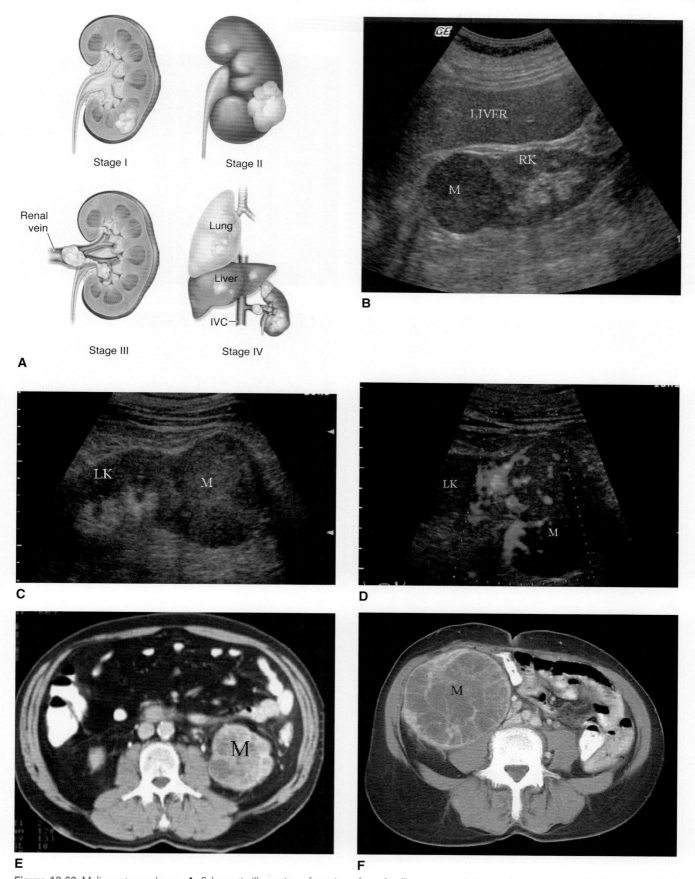

**Figure 10-20** Malignant neoplasms. **A:** Schematic illustration of staging of renal cell carcinoma. **B–F:** Renal cell carcinoma. **B:** This longitudinal image of the right kidney demonstrates a hypoechoic, well-circumscribed mass *(M)* arising from the superior pole. This mass was confirmed to be a renal cell carcinoma. On a different patient, a longitudinal image **(C)** reveals a hypoechoic mass *(M)* arising from the left inferior pole. **D:** Power Doppler demonstrates peripheral and internal vascularity. **E:** Computed tomography (CT) scan of the same lesion *(M)*. The lesion was determined to be adenocarcinoma. **F:** CT scan on a different patient shows a large right renal mass *(M)*. Sonography in longitudinal *(continued)*

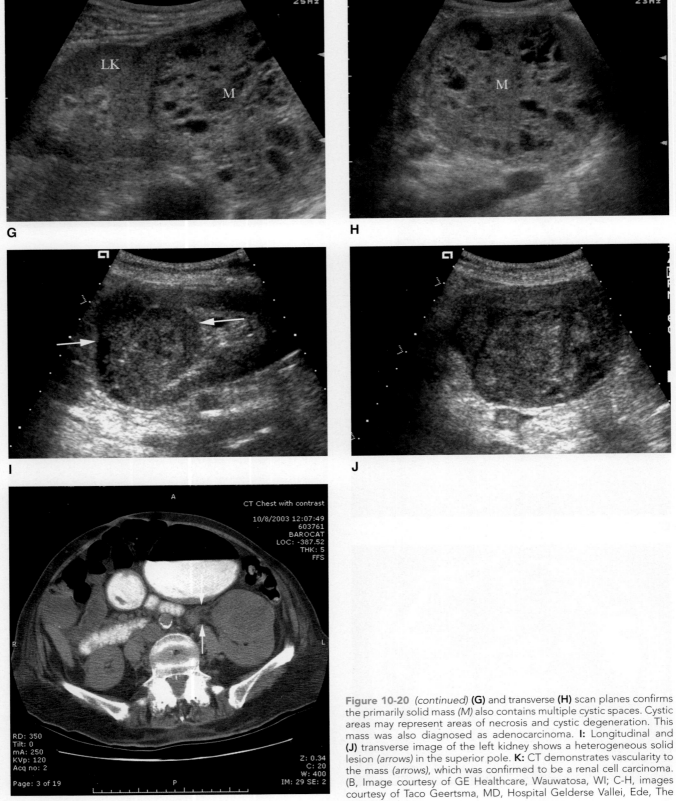

**Figure 10-20** *(continued)* **(G)** and transverse **(H)** scan planes confirms the primarily solid mass *(M)* also contains multiple cystic spaces. Cystic areas may represent areas of necrosis and cystic degeneration. This mass was also diagnosed as adenocarcinoma. **I:** Longitudinal and **(J)** transverse image of the left kidney shows a heterogeneous solid lesion *(arrows)* in the superior pole. **K:** CT demonstrates vascularity to the mass *(arrows)*, which was confirmed to be a renal cell carcinoma. (B, Image courtesy of GE Healthcare, Wauwatosa, WI; C-H, images courtesy of Taco Geertsma, MD, Hospital Gelderse Vallei, Ede, The Netherlands.)

Complex patterns are encountered, with localized areas of hemorrhage, necrosis, or cystic degeneration (Fig. 10-20F–K). These may appear as a unilocular or multilocular mass. A multiloculated RCC has multiple noncommunicating, fluid-filled cystic spaces of various size and is more closely associated with RCC involvement in cases of von Hippel-Lindau disease, discussed previously. RCC may also appear as a cystic renal tumor, unilocular mass, or papillary mass.

Doppler examination of all solid renal masses is useful for tissue characterization. Most malignant renal tumors are characterized by abnormal vascular structures not seen in benign neoplasms. Duplex Doppler examination of renal masses is useful for tissue characterization and assessment of vascular signals from neovascular tissue.

With neovascular renal tissue, there is a high systolic, high diastolic arterial flow (AV shunt pattern) and a high velocity, continuous flow, with little or no systolic-diastolic fluctuations (low-impedance signals probably related to sinusoidal spaces and representing flow within abnormal thin-walled venous structures).

The detection of any solid renal mass requires a concerted effort to visualize the renal vein, the IVC, the renal hilar and para-aortic lymph nodes, and the contralateral kidney to complete the examination. Invasion of the IVC is more common with RCC of the right kidney than with that of the left kidney. Extension of RCC into the renal vein occurs in 20% to 30% of patients, and renal thrombus may extend into the IVC in 5% to 10% of cases (Fig. 10-21A–D). Duplex Doppler

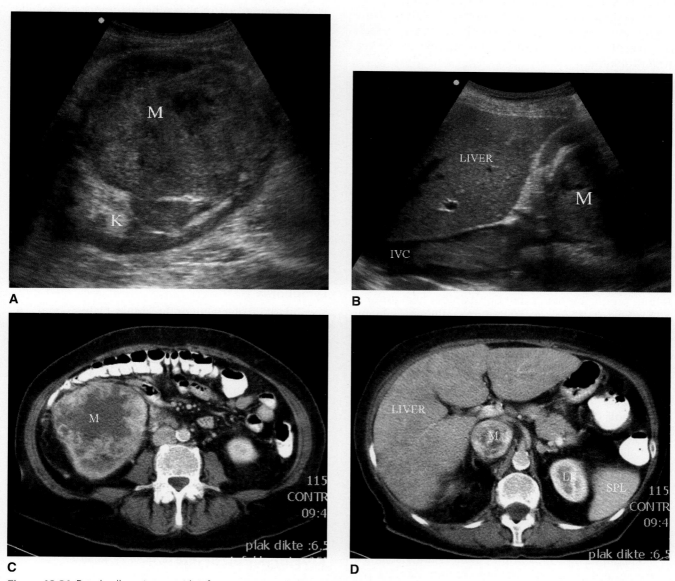

**Figure 10-21** Renal cell carcinoma with inferior vena cava (IVC) invasion. **A:** A large right renal mass *(M)* was found in this 69-year-old woman who presented with hematuria. **B:** Further sonographic evaluation reveals a soft tissue mass within the lumen of the inferior vena cava. **C:** Computed tomography images confirm the renal mass and **(D)** the tumor invasion of the IVC. (Images courtesy of Taco Geertsma, MD, Hospital Gelderse Vallei, Ede, The Netherlands.)

sonography of the normal IVC and a renal vein Doppler waveform illustrate a wide spectrum of low frequencies that are phasic with respiration. In the presence of thrombus or obstruction, the Doppler signal may be damped, absent, or continuous (see Chapter 4). The presence and extent of tumor thrombus within the renal vein and IVC can be detected by color Doppler examination as a color void representing the filling defect within distended veins. Doppler can demonstrate the neovascularity found in a tumor thrombus, which is not seen in hemorrhagic thrombus.

Discrete intraluminal echoes within involved fistula formation, distention by the thrombus, compression secondary to adenopathy, and displacement of the IVC all indicate extension and are readily imaged with real-time sonography. Hilar adenopathy is imaged as solid, hypoechoic masses surrounding the renal pedicle and the aorticorenal junction. Paraaortic nodes obscure the outline of the great vessels or present as solid masses in the midline of the retroperitoneum.

### Wilms Tumor

Wilms tumor, a highly malignant childhood tumor also referred to as a *nephroblastoma,* is discussed in Chapter 20.

### Urothelial Carcinoma[45,46]

Urothelial tumors are malignant tumors of the lining of the renal pelvis, calyces, ureter, and bladder. They account for 8% to 10% of all renal cancers. The majority (90% to 92%) are transitional cell carcinomas (TCCs), and the remaining 10% are squamous cell carcinomas (SCCs) and, rarely, adenocarcinomas. These primary renal tumors become clinically apparent within a relatively short time because their growth causes fragmentation, producing noticeable but painless hematuria in 60% of cases. They are small and usually not palpable but may block urinary outflow, causing palpable hydronephrosis. These tumors are invasive without the bulky mass, infiltrating the wall of the pelvis, calyces, and renal vein. Following surgical removal, the 5-year survival rate is 90%.

### Transitional Cell Carcinoma[6,11,12,17,49]

TCCs represent 7% of all renal neoplasms, 90% of primary renal pelvis tumors, and more than 90% of all cancers of the ureter.[49] The patient usually presents with painless hematuria. The mean age at diagnosis is approximately 61 years, and more common in men than women. The tumor is usually multiple and bilateral. TCCs are usually too small to be detected sonographically and are diagnosed with CT, IVP, and retrograde pyelography.

Sonographically, large, bulky tumors are visualized. The appearance of TCC includes an intraluminal polypoid mass, thickening of the urothelium, and a nonspecific solid mass centered in the renal sinus. Two sonographic patterns have been described: splitting or separation of the central echo complex similar to hydronephrosis and a bulky, hypoechoic mass lesion. The location of the tumor in the renal sinus suggests the diagnosis. Infiltration of the adjacent renal parenchyma can occur, and in such cases it is not possible to distinguish TCC from RCC (Fig. 10-22A–C). The differential diagnosis includes blood clots, fungus balls, fibroepithelial malacoplakia, and calculi. A scanning pitfall is to mistake prominent renal papillae as filling defects in the calyces in the setting of hydronephrosis. The distinction is that papillae appear in all calyces, but other lesions, such as TCC, appear only in one or a very limited number of calyces. Color Doppler is not helpful in evaluating TCC, as the tumor grade, stage, and size are not related to vascularity.[50]

### Squamous Cell Carcinoma[4,6]

The remaining 15% of all urothelial tumors are the highly malignant SCCs. This tumor has an insidious onset, metastasizes early with a poor prognosis, and is associated with renal calculi and infection. Sonographically, the diagnosis is suggested by the presence of faceted calculi and marked hydronephrosis from ureteropelvic junction obstruction.

## METASTATIC RENAL TUMORS[4]

Because of its profuse blood flow, the kidney is frequently the site of metastasis of carcinomas and sarcomas that arise in other organs. Lung and breast tumors are the main sources. RCC of the kidney is the only malignancy that selectively metastasizes to the opposite kidney. There is no specific pattern that distinguishes these lesions from other solid masses, and they may present as hypoechoic to hyperechoic.

### Lymphoma [6,11]

Secondary involvement of the kidney by lymphoma, including Hodgkin lymphoma and leukemia, occurs with significant frequency and is manifested by nonspecific enlargement of the kidney. In Hodgkin disease, the incidence is approximately 10%, whereas in malignant lymphoma it varies from 35% to 60%. Sonographically, most lymphomas present as anechoic or hypoechoic, single or multiple masses. Characteristically, lymphosarcoma is bilateral. The pattern of tumor growth is into the perinephric space so that it surrounds and encapsulates the kidney. It may appear anechoic because it has very few internal reflectors and simulates renal cysts. It is important to document a lack of acoustic enhancement deep to the mass to indicate that it is a solid lesion.

## HYDRONEPHROSIS[12,13,16,29,46,50–57]

Hydronephrosis represents urine dilatation of the renal pelvis, calyceal structures, and infundibula. Pathology Box 10-4 presents the intrinsic and extrinsic causes

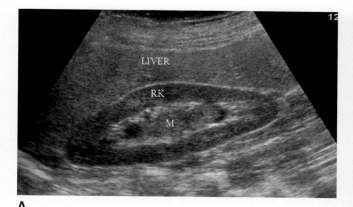

**A**

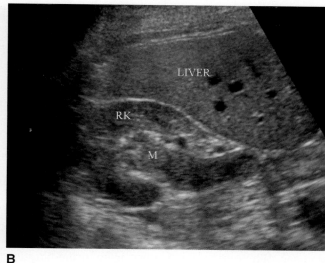

**B**

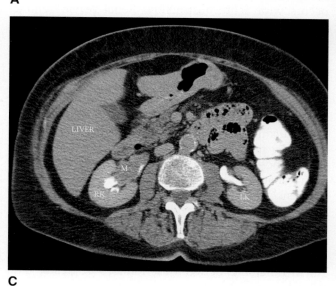

**C**

**Figure 10-22** Transitional cell carcinoma. **A:** Longitudinal and transverse **(B)** sections of a 79-year-old woman's right kidney reveal a hypoechoic mass located within renal sinus. **C:** Computed tomography confirms the presence of a mass in the renal pelvis. The appearance and location is consistent with transitional cell carcinoma. (Images courtesy of Taco Geertsma, MD, Hospital Gelderse Vallei, Ede, The Netherlands.)

---

**PATHOLOGY BOX 10-4**

### *Hydronephrosis*

| Cause | Grade and Extent |
|---|---|

**Cause**

Intrinsic: calculi, hematoma, neoplasm, ureteropelvic stricture or obstruction, ureterocele, sloughed papilla, pyelonephrosis, congenital (aberrant vessels, vesicoureteral reflux, posterior urethral valves, ectopic ureterocele collecting system duplication)

Extrinsic: neoplasm, trauma, neurogenic bladder, surgery (ligation, transection, edema, etc.), bladder outlet obstruction (neoplasm, prostatic hypertrophy, urethral problems), retroperitoneal fibrosis, gynecologic (tubo-ovarian abscess, endometriosis, etc.), pregnancy, inflammatory lesions (pelvic, gastrointestinal, retroperitoneum)

**Grade and Extent**

Grade I (mild): minimal separation of sinus echoes (2 mm); distortion of pelvocaliceal structure with dilated, fluid-filled calyces, infundibula, and pelvis, causing splaying of central echo complex; depending on point of obstruction, may be unilateral or bilateral

Grade II (moderate): anechoic separation of entire central sinus with (1) continuous broad, anechoic band and distention of intrarenal pelvis; (2) oval, anechoic collections along the periphery of central echo complex when calyceal enlargement is greater than renal pelvis enlargement; or (3) mixed pattern with pelvis and calyces enlarged

Grade III (marked): extensive separation of central sinus and calyces, with parenchymal thinning, with (1) a single, blown-out, ellipsoid, anechoic collection spreading central echo complex with loss of individual calyceal structures into markedly distended pelvis; (2) lobulated or large septate, anechoic pattern representing markedly distended individual calyces; or (3) anechoic dumbbell configuration due to a ureteropelvic obstruction with marked extra-renal pelvis and intrarenal infundibulum enlargement leading to dilatation. Depending on the cause, laboratory values and symptoms vary. Patients may be asymptomatic if unilateral, mild or moderate, or associated with other entities (pregnancy); or patients may present with abdomen, back, and flank pain. Hydronephrosis can be caused by intrinsic or extrinsic obstruction, or by postobstruction atrophy, infection (pyelonephritis), post renal failure, overhydration, or high-flow states (polyuria), and reflux.

Obstructive disorders can occur at any age and cause impairment of urine flow by involving any urinary tract structure from the renal tubules to the urinary meatus. In 90% of cases, the obstruction is located below the level of the glomeruli. As the severity and duration of obstruction increase, the kidneys become more susceptible to infection, calculus development, and permanent damage. When urine flow is obstructed, urine filtration continues, the calyces become distended, the renal pelvis dilates, and its pressure is elevated. Transmitted back to the collecting ducts, the elevated pressure causes blood vessel compression. If the obstruction is complete, serious and irreversible kidney damage occurs after about 3 weeks and, if incomplete, after about 3 months.

Hydronephrosis is often found incidentally in asymptomatic patients during routine obstetric sonography. It occurs in 65% to 85% of pregnancies[12]; the incidence is greater in the right kidney (90%) than in the left (67%). The cause of hydronephrosis and the reason for the right-sided preponderance remain controversial. It may be due to mechanical pressure on the uterus or muscular relaxation of the ureters resulting from hormonal factors. There is a wide variation in the extent of dilatation, with an increasing calyceal diameter seen at 10 to 20 weeks and usually peaking at 24 to 28 weeks.[12] Bladder filling, parity, and a history of urinary tract problems are not related to the degree of dilatation. These findings are most often not considered pathologic. The dilatation usually resolves within several weeks postpartum.

The sensitivity of real-time sonography is 100% for the detection of chronic obstruction and 60% to 70% for acute obstruction. Because sonographic examination readily images the presence of hydronephrotic changes, it can be recommended as the initial procedure when obstructive uropathy is a clinical consideration. The sonographic hallmark of hydronephrosis is splaying, spreading, or ballooning of the central echo complex. The extent of hydronephrosis can be graded based on its sonographic appearance (Pathology Box 10-4 and Fig. 10-23A–H). In addition to documenting the extent of hydronephrosis, the sonographer must attempt to document its cause. The examination includes imaging (1) the ureters for dilatation; (2) the prostate for hyperplasia, carcinoma, and prostatitis; (3) the urinary bladder for calculi, tumors, ureterocele, and functional disorders (reflux, neurogenic); (4) pelvic structures and the retroperitoneum for pregnancy, tumors, or retroperitoneal fibrosis; and (5) the urethra for posterior valve stricture and tumors, which are rare.

For patients being evaluated for hydronephrosis due to postrenal failure, the renal pelvic peristaltic wave contractions should be evaluated in real-time to help distinguish obstruction from renal pelvic distention due secondary to diuresis. Normally, two to four contractions occur per minute and are directly related to the amount of urine the kidney produces. Renal pelvic and ureteral peristalsis increases if urine flow rates rise due to pathology, increased hydration, or diuretic use. An irregular rate of peristalsis, with bursts of repeated incomplete contractions followed by aperistaltic periods, occurs with acute obstruction. Renal pelvic contractions usually cease with chronic obstruction.

Several studies have been performed in an attempt to add physiologic information to the anatomic information provided by the sonographic examination. These include successful diuretic ultrasound examination to evaluate upper tract obstruction, determining the role of Doppler in evaluating upper tract renal obstruction, and in evaluating maternal kidneys in asymptomatic pregnancy. In most of the Doppler evaluations, there was no significant difference in the RI of intrarenal arteries with native kidney obstruction; there was a significant difference in the evaluation of normal versus obstructed kidneys and of obstructed versus contralateral nonobstructed kidneys. The mean RI for obstructed kidneys was $0.77 \pm 0.07$ (standard deviation) compared to the contralateral normal kidney, with an RI of $0.60 \pm 0.04$.[57] An RI difference between the kidneys of greater than 0.1 has been shown to be indicative of functionally significant unilateral obstruction. This would indicate the value of utilizing the Doppler examination because obstruction produces hemodynamic changes with intrarenal vasoconstriction and elevation in renal arterial resistance, which may be detectable before pyelocaliectasis can be observed with sonography alone.

False-positive diagnoses include extrarenal pelvis, vesicoureteral reflux, full bladder, high urine flow as seen with overhydration and furosemide use, and parapelvic or peripelvic cysts; and false-negative diagnoses arise from performing the examination before dilatation has occurred. It is difficult to distinguish mild hydronephrosis from conditions that simulate it: (1) normal variants (distensible collecting system, extra-renal pelvis, full bladder, congenital megacalyces, calyceal diverticulum); (2) increased urine flow (overhydration, medications, osmotic diuresis during or immediately after urography, diabetes insipidus, diuresis in nonoliguric azotemia); (3) inflammatory disease (acute pyelonephritis, chronic pyelonephritis); (4) renal cystic disease (single cyst, parapelvic cysts, adult polycystic kidney disease, medullary cystic disease, multicystic dysplastic kidney); and (5) other causes such as postobstructive or postsurgical dilatation, vesicoureteral reflux, papillary necrosis, and renal sinus lipomatosis. It

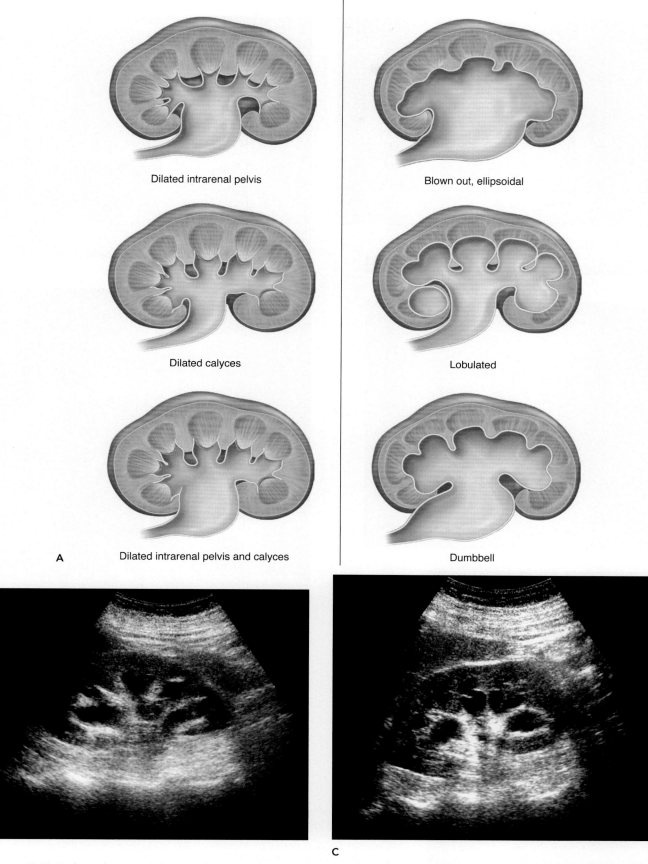

Moderate Hydronephrosis

Dilated intrarenal pelvis

Dilated calyces

**A**  Dilated intrarenal pelvis and calyces

Severe Chronic Hydronephrosis

Blown out, ellipsoidal

Lobulated

Dumbbell

**B**

**C**

**Figure 10-23** Hydronephrosis. **A:** Schematic illustration of the sonographic patterns of moderate hydronephrosis and severe chronic hydronephrosis. **B–D:** Grade I hydronephrosis in a 61-year-old woman who presented with bilateral flank pain. Longitudinal sections of the right kidney **(B)** and left kidney **(C)** demonstrate mild distortion of the pelvocaliceal structures with dilated fluid-filled calyces. *(continued)*

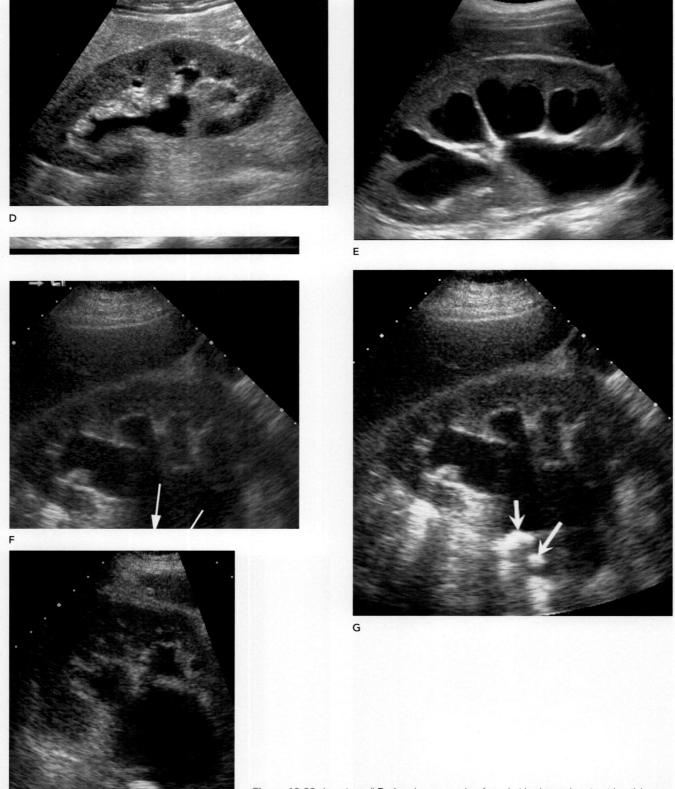

**Figure 10-23** *(continued)* **D:** Another example of grade I hydronephrosis with mild separation of the renal pelvis. **E,F:** Grade II hydronephrosis with dilated calyces and renal pelvis on two different patients. **G,H:** Grade III hydronephrosis in an 82-year-old woman being evaluated for frequent urinary tract infections. **G:** On longitudinal and **(H)** transverse sections of the right kidney there is dilatation of the pelvis, calyces, and proximal ureter. Urolithiasis *(arrows)* is noted within the proximal ureter in both images. (**B,C,** courtesy of Jody Kutney, Columbus, OH; **D–F,** courtesy of Philips Medical Systems, Bothell, WA; **G,H,** courtesy of Mount Carmel West Hospital, Columbus, OH.)

is important to remember that hydronephrosis causes spreading of the calyceal echoes and that some entities that simulate hydronephrosis (cystic disease) compress the central sinus echoes. With hydronephrosis, evaluating the remaining kidney cortex is important, as it indicates how much functioning tissue remains. Identifying a dilated ureter in continuity with a cystic mass of the upper pole is extremely helpful in making a diagnosis. The diagnosis is most likely ureteropelvic junction obstruction, with the presence of either bilateral or unilateral hydronephrosis in the absence of ureteral dilation.

# LITHIASIS

## UROLITHIASIS[4,13,20,29,38,45,46,51–52,58–62]

Calculi can develop anywhere in the urinary system (urolithiasis), but most develop in the kidney (nephrolithiasis). The prevalence of nephrolithiasis is 0.1% to 5% of the population in industrial countries. It is more common in White men aged 20 to 50 years. Because of the increased incidence of urolithiasis, the southeastern part of the United States is referred to as a geographic "stone belt." Hot climates favor stone formation. The prevalence is higher among people new to these areas, owing to unsuspected water loss leading to concentrated urine and increased precipitation of dissolved salts.

A clearly defined cause for urinary calculi has not yet been established. What is known is that their development requires the presence of a nidus for stone formation and an environment that supports the continued precipitation of stone components. Calculus formation is influenced by hereditary and familial predispositions, high concentrations of stone constituents, changes in urinary pH, or the presence of bacteria, but many calculi form in the absence of these factors. The three major theories of stone formation and the four types of urolithiasis are presented in Pathology Box 10-5. Urine cultures, urine analysis, and serum protein, bicarbonate, and uric acid levels help determine the cause of stone formation.

Depending on the size and location of the urolithiasis, clinical symptoms can include hematuria (resulting from tissue damage), oliguria (resulting from obstruction), or renal colic (as calculi are passed). Painful spasms radiating from the costovertebral angle to the flank and from the suprapubic region to the external genitalia are termed *renal colic*. When nephrolithiasis is confined to the renal pelvis and calyces, the pain is more constant and dull. Nausea, vomiting, fever, chills, abdominal distention, and pyuria can also be included in the list of symptoms. Anuria is present only with bilateral obstruction (or unilateral obstruction in a patient with only one kidney). Stones in the right ureter may mimic symptoms of appendicitis.

Unlike cholelithiasis situated in a bile-filled gallbladder, highly reflective nephrolithiasis situated within the highly reflective central echoes of the renal sinus collecting system are difficult to discern unless they are large and cast an acoustic shadow (Fig. 10-24A–D). More than 80% of nephrolithiases contain some form of calcium, the most common being composed of calcium oxalate, calcium phosphate, or a combination of the two. For optimal visualization of an acoustic shadow caused by the difference in acoustic impedance at the interface of the crystalline surface of the stone and adjacent tissue, varying gain settings must be used, usually lower, and the narrow portion of the focal zone is positioned in the region of the suspected calculus.

---

 **PATHOLOGY BOX 10-5**

### *Stone Formation and Types of Urolithiasis*

**Theories Explaining Stone Formation**

1. Saturation theory attributes cause to urine saturated with calcium salts, uric acid, magnesium ammonium phosphate, or cystine.
2. Deficiency of stone formation inhibitors theory states that the kidney lacks a normally produced substance that inhibits stone formation.
3. Matrix theory states that organic materials derived from tubular cells act as a nidus for stone formation and is based on observation that organic matrix materials are found in all layers of kidney stones, although it is not known whether matrix material contributes to initiation of formation or whether material is trapped in stone as it forms.

**Types of Urolithiasis**

Calcium oxalate, calcium phosphate, or a combination of the two (80%–90%), usually associated with increased blood and urinary concentration of calcium predisposed by excessive bone reabsorption caused by immobility, bone disease, renal tubular acidosis, milk-alkali syndrome, hyperparathyroidism, hypervitaminosis D, medullary sponge kidney, and hyperoxaluria.

Struvite or magnesium ammonium phosphate (recur in 27% of susceptible persons) most commonly associated with bacteria (*Proteus* infections) and are caused by urea-splitting action of bacteria.

Staghorn calculus, stone filling the entire renal pelvis, is almost always associated with urinary tract infection, persistent alkaline urine, or both.

Uric acid (8%) caused by high concentration of uric acid (urine pH about 5.5) associated with gout and dehydration.

Cystine formed in acid urine due to an inherited renal tubular defect affecting the absorption of urine amino acids.

When a renal calculus is identified by its characteristic dense echo pattern and by its associated sound attenuation and strong acoustic shadow, observation of associated hydronephrosis enables the examiner to localize the area of obstruction (Fig. 10-24E–G). Ureteral stones are more difficult to visualize sonographically and will be detected only if the ureter is dilated significantly (Fig. 10-23G,H). Traditionally, IVP studies were used to evaluate for urolithiasis, but that study has been largely replaced by CT. The most sensitive imaging modality for evaluation of urolithiasis is a noncontrast helical CT.

Within the resolving capabilities of the equipment and regardless of their chemical composition, sonography images most calculi as echogenic structures (Fig. 10-24H–L). The exceptions are three nonopaque matrix calculi. These nonshadowing calculi are found more frequently in women than in men. They are associated with the presence of urea-splitting bacteria and may coexist with crystalline calculi. The three are (1) uric acid calculi seen with gout and the treatment of myeloproliferative disorders, (2) xanthine calculi, and (3) mucoprotein matrix calculi seen in poorly functioning, infected urinary tracts. The

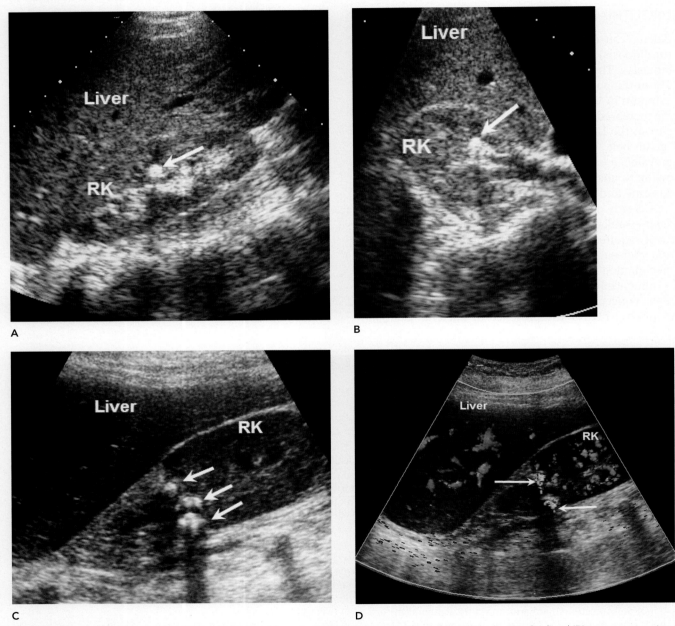

**Figure 10-24** Nephrolithiases. This 24-year-old woman presented with left lower quadrant pain. **A:** The longitudinal and **(B)** transverse sections of the right kidney (RK) demonstrate a single hyperechoic focal lesion (*arrow*) representing nephrolithiasis. Acoustic shadowing is seen posterior to the calculi. **C:** This 42-year-old woman presented with hematuria. Longitudinal image of the right kidney reveal multiple hyperechoic foci (*arrows*) representative of renal calculi. There is acoustic shadowing due to the attenuation of sound by the stone. **D:** A color Doppler image of the same patient, demonstrates the twinkle artifact (*arrows*) posterior to the stones. *(continued)*

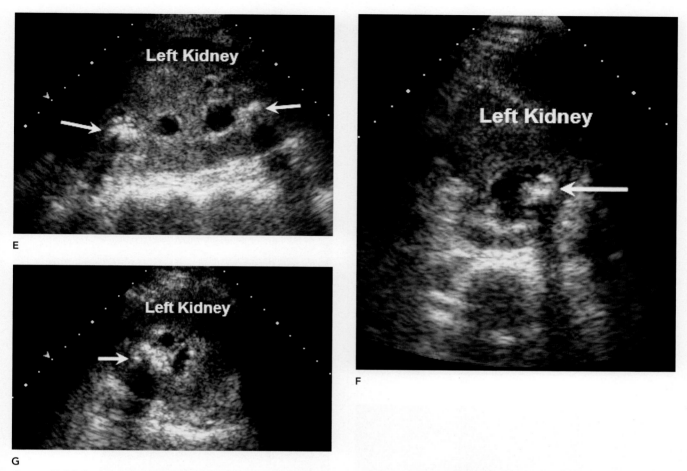

**Figure 10-24** *(continued)* **E–G:** Multiple renal stones *(arrows)* are demonstrated in this 20-year-old patient who was 35 weeks pregnant and complained of flank pain. **E:** Longitudinal section of the left kidney reveals nephrolithiasis in the superior and inferior poles. **F:** Transverse sections of the superior and **(G)** inferior poles in the same patient. *(continued)*

occurrence of xanthine and matrix calculi are rare.[51] The renal matrix calculus has less acoustic impedance mismatch and a lower absorption coefficient, which makes it more difficult to detect sonographically.

Hyperechoic regions within the kidney that lack an acoustic shadow or indistinct areas of echogenicity may be further evaluated with color Doppler. In a study by Lee et al., 80% of renal stones and 88% of ureteral stones displayed the twinkling artifact, suggesting the artifact could be considered as another sonographic criteria for urinary stones. Twinkle artifact is a rapidly changing mixture of colors visualized posterior to rough, highly reflective structures on color Doppler (Fig. 10-25A,B). The pulsed wave spectrum displays close vertical bands with no discernable waveform.

To consistently obtain a twinkling artifact, a high color-write priority should be selected and gray scale gain kept to a minimum. The color Doppler box should be sized over the area of interest and adjacent tissue. For maximum artifact intensity, the focal zone should be placed just below the area of interest.

The key to the twinkling artifact is that the color is produced behind the calcification and the concomitant Doppler spectral analysis tracing shows noise, not flow.

Because most urolithiases are smaller than 5 mm, the treatment of choice is to facilitate natural passage of the stones. Vigorous hydration and administration of diuretics flush the kidneys and ureters. Calculi too large to be passed, usually larger than 7 mm, require a more invasive procedure. Cystoscopy with retrieval instruments can aid in the removal of stones. Removal of calculi confined to the renal pelvis, parenchyma, or calyces may require a flank or lower abdominal incision. Extracorporeal shock wave lithotripsy focuses shock waves on localized renal calculi to disintegrate them so that they can be passed naturally. Prophylaxis to prevent recurrent calculus formation in predisposed patients includes a low calcium diet to prevent hypercalciuria, parathyroidectomy for hyperparathyroidism, allopurinol for uric acid calculi, and daily doses of ascorbic acid to acidify the urine.

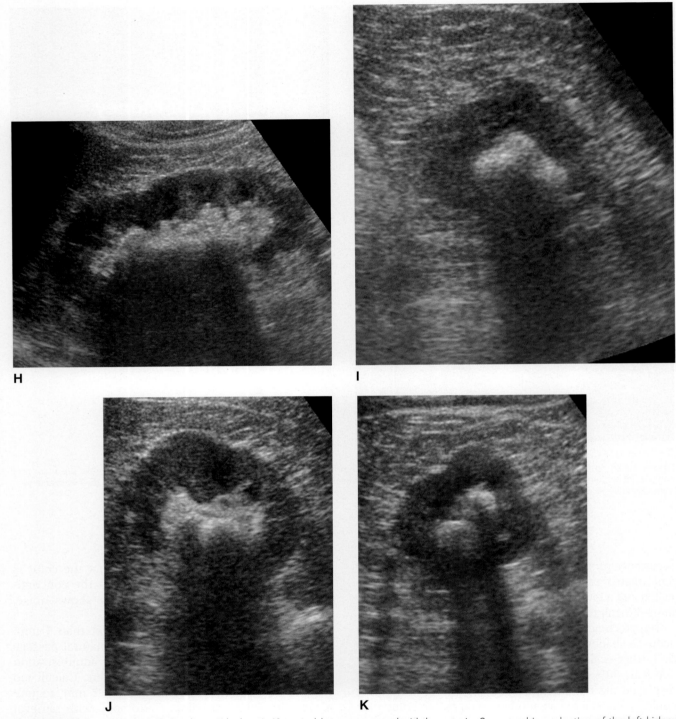

**Figure 10-24** *(continued)* **H–K:** Staghorn calculus. A 40-year-old man presented with hematuria. Sonographic evaluation of the left kidney reveals a staghorn calculus filling the renal sinus. **H:** Longitudinal section of the left kidney demonstrates a strong acoustic shadow emanating from the renal sinus. Transverse sections through the **(I)** superior **(J)** mid, and **(K)** inferior poles confirm the calculus extends the length of the kidney. *(continued)*

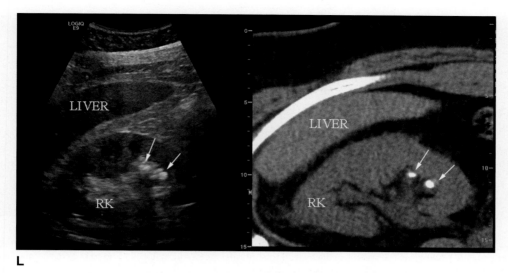

**Figure 10-24** *(continued)* **L:** Fusion image demonstrates a sonogram *(left image)* of the right kidney with multiple renal calculi *(arrows)* in the inferior pole. Computed tomography *(right image)* demonstrates two renal calculi. (**A,B,** Images courtesy of Miranda Bailey, Westerville, OH; **C,D,** Images courtesy of Kala Penney, Cambridge, OH; **E–G,** Images courtesy of Christi Tumblin, Zanesville, OH; **H–K,** Images courtesy of Chris Everett, Columbus, OH; **L,** Image courtesy of GE Healthcare, Wauwatosa, WI.)

## NEPHROCALCINOSIS[16,38,49,63,64]

Renal parenchymal calcium deposition, predominantly cortical or medullary or involving both regions, is commonly called *nephrocalcinosis* (nephrolithiasis occurs in the collecting system). Cortical nephrocalcinosis is usually bilateral and diffuse. The most common cause is cortical calcification identified in the hypercalcemic states associated with malignancy, hyperparathyroidism, or vitamin D intoxication; acute cortical necrosis (ACN); chronic glomerulonephritis; and AIDS cases associated with *Mycobacterium avium-intracellulare* (MAI) infection. The most common

cause of medullary nephrocalcinosis is a metabolic abnormality usually identified in hypercalciuria and hypercalcemic states associated with medullary sponge kidney and papillary necrosis in situ. Medullary nephrocalcinosis can also be caused by other processes affecting hydrogen ion excretion from the distal tubule identified with medullary sponge kidney (distal renal tubular acidosis), Wilson disease, Fanconi syndrome, hyperglobulinemias, and the use of nephrotoxic drugs or acetazolamide administration.

The sonographic appearance of nephrocalcinosis may be difficult to differentiate from large renal calculi (staghorn calculi) or air (emphysematous

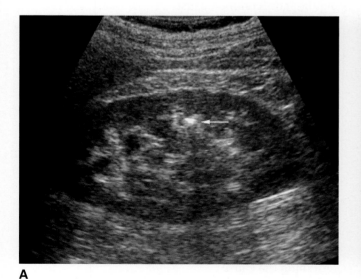

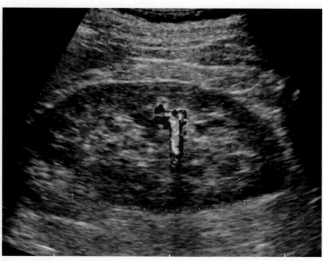

**A**                                    **B**

**Figure 10-25** Twinkle artifact. **A:** A grayscale image of a kidney with an echogenic area *(arrow)* creating minimal shadowing in the midpole. **B:** Color Doppler shows a mix of colors posterior to the hyperechoic area, confirming the diagnosis of nephrolithiasis. (Images courtesy of Taco Geertsma, MD, Hospital Gelderse Vallei, Ede, The Netherlands.)

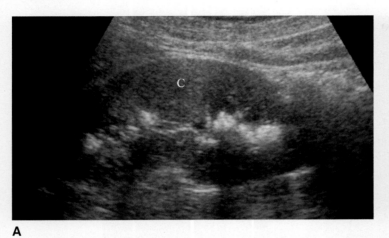

**A**

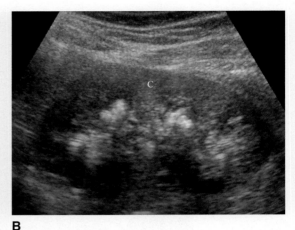

**B**

**Figure 10-26** Nephrocalcinosis. Longitudinal images of the right **(A)** and left **(B)** kidneys reveal multiple hyperechoic medullary calcifications and a normal renal cortex **(C)**. Nephrocalcinosis is usually related to abnormal metabolic states leading to hypercalcemia. (Images courtesy of Taco Geertsma, MD, Hospital Gelderse Vallei, Ede, The Netherlands.)

pyelonephritis). In cases of cortical nephrocalcinosis, calcifications appear as hyperechoic foci with or without acoustic shadowing in the renal cortex, and the corticomedullary junction is not well defined. The appearance may be bilateral or unilateral; the kidney can appear small or normal in size; and the kidney may be diffusely more echogenic and difficult to separate from adjacent tissue. With medullary nephrocalcinosis, the normally hypoechoic renal pyramids appear highly echogenic with acoustic shadowing, but the renal cortex is of normal echogenicity (Fig. 10-26A,B). The presence of hyperechogenic rings in the periphery of renal medullary pyramids was correlated with the earliest signs of nephrocalcinosis in one study; however, in another study,[63] the sonographic sign was nonspecific and showed a poor correlation with the severity of renal disease. In a study conducted by Lucaya and colleagues,[64] renal calcifications were a common finding in older children with autosomal recessive polycystic kidney disease. Hypocitraturia and the urine acidification defect resulting from renal failure are the leading factors in the pathogenesis of bilateral renal calcifications.

## TRAUMA

### RENAL CAPSULE AND PARENCHYMA

Renal injuries are divided into those resulting from blunt trauma (70%) and those resulting from penetrating trauma or secondary to operative intervention. Athletic injuries, automobile or motorcycle accidents, and various types of crush injuries account for the majority of blunt injuries, whereas gunshot and knife wounds account for most penetrating injuries. Even when the traumatic event is mild, preexisting renal abnormalities such as ectopia, anomalies, or tumor predisposes to significant renal damage.

Even though CT is frequently the examination of choice in trauma situations, sonography can provide a quick, real-time, portable evaluation of the kidneys and surrounding areas. A reproducible linear absence of echoes seen in the area of a traumatized kidney suggests renal fracture. Depending on the interval since the trauma, sonography demonstrates either an anechoic or a hyperechoic region in a kidney fracture, with bleeding into the retroperitoneal space. Focal areas of internal hemorrhage and edema are hypoechoic. A blood clot in the collecting system can be identified as a low level echo mass separating the walls of the affected system.

### VASCULAR TRAUMA[11,65]

Chapter 4 discusses AV fistula, which may result from penetrating trauma, with percutaneous renal biopsy being the most common cause.

### Hematomas[11,16]

Renal hematomas may result from a variety of causes and are divided into spontaneous and posttraumatic types. Spontaneous hemorrhage into the subcapsular and perinephric spaces is rare but can be attributed to a variety of pathologies, including RCC, AMLs, segmental renal infarction, AV malformation, hemorrhagic cyst, abscess, and idiopathic causes. Posttraumatic intrarenal hematomas usually occur as the result of a bleeding diathesis, commonly related to anticoagulant drugs such as warfarin or heparin, but they are also associated with renal infarcts, necrotizing arteritis, intratumoral hemorrhage, and hemophilia. Sonography is very sensitive to the presence of hemorrhage and hematoma but, unlike CT, is more problematic in determining the cause.

Depending on the age of the bleed, hematomas have varying echo patterns (Fig. 10-27A,B). Acute hematomas appear echogenic or even hyperechoic and can

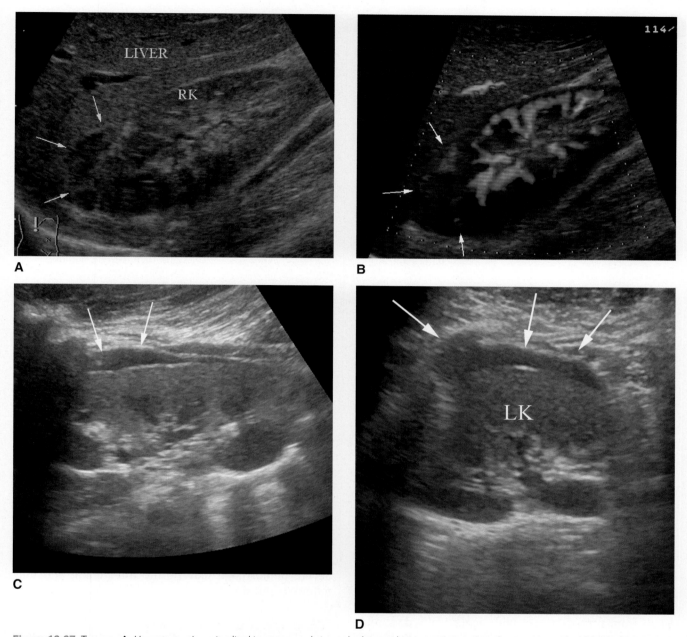

**Figure 10-27** Trauma. **A:** Hematoma. Longitudinal image reveals irregular hypoechoic area *(arrows)* on the superior pole of this kidney in a patient who experienced blunt trauma. **B:** Power Doppler indicates no flow in the hypoechoic area *(arrows)*. Based on the clinical and sonographic information, the diagnosis of hematoma was made. **C,D:** Subcapsular hematoma in 24-year-old patient with a history of blunt abdominal trauma. **C:** Longitudinal image of the left kidney demonstrates a hypoechoic collection anterior to the kidney *(arrows)*. The collection lies between the echogenic renal capsule and the renal cortex. The hematoma follows the contour of the kidney. **D:** Transverse image demonstrates the fluid collection anterior to the kidney. (**A,B,** Images courtesy of Taco Geertsma, MD, Hospital Gelderse Vallei, Ede, The Netherlands.)

mimic a solid renal mass. Gradually, as a hematoma becomes organized and develops a clot, it reveals a complex, heterogeneous pattern of internal echogenic, hypoechoic, and anechoic areas. Eventually, they undergo complete liquefaction and become seromas, reverting to an anechoic pattern. Chronic hematomas may become calcified, producing the characteristic acoustic shadows (Pathology Box 10-6). To rule out an active bleeding process, color Doppler could be performed over the hemorrhage site to determine if blood flow exists.

A subcapsular hematoma lies between the kidney cortex and the capsule. In the acute stage, subcapsular hematomas are difficult to visualize sonographically, as they may be isoechoic to the kidney. The renal capsule's hyperechoic pattern outlines the hematoma as a well-defined linear echo. The renal cortex may appear flattened or distorted by the surrounding fluid collection. Hematomas can also develop along or within any of the spaces surrounding the kidney and usually appear elongated. Whenever a fluid collection following

## PATHOLOGY BOX 10-6

### *Vascular Trauma*

| Lesion | Cause | Clinical Features | Laboratory Values | Sonographic Features |
|--------|-------|-------------------|-------------------|----------------------|
| Hematoma | Disease, pathology, trauma, anticoagulant therapy, bleeding diathesis | Mass may be palpable; unilateral flank pain | Decreased hematocrit | Irregular, thick wall; depending on stage of the bleeding process, varying echo patterns from anechoic to complex masses, with both cystic and solid components; chronic hematoma may develop calcifications with characteristic acoustic shadowing |
| Infarction | Obstruction of blood supply or drainage | Hypertension; lower extremity pulses absent | Elevated LDH, hematuria | Depending on the time frame following occlusion, renal parenchyma appears normal, hypoechoic, or hyperechoic |
| PA | Penetrating trauma | Mass may be palpable; unilateral flank pain | Decreased hematocrit | Anechoic spaces; in presence of AVF, flow usually progresses from artery to PA and then to vein; without AVF, Doppler waveform is "to-and-fro" at neck of PA |

LDH, lactate dehydrogenase; PA, Pseudoaneurysm; AVF, arteriovenous fistula.

the contour of the kidney is identified, the first impression should be a hematoma, and this finding should be considered in the context of the patient's clinical history (Fig. 10-27C,D).

### Infarction[16]

A renal infarction is caused by obstruction of the blood supply or blood drainage by occlusion or stenosis of a vessel. Immediately after an infarction, a little parenchymal loss may not be sonographically evident or the affected area may appear echogenic. Within 24 hours of an arterial occlusion, the infarcted area will typically appear hypoechoic. Within 7 days, echoes begin to appear within the mass, and by 17 days the area will once again appear echogenic, with no appreciable change in cortical echogenicity. Over time, the appearance may be a hyperechoic focal renal mass, which is believed to result from fibrosis mixed with acoustically dissimilar tissues and thinning of the involved cortex (Pathology Box 10-6).

### Pseudoaneurysm[12]

Pseudoaneurysms (PAs), like arteriovenous fistulas (AVFs), are caused by penetrating trauma. Sonographically, they appear as anechoic spaces similar to a renal cyst. Most are associated with AVF and can be identified with Doppler and color Doppler analysis. They can be differentiated from cystic masses by demonstrating pulsatile flow with an internal swirling pattern of blood flow. With an AVF, the flow usually progresses from the artery to the PA and then to the vein. When they are not associated with an AVF, renal PAs display the characteristic "to-and-fro" waveform pattern seen when the Doppler sample volume is placed at the neck of a PA; during systole, there is rapid influx of blood

into the collection through the communicating channel, and during diastole the energy stored in the soft tissues surrounding the collection is sufficient to drive blood back into the native artery. Color Doppler best demonstrates the connection between the PA and the adjacent artery. Artifactual flow is seen when avascular cystic areas show splashes of color. This can be differentiated from true flow in a PA by its random and homogeneous nature, lack of a characteristic pulsed Doppler waveform, and, in most cases, the ability to eliminate the artifact by changing color threshold and gain settings (Pathology Box 10-6). If the PA ruptures, it may produce a subcapsular hematoma, which may lead to renal dysfunction or hypertension because of renal compression. Severe hemorrhage may be life threatening and may require surgical repair.

## RENAL INFECTION AND INFLAMMATORY DISEASES[4,7,29,46,50,66,67]

Upper urinary tract infections (UTIs) and inflammatory diseases cover a wide spectrum. UTIs cause significant morbidity—they are second only to respiratory infections in prevalence. Bacterial infections may remain asymptomatic or localized to the bladder but carry the potential for spread to the kidneys. Their incidence is higher in women: approximately 20% develop at least one UTI during their lifetime. Among all patients receiving dialysis to sustain life, infections are responsible for 13% to 22% of disease.

*Escherichia coli* and *Enterobacter, Klebsiella, Pseudomonas,* and *Proteus vulgaris* species are the gramnegative bacilli responsible for 85% of UTIs. Any interference with normal voiding, incomplete emptying, stasis, or instrumentation leaves residual urine in the bladder and enhances bacterial multiplication. The bacteria ascend the urinary tract through the urethra (urogenous ascending route) or along the lymphatics (lymphogenous). It is believed that lymphogenous spread is facilitated by lymphatic connections between the upper and lower urinary tracts along the adjacent mucosa of the collecting system, and there may be lymphatic channels between the colon and the right kidney.

The incidence of these infections is greatest in women 15 to 24 years of age, suggesting that the shorter female urethra located close to the vagina and rectum, together with associated hormonal and anatomic changes, contribute to the higher incidence. Sexual activity may contribute in predisposed women, but the association with the development of urethritis and cystitis is controversial. The higher incidence during pregnancy is believed to be related to anatomic and physiologic changes and to the fact that estrogen and progesterone play a part in smooth muscle relaxation affecting the normal peristalsis in the ureters. In men, the length of the urethra and the antibacterial properties of prostatic fluid provide some protection from urogenous spread until age 50 years. After this age, prostatic hypertrophy becomes more common, and with it may come obstruction and UTI.

The second pathway for UTI is hematogenous dissemination. *Staphylococcus aureus* organisms from skin furuncles, skin infections, osteomyelitis, or endocarditis can reach the renal and perirenal tissues from remote sites months after initial exposure by hematogenous dissemination. Lymphogenous seeding of *S. aureus* is believed to be responsible for some UTIs.

Once bacteria have gained access to the kidney, the virulence of the infecting organism, host immunity, and other factors determine the extent of UTI involvement. Persons with diabetes and other states of immune compromise are more likely to develop infections than patients with normal immunity.

Laboratory function tests vary with the different renal infections and inflammatory diseases. Most patients have neutrophilic leukocytosis with varying degrees of hematuria, pyuria, bacteriuria, with or without WBC casts. Patients may appear asymptomatic but usually have malaise, tenderness or pain at the costovertebral angle on palpation, and varying degrees of flank pain. Lower urinary tract symptoms may include urinary frequency and urgent urination, with or without dysuria.

CT is the imaging modality of choice for acute renal infections. Sonography provides an excellent modality for assessing the internal renal architecture, but is less sensitive in demonstrating the presence of acute renal pathology, localizing the site of infection (intrarenal, perinephric, pararenal, intraperitoneal, etc.), and determining an etiology. Abnormalities can be recognized early in the course of the disease, diffuse renal inflammatory disease can be differentiated from focal lesions,

and extension into the retroperitoneum may be demonstrated. Sonography is an important examination for patients with urosepsis resulting from pyelonephritis, pyonephrosis, or a large renal or perirenal abscess. Urosepsis represents a true urologic emergency and requires urgent drainage. Serial examinations are easily performed to define different phases of the disease when there is an inadequate clinical response to antibiotic therapy or suspicion of an underlying lesion that predisposes to infection, such as obstruction by a urinary tract anomaly. Sonography does not depend on renal function or expose the patient to the risk of allergic reactions to contrast media. For women of childbearing age, its greatest advantage is its use of nonionizing radiation.

## ACUTE PYELONEPHRITIS[12,29,68,69]

The imaging literature uses inconsistent and ambiguous terminology in describing acute renal infection. Several authors have used the same term to describe different disease states. This textbook incorporates the Society of Uroradiology's recommendation to use *acute pyelonephritis* (APN) to replace the terms *bacterial nephritis, focal bacterial nephritis, acute bacterial nephritis, acute focal bacterial nephritis, lobar nephritis, lobar nephronia, preabscess, renal cellulitis, renal phlegmon,* and *renal carbuncle.*

APN is an acute suppurative bacterial inflammation of renal tubulointerstitial tissues, either unilateral or bilateral, and is associated with ascending UTI. In its earliest stages, the histopathologic appearance is diffuse edema producing renal enlargement with intense inflammatory foci, which may lead to microabscess formation throughout the involved renal interstitium. The onset is usually abrupt. Bladder irritation—along with symptoms such as dysuria, frequency, and urgency—is usually present. Without other symptoms, pyuria is not diagnostic of APN because it is also present in lower UTIs.

APN is most common in women aged 15 to 35 years and occurs in 1% to 2% of all pregnant women. It is postulated that the most common routes of infection are ascent along the lymphatics and urogenous spread facilitated by reflux, obstruction, or congenital renal anomaly. In an estimated 85% of cases, the most common organism is *E. coli,* which usually responds to antibiotic therapy. The widespread use of antibiotics makes hematogenous seeding of *S. aureus* from a remote site a rare cause.

The sonographic appearances of APN are described in terms of the phases of renal infection. Serial examinations are recommended because the sonographic appearance of APN (1) depends on the time the sonographic examination occurred in relation to the onset of infection; (2) may change rapidly (i.e., within hours); and (3) can be modified with

**PATHOLOGY BOX 10-7**

## Renal Infection and Inflammatory Disease

| Disease | Cause | Sonographic Features |
| --- | --- | --- |
| Acute pyelonephritis | Most often gram-negative bacilli by urogenous or lymphogenous ascent; *Staphylococcus aureus* by hematogenous or lymphogenous seeding | Appearance depends on onset, treatment, and examination time. (1) Homogeneous unilateral or bilateral renal enlargement, with or without focal (multifocal) swelling or patchy, disorganized parenchymal pattern; strong back wall compared to normal renal parenchyma; as infection progresses, renal sinus echoes blend into edematous, homogeneous parenchyma. (2) No renal enlargement but focal (or multifocal), indistinct, hypoechoic solid mass without definable wall; normal corticomedullary differentiation disrupted with scattered low-level echoes. |
| Emphysematous pyelonephritis | *Escherichia coli* infection; occurs most often in middle aged or elderly diabetic patients, those with urinary tract obstructions, and immunosuppressed patients | Unilateral hyperechoic foci (gas accumulation) in the renal parenchyma, renal sinus, or both; reverberation causes dirty shadowing; multiple tiny gas bubbles causes ring-down artifact |
| Chronic atrophic pyelonephritis | Recurrent infections superimposed on diffused or localized obstructive lesions or vesicoureteral reflux, resulting in renal scarring and atrophy | Small kidney with increased echoes in the involved area of the cortex and medulla from focal fibrosis; focal or multifocal processes with loss of renal parenchyma; with one or more calyces retracted and not distended, an echogenic zone extends beyond normal area of sinus |
| Xanthogranulomatous pyelonephritis | Chronic infection and obstruction of ureteropelvic junction, staghorn calculus, gram-negative (*Proteus*) infection in women and diabetic patients | Enlarged kidney maintains its reniform shape with a smooth contour; staghorn or other central calculus will cast an acoustic shadow; anechoic to hypoechoic, smooth to irregular bordered masses corresponding to debris-filled, dilated calyces or foci of parenchymal destruction; in diffuse pattern, parenchyma is replaced by multiple circular masses surrounding the central echo complex; in segmental disease, one or more masses surround a single calyx containing calculus |
| Renal abscess | *S. aureus* by hematogenous or lymphogenous seeding; gram-negative bacilli by urogenous or lymphogenous ascent | Anechoic to hypoechoic, complex mass with irregular borders; if present, debris provides numerous interfaces; if chronic, can contain internal septa; gas, if present, may cause acoustic shadowing or may be highly reflective, with microbubbles |
| Perinephric abscess | *S. aureus* by hematogenous or lymphogenous seeding, rupture of renal abscess, renal calculi, stricture, congenital anomaly, or *E. coli* or *Proteus vulgaris* via ascending lymphatics from urinary bladder | Anechoic to hypoechoic, complex mass displacing kidney; normal size and contour separate from the mass; anechoic (hydronephrosis) to hypoechoic, with very fine echoes throughout collecting system; may have a sludge-fluid level that remains in horizontal plane when patient changes position; may present with intense linear echoes, with/without shadow representing air from gas-forming organism |
| Pyonephrosis | Chronic suppurative infection in obstructed system | Enlarged kidney with mild-to-severe hydronephrosis; low-level echoes through dilated renal collecting system; sludge-debris level seen in dependent portion of dilated renal collecting system |
| Fungal infections | *Candida albicans* and others | Distinct focal or multifocal solid mass; change in renal size, abnormal renal cortical echogenicity; fungal balls appear as hyperechoic, nonshadowing masses |
| Renal tuberculosis | Hematogenous spread of *Mycobacterium tuberculosis* associated with pulmonary infection | Normal to several abnormal sonographic appearances which must be correlated with patient history, intravenous pyelogram, and computed tomography findings for diagnosis |
| Malakoplakia | Chronic *E. coli* infection | Unilateral enlarged kidney; multiple poorly defined, hypovascular cortical masses; diffuse disease, poorly defined masses distort and compress the central echo complex; if unifocal, nonspecific echogenic mass |

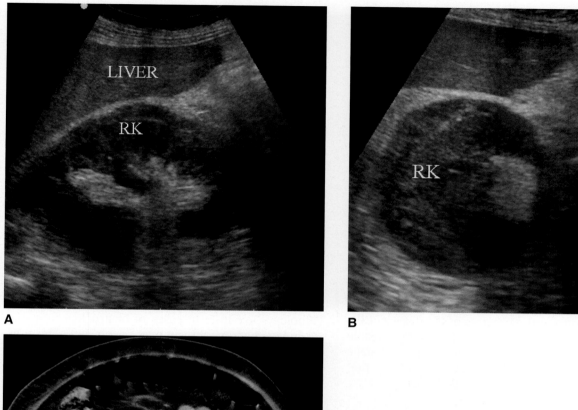

**A**

**B**

**C**

**Figure 10-28** Acute pyelonephritis. This 60-year-old woman presented with severe urosepsis. The longitudinal **(A)** and transverse **(B)** sections through the right kidney reveal a swollen, hypoechoic, heterogeneous right kidney. **C:** Computed tomography demonstrates the enlargement of the right kidney and a normal left kidney. (Images courtesy of Taco Geertsma, MD, Hospital Gelderse Vallei, Ede, The Netherlands.)

antibiotic therapy. Close correlation of the patient's clinical course is vital. Adopting *acute pyelonephritis* to incorporate a list of previously used terms, the sonographic appearance should be described in terms of (1) unilateral or bilateral; (2) focal (multifocal) or diffuse; (3) focal swelling or no focal swelling; and (4) renal enlargement or no renal enlargement. Serial examinations of patients undergoing therapy should show the central sinus echoes reappearing with their normal echogenicity (Pathology Box 10-7 and Fig. 10-28A–C).

## EMPHYSEMATOUS PYELONEPHRITIS[7,11,12,50,70]

Emphysematous pyelonephritis (EPN) is generally considered a life-threatening disease, with a mortality rate as high as 30% to 40%.[7] It occurs most frequently in middle aged or elderly diabetic patients, immunosuppressed patients, and women with urinary tract obstructions. EPN is most commonly caused by *E. coli* infection and because it may not respond to antibiotic treatment due to associated renal ischemia, it is treated with nephrectomy.

The sonographic examination can demonstrate gas accumulations, which appear as hyperechoic foci with sharp and usually flat anterior margins located in the renal parenchyma, renal sinus, or both. The acoustic impedance mismatch between renal tissue and intraparenchymal gas accumulation causes reverberation artifacts on the distal margin resembling a dirty shadow, which can be differentiated from the normal acoustic shadow that results from calculus attenuating sound energy. If there are multiple tiny gas bubbles, a ring-down artifact may occur. The examination may be difficult to obtain if the intrarenal gas or if an intestinal ileus associated with EPN obscures renal tissue (Pathology Box 10-7).

## CHRONIC PYELONEPHRITIS[4,16,20,29]

CPN is a chronic, progressive renal disorder in which renal scarring, either unilateral or bilateral, is associated with pathologic involvement of the calyces and pelvis. The disorder results from recurrent infections superimposed on diffused or localized obstructive lesions or vesicoureteral reflux. These recurrent renal inflammatory bouts eventually scar the kidney, and the obstructions contribute to parenchymal atrophy. Evidence suggests that autoimmune mechanisms may contribute to the pathogenesis of CPN. Many of the symptoms of APN are identified, but its onset may be insidious. Owing to the loss of tubular function and the ability to concentrate urine, polyuria and nocturia with associated mild proteinuria are common. Severe hypertension contributes to the progress of the disease. CPN is a significant cause of renal failure, being responsible for 25% of all cases of renal insufficiency and end-stage renal disease. The sonographic findings of CPN are presented in Pathology Box 10-7 (Fig. 10-29A,B).

### Xanthogranulomatous Pyelonephritis[7–9,11,12,16,17,51,69,71]

Xanthogranulomatous pyelonephritis (XGP) is a rare type of CPN characterized by replacement of normal renal parenchyma with lipid-laden (foamy) macrophages, plasma cells, and multinucleated giant cells. The most common predisposing factors are chronic infection and obstruction of the ureteropelvic junction, generally from a staghorn calculus. It is commonly associated with *Proteus mirabilis* and *E. coli* infections. Women and diabetic patients seem more susceptible.

The pathologic spectrum is variable and depends on the chronicity of the disease process. The process begins in the calyces and pelvis, and subsequently destroys the mucosa and extends into the adjacent medulla and cortex. Distended calyces compromise medullary perfusion, leading to papillary necrosis. Pus-filled, dilated calyces may predominate, or the kidney may be replaced with xanthogranulomatous tissue and less purulent components.

Generally, patients present with malaise, flank pain, a mass, weight loss, and UTI. Patients normally present with this triad: (1) 75% have renal calculi, usually of the staghorn variety; (2) have renal enlargement; and (3) lack of renal function.

The sonographic features of the varying diffuse or segmental patterns of involvement are presented in Pathology Box 10-7. In cases of obstructive uropathy, secondary hydronephrosis may be present. The presence of pelvic calculus, obstructive uropathy, marked hydronephrosis with replacement of the normal renal architecture by multiple fluid-filled masses, poor definition of the central echo complex, or diminished renal function is instrumental in helping to differentiate XGP from other focal complex lesions, including neoplasms, other inflammatory processes, and hematomas. When sonographic findings suggest the diagnosis of XGP, CT is often more specific in determining the full extent of XGP into perirenal and pararenal areas (Fig. 10-30A,B).

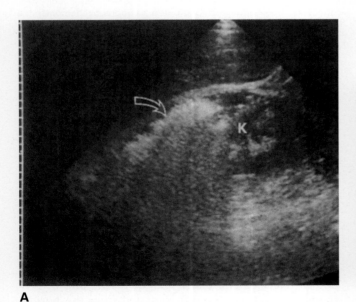

**A**

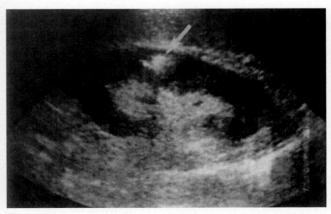

**B**

**Figure 10-29** Emphysematous pyelonephritis. **A:** Longitudinal sonogram reveals gas within the renal parenchyma *(open arrow)*. **B:** A follow-up longitudinal coronal sonogram performed 2 weeks later after therapy with intravenous antibiotics reveals improvement, although there is still some gas *(arrow)* within the renal cortex. (Reprinted with permission from Jeffrey RB, Ralls PW. *Sonography of the Abdomen*. New York, NY: Raven Press; 1995:292.)

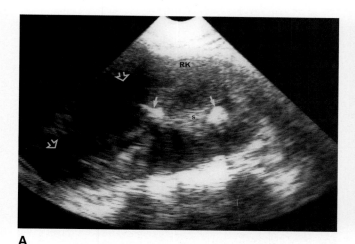

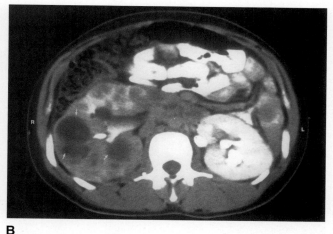

**Figure 10-30** Xanthogranulomatous pyelonephritis. This renal examination was done on a pregnant patient. **A:** The sonogram of the right kidney (RK) demonstrates two hyperechoic focal calcifications (arrows) seen in the renal sinus (s) and hypoechoic areas (open arrows) representing abscess seen in the renal cortex. **B:** On computed tomography (CT) examination, multiple poorly defined low-density areas (arrows) are identified within the renal parenchyma. The patient's history and the sonographic and CT appearances are consistent with XGP. (Images courtesy of Harris Cohen, MD, Brooklyn, NY.)

## RENAL AND PERINEPHRIC ABSCESSES[4,68,71]

The term *carbuncle* originally referred to a cluster of skin or subcutaneous boils but was adopted to describe hematogenously seeded renal abscesses that were usually caused by *S. aureus*. Radiologists, pathologists, and surgeons used the term to describe multiple coalescent intrarenal abscesses, and so *carbuncle* was incorrectly adopted as a synonym for *renal abscess*. Although a true carbuncle can be defined with a distinctive macroscopic appearance, it will not be used in this text because there is no corresponding image finding.

Abscesses, either acute or chronic, are septic conditions that produce unilateral flank pain, chills, fever, and point tenderness in the costovertebral angle. An abscess in the renal cortex may result from the union of several small abscesses and may rupture into the collecting system or through the capsule, causing a perirenal abscess, a pus collection in the space between the kidney and renal fascia.

In 20% of cases of renal or perirenal abscess, it is impossible to isolate the pathogen by urinalysis or culture. Historically, *S. aureus* was the most common agent of renal abscess. Currently, gram-negative bacilli are predominantly found to be the cause of renal abscess formation, spread either by the hematogenous or the ascending route, resulting from infected renal cysts, CPN, tuberculosis (TB), renal trauma, or obstruction. Abscesses most often are confined by the fascia and may extend in several directions, presenting as a draining flank abscess or a subphrenic abscess.

Pathology Box 10-7 presents the variable sonographic appearances of renal and perirenal abscesses. With a perirenal abscess, as with any perirenal mass, displacement is the striking abnormality. A perirenal abscess immobilizes the kidney, so that deep inspiration and

expiration do not produce the normal excursion of the organ (Fig. 10-31A–C).

## PYONEPHROSIS[7,67,68,70,72]

Pyonephrosis (pyohydronephrosis) is the presence of purulent material in a dilated, often obstructed, renal collecting system. When pyonephrosis is suspected, sonography is the imaging procedure of choice. Minimal to marked hydronephrosis, thickness of the renal cortex, and inflammatory extension outside the kidney can be evaluated.

Sonographic findings are variable owing to the stage and duration of inflammation and the extent of proteolysis of the purulent material. The presence of tissue and cellular debris helps make the diagnosis by producing low-level echoes in the dilated collecting system. With tissue and debris, the most common and reliable sonographic finding of pyonephrosis is the presence of a sludge-fluid level in the collecting system that remains in the horizontal plane when the patient's position is changed. Without the tissue and debris, pyonephrosis may present with very fine echoes throughout the dilated collecting system or it may occasionally be anechoic and simulate hydronephrosis. With a gas-forming organism secondary to infection, air in the collecting system may be detected by the presence of intensely echogenic linear densities. Although these echoes are found in the nondependent portion of the dilated system, they may cast a shadow, simulating calculi (Pathology Box 10-7 and Fig. 10-32A,B).

If the pyonephrosis is chronic (symptoms lasting for several months), diffuse XGP may result. Distinguishing pyonephrosis from other causes of urosepsis is important, so that immediate percutaneous or surgical drainage can be instituted.

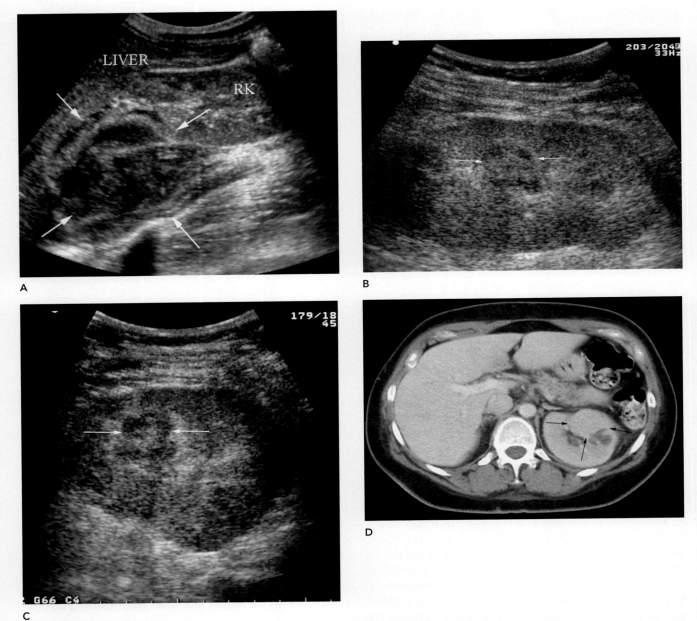

**Figure 10-31** Renal abscess. **A:** The complex mass *(arrows)* seen in the upper pole of the right kidney *(RK)* transverse sonogram was diagnosed as a renal abscess on this patient. **B:** On a different patient, the longitudinal section through this left kidney reveals an edematous, hypoechoic kidney with loss of the corticomedullary definition and a small hypoechoic lesion in the region of the midpole. **C:** A transverse section of the same kidney demonstrates the hypoechoic area. **D:** Computed tomography demonstrates the enlarged kidney and the mass near the midpole. A diagnosis of pyelonephritis with a renal abscess was made. (**A**, Image courtesy of Robert DeJong, Baltimore, MD; **B–D**, Images courtesy of Taco Geertsma, MD, Hospital Gelderse Vallei, Ede, The Netherlands.)

## FUNGAL INFECTIONS[12,69,73]

The most common cause of fungal UTI is *Candida albicans* and, less frequently, *Torulopsis, Cryptococcus, Coccidioides, Phycomycosis, Actinomycosis, Blastomyces,* and others.[74] At risk are premature infants with long-term indwelling catheters used for prolonged hyperalimentation and patients with diabetes, as well as the following conditions: cancer (especially leukemia or lymphoma); indwelling foreign bodies; chronic illness; intravenous drug abuse; prolonged antibiotic,

corticosteroid or immunosuppressive therapy; and immunocompromise from AIDS. The infection may be limited to the upper or lower urinary tract and may be unilateral or bilateral. The affected kidney is usually enlarged, and multiple microabscesses form in the renal cortex, interstitium, and tubules. As the pathology progresses, papillitis and fungus balls are found in the collecting system. Renal obstruction can occur with fungus balls, leading to renal failure and anuria.

The sonographic appearance of fungal infections may be similar or identical to that of APN or an abscess

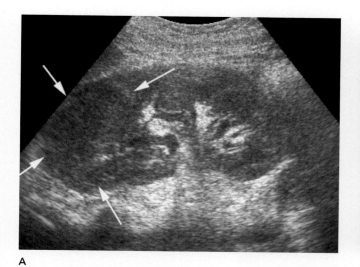
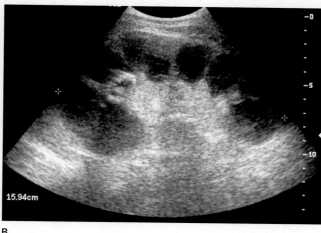

**Figure 10-32** Pyonephrosis. The longitudinal images on these two patients diagnosed with pyonephrosis displays **(A)** focal pyonephrosis (*arrows*) and **(B)** pyonephrosis affecting the entire enlarged kidney. (Images courtesy of Robert DeJong, Baltimore, MD.)

with a distinct focal or multifocal solid mass. Other sonographic appearances are a change in renal size, abnormal renal cortical echogenicity, or renal fungus balls. Fungal balls appear as hyperechoic, nonshadowing masses. The finding of fungal balls may be incidental (Pathology Box 10-7 and Fig. 10-33A–C).

## SCHISTOSOMIASIS[75]

Schistosomiasis is a disease caused by parasitic worms that reside in fresh water in the form of larvae. Although uncommon in the United States, schistosomiasis is prevalent in developing countries. Patients that have been exposed to fresh water in developing countries are at risk for contracting the parasite and developing the disease. Careful attention to patient history can help identify those patients at risk for possible parasitic infection.

The larvae penetrate human skin causing a rash. The larvae shed their tails, enter the lymphatic vessels and capillaries then migrate to the portal system, mesenteric veins, and urinary system. The most common species, *S. haematobium*, affects the urinary tract. Clinical symptoms may include hematuria, dysuria, and renal failure. Sonographically, the kidneys may appear normal or demonstrate ureteral obstruction and hydronephrosis. Calcifications may be present within the bladder and the bladder wall.

Treatment consists of a single-dose oral chemotherapy drug called *praziquantel*. It has been shown to reduce the egg count by 95% and cure the infection in 85% to 90% of patients.

## TUBERCULOSIS[12,69,71,76,77]

Renal TB is acquired by hematogenous spread of mycobacterium TB associated with concurrent or previous pulmonary infection.[71] Patients with renal TB have an abnormal chest radiograph 30% of the time, and only 10% show signs of active pulmonary TB. Usually, renal TB does not manifest itself for 10 to 20 years after the initial infection. Initially, the clinical presentation is often mild and nonspecific, but as the disease advances, more classic findings include night sweats and fever. With renal TB, tubercle destruction occurs that leads to cavitation, ulcer formation, and fistulization—simultaneously, the secondary defense mechanism tries to encapsulate the infection with granuloma formation. The destructive process appears as renal papillary necrosis, and the reparative process results in narrowing from infundibular stenosis, renal pelvis-ureteropelvic junction fibrosis. Treatment usually includes antibiotic therapy, and the overall prognosis is good. In some instances, nephrectomy is required.

Sonographically, renal TB presents with several different appearances, making it very important to correlate the patient's history with the findings of the imaging examination. The infected kidney may appear normal even with absent renal function. More often, the infiltrating pattern shows increased echogenicity secondary to the calcifications and infected debris, with or without abscesses. The corticomedullary distinction may be lost, and calcifications are seen in 25% to 50% of cases.[12] Advanced parenchymal destruction results in a small, calcified, nonfunctioning kidney referred to as a *putty kidney* or *autonephrectomy*. The kidney may simulate the sonographic appearance of other infections and inflammatory processes such as hydronephrosis or pyonephrosis with dilated, clubbed calyces and a small renal pelvis, the tumefactive masses similar to those seen with XGP, and a bacterial abscess, with or without a neoplasm. The diagnosis often depends on a correlation between the sonographic and CT findings (Pathology Box 10-7 and Fig. 10-34).

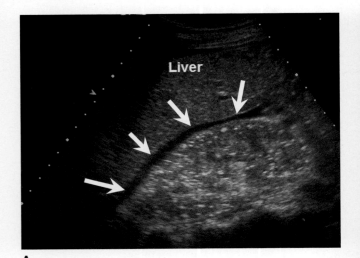

**A**

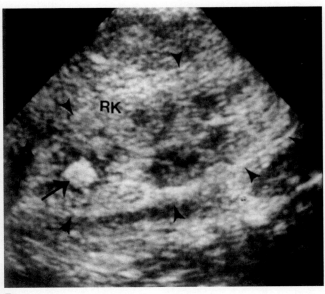

**B**

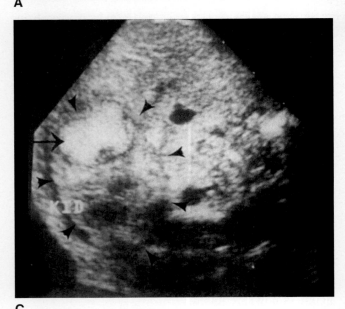

**C**

**Figure 10-33** Fungal infections. **A:** This patient presented with *Pneumocystis jiroveci* pneumonia. The sonogram displays an enlarged, infected kidney *(arrows)* with abnormal echogenicity. **B,C:** These images are on a 3-week-old premature girl who had surgery for peritonitis and bowel rupture. Postsurgical complications included fever, elevated alanine aminotransferase (ALT), aspartate aminotransferase (AST), and alkaline phosphatase, leukocytosis, and pyuria. The sonographic examination of the urinary system demonstrated kidneys of normal size and shape, with echogenic masses appearing in both. On both the longitudinal **(B)** and transverse **(C)** images, loculated, echogenic, nonshadowing masses *(arrow)* are seen in the right kidney *(RK; KID, arrowheads)*. The largest of these measured 5 mm. Other sonographic findings included a markedly enlarged liver and fluid collections. The patient was diagnosed with fungal infection and was treated with antibiotics. Sonographic follow-up within 2 weeks demonstrated less conspicuous fungus balls, and follow-up within 1 month demonstrated normal renal architecture. (**A**, courtesy of Robert DeJong, Baltimore, MD.)

## MALAKOPLAKIA[7,12,69]

Malakoplakia is a rare granulomatous inflammatory disease associated with chronic *E. coli* infection. The disease manifests itself because of the inability of the monocytes to kill and digest the bacteria. The inflammatory process most often affects middle-aged women (4:1 ratio) with recurrent UTI. Although it occurs most often in the lower urinary tract, renal parenchymal involvement occurs in 16% to 33% of cases, and approximately 40% of cases involve immunosuppressed patients.

Sonographically, parenchymal malakoplakia appears as a unilateral enlarged kidney with multiple poorly defined, hypovascular cortical masses. With diffuse disease, poorly defined masses distort and compress the central echo complex. If the disease is unifocal, a nonspecific echogenic mass can be seen. The diagnosis is frequently made after nephrectomy for a presumed renal tumor rather than on the basis of imaging examinations (Pathology Box 10-7).

## RENAL MEDICAL DISEASES[25,63]

When evaluating the kidney for medical disease, correlating the abnormal anatomic presentation with the patient's clinical history and laboratory values is important. Renal pathology involves interrelated nephron, vascular, or interstitial tissues, as (1) nephron changes result from vascular disease; (2) vascular disease causes nephron and interstitial tissue changes; and (3) interstitial tissue changes inevitably accompany and follow vascular and nephron disease. Investigators have had mixed and sometimes conflicting results from studying the echogenicity and thickness of the parenchyma, corticomedullary differentiation, renal

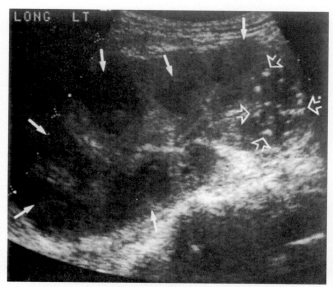

**Figure 10-34** Renal tuberculosis (TB). Longitudinal coronal sonogram of the left kidney. There are multiple dilated, debris-filled calyceal elements *(arrows)*. Multiple small calcifications *(open arrows)* are noted in the lower pole. TB and xanthogranulomatous pyelonephritis can be difficult or impossible to differentiate from one another, both clinically and on images. (Reprinted with permission from Jeffrey RB, Ralls PW. *Sonography of the Abdomen*. New York, NY: Raven Press; 1995:301.)

size, clarity of outline, renal sinus echoes, and prominence of medullary pyramids, with or without duplex Doppler of intrarenal blood flow of native kidneys to find quantitative criteria for renal parenchymal diseases. In the early stage, the sonographic appearance and Doppler examination lack specificity in diagnosing the type of renal parenchymal disease. Over the long term, a seriously injured kidney shows atrophy and scarring and loses the distinguishing features of the specific original disease, regardless of whether it was glomerular, tubular, interstitial, or vascular. In end-stage kidney disease, the primary renal disease often is not identifiable sonographically.

The diagnosis of parenchymal renal disease is based on evaluating (1) renal size, (2) renal contour, (3) cortical echogenicity, (4) distinctness of the corticomedullary junction, (5) detectability of the renal pyramids, (6) size of the renal pyramids, and (7) appearance of the renal sinus. The hallmark of parenchymal renal disease is a diffuse increase in echogenicity throughout the parenchyma of both kidneys (Fig. 10-35).

## RENAL CORTEX[11,78]

The degree of increased echogenicity seen with some renal parenchymal diseases correlates with the severity of the disease but not with the histopathologic change. In the early disease process, histologic changes may be isolated to only one of the three primary components of the renal parenchyma: the nephron, vessels, or interstitium. In the normal adult kidney, the glomeruli occupy

only 8% of the cortex. An early disease process isolated to the glomeruli may not affect cortical echogenicity and corticomedullary differentiation but can affect the biopsy. The following conclusions are drawn from two separate correlation studies of histopathologic and sonographic findings: (1) there is no correlation between the clarity of the corticomedullary junction and any histopathologic finding, type of disease, or laboratory finding; (2) there is no correlation between the nature and severity of the glomerular lesion on renal biopsy and the sonographic findings; (3) there is a correlation between cortical echogenicity and the value of BUN and serum creatinine levels; and (4) there is a definite relation between the nature and severity of the interstitial changes on biopsy and the echo intensity of the cortex. Focal interstitial changes tend to produce a minimal increase in cortical echogenicity, diffuse scarring produces a greater increase in echogenicity, and active interstitial infiltration produces the highest echo level. The lack of sonographic specificity and the limited response of the kidney to various pathologic processes may continue to limit the specific sonographic diagnosis, even when accurate quantitative measurements are made. After the initial diagnosis has been made by biopsy, however, the good correlation between cortical echogenicity and the severity of histopathologic changes indicates that sonography can provide a noninvasive method of monitoring the progression of renal disease.

As disease progresses, sonographic echogenicity is altered from combined changes within the glomeruli, tubules, and interstitium. There is an increase in echogenicity probably related to interstitial diseases because the majority of the cortex is composed of tubules and interstitial tissue. In disease processes with increased

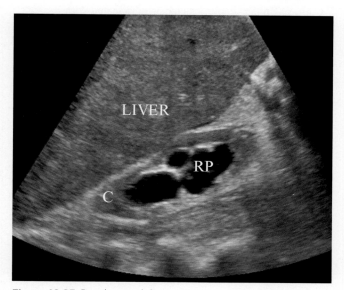

**Figure 10-35** Renal cortical disease. Longitudinal image of the right kidney demonstrates a hyperechoic thin, renal cortex *(C)* consistent with renal cortical disease. Hydronephrosis is also seen. *RP*, renal pelvis. (Image courtesy of Philips Medical Systems, Bothell, WA.)

deposition of collagen or calcium, cortical echogenicity increases but the corticomedullary junction may be preserved (Pathology Box 10-8). With chronic disease, the kidney becomes smaller, the cortex has increased echogenicity, and the medulla eventually becomes equally echogenic.

## RENAL MEDULLARY[74]

If the height of the pyramids exceeds or is thicker than that of the overlying cortex, they are considered enlarged. Medullary echo intensity equal to or greater than that of renal cortex is considered pathognomonic of medullary disease. The clinical history, laboratory values, and biopsy findings all contribute to identifying the pathogenesis of any quantifiable deviation in renal contour, size, or echogenicity.

Three chemical imbalances associated with a hyperechoic medulla are hyperuricemia, medullary nephrocalcinosis, and hypokalemia. The disease entities found in patients with these chemical imbalances and with a diffusely hyperechoic medulla are listed in Pathology Box 10-8. With sickle cell hemoglobinopathies, a larger than normal, diffusely hyperechoic medulla is attributed to vascular dilatation, engorgement of vessels, glomerular enlargement, and interstitial edema. The patient presents with various clinical signs. Symptoms vary and are associated primarily with the type of disease process causing one of the three chemical imbalances.

## RENAL SINUS[78]

Renal parenchymal disease may alter the echogenicity of the renal sinus. If an infiltrative process increases septal thickness, the sinus echoes can appear inhomogeneous and patchy. With fibrosis and atrophy, the loss of adipose tissue results in further loss of distinction between the renal sinus and parenchyma.

---

### PATHOLOGY BOX 10-8

### *Diseases Affecting Renal Parenchyma*

| Disease | Sonographic Features |
|---|---|
| Membranous and chronic glomerulonephritis, hypertensive nephrocalcinosis, leukemic infiltration, amyloidosis, acute tubular necrosis, Alport syndrome, lupus nephritis, diabetic nephrosclerosis, renal transplant rejection, renal cortical necrosis, methemoglobinuric renal failure, and chronic renal failure | Cortical echogenicity increases; preserved or enhanced corticomedullary junction |
| Cysts, calyceal diverticula, renal artery aneurysms, tumors, abscesses, hematomas | Distorted anatomy and obliteration of corticomedullary definition focally or diffusely |
| Oxalosis, metastatic tumors, islet cell neoplasm, and cortical nephrocalcinosis (associated with chronic glomerulonephritis, renal cortical necrosis, and Alport syndrome) | Diffusely increased cortical echogenicity without acoustic shadowing; sparing of renal pyramids; accentuated corticomedullary junction |
| Gout, medullary nephrocalcinosis (associated with hyperparathyroidism, chronic progressive nephropathy, distal renal tubular acidosis with Wilson disease, chronic glomerulonephritis, milk-alkali syndrome, malignant tumors, hypervitaminosis D, primary hypercalcemia, sarcoidosis, and medullary sponge kidney), and renal papillary necrosis (associated with pyelonephritis, diabetes, and obstructive uropathy) | Normal renal cortical echogenicity with focal areas corresponding to renal pyramids; bilateral hyperechoic medullary echogenicity; acoustic shadowing depends on the presence, size, and composition of diffuse calcifications in the medulla |
| AIDS | Normal size; enlarged; normal to increased cortical echogenicity and preservation of corticomedullary junction; focal calcification in cortex, septa, and pyramids (nephrocalcinosis associated with *Mycobacterium avium-intracellulare*); focal hyperechoic areas sparing some parenchyma; diffuse punctate calcifications (associated with *Pneumocystis jiroveci* infection) |
| Diabetic nephropathy | Doppler indeces reflect increased renal vascular resistance; elevated ratio indeces and pulsatility indeces correlate with progression of nephropathy |
| Papillary necrosis | Hypoechoic medullary rims with anechoic spaces (representing fluid dissecting into and around necrotic papillae); calcifications, with or without shadowing, within medullary pyramids (in cases of analgesic nephropathy) |
| Lupus nephritis | Increased cortical echogenicity and either small or large renal size |

## AIDS[7,73,78,79]

Renal failure associated with AIDS cases has many causes and is discussed in this section because of the sonographic changes seen in the renal parenchyma. Kidney disease and renal failure are the fourth leading cause of death in HIV-positive patients. HIV-associated nephropathy now accounts for 10% of new end-stage renal disease cases in the United States. Prerenal failure may be due to dehydration, and postrenal failure may be due to hydronephrosis or AIDS-related nephropathy and nephrotoxic drug use. The sonographic appearance varies with the AIDS-related pathologic process. The most common sonographic findings are increased echogenicity of the cortex, decreased definition of the corticomedullary junction, and decreased renal sinus fat. Glomerular lesions with related nephropathy are thought to increase cortical echogenicity and the kidneys may be enlarged, even with advanced disease. Nephrocalcinosis related to MAI was discussed previously in the section on Nephrocalcinosis. Medications and metabolic disorders put patients with AIDS at a higher risk of developing nephrolithiasis. With AIDS-related disseminated *Pneumocystis jiroveci* infection, diffuse punctate renal calcification may occur, although the finding is more common in the liver, spleen, and lymph nodes (Pathology Box 10-8).

## DIABETIC NEPHROPATHY[79–81]

Diabetic nephropathy is a leading cause of chronic renal failure (CRF) and the cause of diabetic morbidity and mortality. In a diabetic patient, renal disease is defined clinically as the presence of persistent proteinuria with concomitant retinopathy and elevated blood pressure but without UTI, other renal disease, or heart failure. Onset occurs between 10 and 30 years of age in 50% of patients who develop diabetes mellitus in childhood or youth. Glycemic and blood pressure control can slow the progression of diabetic nephropathy. In a study by Brkljacic and colleagues,[80] the Doppler indices reflected increased renovascular resistance in diabetic nephropathy, which correlated with laboratory and clinical parameters (Fig. 10-36A,B).

Elevated RIs and pulsatility indices (PIs) correlated with the progression of nephropathy, and they correlated with the other parameters used to predict diabetic nephropathy (serum creatinine level, creatinine clearance rate, systolic and diastolic blood pressure measurements, and the patient's age); however, RIs and PIs do not provide advantages over these latter parameters in predicting disease progress (Pathology Box 10-8).

## PAPILLARY NECROSIS[78,82]

Papillary necrosis affects the renal medulla and involves sloughed papillae or calcifications in the renal medullary pyramids. It may complicate these other pathologic conditions: phenacetin abuse, obstructive uropathy, diabetes mellitus, APN or CPN, sickle cell disease, renal vein thrombosis, acute tubular necrosis (ATN), and chronic alcoholism. Correlating the clinical and laboratory findings will help distinguish papillary necrosis from other renal abnormalities having a similar sonographic appearance. Based on the sonographic appearance, the differential diagnosis includes postobstructive renal atrophy, hydronephrosis, congenital megacalyces, and diabetes insipidus (Pathology Box 10-8 and Fig.10-37).

## SYSTEMIC LUPUS ERYTHEMATOSUS[78,79,83]

Systemic lupus erythematosus (SLE) is a multisystem, autoimmune connective tissue disease that occurs predominantly in women, with a 9:1 female-to-male ratio. Renal parenchymal involvement ranging from mild proteinuria

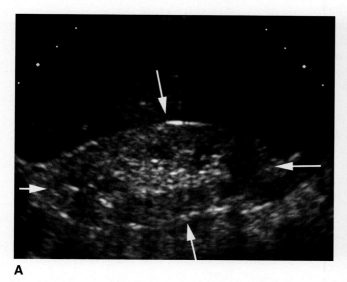

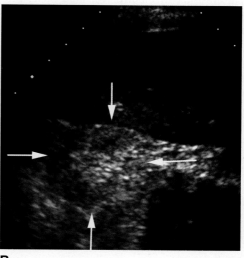

**A**                                    **B**

**Figure 10-36** Diabetic nephropathy. This 46-year-old man has end-stage renal failure and a long history of diabetes. The longitudinal **(A)** and transverse **(B)** images demonstrate a small hyperechoic right kidney *(arrows)*.

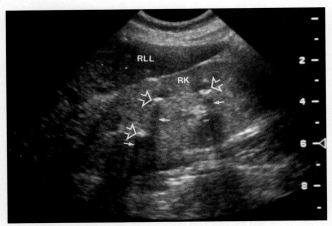

**Figure 10-37** Papillary necrosis. This 70-year-old woman is being evaluated sonographically for renal insufficiency and was diagnosed with papillary necrosis. A longitudinal image of the right kidney (RK) demonstrates multiple calcifications (open arrowheads) within the medullary pyramids associated with acoustic shadowing (small arrows; RLL, right liver lobe). (Image courtesy of Cindy Rapp, Denver, CO.)

to acute fulminant glomerulonephritis occurs in over one-half of SLE cases and is one of the leading causes of morbidity and mortality. The sensitivity of sonographic detection of lupus nephritis is 95%. One study reports a variable correlation between sonographic findings and pathologic findings in lupus nephritis, with a significant number of patients with biopsy-proven lupus nephritis showing a normal cortical echo pattern and normal-sized kidneys. To assist in providing the diagnosis, the sonographic findings must be correlated with the clinical data and laboratory studies, which provide a better estimate of the severity of renal compromise (Pathology Box 10-8).

# RENAL FAILURE[4,20,29,78,84]

Renal failure is the inability of the kidneys to remove accumulated metabolites from the blood. The situation causes alterations in electrolyte, acid-base, and water balance and accumulation of substances that normally are completely excreted. The underlying causes of renal failure are renal pathology, systemic disease, and urologic defects of nonrenal origin attributed to surgery or trauma (43%), various medical conditions (26%), pregnancy (13%), and nephrotoxicity (9%). Renal failure is classified as (1) acute if it develops over days and weeks; (2) chronic if it spans months or years; and (3) acute on chronic if there is a rapid reduction in renal function in patients with previously stable chronic renal disease. Both acute and CRF result in azotemia, which is an overload of nitrogenous wastes (BUN, uric acid, and serum creatinine) in the blood.

## ACUTE RENAL FAILURE[9,20,29,84–86]

Acute renal failure (ARF) affects approximately 10,000 persons annually in the United States, and the mortality rate is about 60%. Pathology Box 10-9 lists the three

major categories. The clinical manifestations of ARF are frequently superimposed on the signs and symptoms of the underlying disease. As ARF is potentially reversible, early signs and symptoms are important to recognize. If it is untreated, the severe reduction in the glomerular filtration rate causes irreversible damage. The two phases of ARF are oliguric and diuretic. In the oliguric phase, urine output is greatly reduced. If there is severe oliguria and associated tissue breakdown, the patient exhibits elevated BUN, creatinine, potassium, and phosphate serum levels causing metabolic acidosis. If this phase is prolonged, hypertension, neuromuscular irritability, muscle weakness, gastrointestinal bleeding, and infection are serious complications of the disease. After a few days to 6 weeks, the diuretic phase of ARF begins, which indicates that the nephrons have recovered to

---

**PATHOLOGY BOX 10-9**

### Etiology of Acute Renal Failure

Prerenal: renal hypoperfusion secondary to a systemic cause
  Acute bilateral renal artery occlusion
  Heart failure
  Hypotension
  Hypovolemia (dehydration, hemorrhage, fluid sequestration)
  Salt depletion
  Septicemia
Intrarenal (intrinsic): result of medical disease
  Acute tubular necrosis
    Ischemic disorders (major trauma; massive hemorrhage; compartmental syndrome; septic shock; transfusion reaction; myoglobinuria; postpartum hemorrhage; cardiac, aortic, and biliary surgery; pancreatitis; gastroenteritis)
    Nephrotoxicities—glomerular membrane injury from exposure to nephrotoxic wastes (aminoglycosides, heavy metals, radiographic opaque materials, organic solvents, pesticides or fungicides, antibiotics)
  Cortical necrosis
  Acute interstitial nephritis—acute infection or inflammatory conditions (pyelonephritis, necrotizing papillitis)
  Intratubular obstruction (uric acid crystals, hemolytic reactions, precipitated proteins from multiple myeloma, rhabdomyolysis)
  Diseases of the glomeruli and small vessels (acute poststreptococcal glomerulonephritis, systemic lupus erythematosus, polyarteritis nodosa, subacute bacterial endocarditis, Goodpasture syndrome, Schönlein-Henoch purpura, rapidly progressing glomerulonephritis, hemolytic uremic syndrome, serum sickness, drug-related vascularities, malignant hypertension, abruptio placentae)
Postrenal: result of outflow obstruction
  Acute bilateral renal vein thrombosis
  Acute urinary tract obstruction (calculi, tumors, prostatic hypertrophy, urethral strictures)

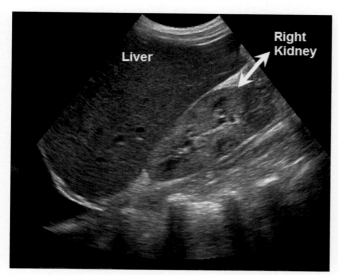

**Figure 10-38** Acute renal failure. Longitudinal sonogram displays an echogenic, normal-sized right kidney. Increased cortical echogenicity is an indicator of diffuse renal parenchymal disease but is not useful in distinguishing acute from chronic causes of renal disease. (Image courtesy of Philips Medical Systems, Bothell, WA.)

are presented in Chapter 4. Postrenal conditions are presented in this chapter as follows: obstruction, hydronephrosis, and pregnancy under Hydronephrosis and Pyonephrosis under Renal Infection and Inflammatory Diseases. Ureteral stricture is presented in Chapter 11 and prostatic hypertrophy, also a postrenal condition, is discussed in Chapter 12.

Real-time renal sonography of the native kidneys is most often normal in the setting of ARF. ARF can occur suddenly or can develop over days or weeks. Once ARF has been established as the diagnosis, sonography's most important role is to provide accurate evaluation of hydronephrosis, distinguish postrenal or obstructive causes, and screen for parenchymal diseases (Fig. 10-38).

Distinguishing the cause is important in relieving obstruction, a feature of 5% of cases of ARF, and in facilitating appropriate treatment of other renal medical disease. Prompt intervention prevents secondary loss of renal parenchyma. Duplex Doppler may allow detection of changes associated with ARF. In a study by Platt and coauthors,[86] duplex Doppler provided significant information to help distinguish between acute prerenal failure and ATN. The mean RI for patients with ATN was 0.85 ± 0.06, and the mean RI for those with prerenal ARF was 0.67 ± 0.09.[86] An elevated mean RI was seen in 91% of patients with ATN but in only 20% of those with prerenal azotemia.[86] Most of the patients with an elevated mean RI coupled with prerenal azotemia had concurrent severe liver disease (Fig. 10-39A,B).

the extent that urine excretion is possible. The diuretic phase often occurs before renal function returns to normal, which explains why BUN, serum creatinine, potassium, and phosphate levels remain elevated or continue to rise even though urine output has increased. Excessive loss of water and electrolytes occurs if the diuresis is associated with impaired nephron function.

The prerenal conditions related to hemorrhage and dehydration, and hyperperfusion due to thrombosis,

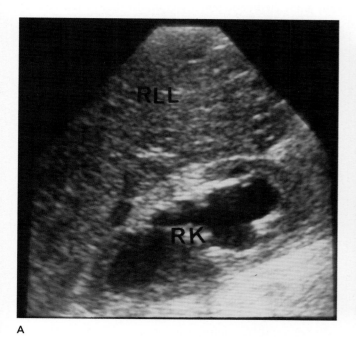

A

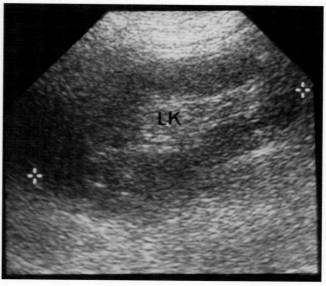

B

**Figure 10-39** Acute renal failure. This 86-year-old woman was diagnosed with acute renal failure based on clinical presentation and laboratory results. **A:** The longitudinal section of the right kidney *(RK)* reveals hydronephrosis; whereas, **(B)** the left kidney *(LK)* is small with increased cortical echogenicity and a small kidney measuring 8.6 cm in length.

## Intrarenal Conditions

The intrarenal conditions that cause renal failure from infantile polycystic disease are presented in Chapter 20. Other intrarenal conditions not discussed in this section but presented in this chapter are adult polycystic disease, medullary cystic disease, and nephronophthisis under Cystic Renal Masses; APN and XGP under Renal Infection and Inflammatory Diseases; and nephrocalcinosis under Lithiasis.

### Acute Tubular Necrosis[20,78,84]

The most common cause of ARF is ATN, which is the mechanism of many forms of renal failure resulting from a variety of toxic and ischemic insults leading to widespread tubular epithelial cell destruction. In such cases, renal insufficiency develops abruptly, although the process may be reversible. Histologically, there is necrosis of tubule cells and cellular casts in the collecting tubules, and grossly the kidneys are often swollen and edematous.

Sonographically, most patients with ATN have normal kidneys, with no changes in renal architecture, cortical echogenicity or thickness, or the appearance of medullary pyramids. Occasionally, increased cortical echogenicity, accentuated corticomedullary definition, and a slightly enlarged kidney are observed. When ATN is secondary to nephrotoxicity, such as in myoglobinuria following renal trauma or ethylene glycol poisoning, sonography demonstrates an increase in bilateral cortical echogenicity with preservation of the corticomedullary definition.

### Acute Cortical Necrosis[68,85]

ACN, a rare form of ARF, is precipitated in patients with shock, sepsis, hemorrhage, burns, renal vein thrombosis, hemolytic uremic syndrome, pregnancy-induced hypertension with abruptio placentae, and severe dehydration. Although the actual mechanism of ACN is uncertain, it may be capillary damage and vasospasm secondary to intravascular thrombus or toxin production, resulting in ischemia. Histologic findings are those of acute ischemic infarction limited to the cortex, necrosis of tubular cells, and cellular infiltration in the interstitium. The medulla and a thin rim of subcapsular tissue remain intact. Punctate or linear calcifications can be identified within 6 days after infarction, at the junction of necrotic and viable tissue, or diffusely throughout the renal cortex.

The sonographic findings are of bilateral, normal sized kidneys. Initially, the renal cortex appears hypoechoic, and there is a loss of normal corticomedullary definition. As the disease progresses to the chronic stage, follow-up studies demonstrate progressive decreases in renal size and various degrees of increased renal cortical echogenicity directly related to the degree of calcification and collagen deposition.

### Myoglobinuria[43,85]

Myoglobinuria is the cause in 5% to 7% of patients with ARF and occurs in 33% of patients with myoglobinemia. Normally, myoglobin is cleared by metabolism to bilirubin. Increased amounts of myoglobin are released into the tissues and bloodstream following rhabdomyolysis (an acute, sometimes fatal disease characterized by destruction of skeletal muscle) or as a result of other causes, including alcohol and drug addiction, crush injuries, strokes, toxins, fever, or myositis. Renal failure is thought to be secondary to nephrotoxicity with tubular obstruction. Histologic findings include ATN, brown casts, interstitial edema, cellular infiltration, and possibly engorgement of medullary and glomerular vessels. Fibrosis and atrophy are seen in chronic cases.

The histologic changes create various sonographic appearances, ranging from completely normal kidneys in ATN to enlarged, echogenic kidneys in cases where changes reflect cellular interstitial infiltration. With enlarged, distended medullary vessels, the pyramids may be prominent and hypoechoic. In end-stage fibrosis, the kidneys may be shrunken and echogenic.

### Acute Glomerulonephritis[84,85]

Acute glomerulonephritis (AGN) is a renal inflammation that may be categorized as (1) a renal inflammatory response caused by an autoimmune reaction resulting in glomerular damage or (2) interstitial inflammation due to infection (by gram-negative bacilli), exposure to toxins and drugs, or infiltration of inflammatory cells into the renal interstitium. Histologically, there is proliferation of endothelial and mesangial cells in glomeruli and exudate of WBCs. The process may reverse or progress to end-stage renal disease. Typically, patients present with hematuria, hypertension, azotemia, and red cell casts in the urine.

The sonographic appearance varies from normal size early in the disease process to enlargement, with markedly increased echogenicity equal to that of the central echo of the renal sinus. On follow-up examination, the kidneys progressively shrink. With reversal of azotemia, renal echogenicity may become more normal.

### Amyloidosis[85]

Amyloidosis, a metabolic disorder, is associated with extensive amyloid deposits in the glomeruli, arterioles, and interstitium that eventually cause complete obliteration of the glomerulus. Patients present with excessive proteinuria or the nephrotic syndrome. As glomerular destruction progresses, the patient dies of uremia. Amyloid deposits are commonly associated with abnormal serum proteins, or with chronic infection or inflammation such as rheumatoid arthritis. At postmortem examination, 14% to 26% of patients have histologic evidence of amyloidosis.

Depending on the stage of amyloidosis, the sonographic appearance of the kidneys may be large, normal, small, and eventually shrunken in end-stage disease. Increased cortical echogenicity and accentuated corticomedullary definition are more pronounced in chronic disease. In patients with a history of collagen vascular disease or chronic illness, these nonspecific findings should suggest the possibility of amyloidosis.

## CHRONIC RENAL FAILURE[20,29,78,84,85]

CRF is an irreversible condition characterized by diminished function of the nephrons resulting in decreased glomerular filtration rate, renal blood flow, tubular function, and resorptive capability. Progressive renal impairment leads to end-stage renal disease. The multiple causes of CRF are summarized in Pathology Box 10-10. Having only a limited number of ways to respond to various insults, the end-stage kidney, regardless of the cause of renal failure, usually has a similar appearance pathologically and sonographically. The sonographic findings are not disease specific, and there is no correlation between the type and severity of glomerular disease and the kidney's echogenicity. Sonographically, a small, shrunken, echogenic kidney is quite definitive of end-stage renal disease, which can be the result of a variety of processes (Fig. 10-40A,B).

When conservative management of end-stage renal disease is no longer effective, dialysis or renal transplantation becomes necessary. The choice is dictated by the patient's age, related health problems, donor availability, and personal preference.

## DIALYSIS PATIENT[85]

During dialysis, blood from an artery moves through an artificial kidney unit designed to assume the physiologic function of the nephrons, after which it is returned to a vein. Sonography is useful for monitoring the kidneys of patients who are receiving long-term hemodialysis.

### Complications

#### Acquired Cysts[85,87]

Many patients with CRF who receive hemodialysis develop bilateral cystic disease: 43% of patients on dialysis for 3 years, more than 79% of patients on dialysis for

---

### PATHOLOGY BOX 10-10

#### Etiology of Chronic Renal Failure

Glomerulonephritis

Chronic pyelonephritis

Renal vascular disease

Metabolic renal disease (diabetes, gout, hypercalcemia, hyperoxaluria, cystinosis, Fabry disease)

Chronic obstructive uropathy

Hereditary or congenital anomalies (polycystic kidney disease, medullary cystic disease, Alport syndrome, cystinosis, hyperoxaluria, chronic tubular acidosis, infantile nephrotic syndrome, dysplastic kidney, oxalosis)

Nephrotoxins

Tuberculosis

Sarcoidosis

Tubular diseases (radiation nephritis, toxic nephropathy, hyperoxaluria)

Infiltrative processes (lymphoma, amyloidosis, glycogen storage diseases)

Infections

Dysproteinemia (myeloma, amyloidosis, mixed IgA-IgM cryoglobinemia, Waldenström macroglobinemia)

Collagen vascular disease (systemic lupus erythematous, polyarteritis nodosa)

Major blood vessel disease (renal artery thrombosis, embolism, or stenosis; bilateral renal vein thrombosis)

Hepatorenal syndrome

Acute pyelonephritis

---

more than 5 years, and 90% of patients on dialysis for more than 10 years. The pathogenesis of these multiple, 0.5 to 3 cm diameter, acquired lesions is unknown. Suggested mechanisms include obstruction secondary to fibrosis or oxalate crystal formation, vascular insufficiency, and direct toxicity of circulating metabolites. The

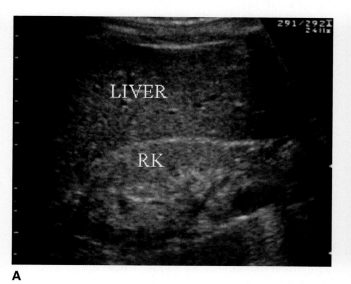

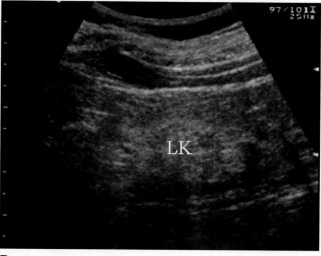

**A**

**B**

**Figure 10-40** Chronic renal failure. **A:** These longitudinal sections of the right kidney and **(B)** left kidney demonstrate small, hyperechoic kidneys in this patient with a history of chronic renal failure. (Images courtesy of Taco Geertsma, MD, Hospital Gelderse Vallei, Ede, The Netherlands.)

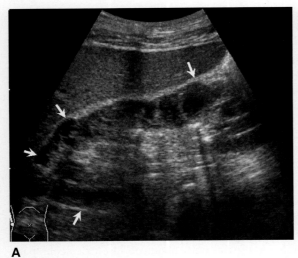
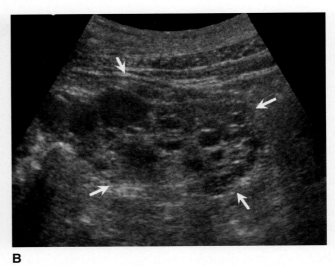

**A**    **B**

**Figure 10-41** Acquired cystic disease of the kidneys, dialysis related. Longitudinal images of the **(A)** right and **(B)** left kidneys reveal shrunken, echogenic, bilateral kidneys *(arrows)* consistent with chronic renal failure. Multiple small bilateral cysts are seen in this hemodialysis patient. (Images courtesy of Taco Geertsma, MD, Hospital Gelderse Vallei, Ede, The Netherlands.)

cysts are located throughout the kidney and involve the cortex, corticomedullary junction, and medulla.

Sonographically, the kidneys may appear somewhat small and echogenic, and cysts are seen throughout the parenchyma. As the cysts grow, the kidney may enlarge. Hemorrhage often occurs into acquired renal cysts, resulting in perirenal and retroperitoneal hematoma, pain, hematuria, and echogenic collections in the cysts on sonography. Hemorrhagic cysts may be indistinguishable from neoplasms. Without a history of dialysis, the differential diagnosis includes hydronephrosis and polycystic disease, although with acquired cysts the kidneys usually are smaller (Fig. 10-41A,B).

### Renal Tumors[38,85]

Renal tumors occur in approximately 7% of patients with acquired cystic disease. The tumors usually measure less than 2 cm and are found incidentally. Sonographically, neoplasms may be multiple and bilateral, arise adjacent to or within cysts, and appear hyperechoic to anechoic, without posterior acoustic enhancement. The sensitivity of precontrast and postcontrast CT is greater than that of sonography. Sonography is less expensive and detects most renal cell cancers before they metastasize; however, whether the dialysis patient population requires a screening examination for renal tumors is questionable.

## OTHER IMAGING PROCEDURES

### CONTRAST-ENHANCED SONOGRAPHY[88–92]

Contrast-enhanced sonography utilizes microbubble contrast agents and specialized imaging techniques to display sensitive blood flow and tissue perfusion. Ultrasound waves directed at the vasculature are scattered upon interaction with intravenously infused contrast agents resulting in a brighter image of the vasculature.

The ultrasound unit requires contrast-specific software that suppresses the signal from the background tissue while enhancing the signal from the microbubbles.

The normal kidney enhances quickly after contrast injection due to the high renal blood flow. Enhancement in the central arteries becomes apparent 10 to 15 seconds after contrast injection. The cortex enhances a few seconds later. The renal pyramids fill in slower, becoming isoechoic to the cortex 30 to 40 seconds after contrast injection. Initially, the kidney appears hyperechoic, and then becomes hypoechoic. The enhancing effect decreases as the contrast concentration decreases. The collecting system does not opacify because the ultrasound contrast media does not show excretion.

Although widely used in Europe and Asia, the U.S. Food and Drug Administration (FDA) has not approved any microbubble contrast agent for radiology imaging. Currently, only cardiac contrast imaging applications have been approved with limitations. Renal applications include evaluation of small indeterminate hypoechoic masses, atypical cystic masses, renal clear cell carcinoma versus angiomyolipoma, perfusion defects related to renal trauma, pyelonephritis, and assessment of pseudotumors. Detection of diffuse lesion enhancement is a significant criterion in the differential diagnosis between benign and malignant lesions. Contrast-enhanced sonography has the potential to become a useful diagnostic tool aiding in the improved visualization of the neovascularity associated with malignancy and perfusion defects associated with infection and trauma.

### RADIONUCLIDE STUDIES[93]

The main advantage of radionuclide imaging is the demonstration of the pathophysiology involved. The vascular, excretory, and drainage phases of the examination permit the evaluation of renal perfusion, renal parenchymal function, and the status of the collecting system. Radionuclide examination plays a significant complementary role in image evaluation of hydrone-phrosis, renal artery stenosis, flank pain, renal mass, pyelonephritis, and transplanted kidney. With cortical agents, radionuclide imaging confirms the diagnosis of fetal lobulations or dromedary humps and hyper-trophied column of Bertin by demonstrating normally functioning tissue. If functioning parenchymal tissue connects a horseshoe kidney, it can be diagnosed with a radionuclide renal examination.

## COMPUTED TOMOGRAPHY[16,17,94–96]

CT, like sonography, is capable of imaging the kidneys in cross-sectional planes. As the slice thickness has de-creased, CT has replaced IVP as the imaging modality of choice in many evaluations of the kidneys. Because of its higher cost and use of ionizing radiation, CT is usually not indicated, however, as the primary modality for assessing abnormalities of renal size. It is an excel-lent adjunctive procedure for the detection, character-ization, and staging of renal masses. CT is excellent in demonstrating both ectopic and horseshoe kidneys. In the case of a horseshoe kidney, CT demonstrates the isthmus regardless of the tissue type. Contrast-enhanced CT is excellent for distinguishing an organizing abscess from inflammatory edema and in evaluating the peri-nephric spaces. In patients with hypertension, CT is the imaging modality of choice to determine if the underly-ing cause is an adrenal or extra-adrenal pheochromocy-toma. In the diagnosis of renal and perirenal abscesses, CT may be more sensitive because it is capable of de-tecting poorly defined, smaller abscesses and defining subtle alterations in perinephric fat. Noncontrast spiral CT is used to evaluate for urolithiasis. Some of the ben-efits of CT over IVP include the speed with which the examination can be performed, the lack of iodinated contrast material, and the ability to detect radiolucent uric acid stones.

## MAGNETIC RESONANCE IMAGING

MRI has advantages in staging RCC because of its abil-ity to clearly demonstrate any perivascular adenopa-thy or tumor thrombus within a vascular lumen with-out the need for intravenous contrast material.[96] Even though abscesses cannot be distinguished from necrotic tumors, MRI is valuable in the detection of fluid-filled processes in the retroperitoneum, and higher specificity has been demonstrated in the case of hematomas.

## SUMMARY

- The urinary system, located in the retroperitoneum, consists of two kidneys, two ureters, the urinary bladder, and the urethra.
- Each normal adult kidney is approximately 10- to 12-cm long, 5- to 7.5-cm wide, and 2- to 3-cm thick;

the normal cortical thickness is greater than 1 cm; and the kidneys are typically within 2 cm or each other in length.

- The nephron begins functioning around 8 weeks ges-tation, it is the smallest renal functional unit, it is capable of producing urine, and it is so important that one-third of the nephrons must function simply to ensure survival.
- The three layers surrounding the kidney are the: in-nermost layer (fibrous renal capsule), the middle layer (mass of perirenal fat and the adipose capsule), and the outermost layer (renal fascia, also referred to as Gerota fascia, the perirenal fat, and the adrenal gland).
- The renal cortex extends from the renal capsule to the bases of the pyramids with an echogenicity nor-mally less than the liver, spleen, and renal sinus.
- The renal medulla is made up of triangular or cone-shaped tissue masses called medullary pyramids, which are hypoechoic to anechoic and are more prominent in children.
- The renal sinus is a homogeneous, hyperechoic re-gion in the central kidney that contains adipose tis-sue, blood vessels, and the collecting system.
- The calyces collect urine and join together to empty into the renal pelvis, which is continuous with the proximal ureter.
- Renal blood vessels, lymphatics, nerves, and the ure-ter enter or exit the kidney at the medially located hilus that occupies the renal sinus.
- The renal arteries arise from the lateral aspects of the abdominal aorta just inferior to the SMA; the right re-nal artery is longer than the left and passes posterior to the IVC.
- The renal veins exit the renal hilum and empty into the lateral aspects of the IVC; the left renal vein crosses anterior to the aorta and posterior to the SMA before entering the IVC.
- Common renal variants include: a dromedary hump, junctional parenchymal defect, hypertrophied col-umn of Bertin, renal sinus lipomatosis, and extrare-nal pelvis.
- Three important nephron functions are controlling blood concentration and volume by removing select-ed amounts of water and solutes, helping to regulate blood pH, and removing toxic wastes from the blood.
- BUN, creatinine, and uric acid are used to evaluate re-nal function along with the urinalysis, which can de-tect the presence of RBCs, WBCs, protein, and bacteria.
- The sonographic evaluation of the kidneys should in-clude longitudinal sections, coronal sections, or both in long axis for the renal length, sinus, and calyces; the lateral margin; and the medial margin and trans-verse sections of the superior pole imaging the upper renal sinus, the midpole imaging the renal artery and vein and making measurements, and the inferior pole.

- An RI of 0.70 is generally considered the upper limit of normal for the adult kidney.

- Congenital anomalies of the kidneys include hypoplasia, unilateral agenesis, bilateral agenesis, which is incompatible with life, complete duplication of the collecting system, ectopic kidney, and horseshoe kidney.

- Cystic masses of the kidney may be hereditary alterations in differentiation, nonhereditary but developmental, or acquired disorders.

- ADPKD is a relatively common disease that usually manifests clinically in the fourth decade and accounts for 8% to 10% of the patients who require chronic dialysis or renal transplantation.

- Patients with ADPKD can also develop cerebral artery aneurysms as well as cysts in the liver, pancreas, lung, spleen, ovaries, seminal vesicles, testes, epididymis, thyroid, uterus, and bladder.

- In patients with ADPKD the kidneys are usually enlarged bilaterally, with numerous discrete cysts in the cortical regions; with age, the cysts enlarge and renal function begins to decrease. The most frequent complications are infection and renal calculi.

- Simple renal cysts are common, usually remain asymptomatic, and increase in incidence with increasing age. Simple cysts must demonstrate a clear, smooth wall, spheric or slightly ovoid shape, absence of internal echoes, and posterior enhancement.

- Atypical cysts are those that do not meet the criteria of simple cysts and require further evaluation including: complex cysts, hemorrhagic cysts, infected cysts, and septated or multilocular cysts.

- Tuberous sclerosis is a multisystemic disorder that presents with mental retardation, seizures, and skin lesions and is associated with renal cyst formation, angiomyolipomas, and an increased incidence of renal cell carcinoma.

- Von Hippel-Lindau disease is an autosomal dominant disorder that predisposes patients to form a variety of visceral cysts and neoplasms including cerebellar or spinal cord hemangioblastomas, retinal angiomas, pancreatic islet cell tumors, pheochromocytomas, and epididymal cystadenomas, renal cysts, and renal cell carcinoma.

- Cortical adenomas are the most prevalent benign kidney tumors and appear sonographically similar to RCC.

- Angiomyolipoma usually presents as a solitary, homogeneous, markedly hyperechoic mass in the renal cortex. In patients with tuberous sclerosis, the masses are typically multiple and bilateral.

- RCC (hypernephroma), accounting for approximately 80% to 90% of all renal malignancies in adults, is the most common malignant tumor of the kidney, occurs after most often age 50, has a 2:1 male-to-female ratio, and has an increased incidence in patients with von Hippel-Lindau disease, ADPKD, tuberous sclerosis, and other diseases and syndromes associated with multiple renal cysts.

- RCC can spread into the perinephric fat and renal vein; lymphogenous and hematogenous spread to the regional nodes, lungs, bone, the contralateral kidney, liver, adrenal, and brain are possible.

- RCC may appear sonographically as a hyperechoic or hypoechoic solid mass, or may present as a complex mass with localized areas of hemorrhage, necrosis, or cystic degeneration.

- Urothelial tumors, malignant tumors of the lining of the urinary tract making up 8% to 10% of all renal cancers, include transitional cell carcinomas (TCC) and squamous cell carcinomas (SCC) and have a 5-year survival rate of 90% due to the fact they become clinically apparent within a short time because their growth produces noticeable painless hematuria in 60% of cases.

- Lymphoma can occur in the kidney and is usually manifested by nonspecific enlargement of the kidney, although lymphoma may present as anechoic or hypoechoic, single or multiple masses.

- Hydronephrosis represents a dilatation of the renal pelvis, calyceal structures, and infundibula and can be caused by intrinsic or extrinsic obstruction, or by postobstruction atrophy, infection (pyelonephritis), postrenal failure, overhydration, or high-flow states (polyuria), and reflux.

- Hydronephrosis occurs in 65% to 85% of pregnant patients, is more common on the right and resolves after delivery.

- The sonographic hallmark of hydronephrosis is splaying, spreading, or ballooning of the central echo complex.

- False-positive diagnoses of hydronephrosis include extrarenal pelvis, vesicoureteral reflux, full bladder, high urine flow as seen with overhydration, and parapelvic or peripelvic cysts.

- Calculus formation, influenced by hereditary and familial predispositions, high concentrations of stone constituents, changes in urinary pH, or the presence of bacteria, can develop anywhere in the urinary system (urolithiasis), but most develop in the kidney (nephrolithiasis).

- Clinical symptoms of nephrolithiasis can include hematuria, oliguria, renal colic, nausea, vomiting, fever, and chills.

- Sonographically, renal calculi present as hyperechoic foci with shadowing located in the renal sinus, which can be difficult to discern unless they are large. Color Doppler can be used to demonstrate a twinkle artifact in the presence of stones.

- Injury to the kidney can occur from blunt or penetrating trauma and a renal fracture presents sonographically as a reproducible linear absence of echoes.

- Renal hematomas results from a variety of causes, are divided into spontaneous and posttraumatic types, and have a variable echo pattern depending on the age of the bleed.

- A subcapsular hematoma lies between the kidney cortex and the capsule and may appear to flatten or distort the kidney.

- Upper urinary tract infections are second only to respiratory infections in prevalence and are commonly caused by gram-negative bacteria such as *E. coli.*

- Upper urinary tract infection is usually the result of spread of bacteria along the ureters from a bladder infection.

- APN may be unilateral or bilateral, focal (multifocal) or diffuse, and may present as enlargement of the kidney.

- Renal infections include emphysematous pyelonephritis, chronic pyelonephritis, xanthogranulomatous pyelonephritis, fungal infections, schistosomiasis, tuberculosis, and malakoplakia.

- Renal and perinephric abscesses have a variable appearance depending on the age of the collection and may occur within the kidney or may rupture into the collecting system or through the capsule, causing a perirenal abscess, which presents as a pus collection in the space between the kidney and renal fascia.

- Renal medical disease may have a normal sonographic appearance in the early stage; over the long term, a seriously injured kidney shows atrophy and scarring and loses the distinguishing features of the specific original disease.

- The hallmark of parenchymal renal disease is a diffuse increase in echogenicity throughout the parenchyma of both kidneys.

- The most common sonographic findings in patients with AIDS are increased echogenicity of the cortex, decreased definition of the corticomedullary junction, and decreased renal sinus fat.

- Diabetic nephropathy is a leading cause of chronic renal failure and the cause of diabetic morbidity and mortality and is defined clinically as the presence of persistent proteinuria with concomitant retinopathy and elevated blood pressure but without UTI, other renal disease, or heart failure.

- Classified as acute or chronic, renal failure is the inability of the kidneys to remove accumulated metabolites from the blood, which then causes alterations in electrolyte, acid-base, and water balance and allows the accumulation of substances that normally are completely excreted and results in azotemia.

- In acute renal failure, the role of sonography is to rule out obstructive causes and evaluate the renal parenchyma.

- CRF is irreversible and, sonographically, a small, shrunken, echogenic kidney is definitive of end-stage renal disease.

- During dialysis, blood from an artery moves through an artificial kidney unit designed to assume the physiologic function of the nephrons, after which it is returned to a vein.

- Patients with CRF on dialysis frequently develop bilateral cystic disease and are at an increased risk of developing renal cell carcinoma.

- CT, MRI, radionuclide studies, and sonography all play a role in the evaluation of the upper urinary tract.

## Critical Thinking Questions

1. A 55-year-old man presents with a history of hematuria and mild flank pain for the last month. The sonography examination reveals a 3.5-cm hypoechoic, solid mass extending off the lower pole of the right kidney. Doppler evaluation of the mass demonstrates an arterial waveform with high systolic and high diastolic arterial flow. What is the most likely diagnosis and what structures should be the focus of the sonography examination?

2. While scanning the left kidney in 30-year-old patient, the sonographer notices a bulging of the lateral kidney that at first glance appears to be a mass. With careful scanning, the sonographer determines the echogenicity is similar to and continuous with the renal cortex and the renal sinus appears to project into the bulging. What is the most likely diagnosis?

3. A 22-year-old woman presents for a renal ultrasound with a history of urinary tract infections. The sonographer documents a normal right kidney but the left kidney cannot be located on left side. What are possible explanations for this, and where else should the sonographer look?

4. A patient presents with a current history of a bladder infection and new onset of right flank pain and pyuria. The sonography examination reveals an enlarged right kidney with a hypoechoic, irregular appearance of the lower pole. What is the most likely diagnosis?

5. A 75-year-old man with diabetes presents for a renal sonogram with a history of chronic renal failure. What do you expect to find on his examination?

## REFERENCES

1. Carlson BM. *Human Embryology and Developmental Biology*. 4th ed. St. Louis, MO: Mosby; 2008.

2. Tortora GJ, Derrickson B. *Principles of Anatomy and Physiology*. 12th ed. Haboken, NJ: John Wiley & Son; 2009.

3. Gray H. *Gray's Anatomy: Anatomy of the Human Body, 30th ed. (American Edition, edited by Charles Mayo Goss)*. Philadelphia, PA: Lea & Febiger; 1973.

4. Netter FH. *The CIBA Collection of Medical Illustrations, Vol. 6, Kidney, Ureters, and the Urinary Bladder*. Rochester, NY: The Case-Hoyt Corporation; 1965.

5. Marieb EN. *Human Anatomy and Physiology*. 8th ed. Redwood City, CA: The Benjamin/Cummings Publishing Company; 2009.

6. Paspulati RM, Bhatt S. Sonography in benign and malignant renal masses. *Ultrasound Clin*. 2006;1:25–41.

7. Vourganti S, Agarwal PK, Bodner DR, et al. Ultrasonographic evaluation of renal infections. *Ultrasound Clin*. 2010;5:355–366.

8. Dubinsky T, Fleischer AC, Dubinsky R. General abdominal sonography. In: Odwin CS, Dubinsky T, Fleischer AC, eds. *Appleton & Lange's Review for the Ultrasonography Examination*. 3rd ed. Norwalk, CT: Appleton and Lange; 2004.

9. Hricak H. Renal ultrasound. In: Sarti DA, ed. *Diagnostic Ultrasound: Text & Cases*. 2nd ed. Chicago, IL: Year Book Medical Publishers; 1987.

10. Craig M. *Pocket Guide to Ultrasound Measurements*. Philadelphia, PA: JB Lippincott; 1988.

11. Middleton WD, Kurtz AB. *Ultrasound: The Requisites*. 2nd ed. St. Louis, MO: Mosby; 2003.

12. Kriegshauser JS, Carroll BA. The urinary tract. In: Rumack C, Wilson S, Charboneau J, Johnson J, eds. *Diagnostic Ultrasound*. 3rd ed. St. Louis, MO: Mosby; 2004.

13. Lin EP, Bhatt S, Dogra VS, et al. Sonography of urolithiasis and hydronephrosis. *Ultrasound Clin*. 2007;2:1–16.

14. Patriquin H, Lafaivre JF, Lafortune M, et al. Fetal lobation. An anatomo-ultrasonographic correlation. *J Ultrasound Med*. 1990;9:191–197.

15. Bhatt S, MacLennan G, Dogra V. Renal pseudotumors. *AJR*. 2007;188:1380–1387.

16. Krebs CA, Giyanani VL, Eisenberg RL. Kidney. In: *Ultrasound Atlas of Disease Processes*. Norwalk, CT: Appleton-Lange; 1993.

17. Hagen-Ansert S. Urinary system. In: Hagen-Ansert S, ed. *Textbook of Diagnostic Ultrasonography*. 6th ed. St. Louis, MO: Mosby; 2006.

18. Richard C. Renal function. In: Copstead L-EC, ed. *Perspectives on Pathophysiology*. Philadelphia, PA: WB Saunders; 1995.

19. Brenner B, Coe FL, Rector FC. *Renal Physiology in Health and Disease*. Philadelphia, PA: WB Saunders; 1987.

20. Bullock BL. Urinary excretion (Unit 9). In: Bullock BL, ed. *Pathophysiology: Adaptations and Alterations in Function*. 4th ed. Philadelphia, PA: Lippincott-Raven; 1996.

21. Emamian SA, Nielsen MB, Pedersen JF, et al. Kidney dimensions at sonography: correlation with age, sex and habitus in 665 adult volunteers. *AJR*. 1993;160:83–86.

22. Halpern EJ. Renal measurements. In: Goldberg BB, McGahan JP, eds. *Atlas of Ultrasound Measurements*. 2nd ed. St. Louis, MO: Elsevier Mosby; 2006.

23. Beland MD, Walle NL, Machan JT, et al. Renal cortical thickness measured at ultrasound: is it better than renal length as an indicator of renal function in chronic disease? *AJR*. 2010;195:W146–W149.

24. Platt JF, Rubin JM, Ellis JH. Examination of native kidneys with Duplex Doppler ultrasound. *Semin Ultrasound CT MR*. 1991;12:308–318.

25. Mostbeck GH, Kain R, Mallek R, et al. Duplex Doppler sonography in renal parenchymal disease: histopathologic correlation. *J Ultrasound Med*. 1991;10:189–194.

26. Fernbach SK, Zawin JK, Lebowitz RL. Complete duplication of the ureter with ureteropelvic junction obstruction of the lower pole of the kidney: imaging findings. *AJR*. 1995;164:701–704.

27. Share JC, Lebowitz RL. The unsuspected double collecting system on imaging studies and at cystoscopy. *AJR*. 1990;155:561–564.

28. Weingardt JP, Townsend RR, Russ PD, et al. Seminal vesicle cysts associated with autosomal dominant polycystic kidney disease detected by sonography. *J Ultrasound Med*. 1995;14:475–477.

29. Porth CM. Pathophysiology. *Concepts of Altered Health States*. 8th ed. Philadelphia, PA: Lippincott; Williams and Wilkins 2008.

30. Weber TM. Sonography of benign renal cystic disease. *Ultrasound Clin*. 2006;1:15–24.

31. Jeffrey RB, Ralls PW. *Sonography of the Abdomen*. New York, NY: Raven Press; 1995.

32. Castagna TL, Michael K. Medullary sponge kidney: an imaging study. *JDMS*. 2005;21:247–252.

33. Frishman E, Orron DE, Heiman Z, et al. Infected renal cysts: sonographic diagnosis and management. *J Ultrasound Med*. 1994;191:7–10.

34. Yeh HC, Mitty HA, Halton K, et al. Milk of calcium in renal cysts: new sonographic features. *J Ultrasound Med*. 1992;11:195–203.

35. Patel U, Huntley L, Kellett MJ. Sonographic features of renal obstruction mimicked by peripelvic cysts. *Clin Radiol*. 1994;49:481–484.

36. Letourneau K, Harrington C, Reed M, et al. Tuberous sclerosis complex: typical and atypical sonographic findings. *JDMS*. 2005;21:491–496.

37. Ruff C, Rumack CM, Wootton-Gorges S, et al. Renal cell carcinoma in tuberous sclerosis: a case report and review. *JDMS*. 1997;13:297–300.

38. Middleton WD. Von Hippel-Lindau disease. In: Siegel BA, Stephens DH, eds. *Diagnostic Ultrasonography (2nd Series) Text and Syllabus*. Reston, VA: American College of Radiology; 1994.

39. Reed AB, Parekh DJ. Surgical management of von Hippel-Lindau disease: urologic considerations. *Surg Oncol Clin North Am*. 2008;18:157–174.

40. Choyke PL, Glenn GMN, Walther MM, et al. The natural history of renal lesions in von Hippel-Lindau disease: a serial CT study in 28 patients. *AJR*. 1992;159:1229–1234.

41. Levine E, Hartman DS, Smirniotopoulos JG. Renal cystic disease associated with renal neoplasm. In: Pollock HM, ed. *Clinical Urography*. Philadelphia, PA: WB Saunders; 1990.

42. Anderson DM, Patwell JM, Plaut K, et al., eds. *Dorland's Illustrated Medical Dictionary*. 31st ed. Philadelphia, PA: WB Saunders; 2007.

43. Thomas CL, ed. *Taber's Cyclopedic Medical Dictionary*. 21st ed. Philadelphia, PA: FA Davis; 2009.

44. Anderhub B. *General Sonography*. St. Louis, MO: Mosby; 1995.

45. O'Connor OJ, McSweeney SE, Maher MM. Imaging of hematuria. *Radiol Clin North Am*. 2008;46:113–132.

46. Stec P. Intrarenal disorders. In: Copstead L-EC, ed. *Perspectives on Pathophysiology*. Philadelphia, PA: WB Saunders; 1995.

47. Dierks PR, Berman MC. Renal cell carcinoma: ultrasound, CT, and MRI correlation. *JDMS*. 1987;3:136–140.

48. Kuijpers D, Kruyt RH, Oudkerk M. Renal masses: value of duplex Doppler ultrasound in the differential diagnosis. *J Urol*. 1994;151:326–328.

49. Leder RA, Dunnick NR. Transitional cell carcinoma of the pelvicalices and ureter. *AJR*. 1990;155:713–722.

50. Scoutt LM, Sawyers SR, Bokhari J, et al. Ultrasound evaluation of the acute abdomen. *Ultrasound Clin*. 2007;2: 493–523.

51. Weissleder R, Wittenberg J. *Primer of Diagnostic Imaging*. 4th ed. St. Louis, MO: Mosby; 2006.

52. Tseng TY, Stoller ML. Obstructive uropathy. *Clin Geriatr Med*. 2009;25:437–443.

53. Hertzberg BS, Carroll BA, Bowie JD, et al. Doppler US assessment of maternal kidneys: analysis of intrarenal resistivity indexes in normal pregnancy and physiologic pelvocaliectasis. *Radiology*. 1993;186:689–692.

54. Nazarian GK, Platt JF, Rubin JM, et al. Renal duplex Doppler sonography in asymptomatic women during pregnancy. *J Ultrasound Med*. 1993;12:441–444.

55. Brkljacic B, Drinkovic I, Matovinovic, et al. Intrarenal duplex Doppler sonographic evaluation of unilateral native kidney obstruction. *J Ultrasound Med*. 1994;13: 197–204.

56. Tublin ME, Dodd GD III, Verdile VP. Acute renal colic: diagnosis with duplex Doppler US. *Radiology*. 1994;193: 697–701.

57. Platt JF, Rubin JM, Ellis JH. Acute renal obstruction: evaluation with intrarenal duplex Doppler and conventional US. *Radiology*. 1993;186:685–688.

58. Sidhu R. Bhatt S, Dogra VS. Renal colic. *Ultrasound Clin*. 2008;3:159–170.

59. Zwirewich CV, Buckley AR, Kidney MR, et al. Renal matrix calculus: sonographic appearance. *J Ultrasound Med*. 1990;9:61–64.

60. Lee JY, Kim SH, Cho JY, et al. Color and power Doppler twinkling artifacts from urinary stones: clinical observations and phantom studies. *AJR*. 2001;176:1441–1445.

61. Turrin A, Minola P, Costa F, et al. Diagnostic value of color Doppler twinkling artifact in sites negative for stones on B mode renal sonography. *Urological Research*. 2007;35: 313–317.

62. Rubens D, Bhatt S, Nedelka S, et al. Doppler artifacts and pitfalls. *Ultrasound Clin*. 2006;79–109.

63. Päivansälo MJ, Kallioinen MJ, Merikanto JS, et al. Hyperechogenic "rings" in the periphery of renal medullary pyramids as a sign of renal disease. *J Clin Ultrasound*. 1991;19:283–287.

64. Lucaya J, Enriquez G, Nieto J, et al. Renal calcifications in patients with autosomal recessive polycystic kidney disease: prevalence and cause. *AJR*. 1993;160:359–362.

65. Araujo N, Mendes R. Postbiopsy arteriovenous fistula in renal transplant: two cases of spontaneous resolution. *JDMS*. 2010;26:290–295.

66. Litza JA, Brill JR. Urinary tract infections. *Prim Care Clin Office Pract*. 2010;37:491–507.

67. Jeffrey RB, Vernacchia FS. The role of sonography and CT in urosepsis. *JDMS*. 1986;2:141–144.

68. Talner LB, Davidson AJ, Lebowitz RL, et al. Acute pyelonephritis: can we agree on terminology? *Radiology*. 1994;192:297–305.

69. Kenny PJ. Imaging of chronic renal infections. *AJR*. 1990; 155:485–494.

70. Chou YH, Tiu CM, Chen TW, et al. Emphysematous pyelonephritis in a polycystic kidney: demonstration by ultrasound and computed tomography. *J Ultrasound Med*. 1990;9:355–357.

71. Kuligowska E. Renal infections. *Clin Diag Ultrasound*. 1986;18:89–112.

72. Huether SE, McCance KL, Tarmina MS. Alterations of digestive function. In: McCance KL, Huether SE, eds. *Pathophysiology: The Biologic Basis for Disease in Adults and Children*. 6th ed. St. Louis, MO: Mosby; 2009.

73. Lebovitch S, Mydlo JH. HIV-AIDS–Urologic considerations. *Urol Clin North Am*. 2008;35:59–68.

74. Zinn DL, Haller JO, Cohen HL. Focal and diffuse increased echogenicity in the renal parenchyma in patients with sickle hemoglobinopathies-observation. *J Ultrasound Med*. 1993; 12:211–214.

75. Stone C. Schistosomiasis. *JDMS*. 2005;21:424–427.

76. Goldman SM, Fishman EK. Upper urinary tract infection: the current role of CT, ultrasound and MRI. *Semin Ultrasound CT MR*. 1991;12:335–360.

77. Vijayaraghavan SB. Ultrasonography of genitourinary tuberculosis. *Ultrasound Clin*. 2010;5:367–378.

78. Huntington DK, Hill SC, Hill MC. Sonographic manifestations of medical renal disease. *Semin Ultrasound CT MR*. 1991;12:290–307.

79. Rajashekar A, Perazella MA, Crowley S. Sytemic diseases with renal manifestations. *Prim Care Clin Office Pract*. 2008;35:297–328.

80. Brkljacic B, Mrzljak V, Drinkovic L, et al. Renal vascular resistance in diabetic nephropathy: duplex Doppler US evaluation. *Radiology*. 1994;192:549–554.

81. Platt JF, Rubin JM, Ellis JH. Diabetic nephropathy: evaluation with renal duplex Doppler US. *Radiology*. 1994;190:343–346.

82. Braden GL, Kozinn DR, Hampf EE Jr, et al. Ultrasound diagnosis of early renal papillary necrosis. *J Ultrasound Med*. 1991;10:401–403.

83. Longmaid HE, Rider E, Tymkiw J. Lupus nephritis: new sonographic findings. *J Ultrasound Med*. 1987;6:75–79.

84. Carlson K. Renal failure. In: Copstead L-EC, ed. *Perspectives on Pathophysiology*. Philadelphia, PA: WB Saunders; 1995.

85. Green D, Carroll BA. Ultrasound of renal failure. *Clin Diag Ultrasound*. 1986;18:55–88.

86. Platt JF, Rubin JM, Ellis JH. Acute renal failure: possible role of duplex Doppler US in distinction between acute prerenal failure and acute tubular necrosis. *Radiology*. 1991;179:419–423.

87. Levine E, Slusher SL, Grantham JJ, et al. Natural history of acquired renal cystic disease in dialysis patients: a prospective longitudinal CT study. *AJR*. 1991;156:501–506.

88. Wilson S, Greenbaum L, Goldberg B. Contrast-enhanced ultrasound: what is the evidence and what are the obstacles? *AJR*. 2009;193:55–60.

89. Christensen JD, Dogra VS. New advances in genitourinary ultrasound. *Ultrasound Clin*. 2007;2:105–114.

90. Kalantarinia K, Okusa M. Ultrasound contrast agents in the study of kidney function in health and disease. *Drug Discov Today Dis Mech*. 2007;4:153–158.

91. Harvey CJ, Sidhu PS. Ultrasound contrast agents in genitourinary imaging. *Ultrasound Clin*. 2010;5:489–506.

92. Setola SV, Catalano O, Sandomenico F, et al. Contrast-enhanced sonography of the kidney. *Abdominal Imaging*. 2007;32:21–28.

93. McBiles M. Correlative imaging of the kidney. *Semin Nucl Med*. 1994;24:219–233.

94. Goldman SM, Sandler CM. Genitourinary imaging: the past 40 years. *Radiol*. 2000;215:313–324.

95. Davidson AJ. Abnormal renal size. In: Eisenberg RL, ed. *Diagnostic Imaging: An Algorithmic Approach*. Philadelphia, PA: JB Lippincott; 1988.

96. Demas BE, Fisher MR. Renal masses. In: Eisenberg RL, ed. *Diagnostic Imaging: An Algorithmic Approach*. Philadelphia, PA: JB Lippincott; 1988.

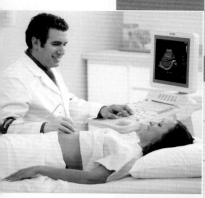

# 11

# The Lower Urinary System

Bridgette M. Lunsford and Christine Schara

## OBJECTIVES

Describe the embryologic development, normal anatomy, and function of the lower urinary tract.

Discuss the various sonographic techniques that can be used for evaluation of the lower urinary tract.

Identify the normal sonographic appearance of the lower urinary tract and common anatomic variants.

List clinical indications associated with lower urinary tract disease.

Describe the sonographic appearance of congenital lower urinary tract abnormalities such as exstrophy, duplication, posterior urethral valves, ectopic ureter, and ureterocele.

List the common causes and sonographic appearance of cystitis.

Identify the sonographic appearance of reflux, neurogenic bladder, and bladder wall abnormalities.

Describe common mechanisms for bladder trauma and the appearance of pathologies related to trauma.

List common causes of bladder wall thickening.

Describe the sonographic appearance of benign and malignant bladder tumors.

Define stress incontinence and describe sonographic techniques used in the diagnosis.

Identify technically satisfactory and unsatisfactory sonographic examinations of the lower urinary tract.

## KEY TERMS

bladder flap hematoma | cystitis | diverticula | ectopic ureter | exstrophy | neurogenic bladder | posterior urethral valves | squamous cell carcinoma | stress incontinence | transitional cell carcinoma | urachal cyst | ureterocele | vesicoureteral reflux

## GLOSSARY

**cystoscopy** procedure in which a scope is used to evaluate the urethra, bladder, and pelvic ureters

**hematuria** presence of red blood cells in the urine; hematuria can be microscopic (not visible with the naked eye) or macroscopic

**trabeculated bladder** thickened, irregular bladder wall frequently seen in patients with long-standing obstruction or neurogenic bladder

**voiding cystourethrogram (VCUG)** a procedure used to evaluate for urinary reflux in which the patient is catheterized and the bladder is filled with a contrast agent; the bladder is examined under fluoroscopy to evaluate for vesicoureteral reflux both before and during patient voiding

The lower urinary tract consists of the pelvic ureters, bladder, and urethra. Whenever a reference is made to the urinary system, the kidneys come to mind first. The ureter, bladder, and urethra are also part of the urinary system and play important roles in transporting, storing, and eliminating urine. The pelvic ureter and urethra are conduits in the process of elimination of urine. The bladder is located anatomically between these two structures and functions as a reservoir for urine storage. The primary focus of this chapter is the urinary bladder. The normal pelvic ureter and the urethra are not usually seen sonographically, but these structures may be visualized with coexisting pathologic conditions.

The urine-filled bladder is one of the most accessible abdominopelvic organs for sonography examinations. Recognition of normal bladder anatomy, including its position, size, shape, and appearance helps the sonographer identify congenital anomalies of the bladder, pathologies, and abnormalities in the surrounding anatomy.

## ANATOMY AND ORGANOGENESIS

During early embryology of the human urogenital system, three sets of kidneys develop—the pronephros (early in the fourth embryologic week), mesonephros (late in the fourth week), and the metanephros (fifth week)—in three successive waves, from cranial to caudal, with the third, most inferior pair of kidneys (metanephros) becoming the permanent kidneys.[1] The caudal end of the hindgut has a dilated chamber, the cloaca. The cloacal endoderm is in close contact with the surface ectoderm, and together, they form the cloacal membrane. An extension from the cloaca into the umbilical cord is the *allantois*. The intermediate mesoderm of the gastrula bulges into the dorsal aspect of the intraembryonic coelom as a urogenital ridge on each side. This further develops into two ridges: a medial genital (gonadal) ridge and a lateral nephrogenic ridge (or cord). A mesonephric (wolffian) duct and paramesonephric (müllerian) duct form in the nephrogenic ridge or cord.[1]

In approximately the seventh gestational week, the urorectal septum between the allantois and hindgut fuses with the cloacal membrane, dividing it into the ventral (anterior) urogenital sinus and a dorsal (posterior) rectum.[2] The upper part of the urogenital sinus is the fusiform bladder. The lower pelvic and phallic parts of the urogenital sinus form the urethra and related glands and structures in each sex. The wolffian ducts give origin to the ureters; they also form the efferent tubules, duct of the epididymis, vas deferens, seminal vesicles, and ejaculatory ducts in males and the epoophoron, paroophoron, and Gartner's duct in females.

The ends of the mesonephric ducts (Wolffian and Müllerian) and the endodermal cloaca form the urinary bladder.[1] The cloaca—the terminal, caudal, blind-ended portion of the hindgut—is the major structure that forms the lower part of the urinary and genital tract. Its primary function is to serve as the primitive receptacle into which the reproductive and excretory tracts empty.

The metanephric duct (future ureter) develops from a ureteric bud growing from the caudal end of the mesonephric duct. In a short time, the metanephric duct shifts anteriorly and makes its own connection with the cloaca/urogenital sinus/bladder.

At 8 weeks gestation, all embryos have identical primordia in the indifferent stage of urogenital development, with gonads capable of developing into testes or ovaries. In males, the paramesonephric (müllerian) ducts degenerate. The mesonephric ducts become the ductus deferens, ejaculatory ducts, and seminal vesicles. The urogenital sinus develops into the urinary bladder, prostate gland, bulbourethral glands (Cowper's gland), paraurethral glands, and prostatic, membranous, and penile (spongy) urethra.[1] In females, the mesonephric (wolffian) ducts degenerate and the paramesonephric ducts develop into the uterine tubes, uterus, and upper part of the vagina. The urogenital sinus forms the bladder, urethra, greater vestibular and paraurethral glands, vestibule, and lower part of the vagina.[1]

Initially, the bladder is contiguous with the allantois, which eventually becomes a fibrous cord, the urachus (known as the median umbilical ligament in the adult).[3] The urachus extends from the apex of the bladder to the umbilicus. In infants and children, the urinary bladder is an abdominal organ until after puberty when it becomes a true pelvic structure.[3,4]

### URINARY BLADDER

The bladder develops into a hollow, smooth, musculomembranous, collapsible sac that acts as a reservoir for urine. The bladder is located in the retroperitoneum on the pelvic floor just posterior to the pubic symphysis.[5] Its size, position, and relationship to other organs vary according to the amount of fluid it contains.[2] The urinary bladder is lined with a mucous membrane of transitional epithelium that allows for expansion. This mucous membrane lining contains rugae or folds. When the bladder is empty, the membrane appears folded or wrinkled.[5] The mucous membrane is loosely attached to the underlying muscle coat except at the trigone region, where it is firmly attached to the muscular coat, appears smooth, and does not expand during bladder filling.

Covering the transitional epithelium, the bladder wall is composed of three layers of smooth muscle fibers: a connective tissue submucosa, a muscle layer, and a fibrous adventitia.[5] The outer fibrous adventitia is continuous except on the superior surface of the bladder, which is covered by the parietal peritoneum.

The inner connective tissue submucosa and the outer fibrous adventitia are arranged in longitudinal layers. They enclose the detrusor muscle, the prominent circular middle muscle layer.[5]

The bladder is capable of considerable distention because of the lining's elasticity and rugae and the wall's elasticity.[5] It is uniquely situated in the pelvic cavity for its function of urine storage. Bladder capacity varies greatly and depends on many factors, including the age and physical condition of the patient. The normal adult bladder is generally moderately full at 500 mL (a pint) of urine, but it may hold nearly double that if necessary.[3,5]

Normally, the bladder is a round-edged tetrahedron with a superior, a posterior, and two inferior surfaces. The superior surface has two regions: the fundus, located posteriorly, and the apex, located anteriorly. The two ureteral orifices are located in the body on the posteroinferior portion. The urethral orifice is located in the neck of the bladder and is the most inferior region.[1]

When the bladder is empty, the anterior surface lies just behind and, rarely, superior to the symphysis in both males and females.[1] The fibrous medial umbilical ligament (obliterated urachus) extends from the apex upward as a blunt cone with a solid, slender continuation in the midline of the abdominal wall and attaches to the umbilicus.[1]

Related anatomy in the pelvis varies depending on the quantity of urine and with the condition of the rectum; being pushed upward and forward when the rectum is distended.[1]

When distended with urine, the bladder can rise approximately 16 cm above the symphysis pubis. It ascends into the abdominal cavity, comes in contact with the lower anterior abdominal wall and, when fully distended, can be readily palpated or percussed. As the bladder enlarges, it loses its ovoid or spherical configuration and becomes more globular. Coils of the small intestine lie adjacent to the upper surface of the bladder and are displaced posteriorly as the bladder enlarges. With overdistention, such as acute or chronic urinary retention, the lower abdomen may visibly bulge.

When the bladder is relatively empty in the female, the fundal region of the bladder lies in contact with the anterior wall of the vagina and cervix (Fig. 11-1A). The uterus and vagina are interposed between the bladder and rectum.[3] When the bladder is empty, the uterus rests on the bladder's superior surface. Female reproductive and pelvic muscular anatomy is greatly enhanced using the traditional full-bladder technique.

In the male, the fundus and the body of the bladder are related to the rectum, separated above by the rectovesical pouch of peritoneum and inferolaterally on each side by a ductus deferens and seminal vesicle.[3] The prostate is a fibromuscular and glandular organ that lies just inferior to the bladder.[3] The base of the prostate is applied to the caudal surface of the bladder.

The greater part of this surface is directly continuous with the bladder wall. The normal prostate encircles the prostatic urethra and prostate gland secretion enters the prostatic urethra via several ducts. The seminal vesicles lie just cephalad to the prostate under the base of the bladder. They are approximately 6 cm long and quite soft. Each vesicle joins its corresponding vas deferens to form the ejaculatory duct (Fig. 11-1B–D).

### Trigone

On the floor of the bladder, a triangular region, the trigone, has no rugae and is firmly attached to the muscular coat.[6] The trigone is outlined by the three openings in the bladder: two from the ureters and one into the urethra (Fig. 11-1C and Fig. 11-2). The ureteral orifices are situated superiorly and laterally at the extremities of the crescent-shaped interureteric ridge that forms the proximal border of the trigone.[1] The urethral opening is located at its anterior, midline, lower corner at the bladder neck.

## URETERS

The ureters are slender tubes that convey urine from the kidneys to the bladder.[6] Each ureter is a continuation of the renal pelvis. From there, they descend in the retroperitoneum and run obliquely through the posterior bladder wall. The average length of the ureter is 30 cm and the diameter is 6 mm.[6] The ureters are constricted in three places: (1) at the ureteropelvic junction, (2) as they cross the iliac vessels, and (3) at the junction with the bladder.

Histologically, the ureter wall is trilayered. The ureter is lined with transitional epithelium—the *mucosa*—that is continuous with that of the renal pelvis superiorly and the bladder inferiorly. The middle layer—the *muscularis*—is composed of two muscle sheets: the internal longitudinal layer and an external circular layer. The composition of circular fibers integrated in the ureter wall contract in peristaltic waves in response to incoming urine, propelling urine toward the urinary bladder.[5,6] The rate of urine formation affects the strength and frequency of the peristaltic waves. An additional smooth muscle layer—the external longitudinal layer—appears in the lower third of the ureter. The outer *adventitia* is made up of fibrous connective tissue.[5]

The distal ureter enters obliquely through the bladder wall by slit-like openings. This anatomic arrangement prevents the backflow of urine. As the bladder fills, the pressure increases causing the upper and lower walls of the terminal portions of the ureter to become closely applied to each other, acting as valves to prevent regurgitation of urine from the bladder. When the bladder is distended, the openings of the ureters are about 5 cm apart; however, the distance between them is diminished by half when the bladder is empty and contracted.

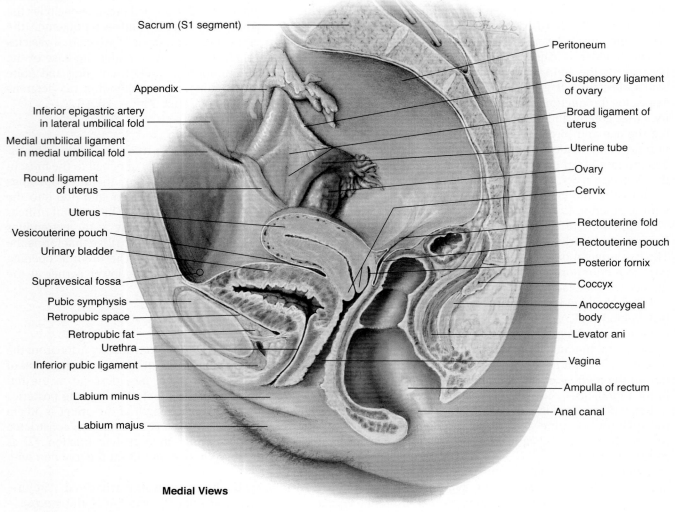

Sacrum (S1 segment)

Appendix

Inferior epigastric artery
in lateral umbilical fold

Medial umbilical ligament
in medial umbilical fold

Round ligament
of uterus

Uterus

Vesicouterine pouch

Urinary bladder

Supravesical fossa

Pubic symphysis

Retropubic space

Retropubic fat

Urethra

Inferior pubic ligament

Labium minus

Labium majus

Peritoneum

Suspensory ligament
of ovary

Broad ligament of
uterus

Uterine tube

Ovary

Cervix

Rectouterine fold

Rectouterine pouch

Posterior fornix

Coccyx

Anococcygeal
body

Levator ani

Vagina

Ampulla of rectum

Anal canal

**Medial Views**

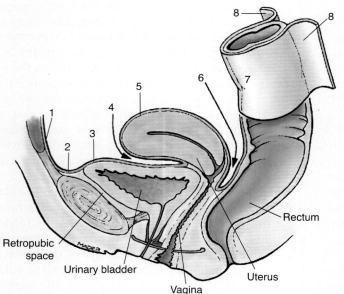

Retropubic
space

Urinary bladder

Vagina

Uterus

Rectum

**Female:**

Peritoneum passes:

- From the anterior abdominal wall (1)
- Superior to the pubic bone (2)
- On the superior surface of the urinary bladder (3)
- From the bladder to the uterus, forming the vesicouterine pouch (4)
- On the fundus and body of the uterus, posterior formix, and all of the vagina (5)
- Between the rectum and uterus, forming the rectouterine pouch (6)
- On the anterior and lateral sides of the rectum (7)
- Posteriorly to become the sigmoid mesocolon (8)

**A**

**Figure 11-1** Normal anatomy. Coronal planes of the female **(A)** and **(B)** male pelvis show the normal anatomic relationship of the bladder with surrounding structures. *(continued)*

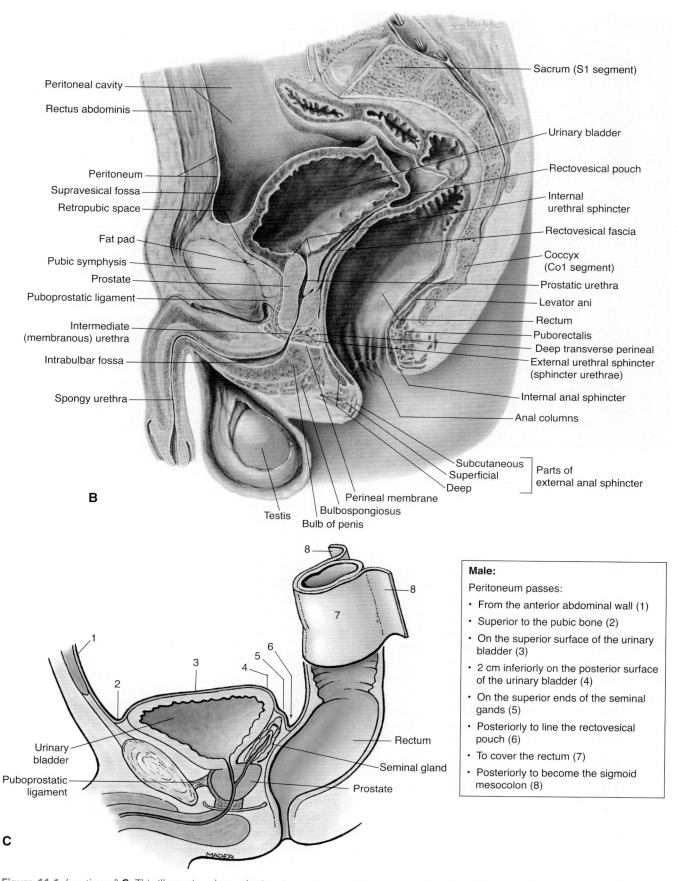

Peritoneal cavity

Rectus abdominis

Peritoneum

Supravesical fossa

Retropubic space

Fat pad

Pubic symphysis

Prostate

Puboprostatic ligament

Intermediate (membranous) urethra

Intrabulbar fossa

Spongy urethra

Sacrum (S1 segment)

Urinary bladder

Rectovesical pouch

Internal urethral sphincter

Rectovesical fascia

Coccyx (Co1 segment)

Prostatic urethra

Levator ani

Rectum

Puborectalis

Deep transverse perineal

External urethral sphincter (sphincter urethrae)

Internal anal sphincter

Anal columns

Subcutaneous
Superficial
Deep
} Parts of external anal sphincter

**B**

Testis

Bulb of penis

Bulbospongiosus

Perineal membrane

8

8

7

1

2

3

4

5

6

Urinary bladder

Puboprostatic ligament

Rectum

Seminal gland

Prostate

**Male:**

Peritoneum passes:

- From the anterior abdominal wall (1)
- Superior to the pubic bone (2)
- On the superior surface of the urinary bladder (3)
- 2 cm inferiorly on the posterior surface of the urinary bladder (4)
- On the superior ends of the seminal gands (5)
- Posteriorly to line the rectovesical pouch (6)
- To cover the rectum (7)
- Posteriorly to become the sigmoid mesocolon (8)

**C**

**Figure 11-1** *(continued)* **C.** This illustration shows the interior cutaway sections of the male urinary bladder and the prostatic urethra and a topographic anatomy of the male pelvic organs.

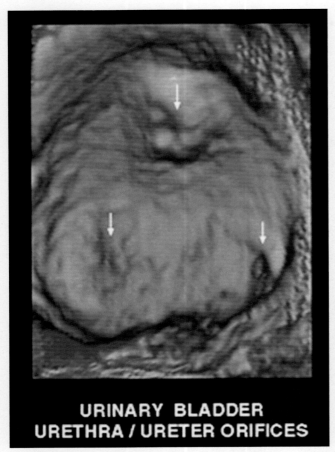

**URINARY BLADDER
URETHRA / URETER ORIFICES**

**Figure 11-2** Trigone. Three-dimensional rendered image of the bladder trigone demonstrating the ureteral and urethral openings *(arrows)*. The three-dimensional rendered image of the inner bladder lining provides a virtual cystogram of the bladder wall. (Image courtesy of Philips Medical Systems, Bothell, WA.)

## URETHRA

The *urethra* is a thin-walled fibromuscular tube that drains urine from the bladder and conveys it outside the body. The urethra represents the terminal portion of the urinary tract. At the bladder–urethral junction, a thickening of the detrusor smooth muscle of the bladder wall forms the *internal urethral sphincter*. This involuntary muscle keeps the urethra closed and prevents leaking between voiding. The sphincter is unique in that contraction opens it and relaxation closes it. The *external urethral sphincter* surrounds the urethra as it passes through the urogenital diaphragm. This sphincter is formed of skeletal muscle and is controlled voluntarily.[5,6]

The length and functions of the urethra differ in males and females. The female urethra is 3 to 4 cm long and functions only to convey urine from the body.[5] It lies directly posterior to the symphysis pubis and anterior to the vagina. The *external urethral orifice*—the external opening of the urethra—lies anterior to the vaginal opening and posterior to the clitoris. The opening of the urethra to the exterior is referred to as the *urinary meatus.*

The male urethra serves a double function: a conduit for eliminating urine and also as the terminal portion of the reproductive system serving as the passage for ejaculate (semen). The male urethra is approximately 20 cm long and has three regions. The *prostatic urethra*, about 2.5 cm long, runs within the prostate.[5] The *membranous urethra,* which runs through the urogenital sinus, extends about 2 cm from the prostate to the beginning of the penis. The *spongy urethra* passes through the penis and opens at its tip—the external urethral orifice.

## PHYSIOLOGY

The mechanism for voiding urine (micturition) starts with involuntary and voluntary nerve impulses.[5] Even though the bladder has a greater capacity, when the volume of urine exceeds 200 to 400 mL, stretch receptors trigger transmission of impulses to the lower portion of the spinal cord, initiating the conscious desire to expel urine and a subconscious reflex, the micturition reflex.[7] The combination of voluntary relaxation of the external sphincter muscle of the bladder, reflex contraction of linear smooth muscle fibers along the urethra, and then contraction of the detrusor muscle squeezes urine out of the bladder.[5] Parasympathetic fibers transmit the impulses that cause contractions of the bladder and relaxation of the internal sphincter.[5,7,8]

Because the external sphincter is under voluntary control, we can choose to postpone bladder emptying. Voluntary contraction of the external sphincter to prevent or terminate micturition is learned and is possible only if the nerves supplying the bladder and urethra—the projection tracts of the cord and brain—and the motor area of the cerebrum are all intact.[7,8] Incontinence—involuntary emptying of the bladder—results from aging or trauma to any of these parts of the nervous system by cerebral hemorrhage or cord injury.[5–7]

*Retention* is an inability to empty the bladder even though the bladder contains an excessive amount of urine.[9] Catheterization may be used to relieve the discomfort accompanying retention. The 30% of patients who are catheterized routinely eventually develop a "ledge" posteriorly at the bladder neck from catheter trauma. The ledge makes voiding difficult and considerably complicates the catheterization process.

## SONOGRAPHIC SCANNING TECHNIQUE

This section includes considerations for optimizing sonographic techniques for examination of the lower urinary tract. This includes the sonographer's role, transducer selection, patient preparation, imaging protocols, patient positioning, and specialized methods used to provide physicians with diagnostic sonographic images.

## PATIENT PREPARATION

Sonographers must obtain and document a thorough patient history, including, but not limited to: previous surgeries; correlation of prior and current results of complementary diagnostic imaging examinations such as computed tomography (CT) and radiographic exams; laboratory results; location and duration of pain; fever; difficult, painful, or frequent urination; and related pelvic history. Sonographers must also analyze patient and clinical findings and be creative in tailoring the examination to produce diagnostic images that best reveal the correct diagnosis. For instance, altering the patient position may enable an optimal imaging plane and/or enhance visibility of diagnostic pathology.

To visualize the bladder with the transabdominal approach, it is important that the patient prepare properly. Bladder distention is absolutely essential to optimal visualization of the bladder, bladder wall, and related anatomy. Filling the bladder can be accomplished by three methods: (1) instructing the patient to drink 16 ounces of water 1 hour before the examination and not to void until the examination is completed; (2) instructing the patient not to void before the examination; or (3) catheterizing the patient and instilling fluid into the bladder through a Foley catheter. Foley catheters are not inserted routinely to fill a bladder unless it is a medical emergency. There have been many studies showing catheter insertion may introduce infectious contaminants into the body. A Foley catheter balloon will appear as a round cystic structure in the filled bladder and may cast shadows in areas of interest.

A fully distended bladder serves as a cystic reference in the abdominopelvic anatomy, pushes adjacent bowel and gas out of the field of view, and provides a sonographic "window" to identify pelvic anatomy. In males, the bladder, seminal vesicles, prostate, and rectum should be imaged routinely; in females, the vagina, bladder, uterus, ovaries, adnexa, and rectum. A full bladder also facilitates identification of dilated ureters. It is not necessary to restrict the diet or use catheters or enemas to reduce intestinal contents or air. Disease processes in pelvic structures can involve or mimic those of other closely related anatomy. Knowledge of pelvic anatomy, including the genitourinary tract, gastrointestinal tract, and pelvic vasculature and musculature is important.

A suitable coupling agent such as ultrasonic gel, is used on the skin surface. The highest frequency transducer possible should be selected for scanning, making sure that penetration is adequate to visualize the posterior aspect of the areas of interest.

## SCANNING TECHNIQUES

The most widely used approach to scan the urinary bladder is the transabdominal method.[3] The patient is usually examined in the supine position. Sometimes, it is necessary to position the patient obliquely or to roll the patient into a lateral decubitus position to better demonstrate bladder wall abnormalities, the movement of debris or stones to the dependant bladder wall, or bladder tumors. Transducer selection should take into consideration body habitus and the examination objectives. The endovaginal, endorectal, and transperineal methods may also be used to a lesser extent.

The lower urinary tract should be scanned in both longitudinal and transverse planes transabdominally, and may be scanned in longitudinal and coronal planes endovaginally and transperineally.[3] Using the endorectal approach, the proximal urethra can be visualized and the distal urethra is identified during penile artery evaluation.[4] Recent studies have also used an endorectal approach to evaluate female urogenital disorders such as stress incontinence.

The normal distended urinary bladder appears anechoic structure with well demarcation of the echogenic smooth bladder walls.[3] The bladder wall is seen as a smooth echogenic interface and should be of uniform thickness. The thickness of the bladder wall will vary from less than 3 mm when fully distended to 5 mm when near empty.[3,4,10,11] A pathologically thickened bladder wall is better visualized when the bladder is fully distended.[4] If larger than 6 mm when empty or partially distended, the bladder wall should be interrogated for a pathologic process. When the bladder is scanned transabdominally, reverberation echoes are often seen anteriorly in the near field of the bladder image.[4,11] Many times, artifacts such as reverberations, side lobes, and shadowing can be eliminated by sonography system controls and/or altering the transducer position to change the angle of the transmitted sound wave to avoid refraction from abdominal musculature[4] (Fig. 11-3A). Equipment manufacturers have added harmonics, speckle reduction, spatial compounding, and other computerized techniques to aid in the elimination of artifact echoes. Although the normal ureters and urethra are not routinely visualized on transabdominal sonography, their location should be examined because they can be identified in some anomalies, diseases, and pathologic processes.

The sonographer should identify the predictable contours of the urine-filled bladder and the smooth echogenic bladder wall. If the patient has never had bladder or pelvic surgery, any deviation from the normal bladder shape, especially asymmetry, should be considered abnormal and a thorough investigation should be performed of the site of the distortion to rule out a mass. This knowledge of normal anatomy provides a baseline comparison when variations in sonographic appearance alert the sonographer to possible pathology. On transverse sections, the bladder should appear symmetric. Superiorly, the bladder appears rounded, but in scanning more inferiorly, it appears square owing to the parallel walls of the acetabulum (Fig. 11-3B,C). On longitudinal

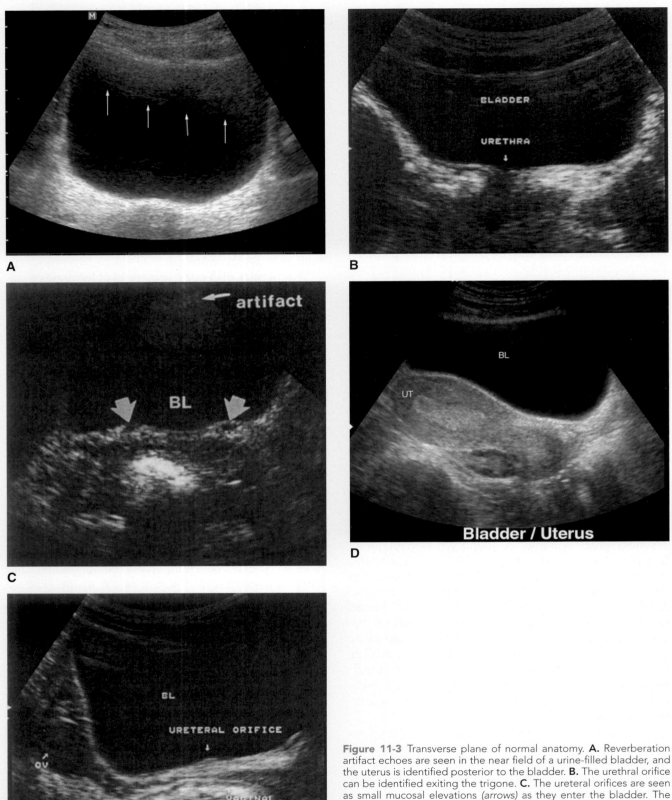

**Figure 11-3** Transverse plane of normal anatomy. **A.** Reverberation artifact echoes are seen in the near field of a urine-filled bladder, and the uterus is identified posterior to the bladder. **B.** The urethral orifice can be identified exiting the trigone. **C.** The ureteral orifices are seen as small mucosal elevations *(arrows)* as they enter the bladder. The anterior wall of the bladder demonstrates the reverberation artifact. **D,E.** Longitudinal plane of normal anatomy. **D.** On the left, near the midline, the left ureteral orifice is seen entering the trigone. **E.** The right ureteral orifice is seen entering the trigone. *BL*, urinary bladder, *OV*, ovary. (Images B and E courtesy of Steven D. Hatch, Logan, UT.)

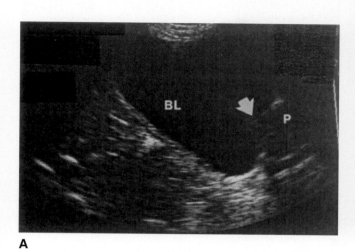

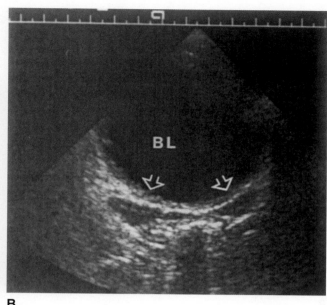

**A**                                                          **B**

**Figure 11-4** Normal male anatomy. **A.** When scanning in a longitudinal plane in the suprapubic region, the relationship between the urinary bladder *(BL)* and prostate *(P)* is visualized. **B.** On a transverse plane of the male urinary bladder *(BL)*, the seminal vesicles can be identified bilaterally as hypoechoic structures inferior to the hyperechoic posterior wall *(arrows)*.

sections, the bladder appears almost triangular, with the base of the triangle parallel with the anterior abdominal wall. In both longitudinal and transverse scans, the lateral walls appear straight or slightly indented by prominent iliopsoas muscles (Fig. 11-3D,E). As the different pelvic structures are encountered, it may be necessary to angle the transducer caudad and cephalad and medial to lateral. The symphysis pubis acts as a point of reference on the body surface, where the transducer can be rocked superiorly and inferiorly on longitudinal scans to better view the superior and inferior aspects of the bladder. Transverse imaging must include tilting or a cross-plane imaging by angling the transducer from side to side while continuing to use the fluid in the bladder as a window. This produces a sharper image of the bladder wall and gives a complete sweep to interrogate the entire bladder. Longitudinal and transverse images are more easily interpreted if they are in a sequential order: right-to-left in the longitudinal plane with the midline image identified and inferior to superior in the transverse plane. Correct labeling must appear on all sonographic images indicating the location of the scan, patient position, and scanning plane.

Frequently, it is possible to visualize the prostate and seminal vesicles in males using the transabdominal approach. When the transducer is angled caudad under the symphysis pubis, the prostate is seen posteroinferior to the bladder. On a longitudinal scan, the prostate appears as a heterogeneous structure at the most inferior aspect of the bladder. On a transverse image, it appears rounded. Although newer transducers with better penetration and resolution enable sonographers to identify the

prostate transabdominally in the adult male, the best way to visualize the prostate is via the endorectal approach (see Chapter 12). The seminal vesicles are seen as two small, oval, hypoechoic structures posterior to the bladder and superior to the prostate (Fig. 11-4A,B).

In patients who are catheterized, the catheter has an anechoic appearance with an echogenic margin and center. If air was used to secure the catheter's position, it may cause a shadow artifact. Sonographically, the symmetry of the catheter is identifiable as an echogenic incomplete circular structure in a urine-filled bladder (Fig. 11-5).

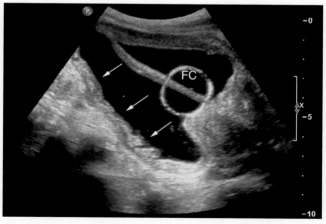

**Figure 11-5** Foley catheter. Longitudinal image of the urinary bladder; a Foley catheter *(FC)* can be identified within the bladder lumen. The catheter appears to be anechoic, with an echogenic exterior. Note the thickened bladder wall *(arrows)*. (Image courtesy of Philips Medical Systems, Bothell, WA.)

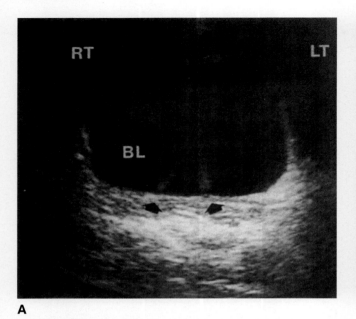
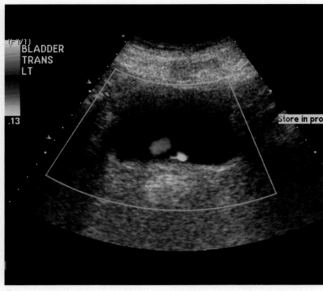

**A**                                                    **B**

**Figure 11-6** Transverse planes of normal ureteral jets. **A.** Simultaneous jets of low-intensity echoes *(arrows)* are visualized entering the urinary bladder *(BL)*. **B.** Color Doppler demonstrates both right and left ureteral jets on the transverse image on a male patient. (Image B courtesy of Natalee Braun, Ogden, UT.)

Routine bursts of echoes—the ureteral jet phenomenon—are seen entering the bladder from the region of the trigone.[1,3] At intervals of 5 to 20 seconds, a jet of low-intensity echoes, which lasts a few seconds, starts at the area of the ureteral orifices and flows toward the center of the bladder. Ureteral jets can occur simultaneously, but more commonly, they are separated (Fig. 11-6). Jets can be individually identified on longitudinal images, but both may be seen simultaneously on a transverse image. Such jets extend up to 3 cm and broaden. After a few seconds, the low-intensity echoes become distributed in the bladder and lose intensity until they can no longer be distinguished. Color Doppler is more sensitive and aids in demonstrating ureteral jets.[3] Although evaluation of ureteral jets with color Doppler is unable to predict reflux, the analysis of ureteral jets with color Doppler has been used successfully to determine the degree of ureteral obstruction with unilateral ureteral calculi, with either no detectable ureteral jets or continuous low-level jets on the symptomatic side.[4] In the case of bladder diverticulum, there is evidence of reversed flow of urine through the communication between the diverticulum and bladder when slight pressure is applied to the lower abdomen.

If either of the ureters is dilated, the dilated ureter can be visualized as a round, anechoic structure posterior to the bladder in the transverse plane. In the longitudinal plane, the dilated ureter can be visualized as a long, linear structure, usually posterior and to the right or left of the midline.

Bladder volume can be calculated using the formula for an ellipsoid (transverse × anteroposterior [AP] ×

length × 0.52).[3] The scanning equipment usually has computerized techniques to calculate volumes. The systems will calculate bladder volume once the three measurements have been entered. Bladder capacity should be noted. The capacity decreases in association with large pelvic masses, in urinary and pelvic inflammatory disease, prostatic hypertrophy, in patients receiving radiation therapy, in advanced stages of tumor infiltration, and after recent surgery.

Frequently, a postvoid residual volume calculation is also indicated.[3] To document the presence of residual urine and calculate its volume, the patient should be asked to empty the bladder. The longitudinal, AP, and transverse measurements must be repeated and another bladder volume calculated for comparison. Determining the amount of residual urine in patients with suspected bladder outlet obstruction has improved the treatment of these patients. Residual volume increases with age, atonic bladders, bladder neck obstruction, long-term cystitis, and advanced invasion by cancer.

Be sure to recheck related pelvic anatomy on postvoid images. What might have appeared as a bladder might not change size postvoid indicating an obstruction or a cystic pelvic tumor not necessarily related to the urinary system.

Three-dimensional (3D) and four-dimensional (4D) sonography has offered a whole new dimension to sonographic imaging. Obstetrical and gynecological 3D and 4D imaging is accepted as routine in the evaluation of fetal and gynecologic anatomy and pathologies. In recent years, the benefits of 3D/4D imaging of the lower urinary tract have been studied. The 3D sonography has some advantages over two-dimensional (2D)

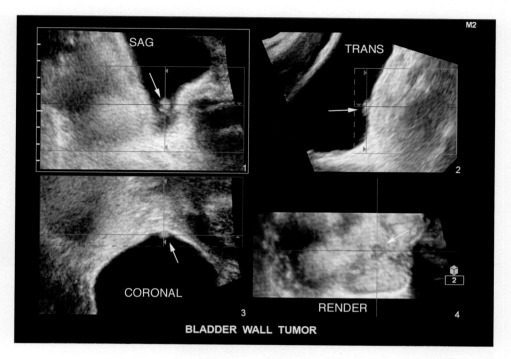

**Figure 11-7** Three-dimensional imaging. Multiplanar reconstruction of the bladder demonstrates a small bladder tumor (arrow) seen simultaneously in the sagittal, transverse, and coronal planes in addition to a rendered image of the bladder lining. The intersecting lines on each image represent the same anatomic location in all three planes.

imaging. An entire volume of data is stored, allowing for manipulation of the data set after the patient has left the exam room and reconstruction of images in all three scan planes. A rendered image of the interior bladder wall can provide a virtual sonographic cystoscopy examination[12] (Fig. 11-7). Three-dimensional bladder volume measurements can be obtained using a 3D technique called *virtual organ computer-aided analysis* (VOCAL), which also creates a 3D model of the organ.[13]

Endoluminal sonography is another imaging technique being investigated and is improving with revolutionary transducer technology. Initial studies using endoluminal sonography is limited by the high-frequency transducer (20 MHz), which allows penetration of only a few centimeters.[14] Although greater penetration is required for the upper urinary tract, the endoluminal transducer may be ideal for examining the urethra, bladder, and pelvic ureters, as researchers develop new technology for transducer construction and may find intraoperative techniques advantageous.

## ABNORMALITIES OF THE LOWER URINARY TRACT

### DUPLICATION

Duplication of the urinary bladder is divided into three types: a peritoneal fold, which may be complete or incomplete; a septum dividing the bladder either sagittally or coronally; and a transverse band of muscle dividing the bladder into two unequal cavities.[1,4] Complete duplication of the urinary bladder is rare. One must be aware that complications may arise from variations of this anomaly. Unilateral reflux, obstruction, or infection may occur secondary to stenosis or atresia of the urethra.

Duplication of the ureters results when the embryonic ureteric bud branches prematurely and leads to partial division and separation of the related blastema.[1] Incomplete duplication includes a bifurcation of the ureter at or near the renal pelvis that unites at a variable distance between the kidney and bladder and enters the bladder as a single ureter in the normal bladder trigone.[1] Duplication is complete when there are two separate renal collecting systems and two separate ureters. The ureter from the lower renal pelvis migrates and enters the bladder in the normal ureteral orifice in the bladder trigone. The ureter from the upper pole of the kidney inserts into the bladder caudad to the ureter from the lower pole. In females, the more caudad ureter may drain ectopically into the trigone, perineum, uterus, vagina, or urethra; in males, the distal insertion can occur in the trigone, urethra, or seminal vesicles.[1,4] Duplications may be unilateral or bilateral and are more common in females than in males.

An accessory or duplicate urethra is an uncommon malformation that occurs almost exclusively in males. True duplication is associated with duplication of the bladder and usually of the genitalia.

### BLADDER AGENESIS

An absent bladder is a rare anomaly. Most infants with bladder agenesis are stillborn and, virtually, all surviving infants are female.[4] During the obstetric scan, it is important to allow adequate time for the bladder to fill and

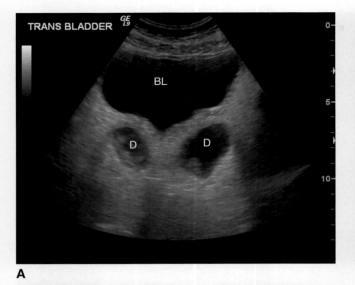

**A**

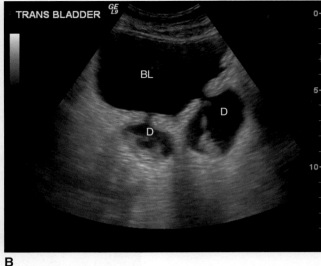

**B**

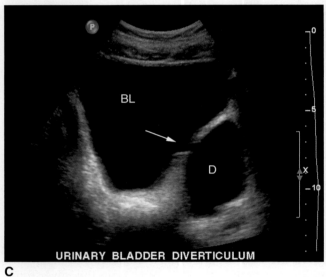

**C**

**Figure 11-8** Bladder diverticulum. **A.** Transverse image of the bladder *(BL)* demonstrates two cystic areas posterior to the bladder *(D)*. **B.** A slight rotation of the transducer reveals a connection between the cystic areas *(D)* and the bladder consistent with bladder diverticula. Note the debris within the diverticula that could indicate infection. **C.** Longitudinal image of the urinary bladder *(BL)* shows a large diverticulum *(D)*. Note the connection between the bladder and the diverticulum *(arrow)*.

empty. In cases of renal agenesis—a lethal anomaly—the bladder is not identified during the obstetric scan.

## DIVERTICULA

Diverticula of the bladder are pouch-like eversions of the wall. Bladder diverticula are produced by mucosal herniation through defects in the muscle wall arising as congenital defects or acquired lesions, usually associated with diseases resulting in bladder outlet obstruction or neurogenic conditions resulting in abnormalities in bladder function with chronically raised intravesical pressure.[3,15] One frequent form is the paraurethral (Hutch's) diverticulum, which forms because the ureter is inserted at an inherently weak point in the bladder wall.[15]

Bladder diverticula are demonstrated sonographically as urine-filled outpouchings.[4,15] Careful scanning may show the narrow communication between the diverticulum and the bladder, which leads to the

diagnosis (Fig. 11-8A–C). Intradiverticular tumors or stones may also be identified. Since diverticula may not empty and, occasionally, actually increase in size with voiding, postvoiding scans can demonstrate urine-filled diverticula.[4] Very large diverticula may be mistaken for the bladder itself, duplication of the bladder, or seminal vesicle or ovarian cysts.[4] Color Doppler provides a cost-benefit, rapid, and noninvasive examination for differentiating bladder diverticula from other cystic masses and fluid collections by evaluating ureteral jets. With color Doppler sonography, the diverticulum is demonstrated as a jet with alternating bidirectional flow between the bladder and the anechoic cystic diverticulum (Table 11-1).

Spontaneous rupture of bladder diverticulum is rare. Without immediate diagnosis, the condition may be mistaken for acute renal failure. Misdiagnosis and mistreatment can be fatal. Transabdominal sonography after injection of saline and air demonstrates extravasation,

| TABLE 11-1 | |
|---|---|
| **Bladder Abnormalities** | |
| **Abnormality** | **Sonographic Appearance** |
| Diverticula | Round, well-defined, thin-walled, fluid-filled masses with acoustic enhancement; variable in size. Color Doppler demonstrates bidirectional flow between bladder and cystic diverticulum. |
| Posterior urethral valve | Dilated, elongated prostatic urethra (peculiar to males); subsequently, thickened bladder wall, hydroureters, or dilated upper urinary tract may develop. |
| Exstrophy | Eversion through anterior abdominal wall; other findings include hydronephrosis caused by ureterovesical obstruction. |
| Bladder neck contracture | Secondary abnormalities include vesicoureteral reflux, vesical diverticula, and large-capacity bladder. |
| Ectopic ureter | More common for ureter to arise from the upper moiety of a duplex kidney; 10% to 20% arise from a solitary renal pelvis; may be massively dilated; may mimic multiseptate, cystic abdominal masses. |
| Ectopic ureterocele | Anechoic, cyst-like, thin-walled mass of variable size and shape projecting into the bladder (sometimes described as a cyst within a cyst). |
| Persistent urachus | Anechoic mass or diverticular outpouching between dome of the bladder and the umbilicus; cyst formation occurs if the ends seal off; adenocarcinoma or calculi may occur in a urachal cyst. |

identifies the injury site, and is more specific than CT or radiographic cystography.

Transperineal and transvaginal scanning is very effective in identifying urethral diverticula in women. The normal urethra can be routinely identified on transvaginal or transperineal scans as a hypoechoic linear structure exiting from the base of the bladder and traveling inferior to the symphysis pubis.[11] The hypoechoic to anechoic appearance of the urethral wall muscles is due to their parallel orientation to the ultrasound beam using these techniques. Variable echogenicity depending on the relative orientation of the transducer and the structure being scanned is called *anisotropy*. Remember this whenever scanning using these techniques of the urethra so that the resulting image is not confused with anechoic urine in the urethra. Urethral diverticula appear as simple or complex collections of fluid intimately related to the urethra. These may involve both lateral aspects of the urethra or wrap around the urethra. They can contain stones or cancer. These may be differentiated from periurethral abscesses with the use of power Doppler. The abscess is not vascular but there is hypervascularity around the abscess. Clinical history is also important in the differential diagnosis if the patient is febrile.

## POSTERIOR URETHRAL VALVES

The most common of bladder outlet obstructions results from the development of abnormal valves in the posterior urethra. The prostatic urethra is markedly dilated because of an obstruction at or just below the *verumontanum* (an elevation on the floor of the prostatic portion of the urethra where the seminal ducts enter). A posterior urethral valve usually consists of a mucosal flap originating from the verumontanum.

Posterior urethral valve syndrome is the most common cause of urinary obstruction in male infants.[4] Almost 75% are discovered during the first year of life. They may present in older children but rarely occur in adults. Approximately 40% of patients have associated vesicoureteral reflux, which is usually due to a periureteral diverticulum.[14]

The sonographic recognition of a dilated and elongated prostatic urethra helps differentiate posterior urethral valves from neurogenic bladder dysfunction. Also, with posterior urethral valves, the bladder wall appears thickened; hydroureters with dilation of the upper urinary tract may be seen (Table 11-1).

Other causes of bladder outlet obstruction include agenesis of the urethra, congenital urethral strictures, urethral tumors, and anterior urethral valves, all of which are rare.[16,17] Thickening of the bladder wall can also occur with cystitis.

Anterior urethral obstruction in males is uncommon but may be secondary to strictures, diverticula, or urethral duplication. Urethral obstruction in females is rare but may be seen in cloacal or female intersex anomalies.[17]

## EXSTROPHY

*Exstrophy of the bladder* is a complete ventral defect of the urogenital sinus and the overlying skeletal system. It is frequently associated with other congenital anomalies.[18] Classically, exstrophy of the bladder represents eversion of the viscus through a defect in the anterior abdominal wall associated with separation of the pubic symphysis.[17,18] The mucosal edges of the bladder and distal ends of the ureters fuse with the skin protruding through the lower central abdominal wall, which has failed to close. Urine spurts onto the abdominal wall from the ureteral orifices. The diagnosis can be made prenatally when no bladder is visualized, a lower abdominal bulge (representing the bladder) is located, and widening of the iliac crests is identified.[18]

The rami of the pubic bones are all widely separated. The pelvic ring thus lacks rigidity, the femurs are rotated externally, and the child duck waddles. Since the rectus muscles insert on the rami, they are widely separated from each other inferiorly. A hernia made up of exstrophic bladder and surrounding skin is therefore present. Bladder exstrophy is almost always accompanied by *epispadias*, a congenital opening of the urethra on the dorsum of the penis in males or by separation of the labia minora and a fissure of the clitoris in females. Renal infection is common, and hydronephrosis caused by ureterovesical obstruction may be found.[1] In this disorder, abnormal persistence of the cloacal membrane acts as a mechanical barrier to mesodermal movement during the first 6 weeks of embryonic life. Since this membrane extends from the hindgut to the allantoic duct, the associated anomalies may involve portions of the urinary, genital, musculoskeletal, and gastrointestinal systems[1] (Table 11-1).

## CONTRACTURE OF THE BLADDER NECK

Narrowing of the bladder neck is a common cause of vesicoureteral reflux, vesical diverticula, large bladder capacity, and the syndrome of irritable bladder associated with enuresis. This contracture has been considered a rare phenomenon. In females, the obstruction is due to spasm of the periurethral striated muscle, which develops secondary to distal urethral stenosis.[1]

## ECTOPIC URETER

The ureteric buds originate from the mesonephric duct instead of the cloaca, and this is often the embryologic basis for an ectopic insertion of the distal ureter in pelvic organs. In both sexes, the mesonephric duct migrates to a lower position on the urogenital sinus before it becomes the vas deferens in the male and disappears in the female. The ureters can be carried with it to open in ectopic locations. An ectopic ureter does not insert near the posterolateral angle of a normal trigone. Most ectopic ureters arise from the superior pelvis (upper moiety) of a duplex kidney and typically insert lower and more medially toward the base of the bladder.[11] In males, ectopic ureters may also insert in the seminal vesicle, vas deferens, or ejaculatory duct. In females, they may insert in the bladder neck, urethra, vestibule, vagina, or uterus[1,4] (Table 11-1).

## URETEROCELE

The *ureterocele* is a cyst-like enlargement of the lower end of the ureter[15] (Fig. 11-9A). Problems arise because (1) the ureteral opening in the wall of the sac is stenotic, and therefore hydroureter, hydronephrosis, and infection proximal to the ureterocele are common; and (2) the ureterocele sac itself may obstruct the bladder outlet or even prolapse through the urethra. An ectopic ureterocele is formed when the ectopic ureter is obstructed in the area where it enters the bladder, causing its anterior wall to balloon into the bladder.

Sonographic diagnosis of ectopic ureters and ectopic ureteroceles must include complete scanning of the kidneys. The duplex kidney may demonstrate two ureters arising from within, although frequently, they are difficult to distinguish. The ectopic ureter may be massively dilated and tortuous in the distal portion and mildly dilated proximally. Many variations are reported.[1] These extremely large ureters sometimes mimic multiseptate, cystic abdominal masses. Ectopic ureteroceles are dynamic structures that change shape and size according to intravesical pressure. Occasionally, a dilated ectopic ureter may indent the lower vesical wall of the bladder, simulating an ectopic ureterocele on sonography.

Simple ureteroceles are easy to see with sonography. In adults, they are usually incidental findings and are located at the expected location of the distal ureteral orifice. Sonographically, they appear as round or oval, thin-walled cystic structure on the posterior wall of a distended urinary bladder.[15,19] Real-time scanning shows these cystic areas as flexible in size as they fill and empty. Color Doppler of the ureteral jets verifies the diagnosis (Fig. 11-9B,C). Pathologic processes such as stones, tumors, or recent manipulation, can cause pseudoureteroceles. Newer transducer technology makes visualization of pseudoureteroceles, which appear thicker walled, possible.

## URACHAL VARIANTS

In the fetus, the bladder is located at the umbilicus and communicates with the allantoic canal, the extension of the cloacae/urogenital sinus, into the umbilical cord. The urachus is an embryonic tract formed as the bladder begins its descent into the true pelvis. As this occurs, the vertex of the bladder elongates, forming a fibromuscular appendage approximately 5 cm long surrounding the allantoic canal. This tract is normally obliterated by the time of birth. If the urachus fails to close, it creates an open channel between the bladder and the umbilicus.

There are four types of urachal anomalies[4]: (1) A patent urachus or fistula (completely patent lumen), occurs in 50% of cases. The urachus fails to close prior to birth and is usually associated with urethral obstruction. In this type, urine may drain constantly from the umbilicus. This serves as a protective mechanism to avoid an obstruction of the urinary bladder that may prevent normal fetal growth. (2) In 30% of cases, a urachal cyst develops when both ends of the urachus close off, trapping a small amount of urine in the canal.

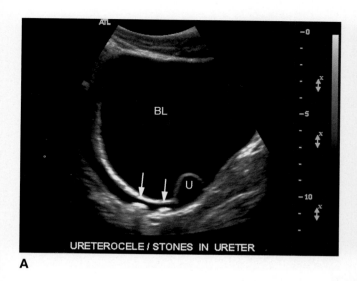

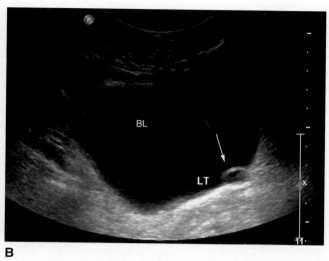

Figure 11-9 Ureterocele. **A.** Longitudinal image of the pelvis demonstrates a dilated ureter containing two echogenic calculi (arrows) and a thin walled ureterocele (U) in the bladder lumen (BL). **B,C.** Transverse image of the urinary bladder shows a small thin walled mass (arrow) projecting into the lumen of the bladder, color Doppler demonstrates the presence of a ureteral jet confirming the diagnosis of a small left ureterocele. (Image A courtesy of Philips Medical Systems, Bothell, WA.)

Clinically, the patient presents with a palpable mass, possible fever, and dysuria. Sonographically, a cystic structure is seen with possible internal echoes near the midline between the bladder and umbilicus. (3) A urachal sinus results, in 15% of cases, when the urachus closes at the bladder but not the umbilicus. (4) Urachal diverticulum, 5% of cases, results when the urachus closes at the umbilicus and remains patent at the bladder.

Urachal variants are easily identified on sonography by their characteristic location adjacent to the dome of the bladder.[4] Sonographically, an anechoic mass or a diverticular outpouching between the dome of the urinary bladder and the umbilicus is identified.

Complications of a persistent urachal sinus include infection, whereas complications of a urachal cyst include adenocarcinoma, calculi formation, or both. When detected, they are easily reexamined due to the easily assessable abdominal wall location.

A urachal remnant near the dome of the bladder can form from neoplasms. Mucinous adenocarcinoma is a leading precursor, and the remnant occurs most commonly in men aged 50 to 60 years. Stones may form in adenocarcinomas (Table 11-1).

# PATHOLOGY OF THE LOWER URINARY TRACT

## CYSTITIS

Urinary tract infections (UTIs) are extremely common, second only in prevalence to respiratory infections. UTI is a frequent cause of hospitalization in the United States and is responsible for significant morbidity and mortality.[20] Six million Americans are infected annually.[9]

Cystitis, inflammation of the bladder, always suggests predisposing risk factors which include urethral obstruction, common rectal or vaginal fistulas, catheterization, surgical instrumentation, bladder calculi, bladder neoplasm, trauma, debilitating illness, pregnancy, sexual intercourse, renal disease, obstructive conditions, radiation therapy, diabetes mellitus, and poor hygiene.[9,20] The most common cause of all urinary tract infections is the gram-negative intestinal bacteria

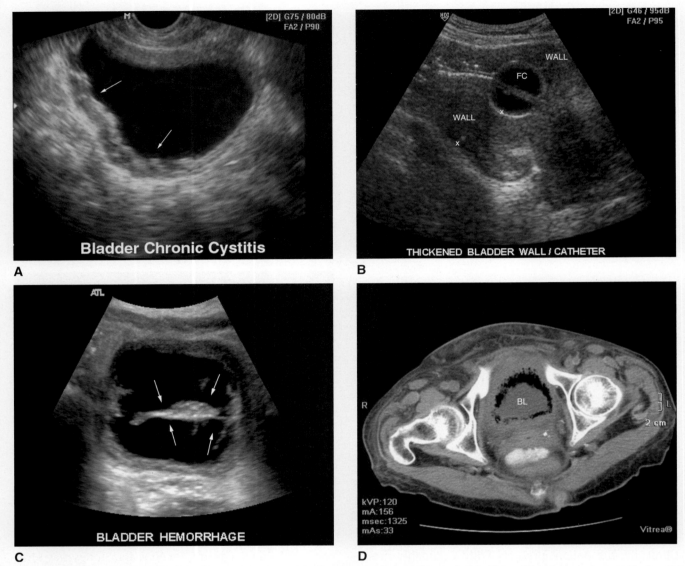

**Figure 11-10** Cystitis. **A.** Endovaginal image of the urinary bladder shows a thickened irregular bladder wall *(arrows)* consistent with chronic cystitis. **B.** Longitudinal image of empty urinary bladder with Foley catheter in place *(FC)*. The bladder wall is extremely thickened *(between calipers)* and collapsed around the Foley catheter. **C.** Transverse image of the urinary bladder in a patient with hemorrhagic cystitis. A blood clot *(arrows)* is seen adhering to the thickened bladder wall. **D.** Computed tomography scan of the pelvis in a patient with emphysematous cystitis shows air within the bladder wall *(BL)*. (Images A–C courtesy of Philips Medical Systems, Bothell, WA.)

*Escherichia coli.* Approximately 85% of all urinary tract infections are caused by *E. coli.*[9,20] Cystitis is more common in females owing to the short female urethra and proximity of the urethral opening and vagina to the anal area. Most infections are *ascending*, arising from organisms in the perineal area and traveling along the *continuous mucosa* of the urinary tract, to the bladder, or possibly even further along the ureter to the kidneys, causing pyelonephritis.[9]

Bullous cystitis, a common finding, is frequently associated with either an infection or catheterization. Constant Foley catheter drainage maintains an empty bladder resulting in continuous contact and irritation of the bladder mucosa with the catheter tip or balloon. Changes are seen: first, thickened bladder mucosa that

is smooth in the early stages and then becomes redundant and polypoid in the later stages (Fig. 11-10A–D). The thickened mucosa is usually hypoechoic, and the outline is often smooth. The underlying muscle wall is always intact. Bladder tumors tend to have shaggier, irregular outlines and are more echogenic. The transition between the tumor and the adjacent normal mucosa is abrupt. Cystitis usually presents as thickened bladder mucosa with hypoechoic or cystic structures along the wall.[3] Pathology Box 11-1 lists the types of cystitis, the most common etiology, and the distinctive sonographic appearance of each type based on histopathology. Diagnosis of the etiology requires correlation of the sonographic appearance with the patient's clinical signs, symptoms, and medical history.

## PATHOLOGY BOX 11-1

### Cystitis

| Type | Common Etiology | Sonographic Manifestations |
|---|---|---|
| Bullous | Infection | Focal bladder wall thickening in early, acute stages; small, contracted bladder in later, chronic stages. |
| *Candida albicans* | Hematogenous, lymphatic, or direct inoculation from anus | Mild thickening of bladder wall; discrete, dense, fluid–fluid-debris interface shifts with changing position. |
| Catheter induced | Irritation to bladder mucosa | Smooth, thickened, hypoechoic mucosa in early stages; redundant and polypoid in later stages. |
| Cystic | Nonspecific inflammatory; associated with chronic cystitis or chronic catheterization | Confined to trigone; thickened, irregular mucosa with cyst-like elevations; associated intravesical mass. |
| Emphysematous | *Escherichia coli* | Echogenic, "dirty" shadowing produced by gas collection within bladder wall. |
| Encrusted | Urinary salts precipitate on bladder surface | Focal bladder wall thickening in early, acute stages; small, contracted bladder in later, chronic stages. |
| Glandularis | Pelvic lipomatosis; chronic infection | Pronounced at ureterovesical junction. Diffuse mucosal thickening. May have echogenic fat surrounding bladder. |
| Hemorrhagic | Prolonged cyclophosphamide therapy | Intraluminal, echogenic debris caused by blood clots or wall thickening; focal calcification possible. |
| Purulent | Neurogenic dysfunction and urine stasis | Pus-urine fluid level. |
| Radiation induced | Radiation therapy | Ulceration, bladder wall sloughing, mucosal irregularity, and fistula formation in later stages. |
| Schistosomiasis | *Schistosoma haematobium* | Polypoid bladder wall thickening; bladder wall calcifications with discrete shadowing; fibrosis and small, contracted bladder in later, chronic stages; vesicoureteral |

## CALCULI

Bladder calculi are usually single and may be asymptomatic. They may cause inflammatory changes or acute bladder neck obstruction. Bladder neck obstruction by a calculus obstructs the flow of urine from the body. Predisposing factors to stone formation include increased concentration of salts in the urine, infection of the urinary tract, and urinary tract obstruction or stasis.[9] Stones usually appear as echogenic foci in the bladder, have an associated acoustic shadow, and shift to the dependent portion of the bladder with patient position changes (Fig. 11-11A C). The anterior fluid-filled bladder provides an excellent acoustic window for the identification of bladder calculi. Stones do not have to be calcified to be identified sonographically. Sonography can distinguish uric acid stones, which have an acoustic shadow and shift position, from a bladder tumor, which appears as a fixed mass without an acoustic shadow. Intradiverticular calculi can also be identified sonographically. In a patient with diverticula, infection and stone formation are common findings due to the stasis of residual urine remaining postvoid.

## REFLUX

Normally, the vesicoureteral junction allows urine to enter the bladder but prevents it from being regurgitated back into the ureter, particularly at the time of voiding. In this way, the kidney is protected from high pressure in the bladder and from contamination by infected vesical urine. When this valve is incompetent, the chance for secondary development of infection in the upper urinary tract is significant.

Reflux may occur as a result of an abnormality of the trigone and secondary to anomalies such as ectopia, posterior urethral valves, paraureteric cyst, prune belly syndrome, and neurogenic bladder.[4]

Vesicoureteral reflux occurs in two distinct groups: neonatal reflux, which is seen more commonly in males; and reflux in older children, which is more common in females. Hydronephrosis, either unilateral or bilateral, can be seen on a prenatal sonography examination. There is a high incidence of contralateral renal abnormalities, including ureteropelvic junction obstruction and duplex kidney.[4] High-pressure reflux (with or without associated UTI) may be a major cause of chronic renal failure with marked scarring and atrophic changes in the kidneys (see Chapter 20).

The sonography examination is valuable in the management of children with reflux, because it is less expensive, employs nonionizing radiation and can identify specific abnormalities. In the transverse plane, the sonographer must scan meticulously in the area where the ureters enter the bladder. Often, the ureter dilates with urine as the reflux is in progress and this may be visualized with real-time sonography.

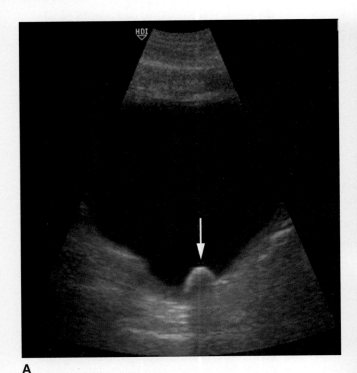

**A**

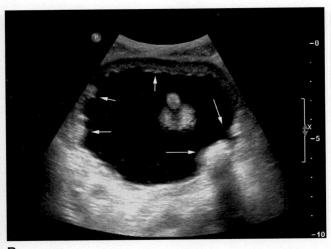

**B**

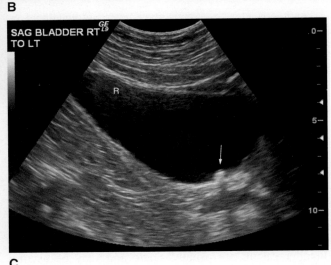

**C**

**Figure 11-11** Bladder calculi. **A.** Longitudinal image of the urinary bladder shows a well-defined, hyperechoic density with an acoustic shadow along the posterior bladder wall consistent with a bladder calculus (arrow). **B.** Transverse image of the urinary bladder shows multiple bladder calculi (large arrows) and a thickened irregular bladder wall (small arrows). **C.** Longitudinal image of the urinary bladder shows a small hyperechoic bladder calculus (small arrow) along the posterior bladder wall. The bladder calculus moved with a change in patient position. Reverberation is seen along the anterior bladder wall (R). (Images **A,B** courtesy of Philips Medical Systems, Bothell, WA.)

## DISTAL URETERAL OBSTRUCTION

Ureterovesical junction obstruction describes an obstruction at the junction of the distal ureter where it enters the bladder. To differentiate a ureterovesical junction obstruction from nonobstructive causes such as reflux, a voiding cystourethrogram (VCUG) may be necessary. The causes of distal ureteral obstruction may be congenital or acquired. Congenital causes include primary megaureter, primary megaureter with coexisting reflux, primary megaureter with coexisting bladder saccule, simple ureterocele, ectopic ureter, and ectopic ureterocele. Acquired causes include ureteral reimplantation procedures, infection, and stricture following the passage of stones. The sonographic findings include megaureter, hydronephrosis, and ectopic ureter, with or without ectopic ureterocele.

## NEUROGENIC BLADDER

A patient with a neurogenic bladder has lost voluntary control of voiding due to a disturbance in the neural pathways. Depending on the nerves involved and nature

of damage, the bladder becomes either overactive (spastic or hyperreflexive) or underactive (flaccid or hypotonic). *Myelodysplasia* (a neural tube defect consisting of defective development of part of the spinal cord) is the most common cause of neurogenic bladder in infants and children. Other causes include: (1) neurologic diseases (multiple sclerosis, syringomyelia, Parkinson disease), (2) congenital anomalies (partial or total absence of the sacrum or meningomyelocele), (3) systemic diseases with neurologic complications (diabetes mellitus, pernicious anemia), (4) infection (herpes zoster, poliomyelitis, spinal cord abscess), (5) trauma (vertebral fractures, operative trauma, disk herniation), (6) brain and spinal neoplasm, (7) central nervous system vascular disease, and (8) heavy metal poisoning. Neurogenic bladder is common in paraplegic patients.[7]

Individuals with overactive bladder have little to no control over voiding functions. Their bladders release urine spontaneously and frequently, although not completely. Their bladders become diminished because they are seldom filled to capacity. Because their bladders tend to retain small quantities of urine, the risk of UTI is significantly increased. Neurogenic *underactive* bladders have the opposite characteristics. Because there is damage to the neural system that informs the brain the bladder is full, the bladder continues to fill and may expand beyond the size and capacity of a normal bladder. At a certain point, the pressure of urine in the bladder will overcome the sphincter muscles ability to retain it and urine will leak out. Like the overactive bladder, an underactive bladder fails to empty completely and retains a small amount of residual urine.

Many patients have a trabeculated bladder and spasm of the external sphincter, causing relative obstruction and narrowing of the urethra as it courses through the urogenital diaphragm. The patient may find it extremely difficult or impossible to void. Because of the obstruction, the pressure in the bladder remains constantly high, which may result in detrusor hypertrophy, the formation of saccules and diverticula, and vesicoureteral reflux[7,21] (Fig. 11-12A–C). Since the urine is chronically infected in such patients, the result may be chronic reflux pyelonephritis, the formation of struvite stones, or bladder debris.[7]

Patients with neurogenic bladder usually undergo serial excretory urography and voiding cystourethrograms. Sonography is performed to aid in the diagnosis of trabeculated bladder, ureterectasis, vesicoureteral reflux, hydronephrosis, or bladder calculi.

## BLADDER WALL ABNORMALITIES

One of the most frequent sonographically observed abnormalities of the bladder is thickening of the bladder wall. This is commonly due to outlet obstruction. Other causes include neurogenic bladder, cystitis, edema from adjacent inflammatory processes, radiation, and primary or secondary neoplasms[10] (Pathology Box 11-2). Patients with inflammatory bladder pathology may have signs and symptoms similar to those of patients with urinary bladder or kidney neoplasm.[11]

Certain pathologic conditions are manifested with extrinsic bladder compression, invasion of the urinary bladder, or both. Endometriosis can present as an intravesical lesion by either direct extension or implantation. Regional enteritis (Crohn disease) has been

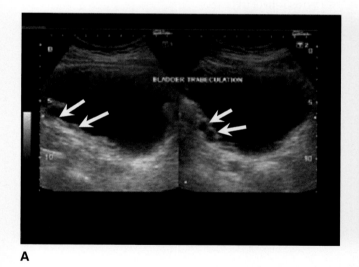

**A**

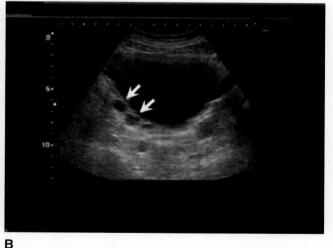

**B**

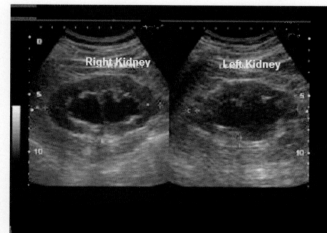

**C**

**Figure 11-12** Neurogenic bladder. **A.** Longitudinal images of the urinary bladder show the presence of bladder saccules *(arrows)*, a sign that bladder outlet obstruction has begun to have adverse effects on the urinary tract. **B.** A postvoid image shows a large postvoid residual within the bladder. Bladder saccules *(arrows)* are seen along the lateral wall. **C.** Longitudinal images of both kidneys show bilateral hydronephrosis.

---

**PATHOLOGY BOX 11-2**

### *Causes of Bladder Wall Thickening*

| Focal | Diffuse |
|---|---|
| **Neoplasm** | |
| Transitional cell carcinoma | Transitional cell carcinoma |
| Squamous cell carcinoma | Squamous cell carcinoma |
| Adenocarcinoma | Adenocarcinoma |
| Lymphoma | |
| **Infectious/Inflammatory** | |
| Tuberculosis (acute) | Cystitis |
| Schistosomiasis (acute); flukes living in the pulmonary venous system and its tributaries or within the veins draining the bladder; serious destruction to surroundung tissue; "swimmers itch" | Tuberculosis (chronic) |
| Cystitis | Schistosomiasis (chronic) |
| Cystitis cystica | |
| Cystitis glandularis | |
| Fistula | |
| **Medical Diseases** | |
| Endometriosis | Interstitial cystitis |
| Amyloidosis | Amyloidosis |
| **Trauma** | **Neurogenic Bladder** |
| Hematoma | Detrusor hyperreflexia |
| Ruptured bladder | **Bladder Outlet** |
| | **Obstruction with Muscular Dystrophy** |

---

reported as a loop of small bowel with thick walls and a narrowed lumen adhering to the bladder dome.[5] Focal or diffuse bladder wall thickening can occur with neurofibromatosis.[4]

In arteriovenous malformation, there is an abnormal connection between the arterial and venous vessels. The higher pressure in the arterial system causes blood to be routed directly from the artery into the vein, which increases blood flow through the veins. A natural response for the vein under increased blood volume is to dilate.

# TRAUMA

## RUPTURE

Bladder rupture follows severe blunt lower abdominal or pelvic trauma or penetrating abdominal or perineal injury. If the bladder was full at the time of blunt injury, rupture is more likely to occur, spilling urine into the peritoneum. Pelvic crush injuries cause bladder rupture in 1% to 15% of cases, four-fifths being extraperitoneal. A urinoma may result from temporary sealing of a small tear. The sonographic appearance of a urinoma is of an anechoic mass with enhanced through-transmission. The mass may have irregular borders and contain septa and may compress surrounding tissue (Fig. 11-13A,B). The best diagnostic procedure for visualizing bladder rupture is cystography.

## BLOOD CLOTS

Blood clots, either from a pathologic process or from trauma, may adhere to the bladder wall, giving a sonographic appearance similar to that of a tumor (Fig. 11-14A–C). They appear as an irregularity along the mucosal surface. Most blood clots are mobile and will move freely with changes in the patient's position and will not demonstrate the presence of vascularity with color Doppler.

## BLADDER FLAP HEMATOMA

During a cesarean section, the surgeon incises the vesicouterine reflection of the peritoneum to obtain access to the lower uterine segment, creating a potential space between the bladder and uterus commonly known as the *bladder flap*.[22] If hemostasis is not obtained after closure of the uterine incision, a hematoma forms between the lower uterine segment and the urinary bladder (bladder flap) or anywhere the surgical scalpel made an incision (abdominal wall, muscle).

A patient with a hematoma can present with fever, a mass, or a dropping hematocrit. An infected hematoma can manifest with the same symptoms, but the patient can additionally have leukocytosis and more pain. The fever can be caused by the infected hematoma alone or by postsurgical complications such as endometritis,

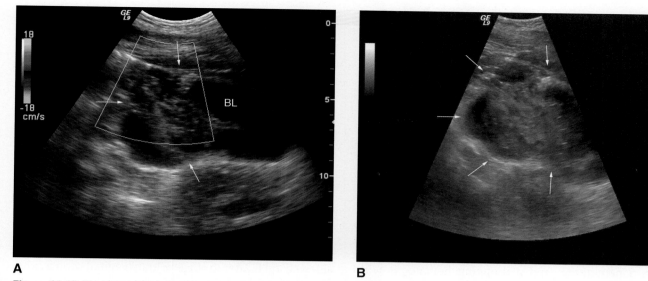

**A**

**B**

**Figure 11-13** Bladder rupture. **A.** Transverse image of the pelvis in a man who experienced recent blunt pelvic trauma. A complex mass *(arrows)* is seen to the right of the urinary bladder *(BL)*. This mass is consistent with a hematoma. No color flow is seen within the mass. **B.** Longitudinal image to the right of the bladder shows the complex hematoma *(arrows)*.

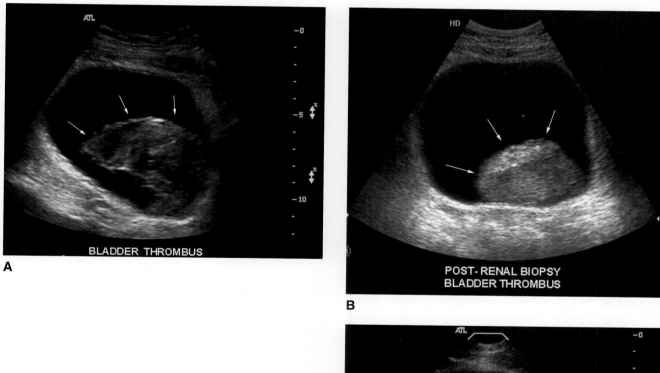

BLADDER THROMBUS

**A**

POST-RENAL BIOPSY
BLADDER THROMBUS

**B**

**Figure 11-14** Blood clot. **A.** Longitudinal image of the urinary bladder shows a large, irregular, echogenic mass *(arrows)* along the posterior abdominal wall. This mass was diagnosed as a blood clot within the bladder. **B.** Transverse image of the urinary bladder shows a large echogenic mass *(arrows)* along the posterior bladder wall. This was diagnosed as a blood clot that developed after a renal biopsy. **C.** Longitudinal image of the urinary bladder shows a large, irregular, echogenic mass *(arrows)* along the posterior abdominal wall. This mass was also diagnosed as a blood clot within the bladder. (Images courtesy of Philips Medical, Bothell, WA.)

**C**

septic thrombophlebitis, abscess, hematoma, or wound infection.[22]

The incidence of bladder flap hematoma is unknown. The sonographic appearances described in the literature vary significantly and include a mass as large as 15 × 12 × 9 cm (length × width × height).[22] The majority of bladder flap hematomas are complex masses with poorly defined borders that are primarily anechoic, with internal septations or debris.[22]

Because it is not possible to differentiate sonographically between a hematoma, an infected hematoma, and an abscess, the patient's clinical presentation is important.[22] A symptomatic patient with a clinical history of leukocytosis suggests an abscess; a dropping hematocrit, a hematoma; and a dropping hematocrit with leukocytosis, an infected hematoma.

If there is a suspected hematoma near the incisional site of the abdominal wall, a high frequency (5 to 10 MHz) linear array transducer and a standoff pad may be required to examine the superficial area. If the incisional site has not healed, sterile gel and a transducer cover must be used to reduce the risk of contamination. This area may be more difficult to examine because of incisional pain and tenderness. To distinguish between a superficial wound and a subfascial hematoma, the rectus muscle must be identified. Superficial hematomas are located anterior to the rectus muscle, and subfascial hematomas are located posterior to it.[23] The typical location for a subfascial hematoma is in the prevesicular space, ventral to the bladder. Based on the sonographic appearance, a superficial hematoma or a subfascial hematoma may appear the same as an abscess or an infected hematoma, making clinical correlation extremely important.

# BLADDER NEOPLASMS

Bladder tumors are frequently found in urogenital imaging, many times in patients having renal sonography for painless hematuria. Bladder tumors are usually epithelial or uroepithelial in origin and are one of the most common tumors of the genitourinary tract. While painless hematuria is the most common symptom, other symptoms may include dysuria, urinary frequency, or urgency.[12,24] An infiltrating tumor disrupts the uniformity of the normal 3 to 5 mm bladder wall thickness (Fig. 11-15A). Hydronephrosis often occurs due to the obstructed outflow of urine. Blood clot, benign prostatic hypertrophy, cystitis, fungal balls, stones, and bladder trabeculae can mimic bladder tumors[3,24] (Fig. 11-15B).

For initial screening of suspected bladder tumor, sonography is an excellent noninvasive, cost-effective, and nonionizing imaging modality. Cystoscopy involves inserting a cystoscope through the urethra into the bladder. Cystoscopy with biopsy is considered the most accurate method for detecting and evaluating bladder tumors, but it is invasive and requires anesthesia.[12,24]

Tumors located in the neck or dome of the bladder are difficult to detect with sonography.[3,24] The ability of sonography to detect the presence or absence of bladder tumors has varied from 33% for tumors smaller than 0.5 cm in diameter to 83% for tumors 1 to 2 cm to 95% for tumors larger than 2 cm.[3,24] Apart from the size and location of the tumor, the degree of bladder distention or obesity may affect the accuracy of tumor detection.

Endovaginal longitudinal scanning has proven effective in the diagnosis of tumors located in any part of the urinary bladder. The endovaginal approach provides good image quality, allowing the tumor to be studied in detail through the anterior wall, the neck, and the apex of the urinary bladder. Bladder tumors situated on the sidewall are harder to stage by transvaginal sonography.

Following the diagnosis of carcinoma of the bladder, sonography can also be helpful in staging tumors. Evidence indicates that the stage of the tumor profoundly influences curability and survival time.[25] The tumor's response to chemotherapy is the primary determinant of whether to continue therapy. Sonography is a useful adjunct to cystoscopy when serial scans of bladder tumors are performed. When sonography and cystoscopy are used together, the staging of bladder tumors is more accurate than when either study is used alone. CT is the imaging modality of choice for identifying contiguous extension of bladder neoplasms and has reduced the number of overstaging and understaging errors.[4,11,25]

## BENIGN NEOPLASMS

*Papilloma*, a benign tumor, is a forerunner of transitional cell carcinoma. Sonographically, papillomas are usually 0.5 to 2 cm in size and have the same appearance as transitional cell carcinoma. The most common location is along the lateral urinary bladder wall; the second most common location is the trigone.

## MALIGNANT NEOPLASMS

According to the National Cancer Institute, each year over 70,000 new cases of bladder cancer are diagnosed and over 14,000 will die from the disease.[26] Bladder carcinoma is the fourth most common type of cancer in men and the eighth most common in women.[26] Men, Caucasians, and smokers have up to three times the risk of bladder cancer than the general population. When diagnosed and treated in a localized stage, bladder cancer is very treatable, with a 5-year cancer-specific survival rate approaching 95%.[26]

Ninety percent are *transitional cell carcinoma* (TCC), a cancer that begins in the cells that normally make up the inner lining of the bladder.[24] Smoking, analgesic abuse, and industrial carcinogen exposure predispose patients to TCC cancer. Five percent are squamous cell carcinomas, the most aggressive of the malignant tumors.[24] They are associated with chronic inflammatory

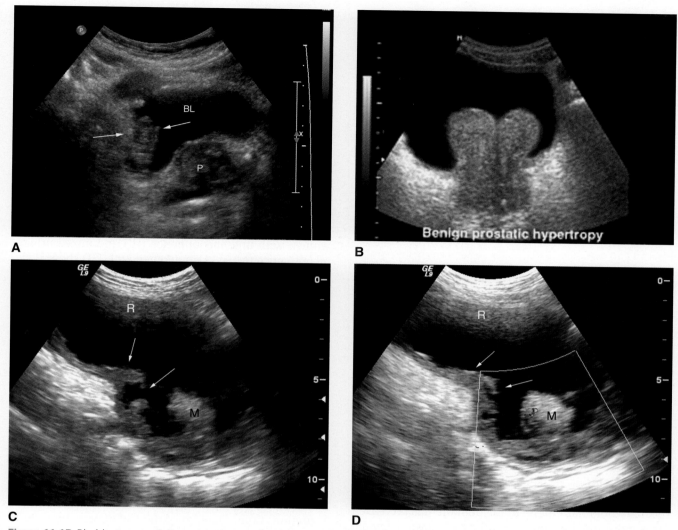

**Figure 11-15** Bladder tumors. **A.** Transverse image of a male pelvis shows a focal irregular thickening of the right lateral bladder wall (arrows) consistent with bladder carcinoma. The prostate (P) is seen posterior to the urinary bladder (BL). **B.** Transverse image of a male pelvis shows a grossly enlarged prostate gland (P) indenting the posterior wall of the bladder. An enlarged prostate gland can be mistaken for a bladder tumor. **C,D.** Longitudinal images of the urinary bladder demonstrate an irregular, echogenic mass projecting into the bladder lumen (M). Note the bladder wall thickening along the bladder wall (arrows). Reverberation is seen along the anterior bladder wall (R). Color Doppler reveals flow within the mass helping to distinguish the bladder tumor from a blood clot. (Images C-D courtesy of Tim S. Gibbs, Anaheim, CA.)

conditions, neurogenic bladder, stones, and patients having bladder schistosomiasis.[25] Two percent of bladder tumors are adenocarcinomas, which are associated with urachal remnants and bladder extrophy.[11,24]

Sonographically, TCC tumors are visualized as an irregular echogenic mass, either polypoid or sessile, that projects into the lumen of the bladder, are fixed to the bladder wall, and may have associated acoustic shadowing.[3,25] Color Doppler shows detectable blood flow in the malignant bladder tumor (Fig. 11-15C,D).

Whenever there is focal thickening of the bladder wall, a malignant primary urinary bladder tumor should be suspected. Sonographically, malignant masses present as echogenic structures protruding into the echo-free bladder lumen. Infiltrating tumors disrupt the normal uniformity of the bladder wall.

## METASTATIC

Metastatic urinary bladder tumors occur most commonly by direct extension from the cervix, uterus, prostate, and rectum, in that order[3] (Fig. 11-16). They may also develop from direct extension from the upper urinary system directly, or by the lymphatic or vascular system. (For a more detailed discussion, see Chapters 9, 10, and 12 and the volume *Obstetrics and Gynecology* in this series.) Prostatic cancer usually metastasizes to the seminal vesicles and perivesical connective tissue.

## STRESS INCONTINENCE

The most common micturition abnormality is stress incontinence. Forty percent of postmenopausal women are affected by incontinence.[27] The condition is caused

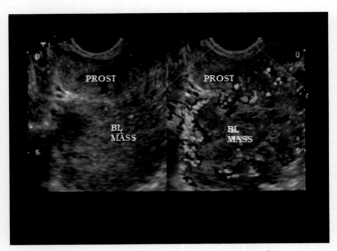

**Figure 11-16** Metastatic invasion. Transrectal image of the prostate demonstrates a large tumor from the prostate invading the urinary bladder. Metastatic tumors of the urinary bladder can occur as a result from direct extension of prostate cancer.

by genuine stress incontinence, detrusor instability, voiding difficulty (overflow), fistulas, and functional or congenital disorders. It may be a temporary condition due to UTIs. Stress incontinence is the leakage of urine from the bladder during acts that increase intra-abdominal and intravesicular pressure, such as Valsalva maneuvers, coughing, or straining.[28]

Incontinence is receiving increased attention by both the public and medical professionals. Many women suffer stress incontinence and are too embarrassed to admit it, seek help, or are unaware of available treatments. As the urogynecology surgical specialty field has emerged, the demand has increased for a more detailed understanding of normal female pelvic floor anatomy.[27–29] Sonography is being used to diagnose and treat incontinence.[28–30] Sonographic evaluation of stress incontinence requires more a detailed pelvic floor assessment. Endovaginal, endorectal, transperineal, and transabdominal methods can all be used to directly observe bladder filling and emptying.[28,30] Three-dimensional sonography is playing an important role in urogynecologic research.[28,29] Transvaginal sonography is sensitive and specific but cannot be used exclusively to determine urinary stress incontinence in females. The pitfalls of using the transperineal method include an overdistended bladder, poor penetration, an excessively small field of view, bowel gas, focal uterine contractions, bladder mistaken for cervix, fluid in the vaginal vault mistaken for cervix, cervical cysts, and pericervical veins.

Stress incontinence is caused by a poorly supported bladder neck (the section between the bladder and the urethra).[28,30] Coughing or bearing down results in the bladder neck moving inferiorly, the urethra opens, and urine is pushed out. Depending on the extent of the findings surgical repair can be an option. A suburethral sling and an anterior repair can be performed and consist of placing a small piece of plastic around the bladder neck to hold it in place, and at the same time, lifting the sagging bladder and stabilizing it.[27,28]

Using dynamic transurethral sonography, Mitterberger et al. showed partial or complete loss of rhabdosphincter function in patients with urethral sphincter deficiency. The findings correlated well with the grade of incontinence.[29] Assessment of intrinsic urethral sphincter deficiency (ISD), bladder neck hypermobility, and urethral diameter has been studied using translabial sonography. Women with the diagnosis of urinary incontinence were examined translabially and showed significantly greater bladder neck descent than continent women and women with urge incontinence (UI) and mixed urinary incontinence (MUI). Also, women with ISD showed significantly larger urethral diameters than control subjects and incontinent women without IDS. This study showed that a simplified method of sonographic imaging was useful in assessing patients with stress incontinence.[28,29]

## SUMMARY

- The lower urinary tract consists of the pelvic ureters, bladder, and urethra and is responsible for transporting and storing urine.

- The bladder wall is composed of three layers: the connective tissue submucosa, a muscle layer, and the adventitia and is lined with a transitional epithelium.

- The trigone is located on the floor of the bladder and contains three openings for the two ureters and the urethra. Color Doppler of the trigone can be used to visualize ureteral jets.

- Congenital bladder anomalies include duplication, agenesis, exstrophy, diverticula, ectopic ureter, ureterocele, and posterior urethral valves.

- Posterior urethral valves are abnormal valves located in the posterior urethra and are the most common cause of urinary obstruction in male infants. A dilated, elongated prostatic urethra is diagnostic of posterior urethral valves.

- An ectopic ureter is usually the result of a duplicated collecting system and typically inserts lower and more medially in the bladder. In males, ectopic ureters may also insert in the seminal vesicle, vas deferens, or ejaculatory duct. In females, they may insert in the bladder neck, urethra, vestibule, vagina, or uterus.

- A ureterocele is a cyst-like enlargement of the lower end of the ureter that can cause hydronephrosis or a bladder outlet obstruction if the structure blocks the ureteral or urethral openings.

- If one or both ends of the urachus fail to close completely, a patent urachus or urachal cyst can develop

## Critical Thinking Questions

1. A 22-year-old woman presents with hematuria, painful urination, and urinary frequency. Sonography of her bladder demonstrates a uniformly thickened bladder wall. What is the likely diagnosis based on the clinical presentation and sonographic findings, and what are some of the common causes of this pathology?

2. A 60-year-old man presents with a history of painless hematuria for a sonography examination of his kidneys and bladder. An echogenic mass is seen projecting into the bladder lumen. What is the likely diagnosis?

3. List the common causes and locations of obstruction in the lower urinary tract.

4. When scanning a female patient for a pelvic sonography examination, the sonographer notices a cystic area adjacent to the bladder. With careful scanning, a connection between the cystic area and the bladder is documented. What does this cystic area likely represent?

5. A 45-year-old patient presents for an evaluation of his bladder with a history of a spinal cord injury 20 years ago. What do you expect to see when scanning his bladder?

and can be seen near the dome of the bladder. The cyst can become infected.

- Cystitis, also referred to as a lower urinary tract infection, has many causes, the most common of which is *E. coli* infection. Sonographically, cystitis presents as a thickened bladder wall.

- Sonographically, bladder calculi usually appear as echogenic foci in the bladder, have an associated acoustic shadow, and shift to the dependent portion of the bladder with patient position changes and may be associated with inflammation or obstruction.

- A patient with a neurogenic bladder has lost voluntary control of voiding due to a disturbance in the neural pathways. The high-pressure environment in the bladder can cause a trabeculated bladder wall, diverticula, and vesicoureteral reflux.

- During a cesarean section a potential space is created between the bladder wall and the uterus known as the bladder flap; a bladder flap hematoma may develop in this space and may become infected.

- The most common presenting symptom of bladder tumors is hematuria; however, dysuria, urinary frequency, urgency, and obstruction can also occur.

- Papilloma is a benign tumor of the bladder that has a similar appearance to transitional cell carcinoma.

- Malignant tumors of the bladder include transitional cell carcinoma (the most common), squamous cell carcinoma, and adenocarcinoma and present sonographically as an echogenic mass that projects into the lumen of the bladder or a focal wall thickening.

- Stress incontinence is defined as a leakage of urine from the bladder during activities that increase intra-abdominal pressure such as coughing or straining and can be caused by a poorly supported bladder neck or urethral sphincter deficiency. Sonography can play a role in the diagnosis and treatment of stress incontinence.

## REFERENCES

1. Cochard L. *Netter's Atlas of Human Embryology*. St. Louis: Elsevier Mosby; 2002.
2. Gray H. *Anatomy of the Human Body*. Philadelphia: Lea & Febiger; 1918.
3. McAchran SE, Hartke DM, Nakamoto DA, et al. Sonography of the urinary bladder. *Ultrasound Clin*. 2007;2:17–26.
4. Rumack C, Wilson W, Charboneau W. *Diagnostic Ultrasound*. St. Louis: Elsevier Mosby; 2005.
5. Marieb EN, Hoehn K. *Human Anatomy and Physiology*. San Francisco: Pearson Benjamin Cummings; 2007.
6. Scanlon VC, Sanders T. *Essentials of Anatomy and Physiology*. Philadelphia: FA Davis; 2003.
7. Samson G, Cardenas DD. Neurogenic bladder in spinal cord injury. *Phys Med Rehabil Clin N Am*. 2007;18:255–274.
8. Bradley CS, Smith KE, Kreder KJ. Urodynamic evaluation of the bladder and pelvic floor. *Gastroenterol Clin North Am*. 2008;37:539–552.
9. Gould BE. *Pathophysiology for the Health Professionals*. St. Louis: Saunders; 2006.
10. Yang JM, Huang WC. Bladder wall thickness on ultrasonographic cystourethrography: affecting factors and their implications. *J Ultrasound Med*. 2003;22:777–782.
11. Middleton WD, Kurtz AB, Hertzberg BS. *Ultrasound: The Requisites*. St. Louis: Mosby; 2003.
12. Kocakoc E, Kiris A, Orhan I, et al. Detection of bladder tumors with 3-dimensional sonography and virtual sonographic cystoscopy. *J Ultrasound Med*. 2008;27:45–53.
13. Suwanrath C, Suntharasaj T, Sirapatanapipat H, et al. Three-dimensional ultrasonographic bladder volume measurement: reliability of the Virtual Organ Computer-aided Analysis technique using different rotation steps. *J Ultrasound Med*. 2009;28:847–854.
14. Goldberg BB, Badgley D, Liu JB, et al. Endoluminal sonography of the urinary tract: Preliminary observations. *Am J Roentgenol*. 1991;155:99–103.
15. Palmer LS. Pediatric urologic imaging. *Urol Clin North Am*. 2006;33:409–423.
16. Henningsen C. *Clinical Guide to Ultrasonography*. St. Loius: Mosby; 2004.
17. Doublet P, Benson C. *Atlas of Ultrasound in Obstetrics and Gynecology*. Philadelphia: Lippincott Williams and Wilkins; 2003.

18. Gearhart JP, Rink RR, Mouriquand P. The bladder exstrophy-epispadias complex. In: Gearhart JP, ed. *Pediatric Urology*. Philadelphia: Saunders; 2010;511–546.

19. Gearhart JP, Jeffs RD. Exstrophy of the bladder, epispadias, and other bladder anomalies. In: Walsh PC, Retik AB, Stamey TA, et al. eds. *Campbell's Urology*. St. Louis: WB Saunders; 1998:1772–1821.

20. Drekonja DM, Johnson JR. Urinary tract infections. *Prim Care Clin Office Pract*. 2008;35:345–367.

21. Crowley L. *An Introduction to Human Disease*. Sudbury, MA: Jones and Bartlett; 2001.

22. Winsett MZ, Fagan CJ, Bedi DG. Sonographic demonstration of bladder-flap hematoma. *J Ultrasound Med*. 1986;5:483–487.

23. Gill K. *Abdominal Ultrasound*. Philadelphia: WB Saunders; 2001.

24. Zhang J, Gerst S, Lefkowitz, RA, et al. Imaging of bladder cancer. *Radiol Clin N Am*. 2007;45:183–205.

25. Eisenberg R, Johnson, N. *Comprehensive Radiographic Pathology*. 4th ed. St. Louis: Mosby; 2007.

26. U.S. National Institutes of Health. *National Cancer Institute*. Available at: www.cancer.gov, 2010.

27. Hall, R. Clinical Update: *Pelvic floor imaging for the urogynecology patient*. Educators' Summit. Milwaukee, WI: Seattle University; 2008–2009.

28. Unger CA, Weinstein MW, Pretorius DH. Pelvic floor imaging. *Obstet Gynecol Clin North Am*. 2011;38:23–43.

29. Mitterberger M, Pinggera GM, Mueller T, et al. Dynamic transurethral sonography and 3-dimensional reconstruction of the rhabdosphincter and urethra: initial experience in continent and incontinent women. *J Ultrasound Med*. 2006;25:315–320.

30. Oliveira F, Ramos J, Martins-Costa S. Translabial ultrasonography in the assessment of urethral diameter and intrinsic sphincter deficiency. *J Ultrasound Med*. 2006;25:1153–1158.

# 12 The Prostate Gland

George M. Kennedy

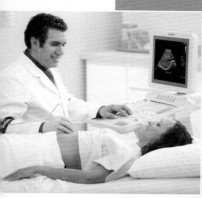

## OBJECTIVES

Discuss embryologic development, differentiation of structures, and hormones influencing the maturation of the prostate gland.

Identify surface, relational, and internal prostate anatomy to include differentiating the four prostate zones.

Demonstrate routine scanning procedure to include the patient preparation; patient instructions; patient positions; transrectal, transabdominal, and biopsy techniques; technical considerations; and common scanning pitfalls.

Describe the pathology, etiology, clinical signs and symptoms, and sonographic appearance of cysts in the male pelvis to include müllerian duct and utricle cysts, seminal vesicle cyst, prostatic cyst (prostatic abscess), and diverticulum of the ejaculatory duct of vas deferens.

Explain the pathology, etiology, clinical signs and symptoms, and sonographic appearance of benign prostatic hyperplasia.

Identify the pathology, etiology, clinical signs and symptoms, and sonographic appearance of prostate calcifications.

Categorize the pathology, etiology, clinical signs and symptoms, and sonographic appearance of prostatitis to include acute bacterial prostatitis, chronic bacterial prostatitis, chronic pain syndrome, and asymptomatic inflammatory prostatitis.

Recognize sonographic characteristics of benign and malignant conditions of the prostate gland.

Discuss the role of prostate sonography in biopsy guidance procedures and evaluation of suspected male infertility.

## KEY TERMS

benign prostatic hyperplasia (BPH) | digital rectal examination (DRE) | infertility | neurovascular bundle | prostate biopsy | prostate cancer | prostate-specific antigen (PSA) | prostatitis | transrectal ultrasound (TRUS) | transurethral resection of the prostate (TURP)

## GLOSSARY

**apex** inferior portion of the prostate gland, which is located superior to the urogenital diaphragm

**base** superior portion of the prostate gland, which is located below the inferior margin of the urinary bladder

**corpora amylacea** calcifications commonly seen in the inner gland of the prostate

**Eiffel Tower sign** is a shadowing created by calcification in the area of the urethra and verumontanum

**ejaculatory ducts** duct that passes through the central zone and empties into the urethra; originates from the combination of the vas deferens and the seminal vesicle

**endogenous calculi** developing or grown from within; calculi formation within the substance of the prostate

**exogenous calculi** developing or originating outside; calculi found in the urethra

**seminal vesicles** a pair of simple tubular glands that extend from outpouching of the vas deferens; they are located superior and posterior to the prostate, between the urinary bladder and rectum

**surgical capsule** a demarcation between the inner gland (central and transitional zones) and the outer gland (peripheral zone), which normally appears hypoechoic but may be echogenic if corpora amylacea or calcifications occur along the line

**vas deferens** reproductive duct that extends from the epididymis to the ejaculatory duct; also known as the ductus deferens

**verumontanum** a longitudinal elevation or ridge within the prosthetic urethral wall where the orifices of the ejaculatory ducts are located on either side

Transrectal ultrasound (TRUS) of the prostate has improved markedly over the past two decades. Equipment technology has progressed from one of the earliest devices, a chair type apparatus with a mechanical probe mounted in the center,[1] to current phased array and three-dimensional (3D) transducers (Fig. 12-1). TRUS is utilized to evaluate the prostate in the setting of malignancy, infertility, chronic pelvic pain syndrome CPPS, and congenital abnormalities. It also plays a significant role in biopsy and treatment guidance.[1] The role of contrast agents in prostate tumor assessment is also being investigated.[1-3]

A sonography examination of the prostate requires a thorough understanding of the anatomy of the prostate and the sonographic characteristics of disease processes.

## ANATOMY AND ORGANOGENESIS

During embryogenesis, all embryos start out with two paired sex ducts, the mesonephric or wolffian ducts and the paramesonephric or müllerian ducts. Each müllerian duct lies lateral to its corresponding wolffian duct.[4] This is termed the indifferent stage.[4] The mesonephric ducts are responsible for development of the male reproductive system, whereas the paramesonephric ducts will form the female reproductive system. A portion of each mesonephric duct will later develop into an ejaculatory duct, vas deferens, and seminal vesicle. In the 11th gestational week, the prostate begins to form from the urogenital sinus, an endodermal derivative. It begins as multiple solid outgrowths of the prostatic portion of the urethra, which form on the posterior

side of the urogenital sinus.[4] As development continues, these penetrate the surrounding mesenchyme to form the five prostatic lobes.[5] Maturation of the gland continues while testosterone levels are high. However, as these levels decrease the gland enters a quiescent state until puberty when testosterone levels rise again.

## GROSS ANATOMY

The adult prostate is a funnel shaped, glandular structure surrounded by a fibrous capsule. In a young adult, it weighs approximately $20 \pm 6$ g and measures on average $4 \times 3 \times 2$ cm. The prostate is composed of glandular and fibromuscular tissue and surrounds the proximal male urethra. The cephalic portion of the gland is referred to as the base, and the caudal end the apex. The base is continuous with the bladder neck, and the apex is adherent to the urogenital diaphragm. Three luminal structures traverse the prostate gland: the right and left ejaculatory duct, and the urethra (Fig. 12-2). The prostatic urethra traverses the central portion of the gland. The duct of the seminal vesicle joins the ampullae of the vas deferens to form the ejaculatory duct at the prostate base. The ejaculatory duct travels within the central zone of the gland to the midline where it joins the urethra at the verumontanum, a longitudinal ridge on the posterior wall of the prostatic urethra.[1,6] This structure is located at the midpoint of the prostatic urethra near the apex and is laterally flanked by openings of the ejaculatory ducts (Fig. 12-3). The utricle is a glandular grouping at the crest of the verumontanum. It is a vestigial of the paramesonephric duct and urogenital sinus and is homologous to the female uterus.[4,6,7] This structure accounts for the "Eiffel Tower" appearance on transverse images of the prostate gland obtained at this level[1,8] (Fig. 12-4).

## VASCULATURE

The prostate is supplied from the internal iliac arteries by the prostaticovesical arteries.[1,9] The arteries course along the medial and inferior surface of the bladder toward the prostate along the neurovascular bundle.[10] The artery on either side bifurcates into the prostatic artery and inferior vesicle artery, which further branch into the urethral and capsular arteries. The capsular vessels are arranged on the surface of the gland in five anterolateral and posterolateral groups. These capsular vessels travel along and supply approximately two-thirds of the glandular tissue.[9,10] The urethral arteries are directed inward and follow the course of the prostatic urethra, supplying the other one-third of the glandular tissue.[9,10]

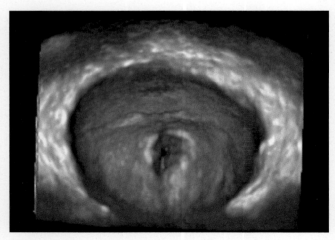

**Figure 12-1** The sonogram is a three-dimensional reconstruction of the prostate gland. (Image courtesy of Philips Medical Systems, Bothell, WA.)

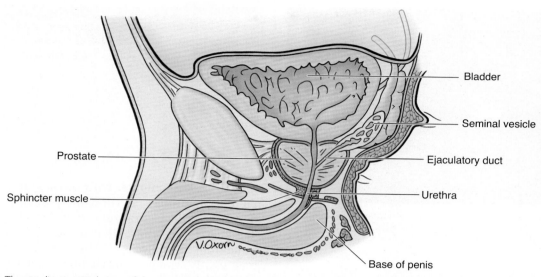

**Figure 12-2** The median sagittal view of the prostate gland and surrounding structures demonstrates the merging of the vas deferens with the seminal vesicle to form the ejaculatory duct. (From Moore KL, Agur A. *Essential Clinical Anatomy.* 2nd ed. Philadelphia, PA: Lippincott Williams & Wilkins; 2002.)

The venous drainage, which occurs laterally to the capsular vessels, consists of irregular venous channels along the anterior, inferior surface. These lead to the veins of the vasa deferentia and ultimately to the vesicle and internal iliac veins.

## PROSTATE ZONES

The urethra is the primary anatomic reference point dividing the gland into an anterior fibromuscular portion and a posterior glandular portion[11] (Fig. 12-5). The glandular tissue accounts for two-thirds of the prostate and contains four zones. Three of the zones—the peripheral zone, the transition zone, and the periurethral zone—have similar embryologic origins from the urogenital sinus. While the fourth zone, the central zone, is derived embryologically from the mesonephric ducts.[1,5,12] The fibromuscular structures account for one-third of the prostate.

The peripheral zone constitutes about 70% of the glandular tissue of the prostate (Table 12-1). It is

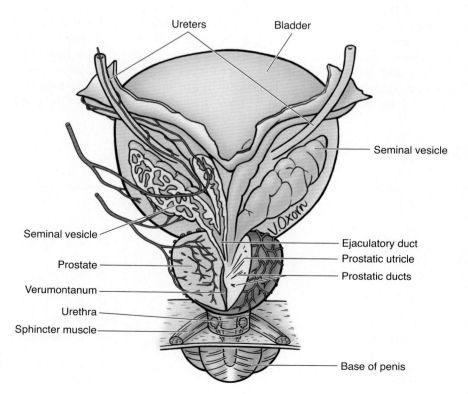

**Figure 12-3** The coronal section illustrates the ejaculatory ducts and urethra joining at the verumontanum.

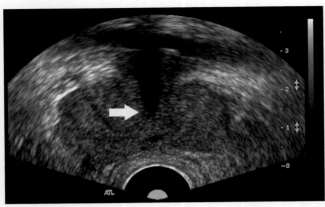

**Figure 12-4** Verumontanum. A coronal sonogram of the normal prostate. The "Eiffel Tower" sign (arrow) is seen at the level of the prostatic utricle.

| TABLE 12-1 | |
|---|---|
| **Prostate Zones** | |
| **Zonal Anatomy** | **% of Glandular Tissue** |
| Peripheral zone | 70% |
| Central zone | 25% |
| Transition zone | 5% |
| Periurethral zone | <1% |

located along the posterior, lateral, and apical portions of the gland, and its ducts drain into the distal segment of the urethra between the verumontanum and the apex. The acini of the peripheral zone are small, round, and simple.[12] The peripheral zone is the most common location for carcinoma[1,13] and prostatitis, with approximately 70% of prostate cancer arising from this area. Sonographically, normal peripheral zone tissue has a homogeneous, isoechoic echotexture. It can be delineated from the central zone by a thin, hyperechoic band separating the two zones. This band, called the *surgical capsule*, is in the shape of a semicircle and borders the central gland laterally and posteriorly.

The central zone accounts for about 25% of the glandular tissue of the prostate and is located at the base of the prostate. It is embedded in the funnel-shaped peripheral zone (Fig. 12-6). This zone narrows to an apex at the verumontanum. It surrounds the ejaculatory ducts and is located between the peripheral zone and the transition zone.[1,2] Microscopically, the central zone acini contrast strikingly in appearance to those in the peripheral zone. They are large and

have irregular contours, with considerable intraluminal folds and ridges.[1,12] These morphologic differences are what set the central zone apart from the rest of the glandular tissue[14] and what presumably make it immune from most disease.[15] The stroma is composed of long, tightly arranged muscle fibers that sweep around the acini. Only about 5% of prostate carcinomas arise in the central zone. Sonographically, the echogenicity of the central zone is normally greater than that of the peripheral zone.

The transition zone accounts for about 5% of the prostate gland in a young man. It consists of two small lobules found lateral to the proximal urethral segment, and is separated laterally and posteriorly from the outer gland by the surgical capsule (Fig. 12-7). It follows the long axis of the urethra toward the bladder neck.[15] The most caudal portion of this zone is at the verumontanum. The acini comprising the transitional zone are similar in appearance to the peripheral zone; however, the stroma are much more compact.[1] As the site of involvement by benign prostatic hyperplasia (BPH), the transition zone may account for a much greater percentage of glandular tissue as men age. Also, because the transitional zone is a common location for BPH, sonographically it becomes more hyperechoic and visible. Approximately 20% of carcinomas occur in this area.[16]

The periurethral glandular tissue composes less than 1% of all prostatic glandular tissue and is embedded

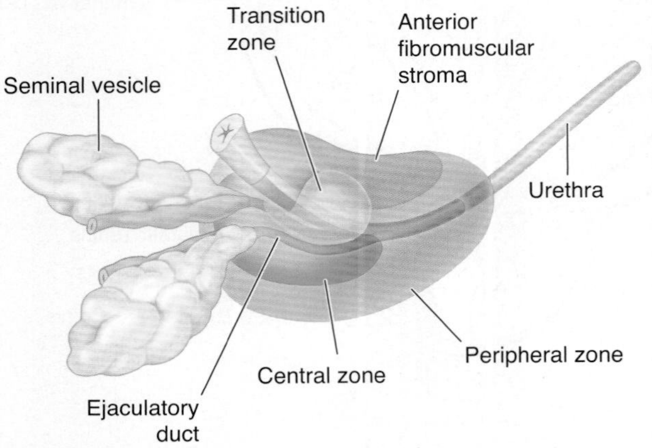

**Figure 12-5** The drawing illustrates the relationship of the prostate zones to the urethra.

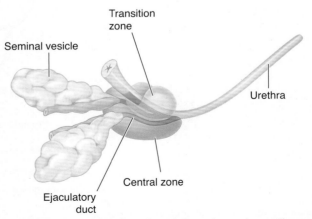

**Figure 12-6** A drawing of the funnel-shaped central zone illustrates the ejaculatory ducts entrance into the prostate.

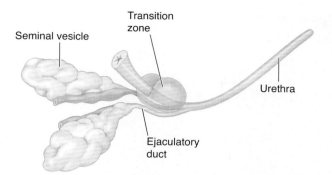

Seminal vesicle

Transition zone

Urethra

Ejaculatory duct

**Figure 12-7** This drawing depicts the saddlebag-shaped transitional zone and its relationship to the urethra.

| TABLE | 12-2 |
|---|---|

## Clinical Role of Prostatic Evaluation

### Advantages

1. High-resolution imaging
2. Complements digital rectal exam
3. No ionizing radiation
4. Cost-effective compared to other imaging techniques
5. Dynamic imaging of blood flow

### Applications

1. Biopsy guidance
2. Complementary to digital rectal examination

### Indications

1. Differentiation of cystic versus solid palpable lesions
2. Abnormal prostate specific antigen blood test
3. Evaluation of inflammatory process
4. Evaluation of male infertility
5. Guidance during biopsy or other invasive procedures
6. Evaluation of patients with a variety of clinical symptoms related to urination and/or ejaculation

in the smooth muscle wall of the urethra. This region runs along most of the prostatic urethral segment.[1] The ducts of this tissue open directly into the urethral lumen. Calculi often appear in this area and are thought to be secondary to reflux of urine into these ducts.

The anterior fibromuscular stroma is a nonglandular region, which is composed mainly of smooth muscle. It is continuous with fibers of the bladder wall and forms the anterior portion of the prostate.[5,17]

## SURROUNDING STRUCTURES

The seminal vesicles are paired saccular structures that lie obliquely and caudally to the prostate. The seminal vesicles are reservoirs for seminal fluid that fluctuate in size and shape secondary to levels of sexual activity. When void of seminal fluid, they appear as curvilinear, hypoechoic structures that flair out laterally. When these structures fill with seminal fluid, they become large, ovoid-shaped cystic structures sonographically, often containing low level echoes within the anechoic fluid.[14,18]

The ampulla of the vasa deferentia are located adjacent and medially to the seminal vesicles. In cross-section, they appear as thick-walled, tube-like structures. The ejaculatory ducts are formed at the junction of the ampulla of the vasa deferentia and the seminal vesicles.

The prostates posterior surface is anterior to the rectum and is separated by connective tissue called the *rectovesical septum*. The anterior surface is connected on either side to the pubic bone by the puboprostatic ligaments and is separated by a plexus of veins of fat. The anterior portions of the levator ani muscles cover the lateral surfaces of the prostate.

## SONOGRAPHIC EXAMINATION

### INDICATIONS AND CONTRAINDICATIONS

Indications for performing a sonographic evaluation of the prostate gland are wide ranging and ever expanding. The examination as a screening tool, however, is still the source of much controversy, particularly in its role of diagnosing prostate cancer (Table 12-2).

TRUS is often utilized in evaluation of patients with an abnormal digital rectal examination (DRE). When a gland feels irregular, sonography is useful in identifying masses, cystic areas, or calcifications. Sonographic characteristics of a disease process may include changes in echogenicity, asymmetry, and a distorted capsule.[19,20] Sonography may also help in identifying nonpalpable lesions as well.

One of the most important uses of sonography is for guidance during biopsy. It is a safe and accurate method of obtaining tissue from a focal area of the gland.[21,22] It also allows for accurate biopsy device placement within a specific zone of the prostate.[5]

A patient presenting with abnormal laboratory values and a negative DRE may also undergo sonographic examination. Prostate-specific antigen (PSA) is the most common blood test utilized to identify men at increased risk of prostate cancer. *PSA* is a protein that is specific to the prostatic epithelium.[23] The higher the value, the more likely malignancy is present.[24,25]

Clinical complaints of hematospermia, pain on ejaculation, dysuria, and perineal pain may also warrant a prostate sonography examination.

Prostatitis is one of the most common causes of these symptoms. Sonographically, color or power Doppler may show increased vascularity secondary to hyperemia when prostatitis is present. The gland may also appear enlarged and less echogenic than usual. Prostatitis may appear as a focal or diffuse process. Sonography is also used to detect BPH, calculi, ejaculatory duct cysts, congenital cysts, or abscesses. Sonography, BPH will demonstrate an enlarged nodular inner gland. The echotexture is heterogeneous, and can contain cystic areas. Calculi appear as echogenic structures and can create a shadow artifact. Cysts and abscess have a spectrum of sonographic appearances ranging from simple and anechoic to a more complex collection of fluids and debris.

Infertility is another indication for TRUS. Male infertility may be related to a congenital abnormality such as agenesis or atresia of the seminal vesicles or ejaculatory duct obstruction secondary to a cyst, mass, or calcification.[20]

A few contraindications to TRUS do exist. Significant rectal lesions such as fissures, obstructing lesions, thrombosed hemorrhoids, or prostatitis may prevent insertion of the rectal probe due to patient discomfort.[26] Additionally, patients with these symptoms are at increased risk of bleeding or infection.

## SCANNING TECHNIQUES

In the early 1970s, a transabdominal approach to visualize the prostate through a full bladder was utilized (Fig. 12-8). This offered limited information due to the limited resolution of low frequency transducers used to penetrate deep enough to reach the prostate gland, and incomplete visualization of the entire gland. The endorectal approach provides close anatomic proximity to the pelvic organs, which results in improved resolution and visualization.

Before beginning a TRUS, pertinent information should be obtained including DRE and PSA results, or clinical symptoms associated with infection or BPH.

TRUS should be performed with the patient's bladder empty to decrease discomfort. The patient is placed in a left lateral decubitus position, with the knees flexed toward the chest similar to the fetal position.

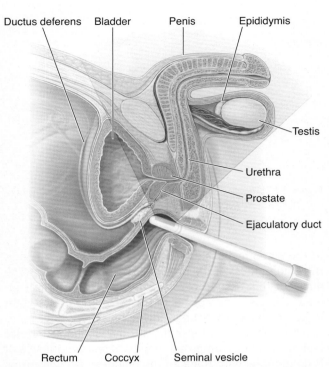

Figure 12-9 Scanning technique of the endorectal approach currently used to evaluate the prostate. An endorectal, end-fire transducer is used to acquire transverse and sagittal images of the prostate.

The transducer is then properly prepared by placing ultrasound gel within a probe cover and then places it over the probe. Currently most transrectal probes are end-fire probes utilizing a frequency range from 6 to 10 MHz.[27] The transducer is then placed within the rectal cavity (Fig. 12-9). When a biopsy is performed, an injection of 2% lidocaine just lateral to the junction of the prostate base and seminal vesicles will significantly reduce pain.

By convention, the orientation of an endorectal scan is slightly different from that of a transabdominal scan and is crucial to understand. The sonography image is inverted so that the near field is at the bottom of the image, and the far field is at the top of the image. In the transverse plane, the right lobe of the gland is at the left side of the image, and the left lobe of the gland is on the right side of the image. On sagittal plane, the base of the gland is at the left side of the image, and the apex of the gland is at the right side of the image. The rectal wall is in the near field, the urinary bladder is in the far field, and the prostate gland lies between these two structures.

Sonographically, the normal prostate appears as a crescent-shaped structure under the bladder base with an intact capsule. It is symmetrical and surrounds the urethra. Both the shape and echotexture of the prostate should be closely evaluated.

The capsule of the prostate should be smooth and without disruption, and the central gland should be contained within that prostatic capsule. Any disruption

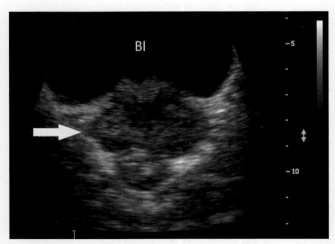

Figure 12-8 A transabdominal, transverse sonogram of the prostate (arrow). The urinary bladder (Bl) was used as an acoustic window to evaluate the gland. Only gross abnormalities were diagnosed using this technique.

of this capsule deserves further exploration for pathology. The internal echo pattern is evaluated by slowly scanning through the gland beginning in a transverse plane at the base of the prostate and moving inferiorly toward the apex. If a lesion is seen within the gland it is important to discern where the lesion is located.

Images are acquired in a transverse plane of the base, mid, and apical region of the prostate. The base of the prostate is located superior to the verumontanum and has a half-moon shape (Fig. 12-10A). It has a homogeneous echotexture and is isoechoic to surrounding tissue. The base of the prostate is predominately made up of the central zone. A hypoechoic arcuate line may be seen within the central portion of the base, which represents the surgical capsule. This demarcates the central gland from the peripheral gland.

The transducer is then moved slightly inferior to the level of the verumontanum, which is seen sonographically as a centrally located shadow (Fig. 12-10). At this level, the urethra passes through the prostate and more of the central gland can be seen. The central gland appears slightly more hyperechoic than the surrounding peripheral gland. This is the level at which the prostate should be measured in both transverse and anteroposterior dimensions. In patients over age 40, the central gland may bulge anteriorly due to BPH, which can change the prostate shape to an ovoid structure.

Located inferior to the verumontanum is the apex of the prostate (Fig. 12-10C). This section is typically more circular and is predominately made up of the peripheral zone. It appears slightly more heterogeneous than the homogeneous base. Since 70% of all prostate cancers occur in the peripheral zone, this is a common location for malignant lesions.

The transducer is then rotated 90 degrees to a sagittal plane. On a midline sagittal image, the urethra can be followed coursing from the bladder neck, through the prostate gland, and toward the apex (Fig. 12-11A). As the transducer is moved to the left or right, more of the central gland comes into view. At this level, the ejaculatory ducts may be visualized. As the transducer is obliqued further, the peripheral zone comes into view (Fig. 12-11B).

The seminal vesicles and vasa deferentia should be imaged in any complete prostate evaluation. These structures are evaluated in transverse and sagittal planes. The seminal vesicles lay laterally and superior to the base of the prostate. They should appear

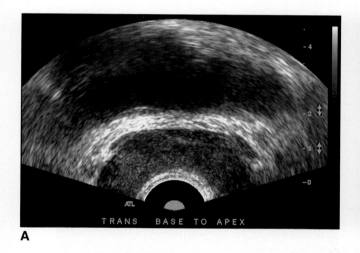

**A**

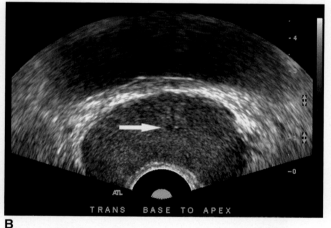

**B**

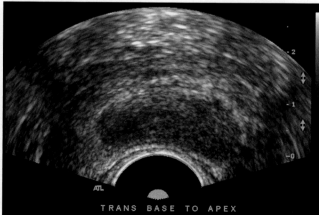

**C**

**Figure 12-10** Transverse sonogram of the normal prostate. **A:** The base of the normal prostate gland is half-moon shaped. **B:** The verumontanum (*arrow*) is visualized at the level of the mid gland. **C:** The apex is the most inferior aspect of the prostate.

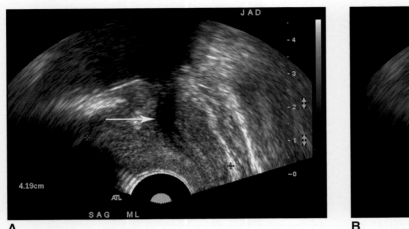

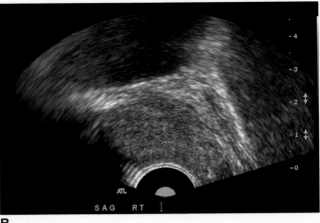

**Figure 12-11** Sagittal sonogram of the normal prostate. **A:** The midline section shows the urethra (arrow) coursing through the gland. **B:** The right lobe of the prostate can be identified.

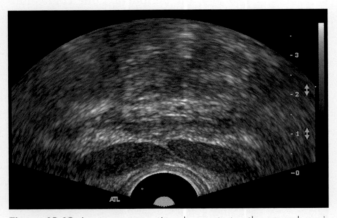

**Figure 12-12** A transverse section demonstrates the normal seminal vesicles.

hypoechoic (Fig. 12-12). If the seminal vesicles appear enlarged, further investigation is required to rule out an obstructive process versus a lack of recent ejaculation (Fig. 12-13A,B). The vasa deferentia are visualized in between the seminal vesicles. They are thick-walled and enter the base of the prostate (Fig. 12-14A,B). In a transverse plane, they appear as two donut-shaped structures, and in sagittal plane, they appear as long tubular structures. They should be free of fluid in the normal setting.

When imaging the prostate in a transverse imaging plane, two groups of blood vessels, the periurethral and the capsular should be visualized. The periurethral vessels will be seen within the center of the prostate gland

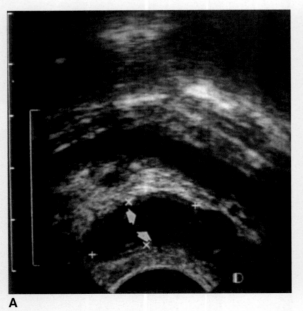

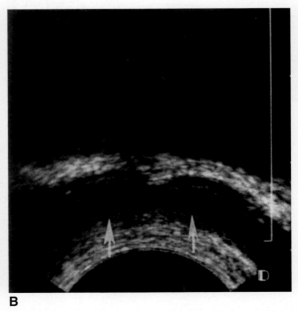

**Figure 12-13 A:** The transverse sonogram shows a dilated seminal vesicle. This patient had not ejaculated for 72 hours. The saccules (arrowhead) of the seminal vesicle are easily appreciated when it is dilated. Distance + = 22.0 mm; distance × = 8.9 mm. (Courtesy of Diasonics, Santa Clara, CA.) **B:** On this transverse sonogram through the base of the prostate, a dilated vasa deferentia (arrow) is seen. (Courtesy of Diasonics, Santa Clara, CA.)

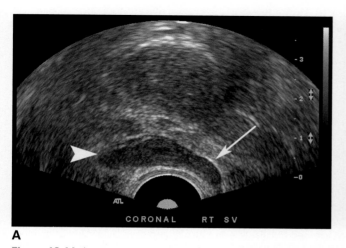

**A**

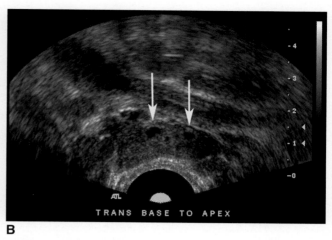

**B**

**Figure 12-14** A transverse sonogram showing normal and abnormal vasa deferentia. **A:** This image shows a normal seminal vesicle *(arrowhead)* and a medially located vas deferens *(arrow)*. **B:** On this transverse sonogram through the base of the prostate, the dilated vasa deferentia *(arrow)* are seen.

at the level of the verumontanum (Fig. 12-15). At the level of the urethra, large vessels will be seen coursing from the apex of the prostate following the urethra up toward the bladder neck. It is not unusual to see an increased amount of blood flow in this region. Color or power Doppler will show capsular vessels penetrating into the parenchyma of the gland (Fig. 12-16A,B). The vessels within the gland travel in a linear progression toward the center of the gland.

Color or power Doppler should also be utilized to identify signs of hyperemia either diffusely or focally within the prostate gland or increased vascularity to an identified lesion (Fig. 12-17A,B).

## CYSTS OF THE MALE PELVIS

Cysts arising in the male pelvis are extremely rare.[28] Patients can present with complex and perplexing clinical symptoms, ranging from urinary retention to perineal pain. There is controversy in the classification and

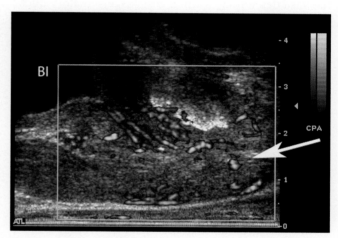

**Figure 12-15** A sagittal, midline sonogram of the prostate gland demonstrates the periurethral vessels displayed by power Doppler. The vessels travel along the course of the urethra through the transition zone from the bladder *(Bl)* toward the apex *(arrow)*. (Image courtesy of Philips Medical Systems, Bothell, WA.)

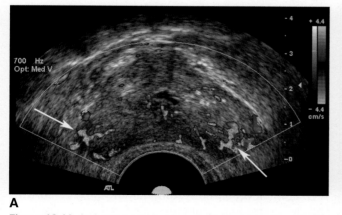

**A**

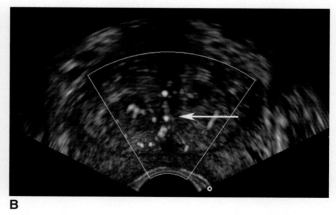

**B**

**Figure 12-16** **A:** A transverse sonogram demonstrates the capsular vessels shown in *red (arrows)*, as displayed by color Doppler. These vessels travel throughout the capsule of the gland. (Images courtesy of Philips Medical Systems, Brothell, WA.) **B:** On this transverse sonogram of the prostate gland, the periurethral vessel *(arrow)* is displayed by power Doppler. (Images courtesy of Philips Medical Systems, Bothell, WA.)

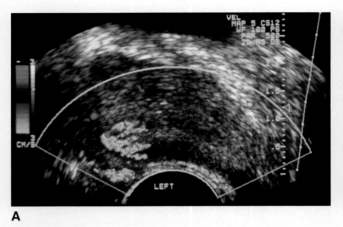

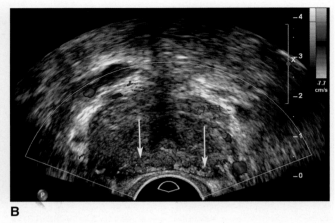

**A** **B**

**Figure 12-17  A:** A sagittal sonogram of the left prostate gland showing increased vascularity in an area of a suspicious lesion. (Image courtesy of Philips Medical Systems, Brothell, WA.) **B:** A transverse image demonstrating abnormal peripheral zone vascularity displayed by color Doppler *(arrows)*. (Images courtesy of Philips Medical Systems, Bothell, WA.)

origination of these cysts due to the close proximity of the vasa deferentia, seminal vesicles, ejaculatory ducts, and prostate, as well as their complex embryologic development.[29]

Sonography is useful in identifying the location of a cyst and its relationship to the prostate. It also offers information about the internal characteristics of the cyst itself. Several different cystic structures may occur in the prostate, seminal vesicles, and vas deferens: müllerian duct (utricle) cysts, seminal vesicle cysts, prostatic cyst, and cysts of the ejaculatory duct or vas deferens[29] (Fig. 12-18).

## MÜLLERIAN DUCT AND UTRICLE CYSTS

Müllerian duct and utricle cysts are the most common of the pelvic cystic masses. These two cystic lesions are often discussed together because of their almost identical locations. There are, however, embryologic differences and clinical findings that suggest these lesions should be considered separately.[15,30]

Müllerian duct cysts are mesodermal in origin and arise from embryonic remnants. They occur because of failure of regression of the müllerian duct structures.[29,30] In contrast to the utricle cyst, genital anomalies are not associated with true müllerian duct cysts. Unilateral renal agenesis, however, may occur. These cysts typically extend above the base of the prostate just off midline and are found between the bladder and rectum. They are attached to the prostate by a stalk-like structure extending into the prostate. The patient will typically present with partial urinary obstruction, hematospermia, low ejaculate volume, infertility, painful ejaculation, and rectal discomfort.[29] Sonographically, the cyst appears slightly lateral from midline and superior to the base of the prostate gland (Fig. 12-19A,B). A müllerian duct cyst does not connect with the urethra or with the seminal vesicle. It is anechoic and may contain debris or calcifications. They can be very large and usually have smooth, regular borders. When aspirated, the fluid may be a brownish red and will not contain spermatozoa. This is because the müllerian system does not communicate with the wolffian duct; therefore, there is no contact between these cysts and the vasa deferentia or seminal vesicles.[29]

A utricle cyst is endodermal in origin and is usually associated with hypospadias, undescended testicles, and renal anamolies.[31] These cysts occur when the prostatic utricle is dilated. They are located directly midline and close to the verumontanum.[30] These cysts are typically smaller in size than müllerian duct cysts. Sonographically, utricle cysts appear midline and are seen at the level of the verumontanum (Fig. 12-20A,B). Utricle cysts may contain calcifications. White or brown fluid is usually aspirated and rarely contains spermatozoa.

Müllerian duct cyst

Cyst of seminal vesicle

Cyst of vas deferens

Utricle cyst

Ejaculatory duct cyst

Retention cyst, abscess

**Figure 12-18** The sagittal cross-section illustration of the prostate gland shows typical locations of various cystic lesions of the prostate gland, seminal vesicle, and vas deferens.

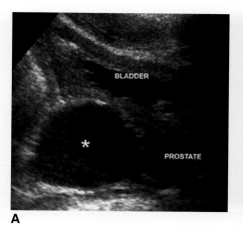
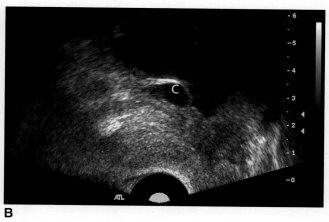

**A**    **B**

**Figure 12-19  A:** A transabdominal sagittal, midline sonogram of the prostate gland demonstrates a müllerian duct cyst as a large midline cystic structure *(asterisk)* superior to the base of the prostate. **B:** This is a different patient with a müllerian duct cyst *(C)*. The aspirated fluid of this cyst was brownish red, but contained no spermatozoa.

## SEMINAL VESICLE CYST

Seminal vesicle cysts are uncommon, occurring in less than 0.005% of the male population.[32,33] Over two thirds of reported cases are associated with ipsilateral renal agenesis.[34] This is explained embryologically by the close proximity of the abnormally developing vesicle and ureteral buds from the mesonephric duct.[34] If a seminal vesicle cyst is noted on a sonagram, both kidneys should be imaged. Sonographically, these cysts typically appear as a paramedian anechoic structure (Fig. 12-21). They are smaller than müllerian duct cysts and are located more lateral. Sometimes, the functioning contralateral seminal vesicle may be enlarged.[35] When a seminal vesicle cyst is aspirated, spermatozoa are typically found, helping to differentiate it from other types of cysts.

## PROSTATIC CYST

There are several different types of cysts within the prostate that fall into this category. These cysts may be congenital or acquired. A retention or inclusion cyst is an acquired cyst of the prostate. It results from occlusion of a prostatic duct causing dilatation of the glandular acini.[29] These cysts are small in size, usually 1 to 2 cm, and typically are not clinically significant. They may occur in any of the three glandular zones. Sonographically, retention cysts are simple, smooth walled, and appear completely anechoic (Fig. 12-22A,B). They do not contain spermatozoa when aspirated.[29]

Cystic changes can be seen in the transition zone due to BPH. These cysts are by far the most common since BPH is a common disorder in the older male population. They occur within the hyperplastic nodules and

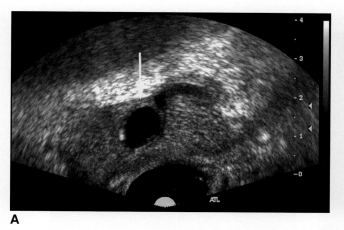
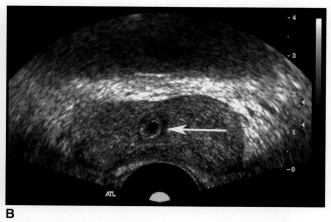

**A**    **B**

**Figure 12-20  A:** A transverse prostate sonogram at the level of the verumontanum shows a midline utricle cyst *(arrow)* with calcifications within the wall of the lesion. The patient presented with the characteristic post-void dribbling. **B:** Another utricle cyst *(arrow)* is seen in this transverse prostate sonogram. This image demonstrates the characteristic location of this cyst.

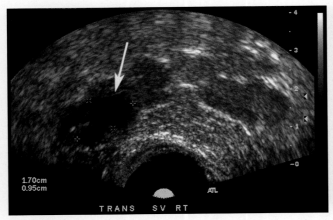

**Figure 12-21** A transverse sonogram showing multiple seminal vesicle cysts as paramedian, anechoic structures *(arrow)*.

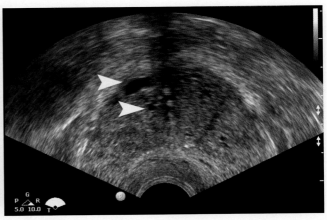

**Figure 12-23** On a transverse sonogram, cystic changes *(arrowheads)* are seen within the hyperplastic nodules in a patient with benign prostatic hyperplasia. (Image courtesy of Philips Medical Systems, Bothell, WA.)

are very small (Fig. 12-23). These cysts are asymptomatic, although the conditions they are seen with causes multiple problems discussed later in this chapter.

There are other cystic lesions of the prostate that are extremely rare. Parasitic cysts, for example, result from secondary spread of echinococcus, or bilharzias, and are typically seen in males living in a region in which these parasites are endemic. Cysts may also be seen in association with carcinoma due to a degenerative process.[29]

### Prostatic Abscess

A prostatic abscess is associated with acute bacterial prostatitis, but can also be seen in diabetic male patients. Early recognition is important, although it can be difficult to distinguish acute prostatitis from an abscess clinically. Symptoms are similar, including fever, chills, urinary frequency, urgency, perineal/low back pain, dysuria, and hematuria. Sonographic findings include focal or diffuse complex areas occurring in any part of the prostate gland.[2] These findings in a patient with the appropriate clinical findings are suspicious for an

abscess. As mentioned previously, color or power Doppler may show hyperemic blood flow. The diagnosis is confirmed by aspiration and microscopic evaluation of the fluid and is treated with antibiotics.

### DIVERTICULUM OF THE EJACULATORY DUCT OF VAS DEFERENS

A diverticulum or cyst of the ejaculatory duct or vas deferens can occur due to a distal obstruction of the spermatic ductal system by a congenital abnormality or inflammation.[29] This lesion may be mistaken for a seminal vesicle cyst; however, sonographic visualization of normal seminal vesicles can distinguish this lesion from a seminal vesicle cyst. Large ejaculatory duct diverticula are associated with perineal pain, dysuria, hematospermia, and ejaculatory pain.[18] These cystic structures are typically seen between the base of the prostate and the seminal vesicles, and can occur along the ejaculatory duct course. If large, these cysts may be confused with a müllerian duct or utricle cyst. Ejaculatory duct cysts can also

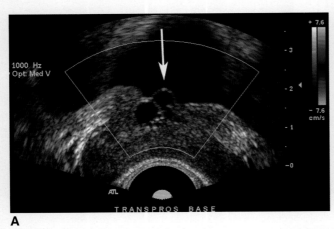

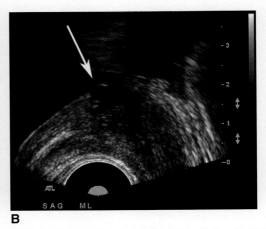

**Figure 12-22 A:** On a transverse sonogram of the prostate, multiple small retention cysts are seen within the base of the gland *(arrow)*. **B:** A sagittal sonogram of the midline shows retention cysts *(arrow)* in the anterior section of an asymptomatic patient. This is characteristic for a retention cyst.

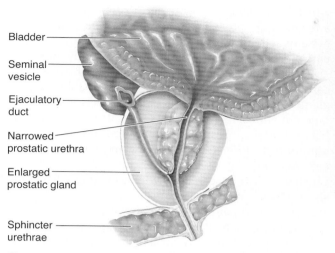

Bladder
Seminal vesicle
Ejaculatory duct
Narrowed prostatic urethra
Enlarged prostatic gland
Sphincter urethrae

**Figure 12-24** This illustration demonstrates the passing of the urethra through the prostate, and how benign prostatic hyperplasia distorts the pathway. (Asset provided by Anatomical Chart Co.)

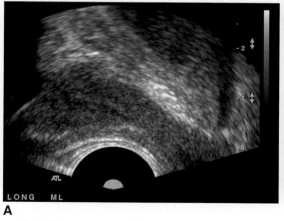

**Figure 12-25** A transverse sonogram on a 57-year-old patient with frequency and nocturia due to benign prostatic hyperplasia demonstrated the central gland as significantly enlarged pushing into the bladder (*Bl*).

contain calculi, and the seminal vesicle on the affected side may be dilated due to the obstruction.[18] Aspiration of these cysts will yield spermatozoa, proving that it does communicate with the spermatic system, which is typically not the case with a utricle or müllerian duct cyst.

## BENIGN PROSTATIC HYPERPLASIA

BPH is the most common symptomatic tumor-like condition in the male population. It is a nodular formation within the transition zone of the prostate. The cause is not well understood but is thought to be similar to leiomyomas of the uterus.[36] This condition is rarely seen in men under the age of 30 but is commonly seen in men over the age of 40 and peaks around the age of 60.[2] BPH is exclusively a disease of the preprostatic region.[15] The nodules typically arise from the transition zone, with some arising from the periurethral zone. Since the urethra passes through this zone, these patients typically present with urinary symptoms (Fig. 12-24). BPH acts as an obstructive process to the flow of urine. Symptoms include frequency, nocturia, dribbling, and difficulty starting a stream. On rectal examination, the prostate feels soft, boggy, and nodular. Sonographically, BPH causes enlargement of the central gland in an anteroposterior direction[5] (Fig. 12-25). In contrast to a normal gland, the prostate no longer has a crescent shape but appears more rounded and can be up to four times its original size (Fig. 12-26A,B). There are three primary types of BPH.

- The first is homogeneous stromal hyperplasia, which is sonographically hypoechoic.
- The second type is glandular hyperplasia, which may look hypoechoic or hyperechoic, depending on the cystic changes and gland size.
- The third is a combination of the aforementioned two types, resulting in a stromal and glandular hyperplasia. This form is the most common and is heterogeneous in appearance.[36]

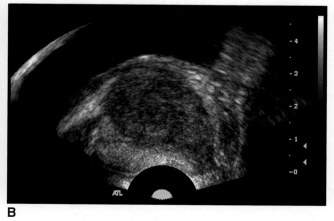

**A**    **B**

**Figure 12-26** The two images demonstrate the contrast between a young, healthy prostate and a prostate affected by benign prostatic hyperplasia. Both sonograms are of the mid gland. **A:** A 22-year-old patient with a normal, crescent-shaped gland. **B:** A 52-year-old with benign prostatic hyperplasia. Notice how the gland is more rounded in comparison.

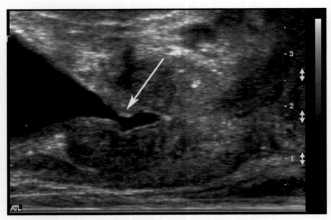

**Figure 12-27** This 65-year-old has a transurethral resection (TURP) defect. The central gland has been removed (arrow) distorting the typical appearance of the mid gland. (Image courtesy of Philips Medical Systems, Bothell, WA.)

As BPH develops, the peripheral gland becomes compressed, making it difficult to evaluate. When BPH is present, the central gland is often easier to visualize with sonography because as the disease develops, the glandular tissue becomes more and more heterogeneous, thus differentiating it from the homogeneous peripheral zone.[20] The heterogeneous pattern is a result of the multiple interfaces between the stromal and glandular tissues of the hyperplastic central gland. BPH is commonly found when performing TRUS on men over the age of 40.

Transurethral resection of the prostate (TURP) is done to relieve the symptoms caused by compression of the prostatic urethra. Using a cystoscope, a surgeon removes the excess tissue, thus creating a large defect. The TURP defect, when seen sonographically, can be dramatic (Fig. 12-27).

## PROSTATE CALCIFICATIONS

Prostatic calculi are frequently encountered in urologic practice and their presence is usually reported as an incidental finding. The exact incidence of these calculi is unknown because most are small, asymptomatic, and difficult to detect by DRE.[37] They are extremely common but rarely give rise to symptoms. However, the conditions they are associated with may cause symptoms. Prostate calculi can be classified into two groups: endogenous and exogenous. Endogenous calculi are found within the substance of the prostate and form from the prostatic fluid. Exogenous calculi are found in the urethra and are derived primarily from urine.[38]

Endogenous calculi are the true prostatic stones. If large enough, they may be felt on DRE and may be mistaken for a tumor because of their firmness. One of the most common causes of endogenous calculi is the consolidation and calcification of the corpora amylacea,

which normally occurs with age. Corpora amylacea are a result of the prostatic acini progressing through their cycle of cell atrophy, degeneration, and death. This occurs most often in the posterior segment of the prostate.

Any pathologic process, such as BPH or prostatitis, can cause endogenous calculi. Inflammation of the gland can cause an imbalance of pH levels in the prostatic secretions.[39] This disrupts the calcium citrate acid balance and causes the condensation of calcium salts onto already formed small stones and corpora amylacea. As these stones get bigger, they block the ducts causing a stasis of secretions within the ducts. This stasis results in stone formation leading to the multiple calculi seen in patients with chronic prostatitis.[39] The association of calculi with BPH can also be explained by this process.[37] As nodular hyperplasia develops, the acini of the prostate may become obstructed resulting in stasis of secretions.

Sonographically, calculi are easily seen (Fig. 12-28). They occur within the parenchyma of the gland and range in size from very small to very large, some becoming as big as 3 cm or more.[39] These are often associated with distal acoustic shadowing. They may appear in clusters or alone. These stones are different from those that occur within the ejaculatory ducts or urethra.

Ejaculatory duct calcifications are often seen during a TRUS (Fig. 12-29). They can be an incidental finding or cause symptoms such as hematospermia or painful ejaculation. These stones can develop for reasons similar to prostate calculi. If a cystic lesion or inflammation obstructs the ejaculatory ducts, stasis may occur resulting in the concretion and calcification of fluid. Hematospermia and painful ejaculations result because of the passage of these stones. On a sonogram, these calcifications can be seen lining the ejaculatory duct. They are best appreciated in a sagittal plane and help to visualize

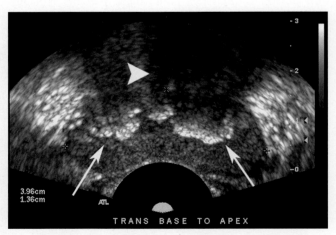

**Figure 12-28** A 41 year old presents with a firm palpable mass. On a transverse sonogram, numerous prostatic calculi (arrows) are seen along the surgical capsule of this mid gland sonogram. Characteristic acoustic shadowing is present (arrowheads).

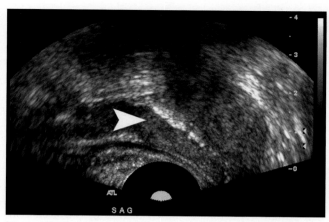

**Figure 12-29** A sagittal sonogram with calculi *(arrowhead)* is identified lining the ejaculatory duct. These calculi provide for excellent viewing of the course of the ejaculatory duct.

**PATHOLOGY BOX 12-1**

*Classification of Prostatitis*

| | Perineal Pain | EPS | Leukocytes (Urine) |
|---|---|---|---|
| Acute bacterial | + | + | + |
| Chronic bacterial | ± | + | + |
| Chronic pelvic pain | | | |
| Inflammatory | ± | + | 0 |
| Noninflammatory | ± | 0 | 0 |
| Asymptomatic inflammatory | 0 | + | 0 |

EPS, expressed prostatic secretion.

the sometimes difficult to image ejaculatory duct. They may or may not cause an acoustic shadow.

Periurethral calcifications involve the urethra, which passes through the prostate. They are exogenous calculi and are derived primarily from urine. Periurethral calculi outline the course of the urethra and are particularly well seen on midline images. They can produce an "Eiffel Tower" appearance if located at the level of the verumontanum, which is best appreciated in a transverse view.

## PROSTATITIS

Prostatitis is a poorly understood condition that is difficult to diagnose both clinically and sonographically. This term refers to an inflammation of the prostate as demonstrated by an increased number of leukocytes in prostatic fluid.[40] Many men are often diagnosed incorrectly with this condition. This is because there is much confusion in the literature regarding its pathogenesis, diagnosis, and treatment. Much of the confusion lies in the variety of organisms that may infect the prostate and the vague symptoms the patient may present with. The clinical diagnosis of prostatitis is made by an evaluation of expressed prostatic secretion (EPS) for either positive bacterial cultures or inflammatory cells. The National Institute of Health (NIH) lists four categories of prostatitis, including acute bacterial, chronic bacterial, CPPS (including inflammatory and noninflammatory pelvic pain syndromes), and asymptomatic inflammatory prostatitis.[41] This classification system is based on a complex clinical and pathologic assessment[41,42] (Pathology Box 12-1).

### ACUTE BACTERIAL PROSTATITIS

The presentation of acute bacterial prostatitis is unique and the diagnosis is usually straightforward. Patients are typically acutely ill, with a fever, low back pain, and perineal pain. The disease is associated with large numbers of gram-negative bacteria present within the urine.[42] This form of prostatitis is easily diagnosed by a urine test. Upon DRE, the prostate will feel hard, swollen, and very tender. Typically, a vigorous examination is contraindicated because it can precipitate bacteremia.[43] Therapy usually consists of a series of bactericidal antibiotics and palliative care.

### CHRONIC BACTERIAL PROSTATITIS

Chronic bacterial prostatitis may be difficult to diagnose and treat due to the wide variety of clinical presentations. The same organisms cause the acute form, yet these patients have not necessarily had an episode of acute bacterial prostatitis. Common complaints include discomfort in the penis, scrotum, and perineum, with irritative voiding symptoms such as dysuria, urgency, and frequency. This disease is characterized by relapsing urinary tract infections.[44] Quite often, physical examination will disclose no findings.

### CHRONIC PELVIC PAIN SYNDROME

CPPS is an inflammation of the prostate of unknown etiology and has an incidence eight times higher than that of bacterial prostatitis.[43] Most studies suggest that it is caused by organisms not detected by conventional cultures.[43] The clinical symptoms are similar to patients with bacterial prostatitis. Patients afflicted with CPPS are difficult to manage because an infectious process is not easily detected, and there is usually no history of urinary tract infections.

Noninflammatory CPPS is typically seen in young to middle-age men, who experience abnormal or irritative urinary flow, lower back, and perineum pain. It has been demonstrated that spasms and narrowing of the prostatic urethra due to neuromuscular dysfunction are responsible for these symptoms.[42,45] Stress is also thought to play a primary role in the etiology of noninflammatory CPPS.

## ASYMPTOMATIC INFLAMMATORY PROSTATITIS

Patients with asymptomatic inflammatory prostatitis are, as the name implies, asymptomatic for prostatitis. However, clinically, they appear to have an inflammatory disease. There is no evidence of bacterial infection or leukocytes in the EPS and the DRE is normal. Infection is usually found in cells from a prostate biopsy, or during evaluation for other disorders.[42] Because the patient is asymptomatic, therapy is warranted only if there is an underlying problem.[43]

## SONOGRAPHIC FINDINGS OF PROSTATITIS

The role of sonography is to differentiate between patients with a genuine inflammation of the gland versus patients with symptoms but no signs of inflammation. Understanding the pathogenesis of this disease helps in make a sonographic diagnosis. The prostate is infected by the ascent of organisms from the lower urethra. Once organisms gain access to the lower prostatic urethra, there is easy access to the ducts of the peripheral zone. Any increase in intraurethral pressure will encourage reflux of urine and organisms into these ducts. Typically, the central zone ducts are not invaded because their oblique entry into the urethra acts like a valve.[44] This accounts for the greater incidence of prostatitis within the peripheral zone.

The sonographic evaluation of patients with symptoms of prostatitis should include gray scale and color Doppler imaging. Grayscale findings are sometimes helpful but not always definitive. One of the most common findings is a hypoechoic halo in the periurethral area.[45] This should not be confused with the cylindrical smooth muscle of the preprostatic sphincter found at the base of the prostate. Another frequent finding is a heterogeneous echo pattern of the peripheral gland (Fig. 12-30A,B). This pattern is most often seen in chronic cases of prostatitis. It is due to areas of scarring and necrosis caused by previous episodes of inflammation. It is also important, when evaluating these patients, to rule out the presence of an abscess because that would require more immediate treatment. Fortunately, these lesions are rare but can occur during an acute episode or in diabetic patients.[42] The sonographic findings of an abscess include focal hypoechoic or anechoic lesions with a thickened wall and/or septations. The sonography examination often causes extreme discomfort for the patient, specifically when scanning the area containing the abscess.

Calculi may be visualized within the gland of a patient with chronic prostatitis. These calculi may be a result of an inflammatory reaction or part of the pathogenesis of the disease, which includes the reflux of urine, as well as organisms, into the prostatic ducts. It has been suggested in the literature that the presence of prostatic calculi may be the cause of recurrent bouts of prostatitis.[46] The calculi may harbor the bacteria that cause prostatitis, making it impossible for antibiotic therapy to be effective.

Color or power Doppler may be useful in detecting a hyperemic flow pattern often associated with infection and abscess. Hyperemia may be diffuse or focal (Fig. 12-31A,B). However, it should be born in mind that increased blood flow is not specific to inflammatory lesions.

## PROSTATE CANCER

Prostate cancer is the most common cancer in American men, and is the second most deadly male cancer.[47] More than 70% of prostate cancers are diagnosed in men over the age of 65.[48] There is an estimated 42% risk for a 50-year-old man to develop occult tumors

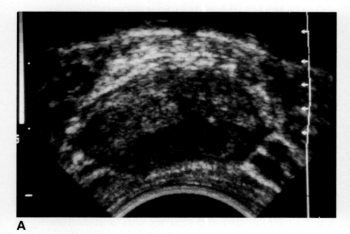

A

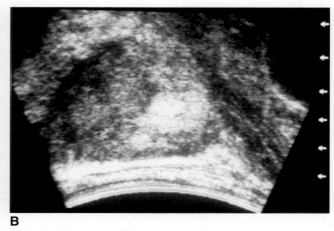

B

**Figure 12-30** Sonograms of the mid gland were obtained on patients with acute prostatitis. **A:** A transverse image showing the heterogeneous echo texture of the peripheral gland. **B:** A sagittal image of the left prostate gland on a patient with known prostatitis.

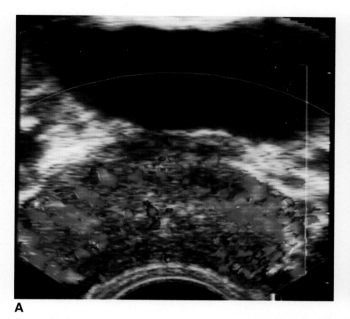
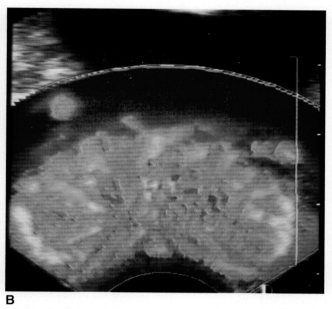

**Figure 12-31** Transverse sonograms of the mid gland were obtained on a 32-year-old with acute prostatitis. **A:** Multiple vessels are seen in the peripheral gland, displayed by color Doppler. **B:** Large parenchymal vessels are seen using power Doppler.

during a lifetime but only a 2.9% risk of dying from the disease.[49] African Americans have a 60% greater risk than Caucasians of developing prostate cancer, with a 2.3 times higher mortality rate.[49] One study performed by Cater et al.[50] to evaluate prostate autopsy data found that 20% of men in the sixth decade of life, and 50% of men in the eighth decade of life had histologic evidence of prostate cancer.[51] According to the National Institute of Health's Surveillance, Epidemiology, and End Results (SEER) study, approximately 75% of all prostate cancers are detected by an abnormal PSA level (>4 ng/ml).[52] The PSA can be reported in several different forms: total PSA, age-adjusted PSA, PSA density, PSA velocity, and free PSA. No specific level is normal or abnormal, although there are charts and guidelines for each test.

The usefulness of early diagnosis of prostate cancer and achieving substantial improvements in patient morbidity and mortality rates remain to be demonstrated. That is why controversy exists in the literature regarding the utility of screening and early detection of this cancer.[20,24]

Most patients referred for TRUS for prostate cancer present with either a bladder outlet obstruction, an abnormal PSA level, or an abnormal DRE. Other symptoms include bone pain, weakness, weight loss, anemia, and azotemia.[53]

DRE was previously considered the gold standard for screening of prostate cancer, but it was found to be very subjective and missed 44% to 59% of cancers.[47] PSA has become the primary test for identifying patients at increased risk of prostate cancer. However, it can be elevated in BPH and prostatitis as well.[23,47,48] Therefore, definitive diagnosis relies on

sonography-guided biopsy. In conjunction with clinical findings, TRUS can be a valuable tool and can serve as an important adjunct to the management of prostate cancer.[47,48,54]

TRUS offers an evaluation of the zonal anatomy and sites through which extracapsular extension (ECE) can occur.[55] Eighty percent of cancers originate in the outer gland (peripheral and central zones) and 20% originate in the inner gland (periurethral and transitional zones).[26] The surgical capsule defines the plane between the inner and outer gland. Prostate cancer behaves differently in each anatomical zone, and is thought to be related to its embryologic derivitative.[12] Although cancer of the prostate may have a variety of appearances, classically it presents as a hypoechoic lesion.[20,26] Adenocarcinoma is the most commonly diagnosed prostate cancer with a vast majority arising from the peripheral zone.[56] Approximately 85% of prostate adenocarcinomas are multifocal in origin, as opposed to a solitary discrete mass.[56] Sonographically, it is not uncommon for adenocarcinoma to appear isoechoic to surrounding prostate tissue. Therefore, TRUS alone has a predictive value of only 6% for prostate cancer diagnosis.

There are several anatomical weaknesses of this gland that result in ECE.[56] The first is within the prostatic capsule of the peripheral zone. Most tumors tend to grow along the prostatic capsule in an oblong fashion.[57] These tumors can easily extend into the subcapsular space. Another area is the trapezoid area, which is located inferior to the apex of the prostate, posterior to the urethra, and anterior to the rectal sphincter. The capsule of the apex can be very thin or absent and provides an excellent escape from

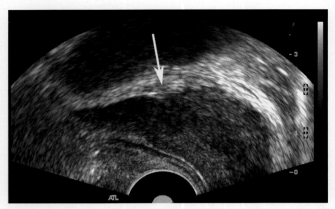

**Figure 12-32** A sagittal sonogram of a normal prostate demonstrates the "beak" (arrow) where the seminal vesicle and vas deferens enters the central zone.

the peripheral zone into the trapezoid area. Seventy-five percent of all tumors occur within 3 to 6 mm of the apex making this a popular tumor location. The seminal vesicle "beak" sign may be visualized when an anatomical weakness occurs in the central zone (Fig. 12-32). This is a defect in the prostatic capsule that occurs where the vas deferens and seminal vesicle enter the central zone to form the ejaculatory duct. This defect provides another potential pathway for tumor extension. On a sagittal sonographic image, this defect looks like a bird's beak. The invaginated extraprostatic space is another weakness of the central zone. This is the location where the vascular-lymphatic channels invaginate the capsule and follow the ejaculatory duct to the verumontanum. This space is in direct contact with glandular tissue of the central gland offering a pathway for tumor spread. The final anatomic weakness of the central zone is a defect of the prostatic capsule at the bladder neck. Tumor may escape from the junction of the bladder neck and the central zone. A sonography-guided biopsy is recommended if a lesion is seen near any of the aforementioned anatomical weaknesses.

The peripheral zone is the location of origin of 70% of prostate cancers.[26] They can be multifocal and typically are either in direct contact or close to the capsule. Most of these cancers involve the apex of the prostate because this is the location of the greatest portion of peripheral glandular tissue. Tumors within the peripheral zone can easily spread to the central zone because of the weak interface separating these two zones. The central zone is the site of origin for 1% to 5% of prostate cancers, likely due to its wolffian duct origin. Cancer may spread to the ejaculatory ducts via the invaginated extraprostatic space. When the ejaculatory ducts are involved, a "halo" sign may be seen on transverse images caused by the surrounding tumor. Tumor may also cause a partial obstruction of the duct resulting in a dilated seminal

vesicle. The remaining 20% of cancers originate in the transitional zone. Cancers of the transition zone commonly arise circumferentially in proximity to the anterior fibromuscular stroma and are most often discovered during TURP.[36] They can originate in either glandular acini or within a hyperplastic nodule. Tumors originating within the glandular acini arise medially, frequently invading the anterior fibromuscular stroma. These tumors tend to remain within the inner prostate gland until they become quite large. Tumors arising from a hyperplastic nodule tend to remain encapsulated. Localized asymmetry and a hypoechoic lesion within the transition zone is highly suspicious.[36]

Attempts have been made to categorize prostate cancer by a specific sonographic characteristic. Most appear as hypoechoic lesions (Fig. 12-33A–C). This appearance is seen because most cancers are composed of a dense mass of cells that differ from the surrounding glandular tissue. Malignant lesions contain fewer sonographically detected interfaces and thus appear hypoechoic.[57] If the lesion is too small, however, it may appear isoechoic with the surrounding tissue. Alternatively, large, diffuse tumors can go sonographically undetected because of total replacement of the gland.[24] The difficulty in evaluating a diffuse lesion is that there is no normal tissue for comparison.

It is important to keep in mind that a hypoechoic lesion is not always specific for cancer. In fact, the majority of suspicious hypoechoic areas within the peripheral zone result from benign causes.[26,56,57] These include inflammation, fibrosis, infarction, smooth muscle surrounding the ejaculatory duct, BPH, atrophy, and lymphoma. Other factors also hinder the specificity of sonography, including the location of the tumor, the presence or absence of an interface with surrounding benign tissue, and BPH. Thus, although sonography is useful in certain cases, it will not detect most cases of prostate cancer. If a suspicious lesion is seen sonographically, further evaluation by biopsy is warranted.

## BIOPSY GUIDANCE PROCEDURES

Sonography is used almost universally for guidance during biopsy of the prostate gland[20] (Fig. 12-34A,B). Sonography guidance offers a safe and accurate placement of the biopsy needle to obtain a tissue sample from the prostate whether it be a random site biopsy or a lesion specific biopsy.

Sonography guided biopsies of the prostate were first described in the early 1980s using a transperineal approach. Currently, the endorectal approach is the method of choice. Both techniques are safe, accurate, and only mildly uncomfortable when certain precautions are taken to correctly perform the examination. Periprostatic nerve block is the most common and

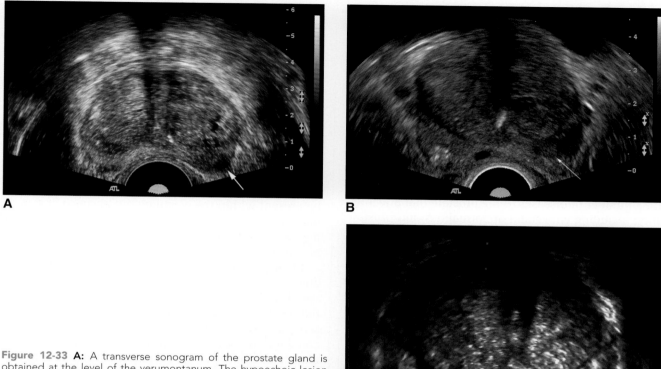

**Figure 12-33 A:** A transverse sonogram of the prostate gland is obtained at the level of the verumontanum. The hypoechoic lesion *(arrow)* is seen within the peripheral zone on the left side of the gland. **B:** This sonogram is an of a hypoechoic malignant lesion *(arrow)* within the prostate. **C:** A classic hypoechoic malignant lesion *(arrow)* is seen on this sonogram. This was a histologically proven cancer. (Images **A,B** courtesy of Philips Medical System, Bothell, WA.)

popular method of anesthesia, as well as the use of lidocaine gel.[58] There is a risk of prostate contamination by fecal material using the endorectal approach. For this reason, a cleansing enema is often given before the biopsy and antibiotics administered prophylactically to minimize the risk of sepsis. This technique may not be appropriate when an abscess is suspected because of the risk of infection with fecal material. The transperineal approach does not require a cleansing enema or antibiotic coverage. It does, however, require extensive use of a local anesthetic directly into the perineum.

Sonographic guidance can be utilized to localize a nonpalpable, sonographically suspicious lesion,[55,59]

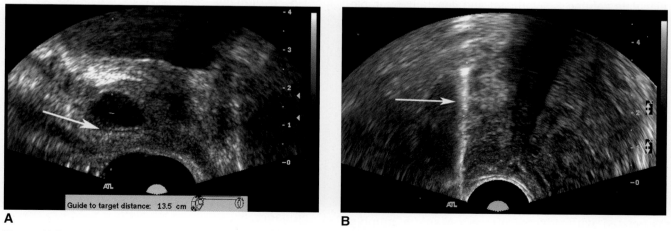

**Figure 12-34 A:** On a sonographically guided endorectal biopsy, the echogenic appearing needle can provide a target distance marker. **B:** The needle is seen as an echogenic, linear structure *(arrowhead)* passing through the prostate gland. (Image courtesy of Philips Medical Systems, Bothell, WA.)

or as guidance for random biopsies of known sites of anatomical weakness: (1) the seminal vesicle beak, (2) the invaginated extraprostatic space which follows the ejaculatory ducts to the verumontanum, and (3) the trapezoid area.[36] Sonographic guidance also assists in staging prostate cancer by obtaining tissue from areas where microscopic ECE is likely to be present.

## INFERTILITY

The use of sonography in the evaluation of male infertility is limited, yet offers valuable information. There are a number of diseases of the prostate that affect fertility, including congenital abnormalities and prostatitis. *Vasography*, the examination for determining the reproductive tract patency, is invasive and can cause scarring of the vasa deferentia.[60] Endorectal sonography is an inexpensive and less invasive examination capable of detecting many abnormalities associated with infertility.

Ten percent of male infertility patients present with azoospermia or lack of spermatozoa within the ejaculate.[60] A minority of these patients with this condition will have an obstructive lesion within the prostate or an endocrine disorder. The remainder have an untreatable testicular defect. A clinical workup involves a DRE to rule out the presence of a mass and to confirm the presence of the accessory organs (seminal vesicles and vasa deferentia). If mature sperm are being produced, a blockage must be occurring to prevent the passage of spermatozoa through the ejaculatory duct, which results in the absence of sperm in the ejaculate. Structural abnormalities of the male pelvis causing azoospermia include congenital or acquired cysts of the prostate or absence or atresia of the vasa deferentia.

Low ejaculate volume is different from azoospermia. In this case, sperm may be present but the overall amount of ejaculate is decreased. Clinically, low ejaculate volume is significant and generally treatable. It occurs in about 7% of male infertility patients. This condition may result from a blockage or congenital anomaly of the seminal vesicles. The seminal vesicles store seminal fluid, which makes up a portion of the ejaculate.[61] A partial obstruction along the ejaculatory duct may be present, allowing some sperm in the ejaculate, but an overall decrease in fluid. Finally, a secretory dysfunction of the gland due to prior infections may result in low ejaculate volume.

Interest has grown, recently, concerning the possible relation of infections of the prostate and male subfertility. Leukocytospermia is typically seen as a clinical sign of genital tract infection and has been associated with adverse effects on sperm number, motility, and sperm velocity.[62] An elevated number of leukocytes in prostatic secretions are typical of acute and chronic bacterial and nonbacterial prostatitis.[63] Acute inflammatory conditions of the prostate gland are often associated with transient disturbances in its secretory function and with changes in sperm quality.

Sonography is most useful in male infertility in the evaluation of the seminal vesicles and the ampullae of the vasa deferentia. Both seminal vesicles and ampullae should be present and free of abnormalities in the normal setting. Absence of the vas deferens and ampulla is a common cause of obstructive azoospermia. Absence of a seminal vesicle may result in low ejaculate volume, although spermatozoa would still be present within the ejaculate.[64] If absence of a seminal vesicle or vas deferens were suspected, the kidneys should be evaluated for associated abnormalities or atresia.[32]

Enlargement of these structures may also be indicative of an obstruction. However, unless the seminal vesicles are grossly enlarged, enlargement may also be the result of sexual abstinence or age. If, however, the seminal vesicles appear grossly enlarged and the above conditions do not apply, a distal obstruction of the ejaculatory duct must be suspected. It is important to rule out cystic structures or calculi that may be obstructing these ducts.[64] These lesions become significant in the presence of fertility issues, such as low ejaculate volume and azoospermia.

## SUMMARY

- The prostate gland is retroperitoneal, anterior to the rectum, and inferior to the urinary bladder.
- The normal prostate gland should appear symmetrical with the majority of the parenchyma appearing homogeneous with medium-level echoes.
- The central and transition zones usually are not sonographically distinct.
- The peripheral zone appears homogeneous and slightly hyperechoic relative to adjacent parenchyma.
- Seminal vesicles should be ovoid structures that are symmetric in size, shape, and hypoechoic echogenicity compared to the prostate.
- If distinguished sonographically, the vas deferens is medial to the seminal vesicles with a similar echo texture and the ejaculatory duct will appear as bright double lines.
- TRUS is the scanning approach of choice.
- Overall, sonography is a useful mechanism of assessing the prostate gland for a variety of abnormalities and for providing biopsy and treatment guidance.
- Its utility as a screening tool for malignant lesions, however, is limited.

## Critical Thinking Questions

1. A 78-year-old man with a history of urinary retention, hematuria, and a PSA level of 8 ng/mL was referred for a TRUS. The sonograms demonstrate enlargement of the central gland and calcifications within the central gland. The prostate volume was greater than 30 mL and there were some mixed echogenic nodules. The peripheral zone was normal. Identify the common condition for this patient based on age, symptoms, and sonographic evaluation.

2. The transverse and sagittal sonograms at the base of the prostate documents a midline 5-mm round, anechoic cystic structure. On the transverse image, the ejaculatory duct is hypoechoic and can be seen on either side of the cyst. On the sagittal image, the cyst measures 8 mm in length and is nearly surrounded by prostatic tissue. The patient has hypospadias with the urethra opening on the underside of the penis and post-void dribbling. Based on this patient's history and sonographic findings, discuss why this is most likely a utricle cyst rather than a müllerian duct cysts?

3. A 52-year-old African American is worried he has prostate cancer. The man's father was diagnosed with prostate cancer at 82 years of age and the brother was diagnosed with benign prostatic hyperplasia (BPH) at 58 years of age. Recently, the man has experienced a more frequent need to urinate and is experiencing some pain while urinating. The sonography examination showed an enlarged gland with increased vascularity affecting the peripheral zone. After a biopsy, the physician diagnosed and treated the man for prostatitis. Explain why the diagnosis is plausible for this patient and why prostatitis and carcinoma primarily affect the peripheral zone.

4. What factors distinguish cancer of the prostate from BPH?

5. A 32-year-old man is scheduled for a sonographic evaluation and has high hopes the examination will detect the cause of azoospermia. What can the sonographer tell the patient regarding the advantages and disadvantages of an endorectal sonography examination?

## REFERENCES

1. Shetty S. Transrectal ultrasonography (TRUS) of the prostate. Urologic Imaging. Available at: http://emedicine.medscape.com/article/457757-overview. Accessed July 31, 2010.
2. McAchran SE, Resnick MI. Prostate ultrasound: past, present, and future. *Ultrasound Clin.* 2006;1:43–54.
3. Frauscher F, Gradl J, Pallwein L. Prostate ultrasound—for urologist only? *Cancer Imaging.* 2005;5:S76–S82.
4. Keith KL, Persaud TVN. The urogenital system. In: *The Developing Human: Clinically Oriented Embryology.* 8th ed. Philadelphia, PA: Elsevier Saunder; 2008:287–328.
5. Muldoon L, Resnick MI. Results of ultrasonography of the prostate. *Urol Clin North Am.* 1989;16(4):693–702.
6. Levin TL, Han B, Little BP. Congenital anomalies of the male urethra. *Pediatr Radiol.* 2007;37:851–862.
7. Dean GE Congenital prostatic abnormalities. *Current Prostate Reports.* 2008;6:39–42.
8. Nghiem HT, Kellman GM, Sandberg SA, et al. Cystic lesions of the prostate. *Radiographics.* 1990;10:635–650.
9. Keener TS, Winter TC, Berger R, et al. Prostate vascular flow. *AJR Am J Roentgenol.* 2000;175:1169–1172.
10. Neumaier CE, Martinoli C, Derchi LE, et al. Normal prostate gland: examination with color Doppler US. *Radiology.* 1995;196(2):453–457.
11. McNeal J. The prostate gland: morphology and pathobiology. *Monogr Urol.* 1988;9:36–54.
12. Laczko I, Hudson DL, Freeman A, et al. Comparison of the zones of the human prostate with the seminal vesicle: morphology, immunohistochemistry, and cell kinetics. *The Prostate.* 2005;62:260–266.
13. Raja J, Ramachandran N, Munneke G, et al. Current status of transrectal ultrasound-guided prostate biopsy in the diagnosis of prostate cancer. *Clin Radiol.* 2006;61:142–153.
14. Fornage BD. Normal US anatomy of the prostate. *Ultrasound Med Biol.* 1986;12:1011–1021.
15. McNeal JE. Normal and pathologic anatomy of prostate. *Urology.* 1981;17(3):11–16.
16. Kaye K. *Prostate ultrasound anatomy: Normal and pathological.* Dallas, TX: American Urological Association Annual Meeting; 1989.
17. Ishidoya S, Endoh M, Nakagawa H, et al. Novel anatomical findings of the prostatic gland and the surrounding capsular structures in the normal prostate. *Tohoku J Exp Med.* 2007;212:55–62.
18. Littrup PJ, Lee F, McLeary RD, et al. Transrectal US of the seminal vesicles and ejaculatory ducts: Clinical correlation. *Radiology.* 1988;168:625–628.
19. Brawer M. Techniques of examination. In: Resnick M., ed. *Prostatic Ultrasonography.* Philadelphia, PA: B.C. Decker Inc; 1990;25–35.
20. Rifkin MD, Dahnert W, Kurtz AB. State of the art: endorectal sonography of the prostate gland. *AJR Am J Roentgenol.* 1990;154:691–700.
21. Vincent R, Sebastien D, Panhard X, et al. The 20-core prostate biopsy protocol—a new gold standard? *J Urol.* 2008;179:504–507.
22. Loch AC, Bannowsky A, Baeurle L, et al. Technical and anatomical essentials for transrectal ultrasound of the prostate. *World J Urol.* 2007;25:361–366.
23. Hernandez J, Thompson IM. Prostate-specific antigen: a review of the validation of the most commonly used cancer biomarker. *Cancer.* 2004;101(5):894–904.
24. Haid M, Rabin D, King KM, et al. Digital rectal examination, serum prostate specific antigen, and prostatic ultrasound: how effective is this diagnostic triad? *J Surg Oncology.* 1994;56:32–38.

25. Jones JS. Prostate cancer: are we over-diagnosing or under-thinking? *Eur Urol.* 2008;53:10–12.

26. Shapiro A, Lebensart PD, Pode D, et al. The clinical utility of transrectal ultrasound and digital rectal examination in the diagnosis of prostate cancer. *Br J Radiol.* 1994;67:668–671.

27. Paul R, Korzinek C, Necknig U, et al. Influence of transrectal ultrasound probe on prostate cancer detection in transrectal ultrasound-guided sextant biopsy of prostate. *J Urol.* 2004; 64(3):532–536.

28. Moukaddam HA, Haddad MC, El-Sayyed K, et al. Diagnosis and treatment of midline prostatic cysts. *Clin Imaging.* 2003;27(1):44–46.

29. Galosi AB, Montironi R, Fabiani A, et al. Cystic lesions of the prostate gland: an ultrasound classification with pathological correlation. *J Urol.* 2009;181:647–657.

30. VanPoppel H, Vereecken R, De GP, et al. Hemospermia owing to utricle cyst: embryological summary and surgical review. *J Urol.* 1983; 129:608–609.

31. Elder JS, Mostwin JL. Cyst of the ejaculatory duct/urogenital sinus. *J Urol.* 1984;132:768–771.

32. Arora SS, Breiman RS, Webb EM, et al. CT and MRI of congenital anomalies of the seminal vesicles. *AJR Am J Roentgenol.* 2007;189:130–135.

33. Labanaris AP, Zugor V Meyer B, et al. A case of a large seminal vesicle cyst associated with ipsilateral renal agenesis. *Scientific World Journal.* 2008;8:400–404.

34. Sheih CP, Hung CS, Wei CF, et al. Cystic dilatations within the pelvis in patients with ipsilateral renal agenesis or dysplasia. *J Urol.* 1990;144:324–327.

35. Anderson W. Anderson's pathology. In: Kissane J, ed. *Anderson's Pathology.* 8th ed. St. Louis, MO: Mosby; 1985.

36. Lee F, Torp P-ST, Siders DB, et al. Transrectal ultrasound in the diagnosis and staging of prostatic carcinoma. *Radiology.* 1989;170(3 pt 1):609–615.

37. Narayan S, Mongha R, Kundu AK. Gross calcification within the prostate gland and its significance and treatment. *Indian J. Surg.* 2008;70:203–204.

38. Suh JH, Gardner JM, Kee KH, et al. Calcifications in prostate and ejaculatory system: a study on 298 consecutive whole mount sections of prostate from radical prostatectomy or cystoprostatectomy specimens. *Ann Diagn Pathol.* 2008;12:165–170.

39. Griffiths G, Clements R, Peeling W. Inflammatory disease and calculi. In: Resnick M. ed. *Prostatic Ultrasonography.* Philadelphia, PA: B.C. Decker Inc.; 1990.

40. Weidner W, Anderson RU. Evaluation of acute and chronic bacterial prostatitis and diagnostic management of chronic prostatitis/chronic pelvic pain syndrome with special reference to infection/inflammation. *Int J Antimicrob Agents.* 2008;31(suppl 1):S91-S95.

41. Naber KG. Management of bacterial prostatitis: what's new? *BJU Int.* 2008;101(suppl 3):7–10.

42. Weidner W, Wagenlehner FM, Marconi M, et al. Acute bacterial prostatitis and chronic prostatitis/chronic pelvic pain syndrome: andrological implications. *Andrologia.* 2008;40(2):105–112.

43. Schaeffer AJ. Prostatitis: US perspective. *Int J Antimicrob Agents.* 1998;10:153–159.

44. Blacklock NJ. The anatomy of the prostate: relationship with prostatic infection. *Infection.* 1991;3:S111–S114.

45. Gulek B, Evliyaoglu Y. Transrectal sonographic findings in chronic prostatitis: a comparative study with an asymptomatic control group. *J Diagn Med Sonogr.* 2008;24:88–92.

46. Shoskes DA, Lee CT, Murphy D, et al. Incidence and significance of prostatic stones in men with chronic prostatitis/chronic pelvic pain syndrome. *Urology.* 2007;70(2):235–238.

47. Dogra VS, Turgut AT. Prostate carcinoma: Evaluation using transrectal sonography. In: Hayat MA, ed. *Methods of Cancer Diagnosis, Therapy, and Prognosis: General Methods and Overviews, Lung Carcinoma and Prostate Carcinoma.* The Netherlands: Springer; 2008:499–520.

48. Pallwein L, Mitterberger M, Pelzer A, et al. Ultrasound of prostate cancer: recent advances. *Eur Radiol.* 2008;18:707–715

49. Crawford ED. Epidemiology of prostate cancer. *J Urol.* 2003;62(suppl 1):3–12.

50. Carter HB, Piantadosi S, Isaacs JT. Clinical evidence for and implications of the multistep development of prostate cancer. *J Urol.* 1990;143:742–746.

51. Franks L. Latent carcinoma of the prostate. *J Pathol Bact.* 1954;68:603–616.

52. Carroll P, Coley C, McLeod D, et al. Prostate-specific antigen best practice policy. Part 1: early detection and diagnosis of prostate cancer. *Urology.* 2001;57:217–224.

53. Carey BM. Imaging for prostate cancer. *Clin Oncol.* 2005;17:553–559.

54. Brawer MK. The diagnosis of prostatic carcinoma. *Cancer.* 1993; 71 Suppl 3:899–905.

55. Matlaga BR, Eskew LA, McCullough DL. Prostate biopsy: indications and technique. *J Urol.* 2003;169:12–19.

56. Hricak H, Choyke PL, Eberhardt SC, et al. Imaging prostate cancer: a multidisciplinary perspective. *Radiology.* 2007;243:28–53.

57. Linden RA, Halpern EJ. Advances in transrectal ultrasound imaging of the prostate. *Semin Ultrasound CT MR.* 2007;28(4):249–257.

58. Mallick S, Humbert M, Braud F, et al. Local anesthesia before transrectal ultrasound guided prostate biopsy: comparison of 2 methods in a prospective, randomized clinical trial. *J Urol.* 2004;171:730–733.

59. Djavan B, Margreiter M. Biopsy standards for detection of prostate cancer. *World J Urol.* 2007;25:11–17.

60. Jarow JP. Transrectal ultrasonography of infertile men. *Fertility and Sterility.* 1993;60:1035–1039.

61. Simpson WL Jr, Rausch DR. Imaging of male infertility: pictorial review. *AJR Am J Roentgenol.* 2009;192:S98–S107.

62. Barratt C, Bolton A, Cooke I. Functional significance of white blood cells in the male and female reproductive tract. *Human Reprod.* 1990;5:639–648.

63. Purvis K, Christiansen E. Infection in the male reproductive tract. Impact, diagnosis and treatment in relation to male infertility. *Int J Androl.* 1993;16(1):1–13.

64. Jarow J: Transrectal ultrasonography in the evaluation of male infertility. In: Resnick M, ed. *Prostatic Ultrasonography.* Philadelphia, PA: B.C. Decker Inc.; 1990.

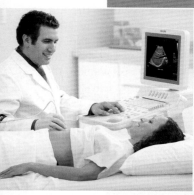

# 13 The Adrenal Glands

Kari E. Boyce

## OBJECTIVES

Identify the sonographic role in the evaluation of the adrenal glands.

Describe the embryologic development of the adrenal glands.

Discuss the anatomy and physiology of the adrenal cortex and medulla.

List the hormones secreted by the adrenal cortex and medulla.

Identify conditions caused by hyposecretion and hypersecretion of adrenal hormones.

Identify the normal sonographic appearance of the adrenal glands.

Describe adrenal gland scanning technique, patient positions, and scanning pitfalls.

Discuss the differential diagnosis for solid adrenal masses.

Discuss alternative imaging modalities used to evaluate the adrenal glands.

## KEY TERMS

Addison disease | adenocarcinoma | adrenal adenoma | adrenal cyst | adrenal hemorrhage | Conn syndrome | Cushing syndrome | hyperadrenalism | hypoadrenalism | myelolipoma | pheochromocytoma | Waterhouse-Friderichsen syndrome

## GLOSSARY

**adrenal cortex** outer parenchyma of the adrenal gland makes up 90% of the organ's weight and secretes corticoids including cortisol and aldosterone

**adrenal medulla** inner portion of the adrenal gland that secretes the catecholamines epinephrine and norepinephrine

**adrenocorticotropic hormone (ACTH)** hormone secreted by the pituitary gland that causes the adrenal gland to produce and release corticosteroids

**endoscopic ultrasound (EUS)** an ultrasound transducer on a thin flexible endoscope is inserted in the mouth or anus to visualize the walls of the upper or lower digestive tract and surrounding organs

**multiple endocrine neoplasia (MEN) syndrome** a group of autosomal dominant disorders characterized by benign and malignant tumors of the endocrine glands

In contrast with other examinations of the abdomen, transabdominal sonographic imaging is not the first choice imaging modality for screening adrenal glands or detecting adrenal pathology. Examination of the adrenal glands challenges the skills of novice and experienced sonographers alike and requires a working knowledge of exact adrenal anatomic locations and landmarks. However, combining planar flexibility and improved beam-resolution capabilities of modern ultrasound equipment with maneuvering the patient into multiple positions increases the likelihood of producing quality sonographic images of the adrenal glands.[1-3] In addition, since the mid-1990s, endoscopic ultrasound (EUS) and intraoperative ultrasound (IOUS) have developed as tools for high-resolution sonography evaluation of suprarenal and retroperitoneal masses. Using a 7.5 MHz transducer positioned 1 to 2 cm from the adrenal gland, EUS and IOUS are particularly useful for detecting adrenal metastases and staging cancer.[4,5] As new technologies are introduced for transabdominal imaging, such as three-dimensional/four-dimensional (3D/4D) imaging and elastography, these tools also become available for EUS and IOUS applications.[6,7]

This chapter provides an overview of relevant anatomy, embryology, scanning techniques, functional and morphologic adrenal pathology, and the sonographic appearance of the normal gland as well as adrenal pathology. As a sonographer, it is important to develop critical-thinking and problem-solving skills for sorting out the origin and extent of abdominal masses, including those of suprarenal and retroperitoneal origin. Related techniques are discussed. In addition, EUS, IOUS, computed tomography (CT), magnetic resonance imaging (MRI), and associated nuclear medicine imaging procedures are presented as related to adrenal imaging. Due to technical improvements in all the diagnostic imaging modalities and the increased use of these modalities, more clinically silent or unexpected masses are being detected. The general term for an unexpected mass detected during an imaging procedure being performed for unrelated disease is "incidentaloma." This term may be applied to any unexpected mass occurring anywhere in the body. Adrenal incidentaloma (AI) has become a common term in the medical literature and represents a diagnostic challenge that includes discovery of masses, which range from benign, nonfunctional lesions to malignant tumors such as pheochromocytomas, adrenocortical carcinomas, or metastases from other primary cancers.[8] Sonographers have a role both in the initial detection of AIs and gathering diagnostic information regarding newly discovered AIs.

# ANATOMY

## EMBRYOLOGY

The adrenal gland consists of two distinct parts: the cortex and the medulla. Each develops from different embryonic tissues, forms different anatomical and functional structures, and combines within a common capsule.[9,10] The result is two endocrine glands in one organ. Most glands of the body develop from epithelial tissue. In contrast, the adrenal cortex is derived from the mesoderm of the same region that gives rise to gonadal tissue.[9,10] The central tissue or adrenal medulla is functionally part of the sympathetic nervous system developed from the neural crest cells that also give rise to postganglionic sympathetic neurons.[9–11] As a result, some adrenal medullary pathology may appear ectopically along the paths of these sympathetic neurons usually near the celiac axis, whereas ectopic adrenocortical tissue may be located inferiorly along the path of gonadal tissue migration.[9–11] In addition, extra-adrenal chromaffin cells also normally deposit near the aortic bifurcation to form the organ of Zuckerkandl.[10–12]

## Cortex

During gestational weeks 5 and 6, the fetal cortex is first recognized bilaterally as a groove between the developing dorsal mesentery and gonad.[9,10] During weeks 7 and 8, the cells arrange into cords with dilated blood spaces, forming a thin capsule of connective tissue that encloses the gland[9,10] and develops an intimate relationship with the superior pole of the kidney. If the kidney does not develop normally, there will be a discoid distortion in the shape of the adrenal gland.[9,10] Initially, the fetal adrenal gland is larger than the kidney and 10 to 20 times the relative size of the adult adrenal gland.[9,10] During the remainder of fetal life, the cortical tissue is composed of two zones comprising 75% to 80% of the bulk of the gland.[10,11] By week 8, the cortex produces precursors to androgen, estriol, and corticosteroids.[9,10] After birth, the inner zone undergoes involution, whereas the thinner outer zone continues to develop into the adult adrenal cortex, which takes on a yellow color.[9–13] By the age of 3 years, the cortex differentiates into three zones: (1) zona glomerulosa, (2) zona fasciculata, and (3) zona reticularis. Each zone develops different cellular arrangements and becomes functionally specialized, producing mineralocorticoids, glucocorticoids, and gonadocorticoids, respectively[9–12,14] (Fig. 13-1).

## Medulla

Specific ectodermal cells ascend from the neural crest, migrate from their origin, and differentiate into sympathetic neurons of the autonomic nervous system.[9–11] Some of these primitive autonomic ganglia differentiate even further into endocrine cells, designated chromaffin cells, and migrate to form a mass on the medial surface of the fetal adrenal cortex.[9–11] Soon these chromaffins, or pheochrome cells, invade the developing cortex, establishing the primordium of the adrenal medulla.[9,10] On cut section, the medulla has a red, brown, or gray color depending on the level of blood perfusion.[15] As mentioned previously, chromaffin cells also form the organ of Zuckerkandl.[10–12]

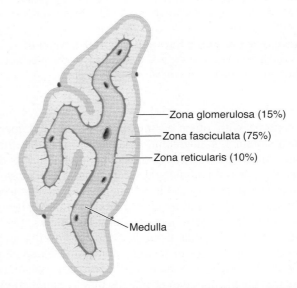

Zona glomerulosa (15%)
Zona fasciculata (75%)
Zona reticularis (10%)
Medulla

**Figure 13-1** Adrenal gland. The anatomic sectional illustration of the adrenal gland demonstrates the medulla surrounded by three differentiated zones of the cortex. (From Premkumar K. *The Massage Connection: Anatomy and Physiology.* 2nd ed. Baltimore, MD: Lippincott Williams & Wilkins; 2004.)

## RELATIONAL ANATOMY

Like the kidneys, the adrenal glands are retroperitoneal. They are generally anterior, medial, and superior to the kidneys.[9,10,13,15] The cortex and medulla are encapsulated by a thick inner layer of fatty connective tissue.[12,13] A thin, fibrous outer capsule attaches to the gland by many fibrous bands, providing the adrenals with their own fascial supports so that they do not descend if the kidneys are displaced or absent.[9,12] The glands are attached to the anteromedial aspect within renal fascia (also referred to as Gerota fascia), and abundant adipose tissue (perinephric fat) surrounds each gland, separating it from the kidneys[11,12,16] (Fig. 13-2).

### Right Adrenal

The right adrenal gland is located posterior and lateral to the inferior vena cava (IVC), medial to the right lobe of the liver, and lateral to the crus of the diaphragm.[9,10,13,15,16] The right adrenal gland has been described as sitting like a triangular cap on the anterior, medial, and superior aspect of the superior pole of the right kidney.

The anterior surface of the right adrenal gland is shaped like a pyramid. Two areas make up the anterior surface: the medial area is narrow and lies posterolateral to the IVC and the lateral, somewhat triangular, portion is in contact with the liver.[9,10,13,15,16] The superior end of the lateral area is devoid of peritoneum as it comes in contact with the bare area of the liver, and the inferior portion is covered by reflected peritoneum from the inferior layer of the coronary ligament[12,13,15] (Fig. 13-3).

A curved ridge separates the posterior dorsal surface into superior and inferior parts. The superior convex portion rests on the diaphragm, and the inferior concave portion is in contact with the superior–anterior surface of the right kidney[15] (Fig. 13-3).

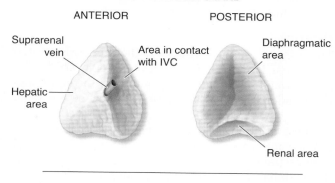

**RIGHT ADRENAL GLAND**

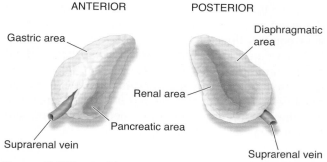

**LEFT ADRENAL GLAND**

**Figure 13-3** Topographic anatomy. There is a difference in the surface anatomy of right and left adrenal glands.

### Left Adrenal

The left adrenal gland appears draped in an elongated, crescent, or semilunar shape on the medial aspect of the left kidney's superior pole.[9–13,15,16] The left gland is larger than the right, and extension to the left renal hilus is a normal variant.

The anterior portion can be separated into superior and inferior parts. The superior area is situated posterior to the peritoneal wall of the lesser sac and is covered by peritoneum of the omental bursa, which separates the gland from the cardiac portion of the stomach.[15] The inferior area is not covered by peritoneum and lies posterior and lateral to the pancreas[9,10,12,13,15,16] (Fig. 13-3). The splenic artery and vein course between the pancreas and the left adrenal gland.

The posterior surface is in close proximity to the splanchnic nerves.[6,15] It is divided into a medial and a lateral area by a vertical ridge. The larger lateral area rests on the kidney and the medial posterior area on the crus of the diaphragm[12,13,15] (Fig. 13-3).

## SYSTEMIC AND LYMPHATIC VESSELS

Similar to other endocrine glands, the adrenals are among the most vascular organs of the body.[13,15,16] The vasculature of the adrenal gland is distinguished from other organs in that the arteries and veins do not actually course together. The abundant arterial supply may contain as many as 50 to 60 small terminal arterioles,

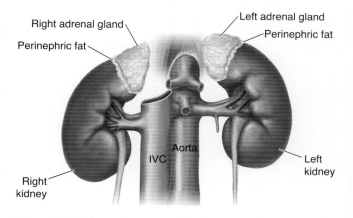

**Figure 13-2** Relational anatomy. The illustration demonstrates the anteromedial relationship of the adrenal glands to the kidneys. (Asset provided by Anatomical Chart Co.)

whereas the venous blood is channeled almost completely through a single, large venous trunk.[12,13,15,16]

## Arteries

Three arteries supply each gland: the superiorly located suprarenal branch of the inferior phrenic artery, the superior and medially located branch of the aorta, and the inferiorly located suprarenal branch of the renal artery[12,13,15,16] (Fig. 13-4).

These arteries are distinctively classified into three types: short capsular arterioles, intermediate cortical arteries (long branches that go through the cortex to the medulla), and the medullary sinusoids.[15]

## Veins

In each adrenal gland, a central vein runs the length of the gland and exits at the hilum.[12] The right suprarenal vein empties directly into the posterior aspect of the IVC as a short (4 to 5 mm) vessel, which exits the gland on the mid-anteromedial surface.[12,15] The left suprarenal vein drains directly inferior and medial into the left renal vein.[12,15] Frequently, the left inferior phrenic vein and the left suprarenal vein join before emptying into the left renal vein[12,15] (Fig. 13-4).

## Lymphatics

Lymph channels drain from the adrenal cortex and medulla to the hilar area.[15] Following the arterial pathways, larger lymphatic vessels drain into para-aortic and lumbar lymph nodes, which drain to the cisterna chyli, thoracic duct, and eventually into the subclavian vein, whereas a few lymphatic vessels drain into the posterior mediastinal lymph nodes.[12,17]

# PHYSIOLOGY

Just as their origin and structure are unique, the function and control of hormones differ for these two different glands in one organ. Adrenal pathology and some medications have the potential to disrupt the level of adrenal hormone secretion and associated regulatory mechanisms.[11,14,18-20] Hormones produced by the adrenal cortex, such as cortisol, are essential to life and must be replaced if both adrenal glands are removed.[11,14,18-20]

## CORTEX

The cortex makes up 90% of the adrenal gland. By 3 years of age, the cortex develops into three epithelial layers, each one evolving functionally into very specialized zones, producing steroid hormones consistent with their mesodermal source. The zona glomerulosa, the outer layer directly beneath the connective tissue covering, makes up 15% of the cortex and produces aldosterone, a mineralocorticoid.[9,10,13,14,16] The zona fasciculata, the middle layer, comprises 75% of the cortex and the zona reticularis, the inner layer, accounts for the remaining 10% of the cortex[9-11,13,16] (Fig. 13-1). Cortisol, a glucocorticoid, and two gonadocorticoids, estrogen and androgen, are produced by the zona fasciculata and zona reticularis.[9,10,13,14,16]

Hormone secretion is often controlled by the negative feedback mechanisms.[14] Low blood concentrations of a hormone trigger the hypothalamus to secrete the primary regulating factor, *corticotrophin-releasing hormone* (CRH), which triggers the anterior lobe of the pituitary to release adrenocorticotropic hormone (ACTH).[14] As blood concentrations of ACTH increase, adrenal hormone activity increases, producing a higher concentration of hormones, such as cortisol, in the bloodstream. This increased concentration of the adrenal hormone inhibits CRH and ACTH and, ultimately, hormone synthesis. When the blood concentration of one or more of the adrenal hormones drop to low levels, the cycle is repeated.[14,18] Adrenocortical hormone secretion, function, and regulation are summarized in Table 13-1.

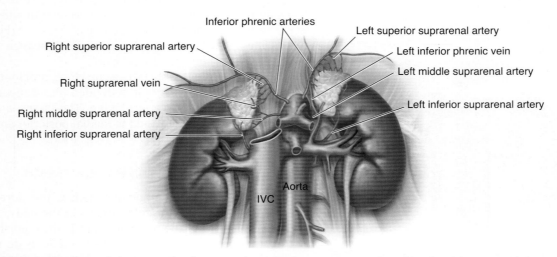

**Figure 13-4** Adrenal gland vascular anatomy. The illustration shows the three arteries supplying blood and the venous drainage for the right and left adrenal glands.

| TABLE 13-1 | | | |
|---|---|---|---|
| **Adrenal Hormone Secretion, Function, and Regulation**[7,11,21] | | | |
| **Layer** | **Hormone** | **Function** | **Regulation** |
| Zona glomerulosa | Aldosterone is responsible for 95% of mineralocorticoid hormone activity | Regulates sodium and potassium levels, which affect fluid and electrolyte homeostasis, including extracellular fluid volumes. Primary activation through the renin-angiotensin system. | Complex process; release triggered by (a) dehydration, sodium deficiency, hemorrhage or (b) elevated potassium levels. ACTH has minor role in stimulation secretion. |
| Zona fasciculata | Glucocorticoids, including cortisol or hydrocortisone (most abundant), cortisone, and corticosterone | Major effect on metabolism of lipids, proteins, and carbohydrates; encourages fat storage. When more energy is required, assists in gluconeogenesis, which helps resist both mental and physical stress. Hormones trigger anti-inflammatory and immune-suppress responses. | High stress or low blood concentration (negative feedback mechanism) |
| Zona reticularis | Regardless of gender, secretes both male and female gonadocorticoids (estrogens and androgens) | Promotes normal development of bones and reproductive organs; affects secondary sex characteristics but not as much as hormones from ovaries and testes | Low blood concentration (negative feedback mechanism) |

ACTH, adrenocorticotropic hormone.

## MEDULLA

Originating from ectodermal cells, the medulla secretes catecholamine hormones, similar to the posterior pituitary and thyroid glands. The medulla's chromaffin (pheochrome) cells, the hormone-producing portion, surround large blood-filled sinuses.[9,10,13,16]

Epinephrine (adrenalin) and norepinephrine (noradrenalin) are the two principal hormones synthesized by the medulla. Epinephrine constitutes about 80% of the total secretion, and its action is more important than norepinephrine. Release of both hormones is usually stimulated through the sympathetic nervous system.[11,14]

Adrenal nerve stimulation results in prompt discharge of medullary hormones without materially influencing cortical secretion.[11,14] Hormone secretion is controlled directly by the autonomic nervous system, and innervation by the preganglionic fibers allows the gland to respond to the neural stimulus.[14] The anticipation or presence of stress or pain causes the hypothalamus to signal the sympathetic preganglionic neurons to stimulate the chromaffin cells to increase output of epinephrine and norepinephrine.[11,14] Functionally, the medulla is a large sympathetic ganglion, which triggers action via hormone release instead of through axons.[11,14] The body responds by (1) accelerating the heart rate and constricting the vessels, causing increased blood pressure; (2) accelerating the rate of respiration and dilating the respiratory passage; (3) decreasing the rate of digestion to make available more blood to the muscles, increasing the efficiency of muscle contraction; and (4) increasing the blood sugar level to provide energy, thus stimulating cellular metabolism.[11,14] This physiologic response to stress is better known as the *fight-or-flight response*.[11,14,18] Hypoglycemia, hypotension, hypoxia, hypovolemia, and exposure to temperature extremes may also stimulate medullary secretion of epinephrine and norepinephrine.[11,14] Like the glucocorticoids of the adrenal cortices, these hormones help the body resist stress; however, unlike the cortical hormones, the medullary hormones are not essential to life.[11,14]

## FUNCTION TESTS

There are many different kinds of laboratory tests to evaluate adrenocortical function. They can be divided into two types: tests that determine the absolute values in serum and urine versus tests that check the interdependency of the various hormones. Table 13-2 summarizes the significance of increased and decreased variance from normal laboratory values for various serum and urine tests.

Of the limited tests available for testing medullary function, 24-hour urine samples are typically used for catecholamines.[11,14,18,20] Metanephrines are measured in urine, whereas dopamines may be assessed via urine or blood samples.[18,20] With hypertension, pheochromocytoma, or neuroblastoma, urine levels of

| TABLE 13-2 | | | |
|---|---|---|---|
| **Tests of Adrenal Function[7,11,21]** | | | |
| **Sample Source** | **Steroid** | **Variation** | **Clinical Implications and Accompanying Conditions** |
| Serum | Adrenocorticotropic hormone (ACTH, corticotropin) | Increase | Addison disease, ectopic ACTH syndrome, pituitary adenoma, pituitary Cushing syndrome, primary adrenal insufficiency, and stress. Drugs causing elevation: amphetamine sulfate, calcium gluconate, corticosteroids, estrogens, ethanol, lithium carbonate, metyrapone, and spironolactone. |
| | | Decrease | Primary adrenocortical hyperfunction (due to tumor or hyperplasia) and secondary hypoadrenalism. Drugs causing suppression: dexamethasone. |
| Serum/urine | Aldosterone | Increase | Adrenal tumor (adenoma), aldosteronism (primary, secondary), bilateral adrenal gland hyperplasia, cirrhosis, chronic obstructive lung disease, congestive heart failure, Conn syndrome (with decreased renin), stress, hemorrhage, hyponatremia, hypovolemia, idiopathic cyclic edema, inadequate renal perfusion causing continual activity of the renin-angiotensin system (renin level is also high), nephrosis (lower nephron), nephrotic syndrome, renovascular hypertension (with hypokalemia), low-sodium diet, and excessive licorice consumption. Drugs causing elevation: corticotropin, diuretics that promote sodium excretion, fludrocortisone, and potassium. |
| | | Decrease | Addison disease, primary hypoaldosteronism, salt-wasting syndrome (high-sodium diet), septicemia, stress, diabetes mellitus, and pregnancy-induced toxemia. Drugs causing suppression: fludrocortisone and methyldopa. |
| Serum/urine | Cortisol | Increase | Pituitary tumor causing ACTH-dependent increase (Cushing disease), Cushing syndrome causing ACTH-independent increase, adrenal gland hyperplasia, pregnancy-induced hypertension, exercise, severe hepatic disease, hyperpituitarism, hypertension, hyperthyroidism, infectious disease, obesity, acute pancreatitis, pregnancy, severe renal disease, burns, shock, stress (severe heat, cold, trauma, psychological), surgery, and amenorrhea (urine). Drugs causing elevation: long-term corticosteroid therapy (virilism), corticotropin, estrogens, oral contraceptives, and vasopressin. |
| | | Decrease | Addison disease from primary hypofunction of the cortex or secondary to hypofunction of the pituitary gland, iatrogenic adrenal insufficiency, adrenogenital syndrome, AIDS, chromophobe adenoma, craniopharyngioma, hyperkalemia, hypoglycemia, hyponatremia, hypophysectomy, hypopituitarism, hypothyroidism, hypovolemia, liver disease, postural hypotension, postpartum pituitary necrosis, renal-glomerular dysfunction (urine), and Waterhouse-Friderichsen syndrome. Drugs causing suppression: withdrawing corticosteroids after long-term administration, dexamethasone, dexamethasone acetate, and dexamethasone sodium phosphate. |
| Urine | 17-Ketogenic steroids (17-KS) | Increase | Adrenogenital syndrome, Cushing syndrome, adrenal carcinoma, burns, hirsutism, hyperadrenalism, infectious disease, obesity, pregnancy, surgery, and virilization. Drugs causing elevation: cephalothin, corticosteroids, digoxin, meprobamate, oral contraceptives, penicillin, phenothiazine, and spironolactone. |
| | | Decrease | Addison disease, cretinism, hypoadrenalism, hypopituitarism, Simmonds disease, postovary or testicle removal, and wasting away diseases in general. Drug intake includes ampicillin, dexamethasone, estrogens, glucose, morphine, phenytoin, prednisone, and prednisolone. |

ACTH, adrenocorticotropic hormone.

catecholamine, vanillylmandelic acid (VMA), or both may be elevated.[11,14,18,20]

Multiple tests are designed to determine the true functions and interdependency of the hypothalamus, pituitary, kidneys, and adrenals, including stimulation and suppression testing for ACTH, aldosterone, and cortisol.[11,14,18,19]

# SONOGRAPHIC SCANNING TECHNIQUE

## PREPARATION

Usually, patients receive no preparatory instructions for sonography of the adrenal glands, but when there is suspicion of a mass or metastases or a need to image any retroperitoneal anatomy sonographically, it is recommended that the patient fast approximately 6 to 8 hours before the examination.

## SCANNING PROTOCOL

Evaluation of adrenals may be approached with the patient in supine or decubitus positions. Common protocols typically begin with transverse scanning, followed by longitudinal and/or coronal assessment. Slight or small scanning maneuvers are used to obtain desired images. One of the imaging goals for adrenal sonography is to document unilateral versus bilateral pathologic involvement. As with most sonographic examinations, width and anteroposterior measurements in transverse sections and length measurements from the longitudinal/coronal sections are required. Various breathing excursions and suspended inspiration may be used to optimize visualization of both adrenal glands.

Select the highest frequency transducer that will provide adequate penetration, given an adrenal depth range of 4 to 12 cm, depending on the patient's size.[21] Selection of a transducer with a small footprint will also facilitate scanning through intercostal spaces.[1,3] Magnifying the field size may improve visualization of small structures. Scanning the patient in a prone position is uncommon, although this method is useful to show the spatial relationship between a large adrenal mass and the adjacent kidney.

### Right Adrenal

For imaging the right adrenal, the liver and sometimes the right kidney are useful acoustic windows (Fig. 13-5). Successful utilization of the liver as an acoustic window depends on hepatic size and attenuation characteristics (Fig. 13-6). Starting with transverse scans using an intercostal approach, find the section of the IVC located medial and anterior to the upper pole of the kidney.[1,2] Direct the plane toward the lateral and posterior aspects of this portion of the

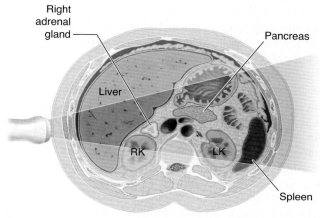

**Figure 13-5** Right adrenal gland scan technique. With the patient in a supine position, a series of transverse images are obtained through the intercostal spaces of the right adrenal gland, using the liver and kidney as acoustic windows. *RK*, right kidney; *LK*, left kidney.

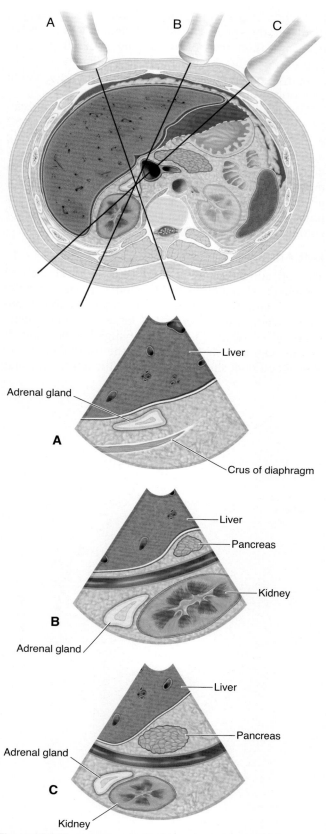

**Figure 13-6** Transverse sectional planes of the right adrenal. The sectional transverse illustration demonstrates the relationship of the adrenal glands to other anatomic structures. Longitudinal images of the right adrenal gland as obtained with the patient in a supine position, using the liver as an acoustic window. **(A)** and **(B)** can be obtained on most patients, whereas **(C)** requires a prominent left liver lobe.

IVC while also keeping the ultrasound beam perpendicular to the spine. The adrenal gland should be seen in this location anterior to the crus of the diaphragm. The entire right adrenal gland is evaluated by scanning transversely from the renal hilus and proceeding superiorly (Fig. 13-5).

Longitudinal or coronal scanning of the right gland can be accomplished with several approaches[1,3] (Fig. 13-6). A higher success rate has been reported when utilizing the liver as an acoustic window and scanning the patient in a left lateral decubitus position.[6,23,24] From an intercostal window, the transducer is angled anterior toward the IVC and posterior toward the right kidney until the entire gland is visualized in the longitudinal or coronal plane (Fig. 13-7).

### Left Adrenal

The left adrenal gland is more difficult to locate and document. Conventionally, the left adrenal has been imaged with the patient in the right decubitus position, using the spleen or left kidney as an acoustic window[21,23,25] (Fig. 13-8). Identifying the left adrenal and its alignment is first done in the transverse plane. The left adrenal should lie between the left kidney and

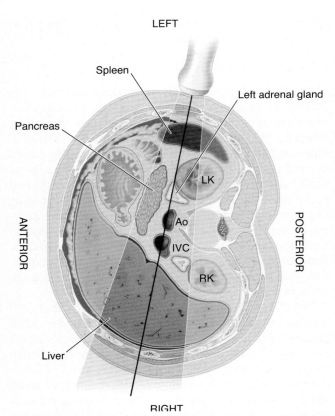

Figure 13-8 Right lateral decubitus technique. Using the spleen or the left kidney (*LK*) as an acoustic window, transverse images of the left adrenal gland can be made with the patient in a right lateral decubitus position. *Ao,* aorta; *IVC,* inferior vena cava; *RK,* right kidney.

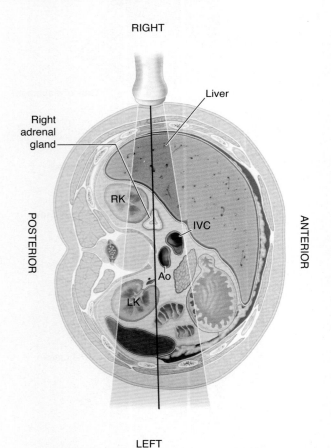

Figure 13-7 Left lateral decubitus technique. With the patient in a left lateral decubitus position, the right adrenal gland may be easier to visualize as the IVC moves forward and the aorta moves over the crus of the diaphragm. *RK,* right kidney; *Ao,* aorta; *LK,* left kidney; *IVC,* inferior vena cava.

the aorta, with the pancreatic tail and splenic vein marking the superior margin of the gland.[26]

Longitudinal or coronal scans may be easier to obtain with the patient in a right anterior oblique position using a left posterior oblique scanning plane. First, in the transverse plane, locate the aorta medial and anterior to the upper pole of the left kidney or the spleen, until the axis of the left kidney and the position of the aorta are determined and the left adrenal gland is identified between these structures[23,24] (Fig. 13-9A). With the patient in the same position, rotate the transducer into the longitudinal/coronal plane. When imaging the left adrenal gland, the transducer may have to be oriented obliquely (Fig. 13-9B).

In the mid-1980s, Krebs and colleagues[21,25] introduced an alternative approach to improve localization and delineation of the left adrenal gland. The patient is placed in a 45-degree left posterior oblique position, termed the *cava-suprarenal line position.*[21,25,27] The transducer is placed on the patient's right side, allowing the acoustic beam to pass through a double vascular acoustic window, the IVC, and the aorta[21] (Fig. 13-10). The protocol starts with transverse scans until the left adrenal gland is located; longitudinal views follow. With this position, the success rate is 90%, compared to 60% in the same patient population using the conventional approach.[21,25]

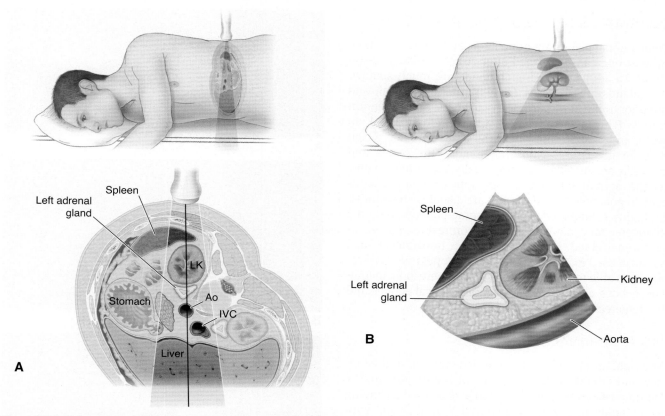

**Figure 13-9** Right anterior oblique technique. **A:** With the patient lying in a right anterior oblique position, the left kidney (*LK*) and aorta (*Ao*) are aligned in a transverse plane until the left adrenal gland is located. *IVC*, inferior vena cava. **B:** After the left adrenal gland is identified in the transverse plane, longitudinal images of the entire gland are easier to obtain.

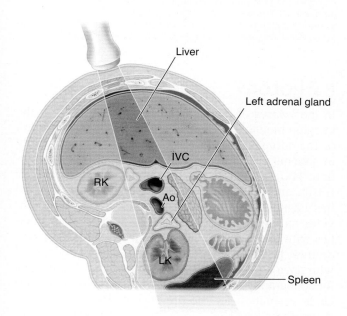

**Figure 13-10** Cava-suprarenal line position. The cava-suprarenal line position uses the inferior vena cava (*IVC*) and aorta (*Ao*) as a double vascular acoustic window for visualizing the left adrenal gland.[35–37] *RK*, right kidney; *LK*, left kidney.

## PITFALLS

The size, location, and pathology of the adrenals and of surrounding structures impose significant limitations on sonographic visualization. Cirrhosis with fatty infiltration of the liver and obesity interfere with adequate penetration. Shadowing from the ribs and narrow intercostal spaces also make this approach challenging.

The right adrenal gland may be obscured by gas and food in the second portion of the duodenum. It is important to differentiate the crus of the diaphragm as a tubular structure located medial to the right adrenal, as it can be mistaken for a normal gland.[28] The right adrenal gland is usually displaced posteriorly when the retroperitoneal fat line is displaced by liver disease.[28,29]

Structures that converge in the area of the left adrenal may mimic this gland: the esophagogastric junction, stomach, gastric diverticula, splenic vessels, portosystemic collateral vessels, tail of the pancreas, prominent hepatic lobes, medial lobulations of the spleen, superior lobulations of the kidney, or adjacent tumors.[1,3,28,30–33] A more posterolateral approach or the cava-suprarenal line position may be indicated for proper visualization of the left adrenal gland.[21,25]

## NORMAL SONOGRAPHIC ANATOMY

Fetal adrenal glands are quite large, and 90% of the time at least one can be imaged after 26 to 27 weeks' gestation.[34] In adults, the adrenal glands are much smaller. The glands are generally located anterior, medial, and superior to the kidneys and vary in shape and configuration.[11,33] Their size varies from 3 to 6 cm long, 2 to 4 cm wide, and 3 to 10 mm thick; the adult adrenals weigh 4 to 14 g.[1,3,23,24,33,35] Transabdominally, the cortex and medulla are usually sonographically indistinguishable, as the normal internal texture appears homogeneous and hypoechoic.[33] The glands are usually surrounded by highly echogenic fat, and in some patients, only the echogenic fat can be identified in contrast to an anechoic adrenal gland.[33] Higher resolution transducers such as those used for endoscopic and intraoperative applications are able to routinely detect the hyperechoic medullary echoes against the hypoechoic cortical echoes and the hyperechoic halo of fatty tissue.[4,17]

### RIGHT ADRENAL

The right adrenal gland is identified superior to the kidney and lateral to the right crus of the diaphragm.[24,33] On transverse sections, the gland is described as having a triangular, trapezoid, or inverted Y or V shape, with the tail extending from the anteromedial aspect of the right kidney[3,31,33,36] (Fig. 13-11A). In a longitudinal plane scanning the medial aspect of the gland, the anteromedial ridge appears as a curvilinear or S-shaped structure and is visualized posterior to the IVC, slightly above or at the level of the portal vein.[1,23,24,33,36] Moving laterally in longitudinal planes through the right adrenal gland, the anterior and posterior wings spread open and the gland takes on an inverted Y or V shape[36] (Fig. 13-11B,C). The anterolateral portion is medial and posterior to the right lobe of the liver and posterior to the duodenum.[33] Care should be taken to differentiate the right adrenal gland from the more medial hypoechoic/anechoic tubular right crus of the diaphragm.

### LEFT ADRENAL

Lateral to the left crus of the diaphragm and lateral or slightly posterolateral to the aorta, the left adrenal gland is visualized superior and medial to the kidney.[23,33,36] This gland is described as having a triangular or semilunar appearance (Fig. 13-12A). Since the stomach lies posterior to the lesser omental sac (a potential space that is usually collapsed), the superior portion of the adrenal gland can appear directly behind the stomach.[1,36] The inferior portion of the gland lies posterior to the pancreas. The splenic artery and vein can be identified passing between the left adrenal gland and the more anterior pancreas.[33,36] On longitudinal sections posterior to the pancreas, the left adrenal has a sonographic configuration similar to that of the right gland[36] (Fig. 13-12B–D).

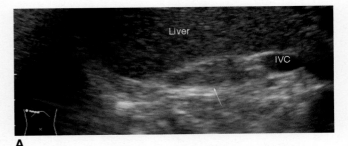

**A**

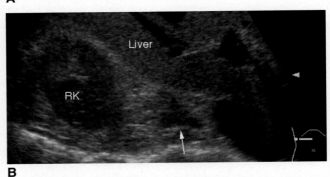

**B**

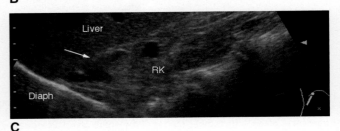

**C**

**Figure 13-11** Sonographic appearance of right adrenal gland. **A:** This transverse section of the normal right adrenal gland (*arrow*) demonstrates its relationship to the liver, inferior vena cava (*IVC*), and diaphragm. **B:** This transverse section of the normal right adrenal gland (*arrow*) demonstrates its relationship to the liver and right kidney (*RK*). **C:** In longitudinal sections moving from lateral to medial, a normal V- or Y-shaped right adrenal gland (*arrow*) is seen in relation to the right kidney (*RK*), liver, and diaphragm (*Diaph*). (Images courtesy of Dr. Taco Geertsma, Gelderse Vallei, Ede, The Netherlands.)

## PATHOLOGY

In most cases of suspected adrenal disease, CT is the imaging modality of choice.[30–32,37,38] Better visualization of the adrenal areas is obtained with CT, particularly in patients with adequate retroperitoneal fat.[38] In addition, MRI, scintigraphy, positron emission tomography (PET), and blood and urine testing are used to refine the diagnoses of adrenal pathologies. Sonography provides an alternative for screening children from families with the multiple endocrine neoplasia (MEN) syndromes, pregnant women, and poor candidates for CT who have a paucity of retroperitoneal fat.[38] Indications for sonography of the adrenals and retroperitoneum include evaluation for the presence of local or regional metastases; localized tumor invasion; origin of retroperitoneal masses; characterization of adrenal hemorrhage, cyst, or tumor for cystic and solid components; patency of local veins and IVC; hypertrophy of the gland; and follow-up on nonresected adrenal masses.

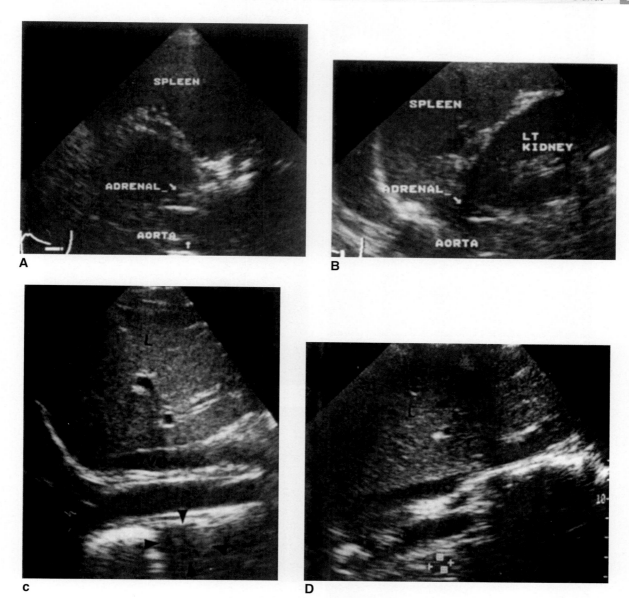

**Figure 13-12** Sonographic appearance of left adrenal gland. **A:** This transverse section demonstrates the triangular shape of a normal left adrenal gland. Its relationship to the aorta and spleen can be identified in this transverse section. **B:** On a longitudinal section made with the patient in a right posterior oblique position, the normal V or Y shape of the left adrenal gland and its relationship to the left kidney, spleen, and aorta can be identified. **C:** The normal left adrenal gland (*arrowheads*) is seen in a coronal section (medial to lateral) using the cava-suprarenal line position. The patient is tilted 45 degrees, and the beam passes through the liver (*L*), inferior vena cava (*IVC*), and aorta (*A*). **D:** On a coronal section obtained by using the cava-suprarenal line position, the normal left adrenal gland measures 1.12 cm (*cursor*) × 0.57 cm (*box*). (Images **A-B** courtesy of Doug Amussen, Hyde Park, UT; images **C-D** courtesy of Linda Reyes, Shreveport, LA.)

Since a mass may be encountered incidentally during routine abdominal or renal scanning, it is important to understand adrenal pathology and its clinical manifestations, to correlate laboratory values, and to identify normal and abnormal sonographic appearances. A change in the normal appearance of the gland's size and configuration is a key indicator for adrenal abnormalities. An increase in size can cause compression or displacement of surrounding structures. With right adrenal disease, the retroperitoneal fat line, IVC, and right renal vein may be displaced anteriorly, whereas the right kidney is displaced inferiorly or posteriorly[29] (Fig. 13-13A,B). An enlarged left adrenal gland may displace the splenic vein anteriorly and the left kidney inferiorly or posteriorly.[29] An adrenal mass should be differentiated from a renal mass by identifying the echo interface separating the mass from the upper pole of the kidney[33,36] (Fig. 13-13B,C). On rare occasions, an adrenal tumor may invade the adjacent kidney (Fig. 13-13D–G). As with other abdominal pathology, adrenal masses may present with irregular outer margins and can indent adjacent organs and vascular structures. Regardless of pathologic origin, large adrenal masses tend to outgrow their vascular supply, potentially producing irregular internal hypoechoic and hyperechoic areas representing central necrosis, liquefaction, or hemorrhage[33] (Fig. 13-14A–F and Pathology Box 13-1).

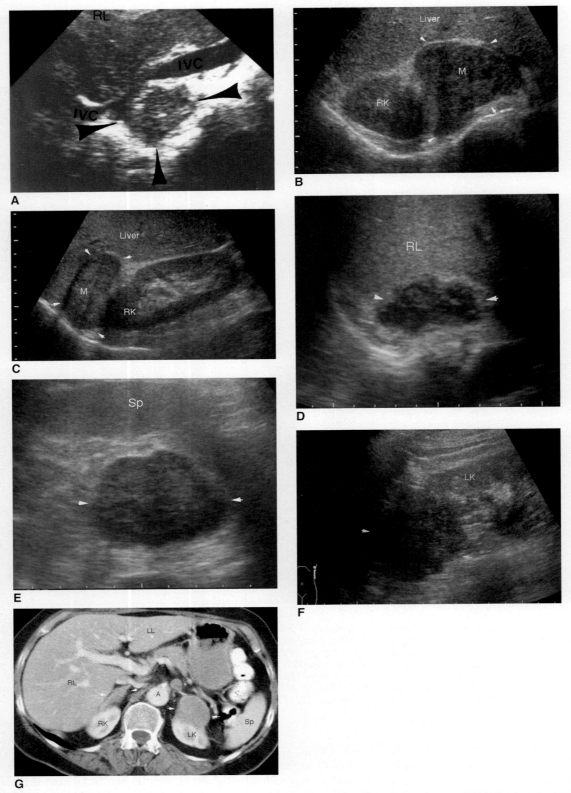

**Figure 13-13** Adrenal metastases. **A:** On a longitudinal section, a right adrenal metastatic mass (*arrowheads*) measuring 4 cm in average diameter is seen posterior to the right liver lobe (*RL*) indenting and displacing the inferior vena cava (*IVC*). The primary site was bone cancer. **B:** On a transverse section of a patient with right adrenal metastases from lung cancer, the adrenal mass (*M, arrowheads*) displaces the liver anteriorly and right kidney (*RK*) laterally. **C:** A longitudinal section on the same patient showing the adrenal mass (*M, arrowheads*) distorting the suprarenal space. An adrenal mass should be differentiated from a renal mass by identifying the echo interface separating the mass from the upper pole of the right kidney (*RK*). **D–G:** These sonograms demonstrate bilateral predominantly hypoechoic solid masses (*arrowheads*), representing metastases to right and left adrenal glands from a lung carcinoma. **D:** A transverse section of the right adrenal mass is identified posteromedial to the right liver lobe (*RL*). **E:** A transverse section of the left adrenal mass is identified medial to the spleen (*Sp*). **F:** A longitudinal section demonstrates the left adrenal mass superior to and infiltrating the left kidney (*LK*). **G:** On the computed tomography image, the location and relational anatomy of the bilateral adrenal masses (*arrowheads*) is demonstrated. *RL*, right liver lobe; *LL*, left liver lobe; *A*, aorta; *RK*, right kidney; *LK*, left kidney; *Sp*, spleen. The appearance of the left adrenal mass on computed tomography gives the impression of a renal mass. (Images courtesy of Dr. Taco Geertsma, Gelderse Vallei, Ede, The Netherlands.)

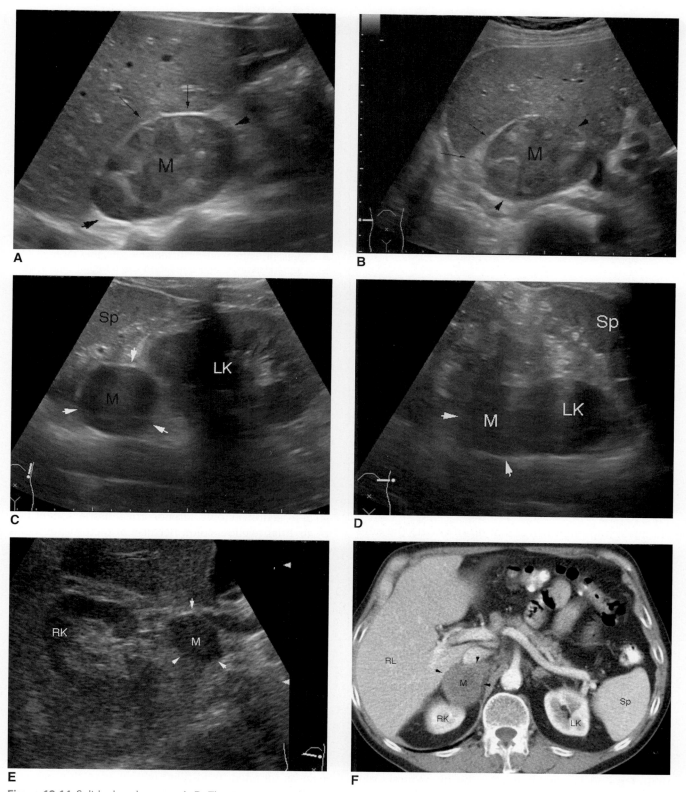

**Figure 13-14** Solid adrenal masses. **A–D:** These sonograms demonstrate solid masses (*M, arrowheads*), representing bilateral metastases to right and left adrenal glands from a melanoma. The longitudinal (**A**) and transverse (**B**) aspects of the right adrenal mass are identified posterior to the right liver lobe, superior to the right kidney (*RK*). Images demonstrate anterior and superior distortion of the Gerota fascia and fat between the adrenal gland and right lobe of the liver (*arrows*). The longitudinal (**C**) and transverse (**D**) aspects of the left adrenal mass are identified medial to the spleen (*Sp*) and superomedial to the left kidney (*LK*). Anterior margin of mass is poorly defined on transverse image (**D**). **E,F:** This patient has a unilateral metastasis to the right adrenal gland. A solid right adrenal mass was identified on both ultrasound and computed tomography (CT) images. The left adrenal gland was unremarkable. **E:** On a transverse section, the adrenal mass (*M, arrowheads*) is differentiated by the echo interface separating the mass from the upper pole of the right kidney (*RK*). **F:** On the CT image, the location and relational anatomy of the right adrenal mass (*arrowheads*) are demonstrated. (*RL*, right liver lobe; *RK*, right kidney; *LK*, left kidney; *A*, aorta; *Sp*, spleen.) (Images courtesy of Dr. Taco Geertsma, Gelderse Vallei, Ede, The Netherlands.)

## PATHOLOGY BOX 13-1

### *Adrenal Gland Pathology: General*

| Pathology | Etiology | Sonographic Appearance |
|---|---|---|
| Metastatic disease | Develops from squamous cell carcinoma of the lung, breast, gastrointestinal tract, thyroid, pancreas, kidney; lymphoma, melanoma | Small masses (4–5 cm); usually bilateral solid, well circumscribed, encased within the adrenal; located anteromedially; may have irregular margins and can indent IVC and displace kidney; necrosis (hypoechoic) or areas of hemorrhage (hypoechoic) may occur within the mass |
| Developmental anomalies | Agenesis–adrenocortical hyperplasia; congenital hypoplasia: anencephalic–cerebral, pituitary, or hypothalamic; cytomegalic unknown; ectopic unknown | Location and size are not commonly identified sonographically |
| Cyst | Develops from hemorrhage, trauma, or idiopathic causes | Rounded, fluid-filled mass with a thin, smooth wall, unilocular or multilocular; calcifications may be present, with acoustic shadowing affecting through transmission; ring calcification has a higher incidence of malignancy; hemorrhage with dense clot presents a thick, hyperechoic area of the pseudocyst type |
| Hemorrhage | Birth trauma or anoxia, systemic disease, anticoagulant therapy, metastases, adrenal trauma | Echo pattern variable, depending on age of hemorrhage; complex mass located anterosuperior to kidney may displace it; may shrink; calcifications, if present, appear as focal, hyperechoic areas, with or without acoustic shadowing |
| Abscess and infection | Opportunistic infections in immunocompromised patients | Both adrenal glands appear enlarged and hypoechoic; hepatosplenomegaly is usually present with lymphadenopathy in patients with HIV/AIDS |

## DEVELOPMENTAL ANOMALIES (PATHOLOGY BOX 13-1)

### Agenesis

The most important congenital disorders are the adrenocortical hyperplasias, which cause alterations and increases in steroid synthesis. These are discussed later in the chapter with hyperadrenalism.

### Congenital Hypoplasia

There are two types of congenital adrenal hypoplasia: anencephalic and cytomegalic. In both types, essential hormone production is altered.

In an anencephalic fetus, usually stillborn, the adrenal gland consists of only a provisional cortex with no fetal zone.[39] The cause of the disorder is either cerebral, pituitary, or hypothalamic.

The cause of the cytomegalic type is unknown. An unusual adrenal cortex is made up histologically of large eosinophilic cells. Usually, the gland weighs less than 1 g and is not identifiable by ultrasound. With early diagnosis, early replacement steroid therapy promotes long-term survival.[39]

### Ectopy

Ectopic adrenal glands consist mainly of accessory cortical material and can occur anywhere from the diaphragm to the pelvis[9–12,39]: in the kidney, liver, retroperitoneal tissues, ovary, testis, and in the tissues accompanying the spermatic cord. The ectopia may have either cortical or cortical and medullary cellular components. On surgical resection, ectopic adrenocortical tissue is identified by its bright yellow color. Because of their location and size, ectopic adrenal glands are not commonly identified with sonography.

## CYSTS

Relatively infrequent and usually asymptomatic, adrenal cysts may be incidental findings. The endothelial type may be subdivided into lymphangiomatous (41%) and angiomatous (3%), pseudocysts (40%) are secondary to hemorrhage into or around the gland, and epithelial cysts (6%) result from cystic degeneration of adenomas and parasitic cysts.[3,33]

Adrenal cysts demonstrate the characteristic sonographic cystic appearance with marked through transmission and posterior enhancement.[1,40] They appear as rounded, fluid-filled masses with thin, smooth walls.[1] They may be unilocular or multilocular, small or large[33] (Fig. 13-15A,B). Calcifications are found in 15% of cases and dense clot retraction may persist, providing a thick, hyperechoic area in the pseudocystic variety[33,36] (Fig. 13-15C). Most adrenal cysts are benign, but adrenal cysts with a "ring" calcification are more often malignant.[36] The calcified cyst wall (aka eggshell)

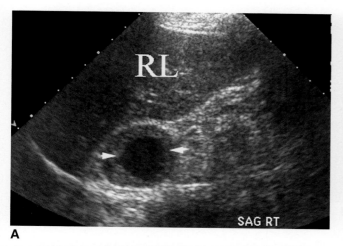

**A**

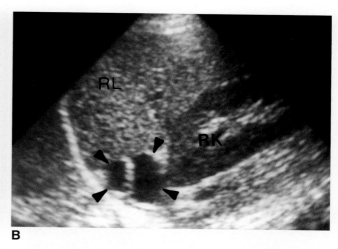

**B**

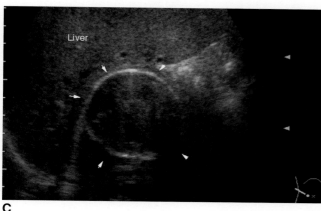

**C**

**Figure 13-15** Adrenal cysts. **A:** A unilocular right adrenal gland cyst (*arrowheads*) posterior to the right liver lobe (*RL*) can be identified in this longitudinal/coronal section. This was an incidental finding. **B:** This patient presented with right upper quadrant pain. The sonographic examination imaged a bilobed, mostly anechoic mass (*arrowheads and cursors*) measuring 4 cm in the anteroposterior dimension. On the longitudinal section, the bilobed mass is identified superior to a normal-appearing right kidney (*RK*) and posterior to the right liver lobe (*RL*). **C:** Calcified cyst (*arrowheads*). The transverse aspects of the right adrenal cyst are identified posterior to the right liver lobe (*RL*), superior to the right kidney. On this patient, a radiograph demonstrated a circumferential calcification of cyst wall. (Image **C** courtesy of Dr. Taco Geertsma, Gelderse Vallei, Ede, The Netherlands.)

produces a thick, hyperechoic ring that may or may not cast an acoustic shadow[3,36,38] (Pathology Box 13-1). For a purely cystic mass, percutaneous fine-needle aspiration may be indicated to examine the contents or relieve symptoms associated with pressure.[33]

## HEMORRHAGE

Hemorrhage of the adrenal gland is seen most often in newborns, especially after a difficult delivery in which fetal oxygen is diminished or cut off for some time (see Chapter 20). Hemorrhage can also be precipitated by adrenal trauma, surgery, stress, anticoagulant therapy, adrenal vein thrombosis, adrenal neoplasms, metastases, or septicemia.[1,3,41,42] The right side is often more involved in the hemorrhagic process, which is probably associated with right adrenal venous drainage directly off the IVC. Trauma-induced hematomas usually resolve without clinical complications, unless the trauma is bilateral; as an Addisonian crisis is a risk associated with bilateral hemorrhage.[1,41]

Depending on the stage of organization, the echo pattern of adrenal hemorrhage varies. The appearance can range from an acute hyperechoic suprarenal mass to the hypoechoic to anechoic pattern of a resolving chronic hematoma[3,33,40,43] (Fig. 13-16A–C). With age, the mass typically shrinks, and calcifications can appear as

focal, hyperechoic areas with associated acoustic shadowing[3,40,41,43] (Pathology Box 13-1).

## INFLAMMATION/INFECTION

### Abscess and Infection

Adrenal abscess is extremely uncommon in adults although less rare with neonates following traumatic delivery or septicemia (see Chapter 20). Adrenal abscess formation in adults has been associated with opportunistic infections (i.e., *Bacteroides*, *Escherichia coli*, histoplasmosis, *Nocardia asteroides*, *Proteus*, *Salmonella*, and tuberculosis) in immunocompromised patients (i.e., HIV/AIDS, hemophilia, or thalassemia minor), direct contamination through an invasive procedure or trauma, as a complication to hemorrhage, and regional contamination from appendicitis.[11,44,45] With percutaneous drainage or aspiration and proper antibiotics, patients can have a full recovery.[44,45]

In patients with HIV/AIDS, focal adrenal lesions are associated with neoplastic changes (lymphoma and/or Kaposi sarcoma) and infections (candida, cryptococcus, cytomegalovirus [CMV], herpes, mycobacterium, toxoplasmosis, and/or tuberculosis).[1,46] Complications of systemic infections including tuberculosis, fungal sources, and viruses can also lead to primary adrenal

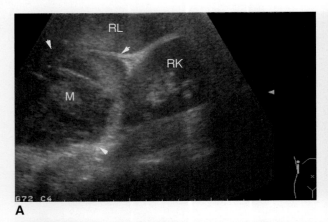

**A**

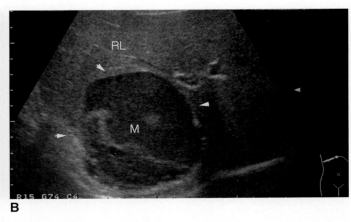

**B**

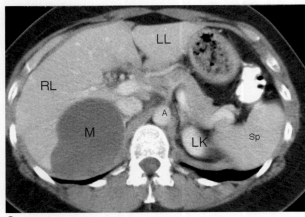

**C**

**Figure 13-16** Adrenal hemorrhage. This case demonstrates an adrenal hemorrhage with septated cystic mass with internal echoes. A complex, predominantly hypoechoic mass measuring 9 cm in maximum diameter was identified in the subhepatic space. Posterior enhancement is noted on the sonograms. **A:** The longitudinal section demonstrates the mass *(M, arrowheads)* superior to the right kidney *(RK)* and inferior and posterior to the right liver lobe *(RL).* **B:** On the transverse section, the primarily hypoechoic, complex mass *(M, arrowheads)* is identified posterior and lateral to the right liver lobe *(RL).* **C:** On the computed tomography image, the location and relational anatomy of the right adrenal hemorrhage *(M, arrowheads)* are demonstrated *(RL,* right liver lobe; *LL,* left liver lobe; *LK,* left kidney; *A,* aorta; *Sp,* spleen.) (Images **A–C** courtesy of Dr. Taco Geertsma, Gelderse Vallei, Ede, The Netherlands.)

insufficiency or hypoadrenalism.[11,14,18] The appearance of Addison disease symptoms may appear gradually, as the adrenal glands are destroyed by these rampant infection processes and deficiencies occur in the production of cortical hormones.[11,14,18] However, the adrenalitis associated with CMV seldom claims more than half of the glandular tissue, so Addisonian crises rarely strike patients with isolated CMV infections.[46] Caution is advised when co-treating CMV-infected HIV/AIDS patients with steroids, as these medications may temporarily disguise impending adrenal insufficiency.[46]

Histoplasmosis, which is disseminated through numerous body systems, requires treatment or it is fatal.[47] Disseminated histoplasmosis (DH) is rare but occurs at higher rates in immunocompromised patients. Both adrenal glands appear enlarged and hypoechoic.[47] Hepatosplenomegaly is usually present along with lymphadenopathy in patients with HIV/AIDS[47] (Pathology Box 13-1). This appearance is also consistent with tuberculosis and is further discussed later.

## CORTICAL PATHOLOGY

Adrenal cortex pathology can be divided into three categories: disorders that diminish steroid output, disorders that increase steroid production, and lesions that have no functional effect. The presentation of cortical disease

categories contributes to an understanding of the range of sonographic appearances of adrenal diseases.

## HYPOADRENALISM (HYPOCORTICISM) (PATHOLOGY BOX 13-2)

Hypoadrenalism or adrenocortical hypofunction may be caused by primary disorders of the cortex or by secondary failure in the elaboration of ACTH. The clinical manifestation, atrophic or necrotic destruction of the cortex, usually is not detectable by ultrasound, but complications such as hemorrhage can be identified.

### Chronic Primary Hypoadrenalism (Addison Disease)

The chronic form of hypoadrenalism (Addison disease) is the most common.[11,18] Insufficient secretion of adrenocortical hormones results from the insidious and profound atrophy of the adrenal glands. Addison disease is uncommon (4 cases per 100,000 population); it becomes evident only when 90% of functioning adrenocortical cells have been destroyed.[11,18] The two major causes of adrenal destruction are idiopathic atrophy (80%) and glandular destruction attributed to an autoimmune disorder, infection, or tuberculosis (20%).[11,18] Females are more often affected by the idiopathic atrophic type and males by the type caused by tuberculosis.[48]

**PATHOLOGY BOX 13-2**

### Disorders of the Adrenal Cortex

| Disorder | Etiology | Sonographic Appearance |
|---|---|---|
| Hypoadrenalism | Addison disease caused by idiopathic atrophy of the adrenal cortex | Unable to identify |
| | Addison disease caused by tuberculosis | Solid, enlarged, and nodular, with hyperechoic capsule; may appear complex, with areas of necrosis |
| | Waterhouse-Friderichsen syndrome | Hemorrhage may occur (see Pathology Box 13-1) |
| Aldosteronoma | Conn disease | Hypoechoic, small (1–2 cm), round masses |
| Hyperplasia | Cushing or Conn disease, adrenogenital disease | Normal or diffusely enlarged; solid, cystic, or complex, with or without focal zones of necrosis within the gland |

Clinical symptoms depend on the degree of hormone deficiency. Because of adrenal atrophy, the steroid response is diminished or absent, causing an increase in the pituitary gland's production of ACTH.[10,11,14,18] Because ACTH has melanin-stimulating properties, about 98% of affected persons present with changes in skin color.[11,14,48] Other clinical manifestations include sodium and potassium retention, renal impairment, and decreases in blood volume, sugar, and lipids.[11,14,18] Symptoms can include fever, fatigue, muscle weakness, hypotension, and gastrointestinal distress such as nausea, vomiting, weight loss, and diarrhea.[11,14,18] The disease may be managed by administration of steroids, but patients are vulnerable to all forms of stress, which may trigger hypoadrenal crisis and shock.[11,14,18]

As mentioned previously, systemic infections including tuberculosis, fungal sources such as histoplasmosis, and viruses such as CMV and AIDS may lead to primary adrenal insufficiency or hypoadrenalism.[11,14,18,46] As the adrenal glands are destroyed by these infections, cortical hormonal deficiencies are revealed.[11,14,18] Sonographic appearances vary depending on the extent of gland destruction and tissue necrosis. During acute stages, there is diffuse glandular enlargement, whereas chronic infection usually leads to patterns of atrophy and calcification.[46]

When Addison disease is caused by tuberculosis, the glands are enlarged, firm, and nodular, with a thick capsule. The sonographic appearance can range from a normal echoic appearance to hyperechoic with areas of necrosis. Small, irregular, and contracted adrenal glands that usually are not identified on ultrasound occur with idiopathic Addison disease.

### Chronic Secondary Hypoadrenalism

Any disorder to the hypophyseal-thalamic axis that reduces the output of ACTH causes atrophy of the adrenal cortex and decreases secretion of cortisol and androgen.[11,18] The most common cause is abrupt cessation of exogenous steroid therapy.[11,18] Other causes include metastatic cancer, infection, infarction, bilateral hemorrhage, bilateral adrenalectomy, and irradiation.[1,11,18] A syndrome of hypoadrenalism similar to

Addison disease results, except that hyperpigmentation is absent with diminished ACTH.[11,18] The adrenal glands may be moderately to markedly shrunken, may appear leaf-like, and become difficult to identify in the periadrenal fat.[39]

### Acute Hypoadrenalism (Waterhouse-Friderichsen Syndrome)

Massive destruction of the adrenals can occur at any age and in a variety of settings, causing acute adrenal insufficiency (Addisonian or adrenal crisis).[39] Hemorrhagic destruction of the adrenal glands occurring due to widespread pneumococcal, meningococcal, or gram-negative septicemia is known as *Waterhouse-Friderichsen syndrome*.[11] Immediate intervention, such as the administration of glucocorticoid therapy and treatment of the underlying infection, is necessary or death will rapidly ensue.[11] Caution should be exercised to avoid treating hyponatremia too fast to prevent additional complications.[11,18]

## HYPERADRENALISM (HYPERCORTICISM)

With hyperadrenalism, the three types of corticosteroids produced by the adrenal cortex result in three distinctive but sometimes overlapping clinical manifestations: Cushing syndrome, Conn syndrome or aldosteronism, and adrenogenital syndrome or congenital adrenal hyperplasia.[11,18]

### Cushing Syndrome

In Cushing syndrome, excessive glucose production results from hypersecretion of cortisol from the adrenal cortex.[11,14] The most common cause is treatment of nonendocrine disorders with long courses of potent glucocorticoid drugs such as prednisone and dexamethasone.[11,18] Three clinically similar forms of Cushing syndrome result from glucocorticoid overproduction.[11,49] Hypersecretion of ACTH by the anterior pituitary (Cushing disease, 68% to 80% of cases) and ectopic ACTH syndrome from adenocarcinoma, oat-cell carcinoma of the lung, or other malignant neoplasms

(8% to 12%) are two ACTH-dependent forms.[11,49] Most patients with ACTH-dependent forms of Cushing syndrome have symmetrically enlarged glands, whereas 30% have normal-sized glands.[49-51] The third form involves ACTH-independent processes, which account for 15% to 20% of Cushing syndrome cases and always are adrenocortical neoplasms, usually hyperfunctioning adenomas, carcinomas, or a few other rare entities.[49,50] A pseudo-Cushing syndrome occurs rarely (<2%) with alcoholism or major depression. In children, tumors are the most common cause, and the child's growth ceases if treatment is not begun before the epiphyses of their bones have sealed.[11]

Cushing syndrome is characterized by increases in cortisol secretion, which trigger increases in gluconeogenesis and results in elevated serum glucose levels.[11,18] Eventually, the islet cells of the pancreas are no longer able to produce sufficient amounts of insulin and diabetes mellitus results.[11] Protein loss occurs almost everywhere except in the liver.[48] This loss results in weakened muscles and elastic tissue, producing a protuberant abdomen and poor wound healing.[11,14] Humoral immunity is impaired, decreasing the threshold for infection.[18] With the loss of collagen in the skin, the tissues become very thin and susceptible to tearing and bruising. Red welts and striae are seen, mostly over the abdomen and thighs.[11] Owing to the melanin-stimulating properties of ACTH, hyperpigmentation may be seen.[11,14] Osteoporosis can result, causing weakness and fractures.[11,18] Hypertension is also evident in most cases.[11,18]

### Hyperaldosteronism (Conn Syndrome)

Primary hyperaldosteronism, or Conn syndrome, is the result of excessive and uncontrolled secretion of the mineralocorticoid aldosterone.[11,14,18] It is uncommon, and in 80% to 90% of patients, it results from a benign aldosterone-producing adrenal adenoma.[8,38,50] Bilateral cortical hyperplasia and rare carcinomas account for the remaining 10% to 20% of the cases. Both categories of tumors are known as *aldosteronomas*.[50] These lesions are difficult to detect because more than 20% are less than 1 cm in size.[50]

Secondary hyperaldosteronism is not a disease process but results from hypersecretion of aldosterone in response to stimulation of the renin-angiotensin system.[11,18] This occurs when almost any factor decreases the blood supply to the kidneys, raising the plasma renin level and increasing subsequent excessive aldosterone secretion.[11,18]

The clinical features of this disorder are a direct result of aldosterone's functions of conserving sodium and losing renal potassium.[11,14,18] Hypernatremia (excess sodium in the blood) and hypokalemia (extreme potassium depletion in the blood) are the principal clinical manifestations.[11,14,18] The condition is suspected whenever a hypertensive patient exhibits concurrent hypokalemia.[11,18] Conservation of sodium leads to water retention, increasing the volume in the extracellular and vascular compartments, causing arterial hypertension.[11,14,18] Potassium loss most commonly results in muscle cramps and weakness.[11] Because the kidneys are the primary site of sodium conservation, renal functional alterations occur.[11,14,18] The sonographic appearance of aldosteronoma is presented in Pathology Box 13-2 and is discussed in the section on cortical tumors.

### Congenital Adrenal Hyperplasia (Adrenogenital Syndrome)

Congenital adrenal hyperplasia encompasses at least six distinctive autosomal recessive syndromes, each characterized by a congenital deficiency of a specific enzyme involved in the biosynthesis of adrenal steroids.[11,18] With bilateral hyperplasia, the enzyme deficiencies may also result from postpubertal adrenal hyperplasia, adrenal adenoma, or adrenal carcinoma.[11] The effect of the deficiencies impairs synthesis of cortisol and distorts other aspects of steroidogenesis.[39] In most cases, this increases levels of ACTH, leading to adrenal hyperplasia and subsequent overstimulation of the pathways of steroid hormone production, particularly those involving the production of adrenal androgens.[11,14] All of these syndromes are adrenogenital, representing an abnormal expression of androgen excess—the ultimate result in most cases is the same: virilization.[11,18]

Newborn girls with congenital adrenal hyperplasia have ambiguous external genitalia resembling those of boys.[11,18] Reconstructive surgery, if indicated, can be performed during the first 2 years of life to reduce the size of the clitoris, separate the labia, and exteriorize the vagina.[11,18] Internal female genitalia are normal. Boys are seldom diagnosed at birth unless they have enlarged genitalia, lose salt, or manifest adrenal crisis.[11,18]

The age and sex of the affected person determine the nature and severity of the disorder when adrenogenital syndromes are caused by benign or malignant tumors. Precocious sexual development and elevated plasma 17-hydroxy-progesterone levels aid in the diagnosis.[11,18] Early diagnosis is important, as the deficiency can often be controlled, allowing normal sexual and physical development.[11,18]

Hyperfunctioning adrenal glands can appear normal or diffusely enlarged but with normal shape.[38] With nodular hyperplasia, a solid, cystic, or complex mass, with or without focal zones of necrosis, may present in the adrenal gland[29] (Fig. 13-17). Since the sonographic appearance is used to describe and characterize, and not to make tissue-specific diagnoses, correlation with the patient's clinical findings and laboratory values expedites interpretation of the sonographic study (Pathology Box 13-2).

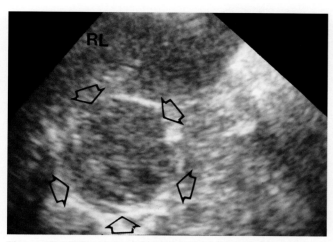

**Figure 13-17** Hyperadrenalism. The right adrenal gland appears as a solid mass (within *arrowheads*) on the transverse section made on a 4-month-old girl displaying clinical signs and symptoms of hyperadrenalism. (*RL*, right liver lobe.) (Image courtesy of Helen Johnson, Salt Lake City, UT.)

## INCIDENTALOMA

The general term for an unexpected mass detected during an imaging procedure being performed for unrelated disease is "incidentaloma." This term may be applied to any unexpected mass, occurring anywhere in the body. AI has become a common term in the medical literature and represents a diagnostic challenge, which includes discovery of masses, which range from benign, nonfunctional lesions to malignant tumors such as pheochromocytomas, adrenocortical carcinomas, or metastases from other primary cancers.[8] These incidental masses are detected on 4% to 5% of CT studies.[52,53]

Diagnoses and treatments for incidentalomas vary based on two important clinical criteria: patient history of cancer and hyperfunction of the mass.[8,11,54,55] Multiple studies have revealed that in patients with a history of extra-adrenal malignancy, 45% to 73% of the incidentalomas are metastases.[35,52,56] This is not surprising since lung cancer commonly metastasizes to the adrenal glands.

In contrast, in recent studies on the general population of patients without a history of cancer, the majority of incidentalomas (60% to 94%) were nonhypersecreting adenomas, 1% to 22% were cysts, 6% to 15% were myelolipomas, 0% to 11% were pheochromocytomas, whereas 0% to 4% were adrenocortical carcinomas and 0% to 2% were metastases.[11,35,52–54,57] Subclinical Cushing syndrome was present in 5% to 20% of patients with incidentalomas, which should account for hypersecreting adenomas.[11]

Unilateral hyperfunctioning lesions (adenomas, aldosteronomas, pheochromocytomas, and adrenal hyperplasias) usually undergo surgical treatment.[8,11,54,55] Laparoscopy is used for small tumors (1 to 2 cm).[11]

Adrenalectomy is also indicated for nonfunctioning masses >4 to 6 cm and lesions that are potentially malignant.[11,55,58] Bilateral masses require alternative or combination treatments to avoid adrenal insufficiency. Gland enlargement, change in appearance on follow-up, or atypical appearance on CT and/or MRI also justify gland removal.[11,59]

## CORTICAL TUMORS

### Adenomas

Adrenal gland nodules measuring less than 3 cm are found in approximately 2% to 9% of patients on autopsy; the majority are nonfunctioning, slow-growing cortical adenomas.[32,39,60] An adenoma may also be one part of the MEN syndromes.[39] Most are benign, poorly encapsulated tumors, 1 to 5 cm in diameter, and consist of lipid-filled cells that do not secrete hormones.[39] Generally, a single-ovoid nodule larger than 1 cm is considered an adenoma; multiple or bilateral nodules located either inside or outside the capsule are considered expressions of nodular hyperplasia.[39] Adenomas greater than 2 cm in size are more likely to be functional and may cause Cushing syndrome (hypercortisolism).[50] Administration of ACTH causes adrenal adenomas to grow in the same way it stimulates adrenal hyperplasia. Adenocarcinoma, however, is independent of pituitary influence and does not respond to ACTH administration.[48]

An adenoma is sonographically difficult to detect because of its anatomic location and the presence of surrounding retroperitoneal fat. Criteria used to support the diagnosis of an incidental adrenal adenoma include a small (less than 5 cm) round or oval mass, clear separation of the margins from adjacent structures, and no evidence of growth on serial examinations[38] (Fig. 13-18A–E and Pathology Box 13-3). Such masses are frequently only 1.5 to 2 cm in diameter, with no calcifications or central necrosis.[49,50,54] Their homogenous,

---

**PATHOLOGY BOX 13-3**

**Adrenocortical Tumors**

| Tumor | Sonographic Appearance |
| --- | --- |
| Adenomas | Hypoechoic, small (1.5–2 cm), round, encapsulated mass; clear separation of the margins from adjacent structures; may have calcifications |
| Myelolipomas | Hyperechoic, well-defined mass with interrupted posterior hemidiaphragm; if small, may blend with perirenal fat |
| Cancer | Hyperechoic, solid, larger masses; echo pattern varies with necrosis or hemorrhage; may invade vasculature and displace surrounding organs |

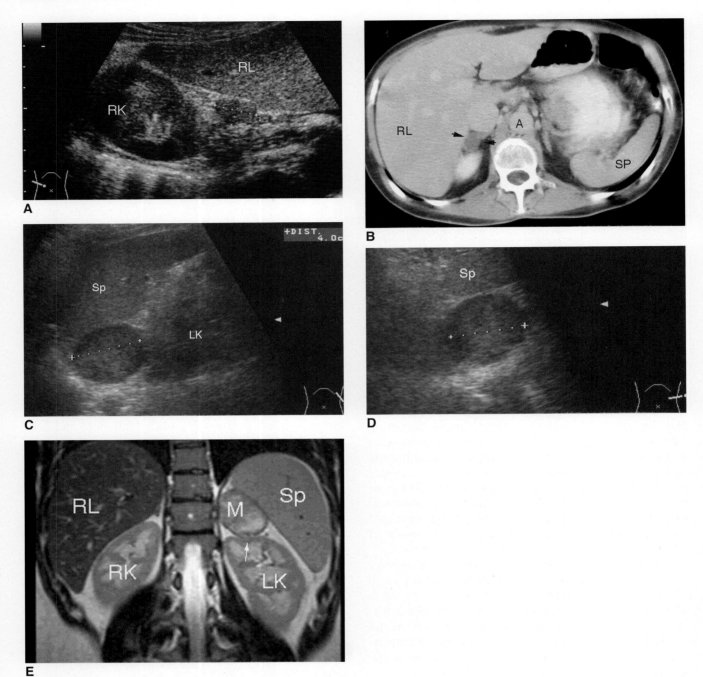

**Figure 13-18** Adrenal adenomas. **A:** On a transverse section, a small right adrenal adenoma appears as an isoechoic mass *(calipers)* measuring 1.9 × 1.3 cm. *RL*, right liver lobe; *RK*, right kidney. **B:** On the computed tomography (CT) image of same patient, the location and relational anatomy of the right adrenal adenoma *(arrowhead)* are demonstrated. *RL*, right liver lobe, *A*, aorta; *SP*, spleen. The mass is posteromedial to the right liver lobe and superomedial to the right kidney. Differential diagnosis includes nonfunctioning adrenal adenoma. Nonfunctioning adrenal adenomas require no special treatment, but the patient should be kept under observation for tumor growth or development of hypersecretory function. Adrenal insufficiency is rarely observed unless both glands are involved. Left gland is normal *(arrow)*. **C–E:** On another patient, this left adrenal adenoma appears as a hypoechoic mass measuring 4 cm in maximum diameter identified in the subsplenic space. **C:** The longitudinal section demonstrates the mass *(calipers)* superior to the left kidney *(LK)* and inferior and medial to the spleen *(Sp)*. **D:** On the transverse section, the primarily hypoechoic mass *(calipers)* is identified posteromedial to the spleen *(Sp)*. **E:** On the coronal magnetic resonance imaging (MRI), the location and relational anatomy of the left adrenal mass *(M)* is demonstrated. (*RL*, right liver lobe; *RK*, right kidney; *LK*, left kidney; *Sp*, spleen.) No mass is identified in the region of the right adrenal gland. The tissue planes between the retroperitoneal organs are clearly delineated and show the adenoma indenting the upper pole of the left kidney on the MRI *(arrow)*. (Images courtesy of Dr. Taco Geertsma, Gelderse Vallei, Ede, The Netherlands.)

hypoechoic sonographic appearance is similar to that of aldosteronomas, which cause Conn syndrome and generally appear sonographically as small, round, relatively anechoic masses.[1]

## Myelolipomas

*Adrenal myelolipoma* is a rare benign tumor of the adrenal cortex. Of uncertain etiology, it is composed of mature lipid rich, macrosomic fatty tissue with a variable proportion of hematopoietic elements resembling bone marrow.[1,3,49,61,62] The lesion is found between the fourth and sixth decades, with an equal incidence in men and women.[27,32] Generally, myelolipomas are unilateral, <5 cm in size, hormonally inactive, and therefore asymptomatic.[1] Large or bilateral lesions may become symptomatic, causing pain or endocrine dysfunction due to hemorrhage, necrosis, or pressure on adjacent structures.[61,62]

A combination of sonography, CT, and angiography can lead to a fairly specific preoperative diagnosis of an adrenal myelolipoma.[61,62] Sonographically, the tumor is usually a well-defined, markedly hyperechoic mass demonstrating an interrupted, posteriorly displaced hemidiaphragm resulting from a velocity artifact caused by the lipomatous content[3,61,63] (Fig. 13-19A–C and Pathology Box 13-3). The sonographic examination is useful in localizing the anatomic origin of these upper quadrant abnormalities, especially on the right side.[61] If it is detected sonographically, the differential diagnosis includes retroperitoneal lipoma, retroperitoneal liposarcoma, renal angiomyolipoma, lymphangioma, increased abdominal fat deposition, and retroperitoneal teratoma.[3,33,61,62] A more complicated appearance is created when an adenoma is imbedded within the myelolipoma or the mass is primarily myeloid tissue.[1,49]

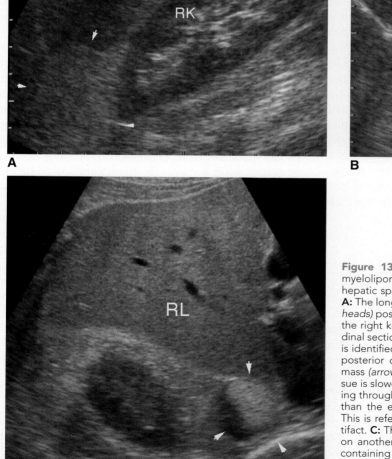

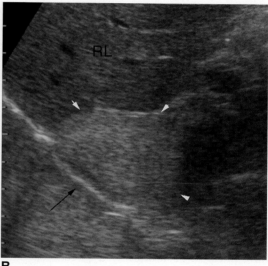

**Figure 13-19** Adrenal myelolipoma. This right adrenal myelolipoma appears as a hyperechoic mass in the subhepatic space and measures 4 cm in maximum diameter. **A:** The longitudinal section demonstrates the mass *(arrowheads)* posterior to the right liver lobe *(RL)* and superior to the right kidney *(RK)*. **B:** On another more lateral longitudinal section, the primarily hyperechoic mass *(arrowheads)* is identified posterior to the right liver lobe *(RL)*. Note the posterior displacement of the diaphragm below to the mass *(arrow)*. The speed of sound through lipomatous tissue is slower than 1,540 m/sec, therefore the echoes passing through this mass return to the transducer a little later than the echoes traveling through adjacent liver tissue. This is referred to as a propagation speed or velocity artifact. **C:** The transverse section of the right adrenal gland on another patient shows a well-defined, complex mass containing a markedly hyperechoic region. This is consistent with a myelolipoma *(arrowheads)* posterior to the right liver lobe *(RL)*. (Images courtesy of Dr. Taco Geertsma, Gelderse Vallei, Ede, The Netherlands.)

CT examination should follow detection of a lipomatous lesion by sonography because CT is capable of identifying the fatty nature of the mass.[62] On CT, a myelolipoma appears as a well-defined, fatty suprarenal mass with negative or low attenuation values compared to the high-attenuating adrenal gland tissue, other tissue types, or hemorrhage.[49,61] These masses also appear hyperintense on T1 weighted in-phase MRI and hypointense on fat-saturated MRI.[49] If present, liposarcomas are nonhomogeneous, poorly defined, and infiltrative.[64] On angiography, an adrenal myelolipoma appears as an avascular mass in the adrenal gland rather than in the kidney or liver.[61] Venography demonstrates displacement of veins around the tumor.

### Cancer

Cortical cancers, such as adenocarcinomas, often produce steroids (36% to 90%) and are usually associated with one of the hyperadrenal syndromes—those that are nonfunctioning are highly malignant.[3,11,33,39] Adrenal carcinomas are rare, accounting for only 2% of cancers in the world.[7,11] They may appear to be encapsulated and many exceed 20 cm in diameter, producing palpable abdominal masses.[11,39] These tumors may show zones of hemorrhage and necrosis.[39] Cortical cancers tend to invade the adrenal vein, IVC, and lymph nodes and commonly metastasize to regional and periaortic nodes, with hematogenous spread to the lungs, liver, bones and other viscera.[1,3,11,33,39] Cortical cancers are solid-looking masses larger than most adrenal masses: 3 to 6 cm for hyperfunctioning tumors and >6 cm for nonfunctioning lesions.[3] The echogenic appearance varies with the presence and degree of hemorrhage and necrosis, with nonfunctioning neoplasms appearing more complex and hyperechoic, whereas hyperfunctioning masses are more likely to be uniformly hypoechoic.[3] Calcifications are seen in 19% of cases.[32] Invasion of the mass into surrounding vasculature and displacement of normal tissue contour and location help identify the mass (Fig. 13-20A–F and Pathology Box 13-3).

# MEDULLARY PATHOLOGY

## PHEOCHROMOCYTOMA

Patients with pheochromocytomas typically present with mild to marked hypertension (90%), headache (80%), sweating (65%), and tachycardia (50%).[11,14,18] Additional signs and symptoms also relate to the excessive and/or intermittent catecholamine secretion from these tumors. The rule of ten describes the incidence of many features: 10% malignant, 10% bilateral or multiple, 10% hereditary syndromes, 10% pediatric, 10% extra-adrenal locations (paragangliomas), and 10% are normotensive nonfunctioning tumors.[11,51,65] Pheochromocytomas are rare (2 to 8 per million) but occur at higher frequency in patients with hypertension (1%), hereditary endocrine tumor syndromes; MEN type 2A and 2B, Von Hippel-Lindau (VHL), and neurofibromatosis (NF-1), as well as neuroectodermal dysplasia syndromes; and von Recklinghausen neurofibromatosis, tuberous sclerosis, and Sturge-Weber syndrome.[11,20] These patients are routinely screened, so the masses are usually smaller when initially detected.[51] For some patients, the incidence of pheochromocytomas is dramatic at 50% to 70% for MEN 2A and 90% and bilateral for MEN 2B.[66] Patients with MEN syndromes are often treated with prophylactic cortical-sparing or complete bilateral adrenalectomies with hormone replacement.[20,37] In addition to these hereditary syndromes, which demonstrate genetic mutations that contribute to a higher risk for pheochromocytomas, there are sporadic genetic mutations, which can be passed by carriers. First-degree relatives should be screened when new cases are discovered.[20,65]

Benign and malignant pheochromocytomas have similar biochemical characteristics, such as elevated levels of urinary catecholamine, plasma free metanephrine, and other metabolites such as VMA.[11,14,20,33,38,48] Clinical manifestations, laboratory values, and metastases to liver, lymph nodes, lungs, or bones help establish a diagnosis of malignancy. The sustained elevation of catecholamine secretion can lead to cardiomegaly, left ventricular failure, cardiomyopathy, and ultimately death due to heart failure.[48] Generally, treatment consists of surgical removal of the gland and epinephrine and norepinephrine substitution therapy.

These tumors are usually well encapsulated, ovoid to round, and may be palpable.[40,51] They are highly vascular masses and, if rupture occurs, massive hemorrhage can be fatal.[48] This tumor occurs in both sexes, usually between ages 25 and 50 years.[39] Pheochromocytomas are usually >2 cm at detection and average 5 to 6 cm in size.[40] Sonographic appearance includes a broad spectrum from (1) hyperechoic, hypoechoic, or isoechoic solid tumors; (2) homogeneous or heterogeneous echogenic solid tumors; (3) complex masses; and (4) cystic masses.[66,67] This variety is attributed to the spectrum of their gross morphologic appearances.[66,67] The well-marginated mass may appear quite large, with purely solid homogenous components or with complex heterogeneous echoes representing hemorrhage and/or necrosis[33,40,66] (Fig. 13-21A,B). Calcification may also be present in an eggshell pattern along the outer margin of the tumor.[40] Larger masses may displace surrounding organs and/or indent vasculature (Pathology Box 13-4).

CT is the imaging modality of choice for the initial detection and localization as indicated by the presence of a soft tissue mass, potential speckled calcifications, and intense contrast enhancement with nonionic contrast media.[51] When central necrosis is present, the peripheral rim of tumor retains the intense enhancement on CT.[51] MRI may also be used to characterize these tumors, which are iso- or hypointense to the liver on T1-weighted images.[66] T2 weighting reveals high intensity in areas of hemorrhage.[51,66] Unfortunately,

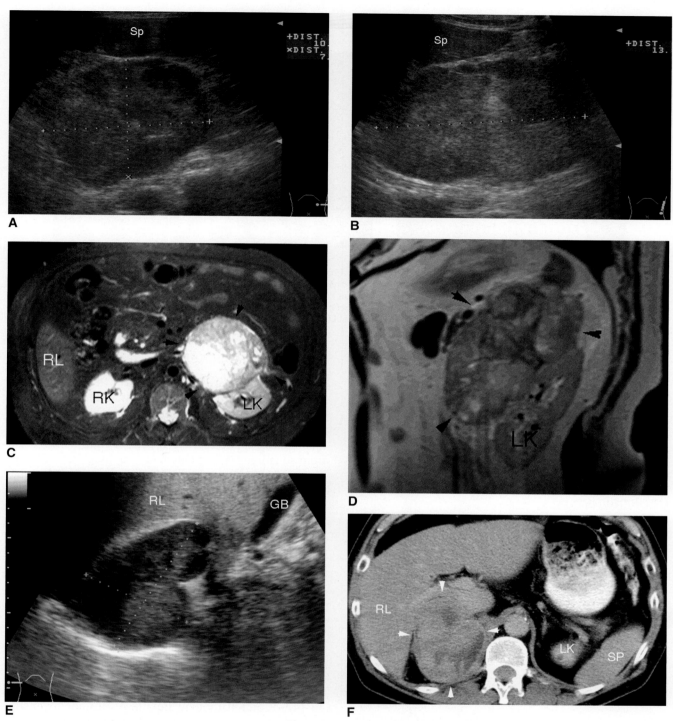

**Figure 13-20** Adrenal carcinoma. Sonographic and magnetic resonance imaging (MRI) examinations documented a very large mass in the subsplenic region consistent with adrenocortical carcinoma. Sonographic characteristics of the mass include fairly well-defined margins with focal areas of increased and decreased echogenicities likely due to hemorrhage and necrosis. The mass measured approximately 11 × 14 cm. The MRI did not demonstrate metastatic spread or involvement of the right adrenal gland. **A:** The transverse section demonstrates the cortical mass (*calipers*), medial to the spleen (*Sp*). **B:** On the longitudinal section, the cortical cancer (*calipers*) displaces the spleen (*Sp*) anteriorly. **C:** On the transverse MRI, the location and relational anatomy of the left adrenal mass (*arrowheads*) is demonstrated. *RL*, right liver lobe; *RK*, right kidney; *LK*, left kidney. No mass is identified in the region of the right adrenal gland. **D:** On the longitudinal section MRI, the mass, spleen, and left kidney appear to be compressed into the left upper quadrant. Tissue variations on the MRI are consistent with the irregular echogenicity seen by ultrasound. The large dimensions and relational anatomy of the left adrenal mass (*arrowheads*) to the left kidney (*LK*) and diaphragm are demonstrated. **E,F:** Sonographic and computed tomography (CT) examinations documented a large mass in the subhepatic region consistent with adrenocortical carcinoma. Sonographic characteristics of the predominantly hypoechoic mass include fairly well-defined margins with focal areas of increased and decreased echogenicities likely due to hemorrhage and necrosis. The mass measured approximately 10 cm. The CT images do not demonstrate metastatic spread or involvement of the left adrenal gland. **E:** On the transverse section, the primarily hypoechoic mass (*calipers*) is identified posterior to the right liver lobe (*RL*) and lateral to the gall bladder (*GB*). **F:** On the transverse CT image, the location and relational anatomy of the right adrenal mass (*arrowheads*) is demonstrated. *RL*, right liver lobe; *A*, aorta; *LK*, left kidney; *Sp*, spleen. No mass is identified in the region of the left adrenal gland. Tissue variations on the CT are consistent with the irregular echogenicities seen by ultrasound. (Images courtesy of Dr. Taco Geertsma, Gelderse Vallei, Ede, The Netherlands.)

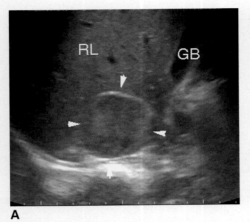

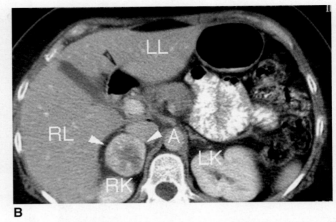

**Figure 13-21** Pheochromocytoma. In the right adrenal gland, a pheochromocytoma *(arrowheads)* approximately 4 cm in maximum dimension. **A:** On the transverse section, the primarily isoechoic round mass with sharply marginated walls *(arrowheads)* is identified posterior to the right liver lobe *(RL)* and lateral to the gall bladder *(GB)*. **B:** On the transverse computed tomography image, the location and relational anatomy of the right adrenal mass *(arrowheads)* is demonstrated. *RL*, right liver lobe; *LL*, left liver lobe; *A*, aorta; *RK*, right kidney; *LK*, left kidney. No mass is identified in the region of the left adrenal gland. (Images courtesy of Dr. Taco Geertsma, Gelderse Vallei, Ede, The Netherlands.)

the appearance of pheochromocytomas on MRI also overlaps with metastases and lipomatous adenomas.[51] A definite benefit of CT and MRI is concurrent detection of additional tumors associated with MEN syndromes.[51] Scintigraphy offers whole body imaging and the ability to simultaneously detect extra-adrenal lesions and metastases.[51] Specific radionuclides used for detection of pheochromocytomas are discussed later in this chapter.

## NEUROBLASTOMA

*Neuroblastoma* is a highly malignant tumor of the adrenal medulla generally found in children (Pathology Box 13-4; see Chapter 20).

---

### PATHOLOGY BOX 13-4

**Tumors of the Adrenal Medulla**

| Tumor | Sonographic Appearance |
|---|---|
| Pheochromocytoma | Broad spectrum (hyperechoic, hypoechoic, echogenic, complex, cystic), marginated or encapsulated; solid components of homogeneous or heterogeneous echoes may represent hemorrhage or necrosis; larger masses displace surrounding organs or indent vasculature; may be bilateral or external to the adrenal |
| Neuroblastoma | Generally affect children (see Chapter 20); hyperechoic, poorly defined borders; focal echogenic areas may be present due to calcifications; hypoechoic areas may be present due to necrosis; inferior and lateral displacement of kidney |

## METASTATIC DISEASE

For patients with a history of cancer, multiple imaging modalities are used for locating new lesions, staging the disease, and treatment planning. Adrenal glands are the fourth most common site of metastases after lungs, liver, and bones.[33,38] Metastases to the adrenal glands occur from squamous cell carcinoma of the lung (33%); breast carcinoma (30%); and lymphoma, leukemia, melanoma; and carcinoma of the gastrointestinal tract, thyroid, pancreas, and kidney (37%) and tend to be bilateral.[3,33,38,40,56,60] There is a 25% incidence of adrenal involvement in non-Hodgkin lymphoma[33] (see Pathology Box 13-1).

Small adrenal metastases characteristically are hypoechoic, round or oval, and are located anteromedial to the upper pole of the kidney[33,36] (Fig. 13-14E,F). Larger metastases (>4 cm) tend to be irregularly shaped, heterogenous in texture, and may show central necrosis. These masses can also indent the posterior wall of the IVC and displace the kidneys inferiorly[33,38] (Figs. 13-3A, 13-14A–D, and 13-22A–C). Hypoechoic and hyperechoic areas within these masses may represent necrosis and/or hemorrhage[33] (Figs. 13-13A–G and 13-14A–F and Pathology Box 13-4). Tumor extension into the IVC is specific for adrenocortical carcinoma.

With nonenhanced CT, the nonnecrotic rim of tissue may show high attenuation. On delayed contrast-enhanced CT, metastases enhance rapidly, but contrast washout is slow.[30,50,54] Although adrenal metastases and lymphomas are often bilateral (50%), this is not unique to the presentation of cancer[30,54] (Fig. 13-13D–G). Hyper- and hypofunctional diseases that commonly occur bilaterally include hyperplasia, infections, and hemorrhage.[54] Less frequently, pheochromocytomas, myelolipomas, and masses replacing normal adrenocortical tissue (adenomas and adrenocortical carcinomas) occur bilaterally.[54] Failure to identify accompanying adrenal insufficiency is life-threatening.[11,18]

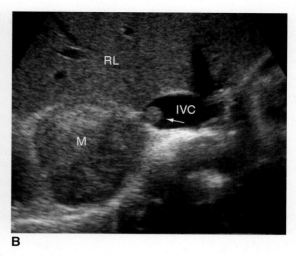

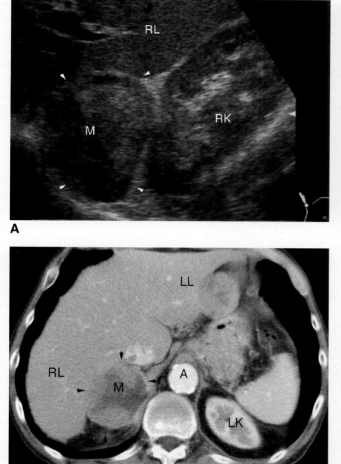

**Figure 13-22** These sonograms demonstrate a predominantly solid mass *(M, arrowheads)*, representing metastases to right gland from a lung carcinoma. The longitudinal **(A)** and transverse **(B)** aspects of the right adrenal mass are identified posteromedial to the right liver lobe *(RL)* and superior to the right kidney (RK). The transverse sonogram also demonstrates direct tumor invasion *(arrow)* into the inferior vena cava *(IVC)*. **C:** On the computed tomography image, the location and relational anatomy of the right adrenal mass *(arrowheads)* is demonstrated. *RL*, right liver lobe; *LL*, left liver lobe; *A*, aorta; *LK*, left kidney. No mass was identified in the region of the left adrenal gland. (Images courtesy of Dr. Taco Geertsma, Gelderse Vallei, Ede, The Netherlands.)

Only about half of the adrenal masses in patients with known primary tumors prove to be malignant on biopsy examination.[38] Therefore, a solitary nonfunctioning adrenal tumor should not be assumed to be metastatic disease without being correlated with other findings.[38] Percutaneous aspiration biopsy is capable of distinguishing metastases from a benign adenoma or a primary adrenal carcinoma.[38] Collision tumor describes an existing adrenal adenoma, which is secondarily infiltrated by a metastasis.[50,68] This tumor produces a mixed-signal MRI anatomically consistent with the adenoma and metastasis components.

## OTHER IMAGING PROCEDURES

### RADIOGRAPHY

With advances in tomographic and volumetric imaging technology, traditional radiographic examinations are no longer the procedure of choice for the adrenal gland; however, incidental radiographic findings may indicate adrenal gland pathology. Calcifications may be visualized on an abdominal radiograph of the kidneys, ureters, and bladder, which is the "scout study" prior to excretory urography, intravenous pyelography (IVP), or nephrotomography (tomography eliminates obscuring overlying structures). The presence of calcifications is not specific as they occur in 10% of adrenal tumors and 15% of adrenal cysts. In adrenal cysts, calcifications are usually located at the periphery and appear more curvilinear, like an eggshell.[36,38] Approximately 70% to 80% of adrenal masses can be detected by combined IVP and tomography, relying on both the delineation of the mass and demonstration of the degree to which it impinges on the kidney. Small adrenal masses, such as aldosteronomas and extra-adrenal pheochromocytomas, are difficult to demonstrate with these modalities.[38]

Angiography is specific in the demonstration of vascular adrenal masses[61] and for defining the vascular supply to the tumor, useful information for the surgical team. Angiography may not be specific, though, in differentiating neoplasms from hyperplasia or delineating hypovascular lesions. Venography demonstrates the displacement of veins around the tumor. Venography with venous blood sampling of circulating hormones is 100% accurate in differentiating between a unilateral adenoma and bilateral adrenal hyperplasia.[41,50] The risks of angiography, venography, and venous sampling include intra-adrenal hemorrhage with pain, infarction, and possibly Addison disease.[41]

## COMPUTED TOMOGRAPHY AND MAGNETIC RESONANCE IMAGING

*Thin-collimation CT* is the first choice imaging modality for evaluating most cases of suspected adrenal disease.[31] In comparison to sonography, CT is superior in detecting normal adrenal glands, especially in obese patients.[30,50,56,66] Several adrenal lesions have inherent tissue characteristics detectable on CT that permit a confident diagnosis based on these images alone.[30,50,54] Use of other imaging modalities (MRI, scintigraphy, and PET) in addition to blood and urine testing contribute to refining the diagnosis in most cases.[35,50,66] MRI offers multiple techniques for evaluating adrenal masses.[59] Both T1- and T2-weighted images may be utilized to obtain a diagnosis, with adenomas producing weak signals, pheochromocytomas strong ones, and carcinomas intermediate signals.[38,59,66]

Diagnostic protocols have been developed and continue to be refined regarding the use of CT and MRI for identifying, characterizing, and treating adrenal lesions. MRI is equal to CT in the identification of a variety of adrenal abnormalities. Diagnosis usually relies on multiple criteria and even after extensive imaging, biopsy may still be required to rule out malignancy.[30] For example, with oncology patients, noncontrast CT is the first step in the diagnostic imaging process. If the attenuation rate of the tumor area is less than 10 Hounsfield units (HU), it is classified as a benign adenoma.[30,50,54] If the mass doesn't meet this criteria, then a delayed contrast-enhanced CT (10 minutes) or chemical shift MRI is the next step. The delayed contrast-enhanced CT provides information about the perfusion of the lesion and the rapidity of washout of the contrast media. Lesion attenuation values less than 30 HU and greater than 50% washout of contrast media at 10 minutes identifies another group of benign adenomas.[30,50] Tumors that do not meet these criteria are destined for biopsy or further evaluation by MRI. Similar to CT, with the more costly contrast MRI, adenomas show rapid enhancement and rapid washout of contrast material. On chemical-shifted MRI, adenomas show signal drop-off, which is not seen with malignant lesions.

The advantages of MRI are multiple acquisition and reconstructed planes and use of nonionizing radiation, while limitations include cost and availability.[32,59] Chemical shift MRI T2-weighted MRI is used for detection of pheochromocytomas. Pheochromocytomas are often, but not always T2 hyperintense.[66] MRI is useful for the detection of recurrence and ectopic pheochromocytomas (aka paragangliomas).[50]

MRI and CT imaging continue to improve and differences occur in technologies and methodologies. For example, single and multiple row helical CT scanners are producing somewhat different image features for some adrenal masses.[54] Further research data will need to be collected to determine how these changes in technology and methodology impact the image characteristics that may eventually become uniquely diagnostic for a variety of lesions evaluated by CT and MRI. When laboratory testing and imaging procedures are not conclusive, biopsy becomes necessary. CT remains the preferred method to provide needle guidance, although these percutaneous procedures are not without complication.[41,50,69]

## RADIONUCLIDE STUDIES

The radiopharmaceuticals are used to locate and differentiate specific types of adrenal masses. The major benefits of nuclear medicine procedures are that the images are based on active tissue physiologic function and can be collected from a whole body perspective, which is particularly useful for identifying ectopic masses and metastases.[66,70] Fusion imaging in the form of SPECT/CT and PET/CT will likely continue to increase because it offers the integration of anatomical and functional data for the diagnosis and treatment of cortical and medullary adrenal disease.[56]

Meta-iodobenzylguanidine ([131]I-MIGB or [123]I-MIGB) and [111]Indium-octreotide (Somastatin analog) are radiopharmaceuticals used to locate adrenomedullary tumors such as neuroblastomas and pheochromocytomas.[50,66,70] Pheochromocytomas are visualized with both radionuclides 50% of the time, 25% of the time only with MIGB, and the other 25% of the time with only In-111.[50] Therefore, using the second radionuclide when there is nonvisualization with the first ensures localization of all adrenal and extra-adrenal pheochromocytomas and paragangliomas of similar embryonic origin when using whole body scans.

An investigational, but very successful radionuclide, [131]Iodine 6-beta-iodomethyl-19-norcholesterol (NP-59) is used to detect and differentiate aldosteronomas from adrenocortical hyperplasia. In patients with ACTH-independent Cushing syndrome, bilateral increased uptake of NP-59 indicates adrenocortical nodular hyperplasia while unilateral increased uptake suggests an adrenocortical adenoma. Absent or faint uptake is considered normal if there are no other signs or symptoms of adrenal disease.[56,70] Currently, NP-59 is not US Food and Drug Administration (FDA)-approved and has limited availability.[50,56,70]

Using a whole body imaging PET approach, the radiopharmaceutical fluorine-18 fluorodeoxyglucose (PET/FDG) is very good at distinguishing benign adrenal masses from malignant adrenal tumors and metastatic disease.[50,56,66,71] Increased costs and reduced availability are limitations for PET/FDG.[71]

## ENDOSCOPIC ULTRASOUND

EUS is a useful tool for assessing the adrenal gland when this invasive procedure is already planned. There is a significant potential to gather additional information regarding presence of adrenal masses, adjacent lymphadenopathy, and for staging lung cancers, which commonly metastasize to the adrenal glands.[5,69] Gastric and duodenal windows are used to image with 5 to 7.5 MHz radial, linear, and/or curvilinear transducers.[5,69] This technique can place the transducer as close as 1 to 2 cm from gland. As a result, the acoustic appearance of a normal adrenal gland is that of seagull-shaped hyperechoic medullary echoes against the hypoechoic cortical echoes and the hyperechoic halo of fatty tissue.[17,69]

Guidance of fine needle aspiration of adrenal lesions can also be performed using this endoscopic approach (EUS-FNA).[69,72] EUS-FNA is used to differentiate benign adrenal masses from metastases or primary adrenal malignancies. This is particularly important for preoperative staging of patients with known malignancies, since adrenal glands are common metastatic sites.[5,69,72] EUS visualization of the left adrenal from a transgastric approach reaches 98%, while it has been reported that imaging the right adrenal gland from a transduodenal window is only successful 30% of the time with a mechanical radial transducer.[73] Others have had improved the success for visualizing and performing EUS-FNA on the right adrenal by instead using a curvilinear transducer.[69,74]

EUS is minimally invasive and has minimal complications for the patient.[5,69,72,74,75] Limitations of EUS for adrenal imaging rests with the experience and motivation of the specialists who use this technology.[5,17,69,72,74]

## INTRAOPERATIVE ULTRASOUND

High-frequency IOUS is also used with a variety of laparoscopic (LIOUS) and open surgery settings.[4,75,76] Benefits of LIOUS concurrent with laparoscopic adrenalectomies are numerous. These include improved localization and guidance of complete and partial adrenalectomies, reduced blood loss due to improved vascular visualization, identification of adjacent tumor infiltration, metastases and lymphadenopathy, fewer complications, and shorter time to recovery.[4,58,75,76] Drawbacks to laparoscopic adrenalectomies with LIOUS are an increase in procedure duration, steep learning curve for physicians, and an increase in patient cost for adding LIOUS.[4,58,76]

## SUMMARY

- The adrenal cortex and medulla develop from different embryonic tissues and are therefore two functionally distinct endocrine glands within one organ.
- The adrenal cortex comprises 90% of the gland and produces corticoids including cortisol, aldosterone, estrogen, and androgen.
- The medulla produces the catecholamines epinephrine and norepinephrine responsible for the body's fight-or-flight response to stress.
- The adrenal glands are retroperitoneal and are located anterior, medial, and superior to the kidneys.
- The right adrenal gland is triangular in shape and is located posterior and lateral to the inferior vena cava, medial to the right lobe of the liver, and lateral to the crus of the diaphragm; the left adrenal gland is larger than the right and is more crescent or semilunar in shape.
- Adrenal cysts are infrequent and usually asymptomatic, whereas most adrenal cysts are benign, and adrenal cysts with a "ring" calcification are more often malignant.
- Hemorrhage of the adrenal gland is seen most often in newborns, especially after a difficult delivery but can also be precipitated by adrenal trauma, surgery, stress, anticoagulant therapy, adrenal vein thrombosis, adrenal neoplasms, metastases, or septicemia. The right side is involved more often than the left.
- Addison disease is a condition caused by hyposecretion of adrenocortical hormones and is characterized by fever, fatigue, muscle weakness, hypotension, and gastrointestinal distress such as nausea, vomiting, weight loss, and diarrhea.
- Cushing syndrome is caused by hypersecretion of the adrenocortical hormone cortisol, which triggers an increase in gluconeogenesis and results in elevated serum glucose levels, protein loss, and hypertension.
- Conn syndrome is caused by hyperaldosteronism and in 80% to 90% of patients, it results from a benign aldosterone-producing adrenal adenoma.
- Adrenal adenomas are typically benign, poorly encapsulated tumors 1 to 5 cm in diameter, and consist of lipid-filled cells that do not secrete hormones. Adenomas greater than 2 cm in size are more likely to be functional and may cause Cushing syndrome.
- Adrenal myelolipoma is a rare benign tumor of the adrenal cortex composed of fatty tissue that sonographically appears as a well-defined and markedly hyperechoic mass.
- Adrenal adenocarcinoma occur in the adrenal cortex, often produce steroids, and are usually associated with one of the hyperadrenal syndromes, those that are nonfunctioning are highly malignant.
- Adenocarcinomas are solid masses larger than most adrenal masses, 3 to 6 cm for hyperfunctioning tumors and >6 cm for nonfunctioning lesions with a variable echogenicity depending on the degree of hemorrhage and necrosis. Nonfunctioning neoplasms appear more complex and hyperechoic, whereas hyperfunctioning masses are more likely to be uniformly hypoechoic.

# Critical Thinking Questions

1. A 40-year-old woman presents with right upper quadrant pain after eating for an ultrasound of the abdomen to rule out gallstones. You notice a 2-cm, round, homogeneous, solid mass superior to the upper pole of the right kidney. This mass appears separate from the kidney. The patient has no other complaints. What is the most likely diagnosis?

2. Which hormones are secreted by the adrenal cortex and which are secreted by the adrenal medulla? What type of symptoms would occur with hypersecretion of the cortical hormones?

3. What can cause adrenal hemorrhage in an adult?

4. A 45-year-old male presents for an abdominal ultrasound with severe hypertension, headaches, and a rapid heart rate. When examining his left upper quadrant you notice a 5-cm complex mass with internal calcifications that is highly vascular. The mass is located superior and medial to the left kidney. What are the differential diagnoses for this mass?

- Benign and malignant pheochromocytomas arise from the adrenal medulla and have similar sonographic and biochemical characteristics. Patients with pheochromocytomas typically present with mild to marked hypertension, headache, sweating, and tachycardia and most have a history of a hereditary endocrine tumor syndrome such as MEN or Von Hippel-Lindau.

- Pheochromocytomas are usually well encapsulated, ovoid to round, and may be palpable. They are highly vascular masses, and if rupture occurs, massive hemorrhage can be fatal. They have a highly variable echogenicity ranging from cystic or complex to echogenic with calcifications.

- Adrenal metastases occur from squamous cell carcinoma of the lung, breast carcinoma, lymphoma, leukemia, melanoma; carcinoma of the gastrointestinal tract, thyroid, pancreas, and kidney; and tend to be bilateral.

- CT is the modality of choice for evaluating the adrenal glands, but MRI, radionuclide studies, endoscopic ultrasound, and intraoperative ultrasound are also utilized.

## REFERENCES

1. Little AF. Adrenal gland and renal sonography. *World J Surg*. 2000;24:171–182.
2. Suzuki Y, Sasagawa I, Suzuki H, et al. The role of ultrasonography in the detection of adrenal masses: comparison with computed tomography and magnetic resonance imaging. *Int Urol Nephrol*. 2001;32:302–306.
3. Wan YL. Ultrasonography of the adrenal gland: a review. *J Med Ultrasound*. 2007;15(4):213–227.
4. Heniford BT, Iannitti DA, Hale J, et al. The role of intraoperative ultrasonography during laparascopic adrenalectomy. *Surgery*. 1997;122(6):1068–1074.
5. Kann PH. Endoscopic ultrasound imaging of the adrenals. *Endoscopy*. 2005;37(3):244–253.
6. Saftoiu A, Vilman P. Endoscopic ultrasound elastography–a new imaging technique for the visualization of tissue elasticity distribution. *J Gastrointestin Liv Dis*. 2006;15(2):161–165.
7. Slapa RZ, Kasperlik-Zaluska AA, Polanski JA, et al. Three-dimensional sonography in diagnosis of retroperitoneal hemorrhage from adrenocortical carcinoma. *J Ultrasound Med*. 2004;23:1369–1373.
8. Nawar R, Aron D. Adrenal incidentalomas—a continuing management dilemma. *Endoc Relat Cancer*. 2005;12:585–598.
9. Barwick TD, Malhotra A, Webb JA. Embryology of the adrenal glands and its relevance to diagnostic imaging. *Clin Radiol*. 2005;60:953–959.
10. Mangray S, DeLellis RA. Adrenal embryology and pathology. In: Blake MA, Boland G, eds. *Adrenal Imaging*. Totowa, NJ: Humana Press; 2009:1–34.
11. Brunt LM, Moley J. The pituitary and adrenal glands. In: Townsend CM, Beauchamp RD, Evers BM, et al., eds. *Sabiston's Textbook of Surgery: The Biological Basis of Modern Surgical Practice*. 17th ed. Philadelphia, PA: Saunders Elsevier; 2004:1023–1070.
12. Banowsky JHW. Surgical anatomy. In: Novick AC, Stewart BH, Pontes JE, eds. *Operative Urology Vol 1: The Kidneys, Adrenal Glands and Retroperitoneum*. Baltimore, MD: Lippincott Williams & Wilkins; 1989.
13. Stephen AE, Haynes AB, Hodin RA. Adrenal Surgery. In: Blake MA, Boland G, eds. *Adrenal Imaging*. Totowa, NJ: Humana Press; 2009:77–90.
14. Genuth SM. The adrenal glands. In: Berne RM, Levy MN, Koeppen BM, et al., eds. *Physiology*. 5th ed. St. Louis, MO: Mosby Elsevier; 2004:949–979.
15. Standring S, ed. *Gray's Anatomy: The Anatomical Basis of Clinical Practice*. 40th ed. London, United Kingdom: Churchill Livingstone Elsevier; 2008.
16. Higham CE, Coen JJ, Boland GWL, et al. The adrenals in oncology. In: Blake MA, Boland G, eds. *Adrenal Imaging*. Totowa, NJ: Humana Press; 2009:65–66.
17. Chang KJ, Erickson RA, Nguyen P. Endoscopic ultrasound (EUS) and EUS-guided fine needle aspiration of the left adrenal gland. *Gastrointest Endosc*. 1996;44(5):568–572.
18. Corbett JV. *Laboratory Tests and Diagnostic Procedures with Nursing Diagnosis*. 7th ed. Upper Saddle River, NJ: Prentice-Hall; 2008.
19. Trikudanathan S, Dluhy RG. Adrenocortical dysfunction. In: Blake MA, Boland G, eds. *Adrenal Imaging*. Totowa, NJ: Humana Press; 2009:35–56.
20. Young WF. Adrenal Medullary Dysfunction. In: Blake MA, Boland G, eds. *Adrenal Imaging*. Totowa, NJ: Humana Press; 2009:57–64.
21. Krebs CA, Eisenberg RL, Ratcliff S, et al. Cavasuprarenal line: New position for sonographic imaging of the left adrenal gland. *J Clin Ultrasound*. 1986;14:535–539.

22. Anderhub B. *General Sonography.* St. Louis, MO: CV Mosby; 1995:107–117.

23. Weinberg K. The retroperitoneum. In: Hagen-Ansert SL, ed *Textbook of Diagnostic Ultrasonography.* 6th ed. St. Louis, MO: Mosby Elsevier; 2006:376–396.

24. Yeh HC. Sonography of the adrenal glands: normal glands and small masses. *AJR Am J Roentgenol.* 1980;135:1167–1177.

25. Krebs CA, Eisenberg RL. Ultrasound imaging of the adrenal glands. *Radiol Tech.* 1985;56:421–423.

26. Krebs C, Rawls K. Techniques for successful scanning: positioning strategy for optimal visualization of a left adrenal mass. *J Diag Med Sonogr.* 1990;5:286.

27. Krebs CA, Giyanani VL, Eisenberg RL. *Ultrasound Atlas of Disease Processes.* Norwalk, CT: Appleton & Lange; 1993.

28. Winter T. Possible Adrenal Mass. In: Sanders RC, Winter T, eds. *Clinical Sonography: A Practical Guide.* 4th ed. Baltimore, MD: Lippincott Williams & Wilkins; 2007: 154–161.

29. Weinberg K. General abdominal sonography. In: Krebs C, Odwin CS, Fleischer AC, eds. *Appleton & Lange's Review for the Ultrasonography Examination.* New York: McGraw-Hill; 2004:187–300.

30. Al-Hawary MM, Francis IR, Korobkin M. Andrenal imaging using computed tomography: differentiation of adenomas and metastasis. In: Blake MA, Boland G, eds. *Adrenal Imaging.* Totowa, NJ: Humana Press; 2009:127–140.

31. Brant WE. Adrenal glands and kidneys. In: Brant WE, Helms CA, eds. *Fundamentals of Diagnostic Radiology.* 3rd ed. Philadelphia, PA: Lippincott Williams & Wilkins; 2007:867–886.

32. Kriegshauser JS, Carroll BA. The adrenal glands. In: Rumack CM, Wilson SR, Charboneau JW, eds. *Diagnostic Ultrasound.* 2nd ed. St. Louis, MO: Mosby; 1997:289–314.

33. Mittelstaedt CA. Retroperitoneum. In: Mittelstaedt CA, ed. *General Ultrasound.* New York, NY: Churchill Livingstone; 1992:714–832.

34. Goldstein RB. Ultrasound evaluation of the fetal abdomen. In: Callen PW, ed. *Ultrasonography in Obstetrics and Gynecology.* 3rd ed. Philadelphia, PA: WB Saunders; 1994: 351–355.

35. Frilling A, Tecklenborg K, Weber F, et al. Importance of adrenal incidentaloma in patients with a history of malignancy. *Surgery.* 2004;136:1289–1296.

36. Yeh HC. Ultrasound and CT of the adrenals. *Semin Ultrasound.* 1982;3:97–113.

37. Goldman SM, Coelho RD, Freire Filho E, et al. Imaging procedures in adrenal pathology. *Arq Bras Endocrinol Metabol.* 2004;48(5):592–611.

38. Mitty HA. Adrenal disease. In: Eisenberg RL, ed. *Diagnostic Imaging: An Algorithmic Approach.* Philadelphia, PA: Lippincott Williams & Wilkins; 1988:373–386.

39. Robbins SL., Cotran RS. *Pathologic Basis of Diseases.* 2nd ed. Philadelphia, PA: WB Saunders; 1979.

40. Hall R. *The Ultrasound Handbook: Clinical, Etiologic and Pathologic Implications of Sonographic Findings.* 3rd ed. Philadelphia, PA: Lippincott Williams & Wilkins; 1999.

41. Lucey BC. Adrenal trauma and intervention. In: Blake MA, Boland G, eds. *Adrenal Imaging.* Totowa, NJ: Humana Press; 2009:193–204.

42. Weissleder R, Wittenberg J, Harisinghani MG. *Primer of Diagnostic Imaging.* 5th ed. Philadelphia, PA: Mosby Elsevier; 2011:231–234.

43. Fleischer AC. Renal and urological sonography. In: Fleischer AC, Kepple DM. eds. *Diagnostic Sonography: Principles and Clinical Applications.* Philadelphia: WB Saunders; 1995:470–557.

44. Dimofte G, Dubei L, Lozneanu L, et al. Right adrenal abscess—an unusual complication of acute appendicitis. *Rom J Gastroenterol.* 2004;13(3):241–244.

45. Kao P, Liu C, Lee C, et al. Non-typhi Salmonella adrenal abscess in an HIV-infected patient. *Scand J Infect Dis.* 2005;37(5):370–372.

46. Uno K, Konishi M, Yoshimoto E, et al. Fatal cytomegalovirus-associated adrenal insufficiency in an AIDS patient receiving corticosteroid therapy. *Intern Med.* 2007;46(9): 617–620.

47. Grover SB, Midha N, Gupta M, et al. Imaging spectrum in disseminated histoplasmosis: case report and brief review. *Australas Radiol.* 2005;49:175–178.

48. Bullock BL. *Pathophysiology: Adaptations and Alterations in Function.* 4th ed. Philadelphia, PA: JB Lippincott-Raven; 1996.

49. Rockall AG, Babar SA, Sohaib SA. CT and MR imaging of ACTH-independent. Cushing syndrome. *Radiographics.* 2004;24(2):435–452.

50. Mayo-Smith WW, Boland GW, Noto RB, et al. State-of-the-art adrenal imaging. *Radiographics.* 2001;21(4):995–1012.

51. Sohaib SA, Rockall AG, Reznek RH. Imaging functional adrenal disorders. *Best Prac Res Clin Endocrinol Metab.* 2005;19(2):293–310.

52. Barzon L, Sonino N, Fallo F, et al. Prevalence and natural history of adrenal incidentalomas. *Eur J Endocrinol.* 2003;149(4):273–285.

53. Song JH, Chaudhry FS, Mayo-Smith WW. The incidental adrenal mass on CT: prevalence of adrenal disease in 1049 consecutive adrenal masses in patients with no known malignancy. *AJR Am J Roentgenol.* 2008;190(5): 1163–1168.

54. Johnson PT, Horton KM, Fishman EK. Adrenal imaging with multidetector CT: evidence-based protocol optimization and interpretive practice. *Radiographics.* 2009;29(5):1319–1331.

55. Zarco-González JA, Herrera MF. Adrenal incidentaloma. *Scand J of Surg.* 2004;93(4):298–301.

56. Gross MD, Avram A, Fig LM, et al. Contemporary adrenal scintigraphy. *Eur J Nucl Med Mol Imaging.* 2007;34(4): 547–557.

57. Kloos RT, Gross MD, Francis IR. Incidentally discovered adrenal masses. *Cancer Treat Res.* 1997;89:286–292.

58. Mansmann G, Lau J, Balk E, et al. The clinically inapparent adrenal mass: update in diagnosis and management. *Endocr Rev.* 2004;25(2):309–340.

59. Kenney PJ. MRI of the adrenal glands. In: Blake MA, Boland G, eds. *Adrenal Imaging.* Totowa, NJ: Humana Press; 2009:141–156.

60. Yeh HC. Ultrasonography of the Adrenal Gland. In: Schwartz AE, Pertsemlidis D, Gagner M. eds. Endocrine Surgery. Informa Healthcare:2003

61. Cintron E, Quntero EC, Perez MR, et al. Computed tomography, sonographic, and radiographic findings in adrenal myelolipoma. *Urology.* 1984;23:608–610.

62. Dieckmann KP, Hamm B, Pickartz H, et al. Adrenal myelolipoma: clinical, radiologic, and histologic features. *Urology.* 1987;29(1):1–8.

63. Richman TS, Taylor JK, Kremkau FW. Propagation speed artifact in fatty tumor (myeloleioma): significance for tissue differential diagnosis. *J Ultrasound Med*. 1983;2:45–47.

64. Friedman AC, Hartman MD, Sherman J, et al. Computed tomography of abdominal fatty masses. *Radiology*. 1981;139(2):415–429.

65. Fernández-Cruz L, Puig-Domingo M, Halperin I, et al. Pheochromocytoma. *Scand J Surg*. 2004;93(4):302–309.

66. Remer EM, Miller FH. Imaging of pheochromocytomas. In: Blake MA, Boland G, eds. *Adrenal Imaging*. Totowa, NJ: Humana Press; 2009:129–126.

67. Schwerk WB, Görg C, Görg K, et al. Adrenal pheochromocytomas: broad spectrum of sonographic presentation. *J Ultrasound Med*. 1994;13(7):517–521.

68. Schwartz LH, Macari H, Huvos AG, et al. Collision tumors of the adrenal gland: demonstration and characterization on MR imaging. *Radiology*. 1996;201(3):757–760.

69. Eloubeidi MA, Morgan DE, Cerfolio RJ, et al. Transduodenal EUS-guided FNA of the right adrenal gland. *Gastrointestinal Endoscopy*. 2008;67(3):522–527.

70. Scott JA, Palmer EL. Single photon imaging of the adrenal gland. In: Blake MA, Boland G, eds. *Adrenal Imaging*. Totowa, NJ: Humana Press; 2009:127–162.

71. Roedl JB, Boland GWL, Blake MA. PET and PET-CT imaging of adrenal lesions. In: Blake MA, Boland G, eds. *Adrenal Imaging*. Totowa, NJ: Humana Press; 2009:173–192.

72. Stelow EB, Debol SM, Stanley MW, et al. Sampling of the adrenal glands by endoscopic ultrasound-guided fine-needle aspiration. *Diagn Cytopathol*. 2005;33(1):26–30.

73. Dietrich CF, Wehrmann T, Hoffmann C, et al. Detection of the adrenal glands by endoscopic or transabdominal ultrasound. *Endoscopy*. 1997;29(9):859–864.

74. DeWitt JM. Endoscopic ultrasound-guided fine-needle aspiration of right adrenal masses. *J Ultrasound Med*. 2008;27(2):261–267.

75. Piccolboni D, Ciccone F, Settembre A, et al. The role of echolaparoscopy in abdominal surgery: five years' experience in a dedicated center. *Surg Endosc*. 2008;22(1):112–117.

76. Lucas SW, Spitz JD, Arregui ME. The use of intraoperative ultrasound in laparoscopic adrenal surgery: the Saint Vincent experience. *Surg Endosc*. 1999;13(11):1093–1098.

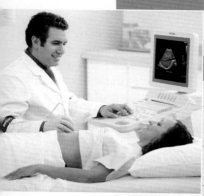

# 14 The Retroperitoneum

Joie Burns

## GLOSSARY

**abscess** a pocket of infection typically containing pus, blood, and degenerating tissue

**adenopathy** also called lymphadenopathy; enlargement of lymph nodes due to inflammation, primary neoplasia, or metastasis

**extravasate** fluid, such as blood, bile, or urine, that is forced out or leaks out of its normal vessel into the surrounding tissues or potential spaces

**fascia** a thin sheet-like tissue that separates muscles

**great vessels** a term used to describe the aorta and inferior vena cava together

**hematoma** an extravasated collection of blood localized within a potential space or tissues

**HIV** human immunodeficiency virus; bloodborne virus that attacks T-lymphocytes resulting in their destruction or impairment eventually leading to AIDS

**mass effect** distortion or displacement of normal anatomy due to a mass, neoplasm, or fluid collection

**metastasis** the spread of cancer from the site at which it first arose to a distant site

**orthogonal** planes that are perpendicular or 90 degrees to each other

**primary neoplasm** a new growth of benign or malignant origin

**urinoma** an extravasated urine collection due to a tear of the urinary collecting system

Sonography plays an important role in the examination of the retroperitoneum, as well as the organs and vessels located within the cavity. Although computed tomography (CT) is the preferred imaging modality for retroperitoneal neoplasms and adenopathy, the radiation dose delivered to the patient over multiple examinations must be considered. Sonography produces high-quality images without ionizing radiation, it can provide real-time biopsy guidance, and it provides safe imaging for follow up of disease progression or resolution. The skill and creativity of the sonographer often dictates the quality of the examination produced. A thorough knowledge of anatomy, pathophysiology, and sonography physics and instrumentation is required to produce the highest quality of sonographic examination. This chapter focuses specifically on the normal anatomy and pathologies found in the retroperitoneum.

## ANATOMY OF THE RETROPERITONEUM

The parietal peritoneum is the outermost of two membranes that enclose most of the intra-abdominal contents, including the intestines, liver, pancreatic head, spleen, and pelvic organs. The other membrane, the visceral peritoneum, lies in direct apposition to the parietal membrane, thus forming a potential space. The area lying behind the peritoneal membrane is referred to as the *retroperitoneum*. The retroperitoneum is a complex abdominal space located between the parietal peritoneum and anterior to the transversalis fascia.[1,2] It extends from the diaphragm superiorly to the pelvic brim inferiorly.[3-5]

### RETROPERITONEAL COMPARTMENTS

The retroperitoneum is divided into three major compartments or spaces by the anterior and posterior perirenal fascia.[6] These retroperitoneal compartments are the anterior pararenal space, the perirenal or perinephric space, and the posterior pararenal space.[1,6,7] The fascial planes are fused superiorly but remain unfused caudally. The literature frequently refers to both the anterior and posterior as Gerota fascia, although it is more correct to reference the anterior renal fascia as Gerota fascia and the posterior renal fascia as Zuckerkandl fascia.[8] The anterior renal fascia courses anterior to the great vessels, kidneys, and adrenal glands and extends across the midline to fuse with the posterior renal fascia laterally. The posterior renal fascia fuses with the anterior renal fascia laterally and tracks posterior to the kidney to blend with the anterior layer of the thoracolumbar fascia and the psoas fascial sheath medially.

An understanding of the retroperitoneal fascia is important to define the retroperitoneal compartments (Fig. 14-1A,B).

### Anterior Pararenal Space

The anterior pararenal space is bordered anteriorly by the posterior parietal peritoneum and posteriorly by the anterior perirenal fascia.[6] The space communicates with the opposite side around the pancreas.[1] Inferiorly, this space communicates with the extraperitoneal space of the pelvis and the posterior pararenal space.[9] The communication is important because it allows cells and fluid to travel between the two spaces. Along with a variable amount of fat, some portions of the digestive organs are embedded in this layer including the pancreas; distal common bile duct; the second, third, and fourth parts of the duodenum; and the ascending and descending colon.[10]

### Perirenal or Perinephric Space

The perirenal space is bordered anteriorly by the anterior renal fascia and posteriorly by the posterior renal fascia. Superiorly, the fascias fuse and attach to the diaphragmatic crura bilaterally immediately superior to the adrenal glands. Inferiorly, the perirenal space is open at the level of the pelvic brim as the fascial perirenal sheaths remain unfused. The perirenal space encloses the kidneys, adrenal glands, perinephric fat, and the prevertebral aorta and inferior vena cava (IVC).[1,10]

### Posterior Pararenal Space

The posterior pararenal space lies between the posterior renal fascia and the transversalis fascia. This space contains no organs, only fat.[10] The retrofascial space is located immediately posterior to the posterior pararenal space and it contains the psoas muscle posteromedially and the quadratus lumborum muscle posteriorly. The retrofascial space is not technically part of the retroperitoneum, but its muscles are frequently referred to in discussions of the retroperitoneal space.

Table 14-1 lists the organs and vessels contained in the retroperitoneum.

## ANATOMY OF THE LYMPHATIC SYSTEM

The lymphatic system extends throughout the body with lymph vessels found immediately adjacent to normal arteries and veins.[7,11] Unlike the vascular system, the lymph vessels end in a blind-ending plexus of tubes at the vascular capillary level. The lymphatic system acts as a fluid recovery system, collecting nearly 3 L of plasma fluid that oozes from the normal vascular capillaries into the extracellular space. The lymphatic system also collects cellular debris and bacteria within the extracellular fluid, as well as absorbing and transporting dietary fat. Since the lymphatic system returns excess fluid to the bloodstream, homeostasis (internal fluid balance) is maintained.

The fluid that enters the lymphatic plexus is referred to as *lymph*. This thin, colorless or slightly yellow

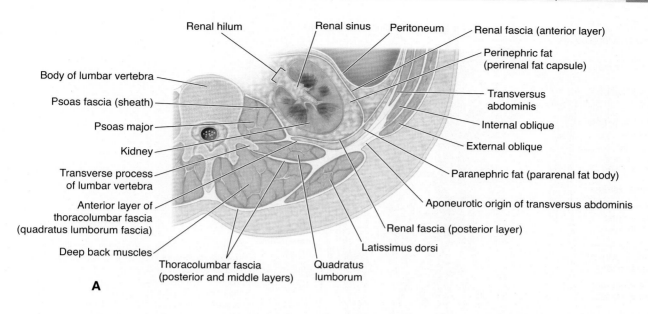

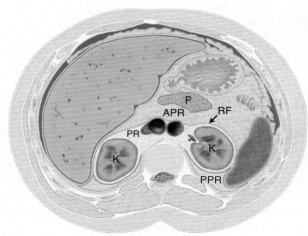

**Figure 14-1** Retroperitoneum. **A:** A transverse sectional retroperitoneum illustration at the renal hilum level demonstrates the fascial planes and musculature relationship. **B:** The transverse drawing illustrates the three major compartments: anterior pararenal space *(APR)*, perirenal space *(PR)*, and posterior pararenal space *(PPR)*. *P*, pancreas; *K*, kidney; *RF*, renal fascia.

fluid has a cellular composition similar to blood plasma. Lymph flows from the lymph capillary plexus toward the great vessels in the abdomen, eventually to the right and left subclavian veins in the thorax. The right lymphatic duct conducts lymph collected from the right head, neck, arm, and chest back into the venous system at the confluence of the right internal jugular and the right subclavian vein. The thoracic duct conducts lymph collected from the rest of the body back into the venous system at the confluence of the left internal jugular and the left subclavian vein. The chyle cistern is a dilated collecting area found in the midretroperitoneum collecting lymph from the lower extremities and pelvis before it ascends to the thoracic duct[7,11] (Fig. 14-2).

Lymph moves through lymphatic vessels, passing through lymph nodes along the way. Each lymph node is a small mass of lymphatic tissue that filters the lymph fluid, phagocytizing foreign proteins and infectious debris, and generating and sending lymphocytes to infected tissues. Lymph nodes are described based on their location. See Table 14-2 for a list of commonly affected abdominopelvic lymph node groups and measurements that indicate abnormal size.

| TABLE 14-1 |  |
| --- | --- |
| Retroperitoneal Organs and Structures |  |
| Diaphragmatic crura | Aorta |
| Pancreas | Inferior vena cava (IVC) |
| Distal common bile duct | Superior mesenteric artery (SMA) |
| Second, third, and fourth parts of duodenum | Superior mesenteric vein (SMV) |
| Kidneys | Hepatic artery |
| Adrenals | Splenic artery |
| Lymphatic vessels and nodes | Splenic vein |

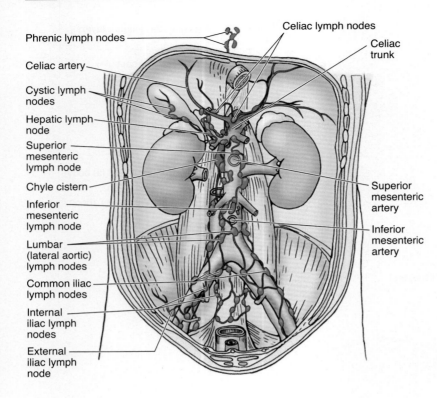

**Figure 14-2** Lymphatic system. This illustration shows the thoracic duct receiving lymph collected from the rest of the body and returning it back into the venous system at the confluence of the left internal jugular and the left subclavian vein. The chyle cistern is a dilated collecting area found in the midretroperitoneum collecting lymph from the lower extremities and pelvis before it ascends to the thoracic duct. (Reprinted with permission from Moore K, Dalley A, Agur A. *Clinically Oriented Anatomy.* 6th ed. Philadelphia, PA: Lippincott Williams & Wilkins; 2010:316.)

In the retroperitoneum, lymph nodes are generally divided into deep abdominal or parietal lymph nodes and superficial abdominal or visceral lymph nodes. Parietal nodes are those lymph nodes found in the retroperitoneum surrounding the principal blood vessels. They are grouped according to the arterial vessel with which they are associated. In the upper retroperitoneum, aggregations can be found around three unpaired vascular branches: inferior mesenteric, superior mesenteric, and celiac. Groups found in the lower retroperitoneum include the external, common, internal iliac, and epigastric.

Nodes are positioned 360 degrees around the aorta and IVC. Those that lie posterior to the main vessels provide the most reliable indicator of lymphadenopathy since they frequently displace the aorta or IVC anteriorly (Fig. 14-3).

Visceral nodes are located within the peritoneal cavity and are generally found at the hilum of organs. The most common groups are gastric, hepatic, pancreatic, splenic, and various groups associated with branches of the colic artery.

A special type of lymph node found along the small bowel and mesentery are called *lacteals*. Lacteals

| TABLE 14-2 | | |
|---|---|---|
| **Abdominopelvic Lymph Node Groups[4,5,7,11]** | | |
| **Retroperitoneum** | **Location** | **Abnormal Size** |
| Retrocrural | Posterior to the diaphragmatic crura | >6 mm |
| Retroperitoneal | Encircling the aorta (periaortic) or inferior vena cava (pericaval) or both (interaortocaval) | >10 mm |
| Mesenteric and celiac | Anterior to the abdominal aorta surrounding the origins of the celiac axis and mesenteric arteries | >10 mm |
| Pelvic | Along the common, external and internal iliac (hypogastric) arteries and veins; also referred to as the *iliac chain* | >15 mm |
| **Intraperitoneal** | **Location** | **Abnormal Size** |
| Gastrohepatic | Within the superior portion of the lesser omentum that suspends the stomach from the liver | >8 mm |
| Perisplenic | At the splenic hilum | >10 mm |
| Parapancreatic | Between the duodenal sweep and the pancreatic head anterior to the inferior vena cava | >10 mm |
| Hepatic hilum | Surrounding the porta hepatis | >6 mm |

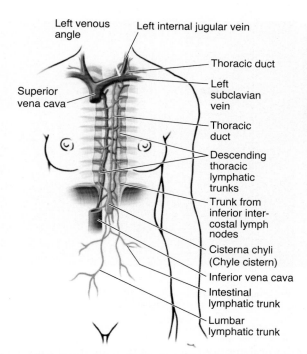

Left venous angle — Left internal jugular vein — Thoracic duct — Left subclavian vein — Thoracic duct — Descending thoracic lymphatic trunks — Trunk from inferior intercostal lymph nodes — Cisterna chyli (Chyle cistern) — Inferior vena cava — Intestinal lymphatic trunk — Lumbar lymphatic trunk — Superior vena cava

**Figure 14-3** Retroperitoneal lymph nodes. The illustration demonstrates the deep abdominal parietal lymph nodes following the course of the major blood vessels. (Reprinted with permission from Moore K, Dalley A, Agur A. *Clinically Oriented Anatomy.* 6th ed. Philadelphia, PA: Lippincott Williams & Wilkins; 2010:316.)

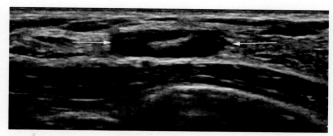

**Figure 14-4** Lymph node. The longitudinal image displays a normal ovoid-shaped hypoechoic lymph node. Note the echogenic central fatty hilum. (Image courtesy of Philips Medical Systems, Bothell, WA.)

take on a milky white appearance as they also absorb dietary fat.

## SCANNING TECHNIQUE AND NORMAL SONOGRAPHIC APPEARANCE

Ideally, patients should be fasting for 6 to 8 hours prior to the examination. This will reduce bowel gas and fluid that may be confused with pathology; however, if needed, an examination of the retroperitoneum may be performed without any patient preparation. Due to the retroperitoneum's deep position, a 3- to 6-MHz sector or curvilinear transducer should offer adequate penetration and a wide field of view for most adult retroperitoneal examinations. Higher frequency transducers should be used on smaller children and a lower frequency transducer will provide better penetration on obese patients.

The retroperitoneum may be scanned using an anterior, coronal, or posterior approach. The anterior approach frequently involves directing the sound beam through the left lobe of the liver in the epigastric region or through a fluid-filled stomach when overlying bowel gas obstructs visualization of deeper anatomy. Coronal scan planes are frequently used, directing the beam through the liver on the right and the spleen on the left, to evaluate kidneys, adrenals, and midline retroperitoneal structures that are not seen well from an anterior approach. The posterior or flank scanning

approach may be employed, directing the ultrasound beam through the deep back muscles (see Fig. 14-1), when the anterior and coronal approach offer less than desirable imaging.

The retroperitoneal examination should include assessment of the kidneys, pancreas, and vasculature for size, relationship, neoplasm, fluid collection, and mass effect. Normal lymph nodes are not seen in the retroperitoneum. Normal superficial lymph nodes may be identified as hypoechoic almond-shaped structures with a bright fat containing hilum (Fig. 14-4). Normal adult adrenal glands are rarely identified, except in extremely thin patients.

A variable amount of fat is identified in the retroperitoneal compartments depending on the patient's body fat composition. Generally, more obese patients demonstrate more pronounced amounts of fat in each space. Typically there is a more generous amount of fat in the perirenal space than in the other retroperitoneal compartments. The anterior and posterior pararenal spaces may not be distinguishable from the perirenal space in average and thin patients. The perirenal fascial planes may be identified only occasionally. When seen, they appear as very fine echogenic lines surrounded by fat. Fat typically appears moderately echogenic and homogeneous in these spaces. In some typically obese patients, the perinephric fat may appear anechoic and should not be mistaken for fluid (Fig. 14-5A,B).

The diaphragmatic crura may be identified fairly routinely. As a muscular structure, the diaphragmatic crura appear as a hypoechoic linear structure surrounded by hyperechoic tissue running obliquely between the aorta and IVC in the transverse epigastric plane and anterior to the longitudinal proximal aorta. Muscles identified during the retroperitoneum examination include the quadratus lumborum and psoas. Both muscles appear hypoechoic with bright linear fibers running along the length of the muscle. Care must be taken not to mistake these muscles for inflammation or fluid collections when they are well developed in very muscular patients. When there is a question, the patient may be asked to flex and extend his or her hip. The muscle can be seen to extend and contract with leg movement.

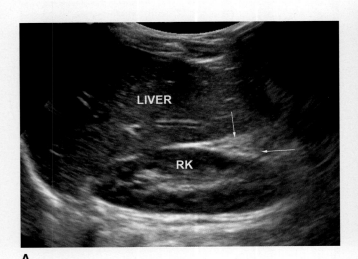

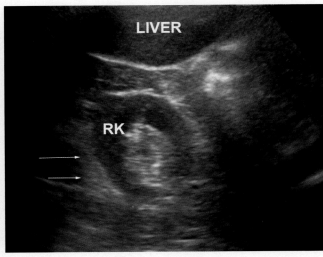

**A**                                                                 **B**

**Figure 14-5** Retroperitoneal fat. The perirenal space contains more fat than the other retroperitoneal compartments. **A:** A longitudinal image of the right kidney *(RK)* and liver with echogenic fat *(arrows)* seen surrounding the kidney. **B:** The transverse image of the right kidney also displays echogenic fat *(arrows)*.

## PATHOLOGY OF THE RETROPERITONEUM

When a mass is identified in the retroperitoneum, the sonographer should demonstrate the following:

- The abnormality in orthogonal planes
- Measurements of the mass in three dimensions
- Mass characteristics (cystic/fluid, solid tissue, air, calcification, borders, wall thickness, septa, etc.)
- The relationship of the mass to surrounding anatomy/mass effect
- The organ or area of mass origin
- Blood flow characteristics and feeding vessel(s) using color, power, and spectral Doppler

### SOLID LESIONS

Solid masses found in the retroperitoneum are usually metastatic and most frequently involve the lymph nodes. Although primary tumors do occur in the retroperitoneum, they are rare. The role of sonography in evaluating retroperitoneal adenopathy is limited. Sonography can detect the presence of solid masses and, in cases where intestinal gas or overlying bony structures do not obscure retroperitoneal imaging, may demonstrate the relationship of these masses to normal structures. The exact histologic nature of solid masses cannot, however, be definitively ascertained by sonography alone. When solid lesions are noted, the patient should be referred for additional diagnostic testing such as CT and possibly fine-needle biopsy of the solid mass.[12]

### Lymphadenopathy

Lymphadenopathy, also called *adenopathy*, describes the enlargement of lymph nodes caused by inflammation, primary neoplasia, or metastasis. The pattern of lymph node enlargement can provide important clues to the origin and type of pathology. Sonographically, enlarged lymph nodes typically appear as oval- to round-shaped masses with a low- to medium-level echo pattern compared to the more hyperechoic fat of the retroperitoneum. Lymphadenitis, describes an enlargement of lymph nodes due to an inflammatory process. Although lymph nodes are enlarged with lymphadenitis, they typically maintain an ovoid shape and fatty hilum. On color or power Doppler, lymphadenitis demonstrates hyperemia within the node (Fig. 14-6A,B). Primary malignant nodes, like those seen with lymphoma, tend to become more hypoechoic to anechoic and round shaped, with a length to width ratio of less than two[5] (Fig. 14-7A,B). Additional node characteristics that increase the likelihood of malignancy include asymmetric cortical widening and a loss of the normal fatty hilum, with color Doppler demonstrating avascular areas within the node or mass effect on normal vascular tree within the node.[5] Metastatic adenopathy tends to appear more echogenic and heterogeneous.[5] Care must be taken to adjust Doppler settings to levels that are sensitive to low flow levels when evaluating lymph nodes.

Enlarged nodes in the retroperitoneum may also fuse together forming a lobulated mantle-like soft tissue mass anterior to the aorta and IVC. Adenopathy may completely encase the abdominal great vessels moving them away from the vertebral column. It may also demonstrate a mass effect on arterial branches displacing them from their normal position while compressing surrounding veins (Fig. 14-8A,B).

Lymphadenopathy is a very common finding in patients with acquired immune deficiency syndrome (AIDS). Patients infected with the bloodborne virus

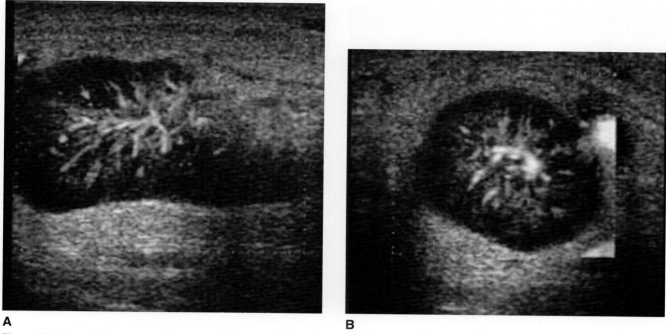

**Figure 14-6** Lymphadenitis. Longitudinal **(A)** and transverse **(B)** images of an infected lymph node demonstrate hyperemia with power Doppler.

human immunodeficiency virus (HIV) experience depression of their immune system due to this virus' destructive effect on T-lymphocytes. Without retroviral medical therapy, the patient's immune system fails and the disease evolves into AIDS. AIDS patients experience multiple opportunistic infections and neoplasms. The more common opportunistic fungal, viral, and bacterial infections include mycobacterium avium complex infection, tuberculosis, candidiasis, cytomegalovirus, and herpes. These infections frequently affect the gastrointestinal tract and are demonstrated on sonography as hypoechoic appearing lymphadenopathy and gut wall thickening. Tuberculosis may demonstrate very low attenuating, anechoic lymph nodes due to necrosis and punctuate echogenicities within the kidneys. Common neoplasms associated with AIDS include Kaposi sarcoma and lymphoma. Kaposi sarcoma is associated with chest and skin neoplasms and adenopathy. The AIDS-related lymphomas are of B-cell origin and include primarily non-Hodgkin lymphoma. AIDS lymphomas tend to affect the central nervous system, gastrointestinal tract, liver, and lungs.

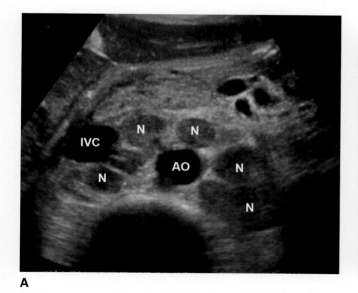

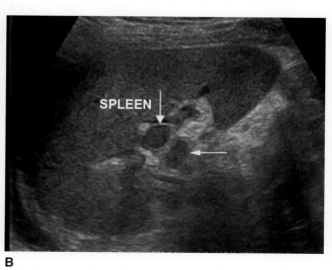

**Figure 14-7** Lymphadenopathy. **A:** Retroperitoneal lymph nodes *(N)* are seen surrounding the aorta *(AO)* and inferior vena cava *(IVC)*. The lymph nodes are more rounded in shape and a normal fatty hilum is not seen. (Image courtesy of Philips Medical Systems, Bothell, WA.) **B:** Rounded lymph nodes *(arrows)* are seen at the splenic hilum. (Image courtesy of Dr. Taco Geertsma, Gelderse Vallei, Ede, The Netherlands.)

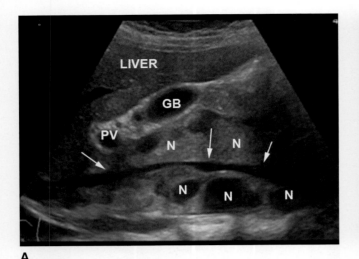

**A**

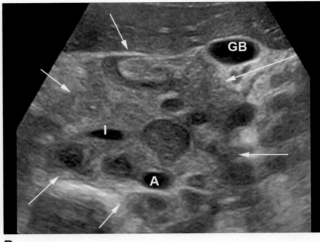

**B**

**Figure 14-8** Midline adenopathy. **A:** Longitudinal image of the abdomen demonstrates compression of the inferior vena cava (IVC; *arrows*) by lymphadenopathy seen anterior and posterior to the vessel. **B:** Transverse midline image demonstrates an echogenic mass encompassing and compressing the aorta *(A)* and IVC *(I)*. The mass is consistent with lymphadenopathy. (Images courtesy of Dr. Taco Geertsma, Gelderse Vallei, Ede, The Netherlands.)

In the abdomen, hypoechoic retroperitoneal adenopathy is frequently seen.[5]

CT is the imaging modality of choice to evaluate retroperitoneal adenopathy because of its ability to generate standard and reproducible views of abnormal nodes without bowel gas interference.[5] Sonography can be used to guide biopsy and assess the effects of lymphadenopathy on vascular and urinary structures of the retroperitoneum during therapy without additional radiation to the patient. Therapies related to lymph node enlargement are dependent on the cause but may include medical therapy to treat infection, chemotherapy, radiation therapy, or surgical removal with malignancies.[12]

### Retroperitoneal Fibrosis

Retroperitoneal fibrosis, also called *Ormond disease* or *chronic periaortitis*, is a chronic inflammatory process that results in fibrous tissue proliferation affecting and encasing the great vessels, ureters, and lymphatics of the retroperitoneum.[13–16] The disease affects middle-aged males twice as often as females.[5] The majority of cases of retroperitoneal fibrosis are idiopathic, thought by some to be autoimmune in nature.[16] Other causes include infiltrating neoplasia of the stomach, lung, breast, colon, prostate, and kidney; methysergide (medication prescribed to treat migraine headaches) use; and less frequently Crohn disease, sclerosing cholangitis, radiation therapy, aneurysm surgery or leakage, retroperitoneal infections, and urine leakage into the retroperitoneum.[5,16]

The ureters are frequently affected demonstrating a characteristic medial deviation or complete stenosis resulting in unilateral or bilateral hydronephrosis.[9,15,16] Additional symptoms include unintended weight loss, nausea, malaise, hypertension, and renal insufficiency.[9]

Although CT is the imaging modality of choice for initial diagnosis, sonography is frequently used to follow this disease process. Sonographically, retroperitoneal fibrosis appears as a hypoechoic smoothly marginated clump or layer in the para-aortic area of the perinephric space and may be mistaken for plaque surrounding the distal aorta (Fig. 14-9A–H). Treatment typically includes corticosteroid therapy with ureteral stenting in cases of ureteral stenosis and medical therapy for concomitant renal insufficiency.

### Primary Neoplasms

Solid retroperitoneal tumors are rare. Primary malignancies include liposarcoma, leiomyosarcoma, rhabdomyosarcoma, myxosarcoma, and fibrosarcoma. Benign retroperitoneal tumors include lipoma, leiomyoma, rhabdomyoma, myxoma, and fibroma. Malignant tumors tend to appear larger and more complex than their benign counterparts. These neoplasms tend to demonstrate mass effect on the vasculature of the retroperitoneum, compressing the IVC, ureters, urinary bladder, and extrahepatic bile ducts. The role of sonography beyond characterizing the neoplasm, evaluating the size, and demonstrating its blood flow characteristics is to demonstrate whether or not the tumor has infiltrated adjacent organs, as complete surgical resection determines prognosis.[5]

Liposarcoma is the most common primary malignancy of the retroperitoneum, representing 95% of all fatty retroperitoneal tumors.[5] This slow growing neoplasm affects middle-aged males more frequently than females. Patient complaints include abdominal pain, unintended weight loss, anemia, and a palpable mass.[17] CT remains the imaging modality of choice; however, sonography may be employed initially due to its noninvasive nature. Sonographically, liposarcoma demonstrates a poorly marginated, lobulated, complex mass that displaces adjacent anatomy rather than

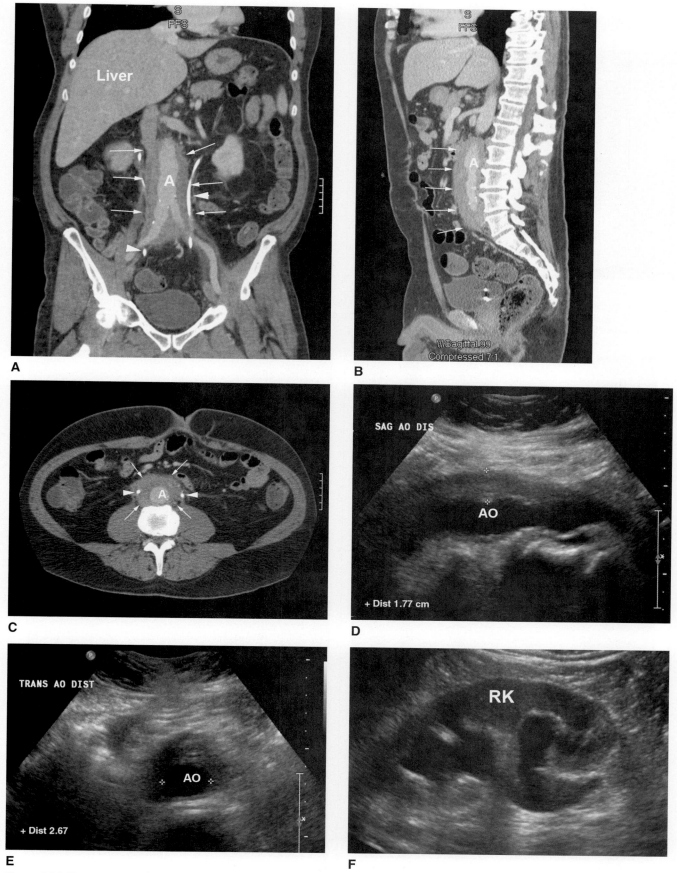

**Figure 14-9** Retroperitoneal fibrosis. **A:** Coronal, **(B)** sagittal, and **(C)** axial magnetic resonance images demonstrate retroperitoneal fibrosis *(arrows)* surrounding the aorta *(A)*. Bilateral ureteral stents *(arrowheads)* are seen on the coronal and axial images. **D:** Longitudinal and **(E)** transverse sonography images of the same patient demonstrate hypoechoic fibrosis seen surrounding the anechoic aorta *(AO)*. **F:** Longitudinal image of the right kidney *(RK)* demonstrates moderate hydronephrosis. Unilateral or bilateral hydronephrosis is a common finding with retroperitoneal fibrosis as the ureters are compressed by the tumor. *(continued)*

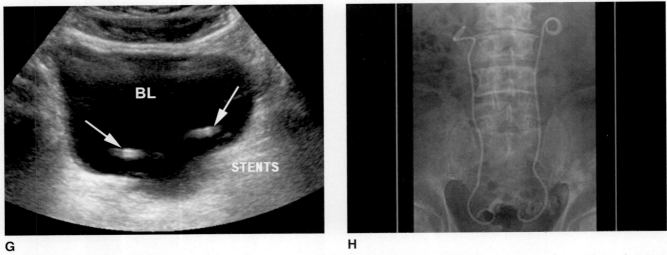

**Figure 14-9** *(continued)* **G:** Transverse image of the urinary bladder *(BL)* demonstrates bilateral echogenic ureteral stents *(arrows)* projecting into the bladder lumen. **H:** The abdominal radiograph demonstrates bilateral ureteral stents. (Image **H** courtesy of Dr. Taco Geertsma, Gelderse Vallei, Ede, The Netherlands.)

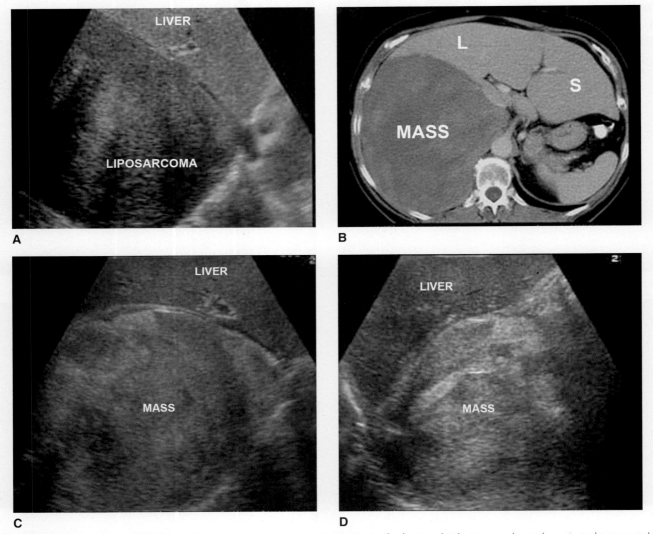

**Figure 14-10** Liposarcoma. **A,B:** A large heterogeneous mass seen posterior to the liver on both sonography and computed tomography. It was diagnosed as a retroperitoneal liposarcoma. (*L*, liver; *S*, spleen.) On this patient, the **(C)** transverse and **(D)** longitudinal images of the right upper quadrant demonstrate a large heterogeneous mass posterior to the right lobe of the liver. The mass was diagnosed as a liposarcoma. (Images courtesy of Dr. Taco Geertsma, Gelderse Vallei, Ede, The Netherlands.)

infiltrating it. One remarkable characteristic of retroperitoneal liposarcomas is the immense size some of them attain before diagnosis.[17] Tumors weighing 20 lb or more are not rare. Liposarcomas occur more frequently anterior to the spine and psoas muscles[5] (Fig. 14-10A–D).

Leiomyosarcoma is the second most common primary retroperitoneal malignancy. This smooth muscle tumor may occur in the uterus, gastrointestinal tract, or in the retroperitoneal cavity and may originate in the wall of the IVC.[18,19,20] Leiomyosarcoma typically affect middle-aged females.[18] Patients complain of an abdominal mass, pain, unintended weight loss, nausea, vomiting, and abdominal distention. Leiomyosarcoma frequently demonstrates bloodborne metastases to the liver, lung, brain, and peritoneum. Approximately 40% of patients demonstrate metastases at the time of diagnosis. Sonographically, these lesions present a mixed echo texture. Internal necrosis and hemorrhage produce fluid-filled areas within a well-circumscribed mass. Erosion of adjacent visceral walls may result in the presence of gas within the mass. This complex solid tumor is indistinguishable from other retroperitoneal neoplasms such as liposarcoma, lymphoma, and adrenal malignancy. Treatment consists of complete surgical resection, chemotherapy, and radiation therapy[5,20] (Fig. 14-11).

Because solid masses cannot displace the musculoskeletal structures of the back, clinical detection may be delayed. Frequently, the tumor must grow large enough to displace intraperitoneal contents before it can be palpated anteriorly. When the mass is finally detected, it is quite large and may have been present for as long as 20 years or more. Typically, the patient presents with a large, protruding abdomen or complains of increasing abdominal girth, weight loss, or abdominal pain. If the tumor has spread to the intestinal tract, symptoms such as nausea, vomiting, anorexia, diarrhea, and altered bowel habits may develop. Involvement of the kidneys or ureters, either by direct invasion or mechanical compression, may lead to hydronephrosis and subsequent pyelonephritis and uremia.

## RETROPERITONEAL FLUID COLLECTIONS

Fluid collections of the retroperitoneum are relatively common and include abscesses, hematomas, urinomas, and lymphoceles. Because they can all have the same sonographic appearance, it is impossible to differentiate the pathologic process on the basis of sonography alone; however, correlation of sonographic findings with the patient's clinical history can frequently provide a presumptive diagnosis. Fine-needle aspiration of suspicious areas provides more specific information on the nature of the mass. Identifying the compartment in which the collection is localized may help narrow the diagnostic possibilities. Fluid collections will conform to the space in which they form, frequently demonstrating sharp corners at organ interfaces. This knowledge may also be helpful in determining the cause and nature of the fluid collection.

The anterior pararenal space is the most common site of retroperitoneal infections. Because the appendix frequently occupies a retrocecal position and lies outside the peritoneal cavity, and because portions of the duodenum and colon also border the anterior pararenal space, perforation by trauma, inflammation, or as a sequela of bowel disease can lead to retroperitoneal infection. In cases of pancreatitis, digestive enzymes are extravasated and cause an inflammatory response in the anterior pararenal space.[13,21,22] Typically, this develops into a pseudocyst. As proteolytic digestive enzymes destroy the cell walls within the pancreas, additional enzymes are released into the interstitial spaces, precipitating further destruction of pancreatic parenchyma. Necrosis of blood vessel walls may also cause hemorrhage into the anterior pararenal space, increasing the fluid content.[22] In some cases, the tissue-dissolving capabilities of the pancreatic enzymes cause further spread of the fluid into the posterior pararenal space.[21,22]

Fluid collections within the perirenal space or contained within Gerota fascia are generally associated with renal abnormalities.[9] Nephritis with subsequent abscess formation, rupture of a renal artery aneurysm, or bleeding from a renal neoplasm may all create a perinephric fluid collection. Sonographically, the fluid collection is contained within the borders of the renal fascia and does not demonstrate significant movement with alterations in patient position.

The posterior pararenal space is bounded anteriorly by the posterior renal fascia and posteriorly by the transversalis fascia. Because it does not contain any

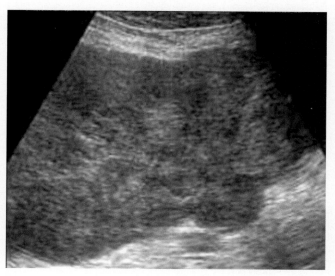

**Figure 14-11** Leiomyosarcoma. This large heterogeneous well-circumscribed mass seen in the retroperitoneum was diagnosed as a leiomyosarcoma. (Image courtesy of Dr. Taco Geertsma, Gelderse Vallei, Ede, The Netherlands.)

specific organs, alterations in anatomic appearance are due solely to processes that originate outside this space. Hemorrhage from trauma or ruptured vessels may dissect along the posterior pararenal space. Postoperative infections from aortic grafts may produce abscess collections, and leaking anastomoses may allow blood to collect there. The most common cause of posterior pararenal fluid collections is aortic disease.

## Hematoma

Bleeding into the retroperitoneum may be the result of trauma, hemophilia, malignant invasion, surgery, or anticoagulant therapy. It may also occur spontaneously.

Spontaneous retroperitoneal hemorrhage is associated with primary renal malignant tumors (30%), benign renal neoplasms (30%), vascular diseases such as aneurysm rupture and arteriovenous malformation (25%), inflammation and infection (10%), anticoagulant therapy, hemodialysis, and primary adrenal neoplasms less frequently. The classic patient complaint is sudden onset of flank pain.[5] CT is the preferred imaging modality;

however, sonography may be requested as an initial imaging modality or to follow up a known hematoma for resolution. Coagulating blood presents a variable appearance depending on the age of the bleed. Initial bleeding appears anechoic, becoming more echogenic with thrombin organization, taking on the echogenicity of splenic parenchyma. As the hematoma ages, it begins to retract and lyse becoming more hyperechoic and complex in its appearance. Eventually, the hematoma is completely resorbed or may deposit a calcification at the hemorrhage site. Treatment is dependent on the cause of the hemorrhage. Thrombus does not contain vascularity and should not be mistaken for a neoplasm (Figs. 14-12A–C and 14-13A,B).

## Lymphocele

Lymphocele is an extravasated lymphatic fluid within the retroperitoneum. These are typically iatrogenically induced following node dissection for cancer staging or following surgery or renal transplant where the lymph vessels are disrupted. They may also occur following

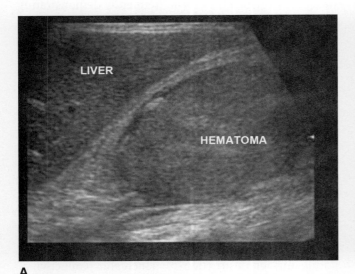

**A**

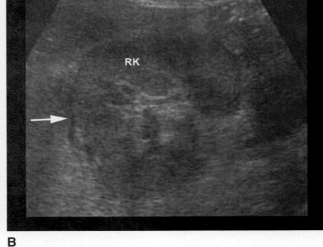

**B**

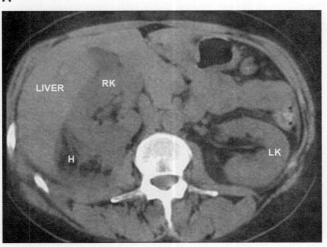

**C**

**Figure 14-12** Perirenal hematoma. Patient with blunt abdominal trauma presents for an abdominal sonogram. **A:** Longitudinal image of the right upper quadrant demonstrates a large homogeneous mass consistent with a hematoma in the right renal fossa. **B:** Transverse image of the right kidney (*RK*) demonstrates a small amount of free fluid around the kidney (*arrow*). The right kidney was displaced anteriorly by the large hematoma. **C:** Computed tomography scan of the same patient demonstrates the right kidney (*RK*) displaced anteriorly with the hematoma (*H*) posterior to the kidney. *LK*, left kidney. (Images courtesy of Dr. Taco Geertsma, Gelderse Vallei, Ede, The Netherlands.)

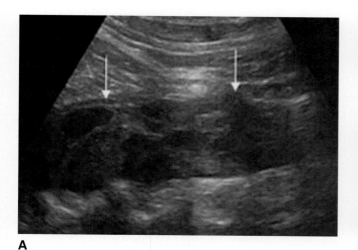

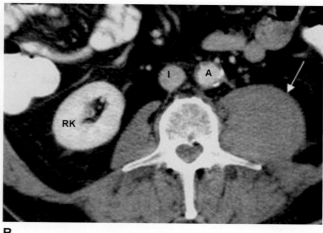

**A**    **B**

**Figure 14-13** Psoas muscle hematoma. **A:** Longitudinal image of the left retroperitoneum demonstrates an ovoid complex mass *(arrows)* consistent with a psoas muscle hematoma. **B:** Computed tomography scan of the same patient demonstrates a left-sided mass *(arrow)* adjacent to the spine. The mass was diagnosed as a psoas muscle hematoma. *A,* aorta; *I,* inferior vena cava; *RK,* right kidney. (Images courtesy of Dr. Taco Geertsma, Ede, The Netherlands.)

trauma. Lymphoceles typically develop within 10 to 21 days following surgery, but may develop up to 8 weeks following renal transplant.[5,9] Typically, these fluid collections are small and resolve on their own. However, if they become large causing hydronephrosis or inducing edema, they will be treated with percutaneous drainage, surgery, or with sclerosing agents.[5] Lymphoceles typically appear similar to a simple cyst but may appear more complex with thin septa seen on sonography.

## Urinoma

Retroperitoneal urinoma is an extravasated urine due to a tear of the urinary collecting system and continued renal function. Urinoma may occur due to nonobstructive causes such as blunt or penetrating trauma, surgery, or infection. Obstructive causes are more common and include ureteral obstruction or bladder outlet obstruction due to neoplasm, calculi, or congenital anomaly. Common patient complaints include fever, nausea, malaise, hematuria, and a compressible tender mass. Treatment includes aspiration of the urinoma and treatment of the primary cause. On sonography, this simple fluid collection is typically confined to the perirenal space (Fig. 14-14). The sonography examination should also include a search for the primary cause. The retroperitoneum should be examined for evidence of retroperitoneal fibrosis, ureteral strictures and calculi, and renal dysplasia.[5]

## Retroperitoneal Abscess

Retroperitoneal abscess may develop as an extension from an adjacent organ such as renal infection, diverticulitis, and Crohn disease or due to an existing retroperitoneal fluid collection that has become infected. Additionally, immunosuppressed patients and those

with diabetes mellitus, ureteral obstruction, recent trauma, or surgery are at an increased risk for developing retroperitoneal abscess.[5] Clinically, abscess presents with an elevated white blood cell count, malaise, and fever. The sonographic appearance of abscess is very nonspecific, ranging from infiltrated solid tissue to a complex or thick-rimmed fluid collection with debris and possibly air (Fig. 14-15). Sonography cannot differentiate a complex fluid collection from an abscess. Aspiration is required to make a definitive diagnosis and may be the primary therapy.[22] Color and spectral Doppler should be used to insure that the complex fluid collection is not an aneurysm before aspiration is performed.

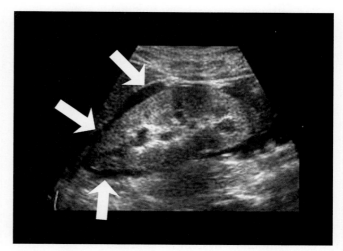

**Figure 14-14** Urinoma. Longitudinal image of the kidney demonstrates an anechoic fluid collection *(arrows)* surrounding the kidney. The fluid collection was diagnosed as a urinoma. (Image courtesy of Dr. Taco Geertsma, Ede, The Netherlands.)

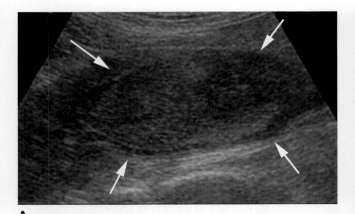

**A**

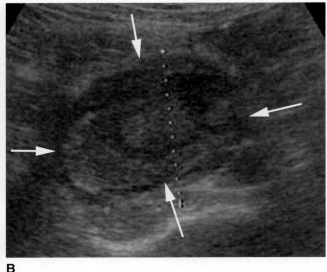

**B**

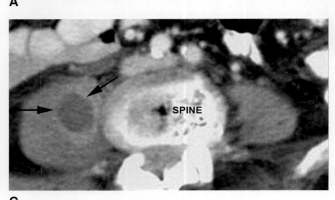

**C**

**Figure 14-15** Psoas muscle abscess. Longitudinal **(A)** and transverse **(B)** images of the right retroperitoneum demonstrate a large hypoechoic mass *(arrows)* in the region of the psoas muscle. **C:** Computed tomography of the same patient demonstrates an abscess of the right psoas muscle. (Images courtesy of Dr. Taco Geertsma, Gelderse Vallei, The Netherlands.)

## SUMMARY

- CT is the primary modality for evaluating the retroperitoneal cavity, but sonography can be used to evaluate the retroperitoneum, guide biopsy or drainage procedures, and can be used for follow-up evaluations for lymphadenopathy, fluid collections, or solid masses.

- The retroperitoneum is located behind the parietal peritoneum, extends from the diaphragm superiorly to the pelvic brim inferiorly and is divided into three major compartments by two fascial planes and the anterior and posterior renal fascia.

- The anterior pararenal space contains portions of the digestive tract, the pancreas, and the distal common bile duct.

- The perirenal space contains the kidneys, adrenal glands, perinephric fat, and the aorta and inferior vena cava.

- The posterior pararenal space lies between the posterior renal fascia and the transversalis fascia and contains no organs, only fat.

- The lymphatic system, comprised of the lymph nodes and lymphatic vessels, functions to return excess fluid from the interstitial spaces to the bloodstream, removes cellular debris and bacteria, and

sends lymphocytes to infected tissues to help fight infection.

- Parietal lymph nodes are found surrounding the principal abdominal blood vessels and are grouped according to the artery with which they are associated, whereas visceral nodes are located at the hila of abdominal organs.

- When evaluating a retroperitoneal mass, the abnormality should be imaged in orthogonal planes; measurements should be obtained in three dimensions, the relationship of the mass to the surrounding anatomy, the origin of the mass, the mass characteristics, and blood flow characteristics should be documented.

- Lymphadenopathy describes the enlargement of lymph nodes caused by inflammation, primary neoplasia, or metastasis.

- Sonographically, enlarged lymph nodes typically appear as oval- to round-shaped masses with a low- to medium-level echo pattern.

- Primary malignant nodes tend to be more hypoechoic to anechoic, more rounded than oval in shape, have an asymmetric cortical widening, and a loss of the normal fatty hilum.

- Enlarged retroperitoneal lymph nodes may fuse together to form a lobulated mantle-like soft tissue mass anterior to the great vessels or may completely

## Critical Thinking Questions

1. Which retroperitoneal compartment is most likely to contain a pancreatic pseudocyst?

2. Which retroperitoneal compartment is most likely to contain a hematoma from a leaking abdominal aortic aneurysm?

3. A 60-year-old patient with a history of renal cell carcinoma presents for an abdominal sonogram. The sonography examination reveals a lobulated hypoechoic mass surrounding the midline abdominal aorta.

The mass appears to displace the aorta anteriorly and displaces the superior mesenteric artery away from the aorta. What is the most likely diagnosis?

4. Name the three retroperitoneal compartments and list the organs located within each.

5. A 45-year-old patient presents for an abdominal sonogram with a recent diagnosis of retroperitoneal fibrosis. Besides evaluating the mass, what other organs must be evaluated?

encase the vessels moving them away from the vertebral column.

- Retroperitoneal fibrosis is typically idiopathic and may affect the ureters resulting in unilateral or bilateral hydronephrosis.

- Although solid retroperitoneal tumors are rare, primary malignancies include liposarcoma, leiomyosarcoma, rhabdomyosarcoma, myxosarcoma, and fibrosarcoma.

- Benign retroperitoneal tumors include lipoma, leiomyoma, rhabdomyoma, myxoma, and fibroma.

- Liposarcoma is the most common primary malignancy of the retroperitoneum.

- Leiomyosarcoma is a smooth muscle tumor and is the second most common primary retroperitoneal malignancy, sonographically appearing as a large complex mass.

- Retroperitoneal fluid collections include abscess, hematoma, urinoma, and lymphocele.

- Retroperitoneal infections most commonly occur in the anterior pararenal space as a result of appendicitis, bowel inflammation, trauma, or pancreatitis.

- Fluid collections within the perirenal space are generally associated with renal abnormalities such as nephritis, ruptured renal artery aneurysm, or bleeding from a renal neoplasm.

- Fluid collections in the posterior pararenal space are most commonly associated with aortic disease and may include hemorrhage from rupture or infection from surgical procedures.

- Hematoma formation in the retroperitoneum may occur as the result of trauma, hemophilia, malignant invasion, surgery, anticoagulant therapy use, or may occur spontaneously.

- A lymphocele typically occurs following node dissection for cancer staging or following surgery such as renal transplant where the lymph vessels are disrupted.

- An urinoma occurs as a result of a tear in the urinary collecting system that may result from trauma, surgery, infection, or obstructive causes.

- Retroperitoneal abscess may develop as an extension from an adjacent organ such as renal infection, diverticulitis, and Crohn disease or due to an existing retroperitoneal fluid collection that has become infected.

## REFERENCES

1. Vanderwerff B, Winter T. Unexplained hematocrit drop: rule out perinephric hematoma; possible perinephric mass. In: Sanders RC, Winter T, eds. *Clinical Sonography: A Practical Guide.* 4th ed. Baltimore, MD: Lippincott Williams & Wilkins; 2007:188–193.
2. Mirilas P, Skandalakis JE. Surgical anatomy of the retroperitoneal spaces part II: the architecture of the retroperitoneal space. *Am Surg.* 2010;76:33–42.
3. Kumar P, Mukhopadhyay S, Sandhu M, et al. Ultrasonography, computed tomography and percutaneous intervention in acute pancreatitis: a serial study. *Australas Radiol.* 1995;39:145–152.
4. Pick TP, Howden R, eds. *Gray's Anatomy: Anatomy, Descriptive and Surgical.* New York, NY: Random House; 1995.
5. Dähnert W. *Radiology Review Manual.* 5th ed. Philadelphia, PA: Lippincott Williams & Wilkins; 2003.
6. Ishikawa K, Idoguchi K, Tanaka H, et al. Classification of acute pancreatitis based on retroperitoneal extension: application of the concept of interfascial planes. *Eur J Radiol.* 2006;60:445–452.
7. Moore KL, Dalley AF, Agur AM. *Clinically Oriented Anatomy.* 6th ed. Philadelphia, PA: Lippincott Williams & Wilkins; 2010.
8. Chesbrough RM, Burkhard TK, Martinez AJ, et al. Gerota versus Zuckerkandl: the renal fascia revisited. *Radiology.* 1989;173:845–846.
9. Lee SL, Ku YM, Rha SE. Comprehensive reviews of the interfascial plane of the retroperitoneum: normal anatomy and pathologic entities. *Emerg Radiol.* 2010;17:3–11.
10. Lee YJ, Oh SN, Rha SE, et al. Renal trauma. *Radiol Clin North Am.* 2007;45:581–592.
11. Moore KL, Agur AM. *Essential Clinical Anatomy.* 3rd ed. Baltimore, MD: Lippincott Williams & Wilkins; 2007.
12. Bertino RE, Saucier NA, Barth DJ. The retroperitoneum. In: Rumack CM, Wilson SR, Charbonneau JW, et al., eds. *Diagnostic Ultrasound.* 4th ed. Vol. 1. Philadelphia, PA: Elsevier Mosby; 2011:447–485.
13. Paetzold S, Gary T, Hafner F, et al. Thrombosis of the inferior vena cava related to Ormond's disease. *Clin Rheumatol.* 2011 April; Epub ahead of print.

14. Moussavian B, Horrow MM. Retroperitoneal fibrosis. *Ultrasound Q*. 2009;25:89–91.
15. Vaglio A, Palmisano A, Corradi D, et al. Retroperitoneal fibrosis: evolving concepts. *Rheum Dis Clin North Am*. 2007;33:803–817.
16. Sinescu I, Surcel C, Mirvald C, et al. Prognostic factors in retroperitoneal fibrosis. *J Med Life*. 2010;3:19–25.
17. Han HH, Choi KH, Kim DS, et al. Retroperitoneal giant liposarcoma. *Korean J Urol*. 2010;51:579–582.
18. Fried AM. Spleen and retroperitoneum: the essentials. *Ultrasound Q*. 2005;21:275–286.
19. Hemant D, Krantikumar R, Amita J, et al. Primary leiomyosarcoma of inferior vena cava, a rare entity: imaging features. *Australas Radiol*. 2001;45:448–451.
20. Al-Saif OH, Sengupta B, Amr S, et al. Leiomyosarcoma of the infra-renal inferior vena cava. *Am J Surg*. 2011;2: e18–e20.
21. Tchelepi H, Ralls PW. Ultrasound of acute pancreatitis. *Ultrasound Clin*. 2007;2:415–422.
22. Rivera-Sanfeliz G. Percutaneous abdominal abscess drainage: a historical perspective. *AJR Am J Roentgenol*. 2008;191: 642–643.

# 15

# The Thyroid Gland, Parathyroid Glands, and Neck

Diane M. Kawamura and Janice L. McGinnis

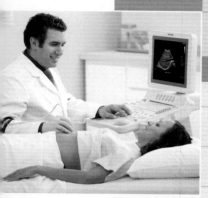

## OBJECTIVES

### The Thyroid Gland

Describe the thyroid gland embryology, surface anatomy, anatomic variants, and the common relational landmarks.

Discuss the physiology of the thyroid gland to include how each of the three thyroid hormones enables thyroid function.

Correlate laboratory values and clinical indications associated with hyperthyroidism and hypothyroidism.

Explain the sonographic evaluation of the thyroid gland to include patient preparation, protocol, and demonstrate the examination procedure.

Differentiate normal from the varying sonographic appearances associated with thyroid gland disease or pathology.

Describe the pathology, etiology, clinical signs and symptoms, and sonographic appearance for thyroid gland cysts, nodules, adenomas, goiters, thyrotoxicosis/ hyperthyroidisms, hypothyroidism, thyroiditis, thyroid disease in pregnancy, and thyroid carcinoma.

Explain the indications and guidelines for fine-needle aspiration.

### The Parathyroid Glands

Describe the parathyroid glands embryology, surface anatomy, anatomic variants, and the common relational landmarks.

Discuss the physiology of the parathyroid glands to include the importance of parathyroid hormone regulating calcium and phosphorus concentrations in extracellular fluid.

Correlate laboratory values and clinical indications associated with hypercalcemia and hypocalcemia.

Explain the sonographic evaluation of the parathyroid glands to include patient preparation, protocol, and demonstrate the examination procedure.

Differentiate normal from the varying sonographic appearances associated with disease or pathology of the parathyroid glands.

Describe the pathology, etiology, clinical signs and symptoms, and sonographic appearance for primary hyperparathyroidism to include adenomas, hyperplasia, and carcinoma.

## Abnormalities and Pathology of the Neck

Differentiate the varying sonographic appearances associated with normal anatomy and disease or pathology of the neck.

Describe the etiology, clinical signs and symptoms, and sonographic appearance of developmental cysts for the thyroglossal duct cyst, branchial cleft cyst, and cystic hygroma.

Identify the usefulness of diagnostic imaging to differentiate between a hematoma and deep neck space infections.

Describe the pathology, etiology, and important sonographic appearance and criteria to differentiate normal versus pathologic cervical lymph nodes.

## KEY TERMS

anaplastic carcinoma | calcitonin (thyrocalcitonin) | elastography | euthyroid | follicular carcinoma | Graves disease | Hashimoto thyroiditis | Hürthle cell carcinoma | hypercalcemia | hyperparathyroidism | hyperplasia | hypocalcemia | hypothyroidism | medullary carcinoma | papillary carcinoma | subacute thyroiditis (de Quervain disease or granulomatous thyroiditis) | thyroiditis | thyrotoxicosis/hyperthyroidism | thyroxine ($T_4$) | triiodothyronine ($T_3$)

## GLOSSARY

**adenoma**

**parathyroid adenoma** a benign, solid tumor of the parathyroid gland that secretes parathyroid hormone, which results in elevated levels of serum calcium

**thyroid adenoma** a benign, solid tumor of the thyroid gland

**adenopathy** enlargement of the glands

**anaplasia** a loss of differentiation of cells that is a characteristic of tumor tissue and occurs in most malignant tumors

**cervical adenopathy** enlargement of the lymph nodes

**cold nodule (photon-deficient area)** seen on a nuclear medicine study as region of thyroid where the radioisotope has not been taken up; the area may correspond to a palpable mass

**euthyroid** the thyroid gland is producing the right amount of thyroid hormone

**fine-needle aspiration** invasive procedure using a small gauge needle to obtain a tissue specimen from a specific lesion

**goiter** focal or diffuse thyroid gland enlargement due to iodine deficiency; multiple nodules may be present

**Graves disease** an autoimmune hyperthyroidism caused by antibodies that continuously activate thyroid-stimulating hormone receptors; it is characterized by enlarge thyroid, protrusion of eyeballs (exophthalmos), a rapid heartbeat, nervous excitability

**Hashimoto thyroiditis (chronic lymphocytic thyroiditis or Hashimoto disease)** most common inflammatory disease of the thyroid gland; usually occurs in genetically predisposed individuals, often presents in patients with other autoimmune disorders that may be associated with the formation of antibodies against normal thyroid tissue, and often accompanied by marked hyperemia

**heterotopic** occurring at an abnormal place or upon the wrong part of the body

**hyperparathyroidism** disorder associated with elevated serum calcium levels; usually caused by benign parathyroid adenoma

**hyperthyroidism** oversecretion of thyroid hormones

**hypophosphatasia** low phosphatase level that can be seen with hyperparathyroidism

**hypothyroidism** underactive thyroid hormones

**indolent** causing little pain (indolent tumor) or slow growing (indolent lesion or tumor)

**isthmus** thin band of thyroid tissue connecting the right and left lobes

**longus colli muscles** wedge-shaped muscle posterior to the thyroid lobes

**microcalcifications** tiny hyperechoic foci that may or may not shadow; sometimes present within a thyroid nodule

**papillary carcinoma** most common form of thyroid cancer

**parathyroid hormone** hormone produced by the parathyroid glands that regulate serum calcium and phosphorus

**primary hyperparathyroidism** oversecretion of parathyroid hormones

**sternocleidomastoid muscles** large muscles located anterolateral to the thyroid

**strap muscles** sternohyoid and sternothyroid muscles located anterior to the thyroid

**thyroglossal duct cyst** developmental fluid-filled spaced; congenital anomaly located anterior to trachea

extending from the base of the tongue to the isthmus of the thyroid

**thyroid inferno** increase in color Doppler vascular flow in the thyroid

**thyroiditis** inflammation of the thyroid

**thyroid-stimulating hormone** hormone secreted by the anterior pituitary gland that stimulates the thyroid gland to secrete thyroxine ($T_4$) and triiodothyronine ($T_3$)

**S**onographic evaluation of the neck provides an important diagnostic screening procedure for the evaluation of both the thyroid gland and parathyroid glands, as well as the soft tissues of the neck. Using a high-resolution, high-frequency transducer, the noninvasive examination provides a fast and an accurate assessment of anatomy without patient preparation. Sonographic guidance is important during such interventional procedures as fine-needle aspiration (FNA) and alcohol ablation of adenomas of the parathyroid glands.[1]

## THYROID GLAND

The thyroid gland is the site of synthesis, storage, and controlled secretion of thyroid hormones.[2] It is the largest endocrine gland in the human and functions to control the basal metabolic rate (BMR).[3] With the development of high-resolution, high-frequency probes designed for small parts scanning, sonography established itself as a superior modality for imaging the thyroid gland.[4] Its greatest clinical value is in confirming mass location, differentiating between cystic and solid lesions, and imaging the biopsy needle during FNA. The thyroid gland is subject to an array of maladaptations, and they and their sonographic appearance are discussed in this chapter.

### EMBRYOLOGY

Emerging between the third and fourth gestational weeks, the thyroid gland is the earliest endocrine glandular structure to appear in the human embryo.[5] The gland develops from an invagination in the floor of the primitive pharynx at the level of the first and second branchial arches, a point in the adult corresponding to the base of the tongue. This invagination is lined by cylindrical epithelial cells and can be distinguished at 16 to 17 days of gestation. These cells separate to form their pharyngeal connections by the fifth gestational week and migrate downward in front of the primitive pharynx and the developing hyoid bone. During this period of growth, the vesicle becomes a solid mass of epithelial cells and severs its connection with the pharyngeal cavity. This journey leaves behind a trace of epithelial cells known as the *thyroglossal tract (duct)*, which normally solidifies

and ultimately atrophies.[6] Dividing into two lobes connected by an isthmus at 7 weeks, the thyroid gland forms a shield over the front of the trachea and thyroid cartilage becoming fully developed by the end of the first trimester.[6]

### ANATOMY

The thyroid gland is located in the anterior neck surrounded by a fibrous capsule. It consists primarily of right and left lobes, and a relatively thin isthmus unites the lobes usually over the second and third cartilaginous rings of the trachea.[7] The superior border of the lateral lobes begins at approximately the thyroid cartilage (*pomum Adami* or Adam's apple) and extends inferiorly (Fig. 15-1A,B).

The thyroid gland weighs 15 to 20 g in the adult.[3,8] The size and shape of the thyroid lobes varies with gender being slightly larger in females, age, and body surface area.[9] On longitudinal sections, the lobes appear elongated in tall individuals and appear more oval on short individuals.[10] The mean length measures 40 to 60 mm, mean anteroposterior (AP) diameter is 13 to 18 mm, and the mean isthmic thickness is 4 to 6 mm.[11] Sonography is very accurate for calculating thyroid gland volume when needed to determine treatment or evaluate response to treatment. The volume can be determined with linear measurements or mathematical formulas for each lobe.[10]

Four arteries provide a rich blood supply to the thyroid gland. The upper poles of the gland receive blood from paired superior thyroid arteries that arise from the external carotids. Two inferior thyroid arteries originate at the thyrocervical trunk of the subclavian artery and supply the lower thyroid poles[12] (Fig. 15-2A). Normal peak velocities from the major thyroid arteries are 20 to 40 cm/sec and normal peak velocities from the intraparenchymal arteries are 15 to 30 cm/sec.[10] On the anterior surface, three pairs of veins normally drain the thyroid plexus of veins.[12] The superior thyroid veins correspond to the superior thyroid artery and drain the superior lobes. The middle thyroid veins drain the middle lobes and the inferior thyroid veins drain the inferior poles. The superior and middle thyroid veins drain into the internal jugular vein and the inferior thyroid veins drain into the brachiocephalic veins[12] (Fig. 15-2B).

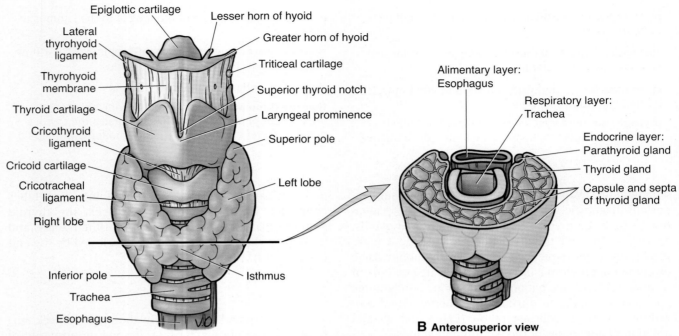

**Figure 15-1** Thyroid gland anatomy. **A:** The illustration demonstrates the relationship of the normal thyroid gland from an anterior view and **(B)** an anterosuperior view, which includes the three layers of cervical viscera. (Reprinted with permission from Moore KL, Agur AM. *Essential Clinical Anatomy.* 3rd ed. Baltimore, MD: Lippincott Williams & Wilkins; 2007:608.)

## Anatomic Variations

Deviations during any stage of development may lead to aberrant configurations or heterotopic locations of the thyroid gland. If the thyroglossal duct fails to involute completely, its persistence is a 1- to 3-cm cystic, fluid-filled remnant located anywhere along the route of the duct.[6] The thyroglossal duct cyst is the most common congenital cyst found in the neck.[13]

The most critical abnormality is the absence of the thyroid gland (athyrosis). This rare condition is associated with cretinism. Early identification and intervention with hormone replacement can stave off the physical and mental retardation associated with the congenital oversight.

More commonly, the gland may differentiate into configurations other than an isthmus and two lateral lobes. The variation occurring most often is a pyramidal lobe, which has been identified to some degree in approximately as many as 50% of normal of patients.[5] Developmentally, the pyramidal lobe arises from the

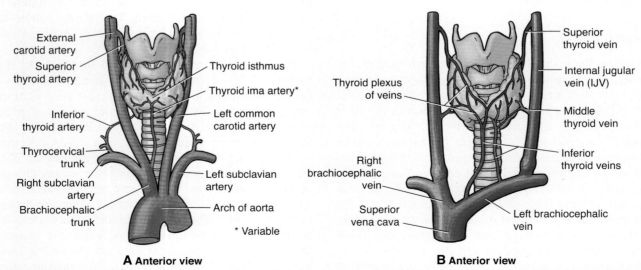

**Figure 15-2** Thyroid gland vascularity. **A:** The anterior view illustration demonstrates the arterial supply to the thyroid gland and **(B)** illustrates an anterior view of the venous drainage of the thyroid gland. (Reprinted with permission from Moore KL, Agur AM. *Essential Clinical Anatomy.* 3rd ed. Baltimore, MD: Lippincott Williams & Wilkins; 2007:609.)

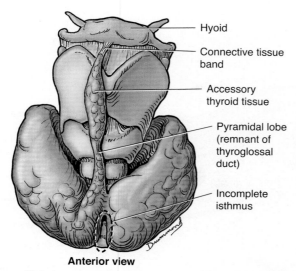

**Figure 15-3** Anatomic variations. An anterior view illustration demonstrates anatomic variations which include accessory thyroid tissue, pyramidal lobe, and incomplete isthmus. (Reprinted with permission from Moore KL, Agur AM. *Essential Clinical Anatomy*. 3rd ed. Baltimore, MD: Lippincott Williams & Wilkins; 2007:612.)

caudal portion of the thyroglossal tract. Usually, this lobe is small extending midline upward from the isthmus, but it can arise from either lobe, more often the left lobe then the right[12] (Fig. 15-3).

Other anatomic variations include the absence of an isthmus with the gland appearing as two independent lobes, the absence of one lobe with enlargement of the remaining lobe, or continuity from one lobe to the other effectively obliterating the isthmus.[5]

Thyroid gland development can occur ectopically at any point along the pathway of descent.[12] A normal gland may also rest entirely above (suprahyoid or prelaryngeal) or below the hyoid bone. Lingual thyroid, although relatively rare (1 in 100,000 cases of thyroid disease), is the most common location for ectopic functioning tissue.[13] This placement is usually identified by an incidental finding of a mass at the back of the tongue.[14]

Other ectopic locations include under the tongue (sublingual), the mediastinum (substernal), and rarely the tracheal or esophageal wall (Fig. 15-4). Small amounts of histologically functioning tissues may also be found along the internal carotid artery, the supraclavicular fossa, adjacent to the aortic arch or between the aorta and the pulmonary trunk, within the upper portion of the pericardium or mediastinum, and even within the interventricular septum.[5,6,15]

## Anatomic Landmarks

Many anatomic landmarks help to define the thyroid gland on a sonogram (Fig. 15-5A). On transverse images, the common carotid artery and internal jugular vein form the posterior lateral border of the gland. The artery is located medial to the vein. These structures are distinguished from the thyroid gland by echogenic walls and anechoic centers. Color Doppler or pulsed

wave Doppler imaging may also assist in clarifying the anatomy. The longus colli muscle appears as a low-level, echogenic structure defining the posterior border of the gland. The air-filled trachea forms the medial border and appears hyperechoic, with posterior shadowing. The sternothyroid, sternohyoid, and omohyoid muscles, collectively called the *strap muscles*, form the anterolateral border of the gland. Directly superficial to the thyroid gland is the sternothyroid muscle, which in turn is bordered by the sternohyoid anteriorly and the omohyoid laterally. The sternocleidomastoid is located lateral and superficial to the omohyoid. The very thin platysma muscle surrounds the neck, but its superficial location and indistinct density make it difficult to image with sonography. The thyroid gland appears as a rounded structure of low- to medium-level echoes, homogeneous in texture (Fig. 15-5B).

When imaged in the longitudinal (parasagittal) planes, the jugular vein and carotid artery appear as long, tubular, anechoic structures located laterally to the thyroid gland. Moving medially from these landmarks, the longus colli muscle, located posteriorly, becomes visible as a low-level, echogenic structure (Fig. 15-5C,D). The thyroid gland again is distinguished by its low- to medium-level, homogeneous echo pattern.

## PHYSIOLOGY

The principal responsibility of the thyroid gland is maintenance of body metabolism.[2] Thyroid hormones modulate oxygen consumption. Protein, carbohydrate, lipid, and vitamin metabolism all rely on or are affected by thyroid hormone action. Normal physical

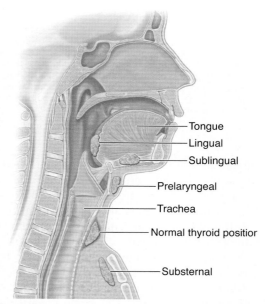

**Figure 15-4** Ectopic thyroid gland locations. The illustration of a lateral view demonstrates the common sites for an ectopic thyroid gland.

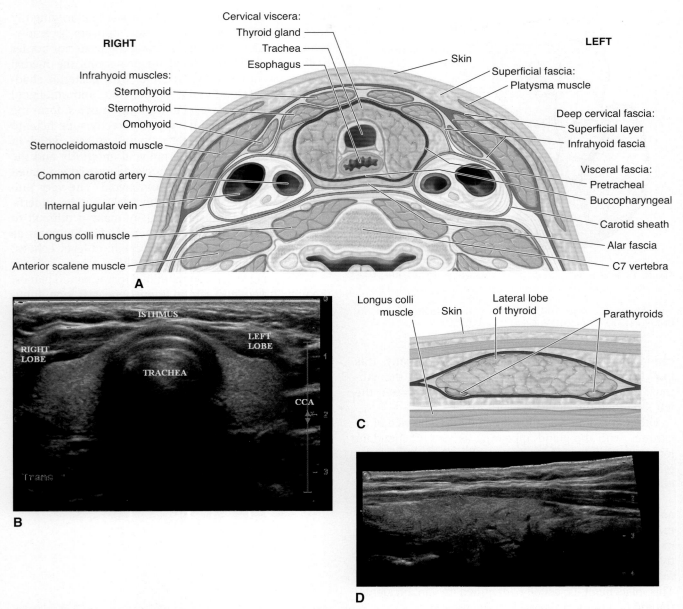

**Figure 15-5** Relational anatomy. **A:** The sectional illustration demonstrates the relationship of the thyroid gland, vasculature, and musculature in the neck. Note: if the colored image is used it should read: (Reprinted with permission from Tank PW, Gest TR. *Atlas of Anatomy*. Baltimore, MD: Lippincott Williams & Wilkins; 2009:305.) **B:** Transverse image of a normal thyroid. Note the homogeneous texture. *CCA*, common carotid artery. **C:** A longitudinal section of either the right or left lobe will show the thyroid gland relationship to the distally located longus colli muscle. **D:** A longitudinal sonogram is performed with a panoramic imaging option and demonstrates a normal right lobe (*cursors*) of the thyroid gland.

and mental growth depends on a healthy, functioning thyroid gland. Thyroid hormones enhance the rate of glucose uptake by fat tissue. Lipolysis and fatty acid mobilization from fat stores are magnified in the presence of thyroid hormone. Blood serum cholesterol levels are generally lowered.[3]

The thyroid gland secretes three hormones: triiodothyronine ($T_3$), thyroxine ($T_4$), and calcitonin, also called *thyrocalcitonin*.[2] The thyroid gland's parafollicular cells, or C cells, secrete calcitonin. Calcitonin lowers the plasma calcium level by inhibiting mobilization of calcium

from the bone. The follicular cells of the thyroid gland chemically process iodine to secrete $T_3$ and $T_4$.[8] The synthesis of these hormones depends on the availability of iodine and the gland's ability to process it properly.[3] When comparing secretion, the thyroid gland produces 90% of the less potent $T_4$ and only 10% of the more potent $T_3$; however, $T_4$ is converted to the more powerful $T_3$, which has the greatest metabolic effect and binds more efficiently to nuclear receptors in target cells.[2]

Maintenance of circulating concentrations of $T_3$ and $T_4$ is achieved by a dynamic regulatory system involving the hypothalamus, the pituitary, and the thyroid gland.[2] Thyrotropin, secreted by the anterior pituitary (adeno-hypophysis) thyrotroph cells, orchestrates thyroid hormone production. The secretion of thyroid-stimulating hormone (TSH) is modulated by both the $T_3$ and $T_4$ hormones and by thyrotropin-releasing hormone (TRH) from the hypothalamus.[2] Utilizing a classic negative feedback system, a drop in circulating thyroid hormones decreases the BMR. The falling BMR stimulates TRH, which in turn provokes the release of TSH. Thus inspired, the thyroid gland liberates the necessary $T_3$ and $T_4$, thereby returning the BMR to normal and retiring the cycle. Because the effects of thyroid hormones represent a complex integration of events at both the cellular and holistic levels, disease states that interfere with this system can have serious consequences.[2]

## LABORATORY TESTS

Thyroid hormones circulate in the blood both free and bound to thyronine-binding globulin (TBG).[6] There are several tests for diagnosing thyroid disease (Table 15-1). The range of values may vary somewhat among laboratories and in different geographic locations. Laboratory tests for calcitonin are done only for known or suspected cases of medullary carcinoma of the thyroid gland.

Diagnosing thyroid disease early is important because most are amenable to medical or surgical management.[6] These include conditions associated with excessive release of thyroid hormones (hyperthyroidism), those associated with thyroid hormone deficiency (hypothyroidism), and mass lesions of the thyroid gland.[6] Normal laboratory values are referred to as an *euthyroid*, which means the thyroid gland is producing the right amount of thyroid hormone.

## SONOGRAPHIC EXAMINATION TECHNIQUE

Sonographic examination is a noninvasive, relatively inexpensive, and objective diagnostic test useful in several settings. For patients with a history of therapeutic radiation to the head and neck, sonographic evaluation may establish pathology in the thyroid gland despite a normal clinical examination. Serial sonographic examinations can follow the size of suspected benign nodules on patients receiving suppressive therapy. If the solitary nodule fails to decrease in size in a

specified period, biopsy or surgery may be necessary for further evaluation. Sonography can reliably distinguish between cystic and solid masses and guide FNA of these and other nonpalpable lesions. Sonographically guided percutaneous ethanol injection has been used as an alternative to surgery for the effective treatment of several benign and malignant conditions.[16] The percutaneous ethanol injection was found to be more effective for thyroid cysts than for solid thyroid nodules.[16]

To begin the examination, review the medical history from the referring physicians and obtain pertinent information from the patient. Information about symptoms, duration, current treatment, history of therapeutic radiation, and locations of any palpable masses are necessary when interpreting the final images. If the patient has had a radioisotope scan, attempt to access and review the images and the report. Included in a complete tailored sonographic examination is an attempt to answer any questions raised by preceding tests. If the patient is able to feel a mass, have the patient identify its location. If the mass is palpable only to the referring physician, obtain a description of the area of interest.

No patient preparation is required for thyroid gland sonography, although some facilities recommend limiting food and drink 1 hour prior to the examination to reduce gastric reflux in patients subject to this problem. With the patient in a supine position, elevate the shoulders and upper back with a pillow or rolled towel, hyperextending the neck.[17] This will permit easier access to the thyroid gland. Be cautious with elderly patients and other patients in whom this position may cause dizziness or neck strain. Do not overextend the neck in any patient, as a comfortable, cooperative patient is important. If this position is not tolerable, request the patient elevate the chin up and back as far as possible and make whatever scanning adjustments are necessary. Turning the patient's head away from the side being examined will also gain surface area for scanning.

Select the highest frequency transducer available, remaining aware that the thyroid gland is a superficial structure and that near-field resolution will be important. Most current sonography equipment offer 7.5- to 15-MHz short-focus linear transducers specifically designed for small parts scanning. Adjust the movable focal zone to the area of interest in the gland. In patients with thick necks, or occasionally in those who have had radiation therapy, a 5-MHz transducer may be needed for penetration. Resolution is diminished at this lower frequency that compromises structural clarity.

Scanning protocol includes multiple transverse, longitudinal, and oblique views. Begin superiorly at the level of the mandible. In the transverse plane, move inferiorly until the characteristic pattern of the thyroid gland is identified. The homogeneously echogenic pattern results from the numerous follicles and surrounding

| TABLE 15-1 | |
|---|---|
| **Thyroid Laboratory Values** | |
| Free thyroxine (T₄ free) | 0.8–2.4 ng/dL |
| Total thyroxine (T₄ total) | 4–11 ng/mL |
| Thyroxine-binding globulin (TBG) | 12–30 mg/L |
| Total triiodothyronine (T₃ total) | 75–220 ng/dL |
| Thyroid-stimulating hormone (TSH) | 0.3–3.04 U/mL |

supportive tissue that constitutes the thyroid gland. Sonographically, it is similar in appearance to normal parenchyma in the liver and testes and it is hyperechoic in appearance relative to adjacent musculature.[7] Stay alert for extra thyroid masses, such as enlarged lymph nodes or parathyroid glands. Proceed slowly through the gland and beyond and pay particular attention to subtle textural or structural changes. Repeat the procedure for the opposite lobe. Most equipment will allow split-screen imaging, which displays two images side by side. This feature provides a method for presenting both thyroid lobes and the connecting isthmus simultaneously. This format may be used if the thyroid gland is small enough to be contained within the display. Panoramic imaging is useful when scanning enlarged glands and in some cases may be the only way to demonstrate the thyroid gland in its entirety. Record as many images as necessary to document normal or abnormal structures. At least acquire representative images from the upper, middle, and lower portions of both lobes, including the isthmus. Measure each lobe in both the anteroposterior and transverse planes, and the isthmus in the anteroposterior plane. Imaging of the lower poles can be enhanced by asking the patient to swallow, which momentarily raises the thyroid gland in the neck.[10]

To scan longitudinal, begin lateral to the thyroid gland, imaging the carotid artery or jugular vein. Move the transducer medially, again noting both the architecture of the gland and any extraglandular structures. Measure the gland in its longest projection, using the split screen or panoramic function if necessary. The examination should also be extended laterally to include the region of the carotid artery and jugular vein in order to identify enlarged jugular chain lymph nodes, superiorly to visualize submandibular adenopathy, and inferiorly to define any pathologic supraclavicular nodes.[10] Color Doppler and pulsed wave Doppler imaging contribute to the thyroid gland sonography examination by revealing internal vascular detail. They are perhaps most helpful when examining ambiguous isoechoic or complex masses. The presence or absence of Doppler flow may help to differentiate among solid vascular masses, simple serous cysts with echogenic fluid, necrotic solid masses, and hemorrhagic cysts.

## PATHOLOGY OF THE THYROID GLAND

The thyroid gland is host to benign, malignant, autoimmune, and metastatic conditions, all of which have varied and often overlapping sonographic appearances. Sonography is most useful in differentiating solid from cystic lesions and in patients in whom there is uncertainty about the origin of a neck mass. The sonography examination for thyroid gland disease should serve to amplify and clarify the clinical, laboratory, nuclear medicine, and cytopathology data obtained for a patient.

## Cysts

Thyroid cysts are common in humans but the term is often used loosely to define thyroid disease.[18] The true epithelium-lined cysts in the region of the thyroid gland are uncommon and are almost always benign.[13] Two true cysts are the thyroglossal duct cyst and the branchial cleft cyst, which can be differentiated from each other by their location. Thyroglossal duct cysts tend to be midline and branchial cleft cysts tend to be lateral to the carotids. More information regarding these two cysts are presented in this chapter with developmental cysts.

Benign nodular thyroid disease is common among adults and the prevalence increases with age.[19] Sonographic evaluation indicates that 15% to 25% of these solitary thyroid nodules are either cystic or predominantly cystic and are sonographically described as either a mixed or a complex lesion.[18,19] The etiology of the cystic portion of the thyroid nodule is usually hemorrhage or is subsequent degeneration of preexisting nodules.[20] FNA cytology provides the diagnosis of benign versus malignant and cystic versus solid lesions.[18] Percutaneous ethanol injection is used to initially treat benign cystic nodules or as follow-up treatment for recurrent thyroid cysts.[19,20] The response rate to the ethanol injection ranges from 72.1% to 93.9%.[18] Malignant cystic nodules are surgically removed.[18]

Sonographically, a simple cyst will be circular or oval, with discrete margins, contain no internal echoes, and exhibit posterior enhancement (Fig. 15-6A). Comet tail artifacts can frequently be encountered in complex cystic thyroid nodules and they are likely related to the presence of colloid substances in the cyst[21] (Fig. 15-6B). A hemorrhagic cyst may contain blood and debris and may appear as a complex mass with irregular borders and internal septa. When more densely echogenic fluid is gravitationally layered in the posterior portion of a cystic cavity, the likelihood of hemorrhagic debris is very high (Fig. 15-6C). Sonographically, papillary carcinomas may present with varying amounts of cystic change, may appear almost indistinguishable from benign cystic nodules, or may appear as uneven cystic structures, with finger-like pedunculated mass(es) of more than 2 cm seen projecting into the lumen[18] (Fig. 15-6D). FNA is important to distinguish these from one another and to obtain a diagnosis.

## Thyroid Nodule

In the United States, thyroid nodules occur between 4% and 7% of adults.[18] They are more common in women and increase in frequency with age and with decreasing iodine intake.[22] Based on the technetium-99m (Tc-99m) radioiodine scintigraphy examination, they are classified either as "hot" (hyperfunctioning/autonomous) or as "cold" (nonfunctioning).[23] A cold nodule is one that does not absorb the radiopharmaceutical used for evaluating the gland and therefore appears as an area of decreased or absent activity on the resulting nuclear image.

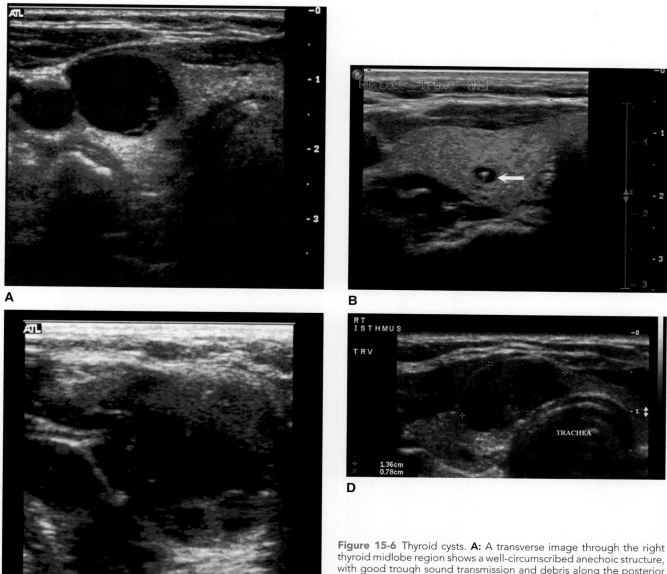

**Figure 15-6** Thyroid cysts. **A:** A transverse image through the right thyroid midlobe region shows a well-circumscribed anechoic structure, with good trough sound transmission and debris along the posterior wall representing colloid elements within the cyst. **B:** A transverse image through the right thyroid lobe shows a small central colloid cyst *(arrow)* with a "comet tail" artifact beneath the small echogenic structure within the colloid cyst. **C:** This transverse image through the right thyroid lobe shows a complex thyroid mass, which on biopsy was identified as a degenerating cyst. **D:** On this transverse image of the right thyroid/isthmus region, the sonographic appearance is similar to Figure 15-6C; however, the cytology report from a sonography-guided biopsy on this 32-year-old woman revealed papillary carcinoma.

In contrast, a hot nodule traps an excessive amount of isotope and presents as a dense collection of activity.

Patients with a thyroid nodule palpated on physical examination, which subsequently appear as cold nodules on a nuclear medicine study, are often referred to sonography for further evaluation. Approximately 80% to 85% of thyroid nodules are cold and 10% to 15% of these are malignant.[24] About 5% to 10% of solitary thyroid nodules are hot nodules, which usually implies benignity.[23] Currently, no single sonographic criterion distinguishes benign thyroid nodules from malignant thyroid nodules

with complete reliability.[10] It is possible to make an accurate prediction of malignancy and recommend FNA when suspicious sonographic signs are seen in combination with multiple signs of thyroid malignancy.

## Adenomas

A thyroid adenoma is a benign, neoplastic growth of thyroid glandular epithelium usually contained within a fibrous capsule.[6] Most adenomas are solitary but they may also develop as part of a multinodular process.[10] Although the terms *adenoma* and *nodule* are used interchangeably, an adenoma is a specific new tissue growth (neoplastic) and a nodule may include a carcinoma, a normal gland lobule, or any other focal lesion. Benign adenomas account for 5% to 10% of thyroid nodules and are seven times more common in females than in males.[10] Most adenomas are derived from follicular epithelium and a small minority of these are toxic and cause hyperthyroidism owing to autonomous function.[13] Based on the degree of follicle formation and the colloid content of the follicles, the rare adenomas make up these histologic subtype classifications: macrofollicular (simple colloid), microfollicular (fetal), embryonal (trabecular), Hürthle cell (oxyphil, oncocytic)

adenomas, and atypical adenomas, and adenomas with papillae.[8] Adenomas grow slowly, remain dormant for years, and are more common in the fifth and sixth decade of life.[6] In order to be palpated on physical examination, an adenoma must reach a size of 0.5 to 1 cm. This explains why sonography has detected small nodules on a thyroid gland that was not detected on palpation. When a hyperfunctioning adenoma suppresses normal thyroid gland tissue, the normal tissue atrophies and the adenoma appears as a hot nodule against a background of minimal uptake on a radionuclide examination.[6] A toxic hyperfunctioning adenoma may provoke thyrotoxicosis. The distinction between

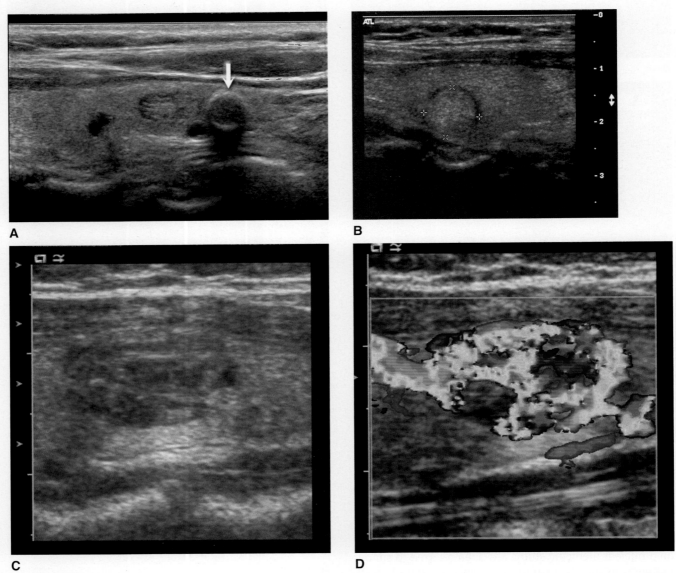

**Figure 15-7** Sonographic appearance of adenoma. **A:** An image from a 71-year-old female of the left thyroid lobe demonstrates three different presentations of adenomatous nodules. The *open solid arrow* points to a calcified nodule. Note the highly echogenic anterior-curved wall and dense shadowing. **B:** This longitudinal image through the left thyroid lobe in a 41-year-old woman demonstrates a hypoechoic halo surrounding the nodule. Fine-needle aspiration of the area marked by cursors returned a diagnosis of a benign hyperplastic nodule consistent with a nodular goiter. **C,D:** On these two images on a 41-year-old woman patient, the fine-needle aspiration results described an adenoma. A longitudinal image **(C)** of the left thyroid gland shows a solitary nodule. On the color Doppler image **(D)**, the circle of color is at the periphery of the nodule and the linear color signals are coursing toward the center. *(continued)*

toxic and nontoxic adenomas cannot be made with sonography. Adenomas are typically asymptomatic but can grow large enough to exert pressure or develop hemorrhage and, thus, they become problematic.

The sonographic features of adenomas are influenced by the amount of structural degeneration and vary widely, ranging from cystic to solid through complex. One other sonographic feature often associated with an adenoma is calcification along the rim (Fig. 15-7A). The most common appearance is that of a solitary, well-circumscribed, oval or circular mass of variable size and echogenicity. Small, solid adenomas with uniformly low echogenicity can be mistaken for cysts. The distinction is made by noting the absence of through sound transmission behind a solid lesion. A peripheral hypoechoic to anechoic halo that completely or incompletely surrounds an adenoma is a relatively consistent finding. The halo, however, cannot be used as the only criteria and additional statistical information is necessary to establish the halo's specificity.[9] A halo in the nodule periphery may be seen with benign or malignant conditions

and suggests that there is an acoustic interface that does not reflect the ultrasound across two different types of histology in the region of the benign or malignant nodule and the surrounding thyroid gland.[25] In the case of an adenoma, this halo is thought to represent the fibrous capsule and the perinodal blood vessels, which can be seen by color Doppler imaging, and mild edema or compressed normal thyroid parenchyma (Fig. 15-7B). Color Doppler performed on an adenoma may have a "spoke and wheel" appearance with peripheral blood vessels extending toward the center of the lesion[10] (Fig. 15-7C,D). Adenomas >2.5 to 3 cm commonly display the sonographic characteristics of a complex cyst. These adenomatous cysts tend to have irregular shapes and borders with thickened walls, an incomplete capsule and are less sharply demarcated from surrounding tissue. Although imaging research is providing increased statistical probabilities to distinguish benign and malignant nodules, imaging procedures cannot be used as the only dependable criteria to specify adenomas from other benign or malignant nodules[21] (Fig. 15-7E–H).

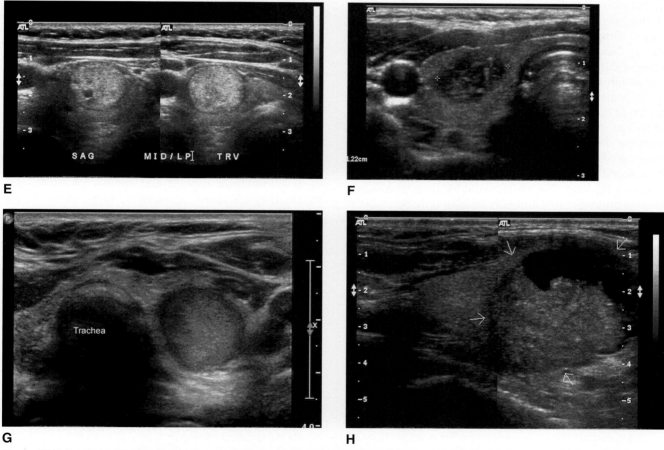

**Figure 15-7** *(continued)* **E–H:** These four images represent biopsy proven benign adenomatous cysts or degenerating adenomas. Although there are some recurrent sonographic appearances associated with benignity, imaging alone cannot definitively predict benign versus malignant biopsy outcomes. **E:** A longitudinal and transverse image through the right thyroid lobe shows a hypoechoic, round to oval mass surrounded by a thin halo. **F:** A transverse scan made through the right thyroid lobe shows a complex mass measuring 1.22 cm *(cursors)*. **G:** A transverse image through the left thyroid lobe shows an oval mass. **H:** A longitudinal image through the left thyroid lobe shows a degenerating adenoma seen as an oval mass with internal cystic components *(arrows)*.

## Goiters

A nontoxic goiter is also termed simple, colloid, or multinodular and refers to an enlargement involving the entire gland without producing nodularity and without evidence of a functional disturbance.[6] The enlarged follicles are filled with colloid.[8] Nontoxic goiter occurs in both an endemic distribution with more than 10% of the population affected and a sporadic distribution.[8] Endemic goiter occurs in geographic areas where the soil, water, and food supply contain low levels of iodine. The decrease or lack of iodine leads to decreased synthesis of thyroid hormone and a compensatory increase in TSH. Increased TSH levels leads to follicular cell hypertrophy, hyperplasia, and goitrous enlargement.[8] *Sporadic goiter* is defined as a benign enlargement of the thyroid gland in euthyroid subjects living in an iodine-sufficient area. The sporadic goiter can be diffuse, uninodular, or multinodular.[26] The cause of sporadic goiter is usually not apparent and may be related to ingestion of substances that interfere with thyroid hormone synthesis or result from hereditary enzymatic defects that interfere with thyroid hormone synthesis.[8] The peak age of subjects with sporadic goiter is between 35 and 60 years and women are three times more likely than men to have the disease.[10]

Due to recurrent episodes of hyperplasia and involution, simple goiters may convert into multinodular goiters. Nodularity of the thyroid gland can be the end stage of diffuse nontoxic goiter. As new follicles develop and outgrow their blood supply, hemorrhagic necrosis of all or part of the nodule results. Scarring then produces an inelastic network into which new follicles are squeezed, resulting in the formation of nodules.[14] Calcifications, fibrosis, degenerative cysts, and hemorrhage result in the heterogeneous sonographic appearance. Multinodular goiters are multilobulated, asymmetrically enlarged gland. The pattern and location of enlargement is unpredictable and may involve only one lobe or may expand growing behind the sternum and clavicles to produce the intrathoracic or plunging goiters.[8] Multinodular goiters may be nontoxic or may induce thyrotoxicosis (toxic multinodular goiters). As is the case of the simple goiter, the incidence of multinodular goiter is greater in females than in males.

The size of nontoxic goiters ranges from a doubling in size (40 g) to a massive enlargement in which the thyroid weighs a few hundred grams.[6] The size of multilobulated goiters may achieve a weight of more than 2,000 g.[8] Symptoms caused by large goiters are usually associated with compressing the esophagus (dysphasia), trachea (inspiratory stridor), neck veins (venous congestion), or laryngeal nerve (hoarseness).[6]

The sonographic appearance may be nonspecific and varies with pathogenesis of the goiter. The sonographic appearance of a dominant nodule, a tender spot, or a region of focal hardness may provide pathologic clues[25] (Fig. 15-8A,B). A second type of pathology may be suggested if one region in a goiter presents an echo pattern distinct from the rest of the goiter, especially if the region is surrounded by an incomplete and irregular anechoic rim, has punctate microcalcifications, or Doppler examination reveals internal vascularity. Sonographic features associated with increased risk for malignancy include hypoechogenicity, the presence of microcalcifications, increased vascular flow, or irregular borders[27] (Fig. 15-8C–F). Neoplasm and lymphomas have been demonstrated in goiters.[25] Table 15-2 lists additional usefulness of the sonographic examinations in goitrous patients.

## Thyrotoxicosis/Hyperthyroidism

Thyrotoxicosis is a hypermetabolic state caused by elevated levels of free $T_3$ and $T_4$.[28] The terms thyrotoxicosis and hyperthyroidism are often used interchangeably because the condition is caused most commonly by hyperfunction of the thyroid gland.[8] Hyperthyroidism is correct to use if elevated levels arise from hyperfunction, as occurs in Graves disease; thyrotoxicosis is correct to use if the increased hormone levels reflect excessive leakage of hormone out of a nonhyperactive gland.[8] Primary hyperthyroidism is a form of thyrotoxicosis in which excess thyroid hormone is synthesized and secreted by the thyroid glands.[8] Secondary hyperthyroidism is rare and is caused by TSH-secreting pituitary adenomas[28] (Pathology Box 15-1).

Pathogenesis of either thyrotoxicosis or hyperthyroidism produces common clinical manifestations (Pathology Box 15-2). Children with Graves disease often have accelerated growth spurts and advanced bone age, symptoms of emotional lability, hyperactivity, difficulty concentrating, and occasionally failure to thrive.

The underlying cause of hyperthyroidism in 50% to 80% of cases is Graves disease.[28] Graves disease is an autoimmune disease and about 75% of autoimmune diseases occur in women, most often during the childbearing years.[29] Graves disease can occur at

| TABLE | 15-2 |
| --- | --- |

### Value of Sonographic Examination for Goitrous Patients[25]

- Differentiate thyroid gland enlargement from adipose tissue or muscle
- Identify large unilateral mass in distinction to an asymmetric goiter
- Confirm pattern and location of enlargement and extensions (substernal, intrathoracic, plunging)
- Provide the correct interpretation to correlate varying clinical impressions among several examiners
- Objectively document volume changes in response to suppressive therapy with thyroid hormone
- Monitor patients undergoing long-term treatment with lithium for mental illnesses (bipolar, depression, schizophrenia)

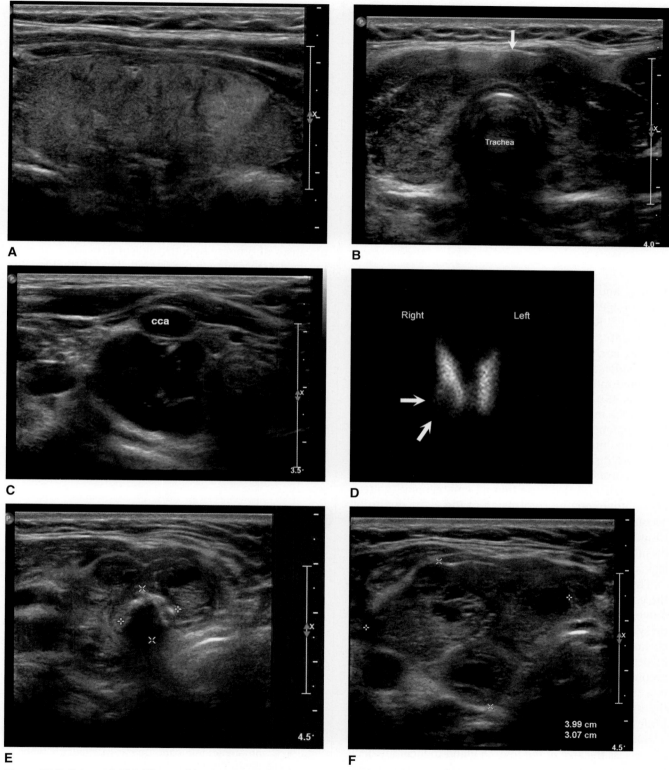

**Figure 15-8** Goiters. **A:** This 79-year-old woman was referred to sonography following a computed tomography diagnosis of a multinodular goiter. The longitudinal image of the right thyroid lobe demonstrates diffuse enlargement and general heterogeneity. **B:** The transverse sonogram on this patient shows a diffusely enlarged, heterogeneous thyroid. There is an increased anteroposterior (AP) diameter of the isthmus when compared to the normal mean diameter measurement of 4–6 mm *(arrow)*. An isthmus measuring >1 cm is a reliable marker for diffuse thyroid enlargement. This patient was diagnosed with a multinodular goiter. **C,D:** A transverse sonogram **(C)** of the right lower thyroid pole in a 30-year-old woman shows a complex mass, which appears as a cold nodule on nuclear imaging. On the scintigram **(D)**, one can see an irregular margin and diminished activity in the lower right pole *(arrow)*. A biopsy cytology report identified a necrosing colloid nodule with associated cyst. **E,F:** These transverse images of the right thyroid lobe obtained on the same patient show diffuse heterogeneity mass with both internal cystic components and calcification. While the presence of calcifications create concern for a malignant process, this mass proved to be a benign adenomatoid multinodular goiter on biopsy.

### Causes of Primary and Secondary Hyperthyroidism[8,28]

**Causes of Primary Hyperthyroidism**

- Graves disease
- Toxic multinodular goiter
- Solitary hyperfunctioning nodules
- Follicular thyroid carcinoma (rare)
- Thyroiditis
- Ingestion of exogenous thyroid hormone administered for hypothyroidism

**Causes of Secondary Hyperthyroidism**

- Secretion of excessive amounts of thyroid hormone by ectopic thyroid arising in ovarian teratomas (struma ovarii)

any age and the peak incidence is between 40 and 60 years of age.[30] The female-to-male ratio is between 5:1 and 10:1.[30] Research indicates a multifactorial etiology where different factors come together to cause Graves disease, such as heredity, the body's immune system, age, gender, and possibly stress.[29] In one study, the concordance rate for Graves disease among monozygotic twins is 35% and the researchers concluded the study supports a major etiologic role for genetic factors in the development of Graves disease but also reported that environmental factors are important.[31]

Graves disease is characterized as a multisystem syndrome consisting of one or more of the following: (1) hyperthyroidism, (2) diffuse thyroid enlargement (goiter), (3) ophthalmopathy (protrusion of the globe due to fat accumulation and inflammation with edema), and (4) Graves dermopathy (pretibial myxedema characterized by subcutaneous swelling on the anterior portions of the legs and by indurated and erythematous skin).[28]

Thyrotoxicosis has a variety of causes. Determining the cause is important because treatment and expected outcomes will vary accordingly. The diagnosis is based on symptoms of thyroid hormone excess and evaluating elevated serum free $T_4$ and $T_3$ variances. TSH is increased in primary hyperthyroidism and TSH is decreased in secondary hyperthyroidism. Radioactive iodine uptake is a good diagnostic tool to determine the etiology of thyrotoxicosis. Treatment will normally focus on controlling excessive thyroid hormone production.[28]

Sonography for thyrotoxicosis and hyperthyroidism can assess the size of the thyroid gland to facilitate decisions regarding treatment.[25] Graves disease can present with either a normal-sized or an enlarged gland. When the gland is enlarged, the echo texture will usually be more heterogeneous compared to a diffuse goiter, which has numerous large intraparenchymal vessels.[10] Normal-sized glands will have a more uniform pattern. Hypervascularity is observed in most patients with Graves disease and has been quantified by the number of

vessels per square centimeter measured on the greatest longitudinal view.[32] The term "thyroid inferno" demonstrating multiple tiny areas of flow in the glandular tissue is often used to describe the hypervascular pattern seen on color Doppler (Fig. 15-9A–E). A bruit or thrill can often be heard over the gland. Spectral Doppler may demonstrate peak velocities exceeding 70 cm/sec.[10]

### Hypothyroidism

Hypothyroidism is the most common occurring thyroid function disorder and affects between 0.1% and 2% of individuals in the United States.[28] It is a clinical syndrome caused by a deficient production of thyroid hormone that results in reduced thyroid hormone action in the peripheral tissues. Hypothyroidism may be primary or secondary. There is a greater incidence and increased number of causes of primary hypothyroidism that arises from an intrinsic abnormality in the thyroid gland (Pathology Box 15-3). Secondary (central) hypothyroidism occurs less frequently than primary hypothyroidism and includes those conditions that cause either pituitary or hypothalamic disease or damage resulting in failure to stimulate normal thyroid function.[28] The conditions contributing to secondary hypothyroidism include pituitary adenoma; tumors impinging on the hypothalamus; irradiation; medication (dopamine, lithium); congenital disorders; and, rarely, Sheehan syndrome.

The most common cause of primary hypothyroidism in areas of the world where iodine levels are sufficient is chronic autoimmune thyroiditis. The literature also

### Clinical Manifestations of Hyperthyroidism[6,8,28]

Cardiovascular system: Increased cardiac output and decreased peripheral resistance; tachycardia at rest; loud heart sounds

Endocrine system: Enlarged thyroid gland (goiter); hypercalcemia and decreased parathyroid hormone secretions

Gastrointestinal system: Weight loss; increased peristalsis leading to diarrhea, nausea, vomiting, anorexia, abdominal pain

Integumentary system: Excessive sweating, flushing, and warm skin; heat intolerance; temporary hair loss; palmar erythema

Musculoskeletal system: Muscular weakness; children experience accelerated growth spurts and advanced bone age

Nervous system: Nervousness; restlessness; short attention span; fatigue; fine hand tremor (particularly when outstretched); insomnia; increased appetite; emotional instability

Pulmonary system: Dyspnea; reduced vital capacity

Reproductive system: Oligomenorrhea or amenorrhea; erectile dysfunction and decreased libido

Sensory system (eyes): Elevated upper eyelid (decreased blinking and staring feature); fine tremor of lid; variable eye changes

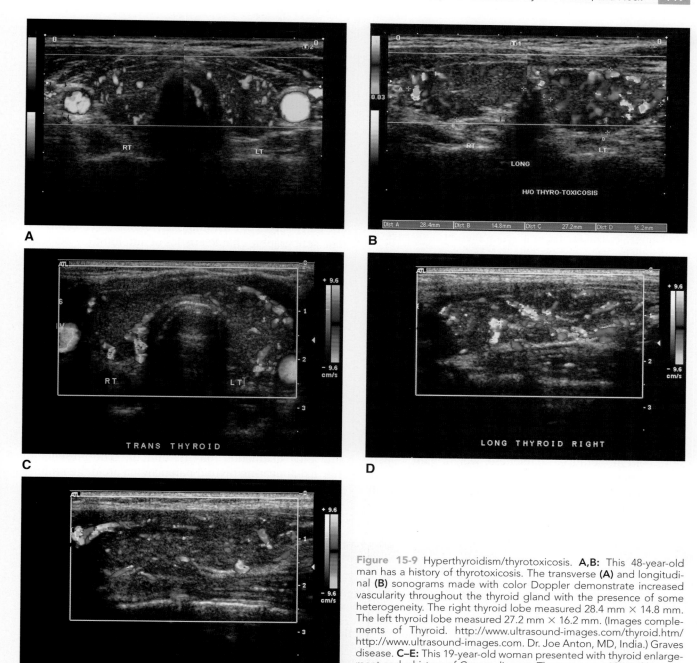

**Figure 15-9** Hyperthyroidism/thyrotoxicosis. **A,B:** This 48-year-old man has a history of thyrotoxicosis. The transverse **(A)** and longitudinal **(B)** sonograms made with color Doppler demonstrate increased vascularity throughout the thyroid gland with the presence of some heterogeneity. The right thyroid lobe measured 28.4 mm × 14.8 mm. The left thyroid lobe measured 27.2 mm × 16.2 mm. (Images complements of Thyroid. http://www.ultrasound-images.com/thyroid.htm/ http://www.ultrasound-images.com. Dr. Joe Anton, MD, India.) Graves disease. **C–E:** This 19-year-old woman presented with thyroid enlargement and a history of Graves disease. The transverse **(C)** and longitudinal of the right lobe **(D)** and left lobe **(E)** made with color Doppler shows markedly increased vascularity and a more heterogenic thyroid gland. (Images courtesy of LaNae Holman, Alamosa, Colorado.)

refers to the disease as chronic lymphocytic thyroiditis, Hashimoto disease, and most commonly as in this chapter as Hashimoto thyroiditis. The name of the disease is derived from a 1912 report where Hashimoto described patients with goiters and intense lymphocytic infiltration of the thyroid gland.[8] It is estimated three-fourths of hypothyroidism cases are due to Hashimoto thyroiditis.[6] The disease occurs in genetically predisposed individuals and is associated with high-iodine intake, selenium deficiency, smoking, and chronic hepatitis C.[28] This disorder is most prevalent between 45 and 65 years of age, has a female predominance of 10:1 to 20:1, and clusters in families with a concordance rate in monozygotic twins between 30% and 60%.[8] Patients with Hashimoto thyroiditis may also present with other autoimmune disorders such as Sjögren syndrome, lupus, rheumatoid arthritis, fibrosing mediastinitis, sclerosing cholangitis, and pernicious anemia and are at an increased risk for the development of B-cell lymphoma (non-Hodgkin).[13] The autoimmune disease can also occur in children to a much lesser extent and is a major cause of nonendemic goiter in children.

### Causes of Primary Hypothyroidism[8,28]

Defective hormone synthesis
  Autoimmune disease (Hashimoto thyroiditis most common); postpartum thyroiditis
Endemic iodine deficiency
Iodine excess
  Iodinated contrast agents used in imaging; amiodarone medication; health tonics
Iatrogenic loss of thyroid tissue
  Radioactive iodine treatment of Graves disease; external neck irradiation (head/neck neoplasm, breast cancer, Hodgkin disease); thyroidectomy
Inflammatory conditions, viral syndromes, or infiltrative disorders
  Neoplasia; leukemia; sarcoidosis; hemochromatosis; amyloidosis; mycobacterium tuberculosis infection; *Pneumocystis carinii* infection; cystinosis
Congenital defect
  Rare inborn errors of thyroid hormone synthesis

The clinical manifestations of hypothyroidism vary, depending on its cause, duration, and severity. The spectrum extends from subclinical hypothyroidism to overt hypothyroidism to myxedema coma.[28] Common signs and symptoms include weakness and fatigue, dry skin, cold intolerance, hoarseness, weight gain, constipation, menstrual irregularities, and decreased sweating (Pathology Box 15-4). The diagnosis is usually made serologically.

The sonographic appearance of Hashimoto thyroiditis changes with the duration of the disease. Over time, the normal homogeneous echo texture is replaced by a coarse and a more heterogeneous texture with multiple ill-defined hypoechoic areas separated by thickened fibrous strands.[13] The thyroid gland is usually diffusely abnormal and no normal parenchyma can be identified (Fig. 15-10A–C). The best imaging clue is a moderately enlarged, lobular thyroid gland without calcifications or necrosis. An indication of diffuse enlargement of the thyroid gland is often best noted by determining if the isthmus measures greater than 1 cm anteroposteriorly. Often, color Doppler demonstrates hypervascularity in the early stages of Hashimoto thyroiditis (Fig. 15-10D,E). The sonographic characteristics of autoimmune diseases seen in Graves disease are also seen in Hashimoto thyroiditis and includes enlargement of the thyroid gland with reduced echogenicity, heterogeneity, and hypervascularity. These sonographic features are more enhanced in Graves disease; however, the sonographic appearance without clinical history, serology reports, and, in some cases, FNA are nonspecific as the same sonographic appearance are also demonstrated in diffusely infiltrative papillary or follicular thyroid cancer.[33] Hashimoto thyroiditis can also cause nodules and other benign and malignant nodules can coexist with Hashimoto thyroiditis.[13] Multinodular goiter and Hashimoto thyroiditis goiter can also have a similar sonographic appearances and their distinction may be difficult. The presence of normal-appearing thyroid parenchyma amid the nodules favors a multinodular goiter, but information regarding the presence of the antithyroglobulin antibodies found

### Clinical Manifestations of Hypothyroidism[6,8,28]

Cardiovascular system: Reduction in stroke volume and heart rate results in lowered cardiac output; increased peripheral vascular resistance to maintain systolic blood pressure; cool skin and cold tolerance; enlarged heart; decreased intensity of heart sounds; EKG changes
Endocrine system: Increased TSH production in primary hypothyroidism; enlarged pituitary thyrotopes, increased serum prolactin levels with galactorrhea; decreased rate of cortisol turnover but with normal cortisol levels
Gastrointestinal system: Constipation, weight gain, and fluid retention; decreased absorption of most nutrients; decreased protein metabolism; edema; decreased glucose absorption and delayed glucose uptake; elevated serum lipid values
Integumentary system: Dry, flaky skin; dry, brittle head and body hair; reduced nail and hair growth; slow wound healing; myxedema; cold skin
Hematologic system: Decrease in red cell mass leading to normocytic, normochromic anemia; macrocytic anemia associated with vitamin B12 deficiency and inadequate foliate or iron absorption in the gastrointestinal tract
Musculoskeletal system: Muscle aching and stiffness; slow movement and slow tendon jerk reflexes; decreased bone formation and resorption, increased bone density; aching and stiffness in joints
Nervous system: Confusion, syncope, slowed speech and thinking, memory loss; lethargy, headaches, hearing loss, night blindness; slow clumsy movements
Pulmonary system: Dyspnea; myxedematous changes in respiratory muscles leading to hypoventilation and carbon dioxide retention contributes to myxedema coma
Reproductive system: In men, decreased androgen secretion; erectile dysfunction, decreased libido, and oligospermia. In women, increased estriol formation; low total hormone values but with increased amounts of unbound hormone; anovulation, decreased libido, and a high incidence of a spontaneous abortion
Urinary system: Reduced renal blood flow and glomerular filtration rate; increased total body water and dilutional hyponatremia; reduced production of erythropoietin

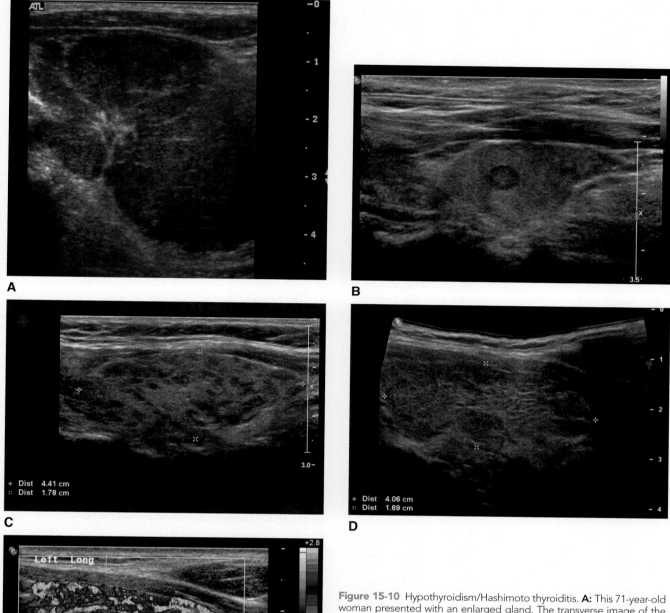

**Figure 15-10** Hypothyroidism/Hashimoto thyroiditis. **A:** This 71-year-old woman presented with an enlarged gland. The transverse image of the left thyroid lobe shows large areas separated with some separation by thickened fibrous strands and no normal parenchyma is identified. The biopsy results describe findings consistent with Hashimoto thyroiditis. **B:** This 53-year-old woman presented with known Hashimoto thyroiditis. A patient presenting with single or multiple nodules makes the distinction between Hashimoto thyroiditis and multinodular goiter difficult to conclude from only the imaging characteristics. This representative longitudinal image of the right thyroid lobe shows an echogenic oval mass. The fine-needle aspiration results were in agreement with the patient's presenting diagnosis. **C:** This 45-year-old woman presented with a palpable thyroid nodule. The longitudinal image of the right thyroid lobe shows multiple small nodules, which give the appearance of a multinodular goiter. The fine-needle aspiration results diagnosed Hashimoto thyroiditis. **D,E:** The images of a left thyroid lobe were made without **(C)** and with **(D)** color Doppler. On this patient with Hashimoto thyroiditis, the image demonstrates the hypervascularity seen in the early stages of the disease.

in Hashimoto thyroiditis is necessary for a definitive diagnosis. In patients who do progress to end-stage Hashimoto thyroiditis, the thyroid gland becomes fibrotic, ill-defined, heterogeneous, and begins to atrophy.[13]

## Thyroiditis

Thyroiditis encompasses a diverse group of disorders characterized by some form of thyroid gland inflammation. Generally, the clinical manifestations and symptoms for this group of disorders vary but most present with hypothyroidism or thyrotoxicosis followed by hypothyroidism (Pathology Box 15-5).

Subacute thyroiditis (de Quervain disease or granulomatous thyroiditis), along with Graves disease and Hashimoto thyroiditis, is one of the more common parenchymal diseases of the thyroid gland.[13] The disorder is most common between the ages of 30 and 50 and the female-to-male ratio is between 3:1 and 5:1.[8] Although it is a nonbacterial inflammation of the thyroid gland, it is often preceded by a viral infection because the majority of patients have a history of an upper respiratory infection just before the onset of subacute thyroiditis.[8,28] There have been reported clusters in association with coxsackievirus, mumps, measles, adenovirus, and other viral illnesses and cases cluster seasonally peaking in the summer.[8]

The gland may be unilaterally or bilaterally enlarged and firm with an intact capsule and it may be slightly adherent to surrounding structures.[8] The sudden or gradual onset of subacute thyroiditis is characterized by neck pain, which may radiate to the upper jaw, throat, or ears and which may be intensified when swallowing. The disease comes to clinical attention when the patient presents with fever, tenderness, fatigue, malaise, anorexia, and myalgia coexisting with inflammation of the thyroid gland.[8] The thyroid gland inflammation and hyperthyroidism are usually transient and resolves in 2 to 6 weeks. Spontaneous recovery of thyroid function usually occurs within 6 to 8 weeks.[8] Aside from some fibrosis, recovery is almost always complete.

The sonographic appearance of either acute or subacute thyroiditis is most often that of a diffusely enlarged, hypoechoic thyroid gland with normal or decreased vascularity due to the presence of diffuse edema compressing the vessels.[13] The presence of hypoechoic and hyperechoic nodules is not uncommon that significantly reduces specificity of the sonographic image (Fig. 15-11).

## Thyroid Disease in Pregnancy

Thyroid diseases are the second most common endocrinopathy that affects women of reproductive age and are well-described complications in reproductive dysfunction, pregnancy, and the puerperium (the 42 days

---

### PATHOLOGY BOX 15-5

#### Types of Thyroiditis[6,8,28]

Acute thyroiditis (suppurative thyroiditis; infectious thyroiditis)
  Rare inflammatory disease usually affecting children
  Cause mainly by bacteria but may be caused by any infectious organism
  Resolves after treating cause
Hashimoto thyroiditis
  Autoimmune with antithyroid antibodies
  Hypothyroidism is permanent
Iatrogenic hypothyroidism
  Caused by radioiodine thyroid ablation (radiation induced), prescription drugs such as amiodarone, lithium, interferons, cytokines (drug-induced) or thyroidectomy
  Depending on cause, hypothyroidism may transient to permanent
Postpartum thyroiditis
  Autoimmune with antithyroid antibodies
  Occurs in up to 7% of all women
  Spontaneous recovery in most women
  Persistent hypothyroidism does occur
Subacute thyroiditis (de Quervain thyroiditis, granulomatous thyroiditis)
  Possibly viral cause
  Inflammation resolves usually in 2 to 8 weeks followed by spontaneous recovery of thyroid function usually in 6 to 8 weeks
Subacute thyroiditis (lymphocytic thyroiditis, painless thyroiditis, or silent thyroiditis)
  Possibly inherited susceptibility
  Incidence from 1% to 10% of all thyroiditis cases
  Course similar to subacute thyroiditis but pathologically identical to Hashimoto thyroiditis
  Thyrotoxicosis followed by hypothyroidism

---

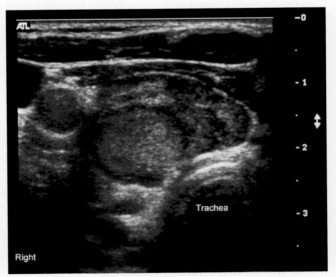

**Figure 15-11** Acute thyroiditis. The 29-year-old woman presented with a short history of sore throat, difficulty swallowing, and tender thyroid. The laboratory data included markedly elevated thyroid-stimulating hormone and decreased free T$_4$. The transverse image of the right thyroid lobe shows a diffusely enlarged, complex echo pattern with an oval nodule. The diagnosis of acute thyroiditis was based on the patient's symptoms, clinical data, physical examination, and complex echo pattern seen on the sonographic images.

following childbirth).[34] The array of thyroid diseases in pregnancy is similar to those in the nongravid population. During pregnancy, a number of physiologic adaptations and hormonal changes alter maternal, fetal, and neonatal thyroid function. Maternal physiologic changes early in pregnancy include an increase in thyroid-binding globulin (TBG), and as human chorionic gonadotropin (hCG) increase and levels peak, there is a partial inhibition of the pituitary gland that yields a transient decrease in TSH between weeks 8 and 14 of gestation.[34] Another physiologic adaptation affecting maternal thyroid function is a reduction in plasma iodine due to fetal iodine usage and increased maternal renal clearance of iodine. The decreased plasma iodide level is associated with a noticeable increase in thyroid size in approximately 15% of women.[34] Early Egyptian and Roman cultures viewed an enlarging thyroid gland in a young woman as a positive sign of pregnancy. The increased size is not correlated with abnormal thyroid function tests. Sonographic measurement of thyroid gland in more than 600 women who did not have thyroid disease confirmed a mean increase in size of 18% with the gland returning to normal size during the postpartum period.[34]

The most common maternal postdelivery thyroid dysfunction that also occurs after an abortion or miscarriage is postpartum thyroiditis (PPT). The prevalence is variable with increased risk reported in women with type 1 diabetes ranging from 3% to 25% incidence and women who previously developed PPT had a 69% recurrence rate with subsequent pregnancy.[35] The classic description includes thyrotoxicosis followed by hypothyroidism and treatment will depend on the phase of thyroiditis and degree of symptoms.

Sonographically, these cases will exhibit the nonspecific decrease in echogenicity and diffuse enlargement of the thyroid gland similar to those seen in other thyroid abnormalities. A definitive diagnosis is made with clinical data.

## Thyroid Carcinoma

Thyroid nodules are very common and are found by palpation in 4% to 7% of an asymptomatic population, with sonography in 13% to 67% of cases, and at autopsy in 50% of cases.[24] Most thyroid nodules are benign and approximately 5% to 6.5% are malignant.[36] Of these, papillary carcinoma accounts for the vast majority of thyroid cancers and it is followed in frequency by follicular, medullary, anaplastic, and Hürthle cell cancer[13] (Table 15-3). Clinical criteria suggestive of a malignant neoplastic thyroid nodule include solitary nodules versus multiple nodules, nodules in younger patients versus older patients, and nodules in males versus in females. The incidence of thyroid malignancy increases in patients with a history of radiation treatment to the head or neck. Although these general trends may favor a malignant diagnosis, they are of little significance without the morphologic evaluation of an FNA

**TABLE 15-3**

### Relative Frequencies of Thyroid Malignant Masses[6,8,47,49]

| Type | % of Cases |
|---|---|
| Papillary carcinoma | 75% to 85% |
| Follicular carcinoma | 10% to 20% |
| Medullary carcinoma | 5% |
| Anaplastic carcinoma | <5% |
| Hürthle cell carcinoma | 3% to <10% |
| Lymphoma | <5% |

biopsy and histologic study of surgically resected thyroid parenchyma.[8] There is no simple noninvasive imaging criteria to diagnose a minority of patients who will prove to have malignant thyroid nodules while reassuring the majority of patients who have benign disease.[37] There are certain sonographic characteristics associated with either an increased risk or with a low risk of thyroid cancer (Table 15-4). The sonographer should be able to identify these sonographic characteristics and must realize they are of limited significance when evaluated independently; however, it is possible to make an accurate prediction when multiple signs of thyroid malignancy appear in combination.[24,33,38,39]

Malignant nodules typically appear solid and hypoechoic compared with normal thyroid parenchyma. This finding is not particularly useful in and of itself since the majority of nodules are benign and a hypoechoic appearance is also noted in approximately 55% of benign nodules.[33] Marked hyperechoic nodules are probably benign,[25] whereas marked hypoechogenic nodules are suggestive of malignancy.[33]

The presence of calcifications within a nodule may occur in both benign and malignant disease and can be classified as microcalcifications (<2 mm) or

**TABLE 15-4**

### Sonographic Characteristics[13,25,33,36–45]

| Associated with Increased Thyroid Cancer Risk | Associated with Low Thyroid Cancer Risk |
|---|---|
| • Hypoechogenicity<br>• Entirely solid<br>• Microcalcifications<br>• Intrinsic hypervascularity (central part)<br>• Incomplete or absent halo<br>• Ill-defined margin<br>• Shape: tall > wide<br>• Local invasion and lymphadenopathy<br>• Elasticity indication of increased tissue stiffness compared to normal tissue | • Hyperechoic or isoechoic<br>• Cystic elements<br>• Large, coarse calcifications (except medullary thyroid cancer)<br>• Eggshell calcifications (few exceptions)<br>• Perinodular hypervascularity (peripheral, circumference) or avascular nodule<br>• Inspissated colloid; comet-tail shadowing |

macrocalcification (>2 mm).[39,40] Microcalcifications present sonographically as punctate hyperechoic foci without acoustic shadowing and may present a twinkling pattern. The presence of microcalcifications is one of the most specific features of thyroid malignancy and may represent calcium salts in the psammoma bodies associated with primary tumors and cervical lymph node metastases.[10] Microcalcifications are commonly found in papillary thyroid cancer (PTC) but have been described in follicular and anaplastic thyroid carcinomas as well as in benign conditions such as follicular adenoma and Hashimoto thryoidits.[33] Kim et al[40] classified these three sonographic patterns of macrocalcifications: (1) solitary calcification that are either linear or round hyperechoic structures >2 mm sonographically presenting with or without acoustic shadowing located in the middle of the nodule or along the margin of the nodule encompassing less than 120 degrees the circumference; (2) eggshell calcifications that are curvilinear hyperechoic structures parallel to the margin of the nodule encompassing 120 degrees or more of the circumference; and (3) all other coarse but not otherwise specified calcifications. The presence of solitary macrocalcifications and peripheral or eggshell calcifications of the thyroid nodule have been an indicator of benignity especially in the absence of other suspicious sonographic findings.[41] The suspicious for malignancy clinical index increases in the presence of at least one or more of the other sonographic characteristics associated with an increased thyroid cancer risk, such as marked hypoechogenicity, irregular or microlobulated margins, and taller than wide shape.[40,41] Macrocalcifications are the most common type of calcifications found in medullary thyroid cancer and may coexist with microcalcifications in papillary cancers. In a person 40 years or younger, calcifications in a solitary nodule is suspicious of malignancy because the relative cancer risk is greater than in a person 40 years or older.[25]

Color or power Doppler sonography should be used to evaluate vascular flow within a thyroid nodule. Intrinsic hypervascularity is defined as flow in the central part of the tumor that is greater than in the surrounding thyroid parenchyma and perinodular flow is defined as the presence of vascularity around at least 25% of the circumference or periphery of a nodule. Marked intrinsic hypervascularity with disorganized vascularity mostly in well-encapsulated forms is seen in 69% to 74% of PTC cases.[33] The intrinsic hypervascularity in and of itself is not specific and can also be seen in more than 50% of benign solid thyroid nodule lesions.[42] Perinodular, circumferential, or peripheral flow is more characteristic of benign thyroid lesions but also has been found in 22% of thyroid malignancies.[33,38] A completely avascular nodule is likely benign.[38]

The halo or hypoechoic rim seen in some thyroid nodules is produced by a pseudocapsule of fibrous connective tissue, a compressed thyroid parenchyma, and chronic inflammatory infiltrates.[33] Although a complete uniform halo around a nodule is highly suggestive of benignity, an absent halo is not significantly associated with either the presence or absence of thyroid cancer because it is not identified sonographically in more than half of all benign thyroid nodules.[39] Approximately 10% to 24% of papillary thyroid carcinomas have either a complete or an incomplete halo.[33,38]

The well-defined margin is typical of benign thyroid nodules but there is an overlap with malignant nodules.[13] An ill-defined thyroid nodule margin is one in which more than 50% of the margin is not clearly demarcated. Sonographically, some papillary thyroid carcinomas have a misleadingly well-demarcated margin but are encapsulated at histologic review.[33] The sonographic appearance of minimally invasive follicular carcinoma may have some features in common with that of follicular adenoma. Without sonographically demonstrating invasion beyond the capsule, the appearance of either a well-defined or poorly defined margin without other criteria is an unreliable basis for determining malignancy or benignity.[33,39,40]

Sonographically evaluating the thyroid nodule to determine if it is taller than wide in shape (greater anteroposterior dimension than transverse dimension) may be potentially useful. The taller than wide shape is thought to be due to a centrifugal tendency in tumor growth, which does not necessarily occur at a uniform rate in all dimension.[33] Kim et al.[40] reported a triple criteria for malignant sonographic features that included (1) solid thyroid nodules with the taller than wide shape, (2) marked hypoechogenicity (decreased echogenicity compared with the surrounding strap muscle), and (3) irregular or microlobulated margins.

Highly specific signs of thyroid malignancy include tumor invasion or lymph node metastasis. Direct tumor invasion sonographically can be identified with subtle extension of the tumor beyond the thyroid gland contours or with frank invasion of adjacent structures. Suspicion of lymph node metastases should be elevated with the sonographic appearance of a rounded bulging shape, increased size, replaced fatty hilum, irregular margins, heterogeneous texture, calcifications, cystic areas, and vascularity throughout the lymph node instead of normal central hilar vessels with Doppler instrumentation.[33] The clinical manifestations of compression and invasion include cough, dyspnea with invasion of the trachea, hoarseness with invasion of the larynx, and dysphagia with invasion of the laryngeal nerve or the esophagus.[8] The pathogenesis of anaplastic thyroid carcinoma, lymphoma, and sarcoma is aggressive local invasion.[33]

Elasticity describes a mechanical tissue characteristic that prevents displacement of stiffer tissue when placed under pressure such as with compression from an ultrasound probe.[43,44] Elastography is an imaging method used to evaluate the stiffness of soft tissues and to display new information about the internal structure of tissue.[45] With further clinical correlations, elastography may become a significant diagnostic technique to help differentiate the malignant nodule, which tends to be harder (stiffer) than normal tissue or the benign nodule. The three primary types of elasticity imaging are (1) strain imaging, (2) color elasticity, and (3) shear-wave imaging. Strain imaging uses a software program with conventional sonography equipment and ultrasound probe to first receive the echo from the tissue; second to lightly compress the tissue with the ultrasound probe along the insonation axis to cause some displacement; and third, to receive a second, postcompression digitized echo from the same tissue.[43] Color elasticity continues to use the push and tract displacement technique of strain image but adds a chromatic scale assigned to different levels of elasticity.[45] Shear-wave elastography is based on the automatic generation and analysis of transient shear waves that are quantitative and reproducible, which sets it apart from other elasticity imaging modes.[45] The preliminary correlation studies between the histologic pattern of thyroid nodules and its elasticity and the ability to quantitatively measure soft tissue stiffness is an important step in differentiating pathology.

## Papillary Carcinoma

Papillary carcinoma is the most common malignant tumor of the thyroid gland, accounting for 75% to 85% of all thyroid cancers. It develops in patients of any age and it occurs most frequently between 20 and 50 years of age. The female-to-male ratio is 3:1 in the adult.[6] Most papillary carcinomas present as (1) a painless, palpable nodule in an otherwise normal gland; (2) a nodule with enlarged cervical lymph nodes; or (3) cervical lymphadenopathy in the absence of a palpable thyroid nodule. Like most benign nodules, a papillary carcinoma tends to move freely during swallowing.[8] More advanced disease is suspected if a patient presents with hoarseness, dysphagia, cough, or dyspnea.

There are a number of variant forms of papillary thyroid carcinomas. The most common variant is the pure papillary carcinoma, which accounts for about 55% to 66% of all well-differentiated thyroid carcinomas.[46] The second most common is the follicular variant of papillary thyroid carcinoma, which accounts for about 9% to 22.5% of all papillary thyroid carcinomas.[46] The encapsulated variant occurs in about 10% of all papillary thyroid carcinomas. The tall cell variant tends to occur in older individuals, has the poorest prognosis, and may be misdiagnosed as Hürthle cell tumors.[8]

A variety of diagnostic tests have been employed to separate benign form malignant thyroid nodules. The FNA biopsy cytology test has a higher diagnostic accuracy than the radionuclide scanning, sonography, or elastography. Treatment varies and may consist of a partial lobectomy, radical neck dissection, or both, followed by suppressive therapy.

Generally, papillary carcinoma is considered the least aggressive of the thyroid tumors. The prognosis is excellent and there is little difference in life expectancy from that of the general population for patients less than 50 years of age. The overall survival rate is 98%.[8] In children, the outlook of recovery is good even in cases with lung metastases.[6] The prognosis is more serious in patients older than 50 years of age and papillary carcinoma is more aggressive in men than in women.[6] The prognosis is poorer in cases where the primary neoplasm is larger, more aggressive, and has a direct extension into the adjacent soft tissues.[6] The proportion of papillary and follicular elements contributes little to the prognosis, but less differentiated papillary carcinomas tend to be more aggressive. The presence of metastases to cervical nodes at the time or surgery does not change the prognosis, and less than 10% of these patients succumb to the tumor. In fatal cases of papillary carcinoma, death is caused principally by metastases to the lungs or brain or by obstruction of the trachea or esophagus.[6]

Sonographic appearance may include one or more of the following: hypoechogenicity (in 90% of the cases) due to closely packed cell contents and minimal colloid substances; microcalcifications owing to deposition of calcium salts in psammoma bodies which appear as tiny, punctate hyperechoic foci, hypervascularity with disorganized vessels, and if there is metastasis to the lymph nodes, tiny punctate calcifications may appear in the affected lymph nodes[10] (Fig. 15-12A–D).

## Follicular Carcinoma

The second most common thyroid cancer is follicular carcinoma, and it accounts for 10% to 20% of diagnosed cases.[8] The female-to-male ratio is 3:1 and most cases affect individuals in the fourth and fifth decades.[6,8] There is an increased incidence in geographic areas of endemic goiter where there is a dietary iodine deficiency,[6] whereas papillary carcinomas are more common in areas of sufficient or excess iodine intake. The pathology comes to clinical attention as a slow growing, enlarging, painless nodule.

Follicular thyroid carcinomas are subdivided into minimally invasive and widely invasive variants, which differ in histology and clinical course.[10] An accurate diagnosis can only be made histologically.[24] The minimally invasive follicular carcinoma is a well-defined, encapsulated tumor. It usually is diagnosed when the tumor extends into but not entirely through the capsule.[6] The widely invasive follicular carcinomas are not well encapsulated and invasion of the vessels and the adjacent thyroid is more easily demonstrated.[10] Unlike papillary carcinoma that has a propensity for invading lymphatics, both types of follicular carcinoma differs in that metastases spreads hematogenously, especially to the bone, lungs, liver, and elsewhere.[6] Metastasis to the neck nodes are distinctly rare with follicular cancer.[13] Distant metastases are present in 5% to 20% of the minimally invasive variant and in 20% to 40% of the widely invasive variant.[13] The prognosis depends on

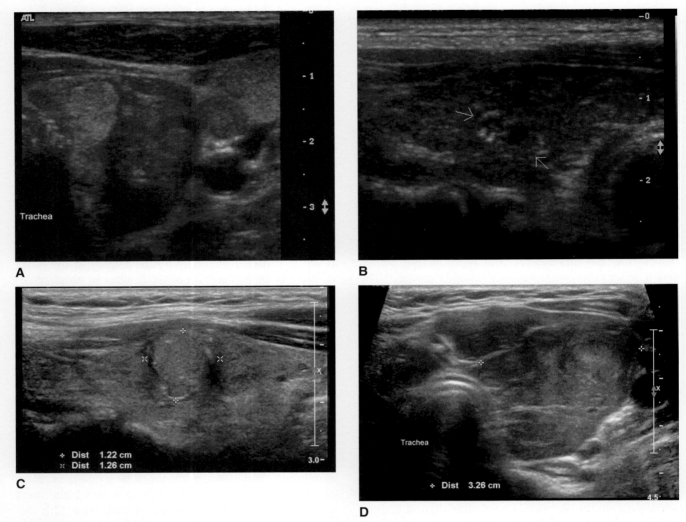

**Figure 15-12** Papillary carcinoma in different patients diagnosed by fine-needle aspiration cytology. Note the variation in appearance, size, and texture. **A:** A transverse image through the left thyroid lobe demonstrates a homogeneous slightly lobulated lesion with tiny hyperechoic punctate calcifications. **B:** A longitudinal image of the right thyroid lobe shows a heterogeneous, but isoechoic mass containing microcalcifications. **C:** A longitudinal image of the left thyroid lobe shows a hypoechoic, homogeneous oval mass with microcalcifications and an irregular thick halo. **D:** A transverse image of the left lobe demonstrates an elongated hypoechoic and heterogeneous mass.

the size of the primary and the presence or absence of capsular and vascular invasion and, to a lesser extent, the level of anaplasia in the lesion.[8] Minimally invasive follicular tumors have a cure rate of at least 95% compared with a survival of about 50% for the widely invasive form.[6] The 20-year mortality for all patients with follicular cancer is approximately 25%.[13]

Follicular carcinomas are treated with lobectomy or subtotal thyroidectomy. Widely invasive tumors are treated with total thyroidectomy, which is usually followed by the administration of radioactive iodine.[8]

The sonographic features of follicular carcinoma overlaps the appearance of follicular adenomas, which is explained with the cytologic and histologic similarities in the two entitities.[10] The two lesions cannot be distinguished on sonography or with FNA.[13] Sonographic features that suggest follicular carcinoma are rarely seen but include irregular tumor margins, a thick irregular halo, and a tortuous or chaotic arrangement

of internal blood vessels on color Doppler images[10] (Fig. 15-13A–C).

### Medullary Carcinoma

Medullary thyroid carcinoma accounts for no more than 5% of all thyroid carcinoma.[6] It is a neuroendocrine neoplasm derived from the thyroid gland's parafollicular cells, which are similar to normal cells but secrete calcitonin (C cells).[8] Serum calcitonin can be used as a tumor marker.[13] The disease occurs in sporadic forms with approximately 80% of cases and in familial forms in approximately 20% of cases.[6] The mean age for sporadic cases is 50 years of age and for familial cases is 20 years of age.[8] The female-to-male ratio in sporadic cases is 1.5:1 with a slight female predominance, but in familial cases, the inheritance is autosomal dominant with an almost equal sex distribution.[6] Sporadic cases of medullary carcinoma come to medical attention most often as a mass in the neck,

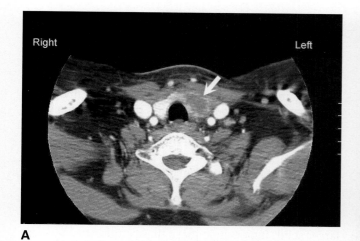

A

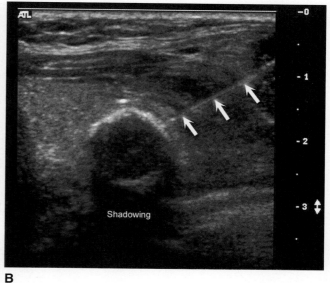

B

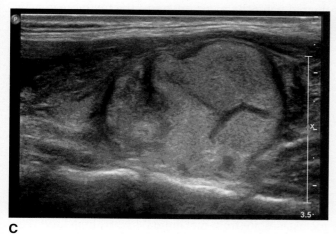

C

Figure 15-13 Follicular carcinoma. **A:** The computed tomography (CT) with contrast image demonstrates the sectional neck anatomy and a heterogeneous area beginning in the isthmus and extending throughout the left thyroid lobe *arrow*. **B:** On the same patient with the CT exam, the transverse sonogram of the left thyroid mass shows a diagonal white line *arrows* entering the image from the right, which is the biopsy needle used during a sonography guided fine-needle aspiration biopsy. The tissue was described as having a smooth calcified rim with difficult gritty penetration. The cytology report diagnosed follicular carcinoma. **C:** The 42-year-old woman in this case presented with a lump in the neck. The longitudinal image of the left thyroid lobe shows a hypoechoic lobular, irregular mass demonstrating some vasculature seen as anechoic vessels. The fine-needle aspiration cytology report diagnosed follicular carcinoma.

sometimes associated with local effects such as dysphagia or hoarseness. Patients often suffer a number of symptoms related to endocrine secretion, which includes carcinoid syndrome (serotonin) and Cushing syndrome with one-third of the patients have watery diarrhea due to vasoactive intestinal secretions.[6,8] Patients with the familial form of medullary carcinoma are often afflicted with multiple endocrine neoplasia (MEN) type 2, which includes hyperparathyroidism, episodic hypertension, and other symptoms attributable to the secretion of catecholamines by pheochromocytoma.[8] Sporadic medullary carcinomas and those arising in patients with MEN type 2 are aggressive lesions with a propensity to metastasize hematogenously and have a 5-year survival rate of 50%.[8] It has a more aggressive behavior than the differentiated carcinomas and it does not respond to either chemotherapy or radiation therapy.[13] In contrast, familial medullary carcinomas not associated with MEN are often fairly indolent lesions.[8]

The sonographic appearance of medullary carcinoma is usually similar to papillary carcinoma although local invasion and metastasis to cervical nodes occurs more often in patients with medullary carcinoma.[13] The features include a hypoechoic solid mass and microcalcifications are common.[10,13] Often, coarse calcification

are seen in the primary tumor, the lymph nodal metastases, and even in hepatic metastases.[10]

## Anaplastic Carcinoma

Anaplastic thyroid carcinoma are undifferentiated tumors of the thyroid follicular epithelium.[8] The thyroid cancer accounts for less than 5% of thyroid malignancies. The female-to-male ratio is 4:1 and it is typically a disease of people over 60 years with a mean age of 65 years.[6] The incidence is greater in endemic goiter areas. Of the patients diagnosed with anaplastic carcinoma, over 50% have a long-standing history of multinodular goiter, approximately 20% have a history of differentiated carcinoma; and another 20% to 30% have a concurrent differentiated thyroid tumor, which is frequently a papillary carcinoma.[6,8] The findings lead some to speculate that anaplastic carcinoma develops from more differentiated tumors as a result of one or more genetic changes.[8]

In striking contrast to the differentiated thyroid carcinomas, anaplastic carcinomas are aggressive tumors, with widespread metastases, and a dismal prognosis with less than 10% of patients surviving for 5 years.[6,8,13] The clinical course for these highly malignant tumors is a rapidly enlarging bulky neck mass that compresses and destroys local structures. Compression and invasion symptoms such as dyspnea, dysphagia, hoarseness, and cough are common.[6,8] In many cases, the disease has already spread beyond the thyroid capsule into adjacent neck structures or has already metastasized to the lungs when the patient presents for the initial examination. There is no effective therapy for anaplastic carcinoma and death results from the aggressive growth and the compromise to vital structures in the neck.[8]

Sonography may not be able to adequately examine the large size of the tumor or extent of tumor invasion and involvement. Computed tomography (CT) and magnetic resonance imaging (MRI) are better imaging modalities to accurately demonstrate the extent of the disease. Sonographically, anaplastic carcinoma usually appears as a large, solid, hypoechoic mass with demonstration of encasing or invading blood vessels and, if present, invasion of the neck muscles.[10,13]

### Hürthle Cell Carcinoma

Hürthle cells are large thyroglobulin-producing epithelial cells and are found in both nonneoplastic and neoplastic thyroid lesions.[47] The Hürthle cell neoplasm is classified as either a benign Hürthle cell adenoma or a malignant Hürthle cell carcinoma, both of which consist of at least 75% Hürthle cells and a paucity of colloid cells.[47,48] The diagnosis of Hürthle cell carcinoma, as with follicular carcinoma, requires histologic identification of capsular or vascular invasion, or nodal and/or distant metastasis.[48] Hürthle cell carcinomas account for approximately 3% but less than 10% of differentiated thyroid malignancies. Although they are uncommon and there is some controversy regarding Hürthle cell carcinoma clinical behavior, they are more aggressive than either papillary or follicular cell carcinomas, which makes their timely diagnosis important for cancer prognosis and therapy.[47] Most studies show that advanced age, male gender, large primary tumor size, degree of invasion, and recurrence are poor prognostic indicators.[48] A total thyroidectomy is usually the treatment of choice with different follow-up therapy.

Sonography is an important tool in evaluation of the thyroid gland but the literature has limited reports regarding the sonographic appearance of either benign or malignant Hürthle cell neoplasms and are clinical descriptions of a single entity.[47] In retrospective studies, researchers concluded there is a wide spectrum of sonographic appearances.[47,48] At this time, sonography can define the size and shape of the tumor, but an accurate diagnosis is only possible with pathologic evaluation of resected tumors.

### Lymphoma

Lymphoma originating in the thyroid gland is distinctly uncommon, accounting for less than 5% of all thyroid malignancies. It can occur as either a manifestation of generalized lymphoma or as a primary abnormality and it is usually a non-Hodgkin variety.[13] Most cases arise in the clinical setting of chronic thyroiditis (Hashimoto thyroiditis) with subclinical or overt hypothyroidism and are

highest in regions where this disorder is frequent. Like chronic thyroiditis, it is more common in women with a female-to-male ratio of 4:1.[6] The mean age at presentation is the seventh decade. The clinical presentation is usually a rapidly growing mass and symptoms of airway obstruction with a history of long-standing thyroiditis. The treatment of choice is usually radiation therapy and chemotherapy. Surgery is often performed to diagnose the primary thyroid lymphoma. Research continues to determine the accuracy of FNA biopsy for diagnosis for subclassification of lymphoma.[49] The 5-year survival rate ranges from nearly 90% in early-stage cases to less than 5% in advanced, disseminated disease.[10]

Sonographically, lymphoma usually appears as a large, solid, hypoechoic mass that compresses adjacent thyroid parenchyma or infiltrates the thyroid parenchyma.[13] The mass may appear lobulated and have large areas of cystic necrosis as well as encasement of adjacent neck vessels.[10] Color Doppler evaluation most likely will demonstrate a mostly hypovascular or a chaotic blood vessel distribution and arteriovenous shunts. If the patient has chronic lymphocytic thyroiditis, the adjacent thyroid parenchyma may be heterogeneous.[10]

### Metastases

Metastases to the thyroid gland are infrequent and occurs late in the course of neoplastic disease and most commonly spreads by hematogenous route and less frequently by lymphatic routes.[10] When it does occur, metastases are from melanoma, breast, lung, and renal cell carcinoma. None of these lesions has a characteristic sonographic appearance; however, metastatic disease should be considered when a solid thyroid nodule is identified in a patient with a known extrathyroidal malignancy[13] (Fig. 15-14).

## FINE-NEEDLE ASPIRATION

Imaging cannot definitively distinguish between benign and malignant thyroid nodules and adenopathy. FNA biopsy is the primary evaluation method of a palpable thyroid nodule.[1] The actual diagnosis of thyroid cancer is made from the cytologic evaluation of the thyroid follicular epithelial cells and minute tissue fragments obtained either from an FNA biopsy or a surgical resection.

### Indications and Guidelines

FNA biopsy of thyroid nodules and adenopathy is a diagnostic adjunct for differentiation and patient management. The FNA is essential to decision making and is able to provide highly accurate information by confirming benignity, confirming suspected malignancies before commencement of nonsurgical treatment such as chemotherapy or radiation therapy, or determining the nature of an indeterminate nodule.[10,24] Sonography-assisted FNA biopsy is a minimally invasive and safe procedure that can be performed on an outpatient basis.[50] Both the Society of Radiologists in

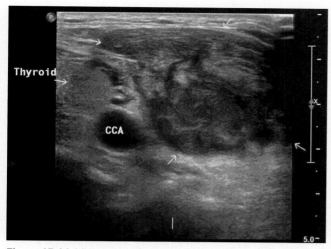

**Figure 15-14** Metastases. The 56-year-old man is undergoing radiation treatment for throat cancer. A transverse image through the left neck adjacent to the thyroid demonstrates a mixed echoic pattern in a large mass *(arrows)* compressing thyroid gland tissue *(arrow)*. The report from the fine-needle aspiration diagnosed metastatic squamous cell carcinoma.

Ultrasound (SRU) and the American Thyroid Association (ATA) provide guidelines for the management of thyroid nodules.[51,52] The physicians writing the ATA and SRU guidelines included endocrinologists and endocrine surgeons and the SRU also included radiologists. The recommendation is to strongly consider FNA when the nodule has microcalcifications ≥1 cm, when the nodule is solid or almost entirely solid, when the nodule has coarse calcifications, and when the nodule is ≥1.5 cm in size. Referencing these guidelines provides a good decision making tool for referring physicians and sonologists to determine which patients should be recommended the FNA biopsy procedure. The benefit for the majority of patients is the assurance of benign disease and for the minority of patients is the diagnosis of malignant disease. Side effects from the FNA biopsy procedure are uncommon but may include bleeding which is especially true in patients using anticoagulants, antiplatelet agents, or those who have a bleeding diathesis.[25] The effect of bleeding can be diminished in some patients if their condition allows discontinuing anticoagulant medication or antiplatelet agents prior to the procedure. Other effects may include hoarseness, infections, and the remote consideration of seeding the needle track with thyroid cancer.[25] In cases where FNA biopsy is to be performed on bilateral masses, the precautionary measure is to schedule separate appointments. Although rare, the development of a post procedure hematoma could compress the trachea which, if present bilaterally, could have catastrophic consequences for the patient.

## Protocol

The outpatient procedure is performed in a sonography room using standard sterile technique. When the patient first enters the room, applying ice to the patient's neck helps anesthetize the skin as well as reduce blood flow to the area. Place the patient in the same position used for a standard thyroid gland examination with a pillow under the patient's knees and place a rolled towel under the neck to gain maximum working space for the procedure. Review any previous sonography examination and reexamine the area to be biopsied. Prior to prepping the patient's neck, demonstrate and discuss the best approach with the physician performing the procedure. A 25-gauge needle is usually used, and since it is small, it can be sonographically visualized best when parallel to the transducer face (perpendicular to the beam). The advantage of performing a sonography-guided FNA biopsy procedure is that the real-time visualization of the needle as it enters the mass better enables the physician to accurately select the intended site. Once in the mass, the physician will pull back slightly on the syringe creating mild suction while collecting tissue by moving the needle within the area of interest. Some physicians prefer to use the natural capillary action of the needle alone for this process. The sampled cells are transferred to laboratory slides and submitted for analysis (Fig. 15-15). The sonographic protocol also provides the physician with guidance for percutaneous treatment of neck pathology such as alcohol ablation of parathyroid adenomas or ethanol injection of benign cystic thyroid lesions.

## Limitations

According to the American Cancer Society, the repeat rate is 2 in every 10 biopsies, a benign diagnosis is made in 7 of 10 biopsies, and a cancer diagnosis is made in 1 of every 20 biopsies.[53] The high repeat rate is due to aspiration of fluid from a cystic lesions and has a higher association with an FNA biopsy procedure performed by palpation versus sonography guidance.[10] Factors that will help decrease the rate of the sample inadequacy include

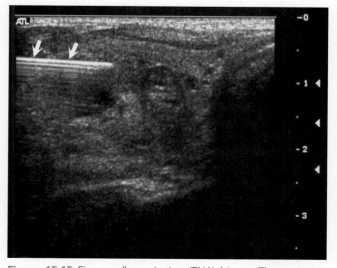

**Figure 15-15** Fine-needle aspiration (FNA) biopsy. The aspiration needle *(arrows)* can be identified during FNA of a complex right thyroid nodule. Note the reverberation artifact from the needle. This needle is correctly positioned perpendicular to the sound beam, which is parallel to the transducer. The needle resolution and the accuracy of the biopsy location are compromised by failure to adhere to this requirement.

an experienced sonographer for lesion targeting and localization, the level of experience of the individual performing the biopsy and obtaining the aspirate, and immediate on-site cytologic examination.[50] With an ample aspirate, cytologic examination is more effective for diagnosing papillary, medullary, and anaplastic carcinoma[54] but lacks specificity in diagnosing follicular carcinoma, Hürthle cell carcinoma, and lymphomas. These cases and other suspicious biopsy aspirates require surgical excision.

# PARATHYROID GLANDS

## EMBRYOLOGY

The embryonic development of the parathyroid glands is a complex process of cell differentiation and migration of the glands from the sites of origin in the pharynx and pharyngeal pouches to the usual anatomic location near the thyroid gland. The pharyngeal pouches (or branchial pouches) form on the endodermal side between the arches. The pharyngeal grooves (or clefts) form from the lateral ectodermal surface of the neck region to separate the arches.[55] The paired superior and paired inferior parathyroid glands have different embryologic origins.[5,56] Between the fifth and sixth gestational weeks, the parathyroid glands derive from the endoderm of the third and fourth pharyngeal pouches.[56]

The superior parathyroid glands arise from the dorsal wing of the fourth pharyngeal pouch.[5,57] At the seventh gestational week, the superior parathyroid glands lose connection to the pharynx and migrate caudally to attach with the posterior aspect of the mid to upper portion of the thyroid gland.[5] At autopsy, the final position for 80% of the superior parathyroid glands are within a 2-cm area located slightly superior to the recurrent laryngeal nerve and slightly inferior to the thyroid artery.[56]

The inferior parathyroid glands arise from the dorsal wing of the third pharyngeal pouch, along with the thymus. The ventral wing becomes the thymus.[5] During fetal development, the "parathymus glands" migrate caudally.[56] The inferior parathyroid glands loses its connections with the thymus and the migration usually stops at the dorsal surface of the thyroid gland, outside of the fibrous capsule.[5] The final position of the inferior parathyroid glands are variable. Usually over 60% come to rest at or just inferior to the posterior aspect of the lower pole of the thyroid gland.[56]

When migration is complete, the normal adult anatomical location of the superior and inferior parathyroid glands, which developed respectively from the fourth and third pharyngeal pouch are now opposite of the pharyngeal rostrocaudal order.

## ANATOMY

Most adults have four parathyroid glands: two superior located posterior to the midportion of the thyroid gland and two inferior located in a slightly more variable position. The inferior parathyroid glands are located posterior or just inferior to the lower thyroid pole in approximately 60% of adults and are located within 4 cm of the lower thyroid pole in approximately 20% of adults[13] (Fig. 15-16). Microscopically, about three-fourths of the parathyroid glands are composed of chief cells and oxyphil cells and the remainder is composed of adipose tissue scattered throughout the parenchyma.[6] Normal parathyroid glands vary from a yellow to a reddish-brown color based on the amount of yellow parenchymal fat and chief cell content.[56] The parathyroid glands are typically somewhat flattened, oval, almond-shaped structures measuring $1 \times 3 \times 5$ mm.[13] Although enlarged, diseased, or cystic parathyroid glands may be differentiated from normal surrounding anatomy, imaging and visualizing the normal parathyroid glands is a challenge due to their variable locations, small size, and isoechoic texture when compared to the normal thyroid gland.

### Anatomic Variants

Accessory or supernumerary "fifth" parathyroid glands are found in approximately 13% of individuals at autopsy.[56] In one study, two-thirds of the supernumerary cases revealed the fifth parathyroid gland inferior to the lower pole of the thyroid gland associated with the thyrothymic ligament or the thymus and one-third had the supernumerary parathyroid gland in the vicinity of the thyroid between the orthotopic superior and inferior parathyroids.[57] Absence of parathyroid glands, defined as less than four, is noted in approximately 3% of individuals at autopsy.[5] In about 25% of cases, the inferior parathyroid glands fail to dissociate from the thymus and continue to migrate lower in the neck or into the mediastinum.[56]

Ectopic parathyroid glands occur in 15% to 20% of patients.[5] Due to the long course of descent during embryologic development, the ectopic locations for the inferior parathyroid glands range from the level of the mandibular angle to the pericardium.[57] The most common ectopic location for the inferior parathyroid glands is in the anterior mediastinum and occurs in approximately 5% of ectopic cases.[57] Other common ectopic locations include the posterior mediastinum and retroesophageal and prevertebral regions.[5,56] It is interesting to note that even in their ectopic locations, the parathyroid glands are symmetrical from side to side when comparing right with left at 80% for the superior and 70% for the inferior glands.[57] The parathyroid glands have also been identified entering the thyroid gland capsule and embedding into the thyroid gland resulting in intrathyroidal parathyroid gland(s).[5]

## PHYSIOLOGY

The chief cells of the parathyroid glands is the primary source for the production of parathyroid hormone (PTH). PTH is the most important endocrine regulator

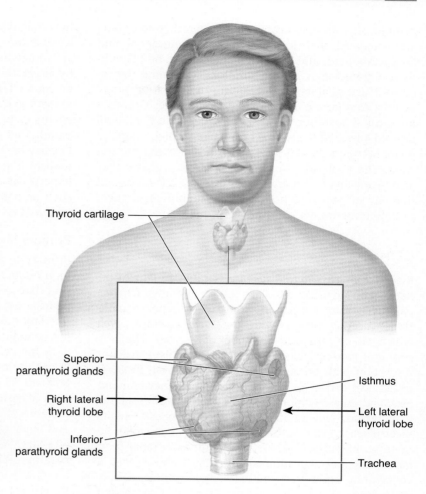

Thyroid cartilage

Superior parathyroid glands

Isthmus

Right lateral thyroid lobe

Left lateral thyroid lobe

Inferior parathyroid glands

Trachea

**Figure 15-16** Anatomic location of the parathyroid glands. The superior and inferior thyroid glands are commonly located on the posterior surface of the thyroid gland surface. When evaluating the parathyroid glands, the scanning area should be large enough to include an investigation lateral and inferior of the thyroid.

of calcium and phosphorous concentrations in extracellular fluid. The major target cells are in the bone and the kidney. The metabolic functions of PTH in supporting serum calcium and phosphorous levels includes activating osteoclasts, which influences the release of calcium by the bones, augmenting the absorption of calcium in the intestinal tract, increasing renal tubular reabsorption of calcium that conserves free calcium, increasing conversion of vitamin D to its active dihydroxy form in the kidneys, and increasing urinary phosphate excretion that lowers the serum phosphate level.[8] These normal metabolic activities act in a classic feedback loop where (1) an increase in the level of free calcium inhibits further PTH secretion and (2) when serum calcium levels are low, PTH secretion increases to act on target organs (skeletal, renal, and intestinal), and to enhance calcium absorption.

## LABORATORY TESTS

A fasting blood PTH test is usually performed with a calcium test to monitor patients with a parathyroid condition or to help diagnose the reason for a variance in calcium levels (hypercalcemia or hypocalcemia).[58] Normal PTH values are 10 to 55 pg/mL and may vary

slightly among different laboratories. Elevated values may occur with chronic renal failure, hyperparathyroidism, and vitamin D deficiency as well as other entities. Decreased values may occur with accidental removal or autoimmune destruction of the parathyroid glands, hypoparathyroidism, and metastatic bone tumors as well as other entities.

## SONOGRAPHIC EXAMINATION TECHNIQUE

The preparation and protocol for a sonography examination of the parathyroid glands are the same as for a thyroid gland examination. To sonographically evaluate, concentrate on the region between the posteromedial thyroid gland and the longus colli muscle.[7] The superior parathyroid glands are slightly more medial than the inferior parathyroid glands. The common ectopic locations for parathyroid glands can also be evaluated. On a transverse section, pay particular attention to the area medial to the carotid artery, posterior to the lateral lobe of the thyroid gland, and anterior to the longus colli muscle. The parathyroid glands normally measure $1.0 \times 3.0 \times 5.0$ mm in size and are similar in echogenicity to the adjacent thyroid gland and surrounding tissues, which makes it difficult to distinguish sonographically.[1] If the parathyroid glands are visualized, their location, size, and number should be documented, and measurements should be made in three dimensions.[17] Minor bundles (containing the recurrent laryngeal nerve and inferior thyroid artery) may be mistaken for a parathyroid adenoma. These bundles are located posteriorly and slightly medial to the lateral thyroid lobes. Note also the esophagus, which often appears between the left lateral thyroid lobe and the trachea. The posteriorly located longus colli muscle may also be mistaken for parathyroid disease. It is important that any suspected pathology can be identified, as such, in both longitudinal and transverse planes.

## PATHOLOGY OF THE PARATHYROID GLANDS

Evidence of parathyroid disease is often sought in patients who present with signs and symptoms of hyperparathyroidism, particularly those with hypercalcemia. Hypercalcemia occurs with excessive calcium levels which can be caused by a number of diseases. The most common causes include hyperparathyroidism; calcium resorption with bone metastases from breast, prostate, or cervical cancer or hematologic malignancy; sarcoidosis; and excess vitamin D.[59] The clinical manifestations may include weight loss, anorexia, dyspepsia, peptic ulcer disease, pancreatitis, and nausea. Renal colic, hematuria, polyuria, and nocturia result from renal tubular dysfunction and diminished ability of the kidney to concentrate urine. Nephrolithiasis and urolithiasis, bone and joint pain, arthritis, and gout may also be present. Other patient history may include short-term memory loss, lack of energy and enthusiasm, and insomnia.

Hypocalcemia occurs with low serum calcium levels and may be either asymptomatic or life-threatening. Mild decreases in calcium can produce paresthesias around the mouth and in the digits, muscle spasms in the hands and feet (carpopedal spasm), and hyperreflexia.[59] Hyperirritability, fatigue, and anxiety are common symptoms. Severely reduced levels may induce dementia, depression, psychosis, and local or generalized seizures. Severe symptoms may include muscle spasm that can interfere with breathing and cause death.[59] Chronic hypocalcemia may affect ectoderm, producing dry skin, coarse hair, and brittle nails. Patients who have undergone partial or complete thyroidectomies may have had an inadvertent removal of all parathyroid glands and are at higher risk for developing hypoparathyroidism and consequently hypocalcemia.

In addition to the inadvertent removal of all parathyroid glands, there are a number of underlying causes of deficient PTH secretion resulting in hypoparathyroidism.[8] Other underlying causes include congenital absence of all glands, primary (idiopathic) atrophy, and familial hypoparathyroidisms.

Hyperparathyroidism is characterized by a greater than normal secretion of PTH. The two major classification of hyperparathyroidism are primary and secondary and a less common tertiary.[8] The pathophysiologic mechanisms are somewhat different for each classification.[28] Primary hyperparathyroidism represents an autonomous, spontaneous PTH overproduction. Secondary hyperparathyroidism generally results as a secondary compensatory enlargement and hypersecretion that usually affects all parathyroid glands in patients with chronic renal insufficiency or vitamin D deficiency.[1] Tertiary hyperparathyroidism is the development of autonomous parathyroid hyperplasia and it is often due to an underlying disease such as parathyroid hyperplasia after longstanding hyperplasia secondary to renal failure.[6]

### Primary Hyperparathyroidism

Primary hyperparathyroidism is one of the most common endocrine disorders and is characterized by inappropriate excess secretion of PTH by one or more of the parathyroid glands.[8,59] Most cases are detected with routine laboratory tests indicating elevated serum calcium levels and inappropriately high levels of PTH compared with the calcium level.[13] Primary hyperparathyroidism is usually caused by a single parathyroid adenoma in 80% to 85%, by parathyroid hyperplasia in 10% to 15% of cases, and by parathyroid carcinoma in approximately 1% of cases.[59] It is usually a disease of adults and tends to affect patients between the ages of 40 and 60 years.[13] Over half of the patients with primary hyperparathyroidism are older than 50 years of age and cases are rare before 20 years of age.[56] The female-to-male ratio is 2.5:1 with an increased incidence in women after menopause.[13,56] Although some cases of primary hyperparathyroidism are associated with prior external neck irradiation, long-term lithium therapy, or an inherited syndrome commonly related to MEN type 1 (MEN 1), most cases of primary hyperparathyroidism are sporadic and related to adenomas or hyperplasia.[56]

Surgery, considered the definitive treatment of primary hyperparathyroidism, is generally reserved for individuals with documented complications (osteoporosis, nephrolithiasis, or gastrointestinal or neuropsychiatric complications), severely elevated serum calcium levels, marked hypercalciuria, or individuals younger than 50 years of age.[28]

### Adenoma

A solitary adenoma is a benign lesion and may involve any one of the four parathyroid glands with equal frequency.[56] Most adenomas are found in the parathyroid glands typical superior and inferior locations, adjacent to the thyroid gland.[1] Approximately 3% of cases are found in the same ectopic locations as the parathyroid glands, which includes the low neck, mediastinum, retrotracheal/retroesophageal, undescended/carotid sheath, and intrathyroidal.[1,13]

Sonographically, the parathyroid adenomas appear as hypoechoic, homogeneous solid masses. The echogenicity is usually less than the thyroid gland and may be so hypoechoic as it simulates a cyst.[13] The vast majority are homogeneously solid and about 2% have an internal cystic components, which is most often due to cystic degeneration or less commonly are true simple cysts.[56] Adenomas are usually oval and less often appear as teardrop-shaped or round lesions. As the parathyroid glands enlarge, the adenoma dissects between longitudinally oriented tissue planes in the neck and acquire a characteristic oblong shape in the craniocaudal direction.[56] Most adenomas range in size from 0.8- to 1.5-cm long, are usually less than 3 cm, but may reach 5 cm.[9,56] Smaller adenomas resected surgically in minimally enlarged, normal appearing parathyroid glands have been found to be hypercellular on pathologic examination[56] (Fig. 15-17A,B). Examining enlarged parathyroid glands with color flow Doppler may demonstrate a hypervascular pattern with prominent diastolic flow, or a peripheral vascular arc that may allow for differentiation from hyperplastic regional lymph nodes, which have a central hilar flow pattern.[1] Sonography may detect an enlarged extrathyroidal feeding artery supplying the adenoma, which often originates from branches of the inferior thyroidal artery.[56]

## Hyperplasia

Primary hyperplasia is the enlargement of all four parathyroid glands; however, the enlargement is frequently unequal and asymmetric with apparent sparing of one or two glands.[8] Hyperplasia may occur sporadically or be associated with MEN syndromes (MEN types 1 and 2A).[6] Approximately 75% of sporadic cases occur in women and are associated with external radiation and intake of lithum.[6] One-third of sporadic cases demonstrate monoclonality, which suggests a neoplastic basis for the proliferation of chief cells.[6] These sporadic cases have both chief cell hyperplasia and multiple small adenomas in the same gland.

Because hyperplasia usually affects more than one gland, it should be suspected when multiple nodules are identified; whereas the sonographically similar parathyroid adenomas should be suspected when a solitary nodule is identified. The sonographic appearances of hyperplasia has these potential pitfalls: (1) misinterpreting hyperplasia as a solitary adenoma; (2) missing hyperplasia when glandular enlargement is minimal; (3) difficulty distinguishing hyperplasia versus adenoma when there is sparing of one or two glands; and

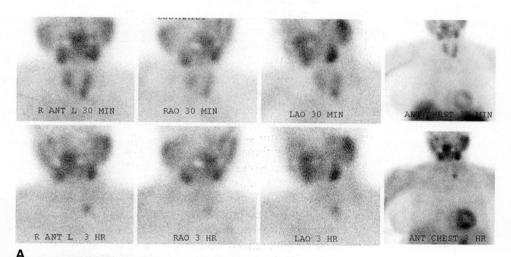

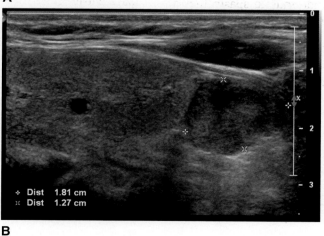

**Figure 15-17** Parathyroid gland adenoma. **A,B:** The 66-year-old woman presented with elevated serum calcium levels. **A:** Images obtained from the radionuclide parathyroid study demonstrates increased focal uptake inferior to the left lower thyroid. **B:** On the same patient with the nuclear medicine exam, the longitudinal sonogram of the left inferior medial thyroid gland area shows a mass with mixed hyperechoic, hypoechoic, and cystic regions in the same left parathyroid gland region. Cursors mark the area corresponding to the focal increased uptake seen on the technetium-99m radionuclide exam. Based on the imaging appearances and the patient's history, the diagnosis was a parathyroid gland adenoma.

(4) misinterpreting normal cervical structures, such as veins adjacent to the thyroid gland, the esophagus, or the longus colli neck muscles, which sonographically may simulate a parathyroid adenoma.[1,56]

### Carcinoma

Parathyroid carcinoma is a functioning tumor found in 1% of patients with primary hyperparathyroidism. These tumors occur equally in both sexes principally between 30 and 60 years of age.[8] They should be included as a diagnostic consideration for patients with primary hyperparathyroidism, particularly when the patient has a very high serum level of calcium, has had an abnormal gland excised, or has a palpable neck mass that is firm and immobile. Parathyroid carcinomas are often slow-growing, indolent masses with a lobular contour measuring more than 2 cm compared to the average 1 cm for adenomas. The mass often adheres to the surrounding soft tissues.[6] Sonographically, carcinomas frequently have a lobular contour with a heterogeneous internal architecture and internal cystic components.[56] The appearance may be similar to a large benign adenoma. A parathyroid carcinoma may demonstrate more attenuation than is normally seen with parathyroid adenomas or hyperplasia but differentiation is difficult prospectively. There is general agreement that a diagnosis of carcinoma based on cytologic detail and appearance is unreliable unless there is evidence of gross invasion to adjacent structures such as vessels or muscle.[8] If gross invasion occurs, it is an uncommon finding that is the only reliable preoperative sonographic criterion for the diagnosis of malignancy.[56] Despite surgical removal of the tumor, local recurrence occurs in one-third of the cases and about one-third of the cases develop metastases to regional lymph nodes, lungs, liver, and bone.[8] In fatal cases, death is most often caused by hyperparathyroidism rather than carcinomatosis.[6]

# NECK

Sonography is excellent for neck anatomy evaluation and can identify intrathyroidal from extrathyroidal pathology, distinguishing between solid and cystic masses, and, when needed, providing biopsy guidance.

## DEVELOPMENTAL CYSTS

The more common developmental cysts that are sonographically identifiable in the neck include thyroglossal duct cysts, branchial cleft cysts, and cystic hygromas.

### Thyroglossal Duct Cyst

A thyroglossal duct cyst is a congenital anomaly that develops within the remnant of the thyroglossal duct, which courses from the base of the tongue to the suprasternal region.[60] Over half of all cases occur in the first decade of life with decreasing incidence from children to adults to rarely occurring in elderly patients.[61] In a study of 40 adult patients, Ahuja and colleagues identified four sonographic appearances: anechoic (28%), homogeneously hypoechoic with internal debris (18%), pseudosolid (28%), and heterogeneous (28%); and in all cases the sonographic images documented posterior enhancement (88%) with midline (63%) and infrahyoid locations (83%).[60] For most patients with thyroglossal duct cyst, surgical excision is curative.[6] The sonographic examination can provide the surgeon with preoperative assessment of the thyroglossal duct cyst size, location, and involvement, if any, of the surrounding musculature and may exclude the need for CT or MRI.[61]

### Branchial Cleft Cyst

In early embryo development, the neck is shaped like a hollow tube with four circumferential ridges termed *arches* which develop into the musculoskeletal and vascular components of the head and neck. During embryonic maturation, the thinner regions between the arches, termed *clefts*, are located on the lateral or skin side and the pouches are located on the medial or pharynx side.[62] The pouches develop into the middle ear, tonsils, thymus, and parathyroid glands. The first branchial cleft develops into the external auditory canal. The second, third, and fourth branchial clefts merge to form a sinus which normally become involuted. The most widely held belief why developmental abnormalities within the branchial cleft occurs is incomplete obliteration of the cervical sinus.[63] With no communication with the inner mucosa or outer neck skin, the trapped arch remnants form a branchial cleft cyst (also known as a *lateral cervical cyst*).[63] On rare occasions, the branchial cleft fails to become involuted and a complete fistula with both external and internal openings forms between the pharynx and skin[62] (Fig. 15-18).

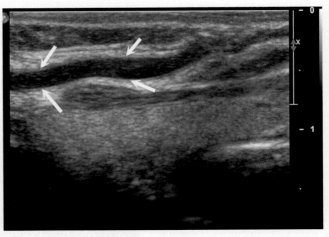

**Figure 15-18** Branchial cleft fistula. This 1-month-old boy presented with an opening in the lateral/anterior neck. A longitudinal image shows a homogeneously hypoechoic structure with some internal debris (*arrows*). A fistula is formed when the cleft fails to involute; whereas, if no communication existed, the trapped arch remnants would form a branchial cleft cyst.

First branchial cleft cysts are usually identified on contrast-enhanced axial CT and are either located in the auditory canal (type I) or in the submandibular area (type II).[62] Second branchial cleft cysts accounts for 95% of branchial anomalies and are identified by sonography along the anterior border of the upper third of the sternocleidomastoid muscle and adjacent to the muscle. Third branchial cleft cysts are rare and extend from the same skin location as a second branchial fistula but is deep to the sternocleidomastoid muscle and extends farther medially between the internal and external carotid artery at the carotid artery bifurcation.[62,64] Fourth branchial cleft cysts are rare and arise from various neck locations including the thyroid gland and mediastinum.[62]

Ahuja and colleagues identified four variable sonographic appearances for second branchial cleft cysts found in 17 adult patients: anechoic (41%), homogeneously hypoechoic with internal debris (23.5%), pseudosolid (12%), and heterogeneous (23.5%).[63] Posterior enhancement was identified in 70% of cases and in all cases, the cysts were located in their classical location posterior to the submandibular gland, superficial to the carotid artery and internal jugular vein, and closely related to the medial and anterior margin of the sternocleidomastoid muscle.[63] There are other benign cystic lateral neck masses that can mimic branchial cleft cysts and abscesses and necrotic adenopathy can be difficult to distinguish from a branchial cleft cyst especially if it has been previously infected.[64]

### Cystic Hygroma

A cystic hygroma is a congenital modification in the cervical lymphatic system. Over 60% are associated with chromosomal abnormality such as Turner syndrome but other aneuploidies are common such as trisomy 21 and trisomy 18.[13] These benign congenital masses occur at many sites but most often appear from the posterior occipital region and are most frequently visualized sonographically as large cystic masses on the lateral aspect of the neck. A cystic hygroma usually appears thin-walled and can be multilocular and multiseptated.

## PATHOLOGY

Sonography is an excellent diagnostic tool used to evaluate masses in the salivary gland, hematomas, deep neck space infections, and cervical lymph node pathology.

### Hematoma

Neck hematomas following trauma or surgery will appear as either cystic, solid, or mixed masses, depending on the degree of coagulation. Because an abscess may present with a similar sonographic appearance, an accurate clinical history is imperative for differentiation. Patients with a hematoma may present with a history of recent surgery or other soft tissue assault, whereas patients with an abscess present clinically with elevated temperature, elevated white blood cell count, and tenderness.

### Deep Neck Space Infections

Once a deep neck space infection is initiated, it may progress to either an inflammation and phlegmon or to fulminant abscess with a purulent fluid collection. The distinction is important because the treatment for these two entities is different.[65] Deep neck space infections are relatively uncommon but are a serious health problem with significant risks of morbidity and mortality.[65] Although the incidence and mortality rates have been reduced with the advancements in antibiotic medication, the diagnosis and treatment of infections in this area is difficult and potentially lethal complication may arise. Deep neck space infections are most commonly odontogenic in origin in adults, and tonsillitis is the most common etiology in children.[65] The infection can be caused by other infections, aspiration, drug use, postbiopsy or surgical procedures, and trauma. The etiology is unknown for 20% to 50% of cases.[65] The patient presents with the signs and symptoms of pain, recent dental procedures, upper respiratory tract infections, neck or oral cavity trauma including surgery or biopsy, respiratory difficulties, immunosuppression or immunocompromised status, or dysphagia. The infectious process can arise or spread to any potential space located between layers of fascia in the neck. The most common spaces that are likely to harbor an abscess are the submandibular space, the retropharyngeal space, and the parapharyngeal spaces.

The usefulness of diagnostic imaging varies and is based on the patient's age and the location of the infection. Sonography is helpful to distinguish between phlegmon and an abscess, give information about the condition of surrounding vessels, guide FNA procedures, and act as a guide to the need for further imaging with CT or MRI. CT is considered the gold standard in the evaluation of deep neck space infections and is capable of imaging infections extending into the chest.[66] MRI increases both the time and expense involved but provides excellent soft tissue resolution to help localize regional involvement.

The sonographic appearance of an abscess, although variable, is most often a partially or fully fluid-filled, thick-walled mass. In the presence of gas forming organisms, small pockets of hyperechoic air can be seen within the collection.[67] Enlarged, hypoechoic lymph nodes may be identified surrounding the abscess.[67]

### Cervical Lymph Node Pathology

Cervical lymph nodes are located along the lymphatic channels of the neck and have been classified for staging of cancers and reclassified for sonographic evaluation that allows the adoption of a systematic protocol for examination.[68] These nodes are also common sites of pathologic involvement with metastases, lymphoma, lymphadenitis, tuberculosis, reactive hyperplasia, and other conditions of benign lymphadenitis.[68,69] Evaluating cervical lymph nodes is an important follow-up on patients with head and neck carcinoma.[70,71] CT and MRI can be used to evaluate cervical lymph nodes; however, CT is less sensitive than sonography in detecting small nodes and MRI is less sensitive than sonography in detecting calcification within lymph nodes that can be identified sonographically.[68] Sonography is sensitive in identifying lymph nodes as small as 2 mm and intranodal calcifications that are useful features to identify metastatic nodes form papillary and medullary carcinoma of the thyroid gland.[68,69]

In healthy people, sonography can identify at least five normal lymph nodes with no racial or gender bias but fewer lymph nodes can be identified with advancing age.[68] Normal cervical lymph nodes are usually found in the submandibular, parotid, upper cervical, and posterior triangle regions, whereas the distribution of cervical lymph nodes is different in patients with metastatic head and neck carcinomas, non-Hodgkin lymphoma, and tuberculosis.[68,70]

Normal cervical lymph nodes are usually found in the submandibular, parotid, upper cervical, and posterior triangular regions.[68] The normal nodes appear hypoechoic when compared to adjacent soft tissue with an echogenic hilus.[70] The echogenic hilus is a hyperechoic linear structure, which is continuous with adjacent soft tissue and is usually considered as a sign of benignity[68] (Fig. 15-19A). The shape of a normal lymph node is predominantly oval, elongated, or elliptical except for the submandibular and parotid regions where the nodes appear round.[68,70] Normal lymph nodes less than 5 mm usually appear avascular as the blood vessels are too small to be detected, whereas, approximately 90% of normal lymph nodes with a maximum diameter greater than 5 mm present with hilar vascularity.[68,70] Using nodal size and vascular resistance has not produced firm criterion to differentiate normal from abnormal.[68,71] Finding a value as a cutoff point using a short axis measurement of 5 mm, 8 mm, and 10 mm increases the sensitivity as nodal size increases but it decreases the specificity as nodal size decreases. Nodal size is not useful as the sole criterion in differential diagnosis; however, it is clinically very useful when the size of lymph nodes in a patient with known carcinoma increases on serial sonography examination, when metastases is strongly suspected, and to evaluate progressive change of nodal size when monitoring treatment response of the patient[70] (Fig. 15-19B).

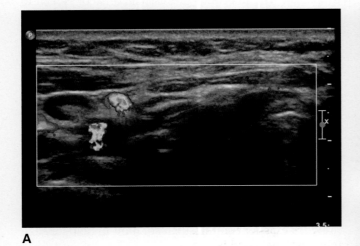

**A**

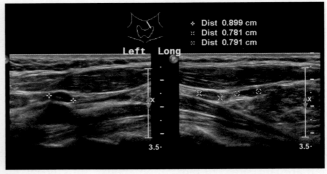

**B**

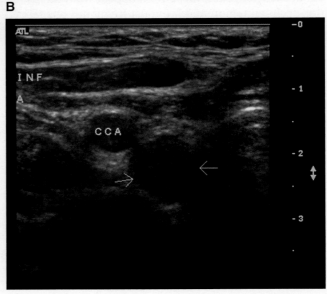

**C**

**Figure 15-19** Cervical lymph nodes. **A:** The sonogram shows an example of a lymph node with a prominent fatty hilum. The blood flow into the hilum is usually seen and will confirm identification of the hilum. **B:** The cursors mark normal lymph nodes seen on the sonograms made in the left lateral neck on a postthyroidectomy patient. **C:** This transverse image through the right inferior thyroid gland between the common carotid artery *(CCA)* and trachea show an enlarged, hypoechoic lymph node without a typical fatty hilum. The sonography examination is on a 25-year-old woman with known thyroid papillary carcinoma. Biopsy confirmed local metastasis of the patient's thyroid cancer. Compare this lymph node with those appearing in Figure 15-19A,B.

The sonographic appearance helpful in differentiating metastatic nodes include hypoechoic nodule except it is hyperechoic when the metastases is from papillary thyroid cancer carcinoma.[68,71] Metastatic nodes tend to be round in shape, the echogenic hilus is absent, there is intranodal cystic necrosis, increasing size on serial examinations, and peripheral or mixed vascularity.[68,70] If the metastasis is from papillary thyroid cancer, intranodal calcification is common.[68] The metastases may also originate from the lung, breast, gastrointestinal tract, or pancreas as well as local head and neck carcinoma (Fig. 15-19C). The differentiation of normal and abnormal cervical lymph nodes is not always possible based on sonographic features and the diagnosis is still based on histology.[69]

## SUMMARY

- The thyroid gland is located in the anterior neck usually over the second and third cartilaginous rings of the trachea.
- The thyroid gland is surrounded by a fibrous capsule and consists primarily of the right and left lobes that are united by a relatively thin isthmus.
- The thyroid gland is responsible for maintenance of body metabolism and secretes three hormones: tri-iodothyronine ($T_3$), thyroxine ($T_4$), and calcitonin (thyrocalcitonin).
- Sonographically, the normal thyroid gland parenchyma appears as a homogeneous gland of medium- to high-level echoes.
- The most common cause of thyroid gland disorders worldwide is iodine deficiency, which may result to goiter formation and hypothyroidism.
- Most thyroid nodules are benign and approximately 5% to 6.5% are malignant.
- Most adults have four parathyroid glands, two superior and two inferior, located on the posterior surface of the thyroid gland.
- The parathyroid glands regulates calcium and phosphorous concentration in extracellular fluid and secretes parathyroid hormone.
- If normal parathyroid glands are visualized, document the location, size, and number and make measurements in three dimensions.

## Critical Thinking Questions

1. The sonography examination was performed on a 52-year-old woman to evaluate and determine if the enlarged area palpated in the left neck is a mass or an enlarged thyroid gland. The gray-scale sonogram demonstrates a well-defined, complex, predominantly solid nodule in the left thyroid lobe with a hypoechoic perimeter. The nodule does not extend beyond the thyroid capsule. On the color Doppler sonogram, there is some blood flow within the nodule with increased blood flow in the region of the hypoechoic periphery of the left thyroid nodule. Based on the clinical presentation and sonographic findings, what is the most likely diagnosis?

2. A sonography examination is requested on a 44-year-old man with an enlarged thyroid gland found on his 6-week clinical follow-up for a viral upper respiratory infection. The patient stated his laboratory tests showed an excessive release of thyroid hormones but his physician stated this would most likely reverse in 6 to 8 weeks. The sonogram showed a diffusely enlarged, hypoechoic thyroid gland with decreased vascularity. The sonography report strongly favored a parenchymal disease of the thyroid gland and the interpreting sonologist reported the disease most likely is subacute thyroiditis. Provide an explanation why the laboratory values suggest thyrotoxicosis/hyperthyroidism but subacute thyroiditis was diagnosed based on his clinical history and the sonographic appearance of the thyroid parenchyma. What is the explanation for the sonographic visualization of decreased vascularity?

3. An 83-year-old woman is diagnosed with papillary carcinoma of the thyroid gland. When reviewing the sonographic examination, it is noted there are several characteristics associated with increased risk of thyroid cancer. The thyroid gland appeared hypoechoic, with the tiny, punctate hyperechoic foci appearance of microcalcifications, and there was hypervascularity and the vessels appeared disorganized. In retrospect, did the sonographic appearance provide enough evidence to make the diagnosis of papillary carcinoma of the thyroid gland?

4. A 38-year-old woman presents with a large palpable, hard mass in the neck region and states she has hoarseness and is uncomfortable when swallowing. The sonography examination shows a 4.5 cm × 6.5 cm complex mass containing both cystic and solid areas in the left thyroid lobe of an enlarged thyroid gland. There is sparing of the right thyroid lobe. Based on the clinical presentation and sonographic findings, what is the most likely diagnosis?

5. On an annual physical examination with laboratory tests, the data was normal except for elevated levels of parathyroid hormones in an asymptomatic 74-year-old woman. Her sonographic evaluation showed a hypoechoic, oval, solid appearing mass located posterior to the left thyroid gland lobe. Based on her laboratory values and the sonographic findings, what is the most likely diagnosis?

- Primary hyperparathyroidism is the most common endocrine disorder.

- Developmental cysts of the neck include thyroglossal duct cyst, branchial cleft cyst, and cystic hygroma.

- Pathology of the neck includes hematomas and deep neck space infections and cervical lymphadenopathy.

- Sonography of the neck, thyroid gland, and parathyroid glands is an excellent diagnostic test for determining the internal architecture and precise location of intrusive pathology.

- The sonography examination relies on the skill, knowledge, and accuracy of the sonographer who must pay attention to the texture, outline, size, and shape of both normal and abnormal structures.

- The patient will benefit most when the sonographic appearance is correlated with patient history, clinical presentation, laboratory function tests, and other imaging modalities to compose a clinically helpful picture.

## REFERENCES

1. Kuntz, KM. Neck mass. In: Henningsen C, ed. *Clinical Guide to Ultrasonography*. St. Louis, MO: Elsevier Mosby; 2004:439–450.

2. Huether SE. Mechanisms of hormonal regulation. In: McCance KL, Huether SE, eds. *Pathophysiology: The Biologic Basis for Diseases in Adults and Children*. 6th ed. St. Louis, MO: Elsevier Mosby; 2010:696–726.

3. Guyton AC, Hall JE. *Medical Physiology*. 10th ed. Philadelphia, PA: Elsevier Saunders; 2000.

4. Baker S, Winter T. Neck mass. In: Sanders RC, Winter T, eds. *Clinical Sonography: A Practical Guide*. 4th ed. Baltimore, MD: Lippincott Williams & Wilkins; 2007:231–239.

5. Kay DJ. Embryology of the thyroid and parathyroids. *Medscape: eMedicine*. January 2010. Available at: http://emedicine.medscape.com/article/845125-overview. Accessed June 4, 2010.

6. Rubin R, Rubin E. The endocrine system. In: Rubin E, Gorstein F, Rubin R, eds. *Rubin's Pathology: Clinicopathologic Foundations of Medicine*. 4th ed. Baltimore, MD: Lippincott Williams & Wilkins; 2005:1125–1171.

7. Tempkin BB, Leonhardt WC. Thyroid and parathyroid glands scanning protocol. In: Tempkin BB, ed. *Ultrasound Scanning: Principles and Protocols*. 3rd ed. St. Louis, MO: Elsevier Saunders; 2009:429–445.

8. Cotran RS, Kumar V, Collins T. The endocrine system. In: Cotran RS, Kumar V, Collins T, eds. *Robbins Pathologic Basis of Disease*. 6th ed. Philadelphia, PA: Elsevier Saunders; 1999:1121–1169.

9. Hagen-Ansert SL. The thyroid and parathyroid glands. In: Hagen-Ansert SL, ed. *Textbook of Diagnostic Ultrasonography*. 6th ed. Vol 1. St. Louis, MO: Elsevier Mosby; 2006:514–528.

10. Solbiati L, Charboneau JW, Osti V, et al. The thyroid gland. In: Rumack CM, Wilson SR, Charbonneau JW, eds. *Diagnostic Ultrasound*. 3rd ed. Vol 1. St. Louis, MO: Elsevier Mosby; 2005:735–770.

11. Needleman L. Thyroid and parathyroid. In: Goldberg BB, McGahan JP, eds. *Atlas of Ultrasound Measurements*. 2nd ed. St. Louis, MO: Elsevier Mosby; 2006:328–332.

12. Moore KL, Agur AM. *Essential Clinical Anatomy*. 3rd ed. Baltimore, MD: Lippincott Williams & Wilkins; 2007.

13. Middleton WD, Kurtz AB, Hertzberg BS. *Ultrasound: The Requisites*. 2nd ed. St. Louis, MO: Elsevier Mosby; 2004.

14. Dempsey R. Lingual thyroid. *J Diagn Med Sonogr*. 2002;18:91–94.

15. Auckland AK. Heterotopic thyroid. *J Diagn Med Sonogr*. 2004;20:120–123.

16. Kim JH, Lee HK, Lee JH, et al. Efficacy of sonographically guided percutaneous ethanol injection for treatment of thyroid cysts versus solid thyroid nodules. *AJR Am J Roentgenol*. 2003;180:1723–1726.

17. American Institute of Ultrasound in Medicine. AIUM practice guidelines for the performance of a thyroid and parathyroid ultrasound examination. October 2007. Available at: http://www.aium.org/publications/guidelines/thyroid.pdf/. Accessed April 3, 2010.

18. Lin JD, Huang BY, Hsueh C. Application of ultrasonography in thyroid cysts. *J Med Ultrasound*. 2007;15:91–102.

19. Sung JY, Baek JH, Kim YS, et al. One-step ethanol ablation of viscous cystic thyroid nodules. *AJR Am J Roentgenol*. 2008;180:1730–1733.

20. Kim DW, Rho MH, Kim HJ, et al. Percutaneous ethanol injection for benign cystic thyroid nodules: is aspiration of ethanol-mixed fluid advantageous? *AJNR Am J Neuroradiol*. 2005;26:2122–2127.

21. Ahuja A, Chick W, King W, et al. Clinical significance of the comet-tail artifact in thyroid ultrasound. *J Clin Ultrasound*. 1996;24:129–133.

22. Hegedüs L. The thyroid nodule. *N Engl J Med*. 2004;351: 1764–1771.

23. Low SCS, Sinha AK, Sundram FX. Detection of thyroid malignancy in a hot nodule by fluorine-18-fluorodeoxyglucose positron emission tomography. *Singapore Med J*. 2005;46:304–307.

24. Yeung MJ, Serpell JW. Management of the solitary thyroid nodule. *Oncologist*. 2008;13:105–112.

25. Blum M. Chapter 6c-Ultrasonography of the thyroid. *Thyroid Disease Manager*. January 2009. Available at: http://www.thyroidmanager.org. Accessed March 28, 2010.

26. Samuels MH. Evaluation and treatment of sporadic nontoxic goiter—some answers and more questions. *J Clin Endocrinol Metab*. 2001;86:994–997.

27. Papini E, Guglielmi R, Bianchini A, et al. Risk of malignancy in nonpalpable thyroid nodules: predictive value of ultrasound and color-Doppler features. *J Clin Endocrinol Metab*. 2002;87:1941–1946.

28. Jones RE, Brashers VL, Huether SE. Alterations of hormonal regulation. In: McCance KL, Huether SE, eds. *Pathophysiology: The Biologic Basis for Diseases in Adults and Children*. 6th ed. St. Louis, MO: Elsevier Mosby; 2010:727–780.

29. Frequently asked questions: Graves' disease. *National Women's Health Information Center*. January 2006. Available at: http://www.womenshealth.gov/faq/graves-disease.cfm. Accessed April 3, 2010.

30. Brent GA. Clnical practice. Graves' disease. *N Engl J Med*. 2008;358:2594–2605.

31. Brix TH, Kyvik KO, Christensen K, et al. Evidence for a major role of heredity in Graves' disease: a population-based study of two Danish twin cohorts. *J Clin Endocrinol Metab*. 2001;86:930–934.

32. Baldini M, Orsatti A, Bonfanti MT, et al. Relationship between the sonographic appearance of the thyroid and the clinical course and autoimmune activity of Graves' disease. *J Clin Ultrasound.* 2005;33:381–385.

33. Hoang JK, Lee WK, Lee M, et al. US features of thyroid malignancy: pearls and pitfalls. *Radiographics.* 2007;27:847–865.

34. Neale DM, Cootauco AC, Burrow G. Thyroid disease in pregnancy. *Clin Perinatol.* 2007;34:543–557.

35. Roti E, Uberti ED. Post-partum thyroiditis—a clinical update. *Eur J Endocrinol.* 2002;146:275–279.

36. Iannuccilli JD, Cronan JJ, Monchik JM. Risk for malignancy of thyroid nodules as assessed by sonographic criteria: the need for biopsy. *J Ultrasound Med.* 2004;23:1455–1464.

37. Hong Y, Liu X, Li Z, et al. Real-time ultrasound elastography in the differential diagnosis of benign and malignant thyroid nodules. *J Ultrasound Med.* 2009;28:861–867.

38. Chan BK, Desser TS, McDougall IR, et al. Common and uncommon sonographic features of papillary thyroid carcinoma. *J Ultrasound Med.* 2003;22:1083–1090.

39. Frates MC, Benson CB, Doubilet PM, et al. Prevalence and distribution of carcinoma in patients with solitary and multiple thyroid nodules on sonography. *J Clin Endocrinol Metab.* 2006;91:3411–3417.

40. Kim MJ, Kim EK, Kwak JY, et al. Differentiation of thyroid nodules with macrocalcifications: role of suspicious sonographic findings. *J Ultrasound Med.* 2008;27:1179–1184.

41. Kim BM, Kim MJ, Kim EK, et al. Sonographic differentiation of thyroid nodules with eggshell calcifications. *J Ultrasound Med.* 2008;27:1425–1430.

42. Frates MC, Benson CB, Doubilet PM, et al. Can color Doppler sonography aid in the prediction of malignancy of thyroid nodules? *J Ultrasound Med.* 2003;22:127–131.

43. Alam F, Naito K, Horiguchi J, et al. Accuracy of sonographic elastography in the differential diagnosis of enlarged cervical lymph nodes: comparison with conventional B-mode sonography. *AJR Am J Roentgenol.* 2008;191:604–610.

44. Sohn YM, Kim MJ, Kim EK, et al. Sonographic elastography combined with conventional sonography: how much is it helpful for diagnostic performance? *J Ultrasound Med.* 2009;28:413–420.

45. Pickerell DM. Elastography: imaging of tomorrow? *J Diagn Med Sonogr.* 2010;26:109–113.

46. Yoon JH, Kim EK, Hong SW, et al. Sonographic features of the follicular variant of papillary thyroid carcinoma. *J Ultrasound Med.* 2008;27:1431–1437.

47. Maizlin ZV, Wiseman SM, Vora P, et al. Hürthle cell neoplasms of the thyroid: sonographic appearance and histologic characteristics. *J Ultrasound Med.* 2008;27:751–757.

48. Lee SK, Rho BH, Woo SK. Hürthle cell neoplasm: correlation of gray-scale and power Doppler sonographic findings with gross pathology. *J Clin Ultrasound.* 2010;38:169–176.

49. Kwak JY, Kim EK, Ko KH, et al. Primary thyroid lymphoma: role of ultrasound-guided needle biopsy. *J Ultrasound Med.* 2007;26:1761–1765.

50. Kim MJ, Kim EK, Park SI, et al. US-guided fine-needle aspiration of thyroid nodules: indications, techniques, results. *Radiographics.* 2008;28:1869–1886.

51. Frates MC, Benson CB, Charboneau JW, et al. Management of thyroid nodules detected at ultrasound: Society of Radiologists in Ultrasound consensus conference statement. *Radiology.* 2005;237:794–800.

52. Cooper DS, Doherty GM, Haugen BR, et al. Revised American Thyroid Association management guidelines for patients with thyroid nodules and differentiated thyroid cancer. *Thyroid.* 2009;19:1167–1214.

53. American Cancer Society. Detailed guide: thyroid cancer. May 2009. Available at: http://www.cancer.org/docroot/CRI/CRI_2_3x.asp?dt=43. Accessed June 5, 2010.

54. Scott AM. Thyroid cancer in adults. *Radiol Technol.* 2009;80:241–261.

55. Graham A, Okabe M, Quinlan R. The role of the endoderm in the development and evolution of the pharyngeal arches. *J Anat.* 2005;207:479–487.

56. Huppert BJ, Reading CC. The parathyroid gland. In: Rumack CM, Wilson SR, Charbonneau JW, eds. *Diagnostic Ultrasound.* 3rd ed. Vol 1. St. Louis, MO: Elsevier Mosby; 2005:771–794.

57. Fancy T, Gallagher D III, Hornig JD. Surgical anatomy of the thyroid and parathyroid glands. *Otolaryngol Clin North Am.* 2010;43:221–227.

58. American Association for Clinical Chemistry. PTH: the test. Sep 2007. Available at: http://www.labtestsonline.org/understanding/analytes/pth/test.html. Accessed June 11, 2010.

59. Huether SE. The cellular environment: fluids and electrolytes, acids and bases. In: McCance KL, Huether SE, eds. *Pathophysiology: The Biologic Basis for Diseases in Adults and Children.* 6th ed. St. Louis, MO: Elsevier Mosby; 2010:96–125.

60. Ahuja AT, King AD, King W, et al. Thyroglossal duct cysts: sonographic appearances in adults. *Am J of Neuroradiol.* 1999;20:579–582.

61. Ducic Y. Thyroglossal duct cysts in the elderly population. *Am J Otolaryngol.* 2002;23:17–19.

62. Branstetter BF. Branchial cleft cysts. *Medscape: eMedicine.* March 2009. Available at: http://emedicine.medscape.com/article/382803-overview. Accessed June 24, 2010.

63. Ahuja AT, King AD, Metreweli C. Second branchial cleft cysts: variability of sonographic appearances in adult cases. *AJNR Am J Neuroradiol.* 2000;21:315–319.

64. Lanham PD, Wushensky C. Second branchial cleft cyst mimic: case report. *Am J Neuroradiol.* 2005;26:1862–1864.

65. Murray AD. Deep neck infections. *Medscape: eMedicine.* November 2009. Available at: http://emedicine.medscape.com/article/837048-overview. Accessed June 27, 2010.

66. Craig FW, Schunk JE. Retropharyngeal abscess in children: clinical presentation, utility of imaging, and current management. *Pediatrics.* 2003;111:1394–1398.

67. Turkington JR, Paterson A, Sweeney LE, et al. Neck masses in children. *Br J Radiol.* 2005;78:75–85.

68. Ying M, Ahuja AT. Ultrasound of neck lymph nodes: how to do it and how do they look? *Radiography.* 2006;12:105–117.

69. Ahuja AT, Ying M. Sonographic evaluation of cervical lymph nodes. *AJR Am J Roentgenol.* 2004;184:1991–1699.

70. Ying M, Ahuja A, Wong KT. Ultrasound evaluation of neck lymph nodes. *ASUM Ultrasound Bulletin.* 2003;6:9–17.

71. Lebouleux S, Girard E, Rose M, et al. Ultrasound criteria of malignancy for cervical lymph nodes in patients followed up for differentiated thyroid cancer. *J Clin Endocrinol Metab.* 2007;92:3590–3594.

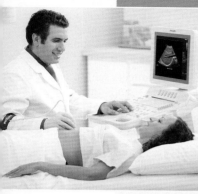

# 16

# The Breast

Catherine Carr-Hoefer

## OBJECTIVES

Discuss sonography's role in the evaluation of the breast.

Explain the indications for sonography of the breast, as well as its advantages and limitations.

Identify other modalities and emerging applications used in breast imaging.

Describe the normal breast anatomy and the corresponding appearance of the sonographic layers.

Demonstrate the sonographic techniques used in evaluating the breast.

Illustrate the annotation methods used in breast sonography.

Explain how patient positioning affects sonomammographic correlation and the techniques used to overcome these differences.

List the characteristics of simple, complicated, and complex breast cysts.

Identify common cystic lesions found in the breast.

Describe inflammatory and traumatic conditions that can affect the breast.

Differentiate the sonographic and mammographic characteristics of benign breast lesions from malignant lesions.

Identify common benign and common malignant breast masses.

Discuss benign and malignant conditions that affect the male breast.

List common sonography guided interventional procedures used to diagnose or treat diseases of the breast.

Discuss the normal appearance and complications that can arise in the augmented breast.

## KEY TERMS

abscess | breast augmentation | breast cyst | breast sonography | colloid carcinoma | complex cyst | complicated cyst | ductal carcinoma in situ | elastography | epidermal inclusion cyst | fat necrosis | fibroadenoma | fibrocystic changes | galactocele | gynecomastia | hamartoma | hematoma | inflammatory carcinoma | intraductal papilloma | invasive ductal carcinoma | invasive lobular carcinoma | lipoma | lobular carcinoma in situ | mammography | mastitis | medullary carcinoma | Mondor disease | Paget disease | papillary apocrine metaplasia | papillary carcinoma | postsurgical scar | sebaceous cyst | seroma | tubular carcinoma | whole-breast sonography

## GLOSSARY

**adenopathy** enlarged lymph nodes

**areola** pigmented skin surrounding the nipple

**axilla** armpit, significant because it contains the lymph nodes that drain the breast tissue

**BI-RADS** Breast Imaging Reporting and Data System; published by the ACR in an effort to promote the use of more consistent terminology when characterizing imaging findings, as well as classifying findings into risk categories for cancer

Recommendations for patient management follow the level of risk

**Cooper ligaments** thin connective tissue bands that connect the breast tissue to the skin and provide structural support to the breast

**desmoplastic reaction** fibroelastic, reactive fibrosis that occurs in the tissues surrounding many malignant breast lesions; often responsible for malignant acoustic shadowing and also contributes to thickening and straightening of the Cooper ligaments that may lead to skin retraction

**echopalpation** a technique used to locate a palpable mass with sonography; the mass is palpated and located between two fingers, the transducer is then placed directly over the palpable area

**elastography** performed in conjunction with two-dimensional sonography; compares the relative "stiffness" of a mass compared to adjacent tissues by measuring the amount of displacement the tissues undergo when compressed; hard lesions (typically malignant) show less deformation (strain) than soft tissues

**in situ noninvasive breast cancer** called carcinoma in situ; the malignant cells are confined within the boundaries of the duct and/or lobule and have not extended past the basement membrane into adjacent tissue, thus virtually eliminating the risk of metastasis

**multicentric breast cancer** coexistent cancers within different quadrants or separated by more than 5 cm within the breast; more likely to be of different histologic types than multifocal cancer

**multifocal breast cancer** the presence of additional malignant lesions within a breast quadrant or within 5 cm of the primary tumor indicating spread of cancer via the ducts

**sentinel node** first node in the drainage basin and at most risk for metastasis; the presence or absence of cancer cells in this node is used in staging the tumor

**spiculation** finger-like extension of a malignant tumor

**terminal ductal lobular unit** the functional unit of the breast; composed of a lobule and its draining extralobular terminal duct; the terminal ductal lobular unit is of histologic importance since most benign and malignant breast diseases arise from this

Sonography is a useful complement to physical examination, mammography, and, more recently, magnetic resonance imaging (MRI) in the assessment of breast disease. The sonography exam provides a real-time tomographic display of the breast without ionizing radiation. Also, the relative comfort of the exam and low cost make sonography an attractive choice for breast evaluation.

Mammography is the most common imaging modality used to evaluate the breast and remains the only widely used screening tool proven effective at reducing breast cancer mortality.[1,2] High-quality mammography is capable of detecting suspicious patterns of microcalcifications, which is typically the first imaging sign of a developing malignancy.[3–6] Early cancer detection and treatment improves long-term survival by decreasing the incidence of lymph node involvement and metastasis to distant sites. Although digital mammography has improved pathology detection in certain breast types, mammography still has some diagnostic limitations. It cannot detect all breast masses. Lesions are more readily detected in a radiolucent, fatty breast and can be obscured in a radiopaque dense breast. Mammography alone cannot directly determine whether a mass is cystic or solid. Localization of a mass is difficult if seen on only one radiographic view. Occasionally, superimposition of a focal area of normal tissues can create a pseudomass, which may be hard to differentiate from a real lesion on standard mammography. Additionally, radiographic features of some breast malignancies are similar to those of benign masses, so the level of diagnostic confidence is reduced.

For these reasons, adjunctive imaging tests are often recommended for breast evaluation in certain patients. When used in addition to mammography or physical examination, high-resolution sonography often improves diagnostic accuracy and assists in appropriate patient management.

## CLINICAL ROLE OF BREAST SONOGRAPHY[4,6–13]

Table 16-1 summarizes the indications and advantages of sonographic evaluation of the breast. Sonography's proven ability to differentiate between cystic and solid masses allows palpable and radiographically indeterminate lesions to be characterized before invasive tests are considered. Dense fibroglandular tissue can hinder mass detection on a mammogram. Conversely, solid lesions are more evident on a sonogram when contrasted against hyperechoic fibroglandular tissue than in a less echogenic fat-replaced breast. Sonography serves as the primary nonionizing imaging modality used to evaluate symptomatic patients who are young, pregnant, or lactating, which are patient groups often associated with increased breast density that compromises radiographic evaluation.

Because sonography allows a tomographic display of the breast without painful compression, it is useful for examining patients with breast trauma, inflammatory changes, augmentation mammoplasty, or postirradiation changes. Sonography can also help evaluate the male breast for physiologic or pathologic changes. Mammography is often difficult to perform on these patients.

Sonographic guidance is highly useful during the performance of interventional and therapeutic breast procedures. High-resolution, real-time sonography can assist needle placement during aspiration or biopsy procedures, affording direct visualization of the needle

**TABLE 16-1**

## Breast Sonography: Clinical Role

| Indications | Advantages |
|---|---|
| • Characterization of palpable breast mass or symptomatic abnormality<br>• Characterization of mass or suspected abnormality detected on recent imaging test (e.g., mammography, magnetic resonance imaging)<br>• Initial imaging test before age 30 and in pregnant or lactating female<br>• Evaluation of breast for clinical concern when mammography is compromised or contraindicated (e.g., dense breast, inflammation, trauma, irradiation, male breast)<br>• Evaluation of augmented breast<br>• Guidance during interventional procedures<br>• Treatment planning for radiation therapy | • Noninvasive, painless<br>• Nonionizing examination<br>• Tomographic display<br>• Real-time imaging and needle-guidance<br>• Cyst versus solid mass differentiation<br>• Mass detection in radiographically dense breast<br>• Chest wall imaging<br>• Doppler capabilities<br>• Mass localization when seen on one mammographic view<br>• No contrast injection (compared to magnetic resonance imaging)<br>• Low cost; widely available |

**Areas of Research[2,27]**

• Supplemental screening in high-risk patient with radiographically dense breast
• Evaluation for occult axillary lymph node metastasis in breast cancer patient

tip as it approaches and enters the mass. Evacuation of cystic lesions, drainage of abscess cavities, and sampling of solid masses can be observed and confirmed. Clip placement to mark the site of mass location after tissue sampling or in conjunction with cancer therapy planning can be performed using sonographic guidance. Additionally, the real-time capability makes sonography a valuable guidance tool during radiofrequency (RF) ablation and other therapeutic interventions.

Although sonography is useful in a number of clinical settings, there are limitations that should be recognized. The diagnostic quality of a sonographic breast examination is very operator and equipment dependent. Some small solid masses that are isoechoic to fat can be missed by sonography although easily seen by mammography. As with other imaging modalities, differentiation between some benign and malignant solid lesions is less reliable when imaging patterns are similar. Even some normal structures and imaging artifacts (e.g., costal cartilage, Copper ligament shadowing) can be mistaken for pathology by an inexperienced breast imager. Newer high-frequency broadband transducers, harmonic imaging, spatial compounding, and advanced processing techniques have increased sonography's ability to assess lesion characteristics and to detect microcalcifications. However, the thin image planes and limitations in resolution restrict sonography's ability to assess the exact size, shape, and distribution patterns of microcalcifications that are readily detectable by mammography. Limitation in detecting suspicious calcifications is a reason why sonography is not approved as a primary breast cancer screening tool; however, sonography and contrast-enhanced MRI are used as supplemental screening

tools to detect occult cancers in high-risk women with radiographically dense breasts when the efficacy of mammography is reduced.[2,14–18]

New and emerging advancements in sonographic imaging such as whole breast scanners, three-dimensional (3D) imaging,[18] elastography,[19] as well as computer-assisted detection (CAD)[20] programs are just some of the progressive changes that hope to enhance sonography's role in breast pathology recognition and diagnosis.

## ANATOMY[3,8,11,21–23]

The breasts, or mammary glands, are paired, dome-shaped structures lying along the anterior chest wall adjacent to the axilla (Fig. 16-1). The primary function of these modified sweat glands is to produce milk to nourish maternal offspring.

The skin, nipple, and areola comprise the external surface of the breast. The outer epidermis and underlying dermis of the skin contain hair follicles, sebaceous, and sweat glands. The nipple is a round fibromuscular papilla projecting from the center of the breast that is encircled by the pigmented areola. Small bumps on the areola mark the sites of sebaceous glands (Montgomery glands), which secrete an oily substance to lessen drying and cracking of the nipple during breastfeeding.

The female breast is primarily composed of glandular, fatty, and fibrous connective tissues that vary in proportion based on the individual's age and hormonal status. The glandular elements of the breast primarily function to produce and transport milk. The stromal elements consist of fat, fibrous connective tissues, as well as blood vessels, lymphatics, and nerves.

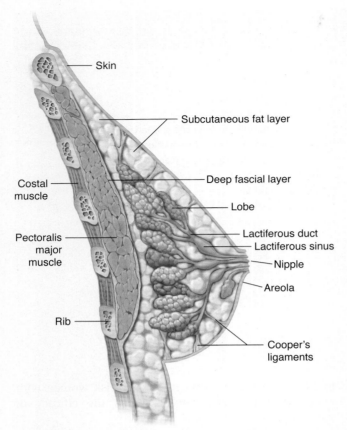

**Figure 16-1** The anatomic sectional illustration demonstrates the major anatomic components of the adult female breast and chest wall.

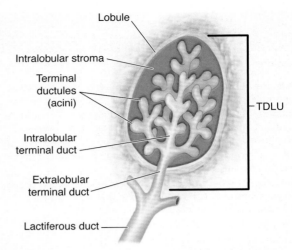

**Figure 16-2** Terminal ductolobular unit (TDLU). A TDLU is composed of an extralobular terminal duct and a lobule. Each breast lobe contains numerous TDLUs. (Reprinted with permission from Carr-Hoefer C. Breast Ultrasound for the Sonomammographer. Corvallis, Sound Imaging Consulting, LLC, 2007.)

Between the skin and chest wall, the breast is subdivided by fascial planes into three layers: the subcutaneous fat layer; the mammary (parenchymal) layer; and the retromammary fat layer. The terms applied to these divisions vary in the literature (Table 16-2).

The parenchyma (fibroglandular tissue) contains the functional glandular elements of the breast and supporting connective tissues. Within this "mammary layer" are 15 to 20 overlapping lobes arranged in a radial fashion around the nipple. Each lobe contains 20 to 40 terminal ductolobular units (TDLUs), which are the functional units of the breast. A TDLU is composed of a lobule and its draining extralobular terminal duct. Each lobule contains an

intralobular portion of the terminal duct that drains numerous, small terminal ductules (Fig. 16-2). During late pregnancy, these ductules transform into tiny sac-like, milk-producing glands called *acini* or *alveoli* that involute after the lactation period ceases. Each lobe has a branching network of lactiferous ducts that transport milk from the TDLUs to the nipple. Smaller subsegmental and segmental ducts join to form a main lactiferous duct that becomes progressively larger. One major lactiferous duct empties each breast lobe and extends radially toward the nipple. Beneath the areola, the main duct focally enlarges at the ampulla or lactiferous sinus, which serves as a reservoir for milk during breastfeeding. Some major ducts from the lobes may join at the sinus level before exiting as excretory ducts through tiny openings at the summit of the nipple.

The ducts are lined by an inner epithelial cell layer and an underlying myoepithelial cell layer. The myoepithelial cells contract to help transfer milk out of the TDLUs during lactation. Breast ducts are surrounded by a basement membrane that separates ductal structures from adjacent tissues.

The TDLU is of histologic importance since most benign and malignant breast diseases arise from this structure. The majority of the glandular tissue lies in the upper outer quadrant (UOQ) of the breast. The TDLUs are typically confined to the mammary layer; however, a TDLU may occasionally project between a Cooper ligament into the superficial breast. A portion of mammary tissue may also extend into the axilla, forming the axillary tail of Spence.

The breast stroma helps provide support to the breast. Adipose tissue (fat) is found in the subcutaneous and retromammary layers and fills out the spaces between the lobes and lobules. Although the breast slides easily over the pectoralis major muscle, the gland itself is firmly attached to the skin by thin connective tissue bands known as *Cooper ligaments*. These suspensory ligaments extend radially from the deep fascia to the skin enclosing fat lobules and

| TABLE 16-2 |
| --- |
| Breast Layers and Major Fascial Planes |

From anterior to posterior beneath skin layer:

- Subcutaneous fat layer = Subcutaneous Zone = Premammary Zone
- *Superficial layer of superficial fascia = anterior mammary fascia = premammary fascia*
- Parenchymal (fibroglandular) layer = Mammary layer = Mammary Zone
- *Deep layer of superficial fascia = posterior mammary fascia = retromammary fascia*
- Retromammary fat layer = Retromammary Zone

providing structural support to the breast. Interlobular stromal tissue and Cooper ligaments make up the dense connective tissue. Hormonally responsive, loose intralobular stroma surrounds the smaller ducts of the lobule. Loose periductal fibrous tissue surrounds the larger ducts.

Posterior to the breast and pectoral fascia are muscles that separate the breast tissue from the chest wall. The pectoralis major muscle lies beneath the upper two-thirds of the breast. The smaller pectoralis minor muscle lies beneath the major muscle. The serratus anterior muscle extends under the lateral breast. The external oblique muscle is beneath a portion of the lower outer breast and the rectus abdominis abuts part of the lower inner breast.

The primary arterial blood supply to the breast is from branches of the internal mammary and lateral thoracic arteries and, to a lesser extent, the thoracoacromial and intercostal arteries. Arterial anastomoses occur beneath the areola.

Venous drainage is through superficial and deep networks. Venous anastomosis occurs in a circular pattern around the base of the areola. Deep veins follow the path of the arteries to drain the breast.

Lymph vessels originate in the connective tissues near the lactiferous ducts and communicate with the subareolar plexus. Lymph drainage is from deep to superficial networks. Numerous lymphatics lie under the skin. Lymph vessels drain into lymph nodes and follow venous drainage pathways out of the breast. Small intramammary lymph nodes are found within the breast, especially in the UOQ and near the axilla. The majority of breast lymph drains into the axillary lymph nodes, with lesser drainage to the internal mammary (parasternal) nodes, interpectoral (Rotter) nodes, and the supraclavicular nodes. Some lymph vessels drain to the opposite breast, toward the diaphragm, or to abdominal nodes. Axillary lymph nodes can be classified by anatomic location or by surgical level (Table 16-3). For surgical and staging purposes, the axillary nodes are subdivided by level relative to the pectoralis minor muscle.

The nerves of the breast are located along the skin and within the glandular tissue. Superficial sensory

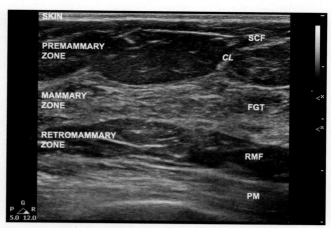

**Figure 16-3** Normal adult female breast. Sonogram demonstrates the skin layer, the subcutaneous fat (*SCF*), and Copper ligament (*CL*) within the premammary zone; fibroglandular tissue (*FGT*) within the mammary zone; retromammary fat (*RMF*) within the retromammary zone; and the pectoralis major muscle (*PM*). The mammary zone is encased within the anterior and posterior mammary fascial planes. (Image courtesy of Philips Medical Systems, Bothell, WA.)

nerves join the cervical, brachial, and intercostal nerves. Glandular nerves are derived from branches of the lateral and anterior cutaneous branches of the second to sixth intercostal (thoracic) nerves.

## SONOGRAPHIC ANATOMY

The anatomic components of the breast are easily demonstrated by high-resolution sonography. The appearance of the normal female breast varies widely from patient to patient and depends on the relative amounts of fat, connective, and glandular tissue in the scanning plane. Unlike mammography, sonography allows sectional evaluation of the breast, one "slice" at a time, from the skin surface to the chest wall allowing delineation of all breast layers (Fig. 16-3).

The skin layer is seen as two thin, reflective bands encasing a band of medium-level echoes representing

| TABLE 16-3 | |
|---|---|
| **Classifications of Axillary Lymph Nodes** | |
| **Anatomic Classification** | **Surgical Classification** |
| • External mammary (**anterior; pectoral**) group: Inferiorly located near lateral thoracic vessels; receives most lymph drainage | • Level I nodes: low axillary nodes lying lateral to the pectoralis minor muscle |
| • Subscapular (**posterior**) group: near posterior margin of axilla and lateral scapula by subscapular vessels | • Level II nodes: midaxillary nodes lying beneath the pectoralis minor muscle |
| • Axillary vein (**lateral**) group: most lateral group; posterior to axillary vein | • Level III nodes: high axillary nodes lying medial to the pectoralis minor muscle |
| • **Central** group: center of axilla medial to axillary vessels; most easily palpated | |
| • Subclavicular (**apical**) group: medial and superior to pectoralis minor muscle near subclavian vessels | |
| • Interpectoral (**Rotter's**) group: between pectoralis major and minor muscles; by pectoral branch of thoracoacrominal artery | |

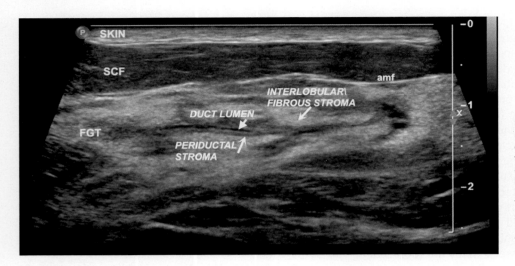

**Figure 16-4** Fibroglandular tissue *(FGT)*. The echogenicity of the peri-ductal tissue and intralobular fibrous tissue is nearly isoechoic to fat. The dense interlobular fibrous tissue is hyperechoic to fat. Anechoic fluid is present within the duct lumen. The anterior mammary fascia *(amf)* separates the FGT in the mammary zone from the subcutaneous fat *(SCF)*. (Image courtesy of Philips Medical Systems, Bothell, WA.)

the dermis. Scanning through an acoustic offset better delineates the skin. Normal skin thickness is usually 2 mm or less but can be slightly thicker near the areola and inframammary fold. The hyperechoic interface between the skin and subcutaneous fat should be intact. Changes in skin contour and thickness may indicate neoplastic, traumatic, postirradiation, or inflammatory changes at or below the skin surface.

The nipple displays a homogeneous texture of medium-level echoes. Connective tissue within the nipple and the irregular contour of the nipple–areolar complex can cause acoustic shadowing. Probe compression and the use of ample scanning gel will flatten the nipple and reduce trapped air pockets to lessen shadowing. Transducer angulation beneath the nipple, the use of spatial compound imaging, or utilizing the two-handed peripheral scanning technique allows better evaluation of subareolar structures.

The subcutaneous fat layer lies between the skin and the mammary layer and does not extend beneath the nipple. When equipment settings are properly set, the echogenicity of fat will be a midlevel gray shade. Blood vessels within the subcutaneous fat layer are easily compressed by transducer pressure. Cooper ligaments are best seen in the subcutaneous layer and imaged as thin, hyperechoic, curvilinear bands ascending toward the skin and encasing the fat lobules. At times, streaks of acoustic shadowing are seen at oblique interfaces from these connective tissue ligaments, caused by refraction of the sound beam.

The mammary (parenchymal) layer lies deep to the subcutaneous fat and is enclosed between the reflective interfaces of the anterior (superficial) and posterior (deep) mammary fascia. The anterior fascia may appear smooth but is often scalloped as leaflets merge anteriorly into Cooper ligaments. In the adult breast, the mammary layer has the greatest variation in echo pattern depending on the distribution of glandular, fibrous, and fatty tissues. Dense stromal fibrous tissue is very

hyperechoic relative to fat, whereas glandular (periductal; lobular) tissue is nearly isoechoic to fat (Fig. 16-4). Tubular fluid-filled ducts may be seen radiating from the nipple and into the breast core (Fig. 16-5). Major lactiferous ducts are best imaged with radial scans. Generally, ducts measure 2 mm or less but are often larger at the lactiferous sinus and during lactation.

The retromammary fat layer lies between the posterior mammary fascia and the pectoralis major muscle. The retromammary layer contains smaller fat lobules and appears thinner on a sonogram than the subcutaneous fat layer.

The pectoralis major muscle lies immediately posterior to most of the breast. The pectoralis minor muscle lies beneath the major muscle in a more superolateral location. These muscles appear as striated hypoechoic to hyperechoic linear bands of echoes parallel to the chest wall. The pectoral fascia planes produce bright, linear echoes on both sides of the muscles. Recognition of the pectoral major muscle is important to confirm ample ultrasound penetration of the breast and to

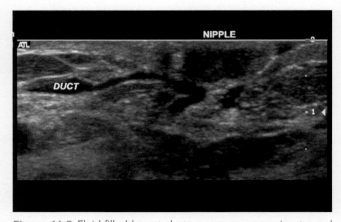

**Figure 16-5** Fluid-filled breast ducts are seen converging toward the nipple. Spatial compounding reduces artifact and helps to better delineate superficial structures. (Image courtesy of Philips Medical Systems, Bothell, WA.)

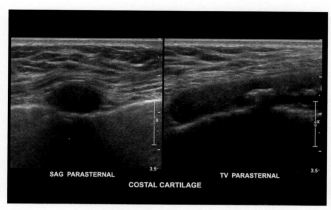

Figure 16-6 Costal cartilage. Rib cartilage can be mistaken for a hypoechoic mass when scanning in the sagittal scan plane near the sternum. Rotating the transducer 90 degrees shows the linear extent of the cartilage and connection to the rib.

help determine whether a deep lying cancer is invading through the pectoral fascia.

Deep to the pectoral muscles are the ribs and intercostal muscle of the thoracic cage. Laterally, the bony portion of the ribs attenuates the sound beam, resulting in acoustic shadowing. Medially, the costal cartilage of the ribs appears as oval structures containing low-level echoes seen best on sagittal scans (Fig. 16-6). Care must be taken not to mistake the cartilaginous portion of the ribs for a breast mass. Rotating the transducer in orthogonal scan planes will confirm the cartilage is not a mass. The hyperechogenic interface beneath the chest wall demarcates total sound reflection from the lung.

Normal lymph nodes can be imaged by sonography, especially in the axilla. Normal intramammary nodes are less often detected. The size of a normal intramammary node is typically less than 1 cm, but axillary nodes can be much larger. Nodes are oval or reniform in shape, well-circumscribed, oriented parallel to the skin, and display a symmetric hypoechoic outer cortex and a hyperechoic fatty hilum (Fig. 16-7). Color

Doppler reveals a main feeding vessel entering the hilum. Axillary nodes containing mostly fat with only a thin hypoechoic cortical rim may be difficult to delineate from adjacent structures. Enlarged lymph nodes may indicate inflammatory or neoplastic change.

## VARIATIONS IN NORMAL PATTERNS

The proportionate amount of stromal and glandular tissues in the female breast depends on the patient's age, parity, and whether she is premenopausal or postmenopausal, pregnant or lactating, or obese. The prepubertal breast is small and fatty. At puberty, estrogen and progesterone stimulate breast development by promoting duct growth and lobular development. The adolescent breast becomes increasingly glandular becoming isoechoic to mildly hyperechoic to fat, while the amount of surrounding fat diminishes.

The adult breast has the greatest range of appearances. Characteristically, the young, nulliparous female breast is densely glandular, with little internal or surrounding fat. Over time, more hyperechoic fibrous stroma is apparent within the mammary zone that can partially attenuate the sound beam. With increasing age and number of pregnancies, fatty replacement of the parenchyma begins to occur. Isolated, hypoechoic fat lobules in the mammary layer may appear "mass like" compared to the more echogenic surrounding fibroglandular tissue; however, fat lobules are very compressible and often merge into other fat lobules on the orthogonal scan plane.

In the breast of the pregnant or lactating woman, glandular tissue practically fills the breast, compressing the surrounding fat. Acini within the breast lobules develop and begin milk secretion in response to hormones that include placental lactose, chorionic gonadotropin, and prolactin. The overall texture of this glandular parenchyma is weakly echogenic. Duct dilatation may be marked during late pregnancy and lactation (Fig. 16-8).

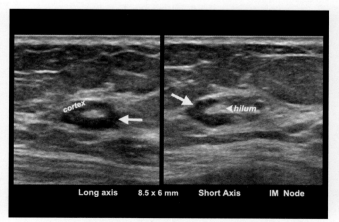

Figure 16-7 Normal intramammary lymph node. This small, circumscribed, oval node displays a hypoechoic cortex and hyperechoic fatty hilum. The cortex has a "C-shape" appearance in cross section.

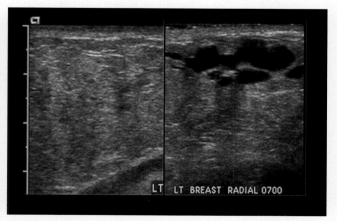

Figure 16-8 Lactating breast. Nearly isoechoic glandular parenchyma fills the breast with little surrounding fat. Dilated milk-filled subareolar ducts are present. (From Carr-Hoefer C. *Breast Ultrasound: A Comprehensive Sonographer's Guide.* Forney, TX: Pegasus Lectures; 2007.)

The postmenopausal breast may show complete or nearly complete fatty replacement as the lobules and ducts atrophy as hormonal influences decline. Cooper ligaments are easily seen encasing the fat lobules. However, older, nulliparous women or those on hormone replacement therapy (HRT) may retain considerable amounts of glandular tissue.

## DEVELOPMENTAL ANOMALIES

In both genders, breast development begins in utero along bilateral ectodermal milk lines that extend from the axilla to the inguinal region.[8,24] Although there are several points along the milk lines for breast tissue to develop, one paired set of breasts grow from mammary ridges located in the thoracic region. Rudimentary ducts arising from epithelial breast buds are present in both females and males at the time of birth. In the neonate, there may be some transient breast enlargement and milky nipple discharge due to residual circulating maternal hormones.

Developmental anomalies of the breast are uncommon.[8-25] Some are associated with abnormal endocrine gland development or hormonal dysfunction and may not become apparent until puberty. Congenital nipple inversion is a normal variant. An accessory nipple (polythelia) is the most common congenital breast anomaly. A complete accessory breast (polymastia) is rare. These supernumerary anomalies can occur anywhere along the milk line. Accessory breast tissue in the axilla (without a nipple) is occasionally present. Underdevelopment (hypoplasia) or excessive growth (hypertrophy) of the breast tissue may affect one or both breasts. Complete failure of the breast tissue to develop is called *amastia*. This rare condition is typically accompanied by congenital absence of the nipple (athelia). Poland syndrome is associated with underdevelopment or absence of the breast, nipple, and chest muscles.[24] *Amazia* refers to absence of breast tissue development although the nipple is present. This acquired condition may be secondary to excessive chest wall radiation or inadvertent excision of premature breast tissue development in a child.

Before the age of 8 years, growth of one breast occasionally occurs before the other. By puberty, however, both breasts are usually comparable in size and development.[24] This variant, referred to as unilateral early ripening or unilateral premature thelarche, should not be mistaken for pathology and do not necessitate excision. Early developing glandular tissue images as a small, mildly hypoechoic region under the nipple corresponding to the palpable region of subareolar nodularity.

If development of both breasts occurs before 8 years of age, precocious puberty is suspected. Causes are varied. Sonographic signs of precocious puberty may include ovarian enlargement with prominent follicular cysts, the presence of a hormone-secreting ovarian tumor (e.g., granulosa-theca cell tumor), a large-for-age uterus, or an adrenal tumor.[24,26]

## BREAST SONOGRAPHIC EXAMINATION AND INSTRUMENTATION

Before scanning, the indication for the exam, as well as any pertinent prior mammograms, breast sonograms, and MRIs are reviewed. The clinical history and the location of palpable masses, biopsy scars, and other changes of the skin, nipple, and breast contour are documented. Correlation of clinical and relevant imaging tests with the sonographic findings is imperative so the interpreting physician can more accurately assign a risk classification, provide a differential diagnosis, and make recommendations for patient management.

The American College of Radiology (ACR) and the American Institute of Ultrasound in Medicine (AIUM) are accrediting organizations that have published practice guidelines and minimum equipment requirements for the performance of breast sonography.[7,27,28] Proper transducer selection, equipment setup, patient positioning, and scanning technique are essential to produce high-quality images.

### Transducer Requirements

Based on current ACR and AIUM guidelines, a high-resolution, linear-array, real-time transducer with a center frequency of at least 10 MHz is suitable for breast sonography.[7,28] Breast sonography systems need to provide excellent spatial and contrast resolution.[6,29] High-frequency, broad bandwidth transducers provide better spatial and contrast resolution than those with lower frequencies and narrower bandwidths. Broad bandwidth transducers with frequency ranges of 8 to 12 MHz are common and provide excellent detail of the breast. Lower frequencies allow better penetration of attenuative tissues and deep lying structures, whereas higher frequencies enhance image resolution and optimize detail of more superficial structures. Some newer transducers offer frequencies up to 17 MHz that further enhance near-field imaging. During the examination, the highest frequency capable of adequate sound penetration of the region of interest should be used.

### Equipment and Gray Scale Settings

Equipment settings must be optimized to display an image that clearly demonstrates all breast tissue from the skin line to the chest wall or for the selected region of interest. Important system controls include output power, time gain compensation (TGC), overall gain, dynamic range, as well as optimization of focal zones, image size, and depth.

Appropriate gray scale setup is important for breast sonography. The gain settings, dynamic range, and processing curves should be set so normal breast fat displays a medium-level gray shade.[4,6,26,29,30] Using accepted ACR lexicon,[30] the echogenicity of other breast structures and masses are described as being hypoechoic, isoechoic, or hyperechoic compared to fat. Correct TCG settings will allow normal breast fat to be displayed with the same

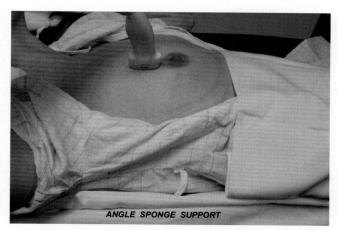

Figure 16-9 Supine-oblique patient positioning. The side to be examined is elevated by a foam support and the patient's arm is positioned near the head. This contralateral oblique position helps flatten the breast tissue over the chest. The transducer is at the 12 o'clock radial position. (Reprinted with permission from Carr-Hoefer C. Breast Ultrasound for the Sonomammographer. Corvallis, Sound Imaging Consulting, LLC, 2007.)

echogenicity within the subcutaneous, mammary, and retromammary breast layers.

## Patient Positioning

Patient positioning during breast sonography can vary depending on breast size, mass location, or as needed for sonomammographic correlation. In general, the patient should be positioned in a manner that minimizes the thickness of the portion of the breast being examined.

The patient is typically placed in a "supine-oblique" or "contralateral-oblique" position[6,10,26,29] (Fig. 16-9). This is accomplished by rolling the supine patient approximately 30 to 45 degrees, allowing placement of a wedge support to elevate the side of the body to be examined. The adjacent arm is extended near the head, which helps to stabilize the breast and provides access to the axillary region. The breast should appear flattened with the nipple centered. The reduction in breast thickness allows sound penetration by higher frequencies and orients major tissue planes more parallel to the face of the transducer optimizing sound beam reflection. This patient positioning can be used to scan the entire breast but is particularly useful when examining the outer breast. Steeper obliquity may be needed to scan large breasts or very lateral lesions. A straight supine position is often preferred when examining medial lesions.

Sometimes, a patient can only feel a mass while in a specific position. Scanning the patient in that position allows correlation of clinical and sonographic findings. For more accurate sonomammographic correlation of breast masses, it may be helpful to scan certain patients in positions that simulate the mammographic views. (See section on Sonographic–Mammographic Correlation.)

## Scan Procedure and Technique

Based on site protocol and indication, either a targeted exam or a whole-breast sonographic examination is performed utilizing a hand-held, high-resolution transducer. A targeted study is limited to the quadrant or region of clinical concern, such as for a palpable mass, or to further characterize a mammographic or MRI finding. Some indications for a whole breast exam include the search for satellite lesions and lymph node involvement in a patient with a known cancer or suspicious lesion, to screen a high-risk patient with radiographically dense breasts, to follow-up multiple masses, or to evaluate implant integrity.

Prior to scanning, the patient is properly positioned and a warm scanning gel is applied to the skin. The breast is methodically surveyed in overlapping orthogonal (perpendicular) scan planes with special attention paid to areas of concern.

The skin overlying a palpable mass can be marked prior to scanning or the location confirmed during the exam by echopalpation.[6,8] During echopalpation, the sonographer secures the palpable area between two fingers while scanning directly over the lump. This allows direct correlation of clinical and sonographic findings. The image should be labeled as the "palpable" region of interest.

Use of an acoustic standoff between the transducer and the breast improves delineation of the skin and superficial breast by optimizing near-field focusing and reducing artifacts. In most cases, extra scanning gel is a sufficient standoff. When a standoff pad is used, the thickness of the acoustic offset should not exceed 1 cm so that the focal plane (elevation focus) is not shifted out of the breast.[6,29]

Besides traditional sagittal and transverse scans, radial and antiradial scan planes are of particular value during breast imaging[6,8,9,29] (Fig. 16-10A,B). Radial scans are often best for examining major lactiferous ducts or for documenting mass location relative to the nipple. Scanning the entire volume of a solid breast mass in both radial and antiradial planes can increase detection of tumor extension coursing toward the nipple within a major duct or branching outward into smaller ducts.

Scanning with a variety of beam angles is needed to fully evaluate the margin characteristics of a mass. This

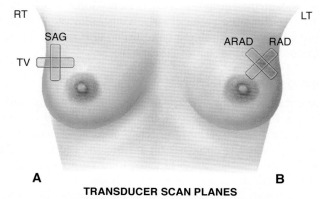

TRANSDUCER SCAN PLANES

Figure 16-10 Orthogonal scan planes. A: Schematic of traditional sagittal (SAG) and transverse (TV) scan planes. B: Radial (RAD) and antiradial (ARAD) scan planes.

can be accomplished by rocking and angling the transducer and by using spatial compounding. Enlarging the image to the region of interest and focusing at the level of the mass allows better inspection of mass features.

During the breast examination, applying variable amounts of transducer pressure to compress the underlying tissues is beneficial for a variety of reasons. Compression decreases breast thickness for better sound penetration by higher frequencies. Applying transducer pressure flattens Cooper ligaments to reduce critical angle shadowing. Compression will also reduce or eliminate false acoustic shadowing beneath a benign lesion or scar tissue, whereas malignant shadowing tends to persist. Applying and releasing transducer pressure assesses the compressibility and the mobility of breast masses, as well as the movement of internal echoes in complicated cysts and dilated ducts. In contrast, too much transducer pressure is detrimental during Doppler evaluation since vessel compression can reduce or ablate blood flow.

Key lesions should be documented with and without caliper measurements.[7,30] Minimally, the maximal dimensions of a mass should be recorded in two orthogonal planes. Maximal dimensions, rather than mean diameter, correlate better with mammographic measurements. Obtaining sonographic measurements in three dimensions (maximal length, height, width) allows for more accurate comparison of lesion size on follow-up imaging or after intervention. For example, three dimensions allow the calculation of volume or mean diameter when assessing an interval change in tumor size following induction chemotherapy. Length-to-height ratios determine if a lesion is "wider than tall" or "taller than wide" when assessing benign and malignant imaging characteristics.

Obtaining a comparison scan of the opposite breast in the same region can be helpful when sorting out questionable findings and helps to contrast inflammatory or traumatic changes with the normal breast.

Based on site protocol, representative images are made of each scanned breast quadrant, the subareolar region, and of all important findings. Images are appropriately labeled and archived on film or in a digital picture archiving and communication system (PACS) for physician interpretation and review. Some PACSs can archive dynamic cine clips showing full sweeps of the breast tissue, pathologic conditions, and needle placement during interventional exams.

## Image Annotation[6–10,29,30]

Accurate labeling of each image should include side (right or left) location in the breast, as well as the transducer scan plane in order to accurately document findings for the interpreting physician. Proper image annotation is also important for follow-up comparison and to relocate a mass prior to intervention.

Common image labeling methods include the quadrant or clock-face position (Fig. 16-11). Many systems provide a breast body marker to document transducer

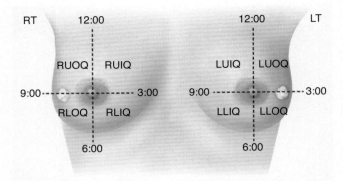

**QUADRANT AND CLOCK-FACE ANNOTATION**

**Figure 16-11** Quadrant and clock-face image annotation. Upper outer quadrant (*UOQ*); upper inner quadrant (*UIQ*); lower inner quadrant (*LIQ*); lower outer quadrant (*LOQ*). Using the clock-face annotation, a mass lateral to the nipple in the right breast is located at 9 o'clock (RT 9:00), whereas a mass lateral to the nipple in the left breast is located at 3 o'clock (LT 3:00).

position and scan plane. Using the clock-face annotation method, a mass directly lateral to the nipple in the left breast can be labeled, "LT 3:00," whereas a mass lateral to the nipple in the right breast can be labeled "RT 9:00." ACR guidelines also recommend including distance from the nipple. Placing a piece of tape with centimeter marks along the side of the transducer can be a useful guide when estimating the distance between the nipple and the center of a mass. An image annotated "RT 9:00 5 cm FN" or "R 9 N+5" would indicate the right breast mass is located 5 cm lateral to the nipple. The scan plane can be added to the annotation: SAG (sagittal) or LONG (longitudinal), TV (transverse), RAD (radial), or AR (antiradial).

Some facilities use the "1-2-3; A-B-C" labeling methods to note the relative distance of a mass from the nipple, as well as the depth within the breast[6,29] (Fig. 16-12).

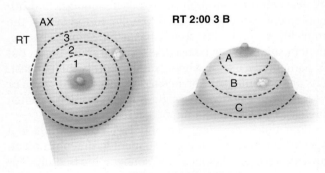

**"1-2-3 A-B-C" ANNOTATION**

**Figure 16-12** 1-2-3–A-B-C annotation. The breast is divided into three concentric rings from the areola to denote the relative distance of a mass from the nipple: *1*, inner third of the breast; *2*, mid third; *3*, outer third of the breast. To denote the relative distance of a mass from the skin to the chest wall, the breast is divided into thirds: *A*, anterior third; *B*, mid third; *C*, posterior third of breast. A peripheral right breast mass at the 2 o'clock position, in the midmammary zone, can be annotated, "RT 2:00 3 B."

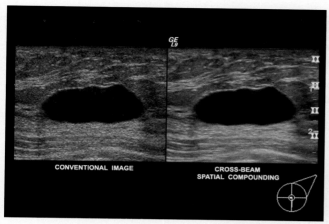

**Figure 16-13** Spatial compounding. Conventional image on the left of a simple breast cyst shows some anterior reverberation artifact. The image on the right is utilizing spatial compounding. Spatial compounding creates a single image from multiple scan angles and improves margin delineation. The reduction in speckle artifact and reverberation produces a smoother image with better contrast resolution. Besides reducing detrimental image artifacts, spatial compounding may also reduce helpful attenuation artifacts. The sonographer should be aware that enhancement beneath a small cyst or subtle shadowing from a cancer may be reduced or eliminated at higher levels of spatial compounding yet be apparent on conventional imaging. Therefore, scanning a region of interest with and without spatial compounding may be necessary. (Image courtesy of GE Healthcare, Milwaukee, WI.)

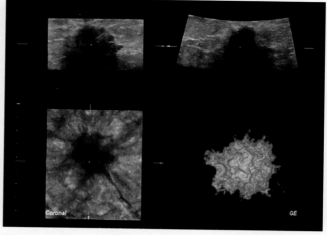

**Figure 16-14** Three-dimensional (3D) sonogram. Malignant spiculation is better appreciated in the coronal plane (bottom left image) that is reconstructed from the 3D data set. A volume rendering of the mass is shown on the bottom right. (Image courtesy of GE Healthcare, Milwaukee, WI.)

## Specialty Techniques

Most current breast sonography systems have split-screen capabilities, extended field-of-view (EFOV), or convex linear (trapezoidal) 2D imaging features that allow larger spans of breast anatomy and masses to be displayed and measured.

Harmonic imaging and spatial compounding are now common features on sonography systems and improve contrast and spatial resolution during breast imaging.[6,29,31] These techniques reduce image artifacts (e.g., speckle, noise, reverberation) and show better margin delineation of masses. These features help make subtle masses, such as small isoechoic lesions, more apparent on the sonogram (Fig. 16-13).

3D imaging provides surface or volume rendering of breast masses that can be further manipulated after completion of the scan. Volume data sets can be viewed in multiple image planes (multiplanar), which is particularly helpful when assessing margin and wall characteristics of solid masses and complex cysts. Reconstructed coronal scans, in particular, can better illustrate some malignant features such as spiculation (Fig. 16-14).

## SONOGRAPHIC–MAMMOGRAPHIC CORRELATION[6,8,29,32–34]

Breast sonography usually follows clinical and mammographic examinations with the hope of providing more specific diagnostic information for appropriate patient management. The breast sonographer must have at least a basic understanding of mammography in order to properly correlate sonographic with mammographic findings. Table 16-4 compares the tissue densities and echogenicities of common breast structures seen on mammography and sonography.

Mammography is performed on asymptomatic patients to screen for occult breast cancer or on symptomatic patients to diagnose a clinical concern. Standard mammographic screening projections are the craniocaudal (CC) and the medial lateral oblique (MLO) views.[4,5,35] Besides these standard views, additional views (e.g., spot compression, magnification, 90 degrees lateral) may be obtained during a diagnostic mammogram to better assess a palpable mass or to further examine an abnormality found on the screening exam.

A mammogram is a superimposed image of breast tissue compressed between the X-ray image receptor and a compression plate. Images are labeled for the specific view and breast side (laterality). For the mammographic CC view, the X-ray tube is oriented vertically over the breast. The breast is positioned so that the X-ray beam enters the superior (cranial) breast and exits the inferior (caudal) breast. With the nipple centered, this view clearly demonstrates the medial, central, and lateral breast (Fig. 16-15). The side marker is always placed by the lateral breast. The MLO view shows the breast in profile from the axilla to the inframammary fold and includes a portion of the pectoralis muscle (Fig. 16-16). Depending on body habitus, the plane of the image receptor for the MLO view is approximately 45 degrees (± 15 degrees) from horizontal to be parallel with the plane of the pectoralis muscle. Unlike a true lateral projection, the X-ray beam passes from the superomedial to the inferolateral aspect of the breast for the MLO projection. The side marker is placed near the axilla at the outer breast. For screening purposes, the

**TABLE  16-4**

## Comparison of Tissue Densities and Echogenicities

| Mammogram Density | Echogenicity |
|---|---|
| **Fat density** (radiolucent–gray) | **Isoechoic/nearly isoechoic** (midlevel gray shade) |
| • Fat | • Fat (reference tissue) |
| • Fat-density mass (e.g., oil cyst; lipoma) | • Lipoma |
| • Fatty hilum of lymph node | • Glandular (epithelial) tissue; adenosis; periductal/lobular tissue |
| | • Certain solid masses and complicated cysts |
| **Water density** (radiodensity greater than fat; described as low, equal, or high density compared to equal volume of fibroglandular tissue) | **Hyperechoic** (more echogenic than normal fat) |
| • Fibroglandular tissues; ducts | • Interlobular stromal fibrous tissue |
| • Blood vessels | • Cooper ligaments |
| • Cooper ligaments | • Skin; fascial interfaces |
| • Cortex of lymph node | • Edematous fat/fibrosis |
| • Solid and cystic masses | • Echogenic pseudocapsule; cyst wall |
| • Pectoralis muscle | • Muscle: striated hyperechoic/hypoechoic bands |
| **Calcium** (appears radiopaque) | **Hypoechoic** (less echogenic than normal fat) |
| • Calcifications | • Nipple |
| | • Complicated fluid; inspissated duct secretions |
| **Special cases: foreign body** (radiopaque) | • Benign/malignant solid mass (some cancers are markedly hypoechoic) |
| • Clip marker | • Lymph node cortex (abnormal nodes may be markedly hypoechoic or nearly anechoic) |
| • Silicone | |
| • Pacemaker | **Anechoic** (without internal echoes) |
| | • Simple cyst; certain fluid collections |
| **Air–VAB Site** (lacks density; appears black) | • Blood; duct secretions; dilated lymphatics |
| **Notes:** | • Saline/silicone implant |
| • Mass density does not differentiate solid from cystic masses | Describe internal characteristics rather than echo drop-out from acoustic shadowing |
| • Mass detection best in fat-replaced breast | |

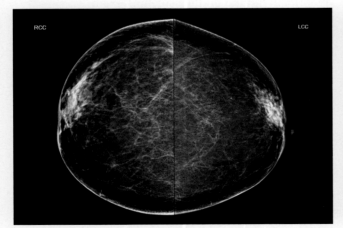

**Figure 16-15** Mammographic craniocaudal *(CC)* view. With the nipple centered, this projection shows the mid, medial, and lateral breast. The side marker is placed by the outer breast.

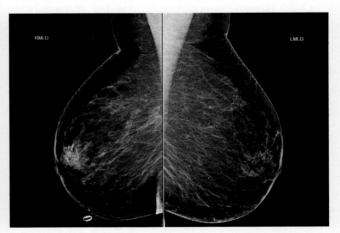

**Figure 16-16** Mammographic medial lateral oblique *(MLO)* view. This projection shows the superior to inferior location of breast structures relative to the posterior nipple line. The lower axilla and radiodense pectoralis muscle is seen on this view. The side marker is always placed by the outer breast near the axilla.

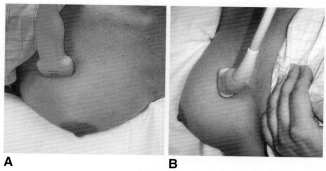

**Figure 16-17** Sonomammographic correlation: positioning options. **A:** Upright positioning can be used to compare the sonography location of a mass to the mammographic craniocaudal view. **B:** Decubital positioning, in this case, is used to access the medial breast to compare relative mass location with the MLO or 90 degrees lateral mammographic views. The patient can be rolled to better access the lateral breast. (Reprinted from Carr-Hoefer C. Breast Ultrasound for the Sonomammographer.)

MLO view shows the greatest amount of UOQ breast tissue and the axillary tail but may exclude some posteromedial tissue. Lower axillary lymph nodes are often visible on this projection.

Differences in technique, patient positioning, and direction of tissue compression between the mammogram and sonogram can affect the relative location, orientation, and shape of a breast mass when correlating imaging findings. During mammographic positioning, breast tissues (and masses) are pulled away from the chest wall. During sonography, structures are pushed toward the chest wall by transducer compression in the anteroposterior (AP) direction.

With the patient supine, it is occasionally difficult to be certain whether a mass seen by sonography is the same mass demonstrated by mammography, especially in larger breasted women. By scanning the patient in a position that simulates the radiographic projection, the sonographic location of a mass can be more accurately correlated with the mammographic findings, although breast tissues will be less compressed. To simulate the CC projection during the sonography examination, the patient can sit upright and use her opposite hand to lift the lower surface of the breast so the nipple is in profile (Fig. 16-17A). The breast can also be lifted and supported on a sponge or tray. After review of the location of the mass on the mammogram, the same area is scanned during the sonography exam. A mass located in the lower quadrants may require scanning from the undersurface of the breast. To simulate the 90-degree lateral or approximate the MLO mammographic views, the patient can lay in a decubital position, so that the breast and nipple is seen are profile (Fig. 16-17B).

## SONOGRAPHIC DESCRIPTORS AND CLASSIFICATION OF FINDINGS

The ACR published the "BI-RADS Breast Ultrasound Lexicon" in an effort to promote the use of more consistent terminology when characterizing sonographic findings[30] (Table 16-5). When applicable, similar terms are applied to mammographic and sonographic findings. The ACR originally developed the Breast Imaging Reporting and Data System (BI-RADS) to standardize the reporting of mammographic findings, as well as classifying findings into risk categories for cancer.[30] The BI-RAD system has more recently been applied to the classification of sonographic and MRI findings. Recommendations for patient management follow the level of risk (Table 16-6).

Breast patients are often referred for sonography examination based on a mammogram report that states: BI-RADS Category 0: incomplete; needs additional imaging evaluation.[30] In such cases, the radiologist will require "more information" before assigning a final risk category. Often, these are cases when a mass or focal asymmetry is present on the mammogram and sonography is needed to further characterize the mass as solid or cystic, as well as provide other diagnostic imaging features that may favor a benign versus a suspicious process.

When a mass is demonstrated by sonography, its imaging characteristics must be carefully examined and documented. A mass occupies space and must be confirmed in orthogonal scan planes.[30] Table 16-5 summarizes these sonographic characteristics. Since mass characterization is also affected by technical factors, adherence to proper scanning technique and equipment setup is critical, as well as recognition of diagnostic pitfalls.

## BREAST DISEASE

A variety of physiologic and pathologic changes affect the breast, many of which have features detectable by imaging techniques. Many of these conditions are reviewed in this chapter.

### BENIGN CYSTIC MASSES AND RELATED CONDITIONS

During the sonographic examination of a breast mass, the first step is to determine if the mass is cystic or solid. Classifying a simple breast cyst is easy when diagnostic criteria are met but can be confusing when cyst fluid is complicated by cellular debris, hemorrhage, or infection. Complex cystic masses that contain solid elements add to diagnostic uncertainty and require additional workup to determine their benign or possibly malignant nature.

#### Simple Cyst

True cysts are epithelial lined fluid-filled masses. Most breast cysts are related to fibrocystic change (FCC) and develop over time from progressive dilatation of small ducts within an obstructed TDLU. Cysts are the most common cause of breast lumps in women 35 to 50 years of age. They can be single or multiple in number and

**TABLE 16-5**

## American College of Radiology BI-RADS Lexicon

**Mass: Occupies space and should be seen in two different projections**
**Terms to describe the dominant features of a mass:**

| Shape | Orientation (relative to skin) | Margin |
|---|---|---|
| ❏ Oval | ❏ Parallel (wider than tall: horizontal orientation) | ❏ Circumscribed |
| ❏ Round | | ❏ Not circumscribed |
| ❏ Irregular (used as a descriptor of shape rather than margin) | ❏ Nonparallel (taller than wide: vertical orientation; or round) | ❏ Indistinct |
| | | ❏ Angular |
| | | ❏ Microlobulated |
| | | ❏ Spiculated |

| Lesion Boundary | Echo Pattern | Posterior Acoustic Features |
|---|---|---|
| ❏ Abrupt interface | ❏ Anechoic | ❏ No posterior acoustic effects |
| ❏ Echogenic halo | ❏ Hyperechoic | ❏ Enhancement |
| | ❏ Complex | ❏ Shadowing |
| | ❏ Hypoechoic | ❏ Combined pattern |
| | ❏ Isoechoic (as compared to fat) | |

| Surrounding Tissues | Calcifications* | Vascularity |
|---|---|---|
| ❏ Duct changes | ❏ Macrocalcifications (≥0.5 mm) | ❏ Not present or assessed |
| ❏ Cooper ligament changes | ❏ Microcalcifications out of a mass (≤0.5 mm; do not shadow) | ❏ Present in lesion |
| ❏ Edema | ❏ Microcalcifications in mass | ❏ Present immediately adjacent to lesion |
| ❏ Architectural distortion | *Calcifications are poorly characterized with ultrasound but can be recognized especially in a mass. | ❏ Diffusely increased vascularity in surrounding tissue |
| ❏ Skin thickening | | |
| ❏ Skin retraction/irregularity | | |

**Special Cases: Those with a unique diagnosis or finding**

❏ Clustered microcysts
❏ Complicated cysts
❏ Mass in or on skin
❏ Foreign body
❏ Lymph nodes—intramammary
❏ Lymph nodes—axillary

Adapted from American College of Radiology BI-RADS US Lexicon Classification Form; 2003. Refer to ACR form for full description of terms: www.acr.org

range from millimeters to several centimeters in size. Ductal secretions and fluid reabsorption contributes to variability in cyst size. With time, most cysts regress or involute. Cysts are uncommon in young or elderly women. However, in postmenopausal women receiving HRT, a cyst may develop, persist, or enlarge.

### Signs and Symptoms

Small and flaccid cysts are often asymptomatic. Tense or enlarging cysts are usually palpable and may be tender. Palpable cysts are typically round or oval, smooth, and freely mobile. Most cysts are compressible unless tense.

Cysts appear as round or oval, smoothly marinated water density masses that may be of slightly higher density than the surrounding parenchyma. These circumscribed masses compress adjacent tissues and are encircled by a thin radiolucent rim referred to as the *halo sign* (Fig. 16-18A). Although findings appear benign, mammography alone cannot tell whether a water-density

lesion is cystic or solid, so a sonography exam is recommended for mass characterization.

### Sonographic Features of a Simple Cyst

The accurate diagnosis of a simple breast cyst is a key role of sonography and important for subsequent patient management. Diagnostic criteria for a simple cyst are summarized in Table 16-7. When strict criteria are met, the diagnosis of a simple cyst can be made with a high level of confidence, allowing for a BI-RADS 2 (benign) ACR classification (Fig. 16-18B). In such cases, no intervention or follow-up is required unless the cyst is symptomatic or enlarges.

### Technical Considerations

Appropriate equipment settings and scanning technique are critical to ensure diagnostic accuracy. Angulation of the sound beam allows all walls to be visualized, helping to exclude wall thickening or an intracystic mass.

**TABLE 16-6**

## American College of Radiology Ultrasound BI-RADS Assessment Categories

| Assessment Category | | Description (Risk for Malignancy) | Recommendation |
|---|---|---|---|
| 0 | Incomplete | | Additional imaging evaluation needed before final assessment |
| **Final Assessment Categories** | | | |
| 1 | Negative | No abnormality or mass found | Routine follow-up |
| 2 | Benign finding | No malignant features | Routine follow-up for age, clinical management |
| 3 | Probably benign finding | Malignancy is highly unlikely (<2%) | Initial short-interval follow-up (usually at 6 months) |
| 4 | Suspicious abnormality<br>*Optional Subdivisions:*<br>*4A-Low suspicion*<br>*4B-Intermediate suspicion*<br>*4C-Moderate suspicion* | Low-to-moderate probability of cancer (3% to 94%): | Tissue sampling (biopsy) should be considered |
| 5 | Highly suggestive of malignancy | Almost certainly cancer (≥95%) | Appropriate action should be taken; biopsy |
| 6 | Known cancer | Biopsy proven malignancy, prior to institution of therapy | Appropriate action should be taken |

Adapted from American College of Radiology BI-RADS US Lexicon Classification Form; 2003.

Proper focusing and the use of spatial compounding and/or harmonic imaging can enhance margin delineation and help reduce internal artifacts. A true simple cyst should be echo-free at normal gain settings and retain a crisp back wall at low gain. Sound enhancement may diminish when a cyst is small, viscous, lies deep near the muscle, or can be related to technical factors (e.g., poor focusing, use of spatial compounding).

## Fibrocystic Change[3,6,8,10,36,37]

FCC is the most common benign diffuse breast condition. Women are typically most symptomatic during late reproductive life (35 to 55 years). FCC is no longer considered a "disease" but rather signifies several changes considered to be aberrations of normal development and involution (ANDI). With aging, female estrogen levels can predominate as menstrual cycles become irregular and ovulatory patterns change. This hormonal imbalance helps induce changes that primarily affect the ducts, lobules, and connective tissues of the TDLUs. Key features of FCC include epithelial hyperplasia, adenosis, stromal fibrosis, and cyst formation. Most FCC findings are nonproliferative do not increase breast cancer risk.

### Signs and Symptoms

At least half of adult women develop some symptoms related to FCC. These include breast tenderness or pain, fullness, and nodularity. Symptoms are usually bilateral

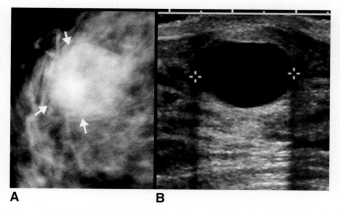

**Figure 16-18** Simple cyst. **A:** Mammogram shows a rounded, circumscribed, water-density mass with a radiolucent halo *(arrows)*. **B:** Sonogram demonstrates a circumscribed, thin-walled, anechoic mass with enhanced sound transmission and refractive edge shadowing.

**TABLE 16-7**

## Benign Simple Cyst Criteria

| Primary Finding | Additional Findings |
|---|---|
| • Round or oval shape<br>• Smooth circumscribed margin<br>• Thin echogenic wall<br>• Absent internal echoes (anechoic)<br>• Distal sound enhancement<br>• Bilateral thin edge shadowing* | • Absent Doppler flow signal<br>• Compressibility with transducer pressure (unless tense cyst)<br>• Mobility with transducer pressure |

*Note: Spatial compounding can reduce edge shadowing and the degree of distal sound enhancement.*

and often increase before menses. Nipple discharge, if present, can be from multiple ducts and tends to be yellow, green, or nearly black in coloration. Symptoms diminish after menopause unless a woman is on HRT.

## Mammographic Features

Common features of FCC include the presence of bilateral, rounded, circumscribed water-density masses, and benign scattered parenchymal calcifications. In some patients, milk-of-calcium sediment within microcysts appears as "teacup-shaped" calcifications. Multiple enlarged lobules (adenosis) can give the parenchyma a "snowflake" appearance. Increased radiodensity of the breast parenchyma can hinder detection of some cysts and lobular changes. Certain FCCs without comma such as sclerosing adenosis, radial scars, and focal fibrosis can occasionally produce suspicious imaging findings.

## Sonographic Features

The most common sonographic finding is the presence of multiple breast cysts of varying sizes in both breasts (Fig. 16-19). Some complicated and septated cysts fall within the spectrum of FCC. Clustered microcysts may show tiny hyperechoic foci reflecting milk of calcium. Stromal fibrosis can increase parenchymal echogenicity and sound attenuation. The fibroglandular tissue may have a basket weave appearance with ductal prominence. High-resolution sonography may detect small solid nodules related to FCC. Enlarged lobules (adenosis) can measure up to 7 mm and appear as isoechoic or hypoechoic solid nodules. Nodular adenosis may appear as a circumscribed mass. Sclerosing adenosis may display an irregular shape, microlobulation, or microcalcifications making differentiation from cancer difficult.

## Complicated Versus Complex Cysts

Some cystic breast masses contain internal echoes or wall changes that are evident with high-resolution sonographic systems. These masses do not meet "simple cyst" criteria

| TABLE 16-8 |
| --- |
| **Causes of Real Echoes within Non Simple Cysts[60]** |
| • Cellular debris |
| • Cholesterol crystals |
| • Epithelial cells; apocrine cells (floating; papillary) |
| • Protein globules; foam cells; fat globules |
| • Blood; pus |
| • Fibrous intervening walls of cyst cluster |
| • Intramural neoplasm (rare) |

and are, instead, classified as complicated or complex cysts. A "nonsimple" breast cyst should be evaluated for signs of acute inflammation or infection and for more worrisome signs of neoplastic change. Possible causes of real echoes within a cystic breast mass along with differential diagnoses are listed in Table 16-8.[6]

Circumscribed, thin-walled complicated cysts are typically benign and often related to FCCs. These are frequently nonpalpable incidental findings and often co-exist with simple cysts. Only rarely is a true intracystic tumor present, which may be benign or malignant. Necrotic tumors can also present as complex lesions.

## Sonographic Features[4,6,8,30,33,38]

Sonography of a nonsimple cystic mass involves assessment of the cyst wall, internal echo pattern, movement of internal echoes, as well as surrounding tissues (Table 16-9). Color or power-mode Doppler assesses for vascularity of the cyst wall and internal contents.

Echoes within complicated breast cysts can present as fluid-debris level, fat-fluid level, or as homogeneous low-level echoes (Fig. 16-20A–C). The mobility of the internal echoes and fat-fluid levels can be assessed by changing the patient's position or by applying and releasing transducer pressure over the mass. Increasing the acoustic power or applying color or power Doppler will often cause lightweight, subcellular particles to

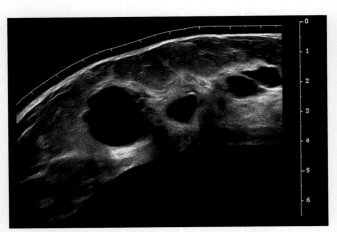

**Figure 16-19** Fibrocystic change showing multiple breast cysts on this extended-field-of-view high resolution scan. (Image courtesy of Philips Medical Systems, Bothell, WA.)

| TABLE 16-9 |
| --- |
| **Sonographic Features of Nonsimple Cysts[11,60]** |

| Complicated Cysts | Complex Cyst, Complex Lesion | Acutely Inflamed or Infected Cyst |
| --- | --- | --- |
| • Mobile internal echoes | • Thick wall (≥0.5 mm) | • Thick isoechoic wall |
| • Fluid-debris level | • Thick septations (≥0.5 mm) | • Hyperemia of wall confirmed by Doppler |
| • Fat-fluid level | • Solid components | • Fluid-debris level |
| • Homogeneous internal echoes |   - Intracystic mass | |
| |   - Mixed solid/cystic | |

*Some authors use the term "complex" cysts to describe nonsimple cysts; others apply the term "complex" for masses containing cystic and solid components.

American College of Radiology lexicon definition for "complex": Mass containing both anechoic and echogenic components.

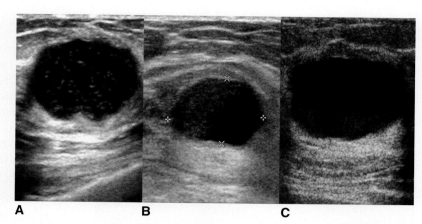

**Figure 16-20** Complicated cyst examples with **(A)** floating internal echoes, **(B)** a partially shifted fat-fluid level, and **(C)** a fluid-debris level. The cyst walls are thin and circumscribed.

A          B          C

move or "stream" away from the transducer. A color flash generated by these moving particles is termed "color streaking." Mobile internal echoes are common in benign cysts of FCC.

An "acorn cyst" displays a nondependent echogenic layer. This pattern can represent a crescent-shaped rim of echogenic papillary apocrine metaplasia (PAM) that is fixed in position, which helps in differentiation from a fat-fluid level. The nondependent echogenic layer of a fat-fluid level can take 5 minutes or longer to shift with positional changes.[6]

Homogeneous internal echoes within a complicated cyst can mimic a solid mass. Inspissated foam or gel cysts are often filled with diffuse low-level internal echoes. PAM, protein, or fat laden fluid can be sources of internal echoes. Compressibility and lack of Doppler vascularity helps differentiate a "solid-appearing" complicated cyst from a true solid mass.

Clustered microcysts represent small cystically dilated acini within an enlarged lobule. These are commonly associated with apocrine metaplasia. Microcyst or macrocyst clusters with thin septations (intervening walls) are typically benign[4,6] (Fig. 16-21).

The presence of thick isoechoic septations or solid components increases the risk of an intracystic papilloma or malignancy.[4]

The term "complex cyst" has more recently been reserved to describe a mass displaying both solid and cystic components, which increases suspicion for neoplastic change. Worrisome sonographic findings include wall thickening ($\geq$0.5 mm), thick internal septations ($\geq$0.5 mm), intracystic nodule, or mixed cystic/solid mass.[4,36] Echoes from proliferative changes along the cyst wall or from an intramural tumor will not shift with positional changes. Both the outer wall and solid intracystic component should be evaluated for suspicious imaging features (e.g., angular margin, microlobulation, duct extension, or invasion past the cyst wall).[6] A true intramural neoplasm, such as an intracystic papilloma or carcinoma, is rare. Doppler confirmation of blood flow within an eccentrically thickened wall or a fibrovascular stalk suggests neoplastic growth. Benign PAM can cause eccentric wall thickening but often has a concave surface and lacks blood flow, unlike a papillary neoplasm. PAM also has a smooth attachment to the inner cyst wall without extension past the cyst border.[6]

Cyst features worrisome for acute inflammation or infection include uniform isoechoic wall thickening, hyperemia of the cyst wall, and possible internal fluid-debris level[6] (Fig. 16-22). Heavier white blood cells tend to settle dependently within an infected cyst and can take longer to shift with positional changes. Color or power mode Doppler can display blood vessels coursing along the wall of a hyperemic inflamed cyst, as opposed to tumoral vessels coursing across the cyst wall. Supportive clinical features of inflammation include focal pain, tenderness, and possible redness and thickening of the overlying skin. Fibrotic cyst wall thickening from prior inflammation typically lacks hyperemic change.

Older hemorrhagic, infected, or oil cysts may develop thin wall (eggshell) calcification causing acoustic shadowing that may obscure all or a portion of the cyst contents.[4,6]

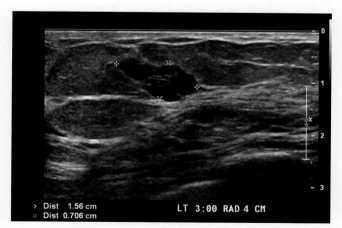

Dist  1.56 cm
Dist  0.706 cm          LT 3:00 RAD 4 CM

**Figure 16-21** Cyst cluster. Sonogram showing a cluster of cystically-dilated acini (ductules) within an enlarged lobule with thin intervening septations. Microcyst or macrocyst clusters are possible depending on the degree of ductule dilatation.

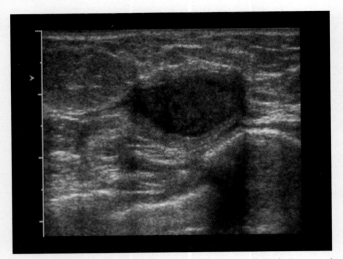

**Figure 16-22** Infected cyst. Uniform isoechoic wall thickening and low-level internal echoes are features of this inflamed cyst.

## Technical Considerations[6,8,29,33]

Before characterizing a cyst as complicated or complex, technical factors and sound beam focusing must be optimized to eliminate as many "false echoes" from artifacts as possible. Common detrimental artifacts include reverberation, slice thickness artifacts, and clutter. The gain settings should be set high enough to visualize true echoes within cyst fluid without introducing false echoes. Harmonics and spatial compounding can help reduce troublesome artifacts.

## Treatment

Patient history and other imaging findings are helpful when considering a differential diagnosis for a complicated or complex cystic mass. In most cases, well-circumscribed, thin-walled complicated cysts are benign and part of the spectrum of FCCs.

Classification of complicated/complex cysts into BI-RADS categories is reported in the literature.[4,6,30] A benign (BI-RADS 2) classification is appropriate for asymptomatic thin-walled, circumscribed, complicated cysts with mobile internal echoes and fluid-debris levels. (Lipid cysts, thinly septated cysts, sebaceous cysts, milk-of-calcium, and calcified cysts can also be classified as benign.) When discovered on a baseline sonography exam or as an incidental finding, asymptomatic complicated cysts with homogeneous internal echoes and clustered microcysts are generally classified as "probably benign" (BI-RADS 3). In such cases, the patient may be offered short-interval follow-up versus aspiration. Aspiration or core biopsy may be needed to differentiate a cyst filled with internal echoes from a solid mass. Cysts filled with PAM will not aspirate.[6]

Aspiration is warranted for symptomatic complicated cysts. A bloody aspirate should undergo cytologic analysis to exclude malignant cells. Cysts that recur after aspiration or cannot be completely aspirated may require excision.

Aspiration can be diagnostic and therapeutic for cysts suspected to be acutely inflamed or infected. A purulent aspirate can be sent for laboratory confirmation, including culture and Gram stain analysis. Antibiotics aid in the treatment of infection.[6]

With suspicious complex lesions (BI-RADS 4+), large core or sonography directed vacuum-assisted biopsy (VAB) is preferred over cyst aspiration since the cyst wall and solid components are of histologic importance. Placement of a clip marker serves as a landmark should excision be required.

## Galactocele[4,6,26]

A galactocele is a milky cyst caused by obstruction of a lactiferous duct in the pregnant or lactating woman. This retention cyst tends to develop after abrupt cessation or suppression of lactation and contains fat, proteins, and lactose. A subareolar location is common but galactoceles also occur in peripheral TDLUs. A galactocele may persist past the lactation period, undergo oily transformation, and become a lipid (oil) cyst. Rupture of an infected galactocele can lead to mastitis and subsequent abscess formation.

### Signs and Symptoms

A galactocele is the most common benign mass to develop in a lactating patient. The presenting mass is usually firm but mobile. Tenderness or mastitis can accompany an infected galactocele.

### Mammographic Features

A galactocele appears as a circumscribed mass containing radiolucent (fat-density) material, which is a benign feature. Radiolucency varies with the fat and protein content. Increased parenchymal density of the lactating breast can hinder mammographic detection of some masses. A thin rim of wall calcification may occur with older lesions.

### Sonographic Features

This round or oval, circumscribed mass can be unilocular or multilocular in appearance. Although galactoceles can be anechoic, variable amounts of internal echoes reflect from milk-laden contents (Fig. 16-23). A fluid-fat level can be present and slowly shifts with positional changes. Doppler confirms absence of internal blood flow. Posterior enhancement may be less than that seen with a simple cyst. Rim calcification, if present, can impede sound transmission. Associated findings in the lactating patient are prominent glandular tissue and dilated ducts.

### Differential Diagnosis

Oil cysts and other complicated cysts can have similar sonographic appearances. If mastitis is present, an infected cyst or localized abscess is considered. A tender mass with a thick hyperemic wall can indicate an infected galactocele.

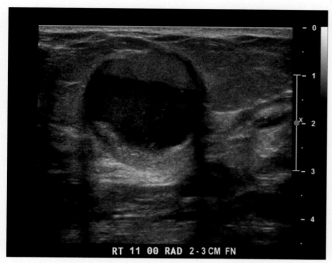

**Figure 16-23** Galactocele. Sonogram shows a unilocular cystic mass of mixed-echogenicity due to milky-fatty contents. An echogenic nondependent fat layer is present in this mass. (Reprinted from Carr-Hoefer C. *Breast Ultrasound: A Comprehensive Sonographer's Guide.* Forney, TX: Pegasus Lectures; 2007.)

## Treatment

Resolution of the galactocele is usually spontaneous, but aspiration using a low-gauge needle is often curative.

## Sebaceous Cyst and Epidermal Inclusion Cyst[4,6,8,9]

Sebaceous and epidermal cysts are small, benign, skin appendage masses that result from obstructed sebaceous glands or hair follicles and contain sebum or keratin. The superficial location is a clue to their origin, residing within or just beneath the dermal layer of the skin. Sebaceous cysts are often located at the inferior or medial margins of the breast or near the axilla. Occasionally, epidermal cysts form after breast trauma (e.g., needle biopsy, reduction mammoplasty). Retention cysts can also develop within the Montgomery glands of the areola. Infected or ruptured sebaceous cysts can lead to abscess formation.

### Signs and Symptoms

Nodules are palpable because of their superficial location. The skin pore overlying the obstructed gland may be darkened. Skin reddening and tenderness overlying the cyst can indicate infection.

### Sonographic Features

Sebaceous and epidermal cysts are round or oval in shape with smooth, thin-walled circumscribed margins. The cyst can be completely or partially located within the dermis or project beneath the skin into the subcutaneous fat. Focal skin thickening usually accompanies the cyst. When a cyst projects into the subcutaneous fat, the surrounding dermis can have a "claw-like" appearance. Although these cysts can be anechoic, the greasy or waxy contents often generate low- to medium-level internal echoes, fluid-fat levels, or produce a multilaminated appearance (Fig. 16-24A,B). Posterior acoustic enhancement is typically preserved. Slight angulation of the sound beam can improve detection of a narrow, hypoechoic, excretory duct or inflamed hair follicle that extends from the cyst to the skin surface. Color Doppler reveals no internal blood flow. Cysts of skin origin can be classified as BI-RADS 2 benign lesions.

Signs of cyst infection or abscess formation are sought when tenderness and skin reddening are present. Over time, sebaceous cysts may develop wall calcification with associated acoustic shadowing.

### Technical Considerations

These superficial lesions are best delineated utilizing high frequency, an acoustic offset (such as extra scan gel), and proper focusing.

## BENIGN INFLAMMATORY CONDITIONS

### Mastitis

Mastitis, or inflammation of the breast, presents most often during pregnancy and lactation but can affect women at any stage of life. Causes are varied. Nonlactational forms of mastitis may result from an infected

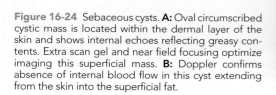
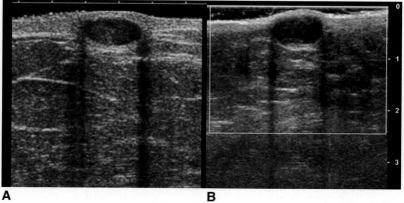

**Figure 16-24** Sebaceous cysts. **A:** Oval circumscribed cystic mass is located within the dermal layer of the skin and shows internal echoes reflecting greasy contents. Extra scan gel and near field focusing optimize imaging this superficial mass. **B:** Doppler confirms absence of internal blood flow in this cyst extending from the skin into the superficial fat.

**A**                    **B**

or ruptured cyst, a ruptured ectatic duct, postsurgical infection, periductal inflammation, or due to granulomatous conditions.

Puerperal mastitis represents breast inflammation related to lactation. It is the most frequent cause of acute mastitis. Bacteria, typically *Staphylococcus aureus*, can enter the ducts through a skin abrasion or cracked nipple or ascend via the ducts. Obstructed lactiferous ducts are susceptible to infection. Dilated infected ducts can show thick isoechoic walls and internal echoes from inspissated milk. With puerperal mastitis, infection can begin centrally within a lactiferous duct or develop more peripherally in a galactocele. Without appropriate treatment, an abscess may develop. Infection may potentially spread by way of the blood and lymph vessels to other parts of the breast.

Mammography is compromised in the woman with acute mastitis due to increased breast density from edema and also from glandular proliferation related to lactation. Breast tenderness can further limit adequate tissue compression. Depending on the patient's age and clinical history, sonography is often the initial imaging exam for patients presenting with mastitis to search for complications such as abscess formation.

Mammary duct ectasia and periductal (plasma cell) mastitis primarily affects subareolar structures. This uncommon, chronic, nonlactational form of mastitis presents closer to menopause although younger women with congenital nipple inversion are also at risk. Symptoms can include subareolar nodularity, a thick sticky nipple discharge, nipple retraction, and discomfort. Clinical features can mimic cancer, however, the ductal ectasia-periductal mastitis complex is usually bilateral in presentation. Subareolar ducts become distended with thick secretions and debris. Irritation and damage to the duct wall can allow secretions to leak into surrounding tissues inciting periductal inflammation. Periductal fibrosis may follow and eventually shorten the ducts resulting in nipple retraction. Mammogram features include an increase in subareolar density from dilated ducts or from a possible abscess. Calcification can develop both within and around the affected ducts.

In patients with periductal mastitis, sonography is primarily used to determine if the cause of subareolar nodularity is from duct ectasia, abscess, or due to a mass. Dilated mammary ducts converging toward the nipple may display thick walls and contain echogenic, inspissated secretions. Color Doppler may show increased blood flow along the duct wall. Rupture of a duct can incite formation of a subareolar or periareolar abscess that may develop fistula tracts. Over time, there can be fibrous obliteration of the duct lumen.

## Abscess

Abscesses are localized areas of pus and necrotic tissue that develop in a small percentage of patients with breast infection. Most often, abscesses form beneath the nipple (subareolar), or they may develop under the skin (subcutaneous), within the gland (intramammary), or deep to the gland in front of the pectoral muscles (retromammary).

### Signs and Symptoms

Acute mastitis presents with varying degrees of fever, pain, skin reddening and thickening, and a purulent discharge. An elevated white blood cell (WBC) count supports infection. In this setting, a palpable mass can indicate an abscess. Axillary nodes may be enlarged and tender.

### Sonographic Features

The sonographic appearance varies with the stage and distribution of the inflammatory process. The inflamed, thickened skin prompts a search for an underlying infected duct or fluid collection. Swollen edematous breast tissues scatter and attenuate the sound beam requiring lower frequencies to adequately penetrate the tissues. Edema can increase the echogenicity of the subcutaneous fat, which reduces delineation of the Cooper ligaments and other tissue planes. Dilated subdermal lymphatic channels or interstitial fluid may be seen (Fig. 16-25). Comparison of the inflamed breast to a similar region in the normal contralateral breast allows the sonologist to appreciate the degree of inflammatory change.

An organized abscess can display varying amounts of liquefaction and tissue necrosis. An abscess appears as a complex fluid collection often with thick, irregular, or indistinct walls (Fig. 16-26). Nonuniform internal echoes, debris levels, and septations are common. Air within an abscess cavity is rare and can cause ring-down artifact. Distal sound enhancement varies with the fluid composition. An abscess can tract to various parts of the breast or peak anteriorly through the superficial fascia forming fistula tracts to the skin.

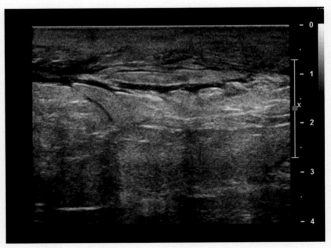

**Figure 16-25** Mastitis. Features of breast inflammation in this patient include marked skin thickening, dilatation of subdermal lymphatics, and increased echogenicity of the subcutaneous fat.

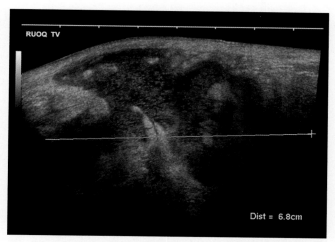

**Figure 16-26** Mastitis abscess. Extended field-of-view image shows a large complex fluid mass in a lactating patient with fever, breast swelling, and skin reddening. The sonogram shows associated skin thickening and increased echogenicity of adjacent tissues.

As an abscess matures, it becomes more encapsulated and well defined. Color or power Doppler documents hyperemic flow to inflamed tissues and the absence of blood flow within the abscess cavity.

### Differential Diagnosis

Depending on the stage of the process, inflammatory change can mimic a hematoma, seroma, infected cyst, degenerating mass, or even cancer.

Both inflammatory carcinoma and acute mastitis can have similar clinical findings and must be differentiated by diagnostic methods if suspicious findings are detected. Cancer can grow rapidly and disseminate diffusely when hormones are elevated in the pregnant or lactating breast.

Skin thickening and edema can also be caused by noninflammatory conditions such as direct trauma, congestive heart failure, lymphoma, and lymphedema. A skin burn or direct radiation exposure can inflame local tissues.

Skin retraction, architectural distortion, fat necrosis, scaring, and fibrosis may indicate residual change from a serious abscess. Clinical correlation is important.

### Treatment

Most inflammatory processes resolve with proper antibiotic therapy. Aspiration of purulent fluid is diagnostic of an abscess when a fluid collection is present. Microbiology studies should include culture and Gram stain. Needle or catheter drainage with irrigation and instillation of antibiotics into the abscess cavity may augment medical treatment. In some cases, biopsy or excision may be needed to exclude an underlying malignancy if a treated abscess does not fully involute.

### Mondor Disease[4,6,8,21,39]

Mondor disease represents acute thrombophlebitis of the superficial veins of the chest wall and breast.

The lateral thoracic, thoracoepigastric, and superior epigastric veins are most often involved. Risk factors for this rare condition include breast injury, surgery, infection, hypercoagulable state, pregnancy, dehydration, and cancer. The presence of a central venous catheter may initiate clot formation and affect the internal mammary vein. Both males and females are affected.

### Signs and Symptoms[39]

A tender, palpable, cord-like superficial mass correlates with the location of the dilated affected vein. The skin overlying the thrombosed vein can be thick and reddened signifying focal inflammation.

### Sonographic Findings

The dilated, tubular, superficial vein may have a somewhat beaded appearance and displays internal echoes from clotted blood (Fig. 16-27). Thrombus is confirmed by showing incomplete compressibility of the vein when applying transducer pressure. Doppler shows absent blood flow in the obstructed vein segment. Edema increases the thickness and echogenicity of overlying skin and the fat surrounding an acutely thrombosed vein. A partially recanalized vein may show fibrous bands within the vessel lumen. Chronic clot may eventually calcify.

The location of the thrombosed vein within the superficial fat layer helps to differentiate the tubular structure from a breast duct located in the mammary zone. Once a clotted breast vein is identified, the course of the thrombus should be traced to its draining vein to exclude extension of clot into the axillary, subclavian, or internal mammary veins.

### Treatment

Symptoms often resolve over a period of several weeks without intervention. Some cases require anticoagulatory therapy. Recurrence is possible.

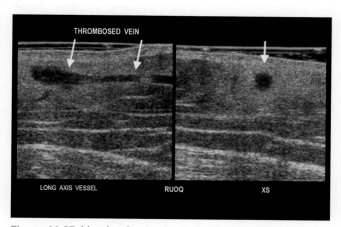

**Figure 16-27** Mondor disease. Internal echoes and noncompressibility are features of this thrombosed superficial breast vein. Edema causes an increase in echogenicity of the fat surrounding the occluded vessel. Doppler will confirm absent blood flow. (Reprinted from Carr-Hoefer C. *Breast Ultrasound: A Comprehensive Sonographer's Guide.* Forney, TX: Pegasus Lectures; 2007.)

## BENIGN TRAUMA RELATED MASSES

The main causes of breast injury include blunt trauma, percutaneous interventional procedures, and surgery. Patient history is very important when establishing a differential diagnosis in a patient following trauma or infection since some residual changes can create clinical and imaging features that simulate cancer.

### Hematoma[6,26,40,41]

Hematomas are blood-filled breast masses that usually result from vessel damage following breast injury. Nontraumatic hematomas may develop in patients with a history of blood disorders or anticoagulant treatment.

### Signs and Symptoms

Bruising and some skin thickening are external signs of hemorrhage. Tenderness is present in varying degrees. A palpable mass following biopsy or trauma suggests a hematoma.

### Mammographic Features

The appearance of hemorrhage varies from mild changes of increased density and skin thickening to an opaque, hemorrhagic cyst or a more sclerotic, retractive mass.[42]

### Sonographic Features

Sonography is usually the preferred imaging modality since it is less painful than mammography and can identify a fluid collection separate from other traumatized tissues. Imaging patterns of hemorrhage depend on the extent, duration, and organization of the bleed. Initially, mild skin thickening and altered echogenicity of subcutaneous fat or other affected tissues may be present. The sonographic appearance of an organizing hematoma is variable and depends on the amount of liquefaction and clotted blood present (Fig. 16-28).

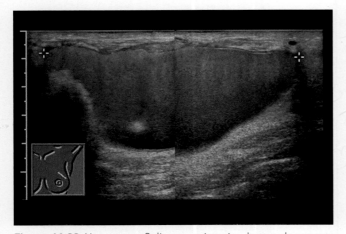

**Figure 16-28** Hematoma. Split-screen imaging better documents this 8-cm, fluid-filled, echogenic mass that resulted from a seatbelt injury. A small area of hyperechoic clotted blood is present. Skin thickening accompanies the area of bruising. (Reprinted from Carr-Hoefer C. *Breast Ultrasound: A Comprehensive Sonographer's Guide.* Forney, TX: Pegasus Lectures; 2007.)

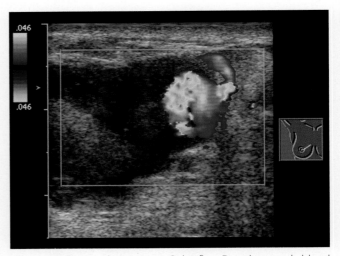

**Figure 16-29** Pseudoaneurysm. Color flow Doppler reveals blood flow within the neck of this postbiopsy pseudoaneurysm. (Reprinted with permission from Carr-Hoefer C. Breast Ultrasound for the Sonomammographer. Corvallis, Sound Imaging Consulting, LLC, 2007.)

A hematoma can appear round, oval, or irregular in shape. Clotted blood along the periphery of the hematoma forms a fibrous wall that helps contain the blood collection. The encapsulated blood may be anechoic, but more often displays diffuse internal echoes, echogenic clot, septations, or fibrous bands. Distal acoustic enhancement is variable.

Doppler confirms the absence of internal blood flow within a hematoma and helps differentiate a postbiopsy hematoma from blood flow jetting into a pseudoaneurysm (Fig. 16-29). Hemorrhage into a simple cyst can occur with trauma.

### Seroma[4,6,8,40]

A seroma is an accumulation of serum that can collect within a surgical cavity or at a biopsy site. A seroma at a lumpectomy site can help reduce contour deformity by allowing breast tissues to reshape as the fluid collection regresses. Drains are more often placed at mastectomy sites to lessen the accumulation of fluids. Seromas help to identify the treatment cavity site for brachytherapy patients undergoing partial irradiation. Axillary seromas can follow lymph node dissections.

### Signs and Symptoms

A seroma is suspected in an afebrile patient with a palpable mass at a surgical site. Larger seromas can cause pain and stretch the overlying skin.

### Sonographic Features

A seroma typically conforms to the shape of the surgical cavity. The fluid may appear anechoic or display low-level internal echoes or septations (Fig. 16-30). Distal sound enhancement is evident. Doppler confirms absence of internal vascularity.

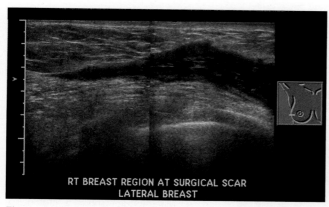

**Figure 16-30** Seroma. Split-screen image shows fluid accumulation with some thin internal septations within the surgical cavity following lumpectomy.

## Differential Diagnosis

Clinical findings and lab values help to differentiate postsurgical fluid collections when imaging features are similar and aspiration is not desired. In the axilla, a lymphocele can mimic a seroma.

## Treatment

Seromas gradually resolve with time, however, therapeutic aspiration is warranted if a seroma is large, persists for a long time, or becomes infected.

## Fat Necrosis[4,6,8,40]

Fat necrosis is an uncommon inflammatory and ischemic process that is a consequence of blunt breast trauma (e.g., seat belt injury), surgery (e.g., reduction mammoplasty), radiotherapy, or inflammation. Trauma can disrupt blood supply causing hemorrhage and liquefaction of a focal area of breast fat, resulting in necrosis and some foreign body reaction.[35] Subsequently, the

traumatized fat may transform into a lipid-filled (oil) cyst or evolve into a fibrous sclerotic mass. Older obese women with large fatty breasts are more prone to fat necrosis, especially within the subcutaneous fat. Large surgical excisions followed by radiation increase risk for ischemic changes. Spontaneous development has been reported in diabetic patients.

### Signs and Symptoms

Palpable findings range from a smooth, mildly compressible lump to a firm, fixed, irregular mass in the region of prior breast injury. There may be associated skin thickening, dimpling, or nipple retraction. Findings are usually painless. Clinical history is important since many of these clinical features mimic signs of cancer. Not all patients recall a history of breast trauma or infection making clinical correlation difficult. Unlike cancer, symptoms typically diminish with time. Some patients are asymptomatic with fat necrosis being initially discovered on an imaging exam.

### Mammographic Features

Findings are variable. An oil cyst appears as a round or oval, radiolucent or mixed fat/water density mass with a radiodense fibrous capsule (Fig. 16-31A). Thin rim (eggshell) calcification may encompass an oil cyst. When a fat density mass is apparent by mammography, sonography is not needed to make a benign diagnosis. Fibrotic changes mimic cancer and include architectural distortion or a spiculated mass with or without calcifications (Fig. 16-32A).

### Sonographic Features

Fat necrosis also has a range of sonographic appearances. Initially, there may be increased echogenicity of the traumatized fat in which an anechoic or hypoechoic area(s) develops. Changes can progress into an oil cyst

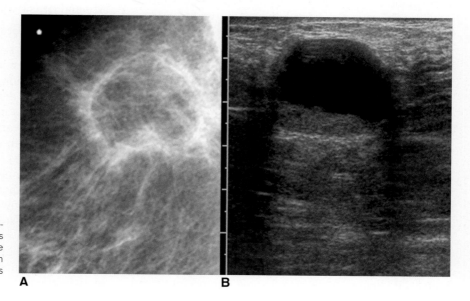

**Figure 16-31** Fat necrosis: oil cyst presentation. **A:** Mammogram of a fatty breast shows a radiolucent rounded mass with a radiodense capsule at an old trauma site. **B:** Sonogram shows a complicated cyst with mixed echoes from fatty contents.

**A**                    **B**

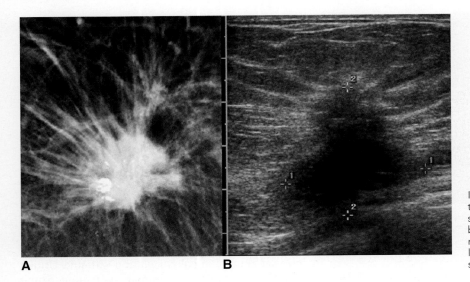

**A**    **B**

**Figure 16-32** Fat necrosis: fibrotic presentation. **A:** Mammogram shows a radiodense spiculated mass with calcification in a fatty breast at the site of prior lumpectomy. **B:** Sonogram shows a poorly circumscribed, spiculated, hypoechoic mass with some acoustic shadowing.

encompassed by a thin or thick wall. Internally, a discrete oil cyst may be anechoic, show a fat-fluid level, display a mixed echo pattern, or mural nodule (fat globule) (Fig. 16-31B). Enhancement is variable. If rim calcification is present, acoustic shadowing may obscure portions of the cyst complicating the diagnosis. Fat necrosis can evolve into a more solid appearance with suspicious features related to fibrosis and granuloma formation. Fibrotic fat necrosis can appear as an irregular or spiculated, hypoechoic, shadowing mass (Fig. 16-32B). Doppler flow shows no associated blood flow as tissues becomes avascular with fibrotic scarring.[6]

### Differential Diagnosis

An appropriate differential factors in the patient's history, the location, and imaging appearance of the mass. Fat necrosis appearing as a fibrotic or granulomatous mass can overlap imaging features of a postsurgical scar, focal fibrosis, radial scar, scirrhous carcinoma, or recurrent tumor. Doppler flow at the site would favor tumor growth. The presence of radiolucent fat within a mass on a mammogram can indicate an oil cyst and should be differentiated from other fat-containing masses.

Patients with Weber-Christian disease can develop multiple oil cysts in the breast, as well as fat necrosis in other parts of the body. Steatocystoma multiplex is manifested by multiple, bilateral, small oil cysts in the axillae, the anterior chest wall, and even the skin layer. These conditions can also be seen in males.

### Postsurgical Scar

A scar forms as connective tissue proliferates at the site of an injury. Postsurgical scarring can affect many tissue layers along the incision site. Scar tissue can also form following involution of a hematoma, seroma, or an abscess. Fat necrosis may complicate scarring. It may take a year for scar tissue to diminish following a benign biopsy. Radiation therapy following lumpectomy can induce significant scarring, which persists longer and potentially obscures early detection of a recurring tumor.

### Signs and Symptoms

Some scars produce minimal, if any, palpable changes. Exuberant scarring at the incision site can cause thickening, firmness, and some retraction of the skin. Deeper scar tissue can present as a breast lump, which may be difficult to differentiate from recurrent tumor in some patients following breast conservation surgery.

### Mammographic Features

A radiodense scar is often better seen on one mammographic view and changes in appearance on a different projection. Patterns include architectural distortion, focal asymmetry, or a spiculated density often with dystrophic calcifications. Compression views show absence of a central mass. Skin changes include thickening, retraction, and fibrous stranding into the underlying fat. Over time, scar tissue tends to diminish in size and density on sequential mammograms.

### Sonographic Features

A postsurgical scar can appear as an irregular hypoechoic area with acoustic shadowing or as architectural distortion at the surgical site. Tissue planes typically show disruption. Associated skin thickening and retraction is common. Unlike a true mass, the linear dimensions and appearance of a scar will change when scanned in orthogonal planes along the incision site (Fig. 16-33). Applying transducer pressure flattens out the connective tissue fibers, which reduces or eliminates the shadowing effect of the scar. In contrast, malignant shadowing will not significantly change with transducer pressure. No Doppler blood flow signal is detected within scar tissue by 6 months following surgery, helping to differentiate it from a recurrent tumor.[6] The effects of a scar typically diminish over time on serial exams.

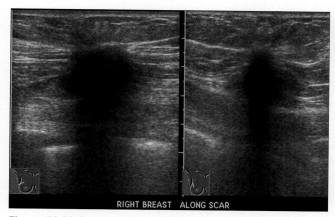

**Figure 16-33** Postsurgical scar. Orthogonal scans along the incision reveal a shadowing, spiculated area and straightening of some Copper ligaments. Note the change in dimension of the scar tissue after the transducer is rotated perpendicular to the long axis of the incision.

| TABLE 16-10 | |
|---|---|
| **Sonographic Characterization of Solid Mass Descriptors (A.T. Stavros, MD)[60,62]** | |
| **Benign Findings** | |
| Marked hyperechogenicity | Uniform hyperechoic tissue that does not contain any "gray" areas larger than normal ducts of terminal ductolobular units (example: benign stromal fibrous tissue) |
| **Solid Mass Features** | |
| Elliptical macrolobulation | Oval, egg-shaped |
| | Three of fewer smooth gentle lobulations (if lobulation is present) |
| Wider than tall | Measures greater in its horizontal dimensions than in anteroposterior dimension. |
| | Long axis of lesion parallels skin line (parallel or horizontal orientation) |
| Thin echogenic pseudocapsule | Well-circumscribed rim of compressed breast tissue encompassing the mass (must completely encompass the lesion) |

Additionally, there must be an absence of any suspicious imaging findings.

## SONOGRAPHIC ASSESSMENT OF SOLID BREAST MASSES

Sonography typically follows clinical exam and mammography and provides additional diagnostic information for risk assessment. In past years, the main role of sonography was to characterize masses as cystic or solid. As the quality of sonography systems have improved, so has sonography's ability to detect more of the morphologic features of masses that correlate with benign or malignant processes. It is reported that about 80% of breast biopsies return benign results. Research studies have shown that sonography can help differentiate benign from malignant solid masses when strict imaging criteria are met.[6,21,42–44] This can impact patient care by allowing certain patients the option of short-interval follow-up imaging when findings correlate with a very high probability of being benign, while expediting biopsy of lesions with suspicious features. However, the development of a new solid mass in a postmenopausal woman is usually treated with suspicion even when circumscribed.

Dr. A.T. Stavros and colleagues developed an algorithm for the sonographic characterization of solid breast nodules based on large-scale research studies. Following strict criteria, solid nodules can be assigned to a risk category based on the presence or absence of specific sonographic findings (Tables 16-10 and 16-11). A recommended approach when examining a solid nodule is to[6,44]:

- First search for the presence of individual suspicious sonographic findings. If one or more suspicious finding is present, the mass is minimally assigned a BI-RADS 4 (suspicious abnormality) classification and biopsy is indicated.
- If no suspicious findings are present, further assess the nodule for the presence of specific benign findings. If benign findings are present, the nodule

can be classified as either BI-RADS 2 (benign) or as BI-RADS 3 (probably benign).

- If benign findings are not present, the nodule is classified as indeterminate with low suspicion of malignancy, BI-RADS 4(A), and biopsy is recommended.

Use of such an algorithm relies on the performance of a high-resolution breast sonography exam by knowledgeable and experienced sonographers and sonologists.

At times, the cause of a palpable lump or an asymmetric mammographic density represents a focal island of fibrous stromal tissue. This is considered a benign finding if the tissue is purely hyperechoic without any gray areas larger than normal ducts or lobules (Fig. 16-34).

Characteristically, a benign mass displaces, rather than invades, adjacent tissues as it grows and display well-circumscribed margins that are sharply demarcated from surrounding tissues (Fig. 16-35A). A benign solid mass assumes an oval shape as it slowly grows within normal tissue planes[45] (Fig. 16-36B). If no suspicious features are present, a circumscribed solid mass with these features meets criteria for a BI-RADS 3 (probably benign) classification. Short-interval follow-up imaging (at 6 months) may be offered as an initial option to biopsy depending on patient factors. Stability of findings over several serial exams reinforces a benign diagnosis.

Several sonographic findings increase suspicion for cancer when evaluating a solid breast mass and these

| TABLE 16-11 | |
|---|---|
| **Sonographic Characterization of Solid Mass Descriptors (A.T. Stavros, MD)[60,62]** | |

| **Individial Suspicious Findings for Malignancy** | |
|---|---|
| **Hard findings:** Most often associated with invasion | |
| Spiculation | Alternating hypoechoic/hyperechoic straight lines radiating perpendicularly from the surface of the mass |
| Angular margins | Variant: thick echogenic halo *(can represent unresolved spiculation)* |
| | Jagged margins; Sharp corners often forming acute angles at points of low resistance to tumor growth |
| Acoustic shadowing | Central, partial, or complete decrease in retrotumoral echoes (often related to degree of desmoplasia and spiculation) |
| **Mixed findings:** Associated with invasive and ductal carcinoma in situ components of lesion | |
| Microlobulation | Multiple small, 1–2 mm, surface lobulations *(ACR-short cycle undulations)* |
| Taller than wide | Anteroposterior dimension > any horizontal dimension *(nonparallel; vertical orientation)* |
| Marked hypoechogenicity | Mass or central part of mass is markedly hypoechoic as compared to fat. |
| **Soft findings:** Associated with ductal carcinoma in situ components of lesion | |
| Microcalcifications | Hyperechoic foci, nonshadowing foci (best seen within mass) |
| Duct extension | Tumor projection from a mass into a single duct directed toward the nipple |
| Branch pattern | Tumor projection into multiple small ducts away from the nipple |

The presence of one or more suspicious finding places mass in either a BI-RADS 4 or 5 category.

findings are summarized in Table 16-11 (Fig. 16-35B). The presence of even one suspicious feature is enough to classify a solid nodule as a suspicious abnormality, although most cancers show multiple findings. Close inspection of a lesion is necessary since a suspicious sonographic feature might affect only a small portion of mass. Cancers vary by tumor type, cellularity, vascularity, growth rate, and effect on surrounding tissues, which influence imaging appearance. Certain findings are more often associated with invasive tumor, whereas others reflect intraductal (DCIS) components. Some invasive cancers are indistinct or clearly spiculated, whereas others may be circumscribed. Some cancers show a combination of findings. (This can also be true for some benign lesions.) Further description of suspicious findings will be discussed in the Breast Cancer section of this chapter.

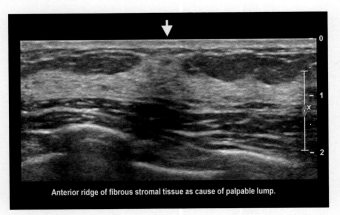

Anterior ridge of fibrous stromal tissue as cause of palpable lump.

**Figure 16-34** Benign fibrous stromal tissue. A focal ridge of hyperechoic fibroglandular tissue is seen extending anteriorly and was confirmed to be the cause of the palpable lump during echopalpation.

## BENIGN SOLID MASSES

### Fibroadenoma[3,4,6,10,26]

Fibroadenoma is the most common benign solid tumor of the female breast. Incidence rate is higher in patients 15 to 35 years of age. Tumors often develop before age 25. This estrogen-induced tumor represents overgrowth of the connective and glandular tissues within a breast lobule. Fibroadenomas may be single or multiple, involving one or both breasts. Large and multiple tumors occur more frequently in young black females. Older fibroadenomas may undergo involution, hyalinization, and calcification.

Fibroadenomas usually grow slowly until reaching a stable size. Most tumors measure less than 3 cm but some grow larger. Accelerated growth can be hormonally stimulated during pregnancy, after initiation of HRT, or during immunosuppression therapy. Rapid growth can lead to infarction.

Juvenile-type or giant fibroadenomas grow quickly during adolescence and account for up to 10% of fibroadenomas in females under age 20. Tumors can grow very large and are usually sol. Histologically, these uncommon tumors display a highly cellular stroma.

### Signs and Symptoms[21,26]

A palpable fibroadenoma presents as a nontender, smooth or lobular, firm or rubbery, movable mass.

### Mammographic Features[4,5,35]

Fibroadenoma appears as a water-density circumscribed, oval, or round mass that may be indistinguishable from a cyst. A thin radiolucent halo supports a benign diagnosis (Fig. 16-36A). Tumors are often isodense to

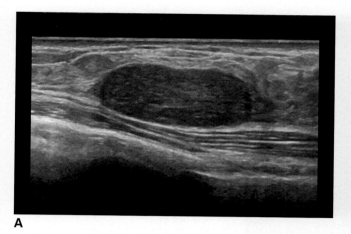
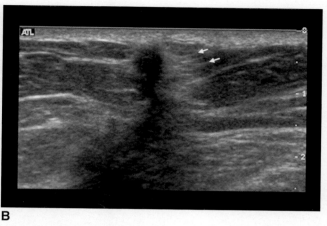

**A**                                                                          **B**

**Figure 16-35** Sonographic characteristics. **A:** Benign features of this solid breast mass (fibroadenoma) include oval shape, smoothly circumscribed margins with a thin echogenic pseudocapsule, wider than tall (parallel orientation). **B:** Malignant features of this mass include spiculation (*arrows*), marked hypoechogenicity and acoustic shadowing. The mass extends through tissue planes and is taller than wide (vertical orientation). There is secondary straightening of Cooper ligaments.

fibroglandular tissue and may show a distinctive notch. Benign, coarse, "popcorn" type calcifications are occasionally seen and help distinguish an older fibroadenoma from a cyst or a circumscribed cancer (Fig. 16-37A).

### Sonographic Features

Typically, a fibroadenoma appears as a smooth, well-circumscribed, oval, wider than tall, homogeneous, solid mass that may be gently lobulated (Fig. 16-36B). The echogenicity is usually isoechoic or mildly hypoechoic compared to fat. On occasion, an echogenic septation may be seen traversing the mass. Normal sound transmission is common although some enhancement or mild shadowing is possible. Color Doppler may show peripheral and feeding vessels.[4]

### Differential Diagnosis

Fibroadenomas account for most circumscribed solid breast masses. Occasionally, internal areas of cystic degeneration, hyalinization, or calcification can cause textural inhomogeneity and alter attenuation effects.[42,43]

Acoustic shadowing from macrocalcifications can obscure portions of the mass (Fig. 16-37B). Findings should be correlated with the mammogram to eliminate confusion with malignant shadowing.

"Complex fibroadenomas" represent a small subset of tumors that contain proliferative changes (cysts >3 mm, epithelial calcifications, sclerosing adenosis, PAM). These complex lesions show a slight increase in relative risk for breast cancer.

A differential diagnosis for circumscribed breast tumors >3 cm are listed in Table 16-12 and tailored to clinical and imaging features. Large, highly cellular juvenile fibroadenomas are usually homogeneous and can demonstrate prominent vascularity and enhanced sound transmission (Fig. 16-38). Pseudoangiomatous stromal hyperplasia (PASH) can mimic fibroadenoma or phyllodes tumor on a sonogram. This benign, solid, mesenchymal tumor contains extensive slit-like spaces that resemble vascular channels. This often large, hormonally stimulated mass can grow quickly and is more prevalent in reproductive age women and those on HRT.

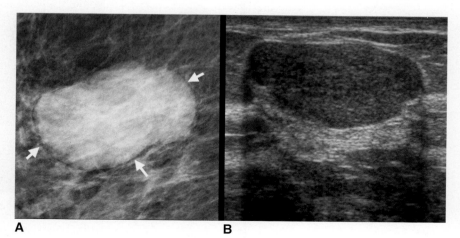

**Figure 16-36** Fibroadenoma. **A:** Mammogram reveals a well-circumscribed, oval, water-density mass with a radiolucent rim (*arrows*). **B:** Sonogram shows an oval, gently lobulated, circumscribed solid mass with a thin echogenic pseudocapsule. This benign-appearing "wider-than-tall" mass is oriented parallel to the skin.

**A**                                    **B**

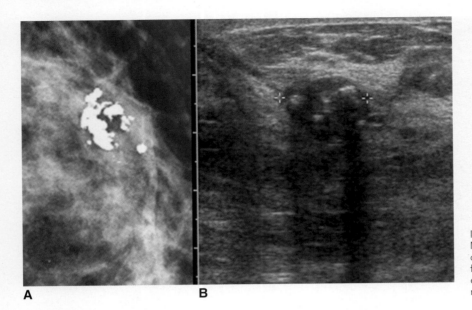

**A**    **B**

Figure 16-37 Calcified fibroadenoma. **A:** Mammogram reveals benign "popcorn" type calcifications consistent with a degenerating fibroadenoma. **B:** Sonogram shows hyperechoic areas with acoustic shadowing from macrocalcification within the mass.

## Adenoma and Secretory Adenoma[3,4,6,10,26]

Adenomas are less common than fibroadenomas and are primarily composed of glandular elements. Slowly growing tubular adenomas can occur in young patients.[9] Secretory (lactating) adenomas present during pregnancy or the lactation period in response to elevated hormones. It is questioned whether a secretory adenoma is a new lesion or represents accelerated growth of an existing fibroadenoma or tubular adenoma during pregnancy.

### Signs and Symptoms

A new palpable, mobile, enlarging mass in a pregnant or lactating patient can indicate a secretory adenoma and should be differentiated from a galactocele.

### Sonographic Features

Sonography is chosen over mammography to evaluate the pregnant or lactating breast. A secretory adenoma is typically an oval, circumscribed solid mass. Internal

areas of increased echogenicity and some fluid-filled slits are likely related to milky secretory products (Fig. 16-39). Prominent vascularity is often a Doppler feature. Lesions can grow large and tend to regress in size after lactation ceases. Tubular adenomas are well-circumscribed, isoechoic to hypoechoic, oval homogeneous breast masses with normal to enhanced sound transmission.

## Phyllodes (Phalloides) Tumor[3,4,6,21,26,46]

A phyllodes tumor is a rare fibroepithelial neoplasm with a "leaf-like" growth pattern. The tumor resembles fibroadenoma but has more stromal cellularity and contains narrow, cyst-like clefts of mucinous, hemorrhagic, or cystic fluid. The median age at presentation for phyllodes is during the late fourth decade, which is later than is typical for a fibroadenoma. The tumor is usually unilateral and can grow to a huge size, sometimes suddenly. Phyllodes represent ≤1.5% of all breast

| TABLE 16-12 | |
| --- | --- |
| **Differential Diagnosis of Large Circumscribed Solid Breast Masses** | |
| **Benign** | **Malignant** |
| Fibroadenoma >3 cm | High-grade invasive ductal carcinoma |
| Juvenile (giant) fibroadenoma | Malignant phyllodes/sarcoma |
| Phyllodes tumor | Medullary carcinoma |
| Pseudoangiomatous stromal hyperplasia | Primary lymphoma |
| Secretory adenoma | |
| Hamartoma | |

Clinical history is taken into account when listing a differential for a mass >3 cm.

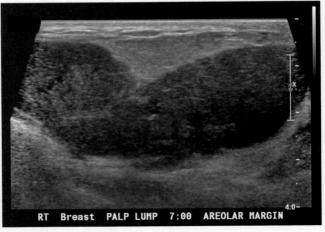

RT Breast  PALP LUMP  7:00  AREOLAR MARGIN

Figure 16-38 Juvenile fibroadenoma. Convex-linear sonogram of a teenage girl with a rapidly enlarging palpable mass reveals a 7.5-cm well-circumscribed, lobulated, hypoechoic solid mass.

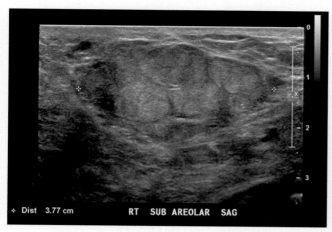

**Figure 16-39** Secretory adenoma. A lactating woman noticed an enlarging breast mass. Sonography displays a large, lobulated, circumscribed mass with isoechoic and hyperechoic internal echoes. The mass diminished in size after cessation of breastfeeding.

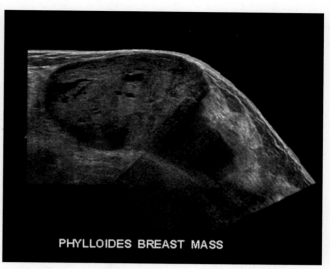

**Figure 16-40** Phyllodes tumor. This fast-growing, lobulated, circumscribed solid mass shows internal cystic areas. (Image courtesy of Philips Medical Systems, Bothell, WA.)

tumors but are the most common breast sarcoma. Although usually benign, a borderline tumor can undergo malignant transformation and has the potential to metastasize. Malignant phyllodes more often metastasize via the blood to the lungs, bones, and liver rather than involving the lymph nodes.[4,21] Chest wall invasion is possible.[4] Treatment includes wide local excision or mastectomy.[4,26] Recurrence is possible if excision is not complete.

### Signs and Symptoms

The palpable mass is discrete, nontender, and mobile. A large mass may bulge and stretch the skin, causing pressure and edema. The axilla is usually clinically normal.

### Mammographic Features[4,46]

The appearance is that of a radiopaque, circumscribed, oval, or polylobulated mass. Calcification is not typical. Veins may be enlarged.

### Sonographic Features[4,45–47]

Imaging features are often similar to those of fibroadenoma. However, demonstration of cystic spaces, especially within a large, discrete, solid lesion, suggests the diagnosis of a phyllodes tumor (Fig. 16-40). Malignant phyllodes tumors tend to be more lobulated, grow larger, and double in size faster than benign lesions.

### Hamartoma[3,4,6,8,21,26]

A hamartoma is an unusual benign mass made up of varying amounts of normal or dysplastic fibrous, epithelial, and fatty breast tissues. Alternative names include fibroadenolipoma, lipofibroadenoma, and adenolipofibroma based on predominating tissue components. This pseudotumor is located within the mammary zone and represents a focal malformation of breast development. Fibrocystic changes, PASH, and rarely cancer may develop within tissues of a hamartoma. A patient with

Cowden disease (multiple hamartoma syndrome) may show increase risk for developing breast cancer.

### Signs and Symptoms

Hamartomas are usually unilateral and often measure over 3 cm when diagnosed. Palpable masses are painless, often with a soft, rubbery consistency, and smooth or lobulated surface. Compressibility varies with the tissue makeup.

### Mammographic Features

A hamartoma appears as a smooth or lobulated encapsulated lesion, containing mixed radiolucent and radiodense areas. This "breast within a breast" pattern has been described as resembling a "piece of cut sausage." Benign calcifications are occasionally present. Mammography is better than sonography at differentiating fat within the lesion.

### Sonographic Features

The circumscribed oval mass displays a mixed echo pattern with isoechoic, hyperechoic and hypoechoic elements reflecting the mixture of tissue makeup (Fig. 16-41). A thin echogenic pseudocapsule of compressed breast tissue surrounds the mass. When fatty or fibrous components predominate, hamartomas may sonographically resemble a heterogeneous lipoma or a fibroadenoma.

### Lipoma[3,4,6,8]

A true lipoma is a benign nodule of mature adipose tissue surrounded by a thin connective tissue capsule. Lipomas can arise in many areas of the body, including the axilla, the breast, and the chest wall. Palpable nodules are slow growing, usually unilateral, and generally range from 2 to 10 cm in size. Large lipomas are susceptible to internal fat necrosis.

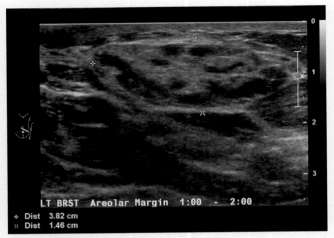

**Figure 16-41** Hamartoma. Sonogram shows a mass within the mammary zone that displays a mixture of echogenicities representing a combination of fibroglandular tissue and fat encircled by a pseudocapsule.

## Signs and Symptoms

When palpable, the painless fatty mass is typically smoothly circumscribed, movable, soft, and compressible.

## Mammographic Features

Delineation of a small lipoma is difficult in the fatty breast. Larger masses displace surrounding tissues. A lipoma appears as a round or oval, circumscribed, purely radiolucent nodule surrounded by a thin radiopaque fibrous capsule (Fig. 16-42A,B). A pure fat-density mass is a benign finding (BI-RADS 2) and does not require sonography for further risk assessment. However, sonography can help differentiate a lipoma from a fat-containing cyst.

## Sonographic Features

On a sonogram, a lipoma is smooth-walled, thinly encapsulated nodule with an echogenicity that is isoechoic or mildly hyperechoic compared to the adjacent normal fat. Lipomas can be homogeneous or may contain multiple fine linear echoes. There may be mild posterior enhancement.

Recognition of a lipoma may be difficult in the isoechoic fatty breast. A lipoma may also be missed if it is larger than the field-of-view of the linear array transducer. Split-screen or EFOV imaging will better display the spatial extent of a large lipoma. Echopalpation allows direct correlation of real-time imaging findings with the clinical findings. A lipoma is soft and usually compresses by at least 30% when overlying transducer pressure is applied and does not indent the pectoralis muscle. This can be documented using dual-screen imaging or with cine clips (Fig. 16-42A).

A small hyperechoic lipoma in the subcutaneous fat is readily discernable (Fig. 16-42B). A differential diagnosis for a hyperechoic subcutaneous lesion may include focal fat edema, fat necrosis, fibrous change, or hemangioma depending on the patient's history.

## Intraductal Papilloma, Intracystic Papilloma, and Papillomatosis

An intraductal (large duct) papilloma is a common neoplasm that most often occurs during late reproductive years.[6] This benign proliferative mass develops from focal overgrowth of duct epithelial and myoepithelial cells and is supported by a fibrovascular stalk.[3,23] A papilloma typically develops centrally, beneath, or close to the areola within a major lactiferous duct, rather than in a TDLU.[6] Central lesions are often solitary and can be too small to palpate. However, some papillomas grow to several centimeters and can extend into duct branches. Malignant degeneration is rare, although the presence of a papilloma slightly increases the risk for developing breast cancer.[21] Because of this, excision is still recommended for a papilloma,

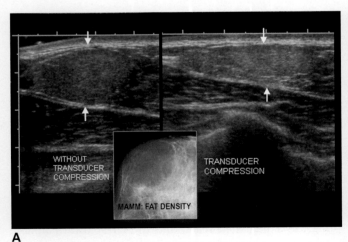

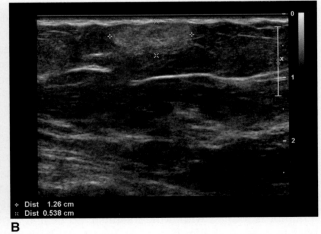

**Figure 16-42** Lipoma. **A:** Transducer pressure confirms compressibility of this soft, palpable, mildly echogenic, circumscribed mass. Mammogram *(insert)* confirms a radiolucent fatty mass. (From Carr-Hoefer C. *Breast Ultrasound: A Comprehensive Sonographer's Guide.* Forney, TX: Pegasus Lectures; 2007.) **B:** Hyperechoic lipoma is present within the subcutaneous fat.

which in some cases may be accomplished utilizing a VAB device.[6,40]

An ingrowing papilloma can obstruct the duct causing a cyst to form that envelops the solid lesion. This variety is termed *intracystic papilloma*. Torsion or infarction of the fibrovascular stalk can cause bleeding into the cyst.

*Peripheral papillomatosis* is a form of epithelial hyperplasia, causing formation of multiple small papillary growths in the small ducts of a TDLU. The occurrence is much less common than large duct papillomas. Papillomatosis can be bilateral and affect multiple lobules in any breast quadrant. This proliferative condition can be associated with radial scars, sclerosing adenosis, atypical ductal hyperplasia, and ductal carcinoma. Papillomatosis carries higher risk for developing breast cancer than a central papilloma.

Juvenile papillomatosis can afflict teens and young women, many of which have a family history of breast cancer. The juvenile form shows papillomatosis with possible severe atypia, extensive cyst formation, and sclerosing adenosis. This uncommon condition also serves as a marker for increased breast cancer risk.

### Signs and Symptoms of Intraductal Papilloma

The patient may be asymptomatic. A bloody or watery (serous) nipple discharge may be the first clinical sign of a developing lesion. A benign papilloma is the leading cause of spontaneous bloody nipple discharge from a single breast duct. Applying pressure over the affected duct can trigger nipple discharge. Occasionally, masses are palpable.

### Mammographic Features[4]

Standard mammography can miss a central papilloma with suspicion raised only by the presence of an asymmetrically dilated subareolar duct. Contrast ductography better delineates the intraductal filling defect.[43]

A solitary papilloma can appear as a subareolar soft-tissue nodule that may have a "raspberry-like" microlobulated appearance. Clusters of soft tissue isodense masses may indicate multiple papillomas. Occasionally, microcalcifications are present.

With an intracystic papilloma, standard mammography does not differentiate the solid component of the round or oval radiodense lesion. Prior to the widespread use of sonography, pneumocystography was used to evaluate the cyst cavity by injecting air into the cyst following fluid aspiration.

### Sonographic Features of Intraductal Papilloma[4,6,8]

A very small papilloma may escape detection. The only clue to its presence may be localized dilatation of a solitary duct.[35,40] Occasionally, the duct dilates enough to allow visualization of a portion of the indwelling soft tissue mass (Fig. 16-43). The soft-tissue mass may extend for a distance within the duct and into duct branches. Color Doppler demonstrates blood flow within the fibrovascular stalk of the lesion allowing differentiation

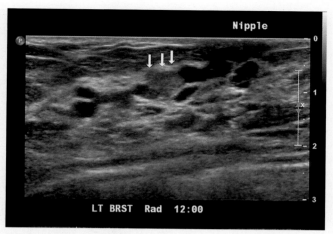

**Figure 16-43** Intraductal papilloma. Fluid within a dilated subareolar duct outlines the indwelling solid soft-tissue mass *(arrows)* in a patient with spontaneous nipple discharge from a single duct.

from echogenic blood or inspissated material within the dilated duct. A papilloma without duct dilatation appears as a circumscribed isoechoic to hypoechoic solid mass often in the subareolar region of the breast. Sonography cannot definitively differentiate benign from malignant intraductal papillary lesions, so tissue sampling or excision is needed.

Radial scans align the transducer along the long axis of a major duct, which allows better detection of intraductal lesions. Performing "two-handed peripheral compression" can also help evaluate dilated subareolar ducts (Fig. 16-44). The "rolled-nipple technique" allows a subareolar intraductal lesion to be followed into the

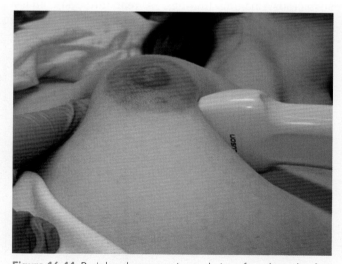

**Figure 16-44** Peripheral compression technique for subareolar duct evaluation. The transducer is oriented in a radial plane along the axis of the duct to be examined. The nonscanning hand is placed on the opposite side of breast to provide counter pressure. The transducer is angled by applying pressure to the peripheral edge of the transducer. This maneuver brings the subareolar duct into a scan plane more parallel to the transducer. Sliding the transducer toward the nipple follows the duct. (Reprinted with permission from Carr-Hoefer C. Breast Ultrasound for the Sonomammographer. Corvallis, Sound Imaging Consulting, LLC, 2007.)

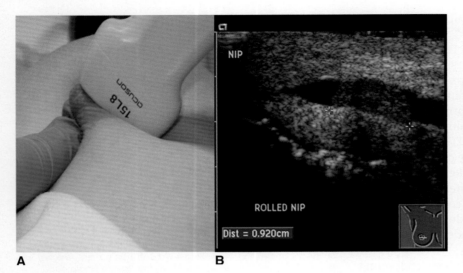

**A**                    **B**

Figure 16-45 Rolled-nipple technique. **A:** The transducer is placed along the nipple and breast in a radial plane parallel to the long axis of the excretory and subareolar duct. The index finger of the sonographer's nonscanning hand is placed on the opposite side of the nipple. Light transducer pressure is applied to roll the nipple over the index finger. This maneuver allows a subareolar duct to be imaged as it passes through the nipple to evaluate for an intraductal mass. **B:** The sonogram shows a nipple adenoma within a dilated excretory duct using the rolled-nipple technique. (Reprinted with permission from Carr-Hoefer C. Breast Ultrasound for the Sonomammographer. Corvallis, Sound Imaging Consulting, LLC, 2007.)

nipple and can also identify a nipple mass, such as an adenoma (Fig. 16-45A,B). Pressing over a dilated duct with the transducer may trigger nipple discharge that correlates with clinical findings.

### Sonographic Features of Intracystic Papilloma

Unlike mammography, sonography delineates both the solid and cystic components of the lesion (Fig. 16-46). A portion of the papilloma is sometimes seen extending past the cyst wall into the duct. Doppler flow within the solid component of the complex cyst differentiates an intracystic papillary tumor from a hemorrhagic cyst with clot, or from FCC with PAM. Both the cyst walls and solid intramural nodule should be evaluated for suspicious imaging findings. A real intracystic mass qualifies for a BI-RADS 4 classification with biopsy or excision to exclude an intracystic cancer since imaging

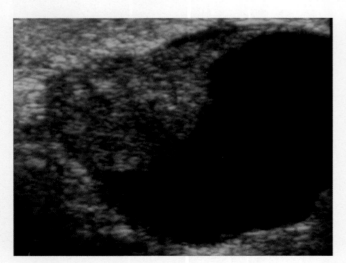

Figure 16-46 Intracystic papilloma. Sonogram documents a solid papillary lesion projecting into a cyst. The cyst is caused by obstruction of the duct by the indwelling mass. (Reprinted with permission form Carr-Hoefer C. Breast Ultrasound for the Sonomammographer. Corvallis, Sound Imaging Consulting,LLC, 2007.)

findings can overlap. VAB facilitates removal of both the cyst fluid and tissue cores for preoperative analysis.

### Sonographic Features of Juvenile Papillomatosis

In young females, a focal, ill-defined, heterogeneous mass containing several small peripheral cysts may indicate juvenile papillomatosis.[48] Multiple small cystic areas within the stroma can give the affected lobe a "swiss cheese" appearance.[6]

### Miscellaneous Solid Nodules[3,4,6,8,23,49]

Mammary fibrosis, radial scar, and granular cell tumor are some uncommon benign processes encountered during imaging that may mimic malignancy. Table 16-13 summarizes the findings in these processes.

### MALIGNANT BREAST MASSES

Excluding skin cancer, breast cancer is the most common malignancy affecting women in the United States. Breast carcinoma ranks second to lung cancer as the leading cause of cancer-related deaths in women over age 50.[1] Approximately one in eight American women develop breast cancer during a lifetime. Rates vary with race or ethnicity. The prevalence of breast cancer is highest in Caucasian women; however, African American women are more likely to die from the disease. Breast cancer is rare in males.[1]

Risk factors for developing breast cancer are well documented.[1,10,26] The majority of breast cancers occur in women over the age of 50 when most are postmenopausal. Occurrence in women under age 40 is less than 5%. Besides gender and increasing age, two major risk factors are a personal or family history of breast cancer and a personal history of biopsy-proven atypical hyperplasia. Only about 5% to 10% of breast cancers are genetically linked. *BRCA1* and *BRCA2* gene mutations significantly increase the risk for developing breast

**TABLE 16-13**

## Miscellaneous Benign Solid Nodules

| Focal Fibrosis | Radial Scar | Granular Cell Tumor |
|---|---|---|
| • Localized area of dense collagenous tissue with absent or sparse ducts and acini<br>• Can cause firm, painless palpable lump<br>• May cause imaging abnormality, ranging from solid hypoechoic mass to shadowing, irregular, spiculated, lesion | • Small, benign, sclerotic lesion affecting the terminal ductolobular unit<br>• Unrelated to breast trauma<br>• Often detected on mammography as an architectural distortion or an irregular mass with long spicules<br>• Sonographic detection is uncommon; may appear as poorly marginated lesion with shadowing<br>• May have increased risk for breast cancer | • Rare nonepithelial lesion; arises from Schwann cells of the peripheral nerves<br>• Occurs in the peripheral upper outer quadrant or inner breast<br>• Painless, palpable tumor; often firm and fixed to adjacent tissues<br>• May appear on sonography as irregular spiculated mass with hypoechoic central nidus and shadowing |

cancer. These gene mutations are also linked to ovarian and colon cancers. Genetically linked breast cancer tends to occur at an earlier age in both females and males and also well documented in those of Ashkenazi Jewish heritage.

The prognosis of breast cancer is greatly affected by the stage and extent of the disease at the time of diagnosis. Breast cancer prognosis is based on histologic type, tumor size, nodal status, evidence of distant metastasis, as well as biologic markers.[3,4,6,26] Lymph node status is a key predictor of cancer survival. The goal of screening is to detect breast cancers early when tumors are small and regional node status is negative, thus improving long-term survival.

Cancers are classified by histologic type and grade. Breast cancers are usually adenocarcinomas that arise from epithelial cells that line the breast ducts. Most cancers likely originate in a TDLU at the junction of the extralobular terminal with the lobule.[6] Malignant cells can further extend along the path of the duct into the lobule and/or migrate into larger ducts and potentially spread within the ductal system to other TDLUs within a breast lobe. Breast cancer has the highest chance (~50%) of developing in the UOQ where there is the greatest amount of glandular-epithelial tissue. Rarer types of malignancies include sarcomas that arise from connective tissues, primary lymphoma, and leukemia, as well as metastases.

Certain cancers are more likely to be multifocal or multicentric, or even bilateral which affects prognosis, surgical management and treatment, and increases recurrence rates. Multifocality describes the presence of additional malignant lesions within a breast quadrant or within 5 cm of the primary tumor, indicating spread of cancer via the ducts (see Fig. 16-54).[6] Multicentricity describes coexistent cancers within different quadrants or separated by more than 5 cm within the breast.[6] Multicentric lesions may be of the same or different histologic types.

This section discusses the pathologic, clinical, and common imaging features of many types of breast malignancies.

## NONINVASIVE CANCER

Noninvasive breast cancer is called carcinoma in situ.[3,23] The malignant cells are confined within the boundaries of the duct and/or lobule and have not extended past the basement membrane into adjacent tissue, thus virtually eliminating the risk of metastasis. Types of noninvasive disease are lobular carcinoma in situ (LCIS) and ductal carcinoma in situ (DCIS).[23]

### Lobular Carcinoma In Situ

LCIS arises in the small ducts of the breast lobule and is often multicentric and bilateral. LCIS is not treated clinically as a true cancer; however, this lobular neoplasia serves as a "marker" of significant increased future risk of developing cancer (ductal or lobular) in either breast.[4,26] LCIS does not usually present with specific clinical, mammographic, or sonographic features to aid detection. Diagnosis is typically made as an incidental finding from histologic analysis of breast tissue from a biopsy or surgical specimen. LCIS has a tendency to affect premenopausal patients.[4]

### Ductal Carcinoma In Situ[4,6,15]

DCIS is the most common noninvasive cancer, accounting for approximately 70% of in situ lesions. DCIS is also called "intraductal carcinoma." The mean age at time of detection in women is about 50 years. This early, node negative cancer is classified as stage 0 disease. The 5-year survival rate approaches 100% in treated patients. Atypical ductal hyperplasia is a precursor to developing DCIS. Like invasive disease, DCIS can be classified by histologic grade, which helps to predict the aggressiveness of the disease and the recurrence risk. Left untreated, high-nuclear grade (comedo) DCIS is more likely,

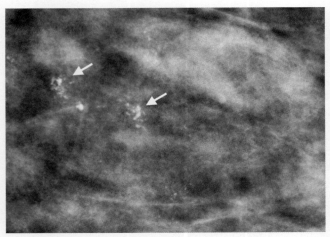

**Figure 16-47** Ductal carcinoma in situ (DCIS). Mammogram shows clustered microcalcifications in a woman with intermediate-to-high grade DCIS.

and more quickly, to progress to invasive cancer than is low nuclear grade (noncomedo) DCIS. High-grade DCIS is also more likely to recur as invasive cancer. High-grade lesions typically distend the duct with malignant cells that usually undergo extensive central necrosis and calcification. The necrotic tumor cells plug the duct with white-to-yellowish paste-like debris.

### Signs and Symptoms

Early stage disease is typically asymptomatic, although some patients may present with nipple discharge. A palpable mass is uncommon.

### Mammographic Features[4,8]

DCIS is the earliest form of breast cancer detected by imaging techniques and best detected by mammography as suspicious calcifications. Microcalcifications can be clustered (>5 within 1 cm$^2$) or follow a linear or branching pattern (Fig. 16-47). DCIS represents approximately 20% to 30% of cancers detected by screening mammography with 70% presenting only as suspicious calcifications. The presence of a focal soft-tissue mass is less common. Stereotactic-guided VAB is often the next step when suspicious calcifications are present, allowing for a histologic diagnosis. In other cases, sonography may be useful to exclude any related mass effect that might be missed in the radiographic dense breast prior to intervention.

### Sonographic Features[4,8,15]

DCIS often goes undiagnosed by sonography. Suspicious calcifications may be missed unless contained within a distended duct or hypoechoic mass (Fig. 16-48A,B). Microcalcifications appear as tiny, hyperechoic foci that do not shadow since they are smaller than the ultrasound beam width. DCIS-filled ducts and cancerized lobules can display microlobulation, duct extension, and branch patterns. Other signs may be an irregular dilated duct with asymmetric thickening or an indistinct wall, or an area of architectural distortion. Doppler flow extending across the duct wall into the lumen differentiates an intraductal neoplasm from inspissated secretions. A microcyst cluster with thick intervening walls or solid components with blood flow can suggest early cancer. Intracystic papillary DCIS appears as a mixed solid and cystic lesion.

### Paget Disease[3,23]

Paget disease is an uncommon cancer involving the epidermis of the nipple often initiated by underlying DCIS within a main subareolar duct. The diagnosis is often suspected clinically based on findings of redness, ulceration, and eczema-like crusting of the nipple and areola, along with nipple discharge and itching. A biopsy of the affected tissues and cytologic analysis of the nipple discharge can yield the diagnosis. Sonography is generally not needed unless to characterize a subareolar mass.

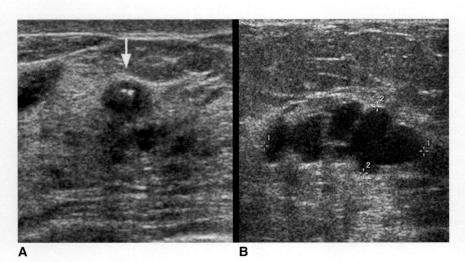

**A**              **B**

**Figure 16-48** Ductal carcinoma in situ. **A:** Sonogram of a dilated duct containing hypoechoic tissue and tiny, nonshadowing hyperechoic microcalcifications. **B:** Microlobulation is a feature of this 14-mm, markedly hypoechoic, intraductal carcinoma. The duct wall is intact.

## INVASIVE CANCER

Invasive cancer describes cases when malignant cells breach the basement membrane of the duct and/or lobule and extend into adjacent tissues.[3,23] Cancer cells can then penetrate nearby blood vessels and lymphatic channels, both pathways for metastatic seeding.

### Invasive Ductal Carcinoma[4,6,19]

Invasive ductal carcinoma, not otherwise specified (IDC NOS) is the most common breast cancer. This designation is used when there are no specific histologic patterns or findings that allow classification as a "special" type. IDC NOS accounts for about 65% of all breast malignancies and about 80% of invasive lesions. The prognosis for IDC NOS patients is usually poorer than for other invasive tumors, especially for high-grade lesions.

IDC NOS typically incites a desmoplastic (fibroelastic) response as tumor cells infiltrate neighboring tissues. Tumors often present as hard, fixed, stellate lesions (scirrhous features). Slow-growing IDCs allow more time for reactive fibrosis to occur, which helps to confine the tumor. Slow-growing lesions are often of lower grade and the fibrous tissue can account for a large percentage of the tumor's makeup. Reactive fibrosis is often responsible for malignant acoustic shadowing and also contributes to thickening and straightening of the Cooper ligaments that may lead to skin retraction. In contrast, fast-growing cancers lack time for much reactive fibrosis to occur, and instead, often incite an inflammatory response causing peritumoral edema. Such tumors are often of higher grade, show expansile growth, and tend to display more circumscribed margins. High-grade lesions typically contain abundant tumor cells, plasma cells, and lymphocytes and show prominent vascularity. High-grade cancers and those with extensive intraductal (DCIS) components are more likely to develop satellite lesions resulting in multifocal disease.

### Signs and Symptoms

When palpable, the carcinoma is usually hard, fixed, and painless. The most common location is the UOQ. Lesions with reactive fibrosis can feel larger on palpation than their actual size. Bloody nipple discharge is a worrisome finding but is rare. Secondary skin dimpling or nipple retraction or breast contour changes may be visible with advanced disease.

### Mammographic Features[4,35]

The principal sign of invasive cancer is an asymmetric, irregular, radiodense mass with spiculated margins (Fig. 16-49A). Associated clustered microcalcifications are common. Thickened and straightened Cooper ligaments and other secondary changes may be seen. A spiculated lesion is classified as BI-RADS 5 being highly suspicious for malignancy with a recommendation for tissue sampling. Sonography is not required to further characterize the mass unless to better assess tumor extent and to search for satellite lesions or adenopathy. However, IDC NOS can display more indeterminate features on mammography and sonographic evaluation is recommended before assigning a final risk classification.

### Sonographic Features[4,6,8,44,50]

As previously discussed, the presence of certain sonographic features allows classification of a mass as "suspicious for malignancy" in the absence of prior site infection or trauma (Table 16-11). Features suggestive of invasive cancer include demonstration of an irregular, hypoechoic, heterogeneous mass with indistinct, angular, or spiculated margins (Figs. 16-49B and 16-50). An echogenic halo surrounding the mass can represent unresolved spiculation. Angular margins occur at points where there is less resistance to tumor growth, such as in fat or at the base of a Cooper ligament. Microlobulation can indicate fingers of invasive

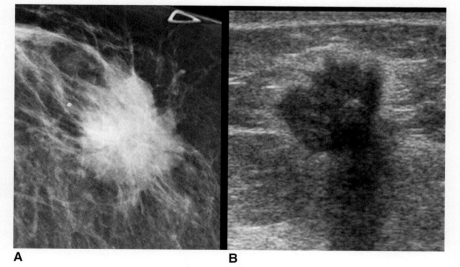

**Figure 16-49** Invasive ductal carcinoma. **A:** Mammogram shows a spiculated, radiodense mass. Skin marker denotes the mass is palpable. **B:** Sonogram of the heterogeneous solid mass shows multiple malignant features including spiculation, thick echogenic halo, irregular shape with angular margins, hypoechogenicity, and partial acoustic shadowing. (From Carr-Hoefer C. *Breast Ultrasound: A Comprehensive Sonographer's Guide.* Forney, TX: Pegasus Lectures; 2007.)

**A**                    **B**

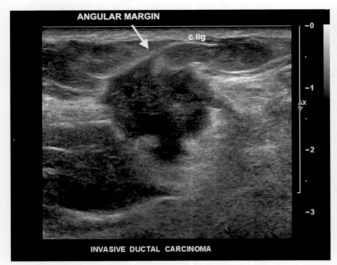

**Figure 16-50** Malignant features. Invasive ductal carcinoma showing an irregular shape. An angular margin *(arrow)* is seen at the junction of the mass with a Cooper ligament. This heterogeneous, hypoechoic mass also displays some spiculation and straightening of Cooper ligaments. (Image courtesy of Philips Medical Systems, Bothell, WA.)

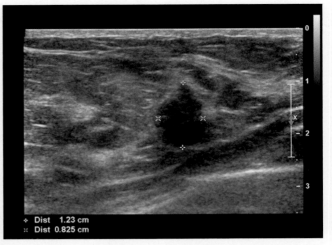

**Figure 16-52** Malignant features. This small (6 × 8.5 × 5.8 mm) markedly hypoechoic, invasive breast carcinoma is growing vertically within a terminal ductolobular unit. The mass is "taller than wide" (nonparallel, vertical orientation) and shows some subtle microlobulation.

tumor or DCIS distended ducts or lobules (Fig. 16-51). Cancers are often markedly hypoechoic compared to fat, especially when imaged using harmonics and spatial compounding. Occasionally, intratumoral microcalcifications are detected with high-resolution scanners. Attenuation shadowing is a worrisome finding and may be central, partial, or complete. The degree of retrotumoral shadowing depends on the amount of fibrous tissue within and around the tumor. Malignant shadowing does not disappear with transducer pressure. A "taller than wide" tumor can represent a small cancer growing within a vertically oriented TDLU or indicate cancer growth across tissue planes (Fig. 16-52). Radial

and antiradial scanning optimizes detection of duct extension from the tumor into a lactiferous duct, leading toward the nipple or branching into smaller peripheral ducts (Figs. 16-53 and 16-54). The entire mass must be carefully inspected since some cancers demonstrate suspicious imaging features involving only a small part of the mass.

A subset of IDC NOS lesions are relatively circumscribed, markedly hypoechoic, and show increased sound transmission (Fig. 16-55). These tend to be higher grade tumors with prominent cellularity and vascularity. Rapid growth can incite an echogenic border of peritumoral edema rather than spiculation. The presence of other suspicious features will lessen confusion with a benign mass. Some high-grade tumors show prominent microlobulations and may extend into main ducts increasing the potential for satellite lesions.

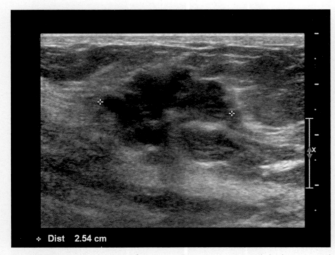

**Figure 16-51** Malignant features. Prominent microlobulation and marked hypoechogenecity are key features of this higher grade invasive breast carcinoma with intraductal components.

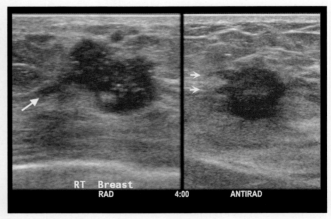

**Figure 16-53** Malignant features. The radial scan shows duct extension *(arrow)* with tumor growing into the duct leading toward the nipple. The antiradial scan shows tumor branching into smaller ducts away from the nipple *(arrows)*.

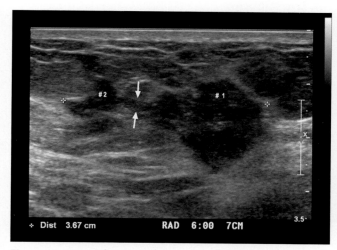

Figure 16-54 Multifocal invasive carcinoma. This high-grade primary tumor *(#1)* shows tumor extending into a major duct *(arrows)* that leads to a smaller satellite lesion *(#2)*. Biopsy confirmed multifocal disease.

Secondary signs of invasion include architectural distortion affecting any level of the breast. Cooper ligaments may appear thickened, straightened, or retracted. The skin may become thickened, flattened, retracted, or bulged. Nipple inversion is possible. Interruption of the fascial planes separating fat, glandular, and muscular structures suggests invasion. Tumors breeching the superficial or retromammary fat layers may eventually penetrate and become fixed to the skin or pectoral fascia. Secondary nodal involvement is possible.

### Differential Diagnosis

Clinical correlation is important, since several benign conditions can display architectural distortion, poorly circumscribed margins, attenuation shadowing, or other

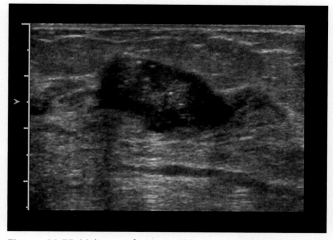

Figure 16-55 Malignant features. This circumscribed high-grade invasive ductal carcinoma, not otherwise specified shows areas of marked hypoechogenicity and distal sound enhancement. Tiny, nonshadowing, hyperechoic foci represent microcalcifications within intraductal components of the tumor.

sonographic features that simulate cancer. A necrotic invasive ductal carcinoma may appear as a complex cystic mass.

### Invasive Lobular Carcinoma[4,6,21,26]

Invasive lobular carcinoma (ILC) is the second most common invasive breast malignancy, representing 10% to 15% of cases. This cancer often shows a diffuse growth pattern and has higher rates of being multifocal, multicentric, and bilateral than invasive ductal carcinoma. Tumor cells tend to line up in "single files" and infiltrate the stroma in a diffuse manner and less often form a solitary discrete mass. Desmoplasia is not a typical feature with ILC.

### Signs and Symptoms

Although ILC can present as a hard fixed palpable mass, this cancer may feel like an area of nonspecific parenchymal thickening making clinical diagnosis difficult. With advanced disease, the affected tissues can retract causing a "shrinking breast."

### Mammographic Features

Mammography can underestimate and even miss ILC, especially in early stages or in the radiographically dense breast. The diffuse infiltrative nature of the disease may have a radiodensity equal to or less than surrounding parenchyma and suspicious calcifications are uncommon. However, some ILCs present as a region of architectural distortion or asymmetric density, or as an ill-defined mass with spiculated or obscured margins.

### Sonographic Features

Sonography is helpful at confirming abnormal tissue patterns at the region of clinical or mammographic concern. Sonographic patterns are variable but ILC often appears as an irregular, ill-defined, hypoechoic solid mass with acoustic shadowing (Fig. 16-56A,B). Subtle findings can include architectural distortion. When ILC is suspected or confirmed by biopsy, bilateral whole breast sonography may be indicated to search for multifocal, multicentric disease (especially if MRI examination is unavailable to evaluate the extent of disease and nodal changes).

### Special-Type Invasive Ductal Carcinomas

Medullary, colloid, papillary and tubular carcinomas represent a small subgroup of invasive ductal carcinomas that have morphologic and histologic features allowing specific classification. Except for tubular cancer, these special-type IDCs are usually highly cellular lesions that tend to display relatively well-circumscribed margins.[8] Compared to IDC NOS lesions, these special-type cancers occur infrequently and usually have better prognoses with lower rates of nodal metastases.

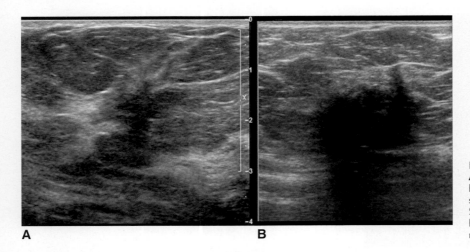

**Figure 16-56** Invasive lobular carcinoma. **A:** Sonogram shows a poorly circumscribed, hyperechoic mass infiltrating the breast tissues. (Image courtesy of Philips Medical Systems, Bothell, WA.) **B:** This markedly hypoechoic, spiculated, invasive lobular carcinoma causes acoustic shadowing.

## Medullary Carcinoma[4,6,8,10,26]

Medullary carcinoma is a well-marinated cellular tumor containing prominent lymphocytes and plasma cells. Pure tumors have been termed "circumscribed carcinoma." This uncommon tumor accounts for 5% to 7% of breast malignancies. Medullary tumors tend to develop earlier than other breast cancers with most occurring before age 50. Medullary cancer represents 10% of invasive cancers in women under age 35. Tumors can occasionally be multiple or bilateral. Medullary cancers compress peripheral tissues as they grow and usually elicit little or no reactive fibrosis. Central necrosis is common in larger lesions. Enlarged axillary nodes may be present that are either reactive or contain metastases. Prognosis is favorable, especially for typical tumors smaller than 3 cm with negative nodes.

### Signs and Symptoms

The discrete, rounded, somewhat soft and mobile palpable mass may simulate a benign mass. A large or rapidly growing mass poses concern with tumors often 2 to 3 cm at time of diagnosis. Most are located in the UOQ.

### Mammographic Features[4]

The round or lobulated radiodense mass is usually circumscribed or partially circumscribed. Patterns may mimic a benign-appearing lesion (Fig. 16-57A). Calcification is not a typical feature.

### Sonographic Features[22,40,42]

Medullary cancer can appear as a round or oval, circumscribed solid mass that can be markedly hypoechoic and often shows distal enhancement. Close inspection of the mass will usually reveal some suspicious finding to warrant biopsy (e.g., microlobulation, multilobulation) (Fig. 16-57B). A thick echogenic halo around the mass from peritumoral edema can make margins less distinct. Color Doppler may reveal prominent vascularity. Central necrosis is relatively common, yielding a complex sonographic appearance.

## Colloid Carcinoma[4,6,10,26]

Colloid (mucinous) carcinoma is uncommon, accounting for less than 2% of breast malignancies. This circumscribed gelatinous lesion contains tumor cells

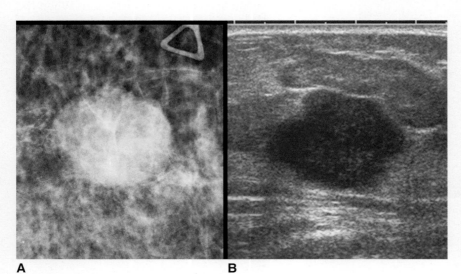

**Figure 16-57** Medullary carcinoma. **A:** Mammogram demonstrates a rounded circumscribed mass. **B:** Sonogram shows a circumscribed, hypoechoic mass with margin lobulations, as well as some distal sound enhancement. (From Carr-Hoefer C. *Breast Ultrasound: A Comprehensive Sonographer's Guide.* Forney, TX: Pegasus Lectures; 2007.)

dispersed in pools of mucin. Pure mucinous tumors more often develop in elderly women. Although slow growing, a colloid carcinoma can attain a large size. Unlike medullary cancer, internal hemorrhage is uncommon. Mixed lesions can display more invasive features.

### Signs and Symptoms

When palpable, the mass can have a soft consistency or feel like an area of thickening. A large lesion may be fixed to the skin or chest wall.

### Mammographic Features

Pure colloid carcinoma can appear as a low-to-high density round, oval, or lobulated circumscribed mass.

### Sonographic Features

Colloid carcinoma can image as a round or oval, circumscribed mass with possible lobulation or microlobulation (Fig. 16-58A,B). Internal echogenicity is often isoechoic or hypoechoic compared to fat, with a homogeneous or mildly heterogeneous echo pattern. Sound transmission is normal or enhanced. Secondary changes are not prominent features with pure forms of this cancer. A colloid cancer may occasionally mimic a fat lobule or lipoma, however, the mucinous tumor will not be as compressible.

### Papillary Carcinoma[4,6,38]

Solid papillary and intracystic papillary carcinomas tend to occur in older women and account for 1% to 2% of invasive breast malignancies. The incidence is slightly higher in men. Papillary carcinoma can occur centrally within the breast from malignant transformation of a large duct papilloma or develop within a peripheral TDLU. Lesions can be focal or multifocal within the breast ducts. Tumor growth is usually slow. Papillary cancers are more often in situ lesions. An absence of myoepithelial cells indicates invasion; however, invasive tumors tend to be low grade. Intracystic variants frequently contain bloody fluid. Clinical and imaging features of intraductal and intracystic papillary carcinomas may not differ significantly from their benign counterparts so histologic evaluation is important.

### Signs and Symptoms

Of concern is bloody nipple discharge from a single duct, which may be associated with a centrally located mass, which may be relatively soft.

### Sonographic Features[4,6,38]

Some in situ lesions may be too small to image. The new development of a circumscribed solid or complex cystic mass in an older patient remains worrisome since imaging features of benign and invasive tumors overlap. Duct dilatation is not always present to outline a papillary lesion. Solid tumors are evaluated for suspicious findings (e.g., microlobulation, duct extension, branch pattern, calcification). Malignant intraductal papillary lesions tend to be larger, extend a greater distance within a duct, branch more extensively into adjacent ducts, and potentially disrupt the duct wall. Radial and antiradial scans better assess ductal patterns. Color Doppler can demonstrate prominent blood flow within the vascular stalk of a papillary cancer, which may show multiple feeding vessels.

An intracystic papillary carcinoma is a complex lesion with solid and cystic components or mural nodule (Fig. 16-59). There may be echoes from bleeding into the cyst fluid. Any loss of wall definition, wall thickening, or extension of the tumor beyond the cyst and duct wall suggests malignant change.

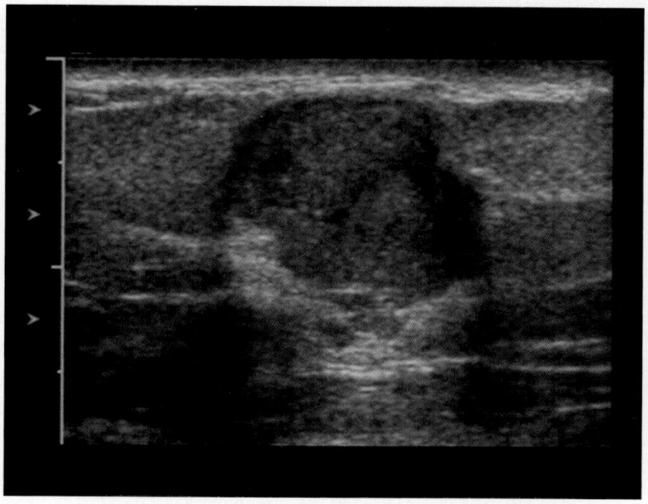

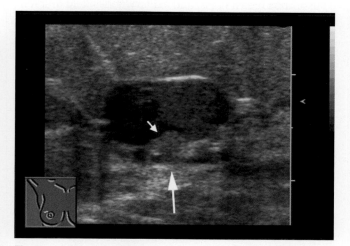

**Figure 16-58** Colloid carcinoma. This circumscribed lesion is mildly hypoechoic compared to fat and shows distal sound enhancement.

**Figure 16-59** Intracystic papillary carcinoma. This complex lesion consists of a small, solid, microlobulated, soft tissue mass *(arrow)* projecting into a cyst. The *larger arrow* shows tumor past the cyst wall extending into the duct. Echoes within the cyst were reflections from blood within the cyst cavity and confirmed during aspiration and biopsy.

## Tubular Carcinoma[4,6,47]

Pure tubular carcinoma accounts for about 2% of all breast cancers. This extremely well-differentiated invasive cancer is typically small, slow growing, and incites prominent reactive fibrosis. Pure tumors rarely exceed 2 cm in size and have an excellent prognosis. Tumors often develop within TDLUs in the peripheral breast and can arise from a radial scar. The median age of women with pure tubular carcinoma is during the late fourth decade, slightly earlier than for most invasive ductal carcinomas. At biopsy, tubular carcinomas are often classified as low grade IDC NOS depending on the percentage of tubular features present. Multicentric and bilateral lesions are often coupled with LCIS in adjacent tissues.

### Signs and Symptoms

Palpable lesions tend to be fixed and may be associated with skin dimpling.

### Mammographic Features

A pure tubular lesion can appear as a small, irregular, centrally radiodense mass often with long spicules (white star appearance).

### Sonographic Features

Tubular cancer is often a small, irregular, centrally hypoechoic mass with frank spiculation or surrounded by a thick echogenic halo (Fig. 16-60). Acoustic shadowing accompanies reactive fibrosis. Adjacent Cooper ligaments can become thick and straight and potentially cause retraction of the overlying skin.

## Inflammatory Carcinoma

Diffuse or inflammatory carcinoma occurs when a highly invasive cancer infiltrates the lymphatics of the skin.[3,21] These are often higher grade invasive ductal carcinomas that may disseminate within the breast. Biopsy of the skin, a suspicious breast mass, and axillary nodes help differentiate inflammatory carcinoma from benign inflammation.

### Signs and Symptoms[3,21]

The skin becomes red, warm, and edematous with an orange peel (peau d'orange) appearance that affects the majority of the breast. The breast is often painful and hard. Axillary lymph nodes are usually palpable.

### Mammographic Features[4]

Patient discomfort and breast swelling limit adequate breast compression. Skin thickening is evident (Fig. 16-61). Parenchymal edema further increases breast density making delineation of a primary tumor difficult in many patients.

### Sonographic Features[4,6,8]

A whole breast exam is warranted to search for underlying suspicious lesions. The inflamed skin appears thick and echogenic. Lymph vessels and veins are often dilated. Doppler reveals hypervascularity of the affected tissues. In some cases, a malignant lesion may interrupt the fat-dermal interface and directly invade the skin. Significant breast edema scatters the sound beam and degrades image detail and sound penetration, thereby allowing primary and satellite lesions to be missed. Scanning at lower frequencies improves sound transmission but reduces resolution. Evaluation of both breasts helps to compare architectural variations. Expanding imaging to the nodal regions may show adenopathy in the axillary and possibly, the internal mammary regions.

The long-term prognosis for inflammatory carcinoma is often poor but has improved in recent years. Some high-grade cancers are initially treated with neoadjuvant chemotherapy in an effort to "down-stage" the cancer prior to surgical resection. In such cases, a mammotomy clip can be placed with imaging-guidance to mark the

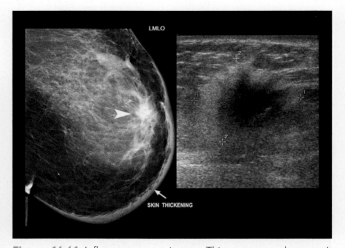

**Figure 16-61** Inflammatory carcinoma. This menopausal woman's breast was swollen, warm and had a peau d'orange appearance. The mammogram shows marked skin thickening primarily involving the mid to lower breast, as well as a suspicious radiodense lesion *(arrow)*. The sonogram showed a spiculated, hypoechoic mass with a thick echogenic rim. Biopsy of the mass and the skin confirmed invasive ductal carcinoma and tumor emboli in the subdermal lymphatics.

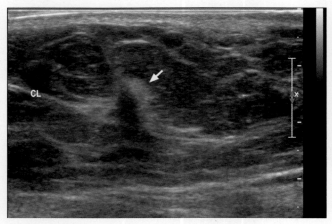

**Figure 16-60** Tubular carcinoma. This small, peripheral, hypoechoic lesion displays a thick echogenic halo from subtle spiculation *(arrow)*, acoustic shadowing, and Cooper ligament *(CL)* straightening.

tumor site. Sonography or MRI can follow the tumor's response to therapy, often showing a marked reduction in skin changes, breast edema, tumor, and nodal size.

Clinical and imaging features of inflammatory carcinoma can mimic acute mastitis. In pregnant and lactating women, breast cancer can grow and disseminate rapidly and should prompt the search for suspicious lesions in these women presenting with breast inflammation.

### Metastatic Carcinoma

The sonographic appearance of metastatic breast disease is variable. Routes for metastasis are via the lymph channels, the blood, or by direct extension. Metastatic disease yields a poorer prognosis and alters patient management based on the extent of disease. MRI and positron emission tomography (PET)-computed tomography (CT) have become particularly helpful in assessing the extent of metastatic changes.

### Spread of Cancer from the Breast

The first site of metastatic spread from a primary breast cancer is usually to the ipsilateral axillary lymph nodes, which receives most of the lymph drainage from the breast. Besides the axillary chain, the internal mammary nodes, as well as the supraclavicular nodes are considered regional lymph nodes for a primary breast cancer. Regional lymph node involvement is a strong predictor of patient survival. For surgical and staging purposes, the axillary nodes are classified as[4,6,8]:

- Level I nodes: low axillary nodes lying lateral to the pectoralis minor muscle
- Level II nodes: midaxillary nodes lying beneath the pectoralis minor muscle
- Level III nodes: high axillary nodes lying medial to the pectoralis minor muscle

(For staging purposes, interpectoral [Rotter] nodes are included as level II.)

The sentinel node is the first node in the drainage basin and at most risk for metastasis, and is typically a low axillary node. A radioisotope (during lymphoscintigraphy), as well as blue dye, can be used to map lymphatic drainage to the sentinel node for subsequent biopsy.

Sonographic features suspicious for lymph node metastasis include nodal enlargement; rounded shape; markedly hypoechoic or heterogeneous cortex; asymmetric cortical thickening; compression, displacement, or loss of echogenic hilar echoes; or indistinct capsule (Fig. 16-62). Transcapsular blood flow on color-flow Doppler and side asymmetry are additional worrisome findings.[6] Spectral Doppler is reported to show a similar waveform pattern in a metastatic lymph node when compared to the primary tumor.[6] Sonography can guide biopsy of a suspicious node since there is an overlap in imaging features with reactive nodes.

Primary breast cancer can also metastasize to distant organs via the bloodstream. The most frequent sites are the bone, liver, lung, and brain.[9,42]

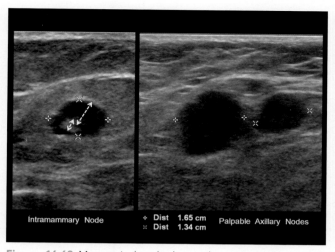

| ÷ Dist | 1.65 cm |
| :: Dist | 1.34 cm |

Intramammary Node        Palpable Axillary Nodes

**Figure 16-62** Metastatic lymphadenopathy. Intramammary node shows an increase in width of the cortical thickness compared to the echogenic fatty hilum. Rounded axillary nodes show marked hypoechogenicity of the cortex (nearly pseudocystic) and absent hilar echoes.

### Spread of Cancer to the Breast

The most common source of metastases to the breast is from a primary cancer in the contralateral breast. Spread to the opposite breast is primarily by way of the lymphatic system and often produces diffuse architectural change without a focal mass similar to inflammatory carcinoma.

Metastatic lesions in the breast from an extramammary primary site are rare. Cancer cells travel to the breast via the blood. Melanoma is the most common distant source, but other cancers such as the lung, ovary, uterus, stomach, and prostate (in men) can seed to the breast. Metastatic lesions most often develop in the UOQ and the superficial breast. Multiple lesions may develop in one of both breasts. Focal metastatic lesions in the breast are often relatively circumscribed without significant shadowing (Fig. 16-63).

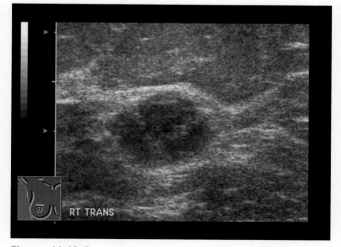

RT TRANS

**Figure 16-63** Breast metastasis. This fairly circumscribed, non-shadowing, mildly hypoechoic, rounded mass is a metastasis from a primary melanoma.

An echogenic halo can represent peritumoral edema. Frank spiculation or calcification is rare.

In rare cases, systemic diseases such as lymphoma and leukemia can also seed to the breast. Secondary disease is more common than primary non-Hodgkin breast lymphoma. On sonograms, primary lymphoma can present as a circumscribed or irregular, markedly hypoechoic mass with distal sound enhancement. Doppler reveals abundant blood flow. Enlarged, lymphomatous nodes can appear pseudocystic with absent or compressed hilar fat. Infiltrative or metastatic lymphoma can diffusely involve the breast and have a clinical and imaging pattern similar to inflammatory carcinoma. Breast changes associated with leukemia can have similar imaging patterns.

## THE IRRADIATED BREAST AND TUMOR RECURRENCE

Alternatives to mastectomy, such as lumpectomy followed by radiation therapy have become more common in recent years because of earlier diagnosis of breast cancer. Sonography can detect changes in the irradiated breast that are not seen in the normal breast. Alterations depend on the extent of surgery, duration of radiation, and time interval since treatment. Initially, skin thickening can be marked. The subcutaneous fat layer may be altered, showing increased echogenicity, interstitial fluid, and dilated lymphatic channels. Cooper ligaments may be thickened and the parenchyma may appear distorted, highly echoic, and attenuative secondary to postirradiation fibrosis or from surgical scarring.[26,40] History helps to differentiate imaging patterns from other inflammatory conditions or underlying malignancy. Residual effects in these radiotherapy cancer patients take longer to diminish than postsurgical changes following a benign biopsy. Scarring can be more pronounced and potentially obscure early tumor recurrence.

Tumor recurrence is suspected when there is an increase in the size of the tumor bed scar or development of a new mass at the surgical site after there has been documented stability of the scar by imaging tests. Additional signs of tumor recurrence can include the interval development of microcalcifications on the mammogram or Doppler blood flow on the sonogram.[4,40]

Contrast-enhanced MRI is reported to be more sensitive than mammography or sonography at differentiating recurrent cancer from scar tissue ≥18 months following breast conserving surgery by detecting early tumor enhancement.[4,8,51]

## THE MALE BREAST

The normal male breast consists mainly of fatty tissue, a small amount of fibrous connective tissue, and some rudimentary subareolar ducts.[26,40] The skin is thicker and the muscles are larger than those usually seen in the female breast.

Males with breast enlargement, nipple discharge, tenderness, or a palpable mass are candidates for sonography. Mammography is often technically difficult and magnification views are recommended for adequate evaluation of smaller breasts. Males can develop many of the types of breast masses seen in women; however, because males typically do not develop breast lobules, masses such as fibroadenomas and lobular carcinomas are rare. The most significant disorders afflicting the male breast are gynecomastia and cancer.

## Gynecomastia[3,4,6,8,52]

Gynecomastia refers to benign male breast enlargement characterized by an abnormal proliferation of ductal and stromal tissues. This is the most common male breast abnormality and is associated with an increased estrogen-to-testosterone ratio. Hormonal imbalances can be linked to physiologic, pharmacologic, or pathologic causes. Depending on the underlying cause, this condition can be unilateral or bilateral, transient or persist for a long time. Physiologic gynecomastia occurs in the neonate, in pubertal boys, and in older men at times of their lives when estrogen levels are elevated or when testosterone levels decline.

*Pseudogynecomastia* refers to male breast enlargement caused by excessive fat deposition without subareolar ductal proliferation. This bilateral condition is a normal variant and common in obese males.

### Signs and Symptoms

Gynecomastia usually presents as a soft-to-moderately firm, mildly tender, area of fullness, or nodularity centered beneath the areola. The abnormality is typically greater than 2 cm in dimension and relatively mobile. Tenderness can subside with chronic forms.

### Mammographic Features

The early "nodular" form appears as a fan-shaped, subareolar density representing glandular tissue that gradually tapers into the surrounding fat. The flame-shape "dendritic" form develops later and radiates deeper into the breast with possible extension into the UOQ (Fig. 16-64). There is more fibrous proliferation with this phase. The "diffuse glandular" pattern results from greater estrogen stimulation and resembles a heterogeneously dense female breast.

### Sonographic Features

Sonography is helpful at determining whether the cause of a subareolar density is due to a mass or gynecomastia (Fig. 16-64). Sonographic patterns of gynecomastia correlate well with mammography. Early changes often show a hypoechoic nodular or triangular region beneath the areola with a somewhat lobulated base. Increased vascularity on Doppler is commonly seen in this early phase of gynecomastia. The more dendritic form shows hypoechoic finger-like extensions radiating further into the breast core surrounded by echogenic

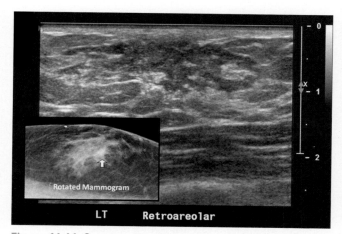

**Figure 16-64** Gynecomastia. This middle-aged male on steroids noted breast enlargement with nodularity beneath the nipple. Sonography shows hypoechoic, subareolar, mass-like tissue with extensions into the breast core, which corresponded to fibroglandular tissue seen on the mammogram (insert).

fibrous tissue. Diffuse gynecomastia can appear similar to the female fibroglandular tissue and occupy more of the mammary zone. Extra breast fat may be present.

Some patients with gynecomastia undergo sonography-guided liposuction as part of their treatment plan.

## Male Breast Cancer[3,4,26,33,52,53]

Breast cancer is rare in men, accounting for about 1% of all breast cancer cases. Most men affected are close to 60 years of age or older, which is much later than in women. Breast cancer can be genetically linked in males and shows a strong association with Klinefelter syndrome (47, XXY). As with gynecomastia, an elevated estrogen-to-androgen ratio increases cancer risk. Because men do not undergo breast screening, cancer is usually invasive by the time of diagnosis, with invasive ductal carcinoma being the most common primary tumor. The relative incidence of intraductal and intracystic papillary carcinomas is higher in men than women.[4,33]

Primary male breast cancer is typically located beneath the areola, usually just eccentric to the nipple, with peripheral lesions presenting less often. Advanced cancer can result in skin ulceration, chest wall invasion, lymph node metastasis, and distant disease.

### Signs and Symptoms

Clinically, cancer often presents as a unilateral, often painless, hard, fixed subareolar, or periareolar mass. Additional suspicious findings include bloody nipple discharge, retraction or ulceration of the nipple or skin, or palpable axillary nodes.

### Mammographic Features

A lesion that is eccentric to the areola increases suspicion when trying to differentiate cancer from gynecomastia. Radiodense lesions can be round, oval, or irregular. Suspicious mammographic findings are similar to those in females, although calcifications are less often present. The close proximity of the mass to the nipple can cause skin and nipple changes. Enlarged low axillary nodes may be seen.

### Sonographic Features

Some male cancers are fairly well-circumscribed or may have a complex appearance (e.g., intracystic papillary carcinoma, necrotic neoplasm), whereas other lesions display definite suspicious features (e.g., irregular shape, spiculation, microlobulation, shadowing) (Fig. 16-65). Feeding vessels may be seen extending into the lesion on Doppler examination. Secondary features include skin thickening, nipple retraction that are best seen when using an acoustic offset.

### Other Male Breast Malignancies

Paget disease of the nipple can afflict men more than women. Other forms of cancer affecting the male breast are rare and include malignant phyllodes, lymphoma, liposarcoma, leukemia, and metastases. Nonmammary primary cancers that can metastasize to the male breast include prostate (most common), melanoma, renal, and lung cancer. Estrogen therapy for prostate cancer increases risk for male breast cancer as well as for gynecomastia.

## DOPPLER EVALUATION OF THE BREAST

Recent advances in transducer design and Doppler capabilities have improved detection of altered blood flow related to breast pathology. Microbubble contrast agents can augment Doppler blood flow detection within breast masses but the practice is not yet approved for routine use in the United States.

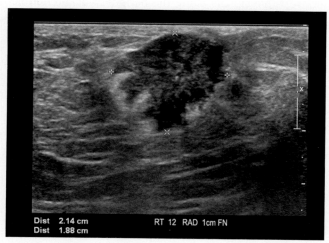

**Figure 16-65** Male breast carcinoma. This elderly male has a family history of breast cancer. The palpable periareolar mass corresponds to an irregular, heterogeneous, nonshadowing mass. A portion of the mass shows microlobulation and an echogenic halo.

Practical uses for color flow or power Doppler during a breast sonography exam include[6,8]

1. Documenting vascular pattern in a solid mass or a complex lesion
2. Differentiating a solid tumor from an echo-filled complicated cyst
3. Documenting a fibrovascular stalk within a intraductal tumor to differentiate from inspissated duct secretions or clotted blood
4. Differentiating hyperemic inflamed tissues from normal tissues
5. Differentiating a blood vessel from a fluid-filled duct
6. Differentiating recurrent tumor from a scar
   a. Differentiating a markedly hypoechoic/pseudocystic solid mass or abnormal node from a cystic mass
   b. Confirming clot within a thrombosed vein
   c. Documenting anatomical structure (e.g., hilar vessel node; internal mammary artery)
   d. Inducing movement of lightweight echoes in a complicated cyst
   e. Differentiating abnormal from normal tissues during performance of vocal fremitus

Doppler has questionable efficacy differentiating benign from malignant solid masses because of overlaps in findings. Current sonography systems have improved Doppler sensitivity, allowing better detection of blood flow in both benign and malignant masses. Researchers have reported vascular patterns that tend to occur more often in cancerous lesions, such as an increased number of blood vessels, penetrating vessels, and vessel tortuosity.[6,18,54,55] Cutoff values for resistive index (RI) using spectral Doppler are not reliable enough to differentiate benign from malignant masses.[6,18] Comparison of RI values from blood vessels along the periphery of the lesion to the interior vessels may provide useful information. Many invasive cancers tend to show higher velocity, more resistive waveforms centrally and lower velocity, less resistive signals along the periphery of the nodule, whereas benign masses tend to show less variation in waveform patterns.[6] When performing a Doppler examination, equipment settings should be optimized for low velocity states. Too much transducer pressure will lessen or ablate blood flow so very light touch is needed. Not all solid masses have detectable blood flow by Doppler techniques, which can limit its utility.

Doppler is being used at some facilities to assess the aggressiveness of a malignant tumor, as well as to monitor the response to therapy. Higher grade lesions tend to show increased vascularity and inflammatory hyperemia, both signs of a more aggressive tumor. A decrease in blood flow can precede tumor shrinkage following neoadjuvant chemotherapy.[6,56]

Some unique roles of Doppler include color streaking and vocal fremitus. During insonation, lightweight echoes suspended within a cyst (e.g., cholesterol crystals) will move toward the back wall when the intensity of the sound beam is increased. This is accomplished

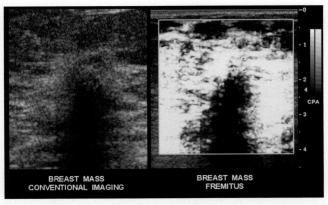

BREAST MASS CONVENTIONAL IMAGING

BREAST MASS FREMITUS

**Figure 16-66** Fremitus. Conventional gray scale image shows a suspicious shadowing breast mass. Power Doppler fremitus image shows a vibratory artifact defect *(color void)* corresponding to the attenuative mass and malignant shadowing. (Image courtesy of Philips Medical Systems, Bothell, WA.)

by using a higher transmit power setting or scanning in color or power Doppler mode. Vocal fremitus is a technique using color- or power-mode Doppler in which the patient is asked to vocalize (e.g., hum "eee") during real-time imaging of an area of interest. Vibrations from the chest wall will transmit through normal breast tissues creating a flash of color artifact. Abnormal tissues and masses will tend to show a "void" of color during vocal fremitus (Fig. 16-66). This vibratory defect can occur with many benign and malignant solid masses, as well as cystic masses. Although not effective at differentiating benign from malignant lesions, there are some situations when Doppler vocal fremitus is helpful.[6]

1. Differentiating an isoechoic solid mass from isoechoic breast tissue/fat lobule
2. Differentiating a fibroadenoma from an isolated fat lobule in the mammary zone
3. Differentiating malignant shadowing from benign artifactual shadowing
4. Delineating an indistinctly marinated mass from adjacent tissues
5. Raising suspicion for multifocal cancer
6. Determining if intracystic echoes are attached to the cyst wall (e.g., intracystic papillary lesion vs. unattached clotted blood)

Technical factors, such as excessive Doppler gain and transducer pressure, can alter the degree of fremitus artifact and hinder demonstration a vibratory defect.

Doppler information must be correlated with the clinical history and other imaging findings before a diagnosis is rendered.

## SONOGRAPHY-GUIDED BREAST INTERVENTIONAL TECHNIQUES[4,6,8,26,27,40,57–60]

Indications for interventional sonographic guidance are both diagnostic and therapeutic and have expanded over the years. The ACR has also published guidelines for the performance of imaging-guided breast interventional exams.[27] Common applications include cyst aspiration; drainage of a fluid collection such as a hematoma or abscess; biopsy of an indeterminate or suspicious mass; lymph node sampling; and preoperative dye or wire localization of a nonpalpable mass. Sonography can guide clip marker placement in a tumor prior to surgery or preoperative chemotherapy. There are a variety of less common applications. Sonography can guide needle placement in a subareolar duct for saline or contrast ductography when nipple cannulation is difficult.[6] In recent years, sonographic guidance has even been used during the performance of sentinel node, brachytherapy, cyrotherapy,[61] and percutaneous tumor ablation procedures.[6]

High-resolution sonography provides an alternative to mammography and MRI for aspiration, biopsy, and localization of certain breast masses. These procedures can be performed on an outpatient basis and are generally well tolerated. After sampling, the histologic or cytologic diagnosis should be compared with imaging findings to assess concordance.

The advantages of sonography often make it the first choice as a guidance tool during biopsy and aspiration procedures. It is widely available and uses no radiation. Sonography is often faster, provides accurate needle guidance, and offers more flexibility in patient positioning than stereotactic or MRI guidance. Real-time sonography systems allow direct visualization of the needle tip as it approaches and enters a mass helping to confirm adequate sampling or aspiration. Masses near the chest wall and those seen on only one mammographic view can often be sampled or localized by sonography. Color Doppler capabilities allow blood flow to be quickly assessed prior to tumor sampling to help limit hematoma formation.

Mammographic stereotactic biopsy is preferred for microcalcifications, especially those not associated with a mass, as well as for suspicious areas of architectural distortion. Also, a small deep solid lesion in a large fat-replaced breast may be better stabilized and more easily visualized during a stereotactic procedure.

Because most breast biopsies yield a benign diagnosis, minimally invasive percutaneous biopsy is preferred over open surgical biopsy for an initial diagnosis. Types of percutaneous biopsy techniques include fine-needle aspiration biopsy (FNAB), automated large core needle biopsy (CNB), and directional VAB, or mammotomy. FNAB is the fastest, lowest cost, and least traumatic biopsy method. However, undersampling and false-negative rates are higher with this cytologic technique. Both CNB and VAB provide multiple tissue cores for histologic analysis, allowing for more accurate diagnosis of benign versus malignant disease, as well as better differentiation of invasive from in situ carcinoma. Chapter 27 covers sonography-guided interventional procedures, including patient preparation and common techniques.

## GUIDANCE TECHNIQUES

The needle approach to the mass is based on the procedure type and the location of the mass within the breast.

### Method 1

A near-vertical approach provides the shortest needle path to the mass (Fig. 16-67A,B). The transducer is positioned so that the largest cross-section of the mass is lying under the center of the probe. The distance from the skin to the center of the mass is measured. The needle is placed alongside the center of the transducer and inserted into the breast with slight obliquity to a depth necessary to intersect the mass. The needle is seen in cross section as it enters the mass (Fig. 16-67C).

For preoperative localization, surgeons often prefer the shortest path to the mass. A drawback to this approach is the difficulty in visualizing the needle shaft and tip as it approaches the mass. This approach should be avoided when performing a spring-loaded biopsy of a deep lesion for fear of puncturing the chest wall or when sampling masses anterior to a breast implant.

### Method 2

The transducer is positioned over the mass. The needle is inserted obliquely under the long axis of the transducer allowing visualization of the needle tip and shaft progressing toward and into the mass (Fig. 16-68A). Using a convex linear format, spatial compounding, or slight rocking of the transducer can aid needle visualization by optimizing beam angle when an oblique needle path is chosen (Fig. 16-68B).

### Method 3

A preferred method is to advance the needle parallel to the long axis of the transducer and chest wall at a depth necessary to intercept the mass (Fig. 16-69A). Because the sound beam is directed perpendicularly, the needle shaft and tip are optimally visualized. This line-of-fire method is recommended for spring-loaded CNB when sampling a deep mass to avoid chest wall puncture and, as well as for sampling a mass anterior to an implant (Fig. 16-70). During VAB, this parallel approach can be used to maneuver the aperture of the biopsy probe underneath the lesion.

As an alternative, the needle can be advanced to the depth of the mass in an oblique approach and then pushed to a more parallel orientation by pressing down on the needle hub. This allows the needle entry site to be closer to the transducer (Fig. 16-69B).

## PROCEDURES[4,6,8,26,37,58,59]

The supplies needed depend on the type of procedure to be performed.

### Directional Vacuum-Assisted Core Biopsy

Handheld VAB devices allow more rapid acquisition of larger, more cohesive, tissue cores through a single needle insertion site. This minimally invasive breast biopsy

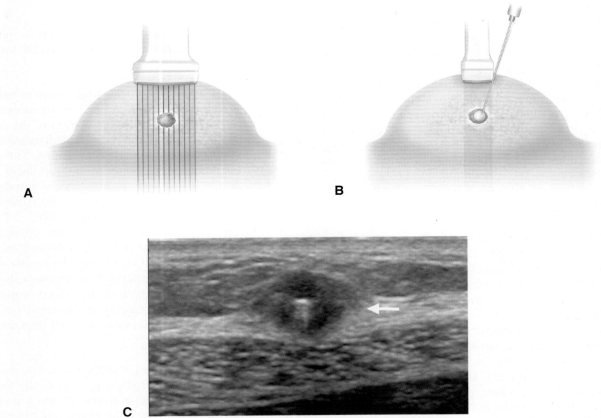

**Figure 16-67** Method 1: Sonographic needle guidance. **A:** Linear-array transducer positioned over the center of the mass. **B:** Side view showing the needle adjacent to the center of the transducer, with a slightly angled insertion path to the mass. **C:** Sonogram showing a cross section of the needle (arrow) within a solid mass.

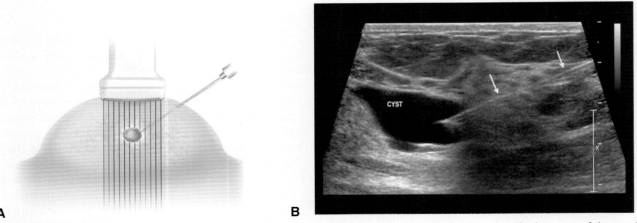

**Figure 16-68** Method 2: Sonographic needle guidance. **A:** Linear-array transducer positioned over the mass. The long axis of the needle shaft and tip can be visualized as the needle is inserted at an oblique angle to intercept the mass. **B:** Convex-linear scanning improves needle visualization (arrows) during oblique needle insertion for this cyst aspiration.

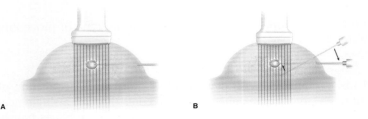

**Figure 16-69** Method 3: Sonographic needle guidance. **A:** The long axis of the needle is inserted parallel to the transducer or chest wall. This optimizes visualization of the needle shaft and tip and avoids needle puncture through the chest wall. **B:** Alternate method is to insert the needle obliquely and then push the needle hub down to a more parallel path. This alternate method allows needle insertion closer to the mass.

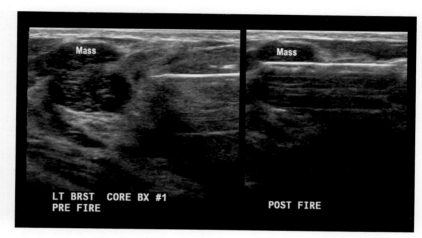

**Figure 16-70** Large-core breast biopsy. A 14-gauge, spring-loaded automated biopsy needle is inserted parallel to the transducer. The hyperechoic needle shaft and tip are well seen. The "pre-fire" image shows the needle in line with the mass. The "post-fire" image documents the biopsy site after real-time tissue sampling.

procedure is also termed *mammotomy*. Several manufacturers produce vacuum-assisted devices. Common biopsy probe sizes are 8- or 11-gauge. Sonographic-guided VAB is usually performed on small suspicious solid lesions (<1.5 cm), sonographically visible suspicious calcifications, some intraductal papillary lesions, as well as to sample complex lesions. VAB is also approved for the excision of small fibroadenomas.

After proper skin prep, there is generous injection of an anesthetic along the intended biopsy path and around the mass. Extra anesthesia can be injected under a deep lesion to help elevate the mass away from the pectoralis muscle. After a small scalpel nick is made, the large-gauge bladed-tip needle probe is inserted into the breast under sonographic guidance. Unlike a spring-loaded core biopsy, the VAB probe is advanced directly under the mass. The needle aperture is opened, producing a "ring-down" artifact that serves as a positioning landmark (Fig. 16-71). Once the aperture is positioned under the mass, vacuum suction is applied to pull the mass into the opening. A rotating cutter then slides across the aperture to obtain

the specimen core. The vacuum pulls the specimen into a collection chamber without removal of the probe. Multiple consecutive cores are quickly acquired, often in a clockwise manner. The cores can be sent for a specimen radiograph if sampling microcalcifications. A metallic clip embedded in a gel foam pledget can be deployed to mark the biopsy site for future localization. Sonographically, the clip marker has an echogenic rod shape appearance. After the biopsy, pressure is applied over the site to reduce bleeding, which is a greater concern with VAB.

Because of the larger tissue cores, there is less chance of undergrading a cancer based on histology from a VAB.

### Preoperative Localization

A spring hook-wire needle is inserted into the lesion under sonographic guidance. Surgeons prefer the shortest path to the lesion. The guide is removed, and a 0.5- to 1-mL mixture of blue dye and Lidocaine is injected along the entire needle track. The syringe is removed, and the hook-wire is inserted through the same needle. The needle is removed, keeping the wire in place. The end of the wire is taped to the skin, and sterile gauze is taped over the site. During subsequent excision, the wire or dye acts as a surgical guide to the nonpalpable mass. A mixture of blue dye and Lidocaine can be injected along a standard fine-needle track to the site of the mass without placement of a hook-wire, but surgery must be performed soon after localization (within 1.5 to 4 hours), before the dye diffuses in the parenchyma.[42]

Sonography can also be used in the operating room to verify complete excision of a localized breast mass. Also, excised specimens can be placed in cellophane wrap[62] or in a saline solution and scanned to confirm removal of the lesion.

## THE AUGMENTED BREAST[6,8,10,26,40,47,63,64]

Although MRI is considered the most accurate imaging tool for assessing implant integrity, sonography is of much lower cost and quite useful when examining

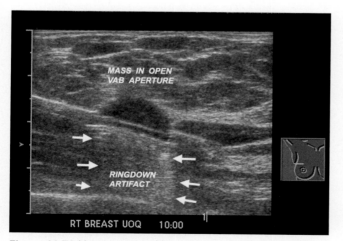

**Figure 16-71** Vacuum-assisted breast biopsy. The biopsy probe is positioned under the mass. The posterior portion of a solid mass is seen within the needle probe aperture. Ring-down artifact emanates beneath the site of the opened aperture.

women who have undergone augmentation or reconstructive mammoplasty. In patients with breast implants, sonography allows evaluation of overlying breast tissues for pathology, as well as for changes within and around the prosthesis. Mammography may be suboptimal and more technically difficult in these patients.

## BREAST IMPLANTS

Over the years, there have been numerous types of implants developed for cosmetic breast augmentation and postmastectomy reconstruction, with saline and silicone being the most common. Silicone gel better simulates the feel of the natural breast than saline, a feature often preferred by women. In 1992, the U.S. Food and Drug Administration restricted the use of silicone implants for breast augmentation due to safety concerns related to leakage. Since then, saline implants have been more widely used. However, in late 2006, the FDA approved the use of certain newer generation silicone cohesive-gel implants with conditions for device monitoring.

When examining the augmented breast, sonographers should understand the imaging differences between common implant types, placement sites, and related complications.

### Placement Sites

For cosmetic breast enlargement, the implants are often placed beneath the glandular tissue in front of the pectoralis muscle (subglandular or prepectoral location). Women with subglandular implants require special mammographic "pushback" (Eklund) views to better visualize the overlying breast tissue. Alternatively, the implants can be inserted beneath the pectoralis major muscle (submuscular or retropectoral location), which may help reduce capsular contracture. A submuscular location is standard for placement of tissue expanders and implants following mastectomy. Implants are less often inserted beneath the pectoralis minor muscle.

### Normal Implant Appearance

Saline implants have a single anechoic lumen and an anterior filling port to allow fluid expansion to the desired size (Fig. 16-72). The fill valve may occasionally be the cause of a palpable lump near the areola (Fig. 16-73). The more gradual filling of a tissue expander allows the skin to stretch prior to placement of a permanent prosthesis.

Silicone gel implants have single or double lumens. Single-lumen silicone gel implants come in prefilled sizes and are generally anechoic. Double-lumen implants have separate silicone and saline chambers. An echogenic membrane separates the chambers. A filling port extends to the expandable saline chamber.

A fibrous capsule naturally forms around an implant, which is an expected response to a foreign body. This fibrous reaction is more pronounced with silicone gel implants. The silicone elastomer shell of a breast implant can be smooth or textured. Texturing of the implant shell

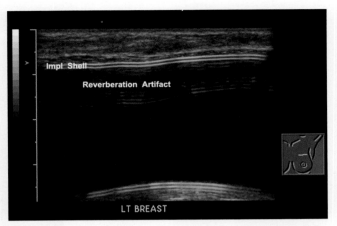

**Figure 16-72** Saline implant. The outer and inner margins of the smooth implant shell are seen as closely spaced parallel lines abutting the fibrous capsule. The implant lumen is anechoic although reverberation artifact is seen within the anterior implant.

helps to reduce the degree of capsular contracture. The inner and outer layers of an implant shell appear as two smooth, thin, parallel, hyperechoic lines when the sound beam is directed perpendicular to implant surface. An intact implant lays adjacent to the fibrous capsule. High-frequency sonography can often delineate three closely spaced echogenic lines, with the outer third line representing the fibrous capsule abutting the implant shell. This has been termed the "capsule-shell-echo" complex is best seen with nontextured implants using a high-frequency transducer. A textured implant shell may have a thicker or fuzzier sonographic appearance.

A common implant finding is a linear infolding of the implant shell, or radial fold, which may extend for a variable distance from the implant margin (Fig. 16-74). Long, wavy folds may mimic a double-lumen or intracapsular rupture (ICR). Some lobulation of the contour of an intact implant, or "wrinkling" of the

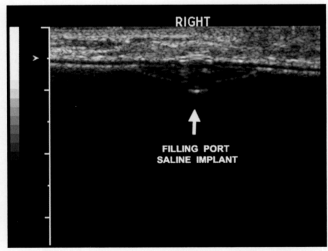

**Figure 16-73** Saline implant. The anterior filling port is the cause of the palpable lump in this patient with a periareolar lump.

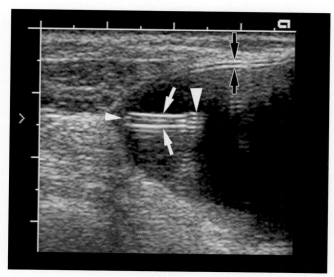

**Figure 16-74** Radial fold. An infolding of the implant shell is seen extending a short distance into the implant lumen. This normal fold is twice the thickness of a single shell layer *(white arrows)*. (Reprinted from Middleton M, McNamara MP Jr. *Breast Implant Imaging.* Philadelphia, PA: Lippincott Williams & Wilkins; 2003.)

implant shell, is occasionally seen. An anterior wrinkle can bulge enough to be palpable in certain positions.

Reverberation artifacts are commonly present and create a band of false echoes across the anterior lumen of the implant (see Fig. 16-72). Harmonic imaging and spatial compounding help reduce imaging artifacts, thereby improving evaluation of the implant shell and reducing error when assessing implant integrity. Lighter transducer pressure can also reduce the amount of near-field reverberation within the implant.

Sound travels much slower though silicone (~1,000 m/s) than through saline or soft tissue (1,540 m/s). This creates a propagation speed artifact (or translation effect), whereby the posterior wall of the implant and distal structures falsely appear to extend deeper into the chest than adjacent tissues. Scanning along the edge of a subglandular silicone implant will show a "step-off" or discontinuity of the chest wall deep to the implant,

which is not seen beneath saline (Fig. 16-75). This artifact is useful when trying to differentiate a silicone from a saline implant in a patient with poor history and when a mammogram is not available for comparison.

A small amount of reactive fluïd may be seen between the implant shell and fibrous capsule, termed *peri-implant effusion*. This normal finding is more common with textured implants and is not to be confused with implant rupture.

## Implant Complications

Sonography can evaluate many of the complications associated with breast augmentation. Changes in implant shape, contour, and size may occur with fibrous or calcific contracture, herniation, rupture, and deflation. Capsular contracture is more often a problem with silicone implants causing thickening and hardening of the fibrous capsule around the implant shell. This causes the implant to become rounded, hard, and immobile. Sonography will demonstrate a thickened capsule-shell complex and poor compressibility of the implant with transducer pressure. A crack in the fibrous capsule can allow focal herniation of the implant through the defect, which may present as a palpable lump. Peri-implant abscess, seroma, or hematoma may result from implant surgery, infection, or trauma. The incidence of silicone implant rupture increases with the age of the prosthesis. Implant rupture may be spontaneous, the result of trauma (including prior closed capsulotomy), or from degeneration over time. Published studies vary on the incidence of silicone implant failure. An MRI study of 344 women, published in 2000, reported a median age for ruptured silicone gel implants to be 10.8 years.[63]

## EVALUATION OF IMPLANT INTEGRITY[4,6,26,40,63–65]

Saline implants are reported to more easily rupture from trauma than silicone implants. Collapse and deflation of a saline implant can be determined by clinical exam and by mammography, without reliance on sonography.

**Figure 16-75** Implant differentiation. Saline implant: There is continuity of the pectoralis muscle *(PM)* beneath the saline implant. A small amount of reactive peri-implant fluid is present *(arrowhead)*. Silicone implant: In contrast, there is discontinuity of the PM and pleural reflection *(large arrows)* beneath the silicone prosthesis (step off sign; translation effect). The slower speed of sound through silicone causes structures beneath the implant to falsely appear deeper in the body than in reality. (Reprinted from Middleton M, McNamara MP Jr. *Breast Implant Imaging.* Philadelphia, PA: Lippincott Williams & Wilkins; 2003.)

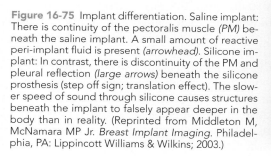
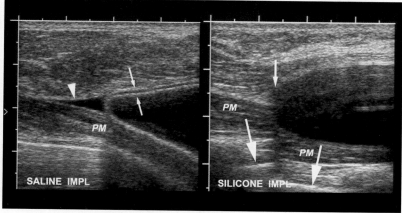

MRI and sonography are more sensitive than mammography when evaluating silicone implant integrity. Unlike saline, silicone blocks the penetration of X-rays, thereby obscuring the implant lumen and underlying tissue. This restricts detection of implant rupture on a mammogram. Sonography is not effective at determining a "gel bleed," which is microscopic passage of silicone fluid from an intact implant due to shell permeability and does not imply rupture.

When scanning the augmented breast for implant failure, it is important to closely inspect the implant lumen, the shell membrane and its proximity to the fibrous capsule, as well as the surrounding tissues and the axilla. High-frequency transducers are utilized to evaluate implants and overlying tissues. However, lower frequencies (5 to 7.5 MHz) may be needed to penetrate the deepest portion of the prosthesis and distal structures or to penetrate significant capsular or calcific fibrosis. EFOV imaging shows a greater extent of the implant. Split-screen imaging allows side-by-side documentation of similar areas in both implants to compare implant integrity or contour changes.

Silicone implant failure is classified as intracapsular or as extracapsular rupture (ECR).

## Intracapsular Rupture

ICR describes when silicone migrates outside the implant through a breach in the implant shell but is contained by the intact fibrous capsule. This type of rupture is most common. Collapse of the implant shell may be minimal, partial, or complete. A very early sign of uncollapsed rupture is silicone trapped within radial folds. On MRI, this early feature is called the inverted teardrop, noose, or keyhole sign and is occasionally detected sonographically. The classic sonographic appearance of ICR is demonstration of the stepladder sign or parallel-line sign seen as multiple, parallel, echogenic curvilinear lines layered within the silicone gel contained by the fibrous capsule (Fig. 16-76). This finding is usually associated with significant rupture. The stepladder sign represents sound reflecting off of the overlapping layers of the collapsed implant shell suspended within the encapsulated silicone and corresponds to the linguine sign seen on MRI scans. Use of spatial compounding or 3D imaging may better display the continuity of the curved edges of the collapsed implant shell.

A diagnostic pitfall is to confuse other band-like echoes within an intact implant with ICR, such as reverberation artifacts, redundant radial folds, or double-lumen membrane interfaces. Anterior reverberation artifact can obscure detection of a minimally collapsed implant shell that might only show a slight separation of the implant away from the fibrous capsule. Overall, noncontrast MRI is more reliable than sonography at diagnosing ICR, especially in patients with double-lumen implants.

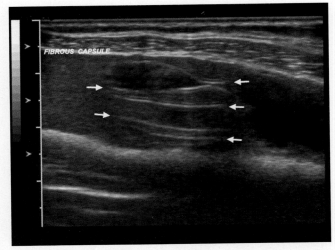

**Figure 16-76** Intracapsular rupture. Silicone implant demonstrates multiple overlapping layers of a collapsed implant shell **(arrows)** suspended in silicone contained by the intact fibrous capsule (*parallel-line sign*). There is increased echogenicity of some of the extruded silicone.

A less reliable sign of ICR is the presence of low-medium level echoes within the extravasated silicone between the implant shell and fibrous capsule. ICR may allow the influx of body fluids, proteins, or organic salts to mix with the silicone, which can increase the echogenicity of the extravasated gel. Other materials injected into the implant to reduce contracture, infection, and to promote symmetry can also cause alterations in the echo pattern of silicone and limit the efficacy of this finding.

## Extracapsular Rupture

ECR indicates silicone leakage into the surrounding tissues through a defect in both the implant shell and the fibrous capsule. The presence of silicone in soft tissues can incite an inflammatory response and granuloma formation. The most specific sonographic finding of ECR is demonstration of the echogenic noise sign, which describes a discrete region of intense hyperechogenicity with dirty distal shadowing emanating from tissue containing free silicone (Fig. 16-77). This distinctive appearance is also termed the snowstorm sign and may result from marked scattering and attenuation of the sound waves when passing through tissues containing microglobules of free silicone. Although usually near the edge of the implant, free silicone can migrate along the chest wall, to the axilla, to the lymph nodes, and even travel to extramammary sites (Fig. 16-78).

With ECR, macroglobules of extruded silicone can appear as anechoic, hypoechoic, or complex cystic masses that may be associated with areas of echogenic noise. Because of the propagation speed variance, the back wall of a silicone gel cyst will falsely appear deeper than its true location. This elongated anteroposterior

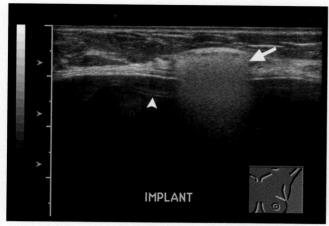

**Figure 16-77** Extracapsular rupture. *Arrow* points to "echogenic noise" from a siliconoma near the fibrous capsule in a woman with silicone implant failure. The implant shell *(arrowhead)* is separated from the fibrous capsule.

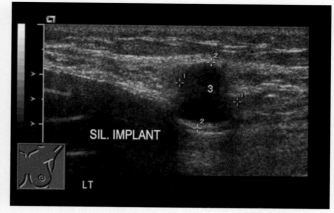

**Figure 16-79** Silicone gel cyst. Extruded silicone gel has the appearance of an elongated cyst in this patient with extracapsular rupture. The propagation speed artifact through silicone increases the cyst's anteroposterior diameter. (From Carr-Hoefer C. *Breast Ultrasound: A Comprehensive Sonographer's Guide*. Forney, TX: Pegasus Lectures; 2007.)

dimension helps to differentiate a silicone globule from a true cyst (Fig. 16-79).

### Nonimplant Presence of Free Silicone

Retained silicone may be detected inside or outside the residual fibrous capsule after explantation of a silicone implant so clinical correlation is needed. Some facilities use sonographic guidance to remove residual silicone granulomas.

Infrequently, a sonographer will encounter a patient that has had substances injected directed into the breast for augmentation purposes rather than use of an implant. Direct injection of silicone oil into the breast tissue has long been discontinued in the United States but the practice continued for a longer period in countries such as Japan and in Asia. These women suffer from complications such as infection, extensive fibrosis,

granuloma formation, and fat necrosis that result in hard, nodular, and even disfigured breasts. Mammographic detection of cancer is severely compromised in these women. On a sonogram, a widespread pattern of echogenic noise correlates with diffuse silicone granulomas (siliconomas). Silicone migration to ectopic sites and lymph nodes is common. Other types of cosmetic augmentation injections have been reported, such as paraffin wax and polyacrylamide hydrogel, which also incite granulomatous reactions.[4]

## AUTOGENOUS BREAST RECONSTRUCTION[4,8]

A patient's own tissues can be used to help reconstruct the shape of the breast following mastectomy. In some patients, an implant is placed in conjunction with a tissue transfer. Autologous tissue transfers can undergo postoperative complications—of most concern is vascular compromise that may lead to possible skin or tissue necrosis. Some of the more common autogenous breast reconstruction procedures involve transferring tissues and muscles from the abdomen or the back.

### TRAM Flap Procedure

The transverse rectus abdominis myocutaneous (TRAM) flap is the most common method of autogenous tissue reconstruction. Keeping the vascular pedicle (superior epigastric vessels) intact, the periumbilical muscle, subcutaneous fat, and skin are excise and tunneled under the skin to the mastectomy site. Closure of the abdominal tissues provides the patient with a "tummy tuck." A free TRAM flap procedure requires microsurgery to attach the vascular supply to the chest wall vessels once the tissue flap is placed at the breast site. A "free flap" procedure often utilizes the deep inferior epigastric vessels and transfers a smaller amount of rectus muscle.

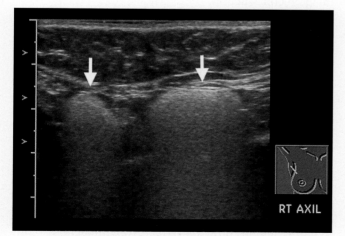

**Figure 16-78** Silicone adenopathy. Axillary nodes display "echogenic noise" from silicone uptake. (From Carr-Hoefer C. *Breast Ultrasound: A Comprehensive Sonographer's Guide*. Forney, TX: Pegasus Lectures; 2007.)

Preoperative duplex Doppler can map and document the size, flow velocities, and resistive indices of the superior and inferior epigastric vessels to help determine their vascular contributions to the rectus abdominis muscle. For a free flap procedure, the surgeon can sever the vessel that contributes a smaller blood supply to the muscle.

### Latissimus Dorsi Myocutaneous Flap Procedure

The latissimus dorsi myocutaneous flap is a reconstruction method in which the muscle and overlying tissue from the upper back is transferred and used to reshape the breast. This method is often used for partial mastectomy defects. In some patients, an implant may be placed under the latissimus dorsi flap.

## EMERGING SONOGRAPHIC TECHNOLOGIES

In recent years, there has been a variety of equipment and software improvements that aide in the detection of breast disorders. 3D imaging is becoming commonplace. Some newer sonography systems incorporate special processing filters to enhance sonographic delineation of microcalcifications. Others apply fusion technology with positional tracking abilities to correlate the location of a breast mass or metastatic lesion with MRI or CT imaging.[66] Elastography and automated whole breast scanners have received much notoriety in the sonography community and are briefly discussed here.

### ELASTOGRAPHY[8,19,60]

Elastography is a newer technique performed in conjunction with conventional 2D imaging and available on some sonography systems. Simply stated, acoustic waves generate an elastogram that displays the relative "stiffness" of a mass compared to adjacent tissues by measuring the amount of displacement the tissues undergo when compressed. Hard lesions show less deformation (strain) than soft tissues. This technique shows potential for reducing the number of unneeded biopsies by better differentiating benign from malignant breast masses. On the elastogram, hues of color or gray scale levels can be used to display the degree of tissue stiffness. A solid mass appears dark (stiff) on an elastogram when not using a color overlay. A "soft" cystic mass appears centrally bright on the elastogram. The size of the mass on the elastogram also indicates relative hardness of the tissues, with most cancers being stiffer than benign masses. A cancer will tend to be larger, whereas a benign mass will tend to be smaller, on the elastogram compared to the lesion's actual size on the conventional 2D image (Fig. 16-80). This, in part, is related to the reactive fibrosis and tumor invasion that causes the cancer to become firm and fixed to adjacent tissues.

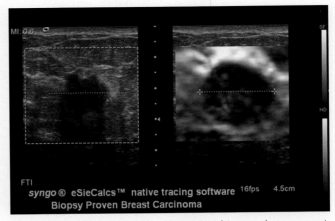

**Figure 16-80** Elastogram. The conventional image shows a suspicious solid mass with acoustic shadowing. The elastogram depicts the mass as "dark" and "larger" than that seen on the conventional image indicating the lesion is "stiff" and suspicious for malignancy. (Image courtesy of Siemens Healthcare, Mountain View, CA.)

### AUTOMATED WHOLE BREAST SCANNER

Handheld breast sonography is very operator dependent and has poorer reproducibility on serial exams than mammography or MRI when scanning the entire breast. This impacts sonography's utility as a screening tool. Dedicated whole-breast sonography systems have been developed to reduce reliance on the operator during image acquisition by automating the scanning process. Equipment design varies by company. In general, the automated systems rapidly acquire image data sets of the entire breast in a preset manner and display standard image planes, as well as reconstructed 3D coronal views (Fig. 16-81). The distance of a mass from the nipple and depth of the lesion can be quickly ascertained. Additional handheld targeted sonography devices can be directed to areas of concern as needed. The volume data set is digitally stored and retrievable on a computer workstation for serial comparison and image reconstruction.

## BREAST MAGNETIC RESONANCE IMAGING[2,4,8,16,42,51,65–68]

Although mammography is the standard screening test for cancer, there are subgroups of patients with dense breast tissue for whom diagnostic efficacy is reduced. MRI is reported to have greater sensitivity at detecting breast cancer than mammography or sonography, although false-positive findings occur from overlaps in benign and malignant breast patterns. Patients lie prone with the breast suspended in dedicated breast coils. Contrast-enhanced MRI is very effective at evaluating the morphologic features of a mass as well as dynamic blood flow patterns. A paramagnetic contrast agent (gadolinium) is given via intravenous (IV) injection. The neovascularity of invasive cancers, in particular, contribute to rapid, moderate-to-marked

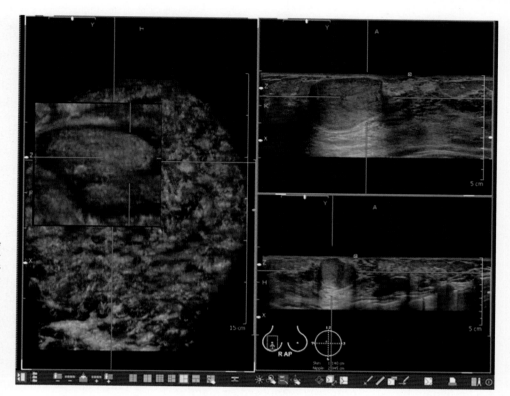

**Figure 16-81** Automated whole breast sonography. After automated image acquisition, images can be displayed in standard scan planes, over a longer scan path, with the nipple location referenced. Three-dimensional data sets can be reconstructed to produce coronal scans, multislice images, and magnification views. These images are of a fibroadenoma. (Image courtesy of Siemens Healthcare, Mountain View, CA.)

tumor enhancement and quick contrast washout on MRI images following contrast injection (Fig. 16-82). Both breasts and adjacent nodal beds can be evaluated with this nonionizing technique. In 2007, the American Cancer Society published guidelines recommending contrast-enhanced MRI be used as an adjunct to mammography to screen for cancer in high-risk patients with a 20% to 25% or greater lifetime risk for the disease.[16] MRI can look for tumor enhancement in regions of DCIS that are often associated with suspicious calcifications on the mammogram. MRI can detect multifocal,

multicentric, and bilateral cancers, as well as for lymph node changes, which can affect surgical and treatment planning. Suspicious masses only seen by MRI can be biopsied with this technique. MRI can also be used to assess tumor response to neoadjuvant chemotherapy prior to surgery, as well as differentiate recurrent tumor from scar in the postsurgical patient. Noncontrast MRI is considered the best imaging tool for assessing implant integrity. Cost, limited availability, exam length, lower specificity, and the need for contrast for most exams are some disadvantages of this technique.

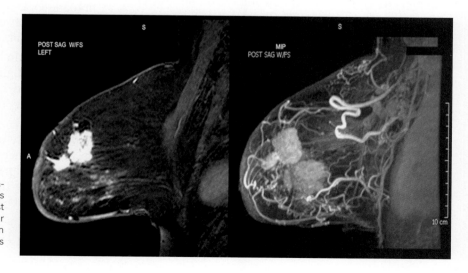

**Figure 16-82** Breast magnetic resonance image. Sagittal scan through the left breast shows marked uptake of the paramagnetic contrast in a patient with multifocal invasive lobular carcinoma. The three-dimensional maximum intensity projection (MIP) of subtracted images shows extensive disease.

# SUMMARY

- Mammography is still the principal technique chosen to localize and biopsy most nonpalpable, solid breast lesions and clustered microcalcifications and remains the only widely used screening tool proven effective at reducing breast cancer mortality; however, when mammography has limited efficacy, as in a dense breast, other imaging modalities, including sonography, can be utilized to detect and localize suspicious masses.

- When used in conjunction, the strengths of sonography offset the weaknesses of mammography, providing greater diagnostic confidence.

- Sonographic evaluation of the breast has proven useful in young, pregnant, or lactating women; helps to differentiate between cystic and solid masses; allows palpable and radiographically indeterminate lesions to be characterized; is better tolerated in patients with breast trauma, inflammatory changes, augmentation mammoplasty, or postirradiation changes; and provides real-time guidance for interventional and therapeutic breast procedures.

- The female breast is primarily composed of glandular, fatty, and fibrous connective tissues that vary in proportion based on the individual's age and hormonal status, whereas the glandular elements of the breast primarily function to produce and transport milk, the stromal elements consist of fat, fibrous connective tissues, as well as blood vessels, lymphatics, and nerves.

- The breast is subdivided by fascial planes into three layers: the subcutaneous fat layer, the mammary (parenchymal) layer, and the retromammary fat layer.

- A high-frequency, broadband, linear transducer with a frequency of 10 MHz or higher is suitable for breast sonography.

- Breast sonography systems need to provide excellent spatial and contrast resolution and the output power, time gain compensation (TGC), overall gain, dynamic range, focal zone placement, image size, and depth must be optimized for each patient.

- Based on site protocol and indication, either a targeted exam or a whole-breast sonography examination is performed. A targeted study is limited to the quadrant or region of clinical concern, such as for a palpable mass, or to further characterize a mammographic or MRI finding. Some indications for a whole breast exam include the search for satellite lesions and lymph node involvement in a patient with a known cancer or suspicious lesion, to screen a high-risk patient with radiographically dense breasts, to follow-up multiple masses, or to evaluate implant integrity.

- Images can be taken in sagittal and transverse planes, as well as radial and antiradial planes.

- Typically annotations include the side being evaluated, the clock-face position, the distance from the nipple, and the scan plane while some institutions include the "1-2-3; A-B-C" labeling methods to note the relative the distance of a mass from the nipple, as well as the depth within the breast.

- The ACR BI-RADS Breast Ultrasound Lexicon is utilized in an effort to promote the use of more consistent terminology when characterizing sonographic findings.

- Most breast cysts are related to fibrocystic change (FCC); other symptoms of FCC include breast tenderness or pain, fullness, and nodularity.

- Cystic breast lesions may be simple, complicated, or complex and include hemorrhagic cysts, infected cysts, galactoceles, and sebaceous cysts.

- Mastitis, or inflammation of the breast, presents most often during pregnancy and lactation but can affect women at any stage of life. Abscess formation is a complication of mastitis.

- Hematoma, seroma, and fat necrosis are related to breast trauma and can be evaluated with breast sonography.

- Characteristically, a benign mass displaces, rather than invades, adjacent tissues as it grows and displays an oval shape and well-circumscribed margins that are sharply demarcated from surrounding tissues. Benign lesions are typically wider than tall.

- Characteristics that make a mass suspicious for malignancy include irregular, indistinct, angular, or speculated margins; a taller than wide orientation; architectural distortion, skin thickening, or nipple retraction; shadowing; and microcalcifications.

- Fibroadenoma is the most common benign solid tumor of the female breast with a higher incidence in patients 15 to 35 years of age; sonographically, a fibroadenoma typically appears as a smooth, well-circumscribed, oval, wider than tall, homogeneous, solid mass that may be gently lobulated.

- Excluding skin cancer, breast cancer is the most common malignancy affecting women in the United States and ranks second to lung cancer as the leading cause of cancer-related deaths in women over age 50.

- Approximately one in eight American women develop breast cancer during a lifetime and early cancer detection and treatment improves long-term survival by decreasing the incidence of lymph node involvement and metastasis to distant sites.

- Breast cancers are usually adenocarcinomas that originate in a TDLU; the majority of cancers develop

## Critical Thinking Questions

1. A 22-year-old woman presents for a targeted breast sonography examination with a large palpable mass. The sonogram shows a 2.5-cm, solid, oval mass that is well-circumscribed and wider than tall. What is the most likely diagnosis?

2. A 40-year-old patient presents with a history of breastfeeding and an acutely painful, swollen, right breast. What is the most likely diagnosis and what complication will you look for as you perform the examination?

3. What are the sonographic characteristics of a simple breast cyst?

4. What are the sonographic characteristics of a malignant breast mass?

5. A 41-year-old woman with a history of silicone breast implants presents for a breast sonogram with a palpable lump. Your examination reveals a highly echogenic area adjacent to the implant. There is a dirty shadow posterior to the area. What is the most likely diagnosis based on your findings?

in the upper outer quadrant where there is the greatest amount of glandular-epithelial tissue.

- Types of noninvasive cancer are lobular carcinoma in situ (LCIS) and ductal carcinoma in situ (DCIS).

- DCIS is the most common noninvasive cancer, accounting for approximately 70% of in situ lesions and frequently presents only as suspicious calcifications on mammography.

- Invasive cancer describes cases when malignant cells breach the basement membrane of the duct and/or lobule and extend into adjacent tissues; cancer cells can then penetrate nearby blood vessels and lymphatic channels, both pathways for metastatic seeding.

- Invasive ductal carcinoma, not otherwise specified (IDC NOS) is the most common breast cancer and invasive lobular carcinoma is the second most common breast cancer.

- Diffuse or inflammatory carcinoma occurs when a highly invasive cancer infiltrates the lymphatics of the skin; frequently, the result of a higher grade invasive ductal carcinomas that may disseminate within the breast.

- With inflammatory carcinoma, the skin becomes red, warm, and edematous with an orange peel (peau d'orange) appearance that affects a majority of the breast. The breast is often painful and hard.

- The first site of metastatic spread from a primary breast cancer is usually to the ipsilateral axillary lymph nodes, which receives most of the lymph drainage from the breast; but breast cancer can also metastasize to the bone, liver, lung, and brain.

- Gynecomastia refers to benign male breast enlargement characterized by an abnormal proliferation of ductal and stromal tissues and is associated with an increased estrogen-to-testosterone ratio.

- Gynecomastia usually presents as a soft, mildly tender, area of fullness or nodularity centered beneath the areola.

- Common sonography guided procedures include cyst aspiration, drainage of a fluid collection such as a hematoma or abscess, biopsy of an indeterminate or suspicious mass, lymph node sampling, and preoperative dye or wire localization of a nonpalpable mass.

- Sonography can be used to evaluate the integrity of saline and silicone implants and complications such as capsular contracture, and intracapsular or extracapsular rupture.

- Advances in instrumentation, as well as future utilization of sonographic contrast agents, computer-aided detection programs may further enhance tissue characterization and blood flow for better discrimination between benign and malignant breast masses.

### REFERENCES

1. American Cancer Society. Breast cancer facts & figures: 2007–2008. Available at: http://www.cancer.org/Research/CancerFactsFigures/BreastCancerFactsFigures/breast-cancer-facts-figures-2007–2008. Accessed January 27, 2011.

2. Berg WA. Tailored supplemental screening for breast cancer: what now and what next? *AJR Am J Roentgenol.* 2009;192:390–399.

3. Bassett LW, Jackson VP, Fu KL, et al. *Diagnosis of Diseases of the Breast.* 2nd ed. Philadelphia, PA: Elsevier Saunders; 2005.

4. Berg WA, Birdwell RL, Gombos EC, et al. *Diagnostic Imaging: Breast.* Salt Lake City, UT: Amirsys; 2006.

5. Cardenosa G. *Breast Imaging Companion.* 2nd ed. Philadelphia, PA: Lippincott Williams Wilkins; 2001.

6. Stavros AT. *Breast Ultrasound.* Philadelphia, PA: Lippincott Williams & Wilkins; 2004.

7. American College of Radiology. *ACR practice guideline for the performance of a breast ultrasound examination.* Reston, VA: ACR; 2007.

8. Carr-Hoefer C. *Breast Ultrasound: A Comprehensive Sonographer's Guide.* 2nd ed. Dallas, TX: Miele Enterprises LLC; 2008.

9. Glenn ME. The breast. In: Hagen-Ansert S, ed. *Textbook of Diagnostic Ultrasonography.* Vol 1. 6th ed. St. Louis, MO: Mosby; 2001.

10. Hagen-Ansert SL, Salsgiver TL, Glenn ME. The breast. In: *Textbook of Diagnostic Ultrasonography*. Vol 1. 2nd ed. St Louis, MO: Mosby Elsevier; 2006.

11. Lanfranchi ME. *Breast Ultrasound*. 2nd ed. New York, NY: Thieme; 2000.

12. Rumack CM, Wilson SR, Charboneau JW. *Diagnostic Ultrasound*. 3rd ed. Philadelphia, PA: Elsevier Mosby; 2005.

13. Demirkazik FB. Palpable and nonpalpable breast masses. *Ultrasound*. 2008;3:277–287.

14. Berg WA. Rationale for a trial of screening breast ultrasound: American College of Radiology Imaging Network (ACRIN) 6666. *AJR Am J Roentgenol*. 2003;180(5):1225–1228.

15. Hashimoto BE. Sonography of ductal carcinoma in situ. *Ultrasound Clin*. 2006;1(4):631–643.

16. Saslow D, Boetes C, Burke W, et al. American Cancer Society guidelines for breast screening with MRI as an adjunct to mammography. *CA Cancer J Clin*. 2007;57(2):75–89.

17. Silverstein MJ, Lagios MD, Recht A, et al. Image-detected breast cancer: state of the art diagnosis and treatment. *J Am Coll Surg*. 2005;201:586–597.

18. Yang W, Dempsey J. Diagnostic breast ultrasound: current status and future directions. *Ultrasound Clin*. 2009;4(2):117–133

19. Varghese T. Quasi-static ultrasound elastography. *Ultrasound Clin*. 2009;4:323–338.

20. Stavros AT. New advances in breast ultrasound: computer-aided detection. *Ultrasound Clin*. 2009;4:285–290.

21. Dahnert W. *Radiology Review Manual*. 6th ed. Philadelphia, PA: Lippincott Williams & Wilkins; 2007.

22. Donegan WL, Spratt JS. *Cancer of the Breast*. Philadelphia, PA: WB Saunders; 1995.

23. Tavassoli FA. *Pathology of the Breast*. 2nd ed. Stamford, CT: Appleton & Lange; 1999.

24. Bock K, Duda VF, Hadji P, et al. Pathologic breast conditions in childhood and adolescence: evaluation by sonographic diagnosis. *J Ultrasound Med*. 2005;24:1347–1354.

25. Harris JR, Hellman S, Henderson IC, et al., eds. *Breast Diseases*. Philadelphia, PA: JB Lippincott; 1987.

26. Carr-Hoefer C. Breast sonography. In: Kawamura D, ed. *Abdomen and Superficial Structures*. 2nd ed. Philadelphia, PA: Lippincott Williams & Wilkins; 1997.

27. American College of Radiology. *ACR Practice Guideline for the Performance of Ultrasound-guided Percutaneous Breast Interventional Procedures*. Reston, VA: ACR; 2009.

28. American Institute of Ultrasound in Medicine. AIUM practice guideline for the performance of a breast ultrasound examination. 2008. Available at: http://www.aium.org/publications/guidelines/breast.pdf. Accessed January 27, 2011.

29. Rapp C. Sonography of the breast. *SDMS 17th Annual Conference Official Proceedings*. Dallas, TX: Society of Diagnostic Medical Sonographers; 2000:57–67.

30. American College of Radiology. Breast imaging reporting and data system. *Breast Imaging Atlas*. 4th ed. Reston, VA: ACR; 2003.

31. Whitsett MC. Ultrasound imaging and advances in system features. *Ultrasound*. 2009;4:391–401.

32. Berg WA, Woel BS. Mammographic–sonographic correlation. *Ultrasound Clin*. 2007;1:567–591.

33. Hashimoto BE, Morgan GN, Kramer DJ, et al. Systematic approach to difficult problems in breast sonography. *Ultrasound Q*. 2008;24:31–38.

34. Leung JW, Sickles EA. The probably benign assessment. *Radiol Clin North Am*. 2007;45:773–789.

35. Tabar L, Dean PB. *Teaching Atlas of Mammography*. 2nd ed. New York, NY: Thieme-Stratton; 1983.

36. Berg WA, Campassi CI, Ioffe OB, et al. Cystic lesions of the breast: sonographic–pathologic correlation. *Radiology*. 2003;227:183–191.

37. Madjar H, Jellins J. *The Practice of Breast Ultrasound: Techniques, Findings, Differential Diagnosis*. New York, NY: Thieme Publishers; 2000.

38. Cardenosa G. Cysts, cystic lesions, and papillary lesions. *Ultrasound Clin*. 2007;1:617–625.

39. Shetty MK, Watson AB. Mondor's disease of the breast: sonographic and mammographic findings. *AJR Am J Roentgenol*. 2000;177:893–896.

40. Esen G, Olgun DC. Ultrasonography of the postsurgical breast including implants. *Ultrasound Clin*. 2008;3(3):295–329.

41. Heywang-Kobrunner SH, Dershaw DD, Schreer I. *Diagnostic Breast Imaging*. New York, NY: Thieme; 2001.

42. Bartella L, Smith CS, Dershaw DD, et al. Imaging breast cancer. *Radiol Clin North Am*. 2007;45:45–67.

43. Muradali D, Kulkarni S. Sonography of the breast: to core or not to core? *J Can Assoc Radiol J*. 2005;56:276–288.

44. Stavros AT, Thickman D, Rapp CL, et al. Solid breast nodules: use of sonography to distinguish between benign and malignant lesions. *Radiology*. 1995;196:123–134.

45. Yang WT. Sonography of unusual breast neoplasms. *Ultrasound Clin*. 2006;1(4):661–672.

46. Liberman L, Bonaccio E, Hamele-Bena D, et al. Benign and malignant phyllodes tumors: mammographic and sonographic findings. *Radiology*. 1996;198:121–124.

47. Carr-Hoefer C. *Breast Ultrasound for the Sonomammographer*. Corvallis, Sound Imaging Consulting, LLC, 2007.

48. Kersschot EA, Hermans ME, Pauwels C, et al. Juvenile papillomatosis of the breast: sonographic appearance. *Radiology*. 1988;169:631–633.

49. Carr-Hoefer C. Granular cell tumor: a benign mimicker of breast carcinoma. *JDMS*. 2003;19:95–100.

50. Mendelson EB. The breast. In: Rumack CM, Wilson SR, Charboneau JW, eds. *Diagnostic Ultrasound*. 2nd ed. St. Louis, MO: Mosby; 1999.

51. Erguvan-Dogan B, Whitman GJ. Breast ultrasound and MRI correlation. *Ultrasound Clin*. 2006;1(4):593–601.

52. Appelbaum AH, Evans GF, Levy KR, et al. Mammographic appearances of male breast disease. *Radiographics*. 1999;19:559–568.

53. Chantra PK, So GJ, Wollman JS, et al. Mammography of the male breast. *AJR Am J Roentgenol*. 1995;164:853–858.

54. Kedar RP, Cosgrove DO, Bamber JC, et al. Automated quantification of color Doppler signals: a preliminary study in breast tumors. *Radiology*. 1995;197:39–43.

55. Madjar H, Prömpeler HJ, Sauerbrei W, et al. Color Doppler flow criteria of breast lesions. *Ultrasound Med Biol*. 1994;20:849–858.

56. Kedar RP, Cosgrove DO, Smith IE, et al. Breast carcinoma: measurement of tumor response to primary medical therapy with color Doppler flow imaging. *Radiology*. 1994;190:825–830.

57. Bassett LW, Mahoney MC, Apple SK. Interventional breast imaging: current procedures and assessing for concordance with pathology. *Radiol Clin North Am*. 2007;45:881–894.

58. Kaplan SS, Racenstein MJ, Wong WS, et al. US-guided core biopsy of the breast with a coaxial system. *Radiology*. 1995;194:573–575.

59. Oktay A. Ultrasound-guided breast biopsies and aspirations. *Ultrasound Clin*. 2008;3(3):289–294.

60. Whitman GJ, Erguvan-Dogan B, Yang WT, et al. Ultrasound-guided breast biopsies. *Ultrasound Clin*. 2007;1:603–615.

61. Littrup PJ, Freeman-Gibb L, Andea A, et al. Cryotherapy for breast fibroadenomas. *Radiology*. 2005;234:63–72.

62. Fornage BD, Ross MI, Singletary SE, et al. Localization of impalpable breast masses: value of sonography in the operating room and scanning of excised specimens. *AJR Am J Roentgenol*. 1994;163:569–573.

63. Brown SL, Middleton MS, Berg WA, et al. Prevalence of rupture of silicone gel breast implants revealed on MR imaging in a population of women in Birmingham, Alabama. *AJR Am J Roentgenol*. 2000;175(4):1 057–1064.

64. Caskey CI, Berg WA, Hamper UM, Hamper UM, et al. Imaging spectrum of extracapsular silicone: correlation of US, MR imaging, mammographic, and histopathologic findings. *Radiographics*. 1999;19:S39–S51.

65. Middleton MS, McNamara MP. *Breast Implant Imaging*. Philadelphia, PA: Lippincott Williams & Wilkins; 2002.

66. Rizzatto G, Fausto A. Breast imaging and volume navigation: MR imaging and ultrasound coregistration. *Ultrasound*. 2009;4:261–271.

67. Berg WA. Beyond standard mammographic screening: mammography at age extremes, ultrasound, and MR imaging. *Radiol Clin North Am*. 2007;45:895–906.

68. Morris EA. Diagnostic breast MR imaging: current status and future directions. *Radiol Clin North Am*. 2007;45:863–880.

# 17 The Scrotum

Wayne C. Leonhardt and Zulfikarali H. Lalani

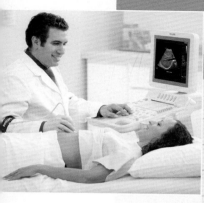

## OBJECTIVES

Illustrate the normal gross and sectional anatomy of the scrotum, including the vascular anatomy.

Describe the sonographic appearance of the normal scrotal anatomy.

Explain the technique and protocol for sonographic evaluation of the scrotum.

State the indications for a sonographic examination of the scrotum.

Identify the common pathologic conditions that can result in an acute painful scrotum.

Differentiate common extratesticular abnormalities from intratesticular abnormalities.

Describe the sonographic characteristics and laboratory values associated with scrotal masses.

## KEY TERMS

choriocarcinoma · embryonal cell carcinoma · epidermoid cyst · epididymal cyst · epididymitis · epididymo-orchitis · hematocele · hydrocele · Leydig cell tumor · microlithiasis · scrotal hernia · seminoma · Sertoli cell tumor · spermatoceles · sperm granulomas · teratoma · testicular torsion · tunica albuginea cyst · undescended testis · varicocele

## GLOSSARY

**AFP** alpha-fetoprotein levels are measured during pregnancy to detect certain fetal anomalies. Blood levels may also be elevated with hepatocellular carcinoma and certain testicular cancers

**beta-hCG** human chorionic gonadotropin is produced during pregnancy but is also secreted by some malignant tumors, including certain testicular cancers

**cryptorchidism** undescended testicle; occurs when one or more of the testis fails to descend into the scrotum before birth

**hyperemia** an increase in blood flow to the tissue

**infarction** tissue death that occurs due to a lack of blood flow

**orchiopexy** a surgical procedure done to fasten an undescended testicle into the scrotum or to repair an acute testicular torsion

**pampiniform plexus** a network of veins that drain the epididymis and testis; located in the spermatic cord and empties into the right and left testicular veins

**Valsalva maneuver** performed during a scrotal sonography examination by asking the patient to bear down like he is trying to have a bowel movement; this increases the intra-abdominal pressure and is helpful in diagnosing varicocele and scrotal hernia

High-frequency gray scale sonography with spectral, color, and power Doppler is the imaging modality of choice and the gold standard for evaluating patients with acute scrotal pain, a scrotal mass, or to assess testicular perfusion when testicular torsion is suspected.[1-5] Compared with other imaging modalities, sonography provides expedient and accurate differentiation of many causes of scrotal pain.[6,7] The diagnosis of scrotal disease is based on many factors, including a thorough clinical history, physical examination, and sonographic findings.[3,8,9] When patients present with scrotal pain or abnormality, clinical evaluation alone is difficult, and the cause of the patient's symptoms frequently remains unanswered. Sonography is used to determine whether a palpable mass is cystic or solid and differentiate between intratesticular and extratesticular abnormalities.[1,9,10] The distinction between an intratesticular lesion and an extratesticular lesion is an important one considering most intratesticular solid masses are considered malignant until proven otherwise.[10,11]

Conversely, extratesticular masses tend to be benign regardless of their cystic or solid nature.[1,3,10] High-resolution gray scale sonography has been shown to be nearly 100% accurate in its ability to characterize the intrascrotal anatomy and distinguish intratesticular and extratesticular abnormalities.[3,10]

Sonography is also useful in the follow-up examination of infection and trauma. Incidentally, 10% to 15% of testicular tumors are identified after an episode of scrotal trauma.[2,12] Due to its speed and efficacy, color Doppler sonography is the most useful imaging technique to establish the diagnosis of testicular torsion in addition to differentiating torsion from epididymo-orchitis.[5,11,13] With an accuracy approaching 100%, sonography is considered the primary imaging modality to assess intratesticular arterial perfusion.[4,5,13,14] Nuclear medicine and sonography are comparable in the detection of reduced or absent intratesticular flow.[14]

When a patient presents with an undescended testis, the evaluation begins with sonography to explore the inguinal canal. In 80% of cases, the undescended testis is located in the inguinal canal.[13,14] Magnetic resonance imaging (MRI) is recommended to locate intra-abdominal testes when sonography fails to locate an undescended testis within the inguinal canal. MRI is 90% to 95% sensitive for identifying intra-abdominal testes.[14]

## SONOGRAPHIC IMAGING TECHNIQUE

Optimal imaging of the scrotum is achieved using a high-frequency, linear transducer (10 to 14 MHz) with spectral, color, and power Doppler capabilities.[2,4] In patients with severe scrotal swelling, a high-frequency curved linear-array transducer increases the field of view (FOV) and is useful for evaluating large segments of intrascrotal anatomy[2] (Fig. 17-1).

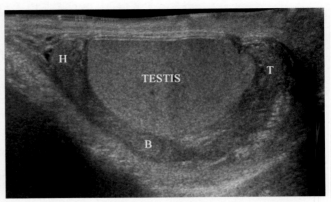

Figure 17-2 Extended field of view. Longitudinal extended field of view image of the scrotum, including the testis and the epididymal head (*H*), body (*B*), and tail (*T*).

Extended FOV imaging is extremely helpful when evaluating large anatomic segments with inflammatory processes and fluid collections as the wider FOV provides a greater understanding of anatomical releationships[3] (Fig. 17-2).

With high-resolution gray scale imaging of greater than 10 MHz, correlating a palpable mass with real-time imaging is easy.[2] High-frequency transducers have excellent spatial resolution and can resolve anatomic structures as small as 0.5 mm.[3,9] Imaging techniques such as harmonics, compound imaging, and multifocal zones are essential to optimizing image quality.[8] Adjusting color Doppler parameters by utilizing a low pulse repetition frequency (PRF), with a low wall filter, and a relatively high color gain output can improve the display of the intratesticular arteries.[3,8,15]

### TECHNICAL CONSIDERATIONS

- When evaluating patients for acute scrotal pain, scan the asymptomatic side first, adjusting the gray scale, color, and power Doppler settings to allow for comparison with the symptomatic side.[15]
- Obtain power, color, and spectral Doppler tracings to confirm the presence or absence of intratesticular arterial and venous flow.
- Gray scale images are often nonspecific for evaluating testicular torsion and often appear normal when torsion is acute.[4]
- Spectral Doppler findings suggestive of partial torsion include asymmetry in resistive indices with decreased diastolic flow or diastolic flow reversal.[4]
- Large hydroceles, hematomas, marked scrotal edema, and epididymo-orchitis are scrotal conditions that decrease intratesticular perfusion, mimicking testicular torsion.
- In patients presenting with acute epididymo-orchitis, spectral Doppler demonstrates decreased

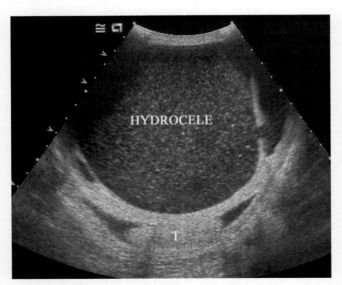

Figure 17-1 Convex transducer. Transverse image of enlarged scrotum best seen with a convex probe. Note the large echogenic hydrocele compressing and displacing the testis (*T*).

vascular resistance (resistive index [RI] <0.5) compared with the normal contralateral testis and epididymis.[2]

- Reversal of the spectral diastolic component of the intratesticular arterial flow in patients with acute epididymo-orchitis suggests venous infarction.[4]
- Use color and power Doppler to differentiate epididymitis from an enlarged, noninflammatory epididymis status postvasectomy.
- Since primary varicoceles may decompress when the patient is supine, perform the Valsalva maneuver or scan the patient in the upright position to increase venous blood flow.
- Large varicoceles can extend posteriorly and inferiorly to the testis, mimicking epididymitis.
- When a right-sided varicocele is detected, scan the upper abdomen for a mass.
- Evaluate the spermatic cord to detect diffuse abnormalities such as hematomas, inflammation, and torsion.
- Use a gel standoff pad to evaluate anterior lesions, such as those in the tunica vaginalis.

## PROTOCOL FOR REAL-TIME SONOGRAPHY

Before scanning the scrotum, review previous studies and obtain a thorough clinical history, including the patient's chief complaint, useful laboratory data, and any pertinent surgical history such as vasectomy, orchiopexy, and hydrocelectomy. Have the patient locate the area of pain, swelling, or palpable mass, and ask if he is currently being treated with antibiotics.[3,8] Once the history is obtained and documented on the anatomy worksheet, explain the procedure to the patient. The scrotal exam is performed with the patient in the supine position. The scrotum is supported on a rolled towel placed between the thighs to isolate and immobilize the anatomy for scanning.[2–4,8] The penis is positioned over the suprapubic region and covered with a second

towel.[2] Generous amounts of warm gel should be applied to the scrotal skin as a couplant.[8]

The spermatic cord, epididymis, testis, and scrotal skin are examined in longitudinal and transverse planes. Oblique scanning planes are useful for demonstrating the intratesticular arteries.[16] Bilateral intratesticular arterial and venous waveforms are obtained. Both testes and epididymides are documented in gray scale and with color Doppler, comparing size, echogenicity, and vascularity.[2] Adherence to a systematic protocol precludes ambiguity and errors of omission.

## PROCEDURE FOR REAL-TIME SONOGRAPHY

Sonographic evaluation of the scrotum begins with longitudinal gray scale and color Doppler images of the spermatic cord (with both quiet respiration and the Valsalva maneuver to evaluate for a varicocele), the epididymis (head, body, and tail), testis, and scrotal skin[9] (Fig. 17-3). Include the body and tail of the epididymis when scanning the mid and lower portions of the testis. The epididymal head is best evaluated in the longitudinal view.[1,2,17]

In the longitudinal scan plane using gray scale at rest and with the Valsalva maneuver, measure the anteroposterior (AP) diameter of the spermatic cord veins. Use color Doppler to assess increased venous flow and reflux with the Valsalva maneuver. Document and measure the AP diameter of the epididymal head and body and superior to inferior diameter of the epididymal tail. With color Doppler, assess epididymal arterial perfusion. Use a linear transducer with a large FOV to scan the testis (midline, medial, and lateral). Document a midline image of the testis and measure the length and AP diameter. Measure the AP diameter of the scrotal wall when measuring the length of the testis. Assess intratesticular arterial and venous flow using color and/or power Doppler imaging. Document intratesticular

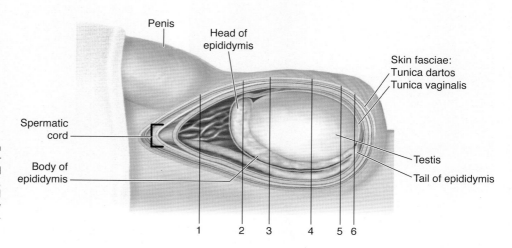

**Figure 17-3** Schematic illustration of longitudinal scanning survey for the testes. *1,* spermatic cord; *2,* head of epididymis; *3,* testis superior; *4,* testis-mid; *5,* testis-inferior; *6,* tail of epididymis. Note that the body of the epididymis is seen in sections 3–5.

Penis

Head of epididymis

Skin fasciae: Tunica dartos Tunica vaginalis

Spermatic cord

Body of epididymis

Testis

Tail of epididymis

1   2   3   4   5 6

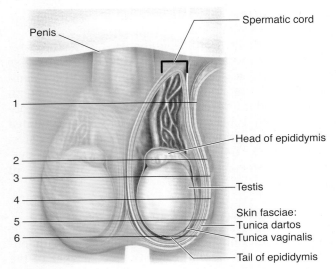

Penis
Spermatic cord
Head of epididymis
Testis
Skin fasciae:
Tunica dartos
Tunica vaginalis
Tail of epididymis

1
2
3
4
5
6

**Figure 17-4** Schematic illustration of transverse scanning survey protocol for the testis. *1*, spermatic cord; *2*, head of epididymis; *3*, testis—superior; *4*, testis—mid; *5*, testis—inferior; *6*, tail of epididymis. The body of the epididymis is seen in sections 3–5.

arterial flow using spectral Doppler and obtain a resistive index.

In the transverse scanning plane, images are obtained of the cord (with both quiet respiration and the Valsalva maneuver), the epididymis (head, body, and tail), testis, and scrotal skin[9] (Fig. 17-4). Include the body and tail of the epididymis when scanning the mid and lower portions of the testis.

In the transverse scanning plane using gray scale at rest and with the Valsalva maneuver, measure the AP diameter of the spermatic cord veins. Use color Doppler to assess increased flow and reflux with the Valsalva maneuver. Image and document the epididymal head, body, and tail. The body and tail of the epididymis are included on the mid and lower portions of the testis. Use color Doppler to assess epididymal perfusion. Obtain transverse images of the testis (upper, mid, and

lower portions). Measure the transverse diameter at the midportion. Assess intratesticular perfusion using color and/or power Doppler imaging. Obtain simultaneous images of both testes in gray scale and with color Doppler to compare the size, echogenicity, and vascularity of the testes[2,3,13,18] (Fig. 17-5A,B).

## NORMAL ANATOMY AND SONOGRAPHIC APPEARANCE

A clear understanding of normal scrotal anatomy and vascular perfusion is paramount. Without a clear concept of normal anatomy, pathologic processes may be missed or a normal variant may be mistaken for disease.

Three major structures are contained in the scrotum: the spermatic cord, the epididymis (head, body, and tail), and the testes. The scrotum is a fibromuscular sac composed of several layers of fascia and muscle, which includes the tunica dartos, external spermatic fascia, middle spermatic fascia, cremasteric muscle, internal spermatic fascia, and tunica vaginalis.[2,10,13,17] The normal scrotal wall thickness is approximately 2 to 8 mm, depending on the state of contraction of the cremasteric muscle.[3,10,13,17] The normal sonographic appearance of the scrotal wall is homogeneous, and slightly echogenic, compared to the testis[9] (Fig. 17-6). The scrotum is divided into two compartments by a midline septum, the median raphe, a fibrous band of tissue that runs ventral to the undersurface of the penis and dorsal along the middle of the perineum to the anus.[3,10,17]

### SPERMATIC CORD

The spermatic cords are paired and pass from the abdominal cavity through the inguinal canal down into the scrotum.[19] Each spermatic cord lies above and parallel to the inguinal ligament and suspends the testis in the scrotum. The spermatic cord is composed of arteries (the testicular, cremasteric, and deferential), veins

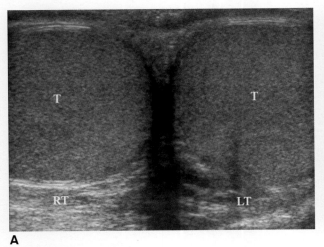

**A**

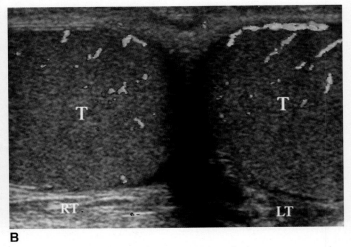

**B**

**Figure 17-5** Comparison. **A:** Transverse image of normal bilateral right *(RT)* and left *(LT)* testes *(T)* demonstrating similar homogeneous echogenicity. **B:** Transverse image of normal bilateral right *(RT)* and left *(LT)* testes *(T)* demonstrating normal flow bilaterally.

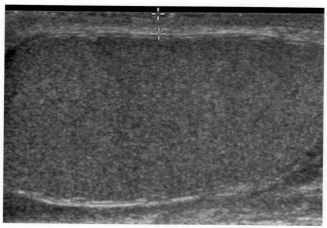

**Figure 17-6** Scrotal wall. Longitudinal image of normal scrotal wall thickness (*calipers*).

of the pampiniform plexus, nerves, lymphatics, vas deferens, and connective tissue.[7,9,10,14,20]

The sonographic appearance of a normal spermatic cord in the longitudinal scan is numerous hypoechoic, slightly tortuous, linear structures measuring up to 2 mm in diameter[9,14,17] (Fig. 17-7A). In the transverse plane, the sonographic appearance of the normal spermatic cord is numerous hypoechoic ovoid structures with echogenic borders representing vascular walls and connective tissue[9,14] (Fig. 17-7B).

Normal veins of the pampiniform plexus measure less than 2 mm in diameter.[14,17] With color Doppler, the normal spermatic cord shows minimal flow within the arteries and veins of the pampiniform plexus at rest (Fig. 17-7C,D). In a normal patient, performing the Valsalva maneuver slightly increases venous flow[9] (Fig. 17-7E,F).

## EPIDIDYMIS

The epididymides store small quantities of sperm prior to ejaculation. Additionally, they act as a conduit for sperm originating in the testis and expressed via the seminal vesicles and secrete a small portion of the seminal fluid.[9,21] The epididymis is divided anatomically into the head, body, and tail.[9] The head of the epididymis, the globus major, is located superolaterally to the testis and measures 10 to 12 mm in AP diameter.[11,18] The body of the epididymis, the corpus, lies adjacent to the posterolateral margin of the testis and measures 2 to

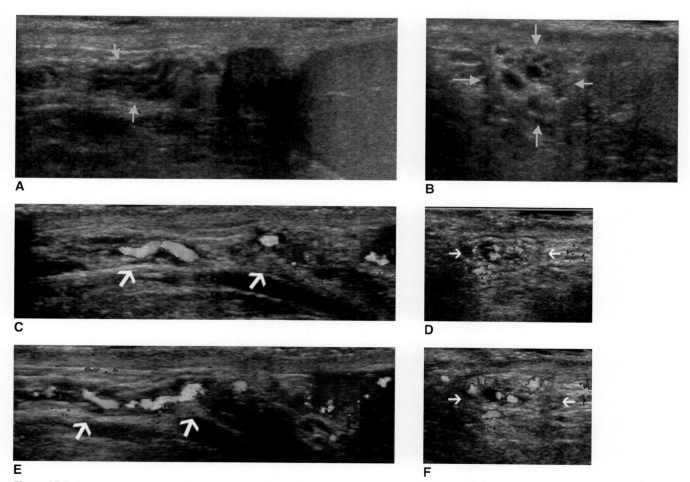

**Figure 17-7** Spermatic cord. **A:** Longitudinal image of the normal spermatic cord (*arrows*). **B:** Transverse image of the normal spermatic cord (*arrows*) with sonolucent ducts and vessels. **C:** Longitudinal and transverse (**D**) images of the normal spermatic cord (*arrows*) with color flow at rest. **E:** Longitudinal and transverse (**F**) images of the normal spermatic cord (*arrows*) with slightly increased venous flow during the Valsalva maneuver.

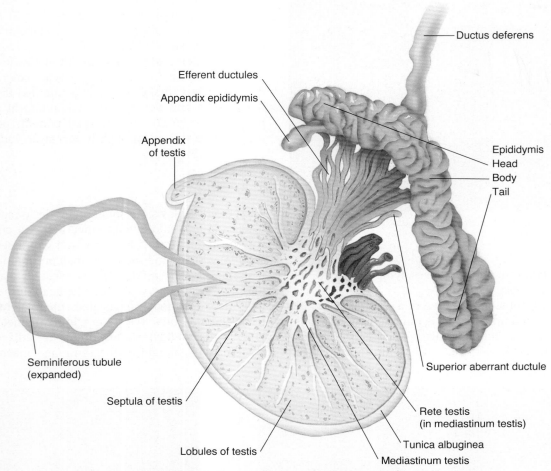

**Figure 17-8** Schematic illustration of the sagittal anatomic section of normal scrotum.

4 mm in AP diameter.[13,22,23] The tail of the epididymis, or globus minor, lies on the inferolateral surface of the testis and measures 2 to 5 mm in superior to inferior diameter.[6,13,17,22,23] The latter continues on to become the vas deferens[9] (Fig. 17-8).

The normal sonographic appearance of the epididymal head is homogeneous and largely isoechoic to or slightly more echogenic than the testis.[6,7,11,15,17,22,23] The epididymal head is best evaluated in the longitudinal scan plane appearing as a triangular, crescent, or teardrop-shaped structure superior to the testis[9,10,11,14,17] (Fig. 17-9A). The echogenicity of the normal body and tail is isoechoic to hypoechoic compared to the testis.[11,22,23] The narrow body and curved tail are smaller, more variable in position, usually posterior and inferior to the testis, and best evaluated in the longitudinal scan plane[6,14,17,22,23] (Fig. 17-9B,C). Color flow imaging of the normal epididymis demonstrates speckled intraepididymal arterial flow[9] (Fig. 17-9D).

### Postvasectomy Changes in the Epididymis

When obtaining a patient history, it is important to know whether the patient has had a vasectomy. Patients with an undiscovered history of vasectomy could be misdiagnosed due to a potential altered sonographic appearance of the epididymis. Epididymal changes occur in 40% of postvasectomy patients and include enlargement of the epididymis, inhomogeneity, spermatoceles, dilatation of the rete testis, and sperm granulomas[9,10,22,23] (Fig. 17-10A–D).

Patients presenting with scrotal pain several years after vasectomy may be suspect for "postvasectomy pain syndrome" resulting from obstruction of the efferent epididymal duct system with concomitant ductal dilatation, interstitial fibrosis, and chronic perineural inflammation.[10]

The sonographic appearance of the postvasectomy epididymis may mimic epididymitis. Clinical history and the use of color Doppler imaging differentiates between the two entities.[9]

### TESTIS

The primary function of the testes is the production of sperm and testosterone. Spermatogenesis takes place within the seminiferous tubules.[21] Testosterone, secreted by the cells of Leydig, stimulates the production of sperm and is the primary sex hormone responsible

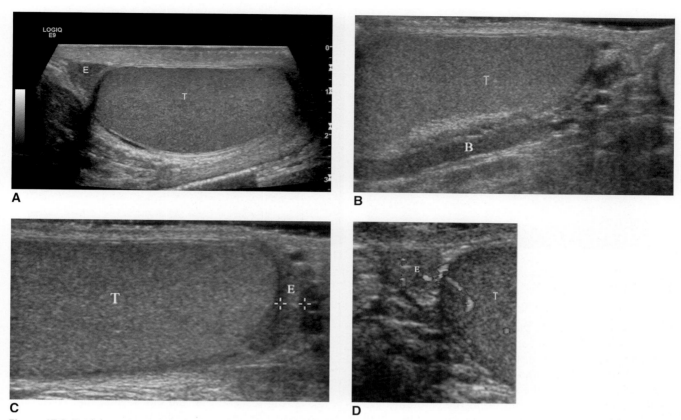

**Figure 17-9** Epididymis. **A:** Longitudinal image of normal testis *(T)* and epididymal head *(E)*. **B:** Longitudinal image of normal testis *(T)* with the body of epididymis *(B)*. **C:** Longitudinal image of normal testis *(T)* and tail of epididymis *(E)*. **D:** Longitudinal color image of testis *(T)* with normal flow in the epididymis *(E)*.

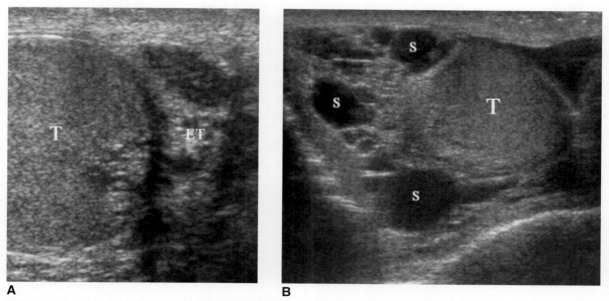

**Figure 17-10** Postvasectomy changes. **A:** Longitudinal image of enlarged heterogeneous epididymal tail *(ET)* in a postvasectomy patient. Normal testis *(T)*. **B:** Longitudinal image of scrotum demonstrating multiple large spermatoceles *(S)* of the head and body of epididymis. *(continued)*

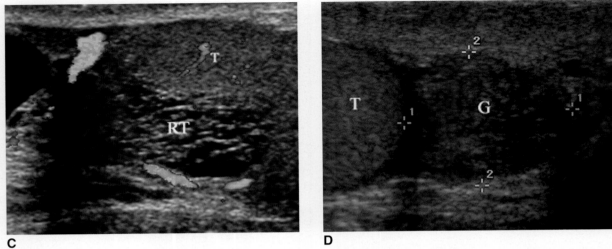

**C** **D**

**Figure 17-10** *(continued)* **C:** Longitudinal image of testis showing cystic changes of dilated rete testis *(RT)*. **D:** Longitudinal image of diffusely enlarged hypoechoic epididymis with sperm granulomas *(G)*. Normal testis *(T)*.

for the development of male reproductive tissues and maintenance of male secondary sex characteristics.[9]

Embryologically, the testes develop between the posterior abdominal wall and the peritoneum. The testes begin to pass through the inguinal ring during the seventh month of gestation and lie in the scrotum by the eighth month. During testicular descent, in the inguinal region, the caudal genital ligament is continuous with a band of mesenchyme that connects the fetal testis to the developing scrotum.[9,24,25] This mesenchyme band is known as the *gubernaculum testis*. The gubernaculum is present only during the development of the urinary and reproductive organs and attaches to the caudal end of the testis.[9] This anchors the fetal testis to the inguinal region to prevent upward movement.[9] In the adult, this gubernaculum testis atrophies and its remnant, the scrotal ligament, extends from the inferior pole of the testis and tail of the epididymis to the skin of the scrotal wall.[9] It secures the testis, tethering it in place and limiting the degree to which the testis can move within the scrotum.[9] The scrotal ligament can be seen in the presence of a hydrocele. The sonographic appearance of the scrotal ligament is an echogenic band extending from the caudal end of the testis to the scrotal wall[9] (Fig. 17-11).

As the testes descend into the scrotum, a peritoneal lining, the processus vaginalis, fuses around the testis to form the tunica vaginalis, whose communication with the peritoneal cavity obliterates after birth.[9,17] The tunica vaginalis is a peritoneal sac, composed of two layers, the visceral and parietal layers, that cover and surround the testis and epididymis except for a small posterior area.[9,14,17] The visceral layer is a serous membrane that produces secretions and covers the testis and epididymis.[8,9,14] The parietal layer is the inner lining of the scrotal wall[8,9,13,14,17] (see Fig. 17-8). The parietal layer contains lymphatics for fluid absorption.[24] Both visceral and parietal layers are separated by a potential space that normally contains a few milliliters of fluid.[3,8,14,17] Bowel (scrotal hernia) and large amounts of serous fluid (hydrocele) or blood (hematocele) can accumulate in the potential space.[9,18] In the normal scrotum, visualizing a small amount of fluid adjacent to the head of the epididymis is common.[9,13,17] This normal amount of fluid should not be misinterpreted as a hydrocele.[13,17]

The tunica albuginea is a fibrous sheath that covers the testis and is seen as a thin echogenic line[2-4,18] (Fig. 17-12).

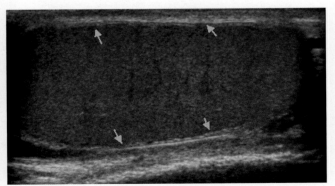

**Figure 17-11** Scrotal ligaments. Longitudinal image of scrotal ligaments *(SL, arrow)* best seen in the presence of a hydrocele. Normal testis *(T)*.

**Figure 17-12** Tunica albuginea. Longitudinal image of testis demonstrating normal tunica albuginea *(arrows)*.

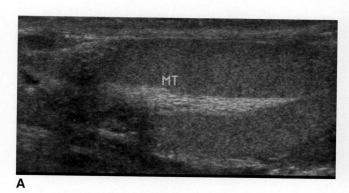
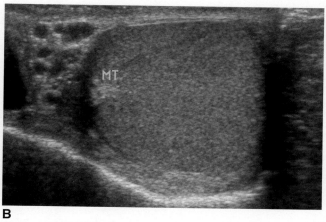

**Figure 17-13** Mediastinum testis. **A:** Longitudinal image of mediastinum testis *(MT)* seen as a bright, echogenic band of fibrofatty tissue across testis. **B:** Transverse image through mediastinum testis *(MT)* seen as a bright, echogenic area in testis at 9 o'clock position.

It invaginates the posterior aspect of the testis at the hilum to become the mediastinum testis.[2,–4,9,11] Sonographically, the mediastinum testis is seen as an echogenic band running in a cephalocaudal orientation within the testis in the longitudinal plane[3,4,14] (Fig. 17-13A). In the transverse plane, it is seen as an ovoid echogenic structure in the 3 or 9 o'clock position[9] (Fig. 17-13B). The mediastinum testis functions as a supporting system for arteries, veins, lymphatics, and seminiferous tubules.[9] Numerous fibrous septa extend radially from the mediastinum into the testis dividing it into 250 to 400 pyramid-shaped compartments called *lobuli testis*.[3,4,9,13] Each lobule contains one to three seminiferous tubules. At the apex of each lobule, the tubules join the tubuli recti, which connect the seminiferous tubules to the rete testis.[2,3,13] The rete testis is a network of epithelial-lined channels embedded within the fibrous stroma of the mediastinum testis. They drain into the epididymis through 10 to 15 efferent ductules[3,4,13] (see Fig. 17-8).

High-frequency sonography can identify the normal rete testis in approximately 18% of patients.[3,13,14] Sonographically, the normal rete testis can be seen as a hypoechoic area with striations, located adjacent to or within the mediastinum testis[3,13,14] (Fig. 17-14). Dilatation of

the seminiferous tubules is refered to as *tubular ectasia* of the rete testis. This is often seen bilaterally and is associated with epididymal cysts and spermatoceles.[24]

The appendix testis and appendix epididymis are embryologic remnants[2,3,9,13] (Fig. 17-15A). They are not routinely visualized by sonography unless a hydrocele is present.[2,3,9] The appendix testis is an ovoid or elongated protuberance about 5 mm in length and is attached to the upper pole of the testis, in the groove between the testis and the epididymis[2,3,13] (Fig. 17-15B,C). The appendix testis has been identified in 92% of testes unilaterally and 69% bilaterally in postmortem studies.[3,13] The appendix epididymis has been identified unilaterally in 34% and bilaterally in 12% in postmortem studies.[3,13] The appendix epididymis is approximately the same size as the appendix testis.[2,3] The shape of the appendix epididymis is more of a stalk-like structure.[2,3] Appendages of the testis and epididymis are visualized sonographically as isoechoic to echogenic protuberances superior to the testis and epididymis.[2,3,9,13] Occasionally, the appendix epididymis may swell or distend forming a cyst-like structure, not to be confused with an epididymal cyst[3] (Fig. 17-15D).

The testes are bilateral symmetrical ovoid glands located within the scrotum. They attain maximum size around puberty. The normal adult testis measures 3 to 5 cm in length and 2 to 3 cm in the transverse and anteroposterior diameters[2–4,13,14] (Fig. 17-16A,B). The size of both the testis and epididymis decrease with increasing age.[9,11] The sonographic appearance of the normal adult testis is homogeneous with medium level echoes similar to the thyroid gland, with a smooth contour.[2,3,9,11,14]

In infants and children, the echogenicity of the testis is hypoechoic compared to that of the adult.[9,24] At birth, the testes measure 1.5 cm in length and 1.0 cm in transverse diameter.[9,14,24] Testicular size increases to 2.0 cm in length and 1.2 cm in transverse diameter by the time the infant is 3 months old.[9,24] During puberty, between 9 and 16 years of age, there is a significant increase in

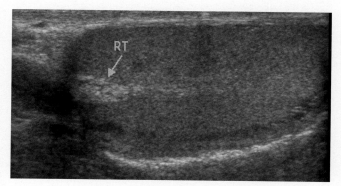

**Figure 17-14** Rete testis. Longitudinal image of normal testis showing echogenic stroma *(arrow)* with tubules of rete testis *(RT)*.

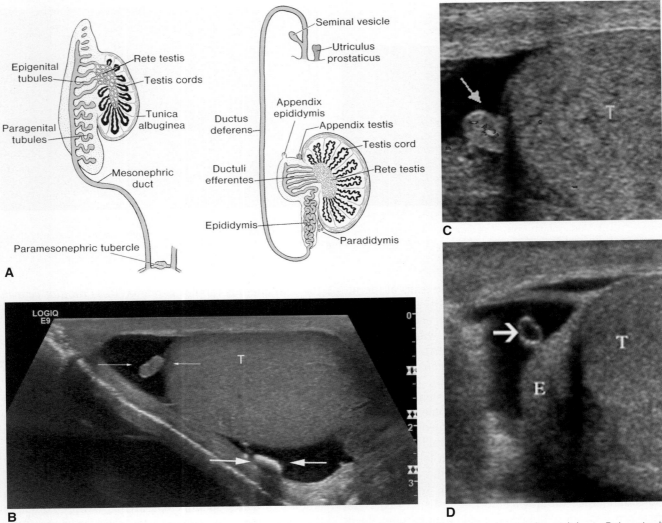

**Figure 17-15** Appendix testis and appendix epididymis. **A:** Schematic illustration of appendix testis and appendix epididymis. **B:** Longitudinal image of testis *(T)* shows hydrocele and appendix testis *(small arrows)*. Scrotal pearl is also seen *(large arrows)*. **C:** Longitudinal image of normal testis *(T)* with appendix testis *(arrow)*. Normal color flow is seen in the appendix. A small hydrocele is present. **D:** Longitudinal image of testis *(T)* with a cyst-like appendix epididymis *(arrow)* arising from the head of the epididymis *(E)*.

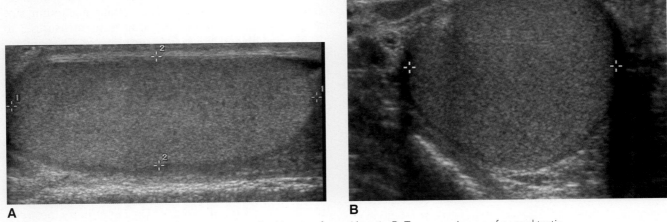

**Figure 17-16** Testis. **A:** Longitudinal image of normal testis. **B:** Transverse image of normal testis.

testicular echogenicity due to the growth of the seminiferous tubules.[9,24]

## Arterial and Venous Anatomy of the Scrotum

Scrotal blood flow is supplied by the bilateral testicular, cremasteric, and deferential arteries.[8,9,11,26] Testicular arteries provide the major blood supply to the testis. They arise from the anterior aspect of the aorta just below the level of the renal arteries and enter the spermatic cord at the internal inguinal ring with the other cord structures.[2,3,9,11,26] In the spermatic cord, the testicular artery is joined by the deferential artery (a branch of the vesicular artery) and the cremasteric artery (a branch of the inferior epigastric artery).[7-9,11,26] The deferential artery supplies the epididymis and vas deferens.[2,3,8,9,11,26] Major blood supply to the epididymis, however, is via the superior epididymal artery, a branch of the testicular artery.[2,4] The cremasteric artery supplies the peritesticular tissues[2,9,11,26,27] (Fig. 17-17A,B). Both the deferential and cremasteric arteries also contribute a variable amount of blood to the testis via anastomoses with the testicular artery[2,9,11,26]

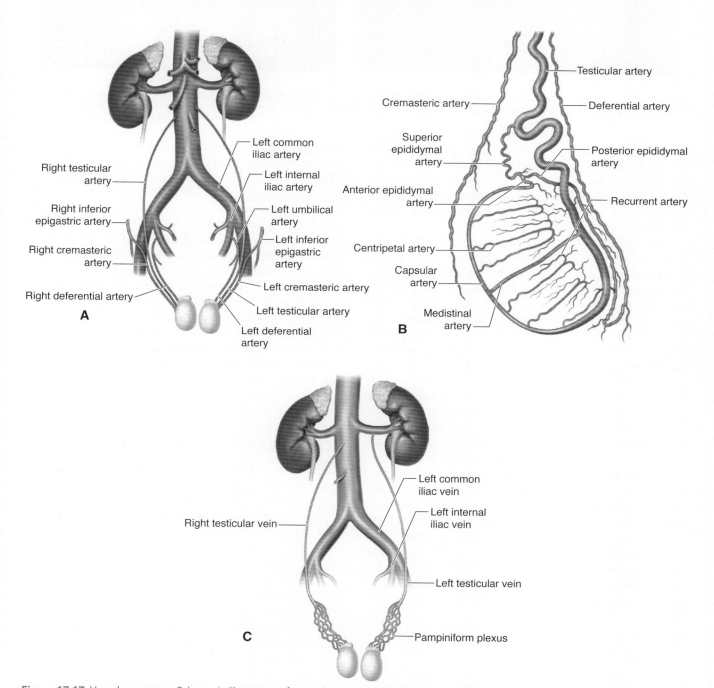

**Figure 17-17** Vascular anatomy. Schematic illustration of normal arterial supply to the scrotum **(A)**, intrascrotal arterial supply **(B)**, and venous drainage form the scrotum **(C)**.

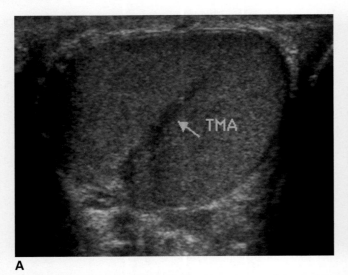
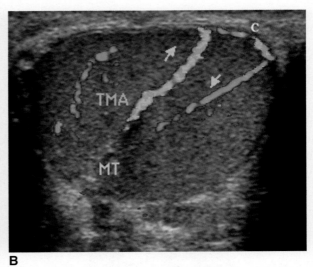

**A**      **B**

**Figure 17-18** Intrascrotal arteries. **A:** Transverse image of the testis showing transmediastinal artery (*TMA, arrow*). **B:** Transverse color image of transmediastinal artery (*TMA*) supplying capsular artery (*C*) and centripetal artery (*blue*) with color flow seen in the opposite direction.

The venous drainage from the scrotum, inclusive of the mediastinum, epididymis, and scrotal wall, is via the pampiniform plexus, which empties into the testicular veins. The right testicular vein drains into the inferior vena cava while the left testicular vein drains into the left renal vein[8,9,11,26] (Fig. 17-17C).

The anatomy of intratesticular arteries is illustrated in Fig. 17-17B. At the posterior superior aspect of the testis, the testicular artery pierces the tunica albuginea to form capsular arteries that run along the periphery of the testis in a layer known as the *tunica vasculosa*. Capsular arteries have centripetal branches that enter the testicular parenchyma and run toward the mediastinum testis. At the mediastinum, centripetal arteries arborize into recurrent rami arteries that course away from the mediastinum testis.[2,3,8,9,11,26] In approximately 50% of normal testes, a transmediastinal arterial branch of the testicular artery enters the mediastinum and courses through the testicular parenchyma in a direction opposite the centripetal arteries to supply the capsular arteries.[2,3,8,9,11,26,27] A transmediastinal vein usually accompanies the artery.[2,3,7–9,11,26,27] The gray scale sonographic appearance of the transmediastinal artery is a prominent hypoechoic band traversing the testis[7,11] (Fig. 17-18A). With color Doppler, the transmediastinal artery is seen as a prominent arterial branch traversing the mediastinum, demonstrating flow toward the periphery of the testis to supply the capsular arteries[3,7–9,26] (Fig. 17-18B). Flow in the transmediastinal artery courses in the opposite direction relative to the centripetal arteries[7,8,26] (Fig. 17-18C).

### Spectral and Color Doppler Sonography of the Intrascrotal Arteries

The testis has low vascular resistance similar to that found in the brain and kidney.[9] The spectral waveform of the testicular artery, and its intratesticular branches,

characteristically have a low-resistance, high-flow pattern, with a mean RI of 0.62 (range: 0.48 to 0.075)[2,3–15,26] (Fig. 17-19A). The normal spectral waveform of the epididymal artery is similar to that of the testicular artery, which is a low-resistance, high-flow waveform, with an RI ranging from (0.46 to 0.68)[2,3,10,14,15] (Fig. 17-19B). Cremasteric and deferential arteries have a high-resistance, low-flow pattern with a mean RI of greater than 0.75.[15,26] Supratesticular arteries (testicular, cremasteric, and deferential) within the spermatic cord demonstrate either low- or high-resistance flow patterns, depending on which artery is insonated[9,26] (Fig. 17-19C). With color Doppler, intratesticular arterial blood flow corresponds well with the described anatomic morphology.

Intratesticular arteries are oriented in vascular planes that intersect the mediastinum.[9,26] Longitudinal oblique views of the testis best demonstrate capsular and intratesticular arteries[9,26] (Fig. 17-19D).

## SONOGRAPHY OF SCROTAL DISEASE

Sonography is used to evaluate the scrotum when patients present with common symptoms such as acute painful scrotum, scrotal mass, and scrotal enlargement. Scrotal pathologies by anatomic region are shown in Table 17-1.

### DECREASE IN SIZE OF THE TESTIS

Decrease in the size of a testis may be a cause of infertility or an indication of a pituitary or hypothalamus gland abnormality, such as hypogonadotropic hypogonadism. Hypogonadotropic hypogonadism results from the absence of the gonadal-stimulating pituitary hormones causing underdeveloped testicles.[9,24] Other causes of testicular atrophy include cryptorchism, "missed torsion" (ischemic damage due to compromised blood

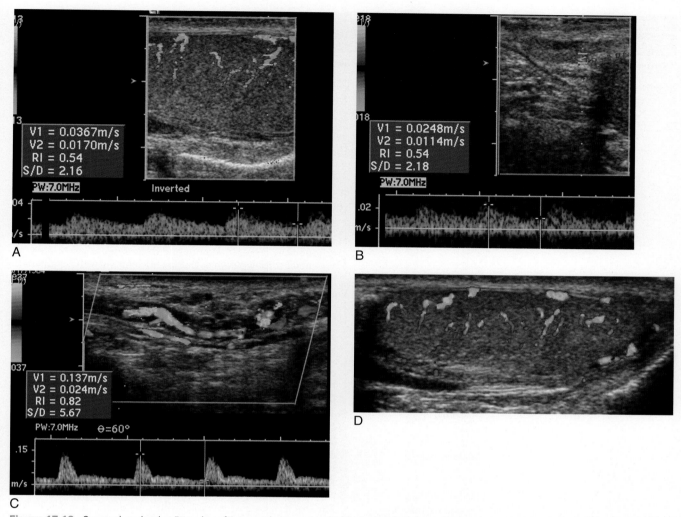

**Figure 17-19** Spectral and color Doppler of intrascrotal arteries. **A:** Normal spectral waveform of intratesticular artery with low-resistance flow. **B:** Normal spectral waveform of epididymal artery with low-resistance flow. **C:** Normal spectral waveform of the spermatic cord with high-resistance flow from either the cremasteric or deferential arteries. **D:** Longitudinal image of testis demonstrating normal intratesticular arteries with color flow Doppler.

flow), postsurgical procedures (i.e., inguinal hernio-plasty, varicocelectomy), epididymo-orchitis due to se-vere inflammation of the spermatic cord, and trauma.[14] The sonographic appearance of testicular atrophy is a small or shrunken heterogeneous testis displaying in-creased echogenicity due to fibrosis.[14] A uniform hy-poechoic testis may be seen with associated concurrent ischemia.[14]

## UNDESCENDED TESTIS

The testicles of the fetus lie in the peritoneal cavity near the inguinal canal. Most boys' testes are descended at birth but occasionally they descend later. The unilateral absence of a testis in the scrotum is an important find-ing since the incidence of malignant degeneration in the undescended testis is 48 to 50 times more likely than in the normally descended testis.[11,13] The incidence of seminoma is 2.5 to 8 times higher in the patient with an undescended testis than in the general population.[3,13,15] The contralateral intrascrotal testis has up to a 20% increased risk of malignancy.[24] An undescended testis is also associated with infertility because sperm are exposed to abnormally high temperatures within the abdomen and/or inguinal canal.[11,17,24] When the unde-scended testis is relocated and orchiopexy is performed before age 2, fertility is preserved.[14] Undescended testes are at increased risk for torsion and commonly associ-ated with malignant degeneration.[24] Torsion becomes more frequent after puberty because the testis is larger than its mesentery. Sixty-four percent of patients with torsion of an intra-abdominal testis are reported to have associated testicular cancer.[24] Congenital inguinal her-nia is also associated with undescended testis.[24] Fail-ure to close the processus vaginalis, which forms the scrotal sac, increases the chance of bowel herniating into the scrotum. Approximately, 90% of patients with undescended testes have herniated sacs.[24]

**TABLE 17-1**

## Sonographic Appearance of Common Scrotal Lesion

| Structure | Lesion | | Sonographic Appearance |
|---|---|---|---|
| Spermatic cord | Varicocele | | Dilated serpiginous veins of the pampiniform plexus (superior, lateral, and posterior) measuring >2 mm with the patient supine (Valsalva maneuver) or when the veins measure >2.5 mm with the patient standing. Color Doppler enhances dilatation and reflux. |
| | Hematoma/hematocele | | Thickening of spermatic cord. Variable echogenicity, depending on duration. Initially hyperechoic, with age the hematoma appears hypoechoic or complex. |
| | Sperm granuloma | | Focal avascular hypoechoic to heterogeneous solid mass. |
| | Hydrocele | | Loculated anechoic fluid collection anterior or posterior to the spermatic cord. |
| | Abscess | | Spermatic cord thickening with areas of increased or decreased echogenicity representing pus and microabscess. Associated spermatic cord hyperemia. Color void centrally with peripheral flow associated with focal abscess. |
| | Torsion | | Enlarged cord with variable echogenicity, hypoechoic to hyperechoic with a "knot" or "whirlpool" mass appearance, representing venous congestion, hemorrhage and arterial occlusion. Color Doppler reveals no flow or partial flow depending on the duration and degree of torsion. |
| | Hernia | | Complex mass with echogenic and anechoic areas representing omentum, air- and fluid-filled segments of bowel. Characteristic haustral appearance and peristalsis (classic appearance). Color Doppler shows blood flow within viable bowel. |
| | Benign Neoplasms | Lipoma | Solid avascular echogenic mass (typical) to uniformly hypoechoic. Variable echogenicity may likely reflect the number of interstices. |
| | | Adenomatoid tumor | Solid mass, variable echogenicity, equal to or greater than the testis. Minimal flow by color Doppler within and in the periphery of the tumor |
| | | Hemangioma, cholesteatoma, leiomyoma | Solid mass, variable echogenicity, hyperechoic to hypoechoic. Minimal flow by color Doppler within the tumor (specifically leiomyoma). |
| | Malignant neoplasms from the mesenchyme | Fibrosarcoma, liposarcoma, rhabdomyosarcoma | Solid ill-defined, inhomogeneous echo texture with echogenic areas and focal anechoic areas representing necrosis. |
| Epididymis | Epididymitis | | Enlargement of the epididymis with variable echogenicity depending on the stage of the disease. The testis is normal. A reactive hydrocele/pyocele is often seen with scrotal wall thickening. |
| | | Acute bacterial | Enlarged hypoechoic epididymis due to edema, with areas of hyperechogenicity, secondary to hemorrhage and infection with hypervascularity. |
| | | Chronic | Epididymis enlarged, focal, or diffuse heterogeneity; tunica is thickened; shadowing from calcifications may be seen. |
| | | Traumatic | Enlarged heterogeneous epididymis, hypervascularity, small hematomas, hematocele. |
| | Spermatocele | | Cystic avascular mass with well-defined walls and few internal echoes secondary to spermatozoa and/or debris in the region of the epididymis, most often located in the head of the epididymis; may be unilocular or multilocular and displaces the epididymal head anteriorly. |
| | Epididymal cyst | | Anechoic avascular mass with well-defined walls occurring anywhere along the epididymis. |
| | Tuberculosis | | Enlarged heterogeneous and nodular epididymis with scanty vascularity seen within or in the periphery of the nodules. |
| | Sarcoidosis | | Enlarged heterogeneous epididymis with hypoechoic nodules. |
| | Sperm granuloma | | Solid avascular hypoechoic or heterogeneous well-circumscribed mass, located throughout the epididymis. |

**TABLE  17-1**  *(continued)*

## Sonographic Appearance of Common Scrotal Lesion

| Structure | Lesion | Sonographic Appearance |
|---|---|---|
| | Abscess | Hypoechoic mass with irregular walls, low-level internal echoes, and peripheral hyperemia. |
| | Torsion | Enlarged heterogeneous epididymal body with only few vascular signals and a highly vascular epididymal head. The testis is normal by gray scale and color Doppler. |
| | Adenomatoid/leiomyoma tumors | Solid well-circumscribed mass, variable echogenicity, equal or greater than the testis. Minimal flow by color Doppler within and in the periphery of the tumor. |
| Tunica vaginalis | Acute hydrocele | Anechoic fluid collection anterolateral to the testis, with strong sound transmission. |
| | Chronic hydrocele | Low-level fluid collection anterolateral to the testis with mobile echoes—that is, cholesterol crystals, fibrin bodies, inflammatory debris, septations secondary to infection and/or trauma, scrotal calcifications, and diffuse scrotal wall thickening. Power Doppler demonstrates movement of internal debris. |
| | Scrotal calcifications/pearls | Highly echogenic spherical focus or foci with associated acoustic shadowing moving freely within the hydrocele. |
| | Acute hematocele | Complex echogenic fluid collection between the parietal and visceral layers of the tunica vaginalis. |
| | Chronic hematocele | Complex echogenic fluid collection with thick internal septa, scrotal wall thickening, calcifications, indistinguishable from chronic hydrocele or pyocele. |
| | Pyocele | Thick hemiscrotal wall; echogenic fluid collection with septations and occasionally focal mural calcifications; similar to chronic hydroceles and hematoceles. |
| | Hematoma | Appearance of hematoma varies with age; acutely, the scrotal wall is thickened; after 2–3 days, hypoechoic areas are seen (liquefaction); extratesticular hematomas can be solid or septated cystic masses. |
| | Abscess | Complex intrascrotal mass with focal hypoechoic low-level echoes or mixed areas, with irregular and hypervascular borders. |
| | Tunica albuginea cyst | Defined anechoic area(s) with posterior enhancement. Meets criteria for a simple cyst. |
| Testicular focal–benign | Hematoma/trauma | Appearance of hematoma varies with age; focal hyperechoic avascular areas are seen in the acute stage and hypoechoic to complex focal areas develop as the hemorrhage ages. |
| | Abscess | Focal complex mass with low-level areas, irregular and hypervascular borders. |
| | Focal orchitis | Ill-defined hypoechoic mass with increased blood flow. |
| | Liquefactive necrosis (seen in subacute torsion) | Focal anechoic areas. Avascular. |
| | Focal ischemic infarction (following infection and torsion) | Focal hypoechoic avascular mass. |
| | Adenomatoid tumor | Solid well-circumscribed mass, variable echogenicity, equal, or greater than the testis. Minimal flow by color Doppler within and in the periphery of the tumor. |
| | Sarcoidosis | Solid, focal hyperechoic mass. |
| | Sperm granuloma | Hypoechoic to heterogeneous solid avascular mass. |
| | Benign gonadal stromal tumors (Leydig, Sertoli) | Focal, variable echogenicity, usually hypoechoic with prominent peripheral flow by color Doppler. |
| | Epidermoid cysts | Well-circumscribed avascular mass with variable echogenicity (hypoechoic to hyperechoic) with an echogenic or anechoic rim. Alternatively, it can contain alternating hypoechoic and hyperechoic concentric rings demonstrating an "onion appearance." |

*(continued)*

| TABLE | 17-1 | (continued) |
|---|---|---|

## Sonographic Appearance of Common Scrotal Lesion

| Structure | Lesion | Sonographic Appearance |
|---|---|---|
| | Dermoid cyst | May simulate simple cyst or may have echogenic areas along periphery; occasionally, cyst itself is echogenic. |
| | Cystadenoma | Multiseptate cystic mass. |
| Testicular diffuse–benign | Orchitis | Enlarged, diffusely hypoechoic testis with hypervascularity. |
| | Infarcts (after trauma, infection, and torsion) | Acutely (within 24 hours), enlarged with normal or decreased echogenicity. After 24 hours, heterogeneous with hypoechoic areas representing necrosis, hemorrhage, and infarction. Absent intratesticular flow by color Doppler. |
| | Granulomatous disease | Enlarged, irregular, heterogeneous testis; may have calcifications. |
| | Sarcoidosis | Enlarged heterogeneous testis with hypoechoic nodules. |
| | Microlithiasis | Multiple small 1–3 mm echogenic foci disseminated throughout the testis without posterior shadowing. The pattern of microliths can vary with cluster calcifications centrally and in the periphery. Bilateral involvement is common. |
| | Acquired atrophy | Small, hypoechoic testis. |
| Testicular focal–malignant | Seminoma | Uniformly hypoechoic mass; well defined (without tunica albuginea invasion), may have scattered hyperechoic areas. Color/power Doppler demonstrates hypervascularity in tumors >1.6 cm. |
| | Embryonal cell | Predominantly hypoechoic mass, poorly marginated, texture is heterogeneous with areas of hemorrhagic necrosis or cystic change. The tumor often invades the tunica albuginea. |
| | Choriocarcinoma | Heterogeneous mass with extensive hemorrhagic necrosis in the central portion, with a mixed cystic and solid appearance. |
| | Teratoma | Large complex mass with multiple cystic areas representing bone, cartilage, smooth muscle, and other tissues. |
| | Yolk sac tumor | Nonspecific inhomogeneous and may contain echogenic foci secondary to hemorrhage or hypoechoic areas due to necrosis. |
| | Lymphoma | Enlarged testis, hypoechoic lesions of various sizes with increased vascularity. |
| | Leukemia | Enlarged testis, hypoechoic mass with increased vascularity. |
| | Metastases | Multiple hypoechoic (less often echogenic) masses; rarely, both are seen together. |
| Testicular diffuse–malignant | Leukemia | Enlarged, hypoechoic testis with hypervascularity similar to orchitis. |
| | Lymphoma | Enlarged, hypoechoic testis with hypervascularity similar to leukemia. |
| | Diffuse embryonal cell | Enlarged, hypoechoic testis with heterogeneous echotexture, irregular margins, and focal echogenic areas due to hemorrhage or necrosis. Tunica albuginea invasion. |
| | Diffuse seminoma | Enlarged, hypoechoic testis with heterogeneous echotexture, lobular or multinodular with hypervascularity similar to diffuse orchitis. The tumor is confined within the tunica albuginea. |

Undescended testes are bilateral in about 10% of cases.[14] Approximately 80% of undescended testes are located within the inguinal canal, and the remaining 20% are intra-abdominal (from the renal hilum to the inguinal canal).[11–15,17,21] The incidence of undescended testis at birth has been reported to be 30.3% for premature infants, 3.4% for fullterm infants, and in 0.28% of adult men.[9,24]

The sonographic appearance of an undescended testis is an oval or elongated well-circumscribed hypoechoic homogeneous soft tissue structure, smaller than the normal descended intrascrotal testis[3,9,11,14,17,24] (Fig. 17-20). Identification of the mediastinum testis helps confirm the presence of the undescended testicle.[3,9,11,14,15,17] Because sonography is relatively inexpensive, delivers no ionizing radiation, and does not require sedation, it should be the initial imaging method for undescended testis, with adjunctive computed tomography or MRI when sonography cannot definitively localize the testis.[24]

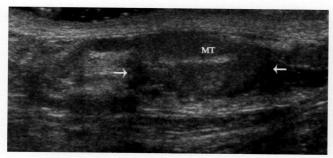

**Figure 17-20** Undescended testis. Longitudinal image of a small, undescended testis (*arrows*) located in the inguinal canal. *MT*, Mediastinum testis.

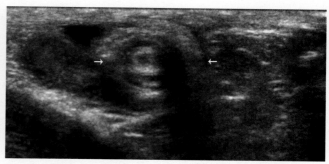

**Figure 17-21** Testicular torsion. Longitudinal image of spermatic cord demonstrating "the knot" or "whirlpool" pattern (*arrows*) seen in testicular torsion. (Image courtesy of Dr. Vijayaraghavan S. Boopathy.)

## ACUTE PAINFUL SCROTUM

Acute scrotal pain is a common clinical problem in both children and adults, and often presents a diagnostic challenge for referring clinicians. Epididymitis and epididymo-orchitis are the most common causes of acute scrotal pain.[1,2,9–11,13,22,26] Differentiating patients with epididymitis from those with suspected torsion is critical. Gray scale sonography combined with color, power, and spectral Doppler increases the diagnostic efficacy in distinguishing inflammatory from ischemic processes.[2,8,14,28] With prompt diagnosis, conditions such as ischemic necrosis and abscess can be surgically corrected to preserve testicular viability and function.[11,16,21,29]

Major causes of acute scrotal pain include epididymitis, epididymo-orchitis, focal orchitis, testicular torsion, abscess, trauma, torsion of the testicular appendices, scrotal wall inflammation, and incarcerated inguinal hernia.[15] With complete testicular torsion, arterial flow is occluded and only surgical restoration of blood flow can prevent loss of the testicle.[11] Abscess is also a surgical emergency since drainage of an abscess can prevent loss of the testicle.[9] Epididymitis is painful, but antibiotic treatment usually resolves the symptoms fairly rapidly.[9] Left untreated, epididymitis may progress to abscess formation, testicular infarction, and necrotizing fasciitis (Fournier gangrene).[2,9,10,30]

## TESTICULAR TORSION

Testicular (spermatic cord) torsion represents 20% of scrotal disease in postpubertal males.[9] Torsion occurs most commonly during adolescence, between 12 and 18 years of age, with a peak incidence occurring at 14 years.[4,9,24] Torsion is caused by a developmental weakness of the mesenteric attachment of the spermatic cord to the testis and epididymis. This faulty development allows the testis to fall forward within the scrotum and rotate freely within the tunica vaginalis, much like a clapper inside a bell.[4,9,11,24] The severity of testicular torsion ranges from 180 to 720 degrees or greater.[2,4,7,11,13,21] Twisting of the spermatic cord results in venous congestion. Initially, this prevents venous drainage and progresses to arterial occlusion, scrotal

edema, hemorrhage, and infarction.[2,4,5,7] Sonographic detection of a spermatic cord "torsion knot" has been described as a whirlpool pattern, manifested by concentric layers with increased and decreased echogenicity at the external inguinal canal above the testis and epididymis. Visualization of the torsion knot is the most specific and sensitive sign of either complete or incomplete testicular torsion[2,4,28] (Fig. 17-21). Pulsed Doppler should always be used in conjunction with color or power Doppler to confirm the presence of arterial and venous flow within the testis as color Doppler can be subject to motion artifacts.[5]

Early diagnosis of testicular torsion is important because it requires orchiopexy, a surgical procedure, to preserve viability and function.[2,4,9,11,24] When surgery is performed within 6 hours after the onset of pain, the salvage rate is between 80% and 100%, as opposed to 70% and 76% when performed within 6 to 12 hours.[11,13,14] After 12 hours, the salvageability drops to 20%.[8,9,13,14,24] Surgery performed after 24 hours almost never results in successful salvage of the testis and is considered a missed torsion.[2,7,9,24]

There are two types of testicular torsion: intravaginal and extravaginal[2,4,9,11,13,14,24,28] (Fig. 17-22 A,B). In the

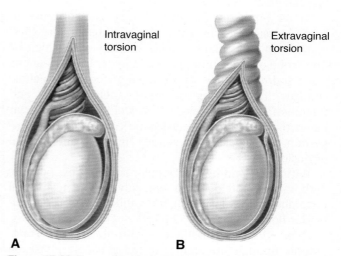

**Figure 17-22** Types of testicular torsion. **A:** Schematic illustration of intravaginal testicular torsion. **B:** Schematic illustration of extravaginal testicular torsion.

intravaginal type, the testis rotates freely within the tunica vaginalis by a long stalk of mesorchium. Intravaginal torsion is the most frequent type of testicular torsion and is seen in 80% of cases.[2,4,11] Extravaginal testicular torsion occurs exclusively in newborns.[2,4,9,11,13,14,24] This type of torsion occurs outside the tunica vaginalis when the testes and gubernacula are not fixed and are able to freely rotate.[2,4,13]

Clinical signs of testicular torsion include a sudden onset of pain, followed by nausea, vomiting, and a low-grade fever.[4] In 50% of cases, the symptoms mimic epididymitis.[24] The cremasteric reflex is usually absent, and pain cannot be relieved by elevating the scrotum.[4] When the spermatic cord twists, the affected testis maintains a higher and horizontal position in the scrotum.[4] After 24 to 48 hours, the pain usually disappears, generally indicating that the testicle is dead. In newborns, testicular torsion may present with only painless swelling and redness.[24]

Torsion can be divided into three phases: (1) acute (within 24 hours), (2) subacute (1 to 10 days), and (3) chronic (more than 10 days).[9,25] Sonographic findings in testicular torsion depend on the duration and degree of spermatic cord rotation.[2,4,11,13]

Gray scale sonographic findings alone of testicular torsion are nonspecific. Differentiation between inflammation and ischemia requires color, power, and spectral Doppler.[2,4,11,13,21,31] Within 1 to 6 hours, the affected testis maybe slightly enlarged, with normal or decreased echogenicity[2,4,9,11,21,24] (Fig. 17-23A). Epididymal enlargement (Fig. 17-23B) is common and is frequently accompanied by the "torsion knot" or "whirlpool" pattern seen in the spermatic cord (see Fig. 17-21), scrotal skin thickening, and a reactive hydrocele (Fig. 17-23C).[2,4,11,13,14,24] Because gray scale sonography findings are often normal in the early or acute phase of torsion, the absence of intratesticular arterial flow by color and power Doppler is diagnostic for ischemia[4] (see Fig. 17-23A).

At 24 hours to 10 days, during the subacute to missed torsion phases, the testis, epididymis, and spermatic cord are enlarged with varying echogenicity.[24] The sonographic findings include a heterogeneous testis and epididymis with diffuse or focal hypoechoic changes representing necrosis, hemorrhage, and infarction[2,4,11,13,14,21,24] (Fig. 17-23D–F). Extratesticular hemorrhage within the spermatic cord is due to congestion and blockage of venous drainage and arterial occlusion.[2,4,11,13,14]

With color and power Doppler sonography, patients with missed torsion or a non-salvageable testis will have absent intratesticular flow and increased peritesticular flow[4,9,11,14] (Fig. 17-23G,H).

After 10 days, classified as chronic torsion, sonographic findings are similar to the subacute phase. In time, ischemic testes become small and hypoechoic.[14,24] In cases of hemorrhage infarction, the testis appear heterogeneous and fibrotic[14,24] (Fig. 17-23I). The epididymis is enlarged and echogenic representing hemorrhage and necrosis.[23]

## TORSION–DETORSION AND PARTIAL TORSION OF THE TESTIS

Acute and intermittent sharp testicular pain and scrotal swelling, interspersed with long asymptomatic intervals, are characteristic of torsion–detorsion.[4] In spontaneous detorsion, there is increased perfusion, manifested by hypervascularity with a low-resistance flow pattern of the testis.[2,4,14]

The testis may be enlarged, and focal infarcts may or may not be present. Cases of partial or transient torsion can present a diagnostic challenge. There are no studies to date that validate the role of spectral Doppler sonography in partial torsion. However, there are few published case reports that suggest its usefulness. Asymmetry of the resistive indices with decreased diastolic flow or diastolic flow reversal may be seen.[2,4,13]

## TORSION OF THE APPENDAGES

Torsion of the appendix testis and appendix epididymis can cause acute scrotal pain mimicking testicular torsion.[2] More than 90% of torsed appendages involve the appendix testis.[2,4,13] Torsion of the appendix testis accounts for 20% to 40% of cases of acute scrotum in pubescent and adolescent males.[8] The peak incidence is between the ages of 7 and 14 years.[2,4,13] With appendiceal torsion, the testis is normal by color duplex sonography.[2,7] The sonographic appearance of a torsed appendage varies, as it may appear as a large circular hyperechoic mass with a central hypoechoic area, or an enlarged circular heterogeneous mass adjacent to a normal testis and epididymis.[2,4,13] Color Doppler of appendiceal torsion shows increased periappendiceal blood flow and absent central appendiceal flow.[2] A testicular appendage larger than 5.6 mm with increased periappendiceal color flow is suggestive of torsion.[2,4] An associated reactive hydrocele and skin thickening are common in these cases.[2,4] Torsed appendages may ultimately atrophy and calcify.[7]

## TESTICULAR RUPTURE

Testicular rupture is rare.[9] It occurs when the capsule, the tunica albuginea, is torn by trauma.[12,18] Testicular rupture is associated with athletic injuries, industrial, and motor vehicle accidents.[2,12,18] Early diagnosis is critical because the surgical testicular salvage rate diminishes from approximately 90% to 45% after 72 hours of onset.[9,14,18] Surgical treatment requires repair of the tunica albuginea or orchiectomy.[2,9] Failure to repair the testis may result in the loss of spermatogenesis and hormonal function, chronic scrotal pain, and secondary anaerobic infection (scrotal gangrene).[9]

Sonographic findings in testicular rupture include a contour abnormality due to an irregular fibrous tunica albuginea, extrusion of the testicular contents into the scrotal sac, hematocele between the tunica vaginalis and parietalis, intratesticular hematoma, and infarction. The latter appears as hypoechoic or hyperechoic focal abnormalities within the testis.[2,12,14,18] The

sonographic appearance of intratesticular hematomas varies with size and duration. Acute hematomas present as avascular echogenic or hypoechoic areas.[2,9,12,18] With time, liquefaction or lysis of the hematoma results in a septated fluid collection containing fine echoes.[9,19]

Disruption of the testicular echogenicity, with focal hyperechoic and hypoechoic areas in the testicle, along with an ill-defined tunica albuginea, must be considered suggestive of testicular rupture. Rupture

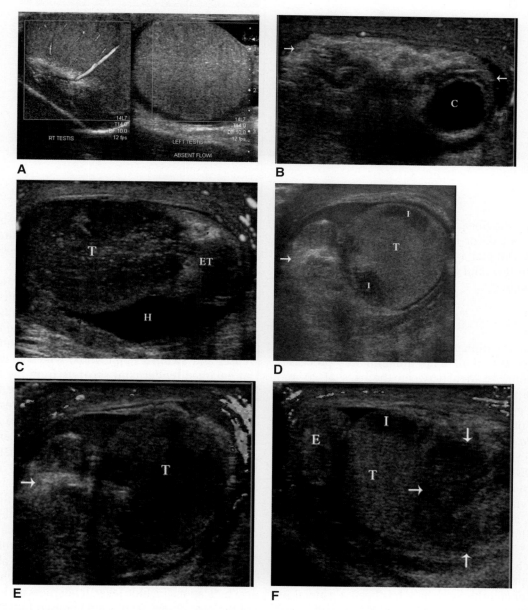

**Figure 17-23** Torsion. **A:** Transverse image of testes with acute torsion in the left testis. Note the enlargement and absence of flow in left testis, whereas the echogenicity remains normal. **B:** Transverse image of enlarged, echogenic, torsed epididymis with hemorrhage (*arrows*). Note absence of flow and cyst (*C*) in the epididymis. **C:** Longitudinal power Doppler image of heterogeneous, infarcted testis (*T*), with absent flow, enlarged epididymal tail (*ET*), and reactive hydrocele (*H*). **D:** Transverse image of testis (*T*) with hypoechoic focal infarcts (*I*) and epididymal hemorrhage (*arrow*) in missed torsion. **E:** Transverse color image of heterogeneous testis (*T*) with diffuse hypoechoic changes and hemorrhage in the epididymis (*arrow*). Absent flow in both the testis and epididymis is consistent with missed torsion. **F:** Longitudinal color Doppler image of testis (*T*) with diffuse hypoechoic changes (*arrows*) representing hemorrhage and infarct (*I*). Absent flow is consistent with missed torsion. Epididymal head (*E*). *(continued)*

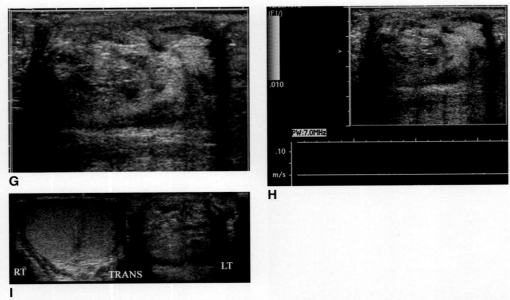

**Figure 17-23** *(continued)* **G:** Longitudinal power Doppler image of a nonsalvageable testis. Note the absent intratesticular flow and increased peritesticular flow consistent with missed torsion. **H:** Longitudinal spectral Doppler of a nonsalvageable testis with missed torsion. Note absence of intratesticular flow. **I:** Transverse image of both testes demonstrating a missed torsion with fibrotic changes in the left testis and a normal right testis.

of the tunica albuginea usually results in hemorrhage, which may occlude or decrease intratesticular arterial flow.[19] Color Doppler imaging is helpful in assessing intratesticular flow and can be used to determine surgical management.[24]

## EPIDIDYMITIS AND EPIDIDYMO-ORCHITIS

Epididymitis (inflammation of the epididymis) represents 75% to 80% of all acute inflammatory processes in the scrotum.[2,9,11] Men between the ages of 20 and 30 years are most often affected.[8] In adolescents and young men, epididymitis often is secondary to sexually transmitted organisms such as *Chlamydia trachomatis* and *Neisseria gonorrhoeae*.[2,13,22] In prepubertal boys and men over 35 years of age, the disease is most frequently caused by *Escherichia coli* and *Proteus mirabilis*.[2,13,22] The infection occurs from direct retrograde extension of pathogens, via the vas deferens, from a lower urinary tract source, such as urethritis, prostatitis, cystitis, and possibly following instrumentation such as catheterization.[2,10,11,14,22] In patients with suppressed immune systems such as those with HIV or those receiving immunosuppression treatment for transplantation or undergoing chemotherapy, there has been a general increase in opportunistic infections of the epididymis.[22] Less frequently, traumatic epididymitis may occur after scrotal trauma or iatrogenic injury to the epididymis during scrotal surgery.[7,12,22] Sonographic findings are similar to infectious epididymitis, including enlargement and hyperemia.[12] Following trauma, the epididymis may also reveal the presence of small hematomas, resulting in enlargement and inflammatory response[12]

(Fig. 17-24A,B). Differentiation between the two entities should be based on the history of trauma since the management of traumatic epididymitis does not require antibiotics.[22]

Epididymitis can affect the head, body, or tail of the epididymis; however, the entire epididymis is affected in 50% of cases.[9,32] Inflammation usually begins in the tail.[2,7,9,11,13,22] Early in the course of the disease, the physical examination may demonstrate an inflamed, tense, and swollen epididymis, which may present as an enlarged tender cord separate from the testis.[22] Epididymitis is usually unilateral but can be bilateral.[9] If epididymitis is left untreated, it can progress to involve the spermatic cord and testis, resulting in a spermatic cord abscess or epididymo-orchitis (inflammation of both the epididymis and testicle).[9] Coexistent orchitis develops in 20% to 40% of patients due to direct spread of infection.[2,7,9,11,13,22] Other complications include pyocele, testicular abscess, infarction, infertility, atrophy, and soft tissue necrosis (Fournier gangrene).[2,7,11,13]

Epididymo-orchitis represents approximately 25% of acute inflammatory processes of the scrotum. Untreated, acute epididymo-orchitis can progress to abscess, gangrene, infarct, pyocele infertility, and atrophy.[2,13,14] Clinical indications include fever, tenderness and enlargement of the epididymis, testis, and hemiscrotum.[9,22]

Gray scale sonographic findings of acute epididymitis, epididymo-orchitis, and orchitis include enlargement and variable echogenicity of the affected structure.[22] The epididymis and/or testis are usually hypoechoic due to edema, with areas of hyperechogenicity, secondary to hemorrhage and infection[22] (Fig. 17-25A–C). Scrotal wall thickening and reactive hydrocele

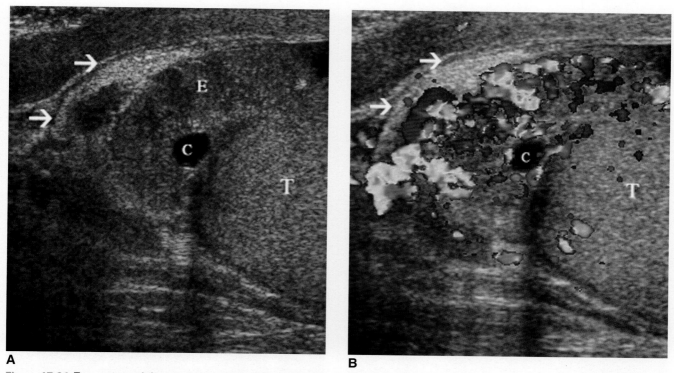

**Figure 17-24** Traumatic epididymitis. **A:** Longitudinal image of epididymis (*E*) with hematoma (*arrows*) and cyst (*C*) in a patient with traumatic epididymitis. Normal testis (*T*). **B:** Longitudinal color Doppler image in the same patient demonstrating hypervascularity in the epididymis *C*, cyst; *T*, testis.

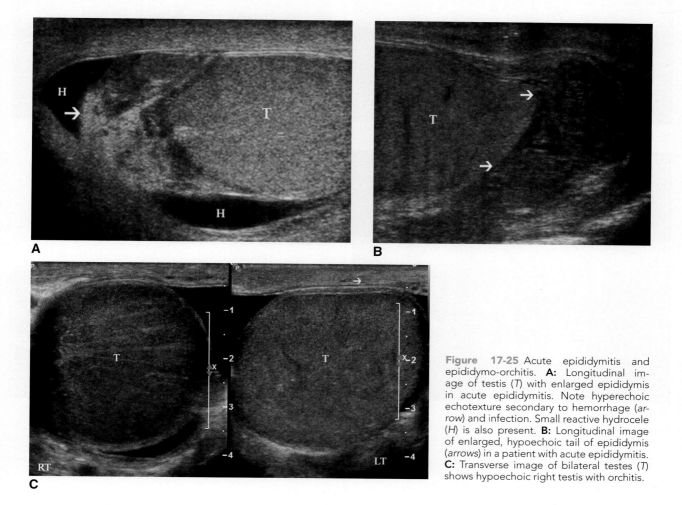

**Figure 17-25** Acute epididymitis and epididymo-orchitis. **A:** Longitudinal image of testis (*T*) with enlarged epididymis in acute epididymitis. Note hyperechoic echotexture secondary to hemorrhage (*arrow*) and infection. Small reactive hydrocele (*H*) is also present. **B:** Longitudinal image of enlarged, hypoechoic tail of epididymis (*arrows*) in a patient with acute epididymitis. **C:** Transverse image of bilateral testes (*T*) shows hypoechoic right testis with orchitis.

(fluid between the parietalis and vaginalis fascia) are common associated findings.[2,11,13,22] The hallmark of scrotal inflammatory disease is color Doppler hypervascularity of the affected structures.[22,32] The sensitivity of color Doppler sonography for the evaluation of scrotal inflammatory disease is close to 100%.[13] In 20% of patients with epididymitis and 40% of patients with orchitis, gray scale findings are normal, and hyperemia may be the only finding.[22] Focal epididymitis occurs in approximately 25% of cases and isolated focal orchitis occurs in 10% of cases.[2,9]

In patients with epididymitis, epididymo-orchitis, and isolated orchitis, color Doppler will show increased hypervascularity within the affected areas[2,22,32] (Fig. 17-26A–E). With focal epididymitis and orchitis, there may be focal hypoechoic and hypervascular areas involving the epididymis and testis[2,9] (Fig. 17-27A,B). Conversely, isolated epididymitis usually demonstrates a sonographically normal testicle.[2] Inflammation of the spermatic cord represents secondary changes associated with epididymitis.[9,14] The gray scale sonographic appearance of an infected spermatic cord is enlargement with areas of increased and decreased echogenicity representing edema and infection[9,23] (Fig. 17-28A). Color Doppler imaging of an infected spermatic cord will show hyperemia of both the pampiniform plexus and the supratesticular arteries[9] (Fig. 17-28B). When inflammation is severe, focal or diffuse testicular infarction may be seen.[2,9,13] Focal testicular infarcts appear sonographically as focal avascular masses[2,14] (Fig. 17-29). Diffuse testicular infarction shows variable echogenicity depending on the time of the ischemic event.[4,9] Color Doppler imaging

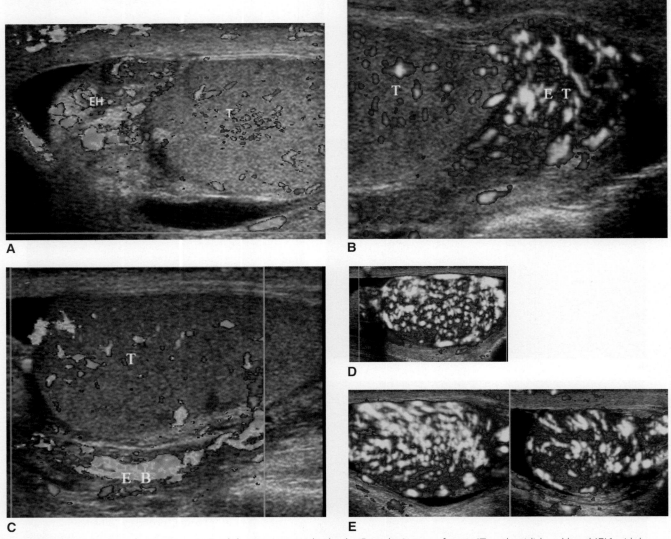

**Figure 17-26** Color Doppler imaging. **A:** Epididymitis. Longitudinal color Doppler image of testis (*T*) and epididymal head (*EH*) with hypervascularity in the epididymal head and a reactive hydrocele. **B:** Epididymitis. Longitudinal power Doppler image of testis (*T*) showing increased vascularity in epididymal tail (*ET*). **C:** Epididymitis. Longitudinal color image of testis (*T*) and epididymal body (*EB*) showing increased flow. **D:** Orchitis. Longitudinal power Doppler image of testis with hyperemia. **E:** Orchitis. Transverse power Doppler image of bilateral testes with orchitis shows diffuse hyperemia. *(continued)*

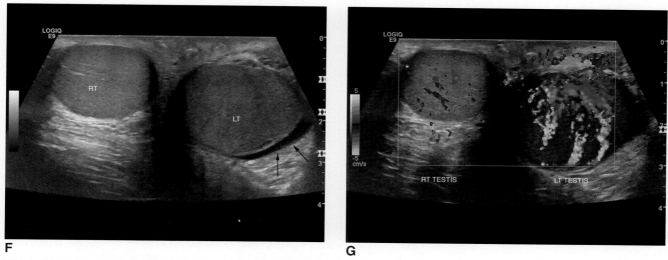

**F**    **G**

**Figure 17-26** *(continued)* **F:** Orchitis. Transverse image of both testes demonstrates a normal right testis (*RT*) and an enlarged, hypoechoic left testis (*LT*). Note small reactive hydrocele (*arrows*). **G:** Orchitis. Color Doppler image of the same patient demonstrates hypervascularity in the left testis (*LT*) consistent with orchitis.

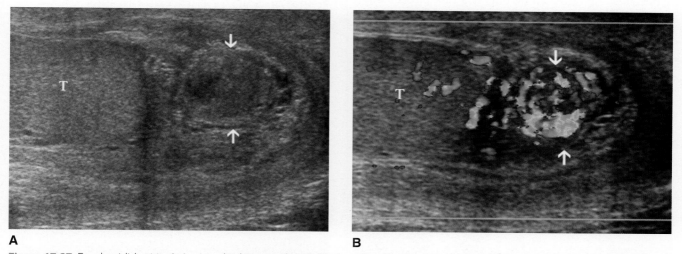

**A**    **B**

**Figure 17-27** Focal epididymitis. **A:** Longitudinal image of testis (*T*) shows focal hypoechoic mass (*arrows*) in epididymal tail. **B:** Longitudinal color image of the same patient shows hypervascularity in focal hypoechoic mass (*arrows*) located in epididymal tail.

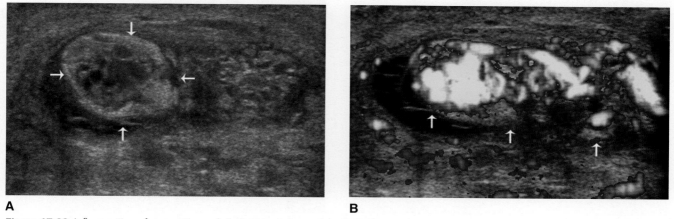

**A**    **B**

**Figure 17-28** Inflammation of spermatic cord. **A:** Transverse image of enlarged spermatic cord (*arrows*) with increased echogenicity secondary to infection and hemorrhage. **B:** Transverse power Doppler image of the same patient shows hyperemia.

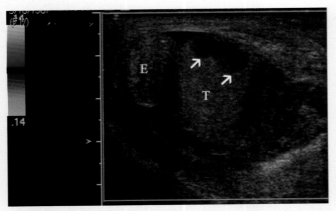

**Figure 17-29** Intratesticular infarct. Transverse color Doppler image of testis (*T*) with focal, avascular, hypoechoic, intratesticular infarct (*arrows*). Epididymis (*E*).

of infarction will show absent flow in the affected parenchyma. With chronicity, the testis may appear small and hypoechoic.[9,14,24] Isolated orchitis is a rare phenomenon and is caused mostly by mumps or AIDS. Sonographically, the testis is enlarged and shows diffuse, focal, or multiple hypoechoic lesions.[2] Color Doppler reveals increased blood flow. Focal orchitis may be difficult to distinguish from testicular tumor.[8]

The appearance of severe untreated epididymo-orchitis resulting in scrotal, testicular, and/or epididymal abscess, is a focal hypoechoic or mixed area, with irregular walls, hypervascular margins, and marked scrotal wall thickening with a reactive hydrocele[2,8,9]

(Fig. 17-30A,B). If the abscess involves the entire scrotum, the epididymis and testis may be replaced by a complex mass and be indistinguishable.[2]

Chronic epididymitis has been classified based on its different etiologies: inflammatory, infectious, and obstructive.[10,22] Patients may also present with a history of recurrent urinary tract infections.[10] Chronic epididymitis is characterized by persistent pain lasting for at least 3 months in the scrotum, testicle, or epididymis.[22] On clinical exam, the epididymis is moderately tender and can be differentiated from the testis.[22] In chronic epididymitis and epididymo-orchitis, the epididymis and testis are enlarged with a heterogeneous echo texture secondary to infection and hemorrhage. Calcifications and epididymal fibrosis are associated findings. The tunica albuginea also becomes thickened[10,22] (Fig. 17-31A,B). Sperm granulomas and calcifications are associated findings in patients with a history of granulomatous disease or obstruction postvasectomy.[9,10]

## SCROTAL AND TESTICULAR MASSES

A scrotal or testicular mass can be an ominous sign. Both benign and malignant disease processes can have similar clinical findings such as pain, swelling, or presence of a palpable mass.[2,3,9] Testicular cancer accounts for approximately 1% of all cancer in men, and most often presents as a painless lump or swelling of the testis.[3] Testicular cancer can present with pain because of associated hemorrhage or infection.[2,3,11] Benign intratesticular masses that can mimic malignancy include

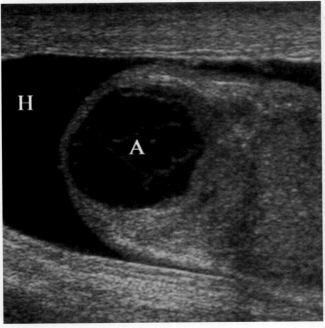

**A**

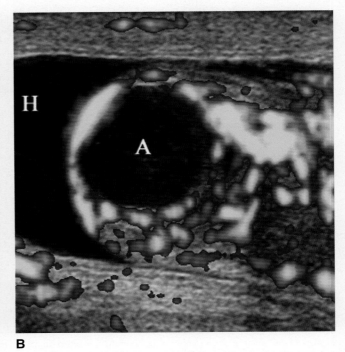

**B**

**Figure 17-30** Epididymal abscess. **A:** Longitudinal image of testis with focal complex abscess (*A*) in head of epididymis. Small hydrocele (*H*) is also present. **B:** Longitudinal power Doppler image of testis with focal complex abscess (*A*) in head of epididymis. Small hydrocele (*H*) is also present.

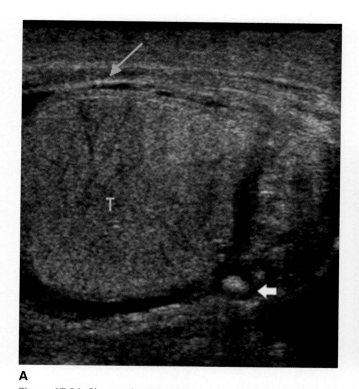

**A**

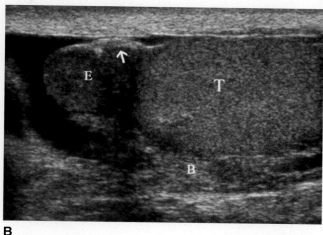

**B**

**Figure 17-31** Chronic changes. **A:** Longitudinal image of testis (*T*) showing thickened tunica (*long arrow*) and scrotal calcification (*short arrow*) in chronic epididymitis. **B:** Longitudinal image of testis (*T*), epididymal head (*E*), and an enlarged, heterogeneous epididymal body (*B*) characteristic of chronic epididymitis. Thickened tunica albuginea (*arrow*) and hydrocele are also present.

hematomas, focal orchitis, infarction, and granuloma.[3,13] Intratesticular solid masses must be considered malignant until proven otherwise.[21] Extratesticular masses are mostly benign, with the prevalence of malignancy being approximately 3%.[10] Having an accuracy approaching 100% in differentiating intratesticular from extratesticular masses, sonography is especially effective in the evaluation of scrotal masses.

## BENIGN SCROTAL MASSES

Benign scrotal masses include hydrocele, spermatocele, epididymal cysts, tubular ectasia, varicocele, scrotal hernia, scrotal abscess, hematoma, hematocele, pyocele, granulomatous disease, tunica albuginea cyst, simple testicular cyst, sperm granuloma, and epidermoid cyst.

### Hydrocele

A hydrocele is an abnormal accumulation of serous fluid in the potential space between the visceral and parietal layers of the tunica vaginalis, which surround the testis.[10,11,14,15,17] Hydroceles are the most common cause of painless scrotal swelling and may be congenital or acquired.[9-11,14] Congenital hydroceles are communicating hydroceles that occur due to failure of the process vaginalis to close, allowing serous fluid to communicate between the abdominal cavity and the scrotum.[10] Congenital hydroceles are present in 6% of male infants

at delivery, but in less than 1% of adults, since most hydroceles resolve within 18 months of age.[9,10]

Acquired or reactive hydroceles are noncommunicating hydroceles that result from impaired fluid reabsorption.[9,10,14] Acquired hydroceles are often associated with infection (epididymitis and epididymo-orchitis), torsion, and are seen with 10% of malignant testicular neoplasms.[2,4,9,11,14] Up to 50% of acquired hydroceles may be secondary to trauma.[2,6,10,18] Rarely, large hydroceles may impede testicular venous drainage, increasing vascular resistance within the intratesticular arteries, and resulting in a decrease or absence of intratesticular arterial diastolic flow[15,17] (Fig. 17-32A).

The clinical sign of hydrocele is a scrotal mass, which may or may not be painful. The classic sonographic appearance of an acute hydrocele is an anechoic fluid collection with enhanced sound transmission, surrounding the anterolateral aspects of the testis[9,11,14,17] (Fig. 17-32B). In patients with acute hydroceles, the testis is usually displaced posteromedially.[14] Chronic hydroceles may contain calcifications that produce acoustic shadowing. These calcifications, known as *scrotal pearls* or *scrotoliths*, may result from inflammatory deposits on the tunica vaginalis that have separated from the lining and/or from calcified missed appendiceal torsion[10,14] (Fig. 17-32C). Scrotal calcifications may be singular or multiple, filling the potential space between the layers of the tunica vaginalis testis.[9,10,14] In chronic inflammatory hydroceles, the sonographic findings may include diffuse

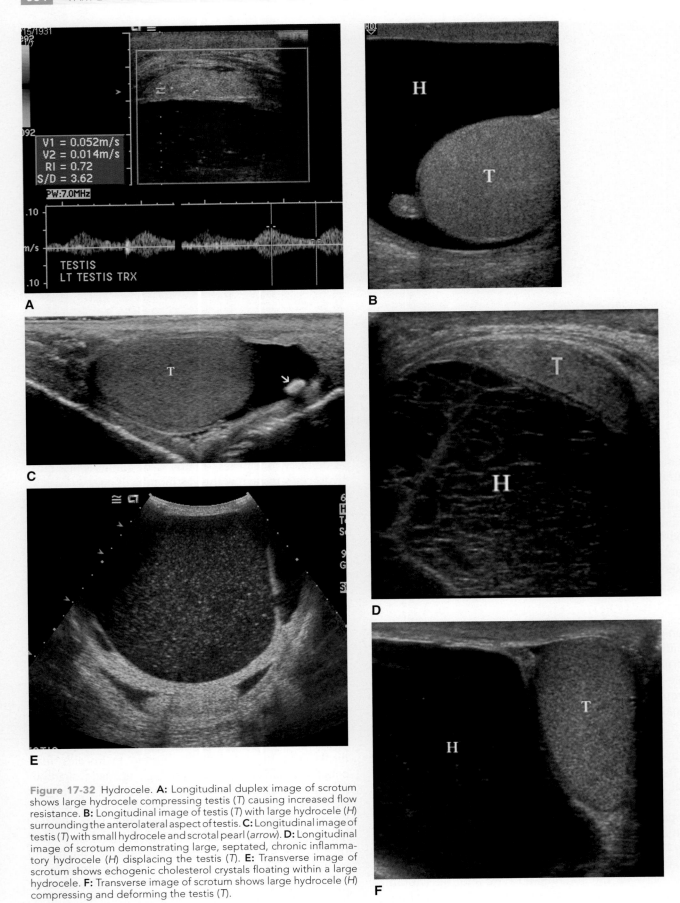

**Figure 17-32** Hydrocele. **A:** Longitudinal duplex image of scrotum shows large hydrocele compressing testis (*T*) causing increased flow resistance. **B:** Longitudinal image of testis (*T*) with large hydrocele (*H*) surrounding the anterolateral aspect of testis. **C:** Longitudinal image of testis (*T*) with small hydrocele and scrotal pearl (*arrow*). **D:** Longitudinal image of scrotum demonstrating large, septated, chronic inflammatory hydrocele (*H*) displacing the testis (*T*). **E:** Transverse image of scrotum shows echogenic cholesterol crystals floating within a large hydrocele. **F:** Transverse image of scrotum shows large hydrocele (*H*) compressing and deforming the testis (*T*).

scrotal wall thickening and echogenic septations resulting from old hemorrhage or infection[9,14,24] (Fig. 17-32D). Fine snowflake-like echoes are occasionally seen moving within the hydrocele representing fibrin bodies or cholesterol crystals[9,11,17] (Fig. 17-32E). In addition, a large chronic hydrocele, can compress the testis causing a contour deformity and atrophy[9,24] (Fig. 17-32F).

## Spermatoceles and Epididymal Cysts

Spermatoceles and epididymal cysts are the most common epididymal lesions. They have been reported in 20% to 40% of asymptomatic patients.[10,11,21] Usually presenting as painless scrotal masses, these lesions vary in size from 0.2 to 9 cm.[9,23,31] Both spermatoceles and epididymal cysts are thought to occur as a result of dilatation of the epididymal tubules, whether secondary to vasectomy, scrotal surgery, trauma, or epididymitis.[10,21-23] The most common location for spermatoceles is in the head of the epididymis, whereas epididymal cysts arise throughout the epididymis[19,21-23,31] (Fig. 17-33A). Spermatoceles usually displace the testis anteriorly, distinguishing them from a hydrocele, the latter of which surrounds the testis.[9,14] They are usually unilocular but can be multilocular[11,22] (Fig. 17-33B,C).

Epididymal cysts are frequently multiple and may contain loculations similar to spermatoceles.[11,23] Spermatoceles generally contain nonviable spermatozoa, cellular debris, and lymphocytes, whereas epididymal cysts are lined with epithelium and contain only serous fluid.[22,31]

Sonographically, a spermatocele is a thin-walled hypoechoic mass located in the epididymal head[22] (Fig. 17-33D). Spermatoceles, characteristically contain low-level echoes, due to the proteinaceous fluid and spermatozoa, and demonstrate posterior acoustic enhancement.[22] The sonographic appearance of an epididymal cyst is typically a well-defined, thin-walled, anechoic mass with good posterior acoustic enhancement and no internal echoes[22,23] (Fig. 17-33E,F).

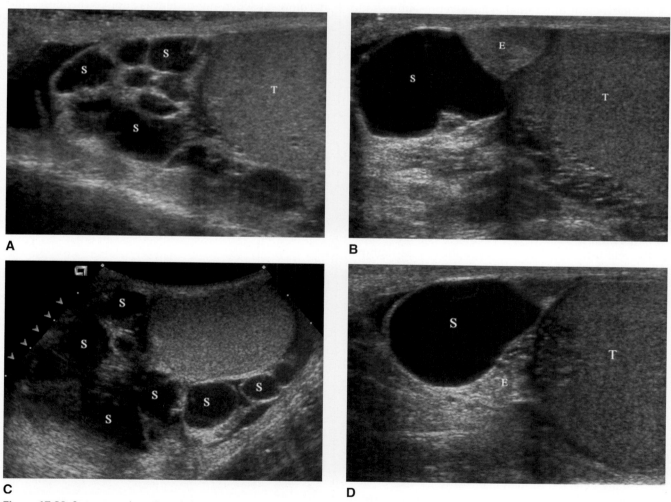

**Figure 17-33** Spermatocele and epididymal cyst. **A:** Longitudinal image of testis (*T*) with multiple spermatoceles (*S*) in the epididymal head. **B:** Longitudinal image of testis (*T*) shows large spermatoceles (*S*) displacing the head of the epididymis (*E*). **C:** Longitudinal image of the testis with multiple spermatoceles (*S*) in the head and body of the epididymis. **D:** Longitudinal image of testis (*T*) shows large thin walled spermatoceles (*S*) in the head of the epididymis (*E*). *(continued)*

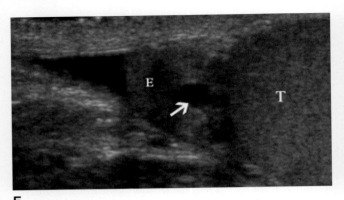

**E**

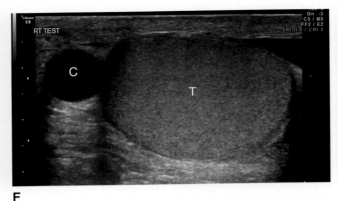

**F**

**Figure 17-33** *(continued)* **E:** Longitudinal image of testis (*T*) shows small cyst (*arrow*) in the epididymal head (*E*). **F:** Longitudinal image of testis (*T*) shows cyst (*C*) in the epididymal head.

Differentiating spermatoceles from epididymal cysts may be difficult if located in the head of the epididymis.[22] Color and power Doppler are useful in improving the accurate diagnosis of a spermatocele by recognition of the "falling snow" sign.[31] This sign is defined as the movement of internal echoes, representing solid particles, within a superficial cystic mass away from the transducer with the application of power or color Doppler imaging. This phenomenon of acoustic streaming or movement of internal echoes helps differentiate echogenic cystic from solid masses.[23,31]

### Tubular Ectasia of the Rete Testis

Dilatation of the efferent ductules is referred to as tubular ectasia of the rete testis. Tubular ectasia is commonly seen in men older than 50 years.[22,23] It is often bilateral and associated with epididymal cysts and spermatoceles, resulting from partial or complete obliteration of the efferent ductules due to inflammation, surgery, or trauma.[22] Tubular ectasia of the epididymis has been described in postvasectomy patients.[22,23] Tubular ectasia of the rete testis manifests sonographically as multiple tiny cystic tubules located within or adjacent to the mediastinum testis.[13,14,22] With color Doppler, dilated tubules are avascular and fluid filled[14] (Fig. 17-34).

### Varicocele

A varicocele is formed by dilatation of the veins of the pampiniform plexus >2 mm.[2,8,10,14] The dilated and tortuous veins are located superior and posterior to the testis and are caused by incompetent valves of the internal spermatic vein.[2,8,10,14] Large varicoceles can extend inferior to the testis.[13] There are two types of varicoceles: primary (idiopathic) and secondary.[2,9,13,14,17] Idiopathic varicoceles are present in approximately 15% of adult men, occur on the left side in 98% of cases, and are usually detected in men aged 15 to 25 years.[2,7,9,11,17] Left-sided predominance has been postulated due to the increased length of the left testicular vein and angulations at the entry of the left renal vein. The left testicular artery sometimes arches over the left renal

vein and causes compression. The right spermatic vein drains directly into the vena cava.[13] Bilateral involvement is seen in 30% of men.[2] Idiopathic varicoceles normally distend when the patient is in the standing position or performs the Valsalva maneuver and may decompress when the patient is supine; therefore, one should perform the Valsalva maneuver with the patient in the supine position or scan the patient in the upright position to detect varices.[7] Varicoceles are the most common correctable cause of infertility, occurring in 21% to 39% of men attending infertility clinics.[9,11,17]

Secondary varicoceles result from increased pressure on the internal spermatic vein or tributaries, caused by an abdominal cavity or retroperitoneal mass, marked hydronephrosis, or cirrhosis[2,7,11,14,17] (Fig. 17-35A,B). The appearance of secondary varicoceles is not affected by patient position.[17] In this situation, the abdomen and pelvis should be scanned carefully to exclude a mass compressing the spermatic vein on the involved

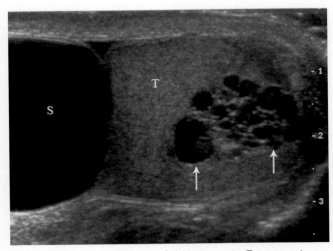

**Figure 17-34** Tubular ectasia of the rete testis. Transverse image of testis (*T*) shows multiple, small cystic areas in rete testes (*arrows*) characteristic of tubular ectasia. Note large cystic mass, consistent with a spermatocele (*S*) adjacent to testis.

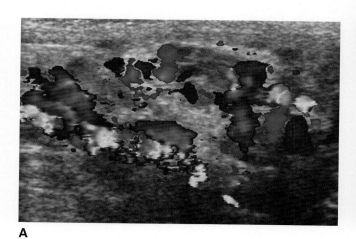

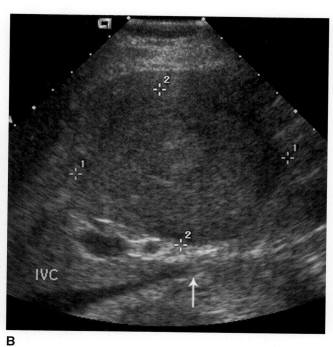

**A**    **B**

**Figure 17-35** Secondary varicocele. **A:** Longitudinal color Doppler image of the spermatic cord with secondary varicocele resulting from abdominal mass. **B:** Longitudinal image of right upper abdomen with hypoechoic hepatocellular carcinoma (*calipers*) compressing the inferior vena cava (*arrow*) causing secondary varicocele.

side.[2,9,11,14] In older men, the detection of a varicocele that cannot be decompressed, on either the right or left side, should prompt the investigation for a retroperitoneal mass.[2] Secondary varicocele and thrombosis of the pampiniform plexus may also occur in the "nutcracker phenomenon," in which the superior mesenteric artery compresses the left renal vein, resulting in stasis and thrombosis.[2,10,11]

Intratesticular varicocele is a rare phenomenon characterized by dilatation of intratesticular veins in the subcapsular location or around the mediastinum testis[2,11] (Fig. 17-36A,B). Most cases are associated with an ipsilateral extratesticular varicocele, suggesting a common pathogenesis.[2,11] Testicular pain is the most common clinical presentation.[2,11] The sonographic findings are similar to those of a pampiniform plexus varicocele.

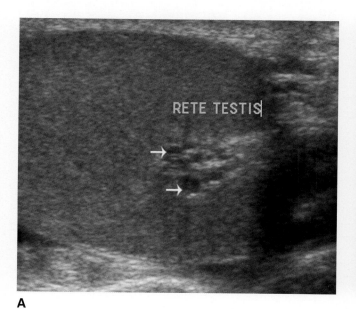

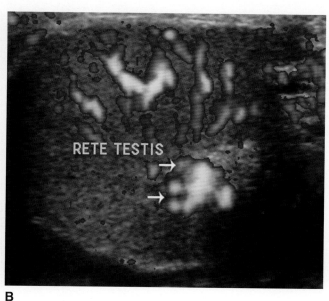

**A**    **B**

**Figure 17-36** Intratesticular varicocele. **A:** Transverse image of the testis with dilated vessels (*arrows*) in rete testis. **B:** Transverse image of testis with power Doppler to confirm intratesticular varicocele (*arrows*) adjacent to rete testis.

Clinical signs of varicocele, in addition to the scrotal mass, may include infertility and an abnormally warm scrotum. Sonographically, the appearance of varicoceles consists of multiple hypoechoic, serpiginous, tubular structures of varying sizes, measuring greater than 2 mm in diameter with the patient in the supine position, present superior, posterior, or lateral to the testis[2,9,14] (Fig. 17-37A,B). When large, a varicocele can extend inferior to the testis[2,13] (Fig. 17-37C). Occasionally, low-level internal echoes can be detected in the varices secondary to slow flow.[13] Color flow imaging has an detection accuracy approaching 100%. Color Doppler confirms the presence of varices when increased flow is visualized within these prominent veins during the Valsalva maneuver.[2,9,11,13,14,17]

## Scrotal Hernia

Scrotal hernias are inguinal hernias that descend into the scrotum. An inguinal hernia is a protrusion of peritoneal contents, usually containing omentum or bowel, through a patent processus vaginalis, the canal that connects the peritoneal cavity to the tunica vaginalis.[2,7,13,17,21] There are two types of inguinal hernias, direct and indirect, which are classified by their relationship to the inferior epigastric artery (IEA).[7,10,13] Direct inguinal hernias

are located medial to the IEA, more common in adults, and occur when abdominal contents herniate through a weak point in the fascia of the abdominal wall and extend into the inguinal canal.[7,10] Indirect inguinal hernias are located lateral to the IEA and are more common in children. The latter is associated with a patent processus vaginalis, which allows abdominal contents to exit through the internal inguinal ring, extending into the inguinal canal and scrotum.[7,10]

Clinical examination can diagnose most scrotal hernias. The clinical sign of scrotal hernia is a persistent or intermittent scrotal mass; the patient may have abdominal pain and there may be blood in the stool. In some cases, a hernia may present as a hard, nonreducible mass, indistinguishable from a primary scrotal mass.[10]

The sonographic appearance of an inguinal hernia depends on the contents. Hernias containing bowel are easier to diagnose than those containing only omentum.[10] Fluid- or air-filled loops of bowel with peristalsis in the scrotum or inguinal canal are diagnostic of a bowel hernia[7,10] (Fig. 17-38A,B) Herniated omentum is seen as a diffusely echogenic paratesticular mass that corresponds to omental fat[2,7,10] (Fig. 17-38C). Strangulated bowel, which is more common with indirect hernias, appears as fluid or air-filled loops of bowel within

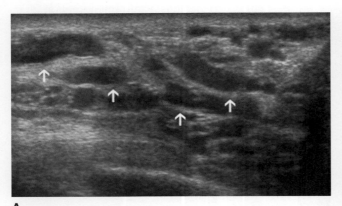

**A**

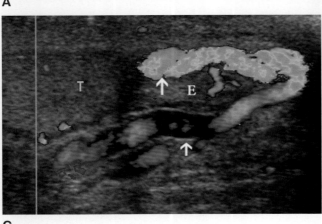

**C**

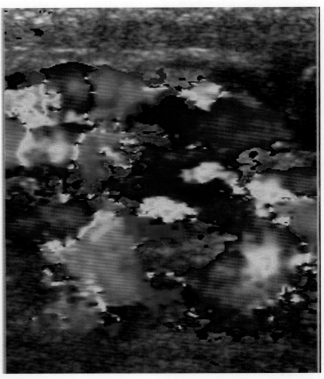

**B**

**Figure 17-37** Varicocele. **A:** Longitudinal image of scrotal varices shows multiple, dilated, hypoechoic tubular structures (*arrows*) along the spermatic cord. **B:** Longitudinal color Doppler image of scrotum with large varicocele in the spermatic cord. **C:** Longitudinal color Doppler image of testis (*T*) with varicocele (*arrows*) adjacent to epididymal tail (*E*).

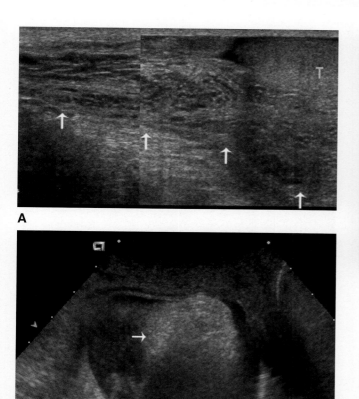

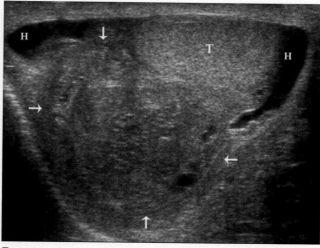

**Figure 17-38** Scrotal hernia. **A:** Longitudinal image of the inguinal canal shows herniated bowel (*arrows*) extending into the scrotal sac. Testis (*T*). **B:** Transverse image of testis (*T*) shows herniated bowel (*arrows*) in the scrotal sac. Hydrocele (*H*). **C:** Transverse image of herniated omentum (*arrow*) in the scrotal sac with shadowing from air. Note small hydrocele in the scrotum.

the herniated sac without peristalsis.[2] Hyperemia of the scrotal soft tissue and bowel wall are associated findings.[2,7] Extratesticular masses such as multiloculated hydrocele and hematocele with fibrous septations may mimic fluid-filled segments of bowel.

## Scrotal Abscess

A scrotal abscess is most often a complication of untreated epididymo-orchitis. Less frequently, a scrotal abscess develops in patients with debilitating underlying disease such as diabetes, human immunodeficiency virus infection, cancer, or alcoholism.[10,30] The clinical presentation is usually a painful, swollen scrotum. There is an association with Fournier gangrene, also known as idiopathic gangrene of the scrotum, which is a potentially life-threatening necrotizing infection occurring in men over 50 years of age. Fournier gangrene is caused by a mixed bacterial infections, most commonly *E. coli*, streptococci, proteus, and enterococci, which spread along well-defined fascial planes.[30] Sonographically, a scrotal abscess appears as a complex fluid collection with irregular borders and hyperemia around the periphery (Fig. 17-39A,B). Gas may be present, causing echogenic shadowing with ring down

artifact[10,30] (Fig. 17-39C). Scrotal wall thickening with hyperemia, in conjunction with a history of immunosuppressive conditions warrants consideration for the diagnosis of Fournier gangrene[2,30] (Fig. 17-39D).

## Scrotal Hematoma

Scrotal hematomas may be intratesticular or involve the extratesticular soft tissues such as the scrotal wall, tunica vaginalis, and epididymis. Both are usually associated with a history of trauma.[2,18] Hematomas are usually focal but may also be multiple or diffuse. In extratesticular hematoma, blood collects beneath the tunica dartos and tunica vaginalis.[24] In intratesticular hematoma, the blood is contained within the scrotum itself. In both conditions, the scrotum is swollen, painful, and sometimes discolored.

The sonographic appearance of scrotal hematomas varies with size and duration. Acute hematomas present as avascular hyperechoic areas compared with adjacent testicular parenchyma. As the hemorrhage ages, the hematoma appears hypoechoic or complex with cystic components.[2,12,18] Hematomas of the scrotal wall may appear as focal thickening of the wall or as fluid collections within the wall.[2,18]

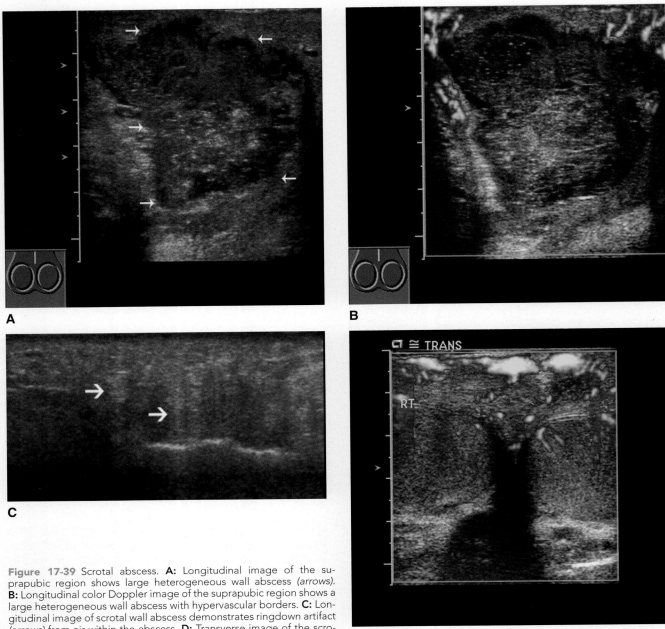

**Figure 17-39** Scrotal abscess. **A:** Longitudinal image of the suprapubic region shows large heterogeneous wall abscess *(arrows).* **B:** Longitudinal color Doppler image of the suprapubic region shows a large heterogeneous wall abscess with hypervascular borders. **C:** Longitudinal image of scrotal wall abscess demonstrates ringdown artifact *(arrows)* from air within the abscess. **D:** Transverse image of the scrotum shows scrotal wall thickening and hyperemia.

Intratesticular hematomas are less common than extratesticular hematomas and may be associated with testicular rupture. Disease processes that can mimic intratesticular hematoma include focal orchitis, testicular infarct, and testicular neoplasm.[2] With focal intratesticular and extratesticular hematomas, color Doppler will show normal perfusion to the testis and peritesticular tissues, with focal areas of absent vascularity.[2]

## Hematocele

A hematocele is an accumulation of blood between the parietal and visceral layers of the tunica vaginalis and generally is the result of trauma, surgery, tumor, or torsion.[10,18] A hematocele may be either acute or chronic.[9,10,12,18] The sonographic appearance of a hematocele is a complex heterogeneous collection within the tunica vaginalis[2,12,14,18] (Fig. 17-40A). Acute hematoceles are usually more echogenic.[2,12] Sonography of chronic hematoceles demonstrate a complex heterogeneous collection with thick septations, debris, scrotal wall thickening, and occasionally focal mural calcifications[2,10] (Fig. 17-40B). Hematoceles, like hydroceles, often exert a mass effect, distorting the contour of the testis.[10] Chronic hematoceles may be difficult to distinguish from chronic hydroceles and pyoceles.[2]

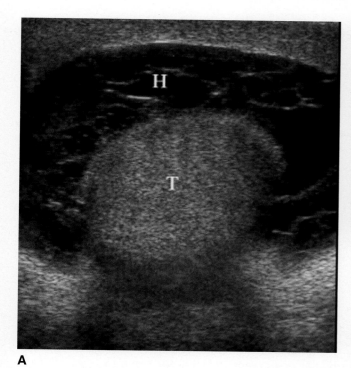

**A**

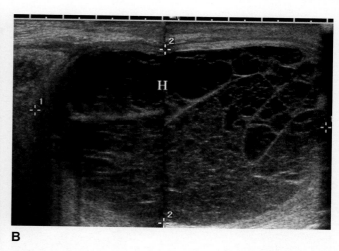

**B**

Figure 17-40 Hematocele. **A:** Transverse image of the scrotum with septated posttraumatic hematocele (*H*). Testis (*T*). **B:** Transverse image of the scrotum shows large hematocele (*H*) containing multiple septations.

## Pyocele

The clinical signs of pyoceles may mimic those of infection and inflammation, with hemiscrotal swelling and pain.[9] Following trauma, iatrogenic contamination, or rupture of a testicular abscess, pus fills the potential space between the parietal and visceral layers of the tunica vaginalis.[24] Sonographic findings of a pyocele include a thick hemiscrotal wall, echogenic fluid collections with septations, and occasionally focal mural calcifications.[9,14,24]

## Granulomatous Disease

Granulomatous disease of the testis and epididymis results from retrograde spread of tuberculosis from the prostate, seminal vesicles, and kidneys or from hematogenous spread. Tuberculosis (TB) infection of the scrotum is rare and occurs in 7% of patients infected with tuberculosis.[20,22] The prevalence of TB has been increasing over the past decade, due to the number of people with HIV and the development of drug resistant strains of *Mycobacterium tuberculosis*.[20] The genitourinary system is the most common affected extrapulmonary site for tuberculosis.[20] The peak incidence of granulomatous disease in the scrotum occurs in men aged 20 to 50 years.[22] Patients present with painful or painless swelling of the scrotum.[22] The epididymis is affected first, causing isolated epididymitis, which in later stages can then spread to the adjacent testes. Isolated testicular infection is rare.[22] TB epididymo-orchitis involvement maybe either unilateral or bilateral.[20]

Sonographically, the epididymis is either diffusely enlarged or nodular and enlarged.[20,22] The gray scale sonographic appearance of nontuberculous epididymitis

is more likely to be homogeneous, whereas TB epididymitis is usually heterogeneous or nodular.[20] Hypervascularity is present with acute bacterial epididymitis, whereas focal linear or spotty blood flow signals may be seen in the peripheral zone of tuberculous epididymitis.[22] Sonographic findings in tuberculous orchitis are similar to those in tuberculous epididymitis.[22] Other associated sonographic findings include scrotal wall thickening, hydrocele, intrascrotal extratesticular calcifications, and scrotal abscess[10,20,22] Focal lesions in granulomatous disease of the testis may mimic a primary testicular mass.[20,22]

Sarcoidosis is a noninfectious, chronic granulomatous disease that affects the genital tract. Intrascrotal sarcoidosis is rare and has been reported in the testes and epididymis. The epididymis is more commonly affected.[10,22] Epididymal sarcoidosis occurs more often in African Americans. It is often asymptomatic, but as the epididymis becomes enlarged, patients may present with a scrotal mass or pain. Testicular granulomas may also be present.[10] The sonographic appearance of intrascrotal sarcoidosis is an enlarged heterogeneous epididymis, with hypoechoic nodules in the epididymis and/or testis.[10,22]

## Tunica Albuginea Cyst

Cysts of the tunica albuginea are uncommon.[33] The etiology of tunica albuginea cysts is unknown, but these cysts are believed to be mesothelial in origin.[13,33] Clinically, tunica albuginea cysts may present as a painless scrotal lump. Tunica cysts are generally seen in men in the fifth and sixth decades.[11,33]

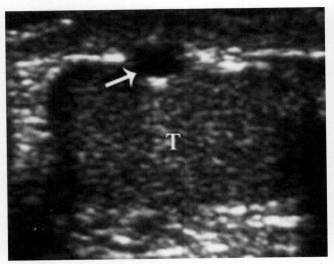

**Figure 17-41** Tunica albuginea cyst. Longitudinal image of testis (*T*) shows anechoic tunica albuginea cyst (*arrow*).

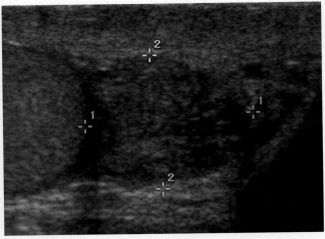

**Figure 17-43** Sperm granuloma. Longitudinal image of enlarged epididymal tail (*calipers*) demonstrates well-defined heterogeneous mass (sperm granuloma) in a postvasectomy patient.

Sonographically, tunica albuginea cysts appear as well-circumscribed anechoic areas measuring 2 to 5 mm in size, which meets all the characteristics of a simple cyst[13,14] (Fig. 17-41). The cysts are small and may be single, multiple, unilocular, multilocular, or septate.[11,33] They are generally located in the anterior and lateral aspects of the testis.[14,33] Tunica albuginea cysts can invaginate into the testicular parenchyma and simulate an intratesticular cystic lesion.[33]

### Simple Intratesticular Cysts

A simple testicular cyst is an incidental finding during routine sonography examination. They appear in approximately 10% of the male population over the age of 40.[11,13,14,17] Simple testicular cysts are asymptomatic and sonographically appear as well-circumscribed anechoic areas in the testis with smooth walls and posterior acoustic enhancement[11,13,14] (Fig. 17-42). Testicular cysts range in size from 2 mm to 2 cm.[14,17] They can be located anywhere within the testis, but are commonly located adjacent to the mediastinum testis.[9,14,17] Suspected causes include trauma, surgery, and prior inflammation.[13] Simple intratesticular cysts are commonly associated with extratesticular spermatoceles.[14]

### Sperm Granuloma

Following trauma, vasectomy, or infection, sperm may extravasate into the surrounding tissues and produce necrosis, resulting in granulomatous formation.[22] Sperm granulomas occur in up to 40% of patients postvasectomy, but only 3% of these patients experience pain.[22] Such granulomas are often found in asymptomatic men, but can present as painful nodules. Sonographically, these lesions appear as well-defined solid hypoechoic or heterogeneous masses located anywhere in the ductal system (Fig. 17-43). They most commonly occur at the cut ends of the vas deferens and can be multiple.[10,11] With improved resolution, echogenic foci noted in sperm granulomas are felt to be secondary to sperm mobility or motion of debris caused by sound waves.[22] Chronic sperm granulomas may contain calcification.[11]

## NEOPLASMS OF THE SCROTUM

### EXTRATESTICULAR NEOPLASMS

Extratesticular scrotal neoplasms are rare and usually involve the epididymis. The vast majority of these masses are benign.[11,23] Only 3% of solid extratesticular masses are malignant.[10]

### Benign Neoplasms

The most common extratesticular neoplasm is the benign adenomatoid tumor. It represents 30% of all

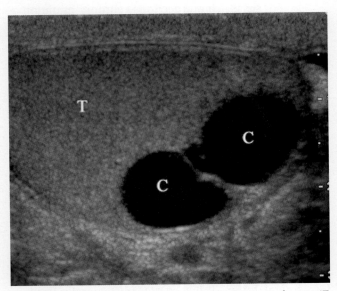

**Figure 17-42** Intratesticular cyst. Longitudinal image of testis (*T*) containing anechoic intratesticular cysts (*C*).

extratesticular benign lesions.[10,11,23,34] These tumors are generally located within the epididymal tail but can occur throughout the epididymis, testis, testicular tunica, and spermatic cord.[10,11,23,34] Adenomatoid tumors usually present as a painless mass or incidental finding. They can occur at any age but are most commonly found in patients aged 20 to 50 years.[11,34]

Sonography of an adenomatoid tumor demonstrates a well-circumscribed solid mass with variable echogenicity compared with the adjacent testis[10,22,23] (Fig. 17-44). With color Doppler, there is minimal flow within and in the periphery of the tumor.[14,23] Their appearance is indistinguishable from other benign tumors such as spermatic granulomas, leiomyomas, fibromas, and lipomas of the spermatic cord.[9,23,34]

Leiomyomas are the second most common primary benign neoplasm of the epididymis. They represent 6% of epididymal tumors reported in a review of the American literature.[22] Generally, asymptomatic, leiomyomas are small, slow-growing painless, firm, intrascrotal extratesticular masses ranging from 1 to 4 cm, which commonly manifest in the fifth decade. Leiomyomas frequently involve the tail of the epididymis and are usually unilateral.[22] An associated hydrocele is seen in 50% of cases.

The sonographic appearance of an epididymal leiomyoma is a well-circumscribed, homogenous, solid mass with variable echogenicity with or without cystic spaces.[14,22] On color Doppler evaluation, there is minimal flow within the mass.[22,23]

Lipomas are the most common extratesticular neoplasm that involve the spermatic cord.[14] The sonographic appearance of a lipoma is a circumscribed, homogeneous, hypoechoic to hyperechoic structure that alters its shape with transducer compression.[10,24] The echogenicity of lipomas varies depending on the ratio of fat cells to interstitial tissue.[24]

## Malignant Neoplasms

Among the malignant tumors involving the epididymis and spermatic cord, rhabdomyosarcomas are the most common, representing 6% of all non–germ cell intrascrotal tumors.[9,24] They occur predominantly in children and adolescents.[24] Other mesenchymal sarcomas arising in the paratesticular soft tissues include leiomyosarcoma, liposarcomas, fibrosarcoma, and malignant mesenchymoma. These malignant tumors most commonly occur in the spermatic cord and in patients more than 40 years of age.[24] Of note, 30% of spermatic cord tumors are malignant.

The sonographic appearance of a leiomyosarcoma, fibrosarcoma, or liposarcoma is a solid, ill-defined, inhomogeneous, disorganized mass with echogenic and anechoic areas representing necrosis.[24] The sonographic appearance of a rhabdomyosarcoma is a circumscribed, unilateral, hypoechoic lesion without a capsule measuring 1 to 2 cm in size.[9,24]

Poorly defined borders characterize invasive malignant tumors of the epididymis. With advancing tumor growth, the epididymis and testicular parenchyma maybe distorted with loss of border delineation.[24]

## INTRATESTICULAR NEOPLASMS

The vast majority of testicular neoplasms are of germ cell origin.[3,8,15,17] As a general rule, all intratesticular masses should be considered malignant until proven otherwise.[11,21]

## Benign Neoplasms

Approximately 4% of testicular tumors are non–germ cell tumors.[13] Leydig cell tumors, also referred to as *gonadal stromal tumors*, are the most common non–germ cell neoplasm of the testis.[11,13] Although considered in the benign group, 10% to 15% of Leydig cell tumors are in fact malignant.[3,11,35] Leydig cell tumors comprise between 1% and 3% of all testicular neoplasms.[3,14] They generally occur in men between the ages of 20 and 50 years.[3,11,35] Clinical features of Leydig cell tumors may include endocrine imbalance, impotence, decreased libido, and gynecomastia.[3,11,24,36]

Sertoli cell mesenchymal tumors account for less than 1% of all testicular tumors.[11,14] The most common clinical presentation is a painless testicular mass. Feminization with gynecomastia may occur, especially with malignant Sertoli cell tumors or those with the large cell calcifying variant type.[11] Sertoli cell tumors may occur in undescended testes and in patients with feminization, Klinefelter syndrome, and Peutz-Jeghers syndrome.[11,36]

The benign Leydig and Sertoli cell tumors are usually small, less than 1 cm, well-circumscribed masses.[3]

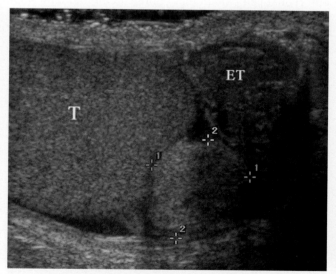

**Figure 17-44** Adenomatoid tumor. Longitudinal image of testis (*T*) and epididymal tail (*ET*) demonstrates a well-circumscribed, hyperechoic solid mass in the tail of the epididymis characteristic of an adenomatoid tumor (*calipers*).

Leydig cell tumors demonstrate prominent peripheral flow by color and power Doppler.[3] The malignant forms of these neoplasms are larger (>5 cm) and have less well-defined borders.[3,14,24] Sonographically, these lesions appear as a solid testicular mass. The echogenicity of the mass varies, but it is usually hypoechoic relative to normal parenchyma.[3,11]

An epidermoid cyst is a benign teratoma with only ectodermal components and squamous metaplasia of the surface mesothelium of the testis.[14] Epidermoid cysts are rare and only account for 1% to 2% of all testicular neoplasms; they generally develop between the ages of 20 and 40 years.[3,37] Reported cases have only occurred in Caucasian and Asian individuals. There is a slightly higher prevalence in the right testis.[37] Epidermoid cysts are usually asymptomatic and present as a painless scrotal mass. Sonographically, these lesions appear as a sharply circumscribed encapsulated mass with variable echogenicity.[14] The lesion can contain a hypoechogenic concentric ring surrounding an echogenic center, with or without a hyperechogenic rim, commonly called a "bull's-eye" or "target" appearance. Alternatively, it can contain alternating hypoechoic and hyperechoic concentric rings demonstrating an "onion ring" appearance.[14,37] Epidermoid cysts are avascular masses.[3,14]

Adenomatoid tumors and leiomyomas are rare benign intratesticular tumors.[9,11,34] The sonographic appearance is the same as their extratesticular manifestations.

Testicular microlithiasis, also referred to as intratubular testicular calcification, is rare. The condition has been associated with a number of other diseases including infertility, cryptorchidism, male pseudohermaphroditism, Down syndrome, testicular torsion, Klinefelter syndrome, intratubular germ cell neoplasia, and granulomatous disease.[11,13,14,36,38] Testicular microlithiasis (TM) is an uncommon condition seen in 1% to 2% of patients referred for scrotal sonography.[11] It is postulated that testicular microlithiasis is due to defective Sertoli cell phagocytosis of degenerating tubular cells, which calcify within the seminiferous tubules.[11,38] TM is defined as multiple intratubular calcifications, within a multilayered envelope containing organelles and vesicles surrounded by stratified collagen diffusely scattered throughout the testicular parenchyma.[14] Bilateral involvement is common. Microlithiasis may be classified as limited if the presence is less than five echogenic foci per transducer field.[11,38] TM has been associated with testicular neoplasms in 18% to 75% of cases, with the largest series reporting a frequency of 40%.[3,13,36] One recent study showed a 21.6-fold increased relative risk for carcinoma in patients who have testicular microlithiasis.[3,36] Because of these high associations and risks, annual follow up sonography exams are recommended for several years after diagnosis.[3,13,39]

The sonographic findings are multiple 1 to 3 mm hyperechoic foci without posterior shadowing, disseminated throughout the testis[3,38] (Fig. 17-45A,B). Patterns of microlithiasis can vary, with cluster calcifications centrally and in the periphery. Color and power Doppler are useful to evaluate if concomitant masses are present.[14]

## Malignant Neoplasms

Approximately 65% to 94% of patients with testicular neoplasms present with a painless unilateral scrotal mass, hardness of the testis, or diffuse testicular enlargement.[11] Ten percent of patients with testicular cancer present with acute pain and fever, usually initially diagnosed as epididymo-orchitis, whereas 10% are detected incidentally following trauma.[3,11,15,18,36] Seminomas and testicular lymphomas may cause orchitis secondary to obstruction of the seminiferous tubules.[3]

Malignant germ cell tumors constitute 90% to 95% of intratesticular primary neoplasms.[11,13–15,17,21,36] Germ cell tumors are divided into seminomas and nonseminomatous tumors. Nonseminomatous tumor include embryonal cell carcinoma, choriocarcinoma, teratoma, yolk sac tumor, and mixed germ cell tumors.[3,11,17,36] Mixed germ cell tumors constitute approximately 40%

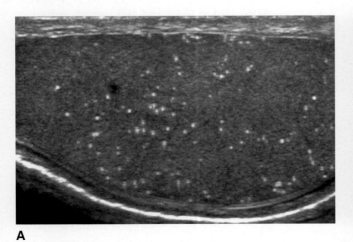

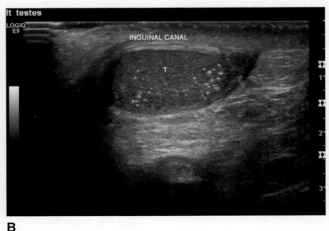

**A**    **B**

**Figure 17-45** Microlithiasis. **A:** Longitudinal image of testis containing multiple, nonshadowing, hyperechoic foci. **B:** Longitudinal image of an undescended testis located within the inguinal canal. The testis contains multiple, nonshadowing, hyperechoic foci consistent with microlithiasis.

to 60% percent of all nonseminomatous germ cell tumors.[3] The most common mixed germ cell neoplasm is a teratocarcinoma. These lesions contain both teratoma and embryonal cells and represent the most frequent tumor after seminoma.[3,17]

Testicular cancer accounts for 1% to 2% of all malignant neoplasms in men.[36] Testicular cancer is the fifth most frequent cause of death in men aged 15 to 34 years.[3,11,14,36] Primary cancer of the testis is 4.5 times more common in Caucasians than African Americans.[3] Patients with cryptorchidism have a 2.5 to 8 times increased risk for developing testicular cancer. Testicular microlithiasis is another risk factor for developing testicular cancer.[3,13,36]

Malignant testicular tumors are predominantly hypoechoic (92%) compared with the normal testicular parenchyma.[17] Less often, neoplasms can appear as focal hyperechoic masses, diffuse infiltration of the testicular parenchyma, or mixed lesions containing focal anechoic areas with echogenic foci.[24] If the tumor is confined to the tunica albuginea, the testis usually retains its oval shape.[24] Invasion of the testis and epididymis distorts the smooth contour of the testis, making it irregular and lumpy.[24] Sonography is sensitive in detecting malignant testicular masses, but it cannot distinguish the cell type of malignancies[24] (Fig.17-46A). Color and power Doppler imaging demonstrates increased vascularity in the vast majority of malignant

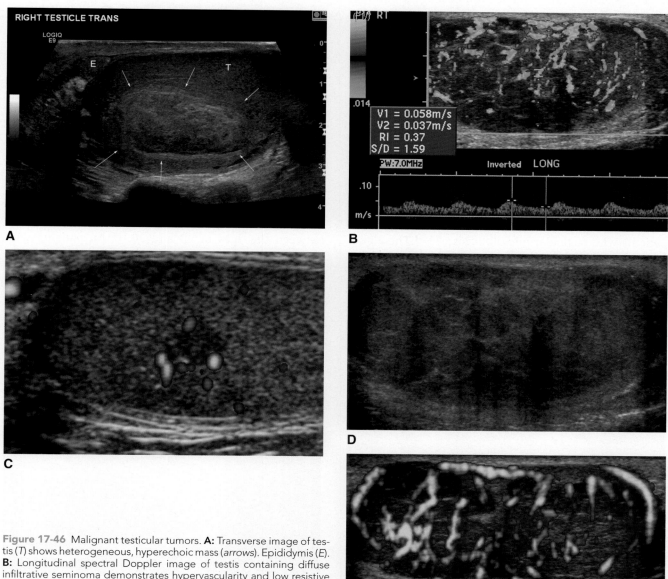

**Figure 17-46** Malignant testicular tumors. **A:** Transverse image of testis (T) shows heterogeneous, hyperechoic mass (arrows). Epididymis (E). **B:** Longitudinal spectral Doppler image of testis containing diffuse infiltrative seminoma demonstrates hypervascularity and low resistive index. **C:** Longitudinal power Doppler image of testis shows a small, focal, hypoechoic mass consistent with a seminoma. **D:** Longitudinal image of testis shows hypoechoic, multinodular, infiltrative seminoma. **E:** Longitudinal power Doppler image of testis demonstrates hypervascularity with infiltrative seminoma.

tumors greater than 1.6 cm and hypovascularity in 86% of those smaller than 1.6 cm.[3,14] The presence of hyper-vascularity is not specific for the diagnosis of malignancy.[3,13] Infiltrating or diffuse malignancies, such as leukemia and lymphoma, exhibit increased vascularity similar to diffuse orchitis, making differentiation difficult[2,3,14] (Fig. 17-46B). In the latter situation, clinical history is extremely important.

Other processes that may mimic testicular neoplasms include abscess, hematoma, focal orchitis, testicular infarcts, and torsion.[2,3] Features that tend to distinguish neoplasms from inflammatory processes are the scrotal wall thickness, the character of the epididymis, the margination of the lesions, and the surrounding testicular parenchyma.[24] In general, with malignancy, the thickness of the scrotal wall is normal as is the epididymis, except in rare cases when the neoplasm invades the epididymis.[24] Inflammatory processes usually show thickening of the scrotal wall and fluid.[24] In 5% to 10% of patients with a testicular neoplasm, there is concurrent epididymitis or epididymo-orchitis; reactive hydroceles accompany 10% of testicular neoplasms.[24]

### Seminoma

Seminoma is the most common pure germ cell tumor and accounts for 40% to 50% of primary testicular neoplasms.[3,11,14,17,36] Seminoma occurs most often in the fourth and fifth decades of life with an average patient age of 40.5 years.[1,15] Approximately 8% to 30% of patients with seminoma have a history of undescended testes. Seminomas are commonly found in patients with testicular microlithiasis.[3,11,13,14] The alpha-fetoprotein (AFP) level is always normal in patients with pure seminomas.[3] If a patient has an elevated AFP with seminoma histology, the tumor is treated as a non-seminomatous lesion.[3]

The sonographic appearance of seminoma is characteristically described as a well-defined homogeneous hypoechoic mass without calcification or tunica invasion[3,8,11,14] (Fig. 17-46C). Ten percent of seminomas present with small cystic areas, which correspond to dilated rete testis caused by tumor related occlusion and liquefaction necrosis. A diffuse echotexture change may be seen secondary to seminomatous infiltration[3,36] (Fig. 17-46D,E). Color and power Doppler is useful in demonstrating hypervascularity in tumors greater than 1.6 cm.[3,14]

### Embryonal Cell Carcinoma

Embryonal cell carcinoma occurs primarily in men between ages 25 and 35 and is the second most common histologic type of testicular tumor after seminoma.[3,36] Often invading the tunica albuginea and distorting the testicular contour, embryonal cell carcinoma is the most aggressive of the primary scrotal malignancies.[3,14,36] The AFP and beta-human chorionic gonadotropin (beta-hCG) levels are elevated in approximately 70% of patients.[3] The sonographic appearance of embryonal cell carcinoma is a hypoechoic mass, more heterogeneous than seminoma, with poorly defined borders[3] (Fig. 17-47A,B). Cystic components are seen in one-third of tumors, and calcifications or echogenic foci are not uncommon.[3,11]

### Choriocarcinoma

Choriocarcinoma is a rare germ cell tumor that is seen in less than 1% patients and usually occurs in men between the ages of 20 and 30.[3,36] All patients with choriocarcinoma have elevated levels of beta-hCG.[3] Choriocarcinoma has the worst prognosis of any of the germ cell tumors, with death occurring within 1 year of diagnosis.[3] Sonographically, choriocarcinomas are

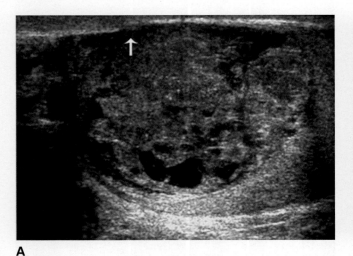

**A**

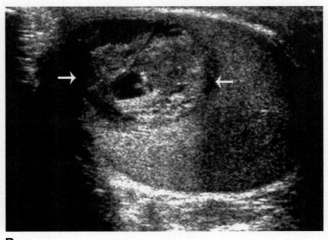

**B**

**Figure 17-47** Embryonal cell carcinoma. **A:** Longitudinal image of testis containing large, heterogeneous mass with cystic areas diagnosed as an embryonal cell carcinoma. Note irregular margins with tunica albuginea invasion (*arrow*). **B:** Longitudinal image of testis demonstrates well-defined heterogeneous mass (*arrows*) with cystic areas characteristic of embryonal cell carcinoma.

heterogeneous and show extensive hemorrhagic necrosis in the central portion of the tumor with a mixed echo pattern.[3,11,14,36]

### Teratoma

Teratoma is the second most common testicular neoplasm in children, usually occurring in children less than 4 years of age. Pure teratomas are rare in adults, but teratomatous components occur in more than 50% of all adult cases of mixed germ cell tumors. Serum AFP (38%) and beta-hCG levels are sometimes elevated.[3] Teratomas contain multiple tissue elements such as bone, soft tissue, skin, and cartilage.[3,11] Sonographically, teratomas tend to be very large and markedly inhomogeneous masses. Cystic components are common. Echogenic foci may or may not shadow, which may represent calcification, cartilage, immature bone, and fibrous tissue.[3,11,36]

### Yolk Sac Tumor

Yolk sac tumors account for 80% of childhood testicular tumors, with most cases occurring before 2 years of age. They exclusively produce AFP in more than 90% of cases. Pure yolk sac tumors are rare in adults, and the presence of any yolk sac tumor element in an adult mixed cell tumor indicates a poor prognosis.[3,36] The sonographic appearance of a yolk sac tumor is nonspecific. These tumors are usually inhomogeneous and may contain echogenic foci secondary to hemorrhage or hypoechoic areas due to necrosis.[3]

### Mixed Neoplasms

Mixed germ cell tumors constitute about 40% to 60% of all germ cell tumors.[3,11] Teratocarcinoma is the most common mixed germ cell neoplasm. It contains both teratoma and embryonal carcinoma cells.[3] Teratocarcinomas are aggressive and the largest of all testicular tumors.[3] The sonographic appearance of teratocarcinoma is a heterogeneous mass with echogenic foci and cystic areas secondary to hemorrhage and calcifications.

### Metastases to the Testis

Metastasis to the testes is rare, with an incidence of 0.68%.[3] The most common primary tumors to metastasize to the testis are prostate (35%), lung (19%), malignant melanoma (9%), colon (9%), and kidney (7%).[3] Metastases are more common than germ cell tumors in patients >50 years and are often multiple and bilateral.[24]

### Lymphoma

Lymphoma accounts for 5% of all testicular neoplasms and is the most common bilateral testicular tumor. Testicular lymphoma occurs in less than 1% of patients who have lymphoma and typically occurs in older patients. Lymphoma is the most common testicular neoplasm in men over 60 years of age.[3,11] Testicular

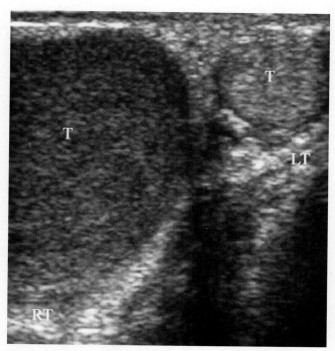

**Figure 17-48** Lymphoma. Transverse image of the scrotum shows diffusely enlarged, hypoechoic right testis with lymphomatous invasion. Left testis is normal.

lymphoma is aggressive and infiltrates the epididymis and spermatic cord in 50% of cases.[3] The scrotal skin is rarely involved. The sonographic appearance of testicular lymphoma is nonspecific.[24] One or both testis may be enlarged, and there are areas of decreased echogenicity, either diffuse or focal as lymphomatous tissue replaces normal testicular tissue[3,11] (Fig. 17-48). Testicular enlargement is bilateral in 50% of cases and is commonly associated with scrotal discoloration.[24] Color Doppler imaging shows increased vascularity regardless of tumor size. Hypervascularity seen with diffuse infiltration may resemble inflammation.[3,11]

### Leukemia

Primary testicular leukemia is rare. The testes may be a sanctuary organ for hematologic malignancies such as leukemia and lymphoma. The blood–testis barrier prevents the accumulation of chemotherapeutic drugs within the testes.[3]

Leukemic infiltration of the testis has been found in 40% to 65% of acute leukemia patients at autopsy and in 20% to 35% of patients with chronic leukemia.[3,13] Leukemia diffusely infiltrates the testis, resulting in hypoechoic enlargement.[3] Unilateral enlargement of the testis with normal echogenicity can also be seen. Focal, sharply marginated, anechoic masses with through transmission and occasional low-level internal echoes have been described in patients with chronic lymphocytic leukemia.[3,11] Color Doppler imaging of leukemic infiltration demonstrates hypervascularity within the affected testis, similar to lymphoma.[3,11]

## *Critical Thinking Questions*

1. A 13-year-old patient presents with an enlarged, painful left scrotum. Sonographic findings demonstrate a diffusely hypoechoic, enlarged left testis with decreased vascular flow. What is the likely diagnosis and treatment option?

2. A 32-year-old patient arrives for a scrotal sonography with a diagnosis of infertility. What pathology will you be looking for and what techniques will help you make the diagnosis?

3. During a physical examination, the pediatrician is only able to palpate a single testicle within the scrotum. He has ordered a scrotal sonogram to evaluate for undescended testis. Where will you begin your evaluation for the undescended testis and what is the clinical significance of a diagnosis of undescended testis?

4. A 28-year-old patient presents with painless unilateral right testicular enlargement. Sonographic findings include a hypoechoic intratesticular mass. What is the likely diagnosis and what lab values could aid in the diagnosis?

5. A 21-year-old patient presents with an enlarged and painful right scrotum. Sonographic findings include an enlarged, heterogeneous epididymal head with increased color Doppler flow when compared to the left epididymis. A fluid collection surrounds the right epididymis and testicle. What is the likely diagnosis and treatment?

## SUMMARY

- Gray scale sonography with color, power, and spectral Doppler is the imaging modality of choice for evaluating patients with acute scrotal pain, undescended testis, or a scrotal mass.

- Sonographic evaluation is always performed bilaterally and should include images of both testes simultaneously to compare size, echogenicity, and vascular perfusion.

- The scrotal sac contains the testis, epididymis (head, body, and tail), and scrotal portion of the spermatic cord.

- The head of the epididymis lies superolaterally to the testes and measures 10 to 12 mm in anteroposterior diameter.

- The tunica vaginalis is a peritoneal sac composed of two layers that surround the testis and epididymis. Serous fluid can accumulate between the layers to form a hydrocele.

- The adult testis is homogeneous with medium level echoes and measures 3 to 5 cm in length and 2 to 3 cm in the transverse and anteroposterior diameters.

- Undescended testes are located within the inguinal canal in 80% of cases. Scrotal malignancy, torsion, and infertility are all associated with undiagnosed undescended testes.

- Causes of acute painful scrotum include epididymitis, epididymo-orchitis, orchitis, testicular torsion, trauma, torsion of the testicular appendices, scrotal wall inflammation, and incarcerated inguinal hernia.

- Color, power, and spectral Doppler are used to distinguish infectious processes from testicular torsion.

- The majority of extratesticular masses are benign, whereas intratesticular masses are considered malignant until proven otherwise.

- Varicoceles are dilated (>2 mm) veins of the pampiniform plexus located superior and posterior to the testis. They usually occur on the left side and are associated with infertility.

- Leydig cell and Sertoli cell tumors are typically benign intrascrotal tumors and are rare.

- Testicular microlithiasis is diagnosed sonographically when more than five echogenic, nonshadowing foci are seen per transducer field. Microlithiasis is associated with an increased risk of scrotal malignancy.

- Malignant germ cell tumors constitute 90% to 95% of primary intratesticular malignancies and are divided into seminomas and nonseminomatous tumors.

- Seminomas are the most common primary testicular cancer.

- Nonseminomatous germ cell tumors include embryonal cell carcinoma, choriocarcinoma, teratoma, yolk sac tumor, and mixed germ cell tumors.

- Knowledge of normal and abnormal scrotal anatomy, consistent use of a methodical protocol, and application of the appropriate imaging parameters are essential for reliable diagnosis of scrotal disease.

## ACKNOWLEDGMENTS

The authors extend their sincere thanks to Michael Martinucci, MD, for providing assistance with the cases and manuscript, and William Pillor, RDMS, for his assistance in acquiring images.

### REFERENCES

1. Thinyu S, Muttarak M. Role of sonography in diagnosis of scrotal disorders: a review of 110 cases. *Biomed Imaging Interv J.* 2009;5:1–10.
2. Turgut AT, Bhatt S, Dogra VS. Acute painful scrotum. *Ultrasound Clin.* 2008;3:93–107.
3. Kocakoc E, Bhatt S, Dogra VS. Ultrasound evaluation of testicular neoplasms. *Ultrasound Clin.* 2007;2:27–44.

5. Dogra VS, Bhatt S, Rubens DJ. Sonographic evaluation of testicular torsion. *Ultrasound Clin.* 2006;1:55–66.

6. Townsend RR, Cheeawai RA, Lee RS. Color evaluation of testicular torsion with subsequent blood flow after immediate manual detorsion. *JDMS.* 1999;15:197–202.

7. Kim W, Rosen MA, Langer JE, et al. US MR imaging correlation in pathologic conditions of the scrotum. *Radiographics.* 2007;27:1239–1253.

8. Chen P, John S. Ultrasound of the acute scrotum. *Applied Radiology.* 2006;8–17.

9. Owen CA, Winter T. Color Doppler imaging of the scrotum. *JDMS.* 2006;22:221–230.

10. Leonhardt WC. Scrotum. In: Berman MC, Kawamura DM, Craig M, et al., eds. *Diagnostic Medical Sonography.* 2nd ed. Philadelphia, PA: Lippincott; 1997:719–766.

11. Woodward PJ, Schwab CM, Sesterhenn IA. Extratesticular scrotal masses: radiologic-pathologic correlation. *Radiographics.* 2003;23:215–240.

12. Gorman B, Carroll BA. The scrotum. In: Rumack CM, Wilson S, Charboneau JW, et al., eds. *Diagnostic Ultrasound.* 3rd ed. St Louis, MO: Elsevier Mosby; 2005:849–848.

13. Bhatt S, Ghazale H, Dogra VS. Sonographic evaluation of scrotal and penile trauma. *Ultrasound Clin.* 2007;2:45–56.

14. Dogra VS, Gottlieb RH, Oka M, et al. Sonography of the scrotum. *Radiology.* 2003;227:18–36.

15. Paunipagar BK. Scrotal sonography. In: Ahuja AT, ed. *Diagnostic Imaging Ultrasound.* Salt Lake City, UT: Amirsys; 2007:1020–1044.

16. Mihmanli I, Kantarci F. Sonography of scrotal abnormalities in adults: an update. *Diagn Interven Radiol.* 2009;5:64–73.

17. Horstman WG, Middleton WD, Melson GL. Scrotal inflammatory disease: color Doppler US findings. *Radiology.* 1991;179:55–59.

18. Pearl MS, Hill MC. Ultrasound of the scrotum. *Semin Ultrasound CT MRI.* 2007;28:225–248.

19. Deurdulian C, Mittelstaedt CA, Chong WK, et al. US of acute scrotal trauma: optimal technique, imaging findings, and management. *Radiographics.* 2007;27:357–369.

20. Ledwidge ME, Lee DK, Winter, TC, et al. Sonographic diagnosis of superior hemispheric testicular infarction. *AJR Am J Roentgenol.* 2002;179:775–776.

21. Muttarak M, ChiangMai WN, Lojanapiwat B. Tuberculosis of the genitourinary tract: imaging features with pathological correlation. *Singapore Med J.* 2005;46:568–575.

22. Futterer JJ, Heijmink S, Spermon JR, et al. Imaging the male reproductive tract: current trends and future directions. *Radiol Clin North Am.* 2008;46:133–147.

23. Lee JC, Bhatt S, Dogra VS. Imaging of the epididymis. *Ultrasound Quarterly.* 2008;24:3–16.

24. Smart JM, Jackson EK, Redman SL, et al. Ultrasound findings of masses of the paratesticular space. *Clinical Radiology.* 2008;63:929–938.

25. Hricak H, Hamm B, Kim B, eds. *Imaging of the Scrotum.* New York, NY: Raven Press; 1995.

26. Feld R, Middleton WD. Recent advances in sonography of the testes and scrotum. *Radiol Clin North Am.* 1992;30:1033–1049.

27. Horstman WG, Middleton WD, Melson GL, et al. Color Doppler US of the scrotum. *Radiographics.* 1991;11: 941–957.

28. Middleton WD, Bell MW. Analysis of intratesticular arterial anatomy with emphasis on transmediastinal arteries. *Radiology.* 1993;189:157–160.

29. Vijayaraghavan SB. Sonographic differential diagnosis of acute scrotum: real-time Whirlpool Sign, a key sign of torsion. *J Ultrasound Med.* 2006;25:563–574.

30. Burks DD, Markey BJ, Burkhard TK, et al. Suspected testicular torsion and ischemia: evaluation with color Doppler sonography. *Radiology.* 1990;175:815–821.

31. Stengel JW, Remer EM. Sonography of the scrotum: case based review. *AJR Am J Roentgenol.* 2008;190: S35-S41.

32. Safriel Y, Cohen HL, Torrisi J. Ultrasound imaging of scrotal wall thickening and its significance in the diagnosis of Fournier's Gangrene in older men. *JDMS.* 2000;16:29–33.

33. Sista AK, Filly RA. Color sonography in evaluation of spermatoceles. *J Ultrasound Med.* 2008;27:141–143.

34. Martinez-Berganza MT, Sarria L, Cozcolluela R, et al. Cysts of the tunica albuginea: sonographic appearance. *AJR Am J Roentgenol.* 1998;170:183–185.

35. Leonhardt WC, Gooding GAW. Sonography of intrascrotal adenomatoid tumor. *Urology.* 1992;39:90–92.

36. Singh V, Srivastava H. Leydig cell tumor of the testis—a case report. *Indian J Urol.* 2004;20:166.

37. Woodward PF, Sohaey R, O'Donoghue MF, et al. Tumors and tumor-like lesions of the testis: radiologic-pathologic correlation. *Radiographics.* 2002;22:189–216.

38. Loya AG, Said JW, Grant EG. Epidermoid cyst of the testis: radiologic-pathologic correlation. *Radiographics.* 2004;24: S243–S246.

39. Cast JEI, Nelson WM, Early AS, et al. Testicular microlithiasis: prevalence and tumor risk in a population referred for scrotal sonography. *AJR Am J Roentgenol.* 2000;175:1703–1706.

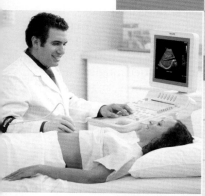

# 18 The Musculoskeletal System

Patrick R. Meyers

## OBJECTIVES

Differentiate when sonography of the musculoskeletal system is the primary versus the adjunct imaging modality in terms of sensitivity, specificity, and accuracy.

List the indications for a musculoskeletal sonography examination for the axial skeletal joints.

Demonstrate transducer position and manipulation techniques to obtain long axis and short axis orthogonal planes.

Identify the normal anatomic location and sonographic signature for tendons, bursa, nerves, ligaments, bone, fibrocartilage and articulate cartilage, fat, and muscle.

Demonstrate the sonographic evaluation for the shoulder, elbow, wrist, knee, ankle, and plantar fascia.

Differentiate between normal and abnormal appearance related to common trauma and acute or chronic pathologic conditions.

## KEY TERMS

amphiarthrosis | anisotropy | articular or hyaline cartilage | diarthrosis | fibrocartilage | orthogonal | paratendinitis | paratenon | pes anserine | retinaculum | synovial | volar flexion

## GLOSSARY

**anisotropy** properties vary with direction. In muscle, the speed of sound differs when propagating parallel to the fibers than when propagating at right angles to the fibers. It is opposite of isotropic

**enthesis** site of attachment of a muscle or ligament to bone

**muscle structure**

    **fascicle** a small bundle or cluster of fibers

    **epimysium** connective tissue surrounds entire muscle

**perimysium** connective tissue surrounds a fascicle (bundle) of muscle fiber

**endomysium** connective tissue surrounds an individual muscle fiber

**paratenon** fatty areolar tissue filling the interstices of the facial compartment in which a tendon is situated

**retinaculum** a general term for a band or band-like structure binding organs or tissue to hold them together for movement or to retain them or in place

Sonographic evaluation of the musculoskeletal (MSK) system is widely practiced by a variety of specialties throughout the world.[1-4] Sonography may be used as the primary diagnostic modality in the evaluation of acute and chronic conditions of joints, tendons, ligaments, synovium, nerves, bone, and soft tissues, as well as an excellent tool for image-guided interventional procedures. A growing body of publications promotes the value of sonography as a cost effective, nonionizing radiation, highly mobile, dynamic modality used as a diagnostic tool, and as an extension of the physical exam, with limitations.[4-11] A multitude of peer-reviewed journal articles by private and academic centers purport the accuracy and sensitivity of sonography for MSK evaluation and promote sonography as an adjunct or primary imaging modality with specificity and sensitivity approaching the gold standards of magnetic resonance imaging (MRI) and computed tomography (CT) and in some cases exceeding accuracy levels when performed by skilled sonographers.[4,7-9] In specific cases, sonography is more sensitive and accurate than standard radiography in detection of chronic and acute inflammatory processes affecting the joints. Successful evaluation of the MSK system, as in any other imaging modality, requires a thorough understanding of the anatomy being evaluated, anatomic variants, and common pathology conditions most frequently encountered as well as artifacts. This chapter on musculoskeletal sonography is not meant to be an exhaustive narrative on all potential normal and pathologic structures and conditions of the appendicular system, but a general explanation of the more commonly encountered structures and conditions and the most typical appearance.

## COMMON IMAGING TERMS AND TECHNIQUES

A description of common imaging terms is essential to provide concise direction while imaging. Evaluation of the MSK system requires the sonographer to evaluate the length and width of anatomy under examination. Although other imaging modalities reference the conventional anatomic sagittal, coronal, and transverse body planes, the references do not translate well into imaging of the MSK system. Although a few structures

in the MSK system are imaged in traditional anatomic planes, evaluation of structures is described using the terms long axis (LAX) and short axis (SAX) referring to the maximum length and maximum width of the structure respectively in orthogonal planes (Fig. 18-1A–E).

Due to histologic composition, varied angles, and challenging location of anatomic structures, manipulation of insonation angle to anatomic structure is critical. As insonation angle to structure exceeds 90 degrees, signal return to the transducer is diminished. *Anisotropy* is the change in the properties of a structure when measured or evaluated in different directions. As structures of the MSK system frequently attach and follow the contour of bone or adjacent soft tissue, congruent transducer positioning must be incorporated. Common transducer manipulation techniques implemented include "heel-toe," "rocking or toggling," transducer "translation," and "fanning or twisting" (Fig. 18-2A–E).

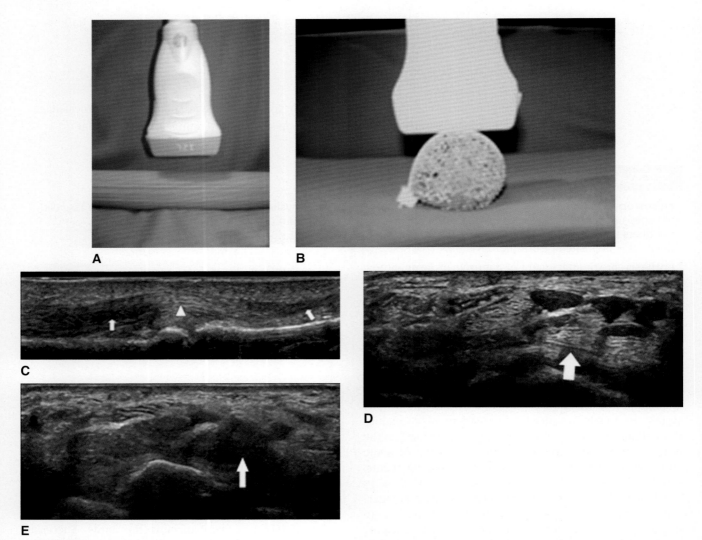

**Figure 18-1** Transducer position and image orientation. **A:** The long-axis (LAX) imaging plane of a tendon is obtained with the transducer face parallel to the tissue. **B:** The tendon is viewed on end using a short-axis (SAX) imaging plane. **C:** The sonogram in the LAX plane of the flexor tendon of the index finger displays normal tendon pattern where the insonation angle is at 90 degrees *(arrowhead)* and where anisotrophy exceeds 90 degrees *(arrows)*. **D:** The SAX projection of flexor tendons of the wrist was obtained with a 90-degree insonation angle *(arrow)*. **E:** The sound properties in the same area as **(D)** changed *(arrow)* as the transducer "toggled" off the perpendicular insonation angle.

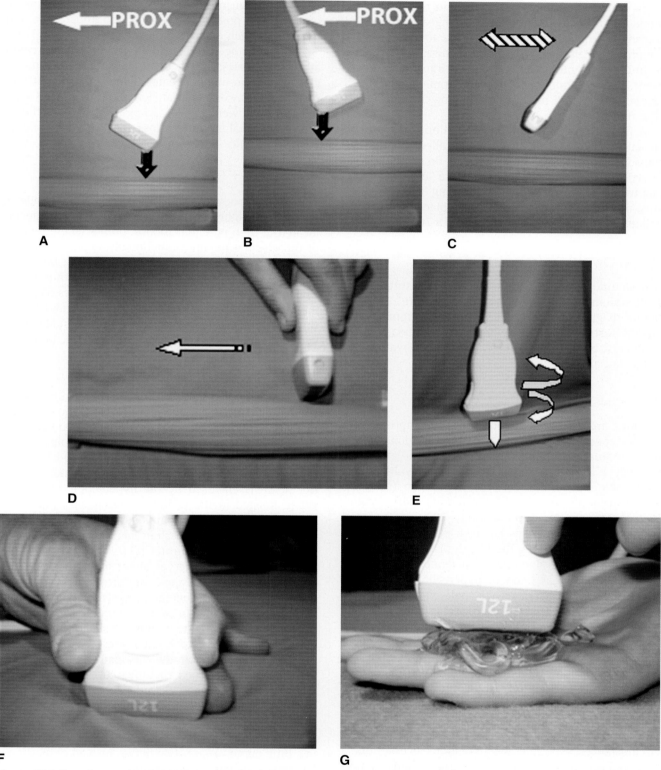

**Figure 18-2** Transducer manipulation. Examples of transducer manipulation to optimize anatomic viewing include **(A)** "heeling" the transducer in the long-axis (LAX) plane; **(B)** "toeing" the transducer in the LAX plane; **(C)** "rocking" or "toggling" the transducer in short-axis (SAX) plane; **(D)** "translation" in the SAX means moving the whole transducer while maintaining the transducer parallel to the anatomy; and **(E)** "fanning" or "twisting" *(curved arrows)* the transducer on the x-axis *(arrow)*. **F:** Tripod technique. Using three fingers to act as a tripod in holding the transducer helps prevent unintended motion. **G:** Gel pad. Using ample amounts of acoustic gel creates a pad (jelly belly) to use for "floating" the transducer. The transducer does not contact or compress the skin or soft tissue.

Typically when imaging, changes in transducer position involve small directional changes. Unintended transducer movement can occur due to the use of a coupling gel, immovable bone structures, or dynamic techniques. To minimize unintended transducer movement, it is recommended the sonographer employs a three-finger, tripod method for holding the transducer (Fig. 18-2F).

A final useful technique in evaluation of superficial structures close to the skin surface is called "floating the transducer." "Floating" the transducer on an abundance of acoustic gel allows the user to make "essential" contact with the skin surface while avoiding excessive pressure resulting in unwanted fluid displacement, vessel collapse, or tissue compression (Fig. 18-2G).

## ANATOMY

A basic understanding of the targeted structures of the MSK system and the specific echo "signature" is essential for diagnostic accuracy. The most commonly evaluated MSK structures include the tendons, bursa, nerves, ligaments, bone, fibrocartilage, articular or hyaline cartilage, fat, and muscle.

### TENDONS

Tendons are extensions of the muscle comprised of a similar specialized cellular structure. Tendons attach bone to muscle and facilitate the flexion and extension through a lever type mechanism. Primary histologic composition of tendons is type II collagen (protein), which accounts for 80% of the tendon's dry weight. Water accounts for approximately 70% of the total weight of the tendon. The collagen fibers are arranged in a linear fashion along the length of the tendon. The sonographic tissue signature of a tendon is that of a tightly bound linear band of hyperechoic strands, fibrillar pattern, interspersed with relatively hypoechoic connective tissue[12] (Fig. 18-3A,B).

In the 90-degree orthogonal SAX plane, the tendon manifests a "whisk-broom" appearance with the collagen fibers displayed as hyperechoic foci throughout the tendon distribution interspersed with hypoechoic connective tissue. The tendon throughout its length should maintain a uniform thickness except at the point where it may broaden at the enthesis, the area where the tendon mineralizes at insertion into the bone. In certain circumstances, especially where tendons lever around a bone projection or in high friction areas where tendons slip between relatively narrow spaces, a functionally active bursa produces fluid to assist in tendon slip. Tendons may have an associated bursa or fibrous sheath that further protects and assists in tendon movement. Tendons that do not have a tenosynovial lining may have a paratenon. The paratenon is a collection of loose connective tissue between the sheath and tendon, which aids in tendon movement (Fig. 18-3C,D). Tendons are often held in position by a band of fibrous tissue, retinaculum, which delimits movement (Fig. 18-3E,F).

Tendon echogenicity, as in all sonographically evaluated structures, is highly dependent on insonation angle. Insonation angles greater than 10 degrees off perpendicular may demonstrate loss of returned signal and therefore a lower level of echogenicity. The deficient returning signal produces a loss of echogenicity and the false appearance of tendon pathology.

### BURSA

The human body contains approximately 150 bursae. Bursae are highly specialized synovial lined pouches located at high-potential friction points where tendons or muscles are required functionally to slip through or around diametrically opposed structures. The bursa produces a viscous fluid that aids in tendon or muscle slip. Depending on location, the bursa may physiologically maintain anywhere from 1 to 3 mm of synovial fluid. Bursa may be indigenous or develop functionally an adventitious bursa based on friction point (Fig. 18-4A–D).

### NERVES

Nerves are divided into sensory and motor function but sonographically they have identical appearance. When imaged in the SAX, the oval or round shaped nerve has a "honeycomb" pattern with the hypoechoic, primarily circular nerve fibers (fascicles) surrounded by the hyperechoic perineuron or connective tissue. The entire nerve is enclosed by the hyperechoic epineuron. When imaged in the LAX, the "fascicular" pattern of the length of the nerve simulates a "railroad track" appearance with the hypoechoic nerve fibers divided by the hyperechoic perineuron[13] (Fig. 18-5A,B).

Normally, healthy nerves either maintain a uniform width and contour or taper from proximal origin to the distal termination. In general, nerves should not increase in diameter or change in contour from origin to termination. Nerves may divide within the sheath into smaller bundles that appear to branch. Nerves may travel in unison with their anatomic compatriots, arteries and veins, in what is termed "neurovascular bundles." Lack of specific knowledge of nerve location should not deter the user from locating a more comfortable vascular or soft tissue landmark and seek the sonographic "fascicle" nerve identifier. Confusion may rein with nerve branching, bifid nerve variant (two nerves instead of the singular nerve), or when surgical intervention has moved a nerve from its native and customary location.

### LIGAMENTS

Ligaments may be described in three ways. The reference in this chapter is to ligaments that attach bone to bone and provide stability and strength to the osseous

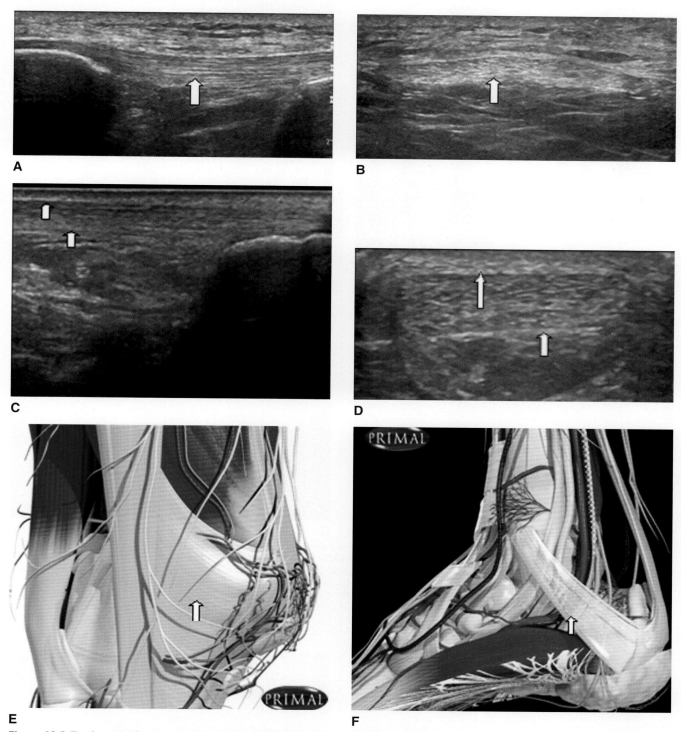

**Figure 18-3** Tendons. **A:** The sonographic signature of the tendon's longitudinal collagen fibers *(white arrow)* are visualized on the long-axis (LAX) image of the patellar tendon. **B:** On a short-axis (SAX) plane, white collagen fibers of the patellar tendon are visualized on end *(white arrow)*. Paratenon **C:** The LAX and **(D)** the SAX image planes of the Achilles tendon area visualizes the paratenon *(white arrows)*. Retinaculum **E:** The illustration of the knee presents the lateral patellar retinaculum *(arrow)*. **F:** On the medial ankle, the medial flexor retinaculum *(arrow)* can be identified. (Images courtesy of Primal Pictures, Ltd., London, England.)

structures and may serve a secondary function in load distribution. They are composed of type I collagen arranged in a basket-weave type pattern. Ligaments may be a narrow cord-like structure like the lateral collateral (fibulocollateral) ligament or a broader thin pattern like the medial collateral (tibiocollateral) ligament. When insonated, ligaments at a 90-degree angle, ligaments are visualized with a similar tissue signature to that of the tendon. However, due to nature of ligamentous attachment angles and sound absorbing osseous

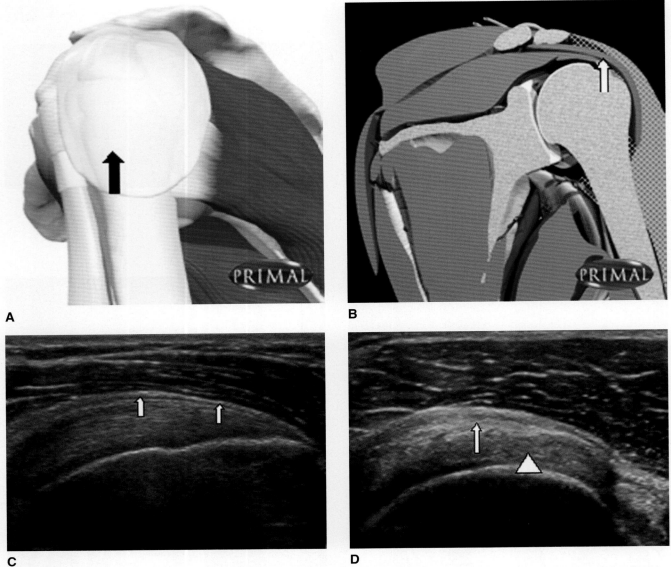

**Figure 18-4** Bursa. **A:** The large subacromial-subdeltoid (SASD) bursa *(black arrow)* can be identified on the illustration of the shoulder. **B:** A sagittal plane through the shoulder illustrates the location of the SASD bursa between the deltoid muscle and the tendons of the rotator cuff *(white arrow)*. **C:** The long-axis sonogram shows the supraspinatus tendon with normal physiologic fluid in the SASD bursa *(white arrows)*. **D:** The short-axis image shows the SASD inferior to the deltoid muscle *(white arrow)* and superior to the supraspinatus tendon *(white arrowhead)*. (Images **A** and **B** courtesy of Primal Pictures, Ltd., London, England.)

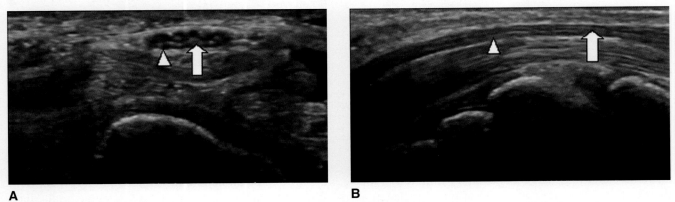

**Figure 18-5** Nerves. **A:** On the short-axis plane of the median nerve proximal to the carpal tunnel, one can see the hyperechoic perineuron *(white arrow)* surrounding the hypoechoic nerve bundles producing a "honeycomb" appearance. The hyperechoic epineuron surround the entire nerve group *(white arrowhead)*. **B:** On the long-axis plane of the median nerve, the "railroad" or track "fascicular" appearance is seen along with both the perineuron *(white arrow)* and the epineuron *(white arrowhead)*.

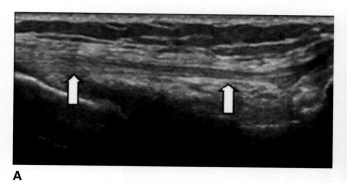

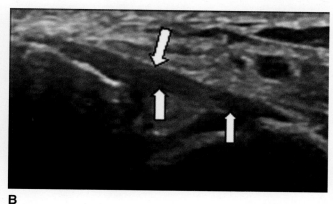

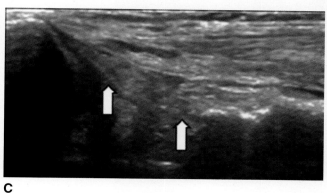

**Figure 18-6** Ligaments. Varied sonographic appearances are seen with ligaments. **A:** The lateral collateral ligament of the knee demonstrates both hyperechoic and hypoechoic components (*white arrows*). **B:** The anterior tibiofibular ligament (ATFL) appears hypoechoic due to the insonation angle (*white arrows*). **C:** The deltoid ligament of the medial ankle appears echogenic (*white arrows*).

structures, ligaments present an imaging challenge due to the lack of a 90 degree acoustic insonation angle. For the latter reason, it may be necessary to evaluate ligaments with a compact linear transducer in conjunction with an acoustic gel pad or "belly of jelly" on the structure (Fig. 18-6A–C).

## BONE

Bone is a living and ever changing mark. Although sonographic evaluation of mineralized bone defies penetration beyond the outer bone structure, acoustic changes in articular (as part of an articulation) and nonarticular bone surfaces may lead the sonographer to focus on soft tissue evaluation in the area adjacent to or at the attachment site of a tendon or ligament. Furthermore, on occasion, attention to changes in bone surface contour may reveal an occult fracture (Fig. 18-7A–C).

Sonography is, by no means, the primary imaging modality in suspected bone pathology but can be a useful tool, in the properly trained hands, for evaluation of areas inconclusive on X-ray or when superior imaging modalities are unavailable or more difficult to use.[14–16]

When nonarticular bone surfaces are insonated at 90 degrees, it manifests a thin, less than 2 mm, echogenic returned signal and reverberation artifact distal to the bone surface. This ring down artifact should not be mistaken for imaging of the internal structure of the bone. Off-axis imaging of bone may produce an irregular, thickened surface (Fig. 18-7D). Changes in the linear appearance of the bone may be a result of occult processes; however, when imaged at the site of an injury, tendon insertion, or ligament insertion, care should be taken in the evaluation of soft tissue in the vicinity of changes to the bone.

## FIBROCARTILAGE AND ARTICULAR CARTILAGE

Fibrocartilage is a matrix of strands of white type I collagen found in the meniscus and intervertebral disk spaces and it functions much like a shock absorber. Type I collagen is the most abundant collagen in the body and is present in scars, tendons, muscle, and bone. It is found in the menisci of the knee, pubic symphysis, and acromioclavicular joint. The sonographic appearance is that of medium echogenicity, homogeneous with minimal changes throughout its structure. Articular or hyaline cartilage lies at the terminal ends of bone in any joint. Comprised of 70% to 80% water by weight, this glistening, white cartilage is closely adhered to and follows the contour of the bone surface. The articular cartilage is segmented into four zones with the deepest zone mineralized and serves as the transition area between bone and cartilage. Its structure allows for minimal friction and excellent weight distribution and compression. In conjunction with the synovial membrane, articular cartilage controls the articular joint fluid level. Sonographically, normal articular cartilage appears as a hypoechoic, noncompressible layer in contact with the bone surface (Fig. 18-8A,B).

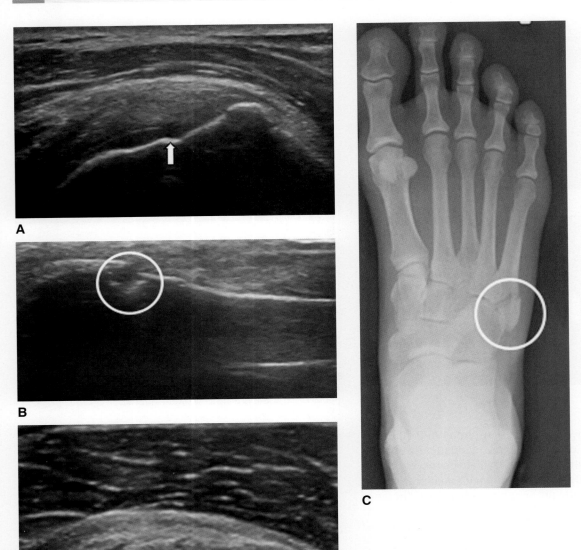

**Figure 18-7** Bone. **A:** The image demonstrates a smooth outline of the humerus with the ideal 90-degree insonation angle *(white arrow).* **B:** The sonogram illustrates the sonographic appearance of a disruption of the bone surface with fracture *(white circle)* and the same patient's radiograph **(C)** of the fifth metatarsal base shows the area of fracture *(white circle).* **D:** The sonogram of the humeral head shows a sharp bone surface *(curved arrow)* compared to an artificially thickened bone surface due to curved surface and off angle insonation *(straight arrow).*

## FAT

Fat presenting without pathology has a unique sonographic signature depending on where it is located. Subcutaneous fat may have a heterogeneous appearance with hypoechoic fat lobules interspaced with connective tissue. Fat pads, commonly found on articular surfaces where bone contacts adjacent bone surfaces are, supplied with nerve endings and capillaries and surrounded by a fibrous capsule are more hyperechoic and homogeneous in appearance (Fig. 18-9A,B).

## MUSCLE

The body is composed of three distinct types of muscles: (1) smooth (involuntary) muscle, (2) cardiac striated muscle, and (3) skeletal striated muscle. Muscle tissue has the unique ability to contract and extend. Sonographic evaluation of the MSK system primarily encounters the skeletal striated muscle. The skeletal muscle cells or muscle fibers are covered by endomysium, a delicate connective tissue membrane.[17] Groups of muscle fibers make up the fascicles, which

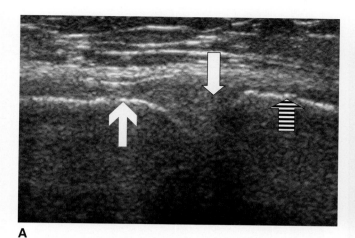
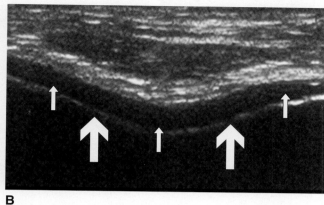

**A**    **B**

**Figure 18-8** Fibrocartilage and articular cartilage. **A:** This long-axis image demonstrates the sonographic appearance of the femoral condyle (*1st white arrow*), fibrocartilage meniscus (*solid arrow*), and tibial condyle (*striped arrow*). **B:** On a short-axis plane, the hypoechoic articular cartilage is seen in the trochlea of the knee (*white arrows*) and bone line (*2nd & 4th white arrows*).

are surrounded and bound together by an envelope of connective tissue known as perimysium or fibroadipose septa.[17,18] The entire muscle group is surrounded by a fibrous epimysium.[17,18] The connective tissues (endomysium, perimysium, and epimysium) are continuous with the fibrous structure that attach muscles to bones or other structures and may be continuous with fibrous tissue that extends from the muscle as a cord-like tendon.[17] The tendons of some muscles form flat sheets, or aponeuroses, that anchor the muscle to the skeleton. A more in-depth discussion to include the six muscle shapes (parallel, convergent, pennate, fusiform, spiral, and circular), attachment of muscles (proximal origin and distal insertion), and muscle actions are beyond the scope of this chapter.

With a 90-degree incident angle, connective tissue appears as echogenic bands, a LAX plane of large muscle fibers appear homogeneous with multiple parallel echoes, and a SAX plane may appear homogeneous with punctate echoes. The sonographer can observe changes in echogenicity with muscle contraction and extension with transducer compression (Fig. 18-10A,B).

## SHOULDER

### JOINT ANATOMY

The shoulder is one of the most common joints evaluated by sonography and requires an understanding of the hard tissue (bone). The major bone anatomy comprising the shoulder girdle is the humerus, scapula, clavicle, and these bone extensions: the spine of the scapula, coracoid process, and acromion process (Fig. 18-11). To successfully evaluate the shoulder, the sonographer should learn the primary attachments of the critical soft tissue structures evaluated in the rotator cuff (Table 18-1).

The shoulder is always a complete study unless contraindicated by patient condition or for interventional procedures. The sonographer may reference Table 18-2 and the useful guidelines it references published by the American

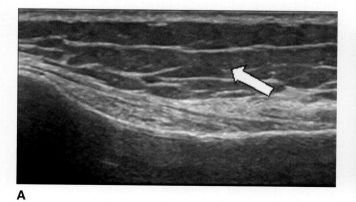
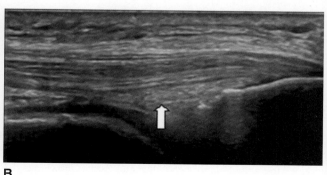

**A**    **B**

**Figure 18-9** Fat. **A:** Without pathology, fat appears heterogeneous with hypoechoic fat lobules interspaced with connective tissue as seen in the long-axis image of subcutaneous fat in the anterior lateral margin of the lower leg (*large white arrow*). **B:** In the knee area, a suprapatellar fat pad (*white arrow*) appears hyperechoic and homogeneous.

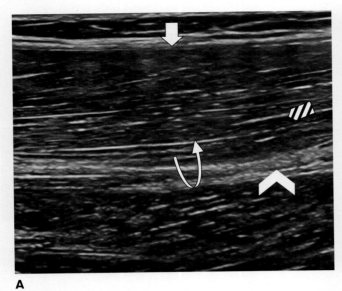

**A**

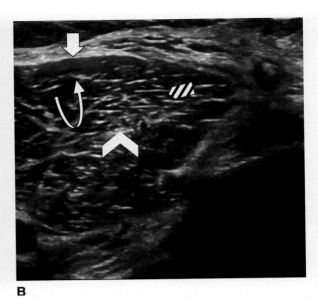

**B**

**Figure 18-10** Muscle. **A:** The long-axis image displays the epimysium *(short solid arrow)*, hypoechoic muscle fascicle *(striped arrow)*, perimysium *(curved arrow)*, and the aponeuroses *(white cursor)*. **B:** The short-axis image shows the epimysium *(short white arrow)*, muscle fascicle *(striped arrow)*, the perimysium *(curved arrow)*, and the aponeurosis *(white cursor)*.

Institute of Ultrasound in Medicine (AIUM) and the European Society of Skeletal Radiology (ESSR)[19,20] (Table 18-2).

## Biceps Tendon

The biceps tendon is a strong supinator and flexor of the arm and elbow. From the biceps muscle of the upper arm, the extra-articular component of the tendon continues proximally between the lesser tubercle and the greater tubercle of the humeral head. The tendon has two heads, "bi," with distinct insertion points. The proximal attachment of the long head of the biceps tendon is on the supraglenoid tubercle in conjunction with the glenoid labrum. The long head has an intra-articular portion that lies superior to the humeral head and is contiguous with the glenohumeral joint and it is an important factor in pathology of the glenohumeral joint and rotator cuff. The short head of the biceps tendon attaches to the lateral and posterior surface of the coracoid process. The proximal insertion of the long head of the biceps tendon cannot be imaged sonographically due to overlying bone (Fig. 18-12A–F).

## Subscapularis Tendon

The subscapularis muscle is an abductor and medial rotator of the humerus and arises from the anterior scapula but is not a single muscle. Its "weave-like" structure from four muscles contributes four to six tendon structures that insert on the capsule, lesser tuberosity, and humeral shaft (Fig. 18-13A–E).

Fibers contributed from the superior aspect of subscapularis tendon form the transhumeral ligament (retinaculum) that restrains translation of the biceps tendon in the bicipital groove. Injury to the transhumeral ligament may result in biceps tendon subluxation or dislocation. The subscapularis tendon has a broad insertion; therefore, interrogation of the tendon requires evaluation from superior to inferior. Due to the medial and posterior location of the tendon in the neutral arm position, the tendon is evaluated in external rotation. A dynamic internal rotation with the arm adducted across the chest and an external rotation is used in evaluation for coracohumeral impingement with a measurement of 12.2 mm ± 2.5 mm (range, 7.8 to 17 mm) in asymptomatic patients and 7.9 mm ± 1.4 mm (range 5.9 to 9.6 mm) in symptomatic patients.[21] The area measured is between the medial aspect of the lesser tuberosity and lateral surface of the coracoid. Close attention is paid to the subacromial-subdeltoid and infracoracoid bursa for impingement (Fig. 18-13F,G).

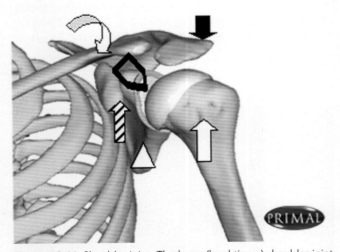

**Figure 18-11** Shoulder joint. The bone (hard tissue) shoulder joint includes the scapula *(arrowhead)*, humerus *(white arrow)*, glenoid fossa of scapula *(black white cursor)*, acromion process of scapula *(black arrow)*, coracoid process of scapula *(striped arrow)*, and the clavicle *(curved white arrow)*. (Image courtesy of Primal Pictures, Ltd., London, England.)

| TABLE | 18-1 |
|---|---|

## Shoulder Protocol[19,20]

| Soft Tissue Structures | Plane | Recommend | Optional/Per Need | Dynamic Clip |
|---|---|---|---|---|
| Biceps tendon | SAX, LAX | Y | N | SAX, LAX |
| Subscapularis tendon | SAX, LAX | Y | N | SAX & LAX |
| Subscapularis tendon | Coracohumeral impingement | Y | Y | LAX |
| Acromioclavicular joint | SAX, LAX | Y | N | SAX cross thorax adduction |
| Supraspinatus tendon: crass position | SAX, LAX | Y | N | SAX, LAX |
| Supraspinatus tendon: modified | SAX, LAX | Y | N | SAX, LAX |
| Supraspinatus-subacromial impingement | LAX | Y | Y | LAX: 20–30 degrees abduction–extension |
| Infraspinatus tendon | LAX | Y | N | LAX |
| Teres minor | LAX, SAX | N | Y | SAX, LAX |
| Spinoglenoid notch/groove | LAX | Y | Y | LAX internal/external rotation |
| Glenoid labrum-posterior superior | SAX | Y | Y | SAX internal/external rotation |
| Suprascapular notch | LAX | N | Y | SAX as needed |
| Supraspinatus/infraspinatus muscle | LAX | Y | Y | Panoramic image/split screen |

LAX, long axis; SAX, short axis.

## Acromioclavicular Joint

The acromioclavicular (AC) joint is an amphiarthrosis, synovial joint formed at the distal clavicle and medial aspect of the acromion process of the scapula (Fig. 18-14A–C). The AC joint supports a complex ligamentous relationship with the acromion and coracoid processes (scapula) that provides stability and strength to the shoulder girdle. The supraspinatus muscle lies inferior to the joint space. The AC joint is a potential source for abnormal fluid collection to form in pathology of the supraspinatus tendon. The joint space is "wedge-shaped" from

| TABLE | 18-2 |
|---|---|

## Shoulder Tendons: Attachment and Function[19,20]

| Tendon | Proximal Attachment | Distal Attachment | Function | Nerve Supply |
|---|---|---|---|---|
| Biceps tendon | Short head-coracoid process long head-supraglenoid tubercle | Dual attachment on the radial tuberosity anterior and posterior | Supinator of the forearm, flexor of the elbow and flexor of the shoulder | Musculocutaneous nerve, C5, C6 |
| Subscapularis | Costal surface of scapula | Lesser tuberosity of the humerus, anterior surface of the humerus, and shoulder joint capsule; multiple muscles woven, provide distal tendinous projections | Adductor and rotator of the humerus | Both subscapular nerves, C5, C6, C7 |
| Supraspinatus | Muscle attachment is supraspinous fossa of the scapula and muscle fascia | Anterior and lateral facet of the greater tuberosity of the humerus | Abduction of the humerus; delimiter of shoulder movement | Suprascapular nerve, C4, C5, C6 |
| Infraspinatus | Posterior infraspinatus fossa of the scapula | Middle facet of the greater tuberosity of the humerus with fibers of the supraspinatus | Lateral rotator of the humerus | Suprascapular nerve, C4, C5, C6 |
| Teres minor | Lateral margin of the scapula | Distal facet of the great tuberosity of the humerus | Adductor and lateral rotator of humerus | Axillary nerve, C4, C5, C6 |

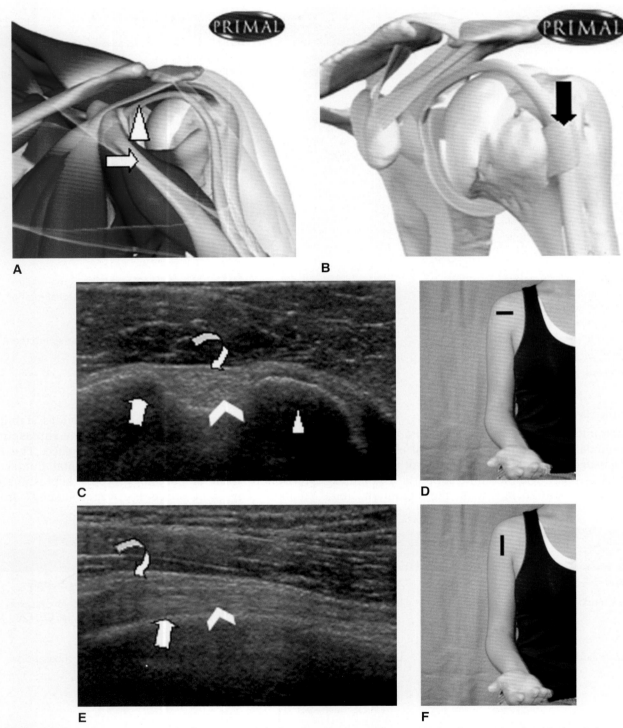

**Figure 18-12** Biceps tendon. Note on the illustrations **(A)** the long head biceps tendon insertion on the superior glenoid tubercle *(arrowhead)*, the short head insertion on coracoid process *(white arrow)*, and **(B)** the transhumeral ligament *(black arrow)*. **C:** The short-axis (SAX) sonogram demonstrates the biceps tendon *(white cursor)*, humeral head with lesser tuberosity *(white arrow)*, the greater tuberosity *(arrowhead)*, and the tendon sheath *(curved arrow)*. **D:** The photo shows the transducer position for SAX plane of biceps tendon. **E:** The long-axis (LAX) sonogram demonstrates the biceps tendon *(white cursor)*, floor of bicipital groove *(solid white arrow)*, and the tendon sheath *(curve arrow)*. **F:** The photo shows the arm and transducer position *(black rectangle)* for LAX plane of biceps tendon. (Images **A** and **B** courtesy of Primal Pictures, Ltd., London, England.)

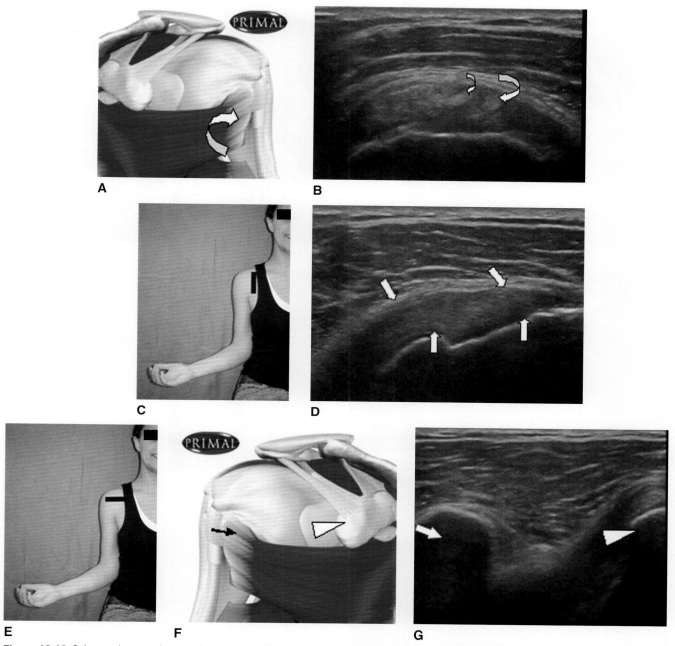

**Figure 18-13** Subscapularis tendon. **A:** The subscapularis tendon is identified on the illustration *(white curved arrow)*. **B:** The short-axis (SAX) sonogram demonstrates the distal tendon heads of subscapularis *(curved arrows)*. **C:** The photo shows the external rotation of the arm and transducer position *(black rectangle)* for the SAX plane of the subscapularis tendon. **D:** The long-axis (LAX) sonogram shows the middle third of subscapularis tendon *(solid white arrows)* at insertion. **E:** The photo shows the external rotation of the arm and the transducer position *(black rectangle)* for the LAX plane of the subscapularis tendon. **F:** The illustration of the subscapularis tendon shows the coracoid process *(white arrowhead)* and subscapularis tendon *(black arrow)*. **G:** The LAX image shows the lesser tuberosity *(white arrowhead)* and coracoid process *(white arrow)*. (Images **A** and **F** courtesy of Primal Pictures, Ltd., London, England.)

posterior to anterior with the anterior aspect wider than the posterior aspect. The space between the acromion and clavicle may support a fibrous disk. The AC joint is a commonly injured joint in lateral to medial crushing injuries and a common site for various types of arthritis and osteophytes. The AC joint is evaluated in neutral position with the arm hanging loosely by the side and in a cross-thorax maneuver with the ipsilateral hand placed on the contralateral shoulder (Fig. 18-14D).

In suspected injuries to the AC joint, the cross-thorax maneuver should be imaged during arm movement. The AC joint may close on adduction and the capsule may bulge superiorly (Fig. 18-14E). However, at no time should the acromion and clavicle abut or should the acromion sublux inferiorly.

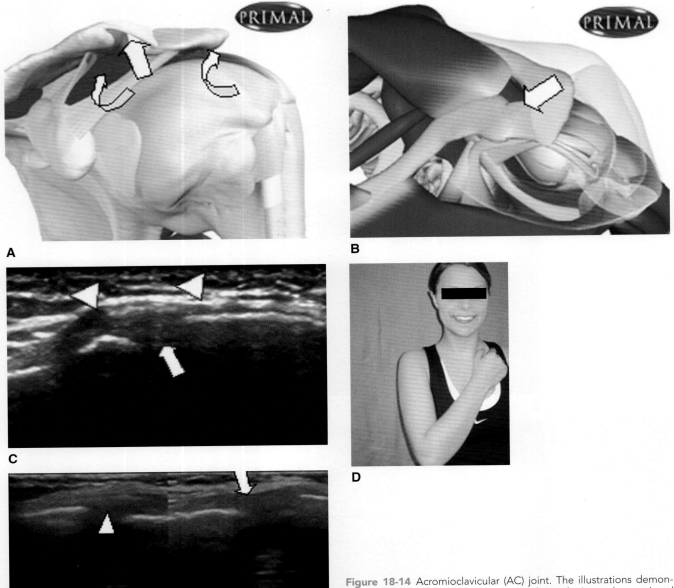

**Figure 18-14** Acromioclavicular (AC) joint. The illustrations demonstrate **(A)** the supraspinatus tendon and muscle *(curved arrows)* and AC joint *(white arrow)* and **(B)** the joint capsule *(white arrow)*. **C:** The LAX image shows the joint capsule *(white arrowheads)* and the AC joint *(white arrow)*. **D:** The photo shows the dynamic cross-thorax maneuver with the ipsilateral hand placed on the contralateral shoulder to evaluate the right AC joint. **E:** The sonogram of the AC joint in dynamic maneuver demonstrates how the joint may close *(white arrowhead)* and the capsule may bulge *(white arrow)*. (Images **A** and **B** courtesy of Primal Pictures, Ltd., London, England.)

A movement of 3 mm or less is considered within normal limits.

### Supraspinatus Tendon

The supraspinatus tendon is the distal projection of the supraspinatus muscle that attaches to the scapula in the supraspinatus fossa. The muscle assists in abduction of the humerus but has a more critical role in stabilization of the humeral head in the glenohumeral joint. In combination with the coracohumeral and superior glenohumeral ligament complex, the muscle strengthens the joint. The distal attachment of the supraspinatus tendon is on the anterior superior facet of the greater tuberosity of the humeral head. It shares a common insertion point with the more laterally positioned infraspinatus tendon with an insertion footprint of approximately 1 to 1.5 cm lateral to the rotator cuff interval (Fig. 18-15A–F).

The infraspinatus and supraspinatus fibers blend at the footprint and share a common area of insertion.

The teres minor, not frequently interrogated, shares the most lateral insertion. A critical area that must be included in the evaluation of the rotator cuff is the rotator cuff interval. Anatomically, this area defines the separation of the subscapularis tendon medially from the supraspinatus tendon laterally by the biceps tendon proximal to the bicipital groove. Insonation of this landmark is essential in differentiation of pathology of the supraspinatus from the subscapularis tendons. A small hypoechoic area, 5 mm in width, medial and lateral to

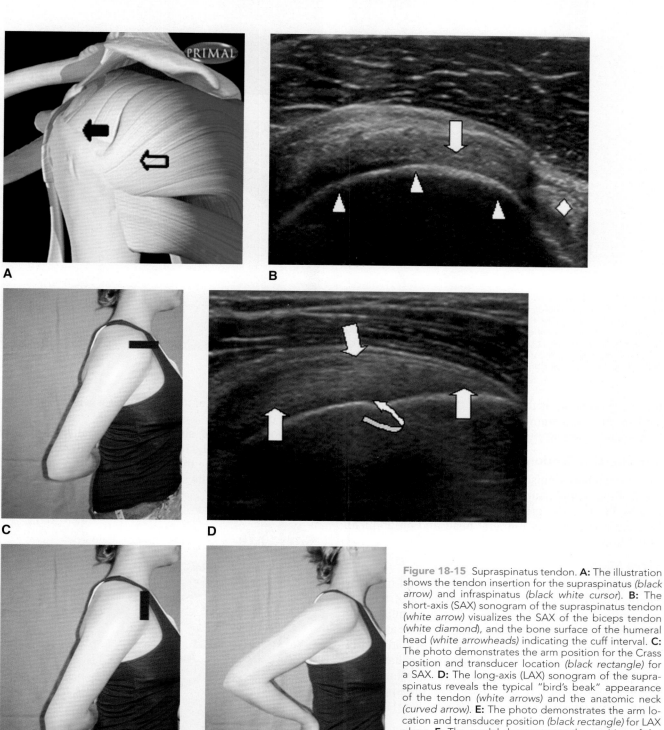

**Figure 18-15** Supraspinatus tendon. **A:** The illustration shows the tendon insertion for the supraspinatus *(black arrow)* and infraspinatus *(black white cursor)*. **B:** The short-axis (SAX) sonogram of the supraspinatus tendon *(white arrow)* visualizes the SAX of the biceps tendon *(white diamond)*, and the bone surface of the humeral head *(white arrowheads)* indicating the cuff interval. **C:** The photo demonstrates the arm position for the Crass position and transducer location *(black rectangle)* for a SAX. **D:** The long-axis (LAX) sonogram of the supraspinatus reveals the typical "bird's beak" appearance of the tendon *(white arrows)* and the anatomic neck *(curved arrow)*. **E:** The photo demonstrates the arm location and transducer position *(black rectangle)* for LAX plane. **F:** The model demonstrates the position of the arm in the modified Crass position, which is used for the LAX and SAX images of the supraspinatus. In this position, it is important that the elbow must be pushed medially. (Image **A** courtesy of Primal Pictures, Ltd., London, England.)

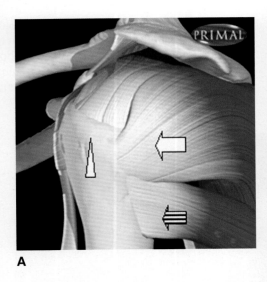

**A**

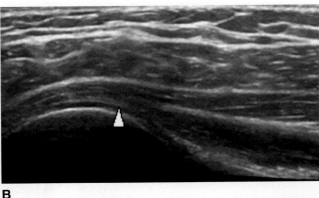

**B**

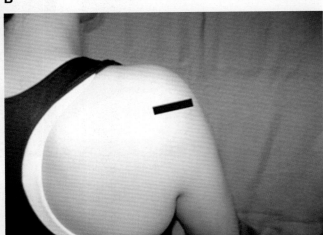

**C**

**Figure 18-16** Infraspinatus tendon. **A:** The illustration shows the location for the infraspinatus tendon *(white arrow)*, greater tuberosity *(white arrowhead)*, and the teres minor *(striped arrow)*. **B:** The infraspinatus tendon *(white arrowhead)* is seen on the long-axis (LAX) image. **C:** The photo shows the correct transducer position *(black rectangle)* for a LAX projection of the infraspinatus tendon. (Image **A** courtesy of Primal Pictures, Ltd., London, England.)

the biceps tendon at the level of the cuff interval created by the coracohumeral ligament and superior glenohumeral ligament may be mistaken for a cuff tear.

## Infraspinatus Tendon

The infraspinatus muscle arises from the infraspinatus fossa of the scapula and the distal tendon inserts on the middle facet of the greater tuberosity. It serves as an external rotator of the humeral head and an abductor of the humerus (Fig. 18-16-A–C).

## Teres Minor

Although anatomically part of the rotator cuff, the teres minor is seldom evaluated in the presence of typically encountered pathology of the cuff. The teres minor is an adductor of the humerus and provides stability to the glenohumeral joint from opposition of the deltoid and biceps brachii. It receives innervations from axillary nerve (C4, C5, C6). The tendon inserts on the lower three facets of the greater tuberosity and arises from the upper two-thirds of the lateral border of the scapula (Fig. 18-17).

## PATHOLOGY

A wide variety of pathologies can be encountered in sonography evaluation of the shoulder. In staying within the scope of this chapter, only frequently encountered

pathologies of the rotator cuff and associated anatomy will be described.

Pathology of the shoulder is generally associated with conditions of the tendons of the rotator cuff. However, shoulder pain, the primary symptom associated with evaluation of the shoulder, can be associated with

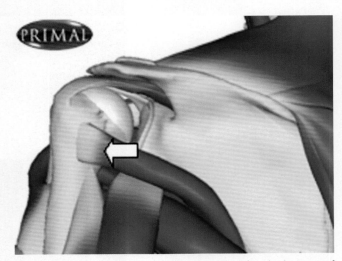

**Figure 18-17** Teres minor. The illustration identifies the location of the teres minor insertion *(white arrow)*. (Image courtesy of Primal Pictures, Ltd., London, England.)

disease of the rotator cuff, tendinopathies, and chronic and acute shoulder instability as well as neuropathies.

Sonographic evaluation of the rotator cuff can be descriptively categorized into major and minor findings that lead to accuracy and sensitivity of results[22-28] (Pathology Box 18-1). The major and minor criteria presented can be used as a guide in the presence of pathology. Although incomplete and certainly overlap exists, this categorization is provided as a useful guide. In inflammatory condition, color flow Doppler (CFD) and/or power Doppler imaging (PDI) can be used to verify abnormal flow characteristics in inflammatory conditions (Fig. 18-18). Equipment instrumentation parameters and imaging technique have substantial impact on the accuracy of Doppler imaging. Improper Doppler frequency, scale, wall filter settings, and/or excessive compressive force can alter outcomes.

The most commonly found pathologies of the tendons of the rotator cuff proper are presented in Figure 18-19. In cases of gross pathology or surgery, the typical hard and soft tissue landmarks can be altered making evaluation more difficult. Pain in the lateral deltoid area is a common finding in rotator cuff pathology.

Pain in the AC Joint can be a source of referred pain in the shoulder. A "Geyser" sign may be found in association with a tear of the supraspinatus tendon (Fig. 18-20A,B).

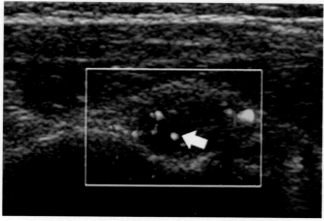

**Figure 18-18** Power Doppler. An abnormal amount of intratendinous vascularity (arrow) is identified when using power Doppler imaging on the short-axis (SAX) plane of the biceps tendon.

# ELBOW

## ANATOMY

The elbow is a medium-sized synovial, and complex hinge joint often involved in overuse injuries. Unlike the shoulder, the elbow is often a targeted evaluation based on clinical history. The primary bone structure of the elbow is the distal humerus and the proximal radius and ulna (Fig. 18-21). The soft tissue structures including tendons, muscles, and nerves will be discussed as a regional evaluation. The entire joint is synovial lined and surrounded by a fibrous capsule.

## ANTERIOR ELBOW

The anterior elbow soft tissue structures include the median nerve, distal biceps tendon, brachial artery, and brachialis muscle. Hard tissue anatomy will include the coronoid fossa, radial fossa, and the articular surfaces of the radius, ulna, and humerus. The median nerve, though seldom pathologic at this level is found adjacent to the brachial artery and biceps tendon (Fig. 18-22A).

The median nerve displays the typical "honeycomb" or "fascicular" pattern. A detailed description of the median nerve will be discussed in the section on the wrist. The two heads of the biceps tendon join separate distally and have a dual insertion on the radial tuberosity of the radius. The biceps muscle has a trifold function. It serves as a supinator of forearm, a flexor of the elbow, and, when supinated, a flexor of the shoulder. The distal insertion of the biceps tendon can be difficult to evaluate due to its insertion on the medially located radial tuberosity.

A SAX at the level of the antibrachial crease images the biceps tendons as a hyperechoic oval lateral to the brachial artery. In LAX with the arm in full extension and hypersupination with distal heeling of the transducer, the fibrillar pattern of the distal biceps tendon can be seen at the insertion (Fig. 18-22B,C).

Two recent techniques described by Smith et al.[29] using a medial approach with the arm in 90 degrees flexion and Tagliafico et al.[30] using a lateral oblique through the supinator has greatly improved the evaluation of the distal insertion integrity. With the supinator approach described by Tagliafico et al.,[30] the biceps tendon insertion is not visualized but movement of tendon signifies at least partial attachment (Fig. 18-22D–F).

The radial fossa and coronoid fossa of the distal humerus are commonly evaluated for joint effusions. The fossas contain intra-articular fat pads that can be seen resting on the bone surface at the bottom of the fossa. The fat pads provide cushioning of the radial head and coronoid process, respectively, and delimit hyperextension of the forearm (Fig. 18-22G–J).

Excessive fluid in the joint results in the fat pads being displaced anteriorly away from the bone. The articular surface of the bone is lined by hyaline cartilage on

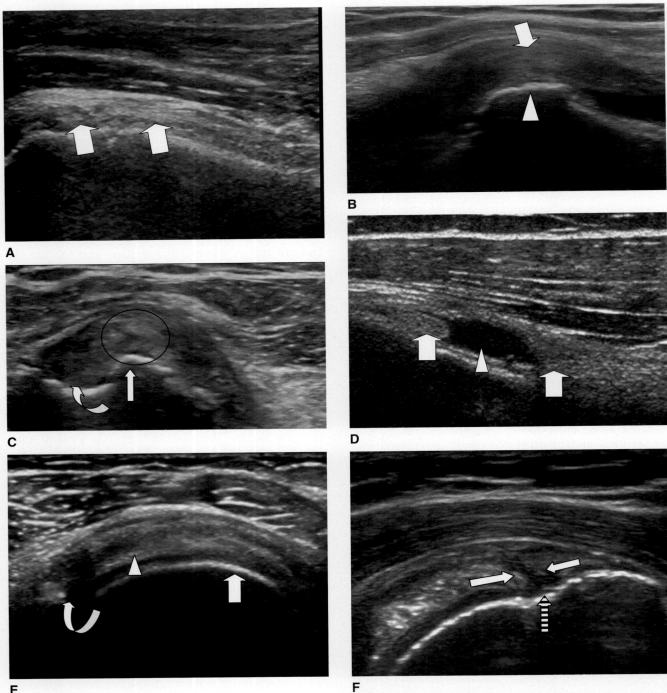

**Figure 18-19** Rotator cuff pathology. **A:** The long-axis (LAX) sonogram reveals a horizontal split of the biceps tendon *(white arrows)*. **B:** This LAX image shows a dislocated biceps tendon *(white arrow)* resting on top of the lesser tuberosity *(white arrowhead)*. **C:** On the same patient as **(B)**, the short-axis (SAX) plane shows the biceps tendon *(black circle)* resting on top of the lesser tuberosity *(white arrow)*, and the vacant bicipital groove *(curved arrow)*. **D:** This image in the LAX plane demonstrates a complete tear of the biceps tendon *(white arrows)* with intervening fluid *(white arrowhead)* between the retracted ends of the tendon. **E:** The SAX plane of the supraspinatus tendon at the cuff interval *(curved arrow)* demonstrates tendinosis lateral to the cuff interval *(white arrowhead)* and humeral head *(white arrow)*. **F:** This LAX image displays a tear of the supraspinatus tendon with bone irregularity *(striped arrow)* and the cleft *(white arrows)* through the tendon approaching the articular cartilage. *(continued)*

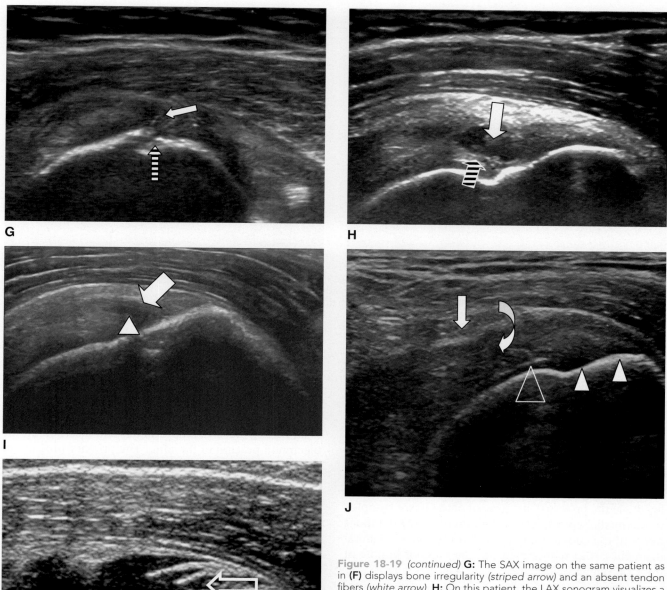

**Figure 18-19** *(continued)* **G:** The SAX image on the same patient as in **(F)** displays bone irregularity *(striped arrow)* and an absent tendon fibers *(white arrow)*. **H:** On this patient, the LAX sonogram visualizes a deep bursal-side tear *(white arrow)* with a few residual fibers *(striped arrow)* covering the articular cartilage. **I:** This LAX sonogram is of a less common intrasubstance tear *(white arrowhead)* of the supraspinatus tendon with fibers covering the tear *(white arrow)*. **J:** The LAX image shows a full-thickness, nonretracted tear of the supraspinatus tendon *(curved arrow)* with "dipping" of the subacromial-subdeltoid (SASD) bursa of deltoid muscle *(white arrow)* and articular cartilage interface sign *(white open arrowhead)* with normal bone surface on the greater tuberosity *(white arrowheads)*. **K:** The LAX image shows a traumatic full-thickness tear of the supraspinatus tendon with tendon fragments *(white open arrow)* and fluid in the devoid tendon space *(white arrow)*. *(continued)*

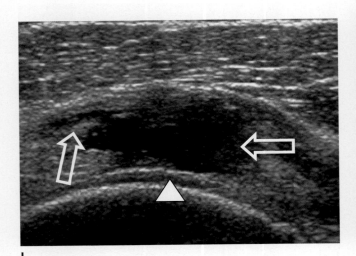

L

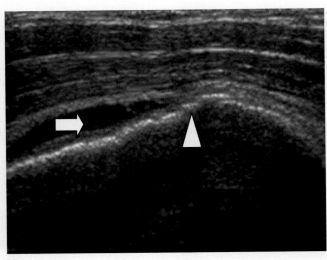

M

**Figure 18-19** *(continued)* **L:** This image on the same patient as in **(K)** is the SAX plane that demonstrates retracted tendon *(white open arrow)* and articular cartilage interface sign *(white arrowhead)*. **M:** This image demonstrates the "naked tuberosity" with no tendon fibers seen over insertion point of supraspinatus tendon *(white arrowhead)* and fluid in the SASD bursa *(white arrow)*.

the humeral capitellum, trochlea, radial head, and coronoid process of the head of the ulna (Fig. 18-22K,L).

Color Doppler can be used to identify the vascular structures. Although nerve entrapments may occur in the antebrachial area, evaluation techniques for this area are beyond the scope of this chapter.

## MEDIAL ELBOW

On the medial elbow, three areas are commonly imaged: (1) the proximal attachment of the flexor complex to the medial epicondyle of the humerus, (2) the ulnar nerve in the cubital tunnel, and (3) the ulnar collateral ligament (UCL) with a focus on the anterior bundle of the UCL (Fig. 18-23A–G).

## POSTERIOR ELBOW

The posterior elbow has three primary areas of interest which include the (1) triceps tendon, (2) olecranon bursa, and (3) olecranon fossa. The triceps tendon is a confluence of three muscles: the medial, lateral, and long head triceps muscles that form a broad insertion on the olecranon process of the ulna. The primary function of the triceps is extension of the elbow (Fig. 18-24A–C).

## LATERAL ELBOW

The extensor carpi radialis brevis, extensor digiti minimi, extensor carpi ulnaris, and the extensor digitorum comprise the common extensor tendon (Fig. 18-25A,B). The common extensor mechanism inserts onto the lateral epicondyle.

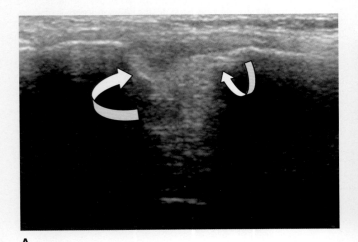

A

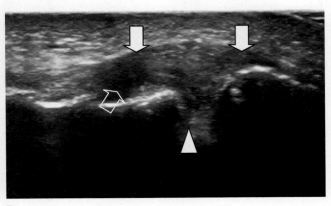

B

**Figure 18-20** Acromioclavicular (AC) joint pathology. **A:** Osteoarthritis is seen at the ends of the acromion and clavicle in AC joint *(curved arrows)*. **B:** The "Geyser" sign is visualized in the AC joint *(white arrowhead)*, fluid is ejected through the joint *(white open arrow)*, and there is distention of the capsule *(white arrows)*.

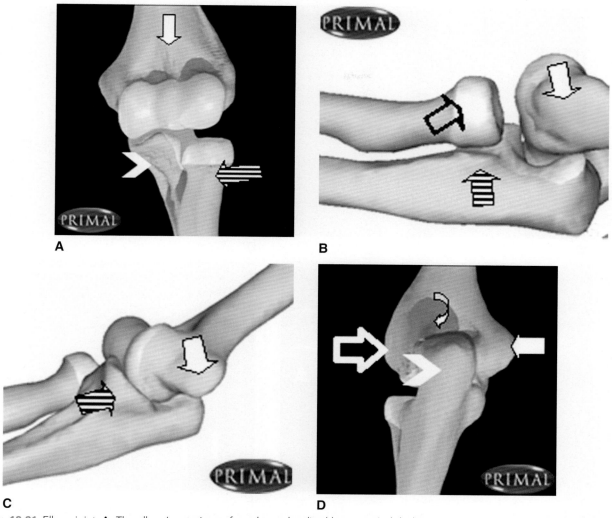

**Figure 18-21** Elbow joint. **A:** The elbow's anterior surface shows the distal humerus *(solid white arrow)*, proximal radius *(striped arrow)*, and proximal ulna *(white cursor)*. **B:** The elbow's lateral surface shows the lateral humeral condyle *(white arrow)*, radial head *(black open arrow)*, and the ulna *(striped arrow)*. **C:** The medial surface of the elbow demonstrates the coronoid process of the ulna *(striped arrow)* and the medial condyle of the humerus *(white arrow)*. **D:** From the posterior surface, the anatomy seen includes the olecranon process of the ulna *(white cursor)*, the lateral condyle *(black-filled arrow)*, medial condyle *(white arrow)*, and the olecranon fossa of the humerus *(curved arrow)*. (Images courtesy of Primal Pictures, Ltd., London, England.)

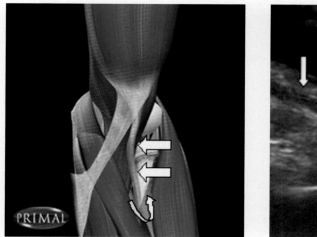

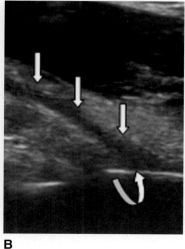

**Figure 18-22** Anterior elbow. **A:** The illustration shows the biceps tendon *(white arrows)* inserting on the radial tubercle *(curved arrow)*. **B:** The long-axis (LAX) image of the insertion of the biceps tendon *(white arrows)* inserting on the radial tubercle *(curved white arrow)*. *(continued)*

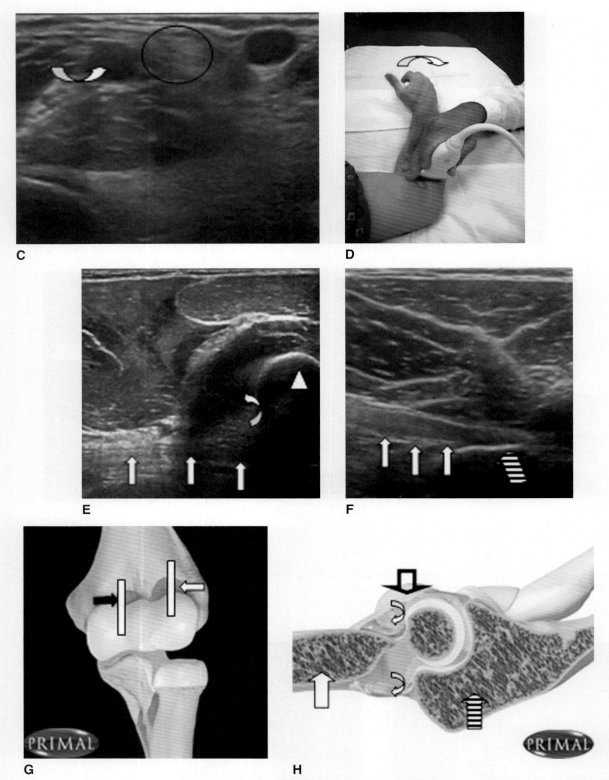

**Figure 18-22** (continued) **C:** The short-axis (SAX) image of the anterior elbow displays the brachial artery (curved arrow) adjacent and medial to the biceps tendon (black circle). Alternative method. Using an alternative method for imaging the distal biceps tendon **(D),** the transducer is placed anterior-lateral using dynamic pro-supination (curved arrow). **E:** The image through the supinator muscle (curved arrow) shows the LAX of biceps tendon projecting under the radius (white arrowhead). **F:** Using the medial approach, the LAX image shows the distal biceps tendon (white arrows) insertion on the radial tuberosity (striped arrow). Radial and coronoid fossa. **G:** The illustration of the anterior elbow surface indicates the transducer placement (white rectangles) over the radial fossa (white arrow) and the coronoid fossa (black arrow). **H:** A sagittal section shows the fat pads (curved arrows), humerus (solid white arrow), ulna (striped arrow), and the anterior capsule of the elbow (black open arrow). (continued)

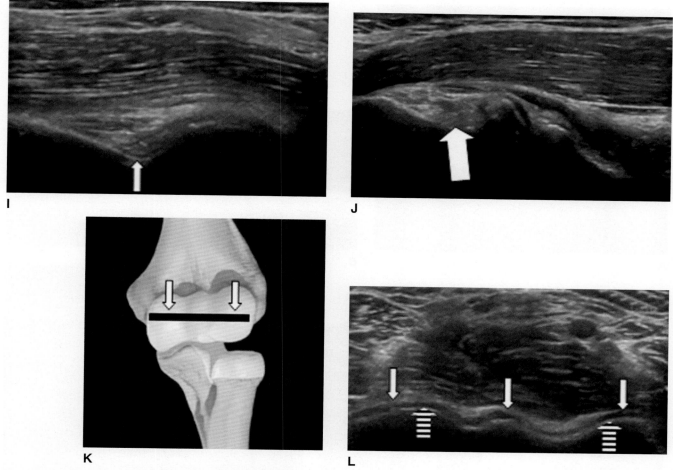

Figure 18-22 *(continued)* **I:** The LAX image over the radial fossa *(white arrow)* shows the echogenic fat pad lying on the bone. **J:** The LAX image of the distal humerus shows the coronoid fossa *(white arrow)*. Distal humerus. **K:** Illustrated is the transducer placement *(black rectangle)* for an SAX plane of the distal humerus and the articular cartilage of distal humerus *(white arrows)*. **L:** An SAX image of the anterior elbow demonstrates the distal humeral surface *(striped arrows)* and the articular cartilage *(white arrows)*. (Images **A, G, H, K** courtesy of Primal Pictures, Ltd., London, England.)

The primary function of the extensor tendons is powerful extension of the wrist, hand, and digits. Evaluation of the common extensor mechanism of the hand and wrist is completed in long and short axis of the lateral elbow.

## PATHOLOGY

### Common Flexor Osteotendinopathy (Golfer Elbow)

The common flexor insertion is a combination of superficial flexor tendons, pronator teres, flexi carpi ulnaris, palmaris longus, and the flexor carpi radialis. Separation into individual tendons at the insertion is difficult as tendon bundles intertwine.

Osteotendinopathy of the flexor complex refers to pathology of the superficial flexor tendons and the pronator teres at insertion. Inflammation and point tenderness over the medial epicondyle of the humerus may signify pathology. Ipsilateral to contralateral comparison of tendon insertion can facilitate evaluation. With osteotendinopathy, changes in echo texture of the

tendon accompanied by increased vascularity evaluated with color flow (CF) Doppler appearance may be observed (Fig. 18-26). Contralateral comparison is common; however, pathology may exist in a subacute stage and manifest in an abnormal tendon in comparison.

### Common Extensor Tendinopathy (Tennis Elbow)

The common extensor tendon is composed of a combination of the extensor carpi radialis brevis, extensor digitorum (communis), extensor carpi ulnaris, and extensor digiti minimi. Like the common flexor insertion, distinguishing separate tendon structure at the lateral epicondyle is difficult. The superficial fibers of the extensor carpi radialis brevis is the most commonly affected section of the common extensor mechanism insertion.[31] The common extensor insertion is a broad-based insertion with fibers of the lateral collateral ligament (LCL) blending in with the extensor complex. The common extensor tendon insertion is longer than the flexor component and exhibits the common fibrillar signature of a tendon.

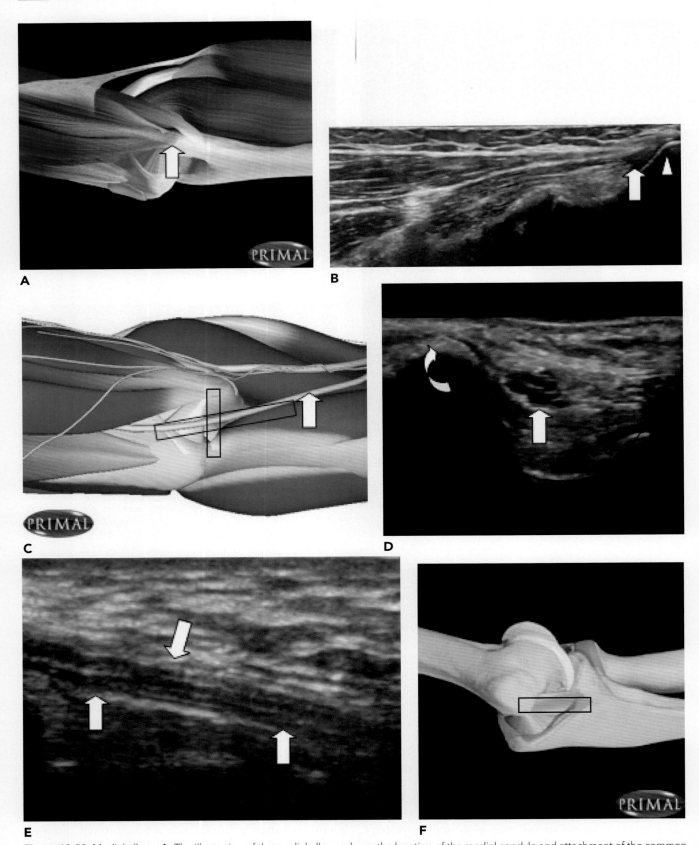

**Figure 18-23** Medial elbow. **A:** The illustration of the medial elbows shows the location of the medial condyle and attachment of the common flexor tendon *(white arrow)*. **B:** A long-axis (LAX) image demonstrates the fibrillar pattern of the short flexor tendon *(white arrow)* and the medial epicondyle *(white arrowhead)*. **C:** The illustration of the posteromedial elbow indicates the LAX and short-axis (SAX) transducer position *(black rectangles)* over the ulnar nerve *(black rectangles)*. **D:** An SAX image shows the cubital tunnel with the medial condyle *(curved arrow)* and the honeycomb appearance of the ulnar nerve *(white arrow)*. **E:** An LAX image of the ulnar nerve *(white arrows)* demonstrates the "fascicular" pattern of a normal nerve. **F:** The illustration of the anterior bundle of the ulnar collateral ligament shows the transducer position *(black rectangle)* across the bone surfaces. *(continued)*

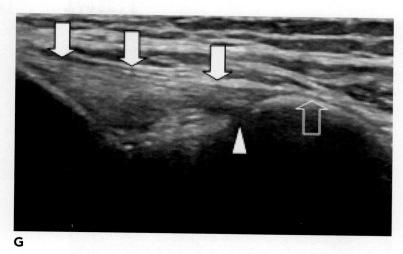

**Figure 18-23** *(continued)* **G:** The image shows the anterior bundle of the ulnar collateral ligament *(white arrows)* bridging the ulnar-humeral joint *(white arrowhead)* and attaching distally on the sublime tubercle of the ulna *(open arrow)*. (Images A, C, and G courtesy of Primal Pictures, Ltd., London, England.)

**G**

The contour of the lateral condyle and its relationship to the radiocapitellar joint resembles a "ski-jump." Placing the transducer on top of the lateral epicondyle in LAX is a typical starting point in evaluation.

The sonographer should be familiar with the most common findings of extensor mechanism osteotendinopathy (Fig. 18-27A–D). The process of insult to the tendon is not clearly understood; however, excessive loading and unloading of the extensor complex combined with vascular insult due to compression of the vessels is suspect. Extensor tendinopathy may also involve bone changes at the insertion. Evaluation of the extensor mechanism on the lateral epicondyle should include the bone surface for enthesophyte.

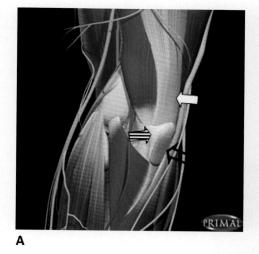

**A**

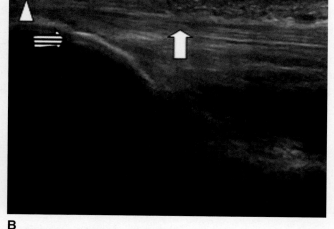

**B**

**Figure 18-24** Posterior elbow. **A:** The illustration depicts on the posterior elbow the olecranon process *(striped arrow)*, the triceps tendon *(white arrow)*, and the olecranon bursa *(open black arrow)*. **B:** A long-axis image demonstrates the fibrillar pattern of the triceps tendon *(solid white arrow)*, the olecranon process *(striped arrow)*, and the potential space for the olecranon bursa *(arrowhead)*. **C:** A short-axis image of the triceps tendon insertion demonstrates the multiple, round, hyperechoic tendons *(white arrows)* inserting on the olecranon process *(striped arrow)*. (Image **A** courtesy of Primal Pictures, Ltd., London, England.)

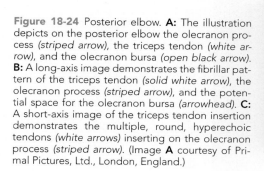

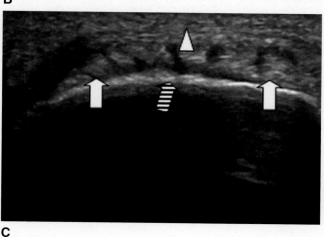

**C**

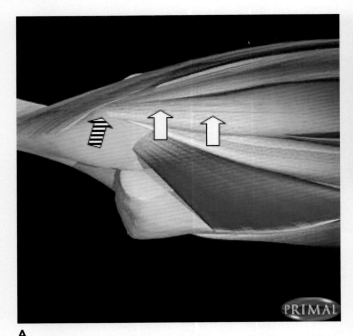

**A**

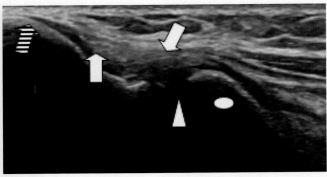

**B**

**Figure 18-25** Lateral elbow. The insertion of the common extensor *(white arrows)* onto the lateral epicondyle *(striped arrow)* can be seen in this illustration of the lateral elbow. **B:** The long-axis sonogram shows the insertion of the common extensor tendon *(white arrows)* onto the lateral epicondyle *(striped arrow)* of the humerus. The common extensor tendon spans the radial-humeral joint *(white arrowhead)* across the radial head *(white oval).* (Image **A** courtesy of Primal Pictures, Ltd., London, England.)

## Biceps Tendon Pathology

The distal biceps tendon inserts medially on the radial tuberosity of the radius. The tendon does not have a tendon sheath. Pathology of the distal biceps tendon primarily involves partial and full thickness tears. Techniques described by Jacobson[23] and Smith[29] and published guidelines[19,32] can be useful in evaluation. Jacobson's dynamic evaluation can separate partial attached tears from full thickness detached tears.[23] Smith's technique can be used with pronation-supination and provides an improved method for distal insertion[29] (Fig. 18-28A–C).

## Medial Elbow–Ulnar Collateral Ligament

The UCL is composed of three sections that include (1) the anterior band, (2) the transverse or oblique fibers, and (3) the posterior band. The UCL provides 50% of stability to the medial elbow and is a critical function in providing torque for the throwing athlete (Fig. 18-29A).

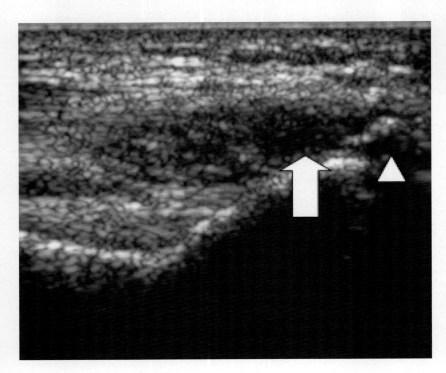

**Figure 18-26** Common flexor osteotendinopathy. A long-axis sonogram of the medial elbow and the common flexor insertion demonstrates a hypoechoic area *(white arrow)* in the tendon consistent with tendinosis and a spur *(white arrowhead)* on the medial epicondyle.

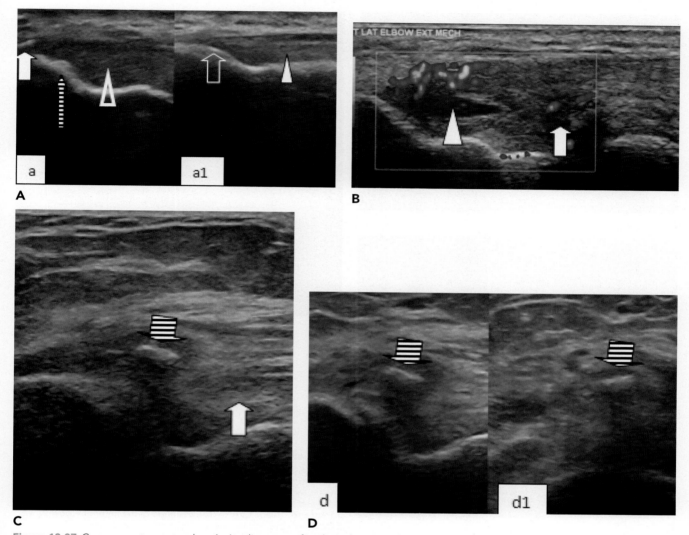

**Figure 18-27** Common extensor tendon. **A:** A split screen of ipsilateral to contralateral comparison: *(a)* The image on the left demonstrates the enthesophyte *(white arrow)*, the hypoechoic tendon with loss of fibrillar pattern *(white arrowhead)*, and irregular bone surface *(striped arrow)*; *(a1)* The image on the right is the contralateral side that demonstrates normal bone surface *(open arrow)* and the normal tendon *(white arrowhead)*. **B:** A long-axis power Doppler image of the same region illustrates neovascularity, a tear of the tendon *(arrowhead)*, and the edematous, hypoechoic tendon *(white arrow)*. **C:** In traumatic tendinopathy, an avulsion fracture *(striped arrow)* can be seen inside the extensor tendon *(white arrow)*. **D:** *(d)* and *(d1)* are short-axis images of the avulsion fracture with distal shadowing.

The anterior bundle is the most critical segment of the UCL and integrity of anterior bundle requires dynamic valgus stressing of the affected area. With practice, one can learn the technique and transducer position used in the evaluation of the anterior bundle (Fig. 18-29B).

Ipsilateral to contralateral comparisons can be useful in both the elite and casual athlete. Recognizing the normal anatomy provides the needed foundation to recognize sonographic evidence of pathology of the anterior bundle of the UCL of the elbow (Fig. 18-29C–E).

## Olecranon Bursitis

Olecranon bursitis can result from trauma, systemic and autoimmune conditions, gout, rheumatoid arthritis, sustained pressure, and infection. Exquisite pain, swelling, and erythema are typical clinical findings in any bursitis. Sonographically, the normal olecranon bursa is indistinguishable from the surrounding tissue. In bursitis, light transducer pressure or "floating" the transducer may be required to adequately interrogate bursa and diminish patient discomfort (Fig. 18-30).

## Triceps Tendon

Injury to the triceps tendon involves the full spectrum of tendinopathy, including partial and complete tears. The inability to extend the elbow against pressure may be a sign of disruption (Fig. 18-31A,B).

## Loose Bodies and Joint Fluid

Loose bodies in the elbow commonly migrate to the largest and deepest fossa of the elbow, the dorsally located olecranon fossa. The olecranon fossa of the distal humerus accommodates articulation of the olecranon process of the ulna with the distal humerus with arm extension.

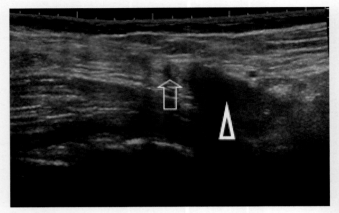

**A**

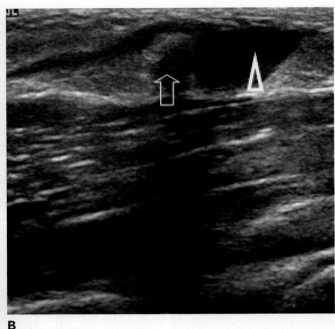

**B**

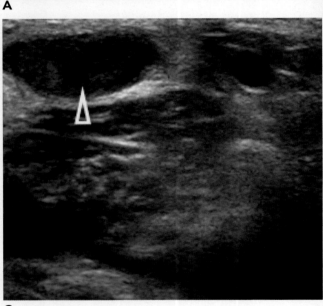

**C**

**Figure 18-28** Biceps tendon. **A:** The panoramic sonogram demonstrates a full thickness tear of the distal biceps tendon with retraction and with the proximal stump *(open arrow)* and fluid in the void left by the tendon *(open arrowhead)*. **B:** A long-axis zoomed image demonstrates the retracted stump *(open arrow)* and the fluid in the void *(open arrowhead)*. **C:** A short-axis image of the anterior elbow shows a fluid-filled void and tendon stump *(white open arrowhead)*.

In acute and chronic degenerative pathology and trauma, bone, articular cartilage, or loose bodies can accumulate in recesses and fossa of the joint (Fig. 18-32).

### Ulnar Nerve

Ulnar nerve subluxation over the medial condyle of the humerus is not uncommon. With entrapment neuropathies, the nerve may increase in size, become inflamed, and exhibit contour changes with loss of the typical fascicular pattern (Fig. 18-33A–E).

## WRIST

### ANATOMY

The wrist is an example of a diarthrosis—a freely movable joint. The complex and detailed anatomy of the ligaments, articulations, and compartments are beyond the scope of this chapter. To begin scanning, however, understanding the basic anatomy is important and expanding that knowledge base will increase confidence and scanning accuracy (Fig. 18-34). In general, sonographic

evaluation is divided into the dorsal and palmar aspect. The wrist is a targeted study based on clinical symptoms and history. Depending on need, refinement of the evaluation process is divided into the extensor compartments, flexor tendons, carpal joints, and carpal-metacarpal joints and will determine the different wrist positions (pronation and supination) and the degree of dynamic imaging (flexion and extension, radial and ulnar deviation).[18,33]

### Dorsal Wrist

Located on the dorsal aspect of the wrist is the extensor mechanism, which is responsible for extension of the wrist, digits, and thumb (Fig. 18-35A). The extensor mechanism is divided into six compartments and is subject to overuse and traumatic injury. The extensor tendons action is to extend, adduct, and abduct the wrist and digits of the hand. Compartments containing more than a single tendon are surrounded by a common sheath that is subject to inflammation. Compartment one on the lateral volar aspect of the wrist is commonly subject to pathology. The compartment contains the extensor pollicis

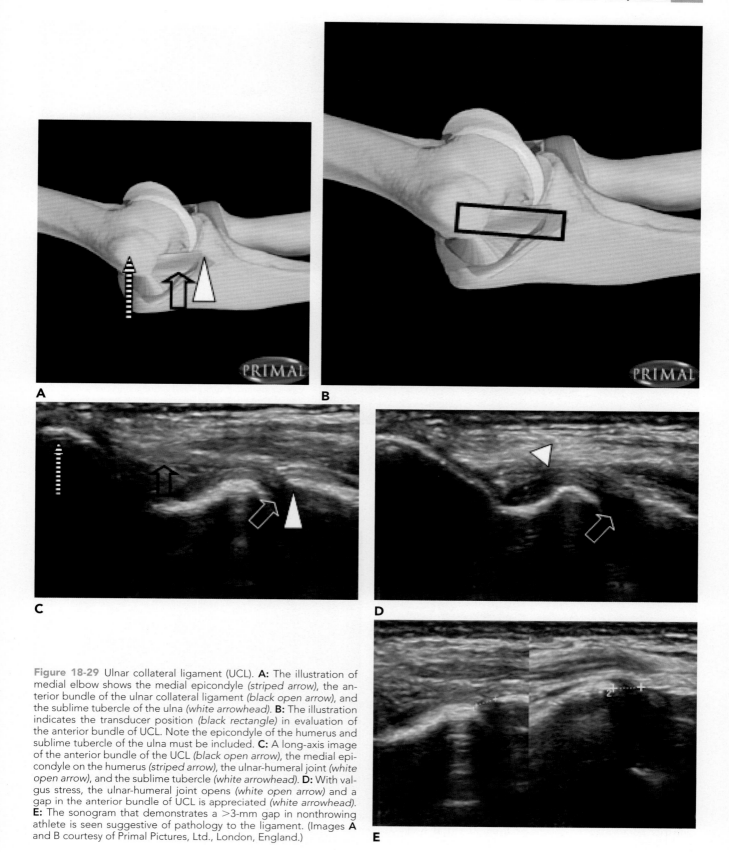

**Figure 18-29** Ulnar collateral ligament (UCL). **A:** The illustration of medial elbow shows the medial epicondyle *(striped arrow)*, the anterior bundle of the ulnar collateral ligament *(black open arrow)*, and the sublime tubercle of the ulna *(white arrowhead)*. **B:** The illustration indicates the transducer position *(black rectangle)* in evaluation of the anterior bundle of UCL. Note the epicondyle of the humerus and sublime tubercle of the ulna must be included. **C:** A long-axis image of the anterior bundle of the UCL *(black open arrow)*, the medial epicondyle on the humerus *(striped arrow)*, the ulnar-humeral joint *(white open arrow)*, and the sublime tubercle *(white arrowhead)*. **D:** With valgus stress, the ulnar-humeral joint opens *(white open arrow)* and a gap in the anterior bundle of UCL is appreciated *(white arrowhead)*. **E:** The sonogram that demonstrates a >3-mm gap in nonthrowing athlete is seen suggestive of pathology to the ligament. (Images **A** and **B** courtesy of Primal Pictures, Ltd., London, England.)

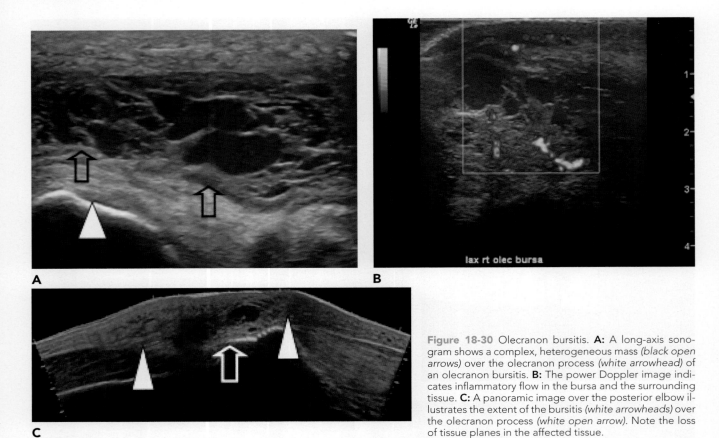

**A**

**B**

**C**

**Figure 18-30** Olecranon bursitis. **A:** A long-axis sonogram shows a complex, heterogeneous mass *(black open arrows)* over the olecranon process *(white arrowhead)* of an olecranon bursitis. **B:** The power Doppler image indicates inflammatory flow in the bursa and the surrounding tissue. **C:** A panoramic image over the posterior elbow illustrates the extent of the bursitis *(white arrowheads)* over the olecranon process *(white open arrow)*. Note the loss of tissue planes in the affected tissue.

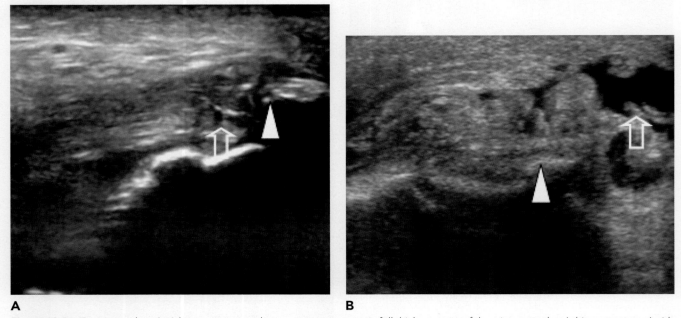

**A**

**B**

**Figure 18-31** Triceps tendon. **A:** A long-axis image demonstrates a traumatic full thickness tear of the triceps tendon *(white open arrow)* with olecranon bone surface irregularity *(white arrowhead)*. **B:** A short-axis image on the same patient as image A demonstrates the bone irregularity *(white arrowhead)* with tendon fiber disruption and fluid *(white open arrow)*. (Images **A** and **B** courtesy of Tony Bouffard, MD, Detroit, MI.)

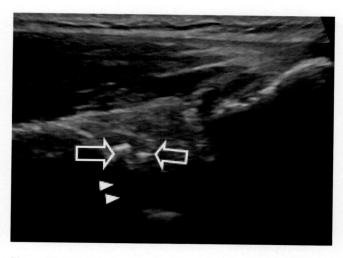

**Figure 18-32** Loose bodies. The long-axis image of the olecranon fossa demonstrates hyperechoic loose bodies *(open white arrows)* with posterior acoustic shadowing *(white arrowheads)*.

brevis (EPB) and the abductor pollicis longus (APL). The EPB primary action is extension of the proximal phalanx of the thumb. The APL is responsible for extension and abduction of the distal phalanx at the first metacarpal-phalangeal joint. Together, the APL and EPB form the volar "anatomic snuff box" (Fig. 18-35B–D).

### Palmar Wrist

The flexor tendons, median nerve, ulnar and radial nerves and their branches, restraining retinacula, and major vascular structures are primarily found in the volar aspect of the wrist. The most commonly evaluated area on the volar wrist is the carpal tunnel. The carpal tunnel is a restricted space delimited by carpal bones dorsally and fibrous capsule and transverse carpal ligament or retinaculum on the volar aspect. The carpal tunnel may be smaller in females than males resulting in greater potential for carpal tunnel syndrome (CTS) in females. The

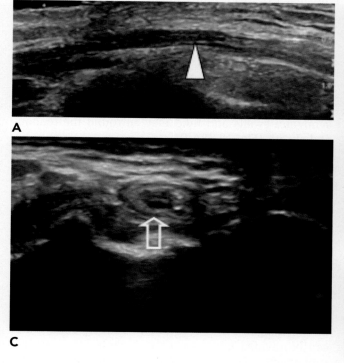

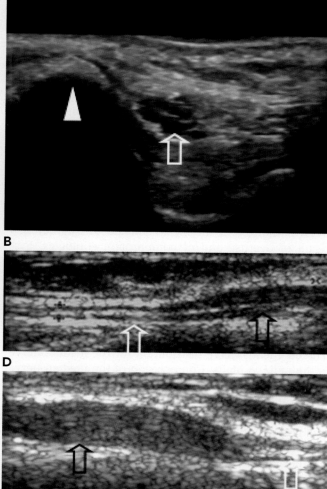

**Figure 18-33** Ulnar nerve. **A:** A long axis of a normal ulnar nerve is seen in the cubital tunnel *(white arrowhead)* and **(B)** a short-axis (SAX) image on the same patient as **(A)** presents with a honeycomb appearance of the ulnar nerve *(white open arrow)* and the medial epicondyle *(white arrowhead)*. **C:** A SAX image of ulnar nerve neuritis is seen as a hypoechoic rim surrounding the nerve *(white open arrow)*. **D,E:** The panoramic images demonstrate the contour change in the ulnar nerve. Normal nerve contours *(white open arrows)* and enlarged nerve *(black open arrows)* with loss of fascicular pattern. (Images **D** and **E** are courtesy of Tony Bouffard, MD, Detroit, MI.)

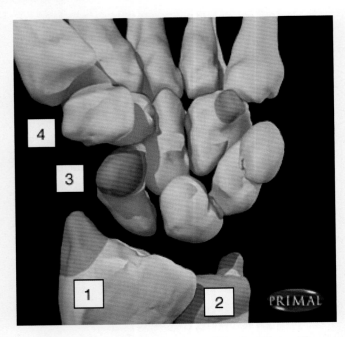

**Figure 18-34** Dorsal wrist bone anatomy: (1) radius; (2) ulna; (3) proximal row from left to right: scaphoid, lunate triquetrum, and pisiform; (4) distal row from left to right: trapezium, trapezoid, capitate, and hamate. (Image courtesy of Primal Pictures, Ltd., London, England.)

proximal carpal tunnel lies between the pisiform on the ulnar side to the scaphoid on the radial side. The distal margin can be defined as the region from the hook of the hamate to the tubercle of the trapezium on the radial side. Through this semirigid tunnel run the flexor tendons of the hand and wrist as well as the median nerve (Fig. 18-36A–D). Any increase in volume in this restricted space may result in compression of the median nerve.

## PATHOLOGY

Most pathology of the wrist, outside of trauma, is a result of overuse and/or compression etiologies. Systemic disease processes that have implications in the wrist include diabetes, lupus, and osteogenic processes such as osteoarthritis, psoriatic arthritis, and rheumatoid arthritis.

### Median Nerve

The cutaneous nerve distribution for the median nerve is the radial 3 digits. Compression of the median nerve may result in nerve paresthesias, although neuropathies may result from systemic pathologies. CTS is the most common entrapment syndrome of the upper extremity and may result from a variety of conditions and anatomic variants. Diagnosis of CTS is generally not an imaging diagnosis, although imaging with dynamic maneuvers may provide insight into the etiologies. Imaging signs of mechanical compressions include (1) a median nerve that is three times greater in one axis compared to an orthogonal plane, (2) loss of the "honeycomb" appearance in SAX, (3) abruptly decreases/increases in contour in

LAX, or (4) display changes in a cross-sectional area when compared to an adjacent section of the same unbranched nerve. Old criteria of overall nerve area are >9 cm$^2$ with a gray area between 1.0 and 1.2 cm$^2$ at the entrance to the carpal tunnel is diagnostic of median nerve compression. Klauser et al.[34] describe a ratio of median nerve cross-sectional area (CSA) at the level of the pronator quadratus (CSAp) and at the carpal tunnel (CSAc). A CSAp-CSAc calculation >2 mm$^2$ defines median nerve compression with great sensitivity (99%) and specificity (100%).[34] A sonographer should be able to identify common imaging manifestations of median nerve compression and have an understanding of the measurement techniques (Fig. 18-37A–F).

### Tendinopathies

Overuse, anatomic variants, systemic diseases, and microvascular insults, individually or in combination may result in pathology of tendons. The histologic disease process resulting in tendinopathies is debated. The most common tendinopathy of the wrist involves the first extensor compartment. De Quervain tenosynovitis involves the APL and extensor pollicis brevis (EPB). Patients complain of focal pain over the distal radius with exaggerated movements of the thumb and wrist. Color or power Doppler can be useful in detecting the associated inflammatory process. Typically, the associated retinaculum bulges, the tendons become hypoechoic and may splinter into several slips. The synovium swells and fluid may surround the tendons and sheath (Fig. 18-38A,B).

## KNEE

### ANATOMY

The knee is a hinge, diarthrosis, synovial lined joint. Pertinent bone anatomy consists of the distal femur, proximal tibia, and the largest sesamoid bone, the patella (Fig. 18-39A,B). Sonographic evaluation of the knee, in most institutions, is a targeted study. However, full evaluation of the knee can lead to a better understanding of anatomy and improve the overall confidence of the novice imager. Protocol-driven evaluation of the knee can be divided into sections to include (1) anterior – suprapatellar, (2) anterior – infrapatellar, (3) lateral, (4) medial, and (5) posterior. In keeping with the focus of this chapter, only commonly sonographic imaged anatomy will be discussed in conjunction with pathology.

### Anterior Knee
#### Suprapatellar

The major soft tissue structures in anterior suprapatellar region are the quadriceps tendon, the contributing muscles of the quadriceps tendon, the suprapatellar fat pad, prefemoral fat pad, and suprapatellar recess or pouch. The quadriceps tendon is an important extensor of the lower extremity. The vastus medialis,

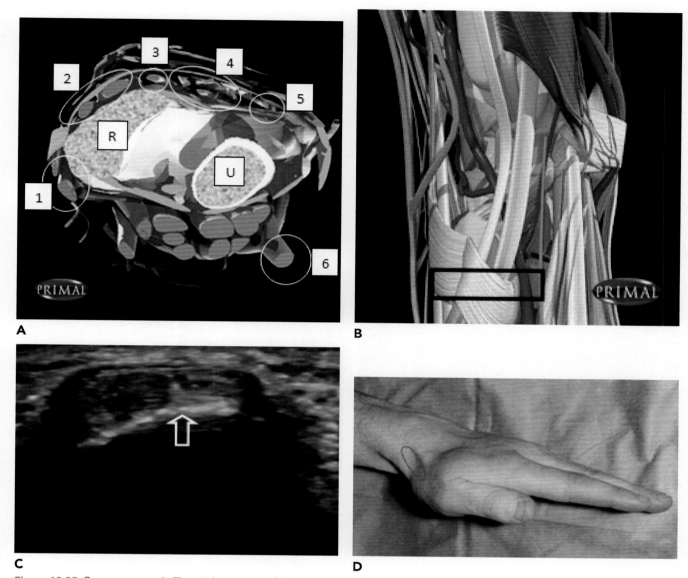

**Figure 18-35** Compartments. **A:** The axial projection of the extensor tendon compartments are labeled 1–6 and begin from the radius. Compartment 1: abductor pollicis longus and extensor pollicis brevis. Compartment 2: extensor carpi radialis longus and brevis. Compartment 3: extensor pollicis longus. Compartment 4: extensor digitorum communis. Compartment 5: extensor digiti minimi. Compartment 6: extensor carpi ulnaris. R, radius; U, ulna. **B:** The illustration shows the transducer location (*black rectangle*) for a short-axis (SAX) plane over the first compartment. **C:** A SAX image shows the normal abductor pollicis longus and extensor pollicis brevis superior to the radius (*white open arrow*). **D:** The photo shows the depression created by the tendons on the lateral side of the wrist at the base of the thumb known as an anatomic "snuff box" (*red circle*). (Images **A** and **B** courtesy of Primal Pictures, Ltd., London, England.)

vastus lateralis, vastus intermedius, and rectus femoris muscles of the anterior, medial, and lateral thigh contribute distal tendons to form the quadriceps (quad = 4) tendon. Over 95% of the fibers of the quadriceps tendon insert on the base of the patella. A small percentage of fibers continue over the anterior surface of the patella and contribute to the more distal patellar tendon (Fig. 18-40A–E).

### Infrapatellar

The infrapatellar region consists of the patellar tendon and the pes anserine. The patellar tendon (patellar ligament) is a 4 × 2 × 6 cm structure attaching

the apex of the patella to the tuberosity of the tibia and medial and laterally to the patellar retinaculum. Posterior to the patellar tendon is Hoffa fat pad, an inhomogeneous, thick layer of intracapsular (an intra-articular inclusion) but is extrasynovial fat (Fig. 18-41).

### Prepatellar

The anterior suprapatellar region primary bone anatomy is the patella and femur. In the prepatellar regions, the proximal and distal insertion of the patellar tendon is broad. The prepatellar bursa lies anterior to the patella and patellar tendon (Fig. 18-42A–E).

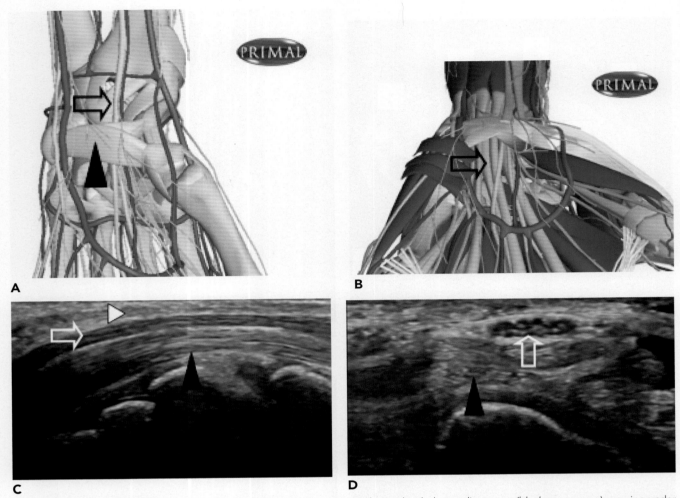

**Figure 18-36** Carpal tunnel. **A:** The illustration shows the dorsal wrist carpal tunnel with the median nerve *(black open arrow)* coursing under the flexor retinaculum *(black arrowhead)*. **B:** The position of the flexor tendons *(black open arrow)* is seen on this illustration. **C:** A long-axis image on of the proximal carpal tunnel shows the echogenic flexor retinaculum *(white arrowhead)*, the honeycomb pattern of the normal median nerve *(white open arrow)*, and the fibrillar pattern of the flexor tendons *(black arrowhead)*, beneath the median nerve. **D:** The short axis sonogram image on of the carpal tunnel shows the fascicular pattern of the normal median nerve *(white open arrow)* and the fibrillar pattern of the flexor tendons *(black arrowhead)*, beneath the median nerve. (Images **A** and **B** courtesy of Primal Pictures, Ltd., London, England.)

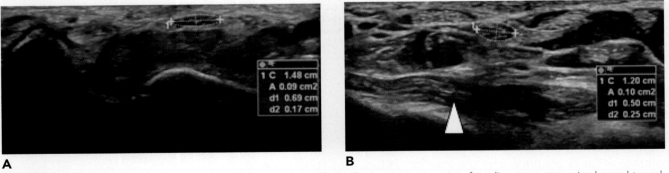

**Figure 18-37** Median nerve. **A:** The short-axis (SAX) sonogram indicates the area measurement of median nerve at proximal carpal tunnel. **B:** The SAX image is proximal to the measurement in **(A)** at the level of pronator quadratus *(white arrowhead)*. *(continued)*

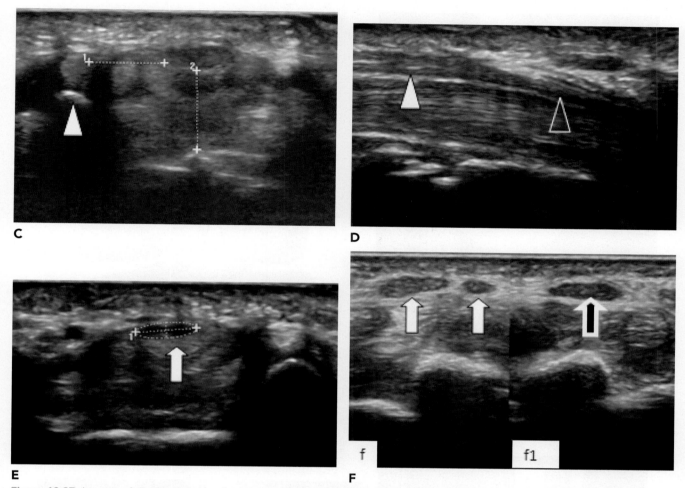

**Figure 18-37** *(continued)* **C:** The technique for locating proximal carpal tunnel by location is to locate the scaphoid *(white arrowhead)* and flexi carpi radialis in a SAX plane dorsal to the scaphoid. Measurement two is from anterior surface of median nerve to carpal bones. **D:** A long-axis (LAX) image of the median nerve illustrates a change in contour from a normal nerve *(white arrowhead)* to a compressed nerve *(open arrowhead)*. **E:** On the same patient as **(D)**, the nerve is compressed and is three times wider than in anterior-posterior measurement. **F:** The image on the left *(f)* is a common anatomic variant with bifid median nerve *(white arrows)* compared to the image on the right *(f1)* showing the contralateral single nerve *(black-and-white arrow)*.

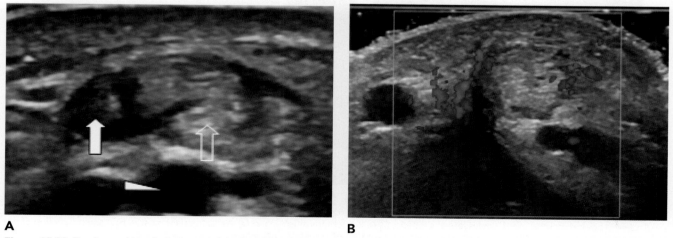

**Figure 18-38** Tendinopathies. **A:** An image of the first extensor compartment in a patient with de Quervain disease shows how the tendon can split into multiple slips *(open white arrow)* or be singular *(white arrow)*. The radial artery *(white arrowhead)* can also be identified. **B:** A power Doppler image illustrates the inflammation of the tendons.

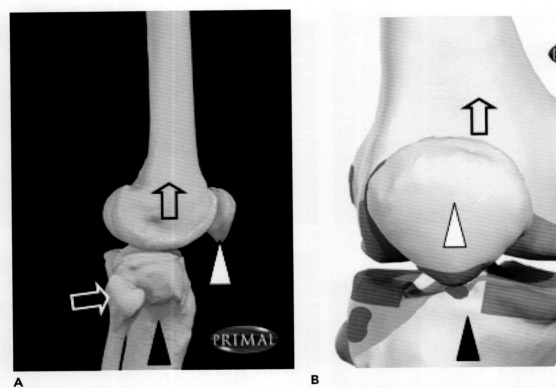

**Figure 18-39** Knee joint. **A:** The lateral knee illustration shows the distal femur *(black open arrow)*, the proximal fibular head *(white open arrow)*, and the patella *(white arrowhead)*. **B:** An anterior knee illustration shows the patella *(white arrowhead)*, distal femur *(black open arrow)*, and proximal tibia *(black arrowhead)*. (Images A and B courtesy of Primal Pictures, Ltd., London, England.)

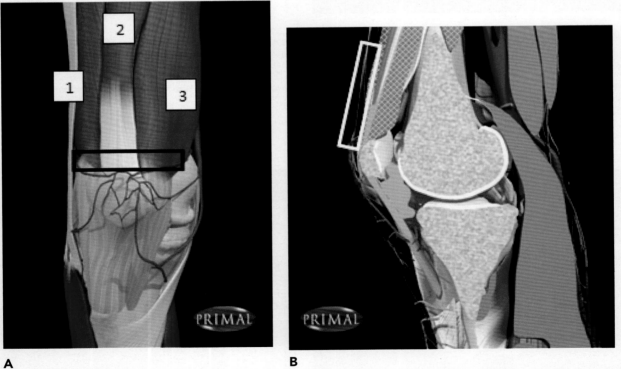

**Figure 18-40** Normal quadriceps tendon. **A:** The anterior knee illustration shows the transducer position *(black rectangle)* for the short-axis (SAX) plane. Labeled muscles are *(1)* vastus lateralis muscle, *(2)* rectus femoris muscle, and *(3)* vastus medialis muscle. **B:** A sagittal section of the knee shows with transducer position *(white rectangle)* in a long-axis (LAX) plane of quadriceps tendon. *(continued)*

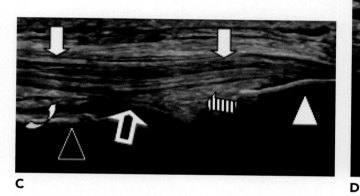

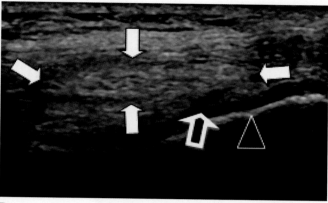

C

D

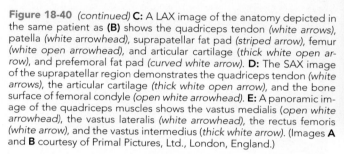

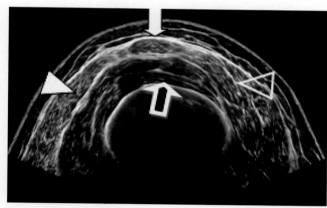

E

**Figure 18-40** *(continued)* **C:** A LAX image of the anatomy depicted in the same patient as **(B)** shows the quadriceps tendon *(white arrows)*, patella *(white arrowhead)*, suprapatellar fat pad *(striped arrow)*, femur *(white open arrowhead)*, and articular cartilage *(thick white open arrow)*, and prefemoral fat pad *(curved white arrow)*. **D:** The SAX image of the suprapatellar region demonstrates the quadriceps tendon *(white arrows)*, the articular cartilage *(thick white open arrow)*, and the bone surface of femoral condyle *(open white arrowhead)*. **E:** A panoramic image of the quadriceps muscles shows the vastus medialis *(open white arrowhead)*, the vastus lateralis *(white arrowhead)*, the rectus femoris *(white arrow)*, and the vastus intermedius *(thick white arrow)*. (Images **A** and **B** courtesy of Primal Pictures, Ltd., London, England.)

## Medial Knee

The medial collateral ligament (MCL) or tibial collateral ligament, which is the primary ligamentous support structure for the medial knee. A broad, thin, fibrous complex attaches to the medial condyle of the femur and to the anterior medial aspect of the tibia. The deep fibers of the MCL attach to the medial meniscus. Sonographic evaluation of the MCL in LAX produces a trilaminar appearance with a hyperechoic leading edge, hypoechoic center portion followed by a hyperechoic portion closer to the bone. The pes anserine (goose foot) is a conjoined tendon of sartorius, gracilis, and semitendinosus muscles. Distal attachment of the pes anserine is on the anterior medial aspect of the proximal tibia in close association with the MCL. Inflammation of the pes anserine bursa can be a cause of medial, inferior knee pain and weakness and may be a result of overuse. The external portion of the medial meniscus anterior and posterior horn can be seen. A fibrous, thin, retinaculum on the medial and lateral aspect of the patella stabilizes the patella (Fig. 18-43A–G).

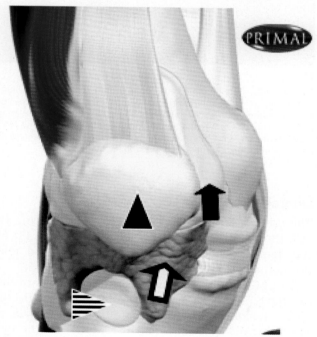

**Figure 18-41** Infrapatellar region. The illustration of the anterior knee shows the patella *(black arrowhead)*, Hoffa fat pad *(black and white arrow)*, retropatellar bursa *(striped arrowhead)*, and the synovial lining of the knee *(black arrow)*. (Image courtesy of Primal Pictures, Ltd., London, England.)

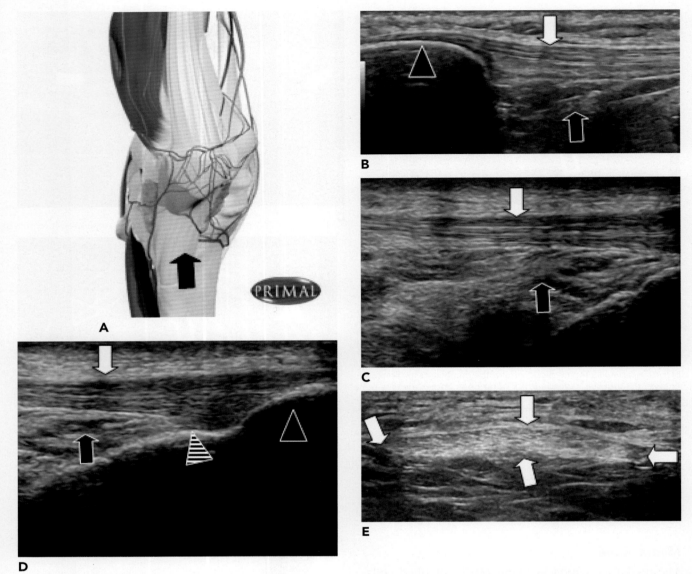

**Figure 18-42** Patellar tendon. **A:** The illustration shows the location and surrounding anatomy of the patellar tendon *(black arrow)*. **B:** A long-axis image of the patellar tendon documents the proximal insertion on the patella *(black arrowhead)*, fibrillar pattern of the proximal patellar tendon *(white arrow)*, and Hoffa fat pad *(black arrow)*. **C:** The image shows the distal insertion *(white arrow)*, trumpet shaped with Hoffa fat *(black arrow)*. **D:** On this image, the distal tendon *(white arrow)*, Hoffa fat pad *(black arrow)*, the anterior tibial tuberosity *(black arrowhead)*, and the potential area for the retropatellar bursa *(striped arrowhead)*. **E:** The short-axis image shows the patellar tendon *(white arrows)*. (Image **A** courtesy of Primal Pictures, Ltd., London, England.)

## Lateral Knee

The primary structures of lateral knee include the (1) LCL (fibulocollateral), (2) iliotibial band (ITB), (3) biceps femoris tendon (BF), and (4) posterior and anterior horns of the lateral meniscus (Fig. 18-44A–C).

The LCL (fibular collateral ligament), a cord-like ligament, shares a common attachment with the biceps femoris on the lateral and medial surface of the fibula distally. Proximal insertion is on the epicondyle of the lateral condyle of the femur. The biceps femoris is a component of the hamstrings and its function is to flex the knee and extend the hip. The two heads of the biceps tendon fuse as they

approach the head of the fibula and primary insertion is on the lateral and anterior head of the fibula (Fig. 18-44D,E).

The ITB, a broad, thin fibrous band, attaches distally to the tibial tubercle (Gerdy tubercle) on the lateral tibial condyle. The ITB is the distal extension of the tensor fasciae latae and supports several functions including internal hip rotation and flexion, flexion and extension of the lower extremity during running, and support of the knee with the gluteus maximus when standing erect. The ITB extends over the lateral condyle of the femur, which is a common friction point and susceptible to inflammation with overuse, which

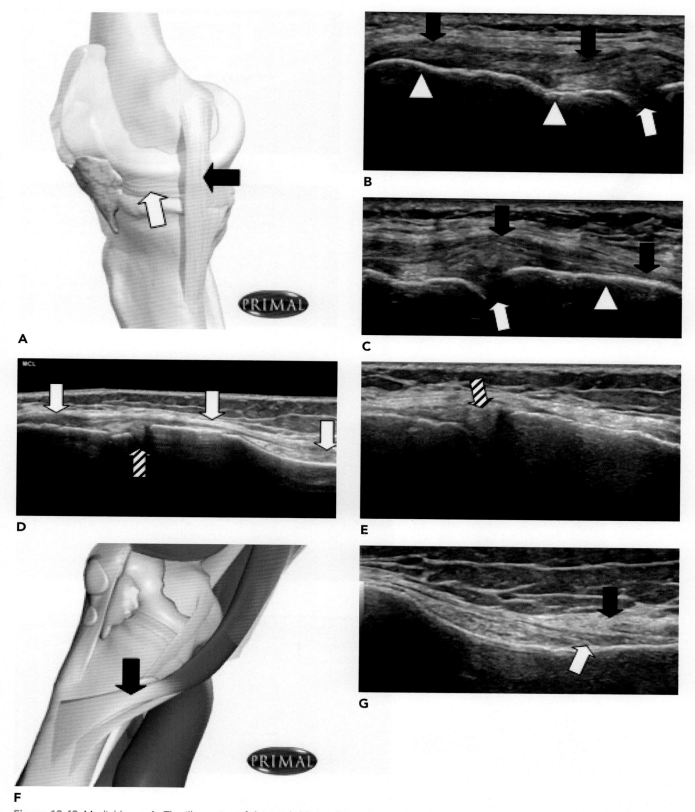

**Figure 18-43** Medial knee. **A:** The illustration of the medial knee shows the medial meniscus *(white arrow)* and medial collateral ligament *(black arrow)*. **B:** A long-axis image visualizes the proximal insertion of the medial collateral ligament *(black arrows)* on to the medial femoral condyle *(white arrowheads)* and joint space with medial meniscus *(white arrow)*. **C:** The sonogram shows the medial collateral ligament *(black arrows)* at the joint space *(white arrow)* and the tibial condyle *(white arrowhead)*. **D:** A panoramic image shows the medial collateral ligament *(white arrows)* and the joint space *(striped arrow)*. **E:** The sonogram reveals the medial meniscus *(striped arrow)*. **F:** The illustration depicts the pes anserine *(black arrow)*. **G:** The sonogram shows the distal insertion of the medial collateral ligament *(white arrow)* with short-axis plane of the pes anserine *(black arrow)*. (Images **A** and **F** courtesy of Primal Pictures, Ltd., London, England.)

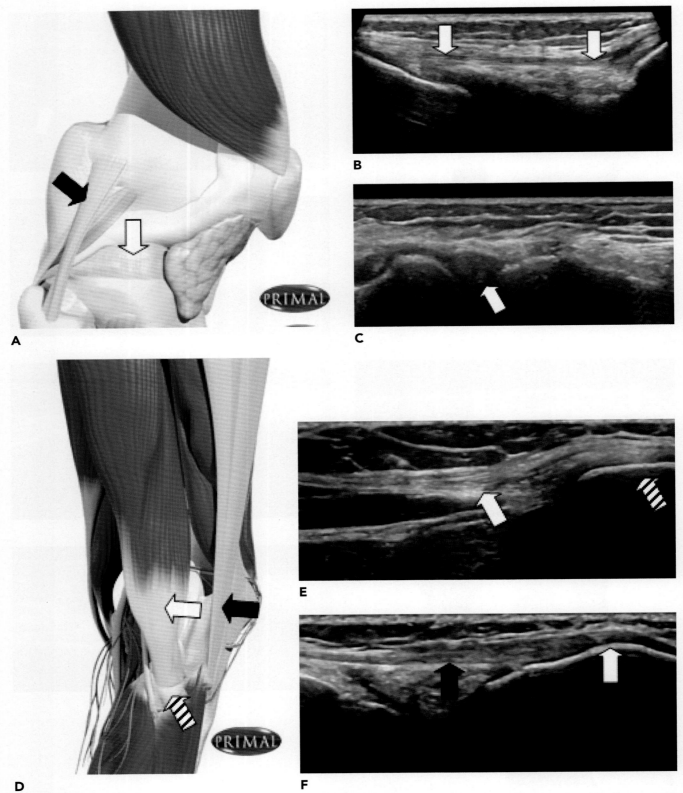

**Figure 18-44** Lateral knee. **A:** The illustration of the lateral knees shows the lateral collateral ligament (*black arrow*) and the lateral meniscus (*white arrow*). **B:** A long-axis (LAX) image visualizes the lateral collateral ligament (*white arrows*). **C:** This LAX sonogram documents the joint space with the lateral meniscus (*white arrow*). **D:** The illustration shows the conjoined long head and short head of the biceps femoris (*white arrow*), fibular head (*striped arrow*), and the iliotibial band (*black arrow*). **E:** A long-axis (LAX) sonogram shows the biceps femoris tendon (*white arrow*) and the fibular head (*striped arrow*). **F:** This LAX image shows the iliotibial band (*black arrow*) inserting on Gerdy tubercle of the tibia (*white arrow*). (Images **A** and **D** courtesy of Primal Pictures, Ltd., London, England.)

is found when runners suddenly increase mileage (Fig. 18-44A–C).

## Posterior Knee

Evaluation of the posterior knee is focused on the gastrocnemius-semimembranosus bursa, more common vernacular is the "Baker" cyst. Recognition of the acoustic landmarks minimizes the risk of misdiagnosis (Fig. 18-45A–D).

Identification of the posterior medial condyle of the femur and the articular cartilage is the most anterior landmarks. Posterior to the medial condyle is the semimembranosus tendon. Implementing "toggling or rocking" of the transducer when in SAX may help identify the tendon. Lateral to the medial condyle and the semimembranosus tendon is the SAX of the medial head of the gastrocnemius muscle. Between the tendon and the muscle lies the potential space for the bursa. The popliteal artery, vein, as well as the tibial nerve lie lateral to the bursa. A communication between the joint space and the suspected bursa is essential to correctly diagnose a Baker cyst.

## PATHOLOGY

Painful or painless swelling of the knee may be one of the most common clinical histories encountered in evaluation of the knee. Evaluation should include the suprapatellar pouch or recess. The suprapatellar pouch, often referred to as the suprapatellar bursa communicates with the joint. Excessive fluid in the joint space may give the patient a feeling of fullness in the knee (Fig. 18-46).

Quadriceps tendon rupture is a relatively rare condition and is usually a result of excess force injuries. In general, there is underlying systemic condition such as diabetes, gout, or rheumatoid arthritis that precipitates tendon failure. The tendon can tear partially or completely and may involve all or any one of the contributing tendons from the quadriceps muscles. Tears generally occur 1 to 2 cm from the insertion on the patella. Clinical management changes depending on whether the tear is complete or partial (Fig. 18-47A,B).

## Collateral Ligaments/Iliotibial Band

Most tears of the collateral ligaments are managed conservatively with the exception of the elite athlete. The MCL tears generally occur from the joint space superiorly, whereas the LCL tears can occur anywhere along the length of the tendon (Fig. 18-48A–C).

Friction tendinopathies of the ITB generally occur at the lateral condyle of the femur. However, pathology of the ITB may occur at the distal insertion on Gerdy tubercle (Fig. 18-49A,B).

## Meniscus

Sonographic evaluation of the menisci is limited to the peripheral portion. Tears, meniscal cysts, and extruded meniscus, common in degenerative disease, can be diagnosed (Fig. 18-50A–D). The internal portion of the meniscus, where most tears occur, cannot be evaluated due to the limited acoustic window. Currently, MRI remains the gold standard for meniscal tears.

## Patellar Tendon

One of the most commonly encountered pathologies of the knee is pathology of the patellar tendon. Tendinopathies include jumper's knee, degenerative changes of the proximal deep fibers of the tendon in association with calcific enthesopathy, as well as partial or full thickness tear. Color or power Doppler can be helpful in inflammation. Multiple bursae surround the tendon. Inflammation of the bursa may cause pain and limited movement (Fig. 18-51A–D). Complete rupture of the tendon is rare.

## Gastrocnemius-Semimembranosus Bursa: Baker Cyst

The most frequently encountered pathology of the knee is the Baker cyst. It is common sequelae of surgical intervention in the knee, obesity, trauma, and advancing age. A palpable mass in the popliteal crease with or without pain is a common clinical symptom. The distal aspect of the unruptured cyst tends to be teardrop shaped and smooth. When the cyst ruptures, the distal aspect may become pointed. Ruptured fluid may extravasate between the fascial planes of the lower leg muscles, commonly in the medial aspect of the lower leg.

Great care must be taken in the evaluation for Baker cyst that a neck or connection to the joint space is observed. If no connection to the joint space can be discerned, other neoplastic processes and vascular abnormalities must be considered. Color or power Doppler should always be employed in the evaluation of the posterior knee. When a meniscal cyst is encountered on the medial knee, the posterior knee should be evaluated for Baker cyst (Fig. 18-52A–G).

## Limitations of Pathology Evaluation

Sonography has limitations in evaluation of the meniscus and cruciate ligaments. The central portion of the meniscus, where many tears occur, is inaccessible by sonography. Dynamic maneuvers with imaging may benefit but techniques for this evaluation are challenging. The anterior and posterior cruciate ligaments may be difficult to evaluate with acute injury. Secondary findings of anterior cruciate injury can be found by performing a SAX projection over the posterior popliteal notch on the medial aspect of the lateral condyle. A hematoma can be seen in this area.

# ANKLE AND PLANTAR FASCIA

## ANATOMY

The ankle is the most frequently injured joint of the body. It is a complex diarthrosis joint with multiple articulations, ligaments, tendons, retinacula, and

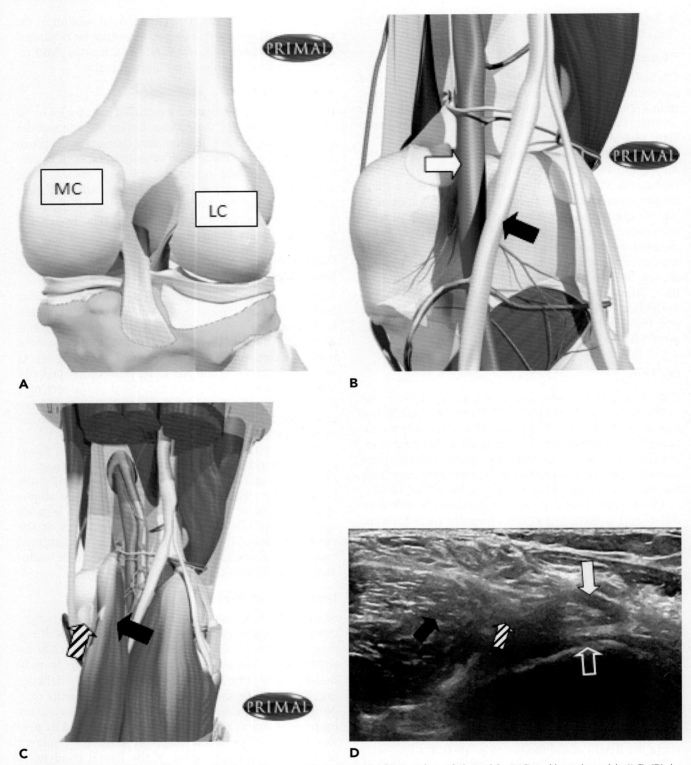

**Figure 18-45** Posterior knee. Shown on the illustrations are **(A)** the posterior knee with medial condyle (*MC*) and lateral condyle (*LC*), **(B)** the tibial nerve (*black arrow*) and tibial artery (*white arrow*), and **(C)** the medial head of the gastrocnemius muscle (*black arrow*) and the potential gastrocnemius-semimembranosus bursa (*striped arrow*). **D:** A short-axis image shows the posterior knee with the gastrocnemius muscle (*black arrow*), the semimembranosus tendon (*white arrow*), the area of bursa (*striped arrow*), and the medial condyle of the femur (*white open arrow*). (Images **A**, **B**, and **C** courtesy of Primal Pictures, Ltd., London, England.)

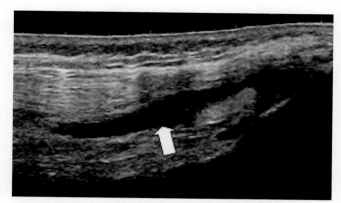

**Figure 18-46** Excess fluid. The long-axis sonogram of the suprapatellar bursa *(white arrow)* shows excessive fluid.

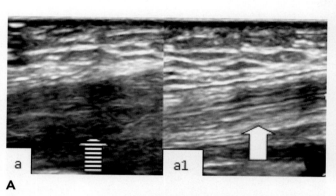

**A**

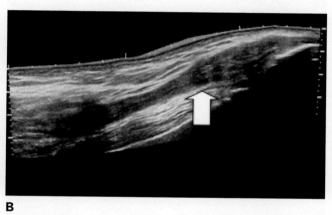

**B**

**Figure 18-47** Torn quadriceps tendon. **A:** A split screen long-axis image shows on the left *(a)* a torn quadriceps tendon *(striped arrow)* and on the right *(a1)*, a contralateral normal tendon *(white arrow)*. **B:** The panoramic long-axis image shows a torn and retracted quadriceps tendon *(white arrow)*.

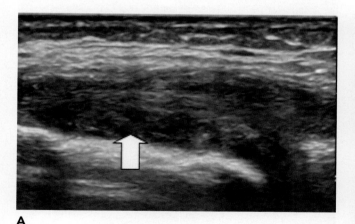

**A**

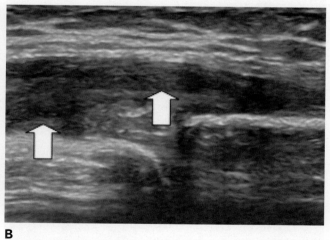

**B**

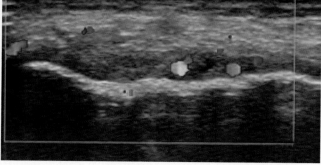

**C**

**Figure 18-48** Collateral ligaments. **A:** A long-axis image shows a tear of the medial collateral ligament at the femoral insertion *(white arrow)*, with ligament lifting off the bone. **B:** At the mid portion, the image shows an edematous ligament *(white arrows)* and **(C)** the color flow Doppler evaluation is on posttraumatic inflammation.

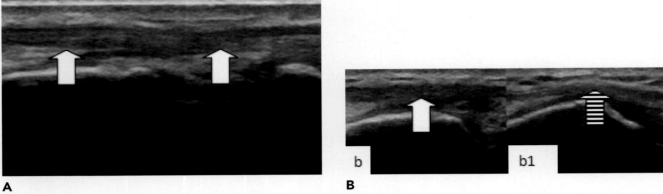

**A**

**B**

**Figure 18-49** Iliotibial band. **A:** The long-axis lateral image over the lateral condyle of femur shows a hypoechoic, thickened iliotibial band *(white arrows)*. **B:** On the image to the left *(b)*, an ipsilateral thickened iliotibial band *(white arrow)* can be compared to the contralateral image to the right *(b1)*, which shows a normal iliotibial band *(striped arrow)*.

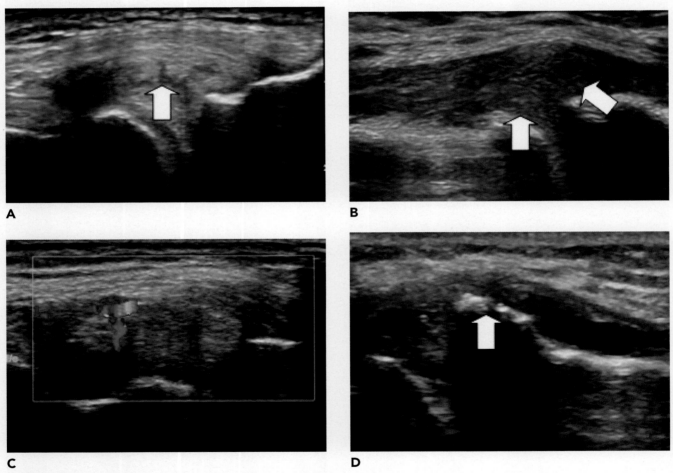

**A**

**B**

**C**

**D**

**Figure 18-50** Meniscus. **A:** A long-axis (LAX) image shows a hypoechoic radial tear in the meniscus *(white arrow)*. **B:** This LAX image demonstrates an extruded, intact meniscus *(white arrows)*. **C:** Directional power Doppler flow is used to evaluate a pathologic meniscus. **D:** An LAX image displays a degenerative spurring of the tibial condyle *(white arrow)*.

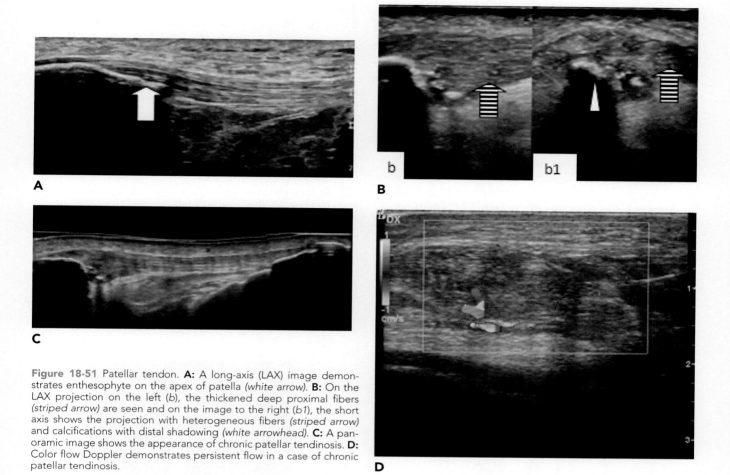

**Figure 18-51** Patellar tendon. **A:** A long-axis (LAX) image demonstrates enthesophyte on the apex of patella (*white arrow*). **B:** On the LAX projection on the left (*b*), the thickened deep proximal fibers (*striped arrow*) are seen and on the image to the right (*b1*), the short axis shows the projection with heterogeneous fibers (*striped arrow*) and calcifications with distal shadowing (*white arrowhead*). **C:** A panoramic image shows the appearance of chronic patellar tendinosis. **D:** Color flow Doppler demonstrates persistent flow in a case of chronic patellar tendinosis.

neurovascular structures. A brief description of the bone anatomy followed by soft tissue structures is described in regional correlation. The plantar fascia is included in this section.

## Bone

The primary long bone structures of the ankle are the tibia and fibula, which articulate distally with the talus and calcaneus. The tibia is the more medial of the two bones. The foot has seven tarsal (flat basket) bones, (calcaneus, talus, cuboid, medial cuneiform, intermediate cuneiform, lateral cuneiform, and navicular), which lie between the tibia and fibula and the metatarsal bones of the forefoot. The calcaneus is the largest of the tarsal bones with multiple facets for articulation with the most plantar section forming the heel. The talus, the second largest bone, forms the summit of the foot and in articulation with the tibia and fibula form the ankle joint proper. The talus and calcaneus are termed the hind foot, whereas the remaining five tarsal bones are considered the shock absorber of the foot and collectively form the mid foot. The distal surfaces of the tarsal bones articulate with the five metatarsal bones. All articulating surfaces of the bone structures are covered with articular cartilage.

The bones in combination with a vast array of ligaments and connective and fibrous capsular tissue form the many joints of the ankle and foot (Fig. 18-53A,B).

### Anterior Ankle

The anterior ankle is seldom involved in minor traumatic injuries. The primary structures of the anterior ankle are the extensor mechanism of the foot and ankle. The tibialis anterior is the largest and most medial of the extensor complex. The distal attachment of the tibialis anterior is on the medial aspect of the medial cuneiform and the base of the first metatarsal. The action of the tibialis anterior is dorsiflexion of the ankle and inversion of the foot. The tendon is the dorsal, soft tissue landmark for the anterior medial recess of the ankle (Fig. 18-54A–D).

Lateral to the tibialis anterior is the extensor hallucis longus (EHL) tendon. The extensor hallucis tendon is smaller than the tibialis anterior and distal insertion is dorsal on the aspect of the distal phalanx of the hallux (great toe). The primary action of the extensor hallucis is dorsiflexion of the great toe. Lateral to the extensor hallucis is the tendons of the extensor digitorum longus. The common tendon splits into individual slips for the lateral four toes and glides underneath the extensor retinaculum inserting on the dorsal base of the distal and middle phalanges. The primary responsibility of the extensor digitorum longus is dorsiflexion middle and distal phalanges of the lateral four toes.

## Lateral Ankle

The lateral ankle is the most often injured area of the ankle due to inversion foot injuries. There is a complex arrangement of ligaments, tendons, and muscle throughout the ankle; however, the most commonly imaged bone structure of the lateral ankle is the lateral malleolus of the fibula, the calcaneus, and talus. The soft tissue structures of the lateral ankle amendable to consistent sonograph evaluation are the anterior talofibular ligament (ATFL), calcaneal fibular ligament (CFL), and the anterior tibiofibular ligament (TFL) (Fig. 18-55A–D).

The tendinous elements evaluated of the lateral ankle can be very complex with many variations. The most common is the peroneus longus and peroneus brevis and the restraining superior peroneal retinaculum. The peroneus brevis distal attachment is on the styloid process of the base of the fifth metatarsal. The distal attachment for the peroneus longus is on the plantar base of the first metatarsal and the lateral surface of the medial cuneiform. The primary action of the peroneus longus and brevis tendons is eversion of the foot. The peroneus tendons are covered in a protective sheath that reduces tendon friction (Fig. 18-55E–H).

## Medial Ankle

The medial ankle is a complex of tendons, neurovascular structures, and ligaments. The primary hard tissue landmarks are the medial malleolus of the tibia, calcaneus, talus, and navicular bones.

A pneumonic devised to identify the relevant soft tissue structures of the medial ankle is "Tom, Dick, and a very nervous Harry." The pneumonic identifies anatomy from the medial malleolus posteriorly. The first, and most

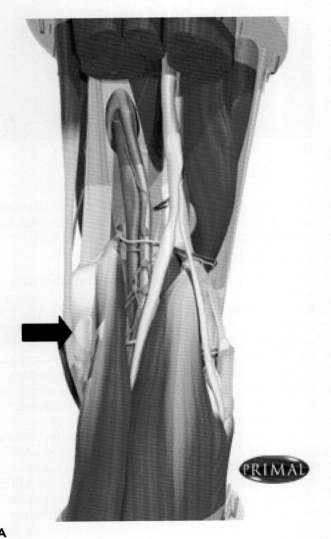

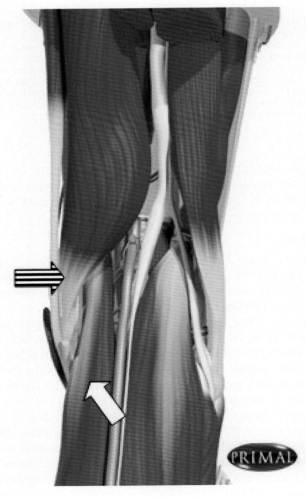

**A**　　　　　　　　　　　　　　　　　　　**B**

**Figure 18-52** Posterior knee pathology. The illustrations show **(A)** the posterior knee gastrocnemius-semimembranosus bursa *(black arrow)* and **(B)** semimembranosus muscle and tendon *(striped arrow)* and medial head of gastrocnemius muscle *(solid white arrow)*. *(continued)*

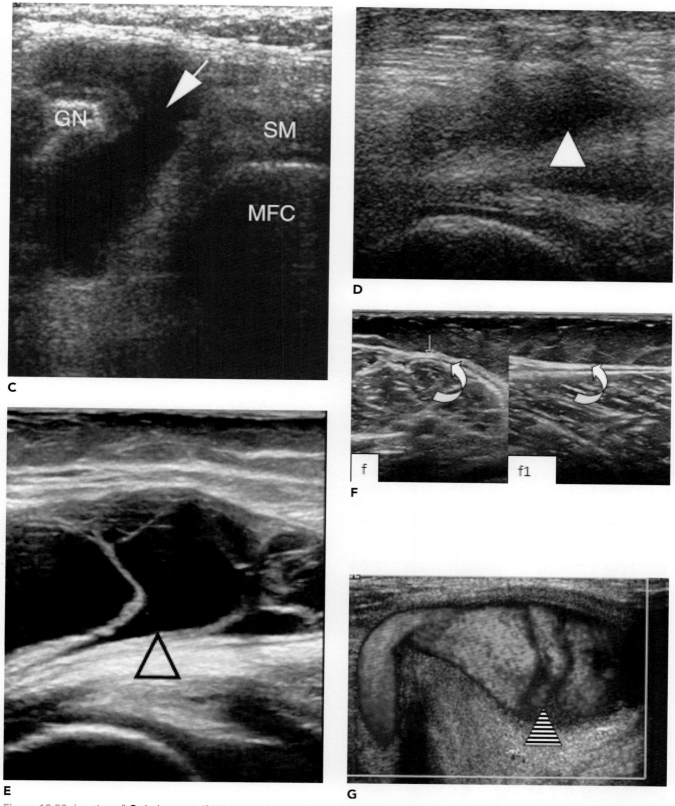

**Figure 18-52** *(continued)* **C:** A short-axis (SAX) image shows a Baker cyst *(arrow)*. *GN,* gastrocnemius; *SM,* semimembranosus; *MFC,* medial femoral condyle. **D:** The SAX image demonstrates a Baker cyst *(white arrowhead)*. **E:** A long-axis (LAX) image displays a complex Baker cyst *(black open arrow)* with septae. **F:** The SAX split image shows on the left *(f)* fluid tracking calf muscles *(curved arrow)* and on the right *(f1)* a LAX of fluid *(curved arrow)* adjacent to calf muscles. **G:** An image obtained with power Doppler demonstrates a popliteal artery aneurysm *(striped arrow)*. (Images **A** and **B** courtesy of Primal Pictures, Ltd., London, England.)

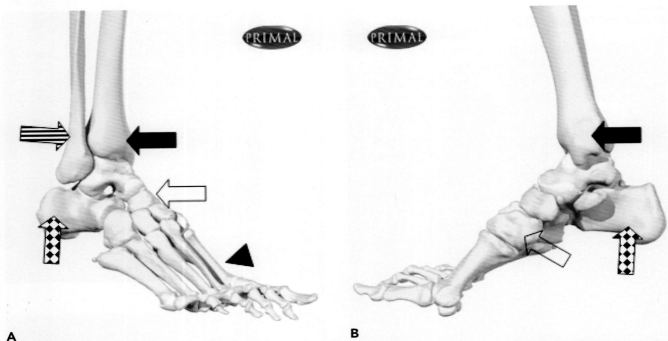

**Figure 18-53** Ankle and foot. **A:** The illustration of the lateral ankle shows the fibula *(striped arrow)*, calcaneus *(diamond arrow)*, tibia *(black arrow)*, tarsal bones *(white arrow)*, and metatarsals *(black arrowhead)*. **B:** On the medial ankle, the illustration shows the tibia *(black arrow)*, calcaneus *(diamond arrow)*, and tarsal bones *(open arrow)*. (Images **A** and **B** courtesy of Primal Pictures, Ltd., London, England.)

important, tendon of the medial ankle is the posterior tibialis tendon (PTT). The PTT is closely associated with the medial malleolus with a distal attachment primarily on the tuberosity of the navicular but has portions attaching to all tarsal bones except the talus and small segments to the base of the second, third, and fourth metatarsals. The primary role of the PTT is to support or maintain the medial longitudinal arch during weight-bearing, thus

acting as a major stabilizer of the hindfoot. Stretching of the PTT and muscle leads to adult flatfoot and a dorsiflexed talus. Surgical intervention is required if there is a poor result of conservative measures to correct flatfoot and a dorsiflexed talus. Directing posteriorly, the second part of the pneumonic, "Dick," refers to the flexor digitorum longus (FDL) tendon. Compared to the PTT, the FDL tendon is one-third to one-half the size. The FDL

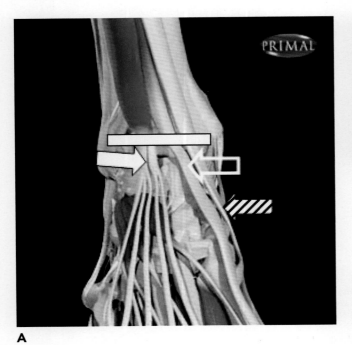

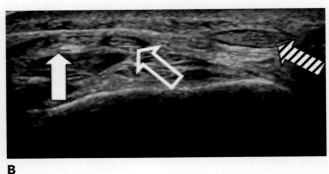

**Figure 18-54** Anterior ankle. **A:** The illustration of the anterior ankle shows the transducer position *(white rectangle)*, extensor digitorum *(white arrow)*, extensor hallucis longus *(open arrow)*, and anterior tibialis *(striped arrow)*. **B:** The short-axis image shows the anterior ankle, tibialis anterior *(striped arrow)*, extensor hallucis *(white open arrow)*, and extensor digitorum *(solid white arrow)*. *(continued)*

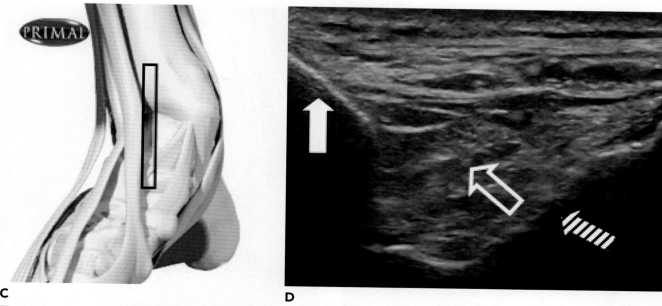

**Figure 18-54** *(continued)* **C:** The illustration shows the transducer position *(black rectangle)* to evaluate the anterior recess. **D:** The long-axis image shows the anterior recess, tibia *(white arrow)*, fat pad *(open arrow)*, and talar dome *(striped arrow)*. (Images **A** and **C** courtesy of Primal Pictures, Ltd., London, England.)

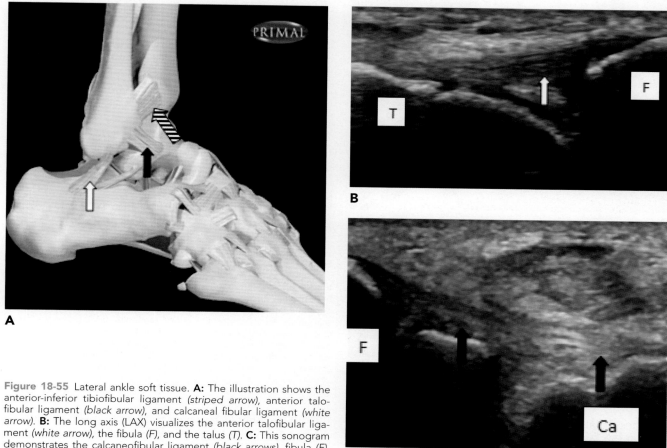

**Figure 18-55** Lateral ankle soft tissue. **A:** The illustration shows the anterior-inferior tibiofibular ligament *(striped arrow)*, anterior talofibular ligament *(black arrow)*, and calcaneal fibular ligament *(white arrow)*. **B:** The long axis (LAX) visualizes the anterior talofibular ligament *(white arrow)*, the fibula *(F)*, and the talus *(T)*. **C:** This sonogram demonstrates the calcaneofibular ligament *(black arrows)*, fibula *(F)*, and calcaneus *(Ca)*. *(continued)*

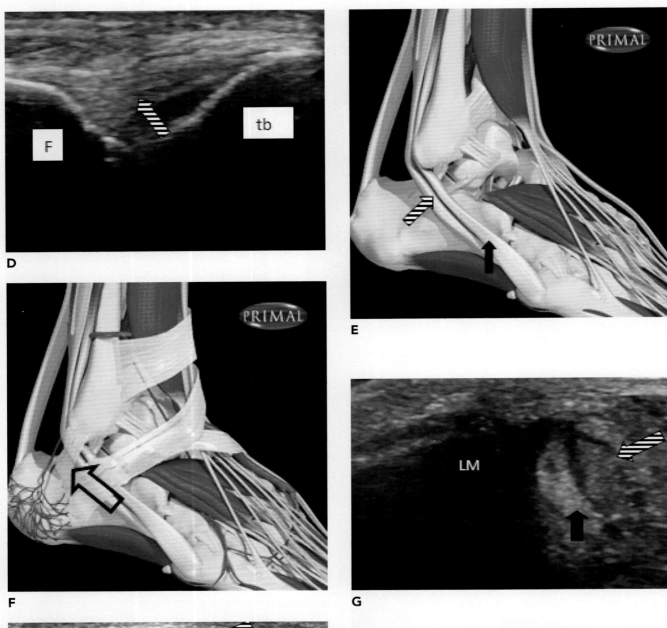

**Figure 18-55** *(continued)* **D:** Seen on this image is the tibiofibular ligament *(striped arrow)*, the fibular *(F)*, and the tibia *(tb)*. Lateral ankle tendons. The illustrations of the lateral ankle show **(E)** the peroneus brevis *(black arrow)* and peroneus longus *(striped arrow)* and **(F)** the peroneal retinaculum *(black arrow)*. **G:** The short-axis image of the lateral ankle demonstrates the lateral malleolus *(LM)*, peroneus brevis *(black arrow)*, and peroneus longus *(striped arrow)*. **H:** The LAX image demonstrates the peroneus longus *(striped arrow)*, the peroneus brevis *(solid white arrow)*, and lateral malleolus *(LM)*. (Images **A**, **E**, and **F** courtesy of Primal Pictures, Ltd., London, England.)

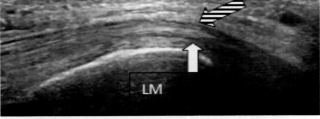

attaches distally to the plantar surface of the distal phalanx of the four lateral toes allowing flexion of the phalanges. A secondary function includes plantar flexion of the ankle joint and delimiting dorsiflexion of the digits during walking. With rupture of the PTT, the FDL may slide medially into the vacated position of the ruptured PTT. Care should be taken to identify this condition by using flexion and extension of the digits to distinguish the abnormally displaced FDL into the event of suspected PTT rupture. Continuing posterior, the sonographer encounters the sustentaculum tali, a horizontal eminence of the calcaneus, which supports part of the talus. The sustentaculum tali serves as a hard surface for the insertion of elements of the deltoid ligament and can be used to locate the position of the third part of the pneumonic, "very nervous," which demarcates the tibial artery, commonly paired veins and tibial nerve (Fig. 18-56A–D). The final, and most posterior located element of the pneumonic, "Harry," is the flexor hallucis longus (FHL). The primary action of the FHL is flexion of the hallus with a secondary action of flexion of the foot at the ankle. Distal attachment of the FHL is primarily on the distal phalanx of the hallux or great toe. Smaller attachments insert onto the base of the second and third toe.

## Posterior Ankle

The most prominent and commonly affected anatomic structure of the posterior ankle is the Achilles tendon. The relevant hard tissue structure is the calcaneus. The Achilles tendon has a broad insertion on the most posterior surface of the calcaneus (Fig. 18-57A–F).

The Achilles tendon (tendo calcaneus) is the largest and strongest of the tendons of the body measuring approximately 14 to 15 cm long and 5.4 to 6.2 mm in anteroposterior (AP), and 9 to 13 mm coronal.[35] It receives contributory fibers from the aponeurosis of the gastrocnemius and the soleus muscles. Due to the nature of

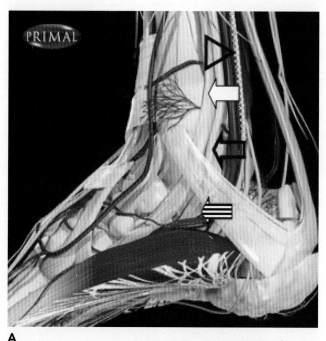

A

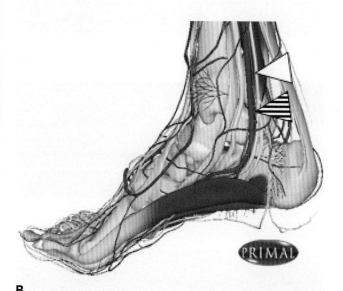

B

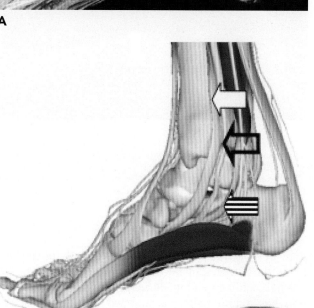

C

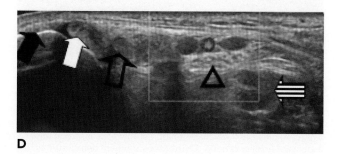

D

**Figure 18-56** Medial ankle. **A.** The cut-down illustrations show the medial ankle, the posterior tibialis tendon (*solid white arrow*), flexor digitorum longus (*black open arrow*), flexor hallucis longus (*striped arrow*), and tibial nerve (*black open arrowhead*). **B:** The tibial veins (*white arrowhead*) and tibial artery (*striped arrowhead*); and **(C)** the close proximity of the posterior tibialis (*white arrow*), flexor digitorum longus (*black open arrow*), and flexor hallucis (*striped arrow*) to bone. **D:** The short-axis image of medial ankle demonstrates the medial malleolus (*black arrow*), posterior tibialis (*white arrow*), flexor digitorum longus (*black open arrow*), tibial artery with power Doppler, tibial nerve (*black open arrowhead*), and the flexor hallucis longus (*striped arrow*). (Images **A**, **B**, and **C** courtesy of Primal Pictures, Ltd., London, England.)

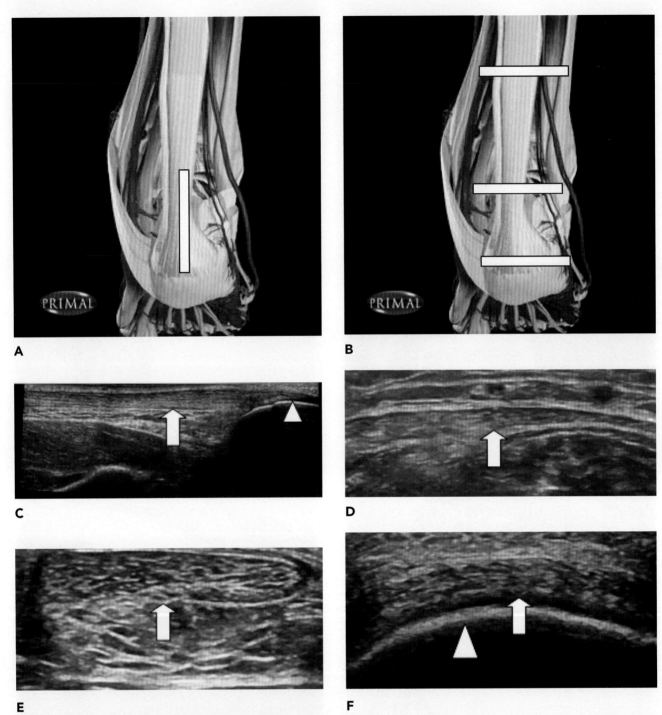

**Figure 18-57** Posterior ankle. The illustrations of the posterior ankle shows the transducer placements (*white rectangular box*) for **(A)** the long-axis (LAX) plane of the Achilles tendon at the distal insertion midline section and **(B)** the short-axis (SAX) plane at the proximal, mid, and distal aspects of Achilles tendon. **C:** The LAX sonogram demonstrates the distal Achilles tendon (*white arrow*) at the insertion of posterior calcaneus (*white arrowhead*). **D:** The proximal SAX sonogram shows the aponeurosis (*white arrow*) where the flattened broad tendon gives way to muscle. **E:** The SAX displays the vascular watershed area (*white arrow*). **F:** The distal SAX sonogram shows the insertion on calcaneus (*white arrowhead*) of the Achilles tendon (*white arrow*). (Images **A** and **B** courtesy of Primal Pictures, Ltd., London, England.)

the insertion of the soleus fibers on the medial aspect of the calcaneus and the gastrocnemius fibers inserting on the lateral aspect, a SAX transducer translation from proximal to distal will demonstrate a swirling motion of the fibers which should not be mistaken for pathology. The plantaris tendon inserts on the medial aspect of the calcaneus. In 20% of normal individuals, the plantaris

may be absent.[36] It should be noted that the normal plantaris tendon can be difficult to separate from the normal Achilles tendon. Structurally, the Achilles tendon has a minimally vascularized area, the vascular watershed section, which is located 2 to 6 cm proximal from the insertion on the calcaneus. The vascular watershed area is the most common site for rupture. Anterior to and adjacent to the posterior surface of the calcaneus is the retrocalcaneal bursa. Anterior and proximal from the Achilles tendon is the extra-articular Kager fat pad. In rupture of the Achilles tendon, Kager fat may inject posterior into the area of disrupted tendon fibers.

## Plantar Fascia

The plantar fascia is a relatively thick fibrous band of connective tissue extending from the tubercles of the calcaneus to the base of all five digits on the plantar surface of the foot. It is composed of three cords—medial, central, and lateral—and the central cord is the thickest and most commonly affected in plantar fasicitis. The primary function of the plantar fascia is the distribution of weight, arch support, and a function in gait. The medial band of the plantar fascia is the most commonly affected section in plantar fasciitis (Fig. 18-58A-D).

## PATHOLOGY

### Ankle Sprain

The ankle sprain is the most common injury of the ankle and up to 80% of all ankle sprains involve the lateral ligament complex caused by ankle inversion with the foot in plantar flexion.[37,38] A simple classification is as follows: grade 1, mild (microscopic without

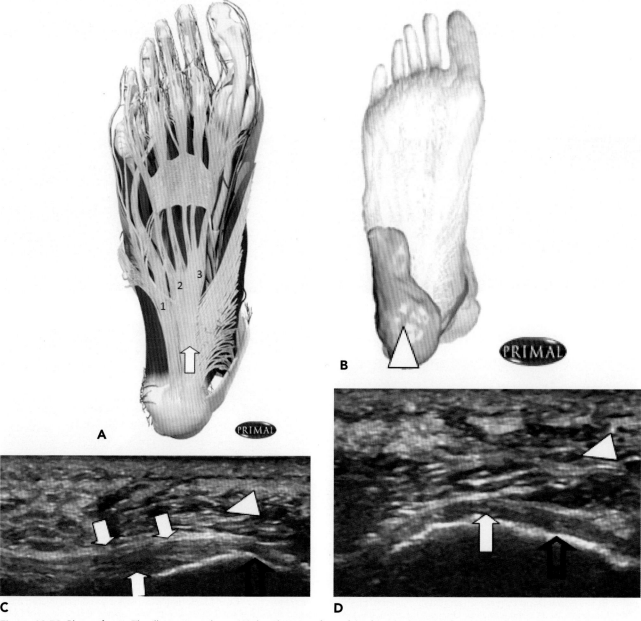

**Figure 18-58** Plantar fascia. The illustrations shows **(A)** the plantar surface of the foot the lateral *(1)*, mid *(2)*, and medial band of plantar fascia *(white arrow)* and **(B)** a thick heel pad *(white arrowhead)*. **C:** The long-axis image displays the plantar fascia *(white arrows)* insertion on the calcaneus *(black open arrow)* and the heterogeneous heel pad *(white arrowhead)*. **D:** The short-axis image displays the plantar fascia *(white arrow)* insertion on the calcaneus *(open black arrow)* and thick heel pad *(white arrowhead)*. (Images **A** and **B** courtesy of Primal Pictures, Ltd., London, England.)

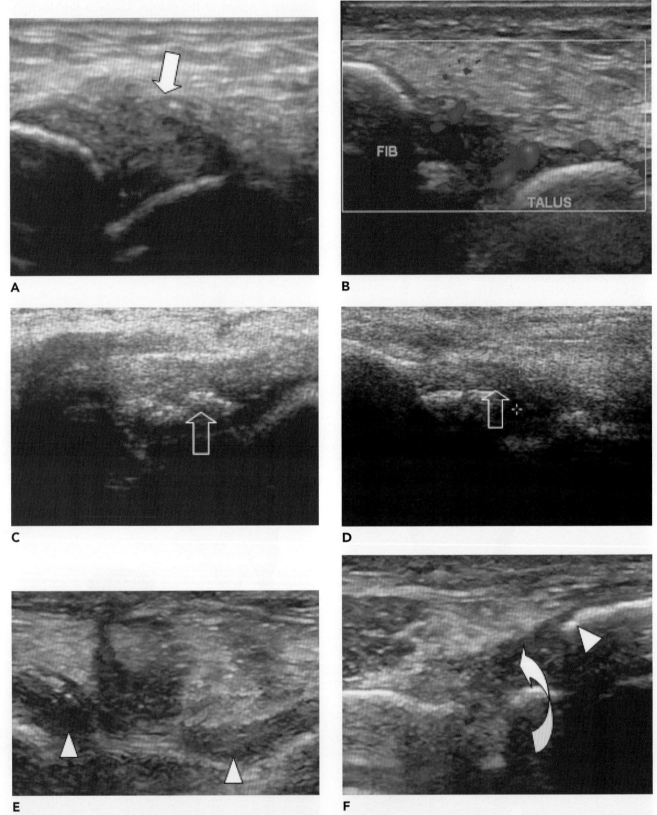

**Figure 18-59** Anterior talofibular ligament (ATFL). **A:** The sonogram shows a disrupted ATFL with no fibers seen and extrusion of fat (*white arrow*). **B:** The power Doppler image on an acutely injured ATFL shows inflammatory flow. **C:** The sonograms displays a chronically injured ATFL with calcification (*white open arrow*). **D:** On this sonogram, there is a thickened ATFL in chronic injury (*white open arrow*). *CFL*, calcaneofibular ligament. **E:** The long-axis image displays an acute rupture with hypoechoic thickened stumps (*white arrowheads*). **F:** The sonogram displays a thickened heterogeneous CFL (*curved arrow*) acute injury with small avulsion fracture (*white arrowhead*).

stretching on the macroscopic level); grade 2, moderate (macroscopic stretching but the ligament remains intact); and grade 3, severe (complete rupture of ligament).[38,39] Chronic instability occurs in 20% of ankle sprains. The most commonly affected ligaments in order of injury are as follows: ATFL, the CFL, and in high ankle sprains, the most serious, TFL (Fig. 18-59A–F).

## Lateral Ankle

Tendon pathology of the lateral ankle involves the PB and longus (PL) injuries, which may be a result of acute trauma or chronic overuse. Tendinopathies range from acute and chronic tendinous, horizontal splits, rupture with tendon retraction, subluxation, and dislocations. The spectrum of sonographic manifestations range from thickening, thickening with areas of focal hypoechoic sections, splits, rupture, and disassociation (Fig. 18-60A–D).

## Medial Ankle

There are numerous pathologies in the medial ankle. The most commonly affected is the PTT. Pathology is more prevalent in obese females. Degrees of pathology range from simple enlargement to disruption. PTT pathology is associated with systemic disease processes such as rheumatoid arthritis. A SAX PTT evaluation from the proximal muscle through insertion assists in making the correct diagnosis. Stretching or disruption of the tendon can lead to flatfoot and excessive pronation[40] (Fig. 18-61A–G). Split screen ipsilateral to contralateral comparison is a "best practice" when unsure. In situations of suspected complete rupture of PTT, it is advised that the sonographer assures all three medial tendons can be visualized. Translation of the FDL toward the medial malleolus is not uncommon in complete disruption of the posterior tibialis. If suspect, flex

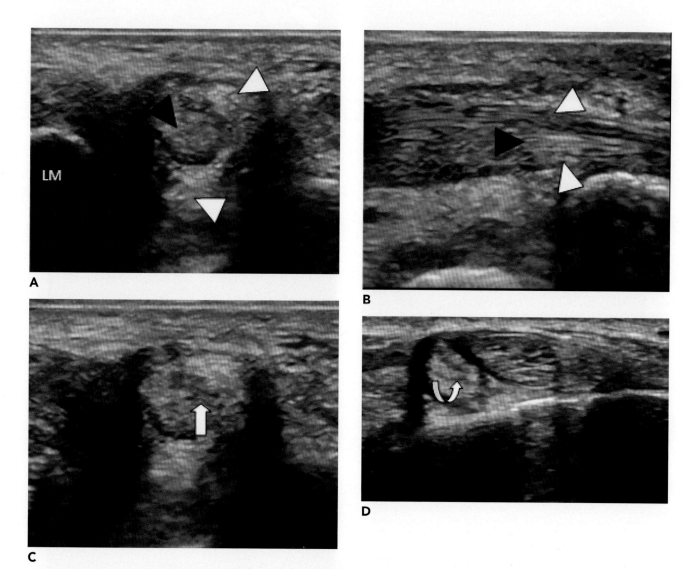

**Figure 18-60** Peroneus longus (PL) and peroneus brevis tendons (PB). **A:** The short-axis (SAX) sonogram shows the posterior lateral malleolus illustrating a split of PB *(white arrowheads)* with PL within *(black arrowhead)*. **B:** The long axis on the same patient as in image **(A)** shows the PL *(black arrowhead)* within the split PB *(white arrowheads)*. **C:** The SAX image shows a vertical split *(white arrow)* in the PB. **D:** The SAX sonogram visualizes multiple splits in the PB *(curved arrow)*.

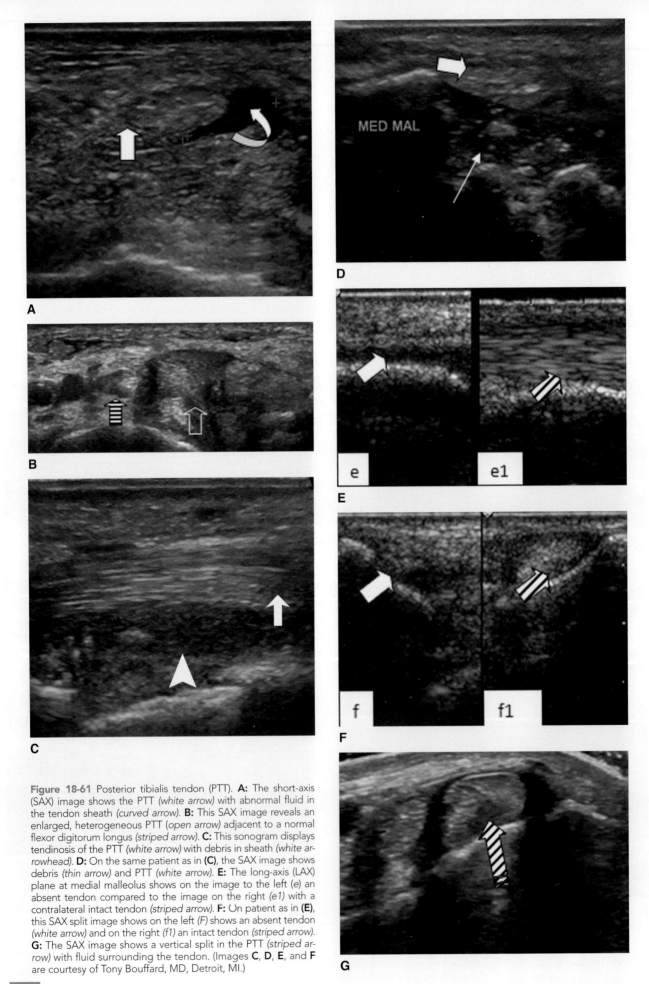

**Figure 18-61** Posterior tibialis tendon (PTT). **A:** The short-axis (SAX) image shows the PTT *(white arrow)* with abnormal fluid in the tendon sheath *(curved arrow)*. **B:** This SAX image reveals an enlarged, heterogeneous PTT *(open arrow)* adjacent to a normal flexor digitorum longus *(striped arrow)*. **C:** This sonogram displays tendinosis of the PTT *(white arrow)* with debris in sheath *(white arrowhead)*. **D:** On the same patient as in **(C)**, the SAX image shows debris *(thin arrow)* and PTT *(white arrow)*. **E:** The long-axis (LAX) plane at medial malleolus shows on the image to the left *(e)* an absent tendon compared to the image on the right *(e1)* with a contralateral intact tendon *(striped arrow)*. **F:** On patient as in **(E)**, this SAX split image shows on the left *(F)* shows an absent tendon *(white arrow)* and on the right *(f1)* an intact tendon *(striped arrow)*. **G:** The SAX image shows a vertical split in the PTT *(striped arrow)* with fluid surrounding the tendon. (Images **C**, **D**, **E**, and **F** are courtesy of Tony Bouffard, MD, Detroit, MI.)

and extend the digits of the foot and check for tendon slip for a displaced FHL.

Less frequently encountered pathologies include entrapment or compression of the tibial nerve in the tarsal tunnel.

### Posterior Ankle

Pathology of the posterior ankle will focus on the Achilles tendon and retrocalcaneal bursa. Intrinsic tendon pathology may be a result of systemic disease such as gout and diabetes. Pathology may occur anywhere in the tendon. For brevity, a focus on the distal insertion on the calcaneus, enthesopathy, and the vascular watershed area will be discussed. The vascular watershed area is located 2 to 6 cm proximal to the Achilles tendon insertion is a common site for the full spectrum of tendinopathy. It is rare to observe any vascularity in the vascular watershed area as this area is devoid of large caliber vessels. Leung et al.[41] described sonographic findings in tendinopathy of the Achilles as enlargement in both the AP and cross-sectional area in the mid and distal portions of the tendon, disruption of the fibrillar pattern, and increased vascularity.[41] Increased echogenicity in Kager fat was observed as a secondary sign. Retrocalcaneal bursitis, manifests as an enlargement of the normal bursa with excess fluid, >1 to 2 mm. Imaging must be correlated with clinical symptoms as in any disease process. Inflammation of the tissue surrounding the tendon, the paratenon, may cause pain without rupture. In paratendon disease, the tendon essentially maintains the fibrillar signature while the paratenon enlarges and becomes hypoechoic and may become hypervascular (Fig. 18-62A–I).

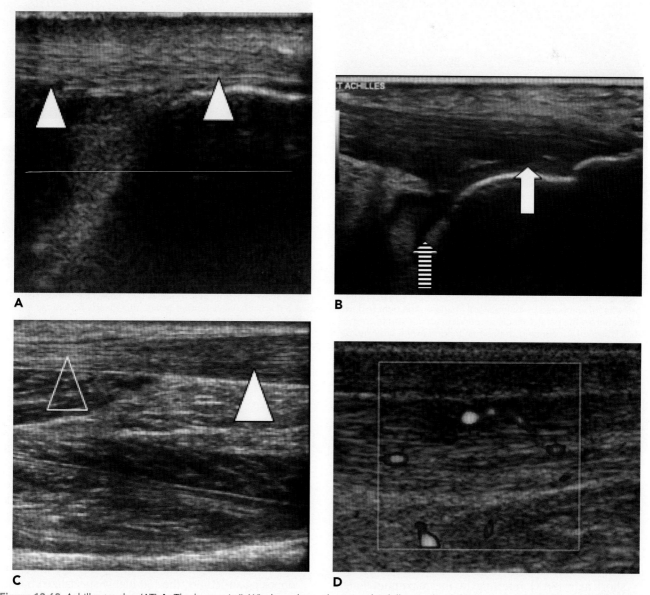

**Figure 18-62** Achilles tendon (AT) **A:** The long-axis (LAX) plane shows the normal Achilles tendon (*white arrowheads*). **B:** This image displays Achilles tendinosis (*white arrow*) with edematous, hypoechoic tendon, and retrocalcaneal bursitis (*striped arrow*). **C.** The LAX image shows tendinosis (*white arrowhead*) and adjacent normal tendon (*open arrowhead*). **D:** The power Doppler evaluation demonstrates inflammation of the Achilles tendon. (*continued*)

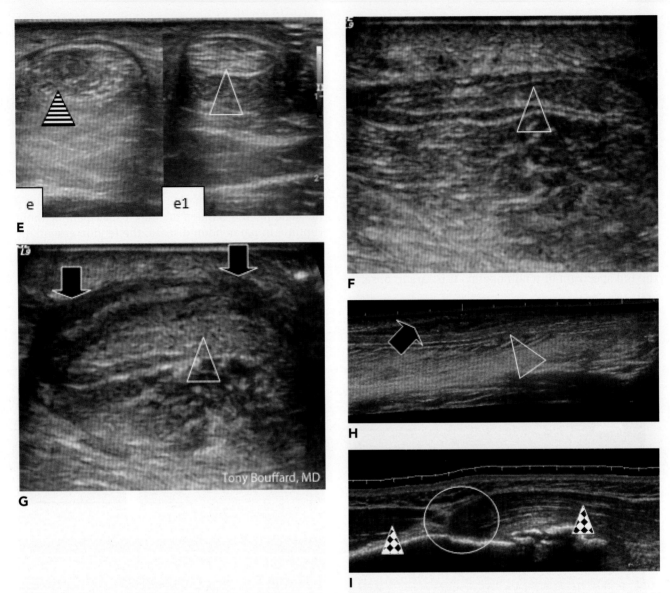

**Figure 18-62** *(continued)* **E:** A short-axis (SAX) split screen image on the left (*e*) shows a hypoechoic region within the Achilles tendon (*striped arrowhead*) compared to contralateral image on the right (*e1*), which shows a normal Achilles tendon (*white arrowhead*). **F:** A proximal SAX image shows the paratendinitis surrounding tendon (*white arrowhead*). **G:** This SAX distal from the image in illustrates a thickened paratenon (*black arrows*) surrounding the normal tendon (*white arrowhead*). **H:** The panoramic image shows paratendinitis with thickened paratenon (*black arrow*) and normal tendon (*white arrowhead*) and **(I)** the LAX panoramic image shows complete rupture of Achilles tendon (*white circle*) and distal a proximal stumps (*diamond arrowheads*). (Images **G** and **H** are courtesy of Tony Bouffard, MD, Detroit, MI.)

## SUMMARY

- The accuracy and sensitivity of sonography for musculoskeletal evaluation as an adjunct or primary imaging modality with specificity and sensitivity approaches and in some cases exceeds the accuracy of the gold standards in imaging when performed by skilled sonographers.

- Sonography evaluation of the musculoskeletal system are described in terms of long axis (LAX) and short axis (SAX) referring to the maximum length and maximum width of the structure respectively in orthogonal planes.

- Anisotropy is the change in the properties of a structure when measured or evaluated in different directions.

- Common transducer manipulation techniques for musculoskeletal evaluation include "heel-toe," "rocking or toggling," transducer "translation," "fanning or twisting," and "floating" the transducer.

- Located at high-potential friction points where tendons or muscles are required to slip through or around opposing structures, the 150 highly specialized bursae are synovial lined pouches that produce and maintain a viscous fluid to aid in tendon and muscle slip.

- Although nerves are divided into sensory and motor function, sonographically, they have identical appearances.

- Ligaments have a similar tissue signature as tendons when scanned at a 90-degree angle but an imaging challenge is created due to their attachment angles and sound absorbing osseous structures.

- Sonographic evaluation of mineralized bone defies penetration beyond the subchondral bone structure but acoustic changes in articular and nonarticular bone surfaces may lead the sonographer to focus on soft tissue evaluation in the area adjacent to or at the attachment site of a tendon or ligament.

- Fibrocartilage found in the menisci of the knee, pubic symphysis, and acromioclavicular joint displays a medium echogenicity and is homogeneous with minimal changes throughout its structure, whereas articular or hyaline cartilage located at the terminal ends of bone in any joint displays a hypoechoic, noncompressible layer in contact with the bone surface.

- Normal subcutaneous fat may have a heterogeneous appearance with hypoechoic fat lobules interspaced with connective tissue, whereas fat pads found on articular surfaces surrounded by a fibrous capsule are more hyperechoic and homogeneous in appearance.

- The shoulder joint is one of the most common joints evaluated by sonography and requires an understanding of the hard tissue (bone) and the primary attachments of the critical soft tissue structures evaluated in the rotator cuff.

- The shoulder is always a complete study unless contraindicated by patient condition or for interventional procedures.

- Pathology of the shoulder is generally associated with conditions or disease of the rotator cuff tendons, which may include tendinopathies, chronic and acute shoulder instability, neuropathies, and pathologies of the AC joint.

- The elbow is a medium-sized complex synovial joint, is often involved in overuse injuries, and is often a targeted evaluation based on clinical history.

- The wrist is a complex diarthrosis, freely movable joint and is sonographically a targeted study based on clinical symptoms and history.

- Most pathology of the wrist, outside of trauma, results from overuse and/or compression etiologies.

- Sonography evaluation of the hinge, diarthrosis, synovial lined knee joint is a targeted study in most institutions.

- Sonography has limitations in evaluating the pathology of the meniscus and cruciate ligaments.

- The ankle is a diarthrosis, complex joint, which is the most frequently injured joint in the body.

- The plantar fascia is a thick fibrous connective tissue band extending from the calcaneus to the base of all five digits and functions to distribute weight, provide arch support, and gait.

- The chapter is an abbreviated description of commonly encountered structures and pathologies of the larger joints and is not comprehensive or conclusive.

- Successful evaluation of the musculoskeletal system requires the sonographer to be able to obtain an adequate history, understand the hard (bone) and soft tissue structure of the joint being evaluated, and to adequately image the suspect area.

- Implementing dynamic imaging, dynamic clips, and master tissue-insonation angles are practical techniques that will encourage successful imaging of the desired anatomy.

## Critical Thinking Questions

1. Explain the musculoskeletal imaging planes and annotation and a rationale for using LAX and SAX versus sagittal, coronal, or transverse.

2. If a sonographer is having difficulty visualizing the ligaments, what technique should be employed before terminating the examination?

3. A 17-year-old girl presents with an ankle injury by "rolling" over the outside of her ankle. She has swelling, hemorrhage, and tenderness over the right ankle. The orthopedist notes there is functional loss with marked abnormalities in joint motion and joint instability. The gray scale sonogram shows a complete ligament rupture. Based on the clinical presentation and sonographic findings, what is the most likely diagnosis?

4. A 52-year-old woman presents with a dull chronic shoulder pain, rotational pain, diminished range of motion, and general arm weakness with elevation. Based on her clinical presentation, list a minimum of two differential diagnoses.

5. What term describes exhibiting sound properties that vary with direction from a 90-degree perpendicular, incident angle and how can the sonographer correct for the artifact?

## REFERENCES

1. Roberts CS, Beck DJ Jr, Heinsen J, et al. Review article: diagnostic ultrasonography: applications in orthopaedic surgery. *Clin Orthop Relat Res.* 2002;401:248–264.

2. Naredo E, D'Agostino MA, Conaghan PG, et al. Current state of musculoskeletal ultrasound training and implementation in Europe: results of a survey of experts and scientific societies. *Rheumatology (Oxford).* 2010;49:2438–2443.

3. Nofsinger C, Konin JG. Diagnostic ultrasound in sports medicine: current concepts and advances. *Sports Med Arthrosc.* 2009;17:25–30.

4. Broadhurst NA, Simmons N. Musculoskeletal ultrasound–used to best advantage. *Aust Fam Physician.* 2007;36:430–432.

5. Buchberger W, Judmaier W, Birbamer G, et al. Carpal tunnel syndrome: diagnosis with high-resolution sonography. *AJR Am J Roentgenol.* 1992;159:793–798.

6. Miller TT, Shapiro MA, Schultz E, et al. Comparison of sonography and MRI for diagnosing epicondylitis. *J Clin Ultrasound.* 2002;30:193–202.

7. Nallamshetty L, Nazarian LN, Schweitzer ME, et al. Evaluation of posterior tibial pathology: comparison of sonography and MR imaging. *Skeletal Radiol.* 2005;34:375–380.

8. Teefey SA, Rubin DA, Middleton WD, et al. Detection and quantification of rotator cuff tears. Comparison of ultrasonographic, magnetic resonance imaging, and arthroscopic findings in seventy-one consecutive cases. *J Bone Joint Surg Am.* 2004;86:708–716.

9. Kang CH, Kim SS, Kim JH,, et al. Supraspinatus tendon tears: comparison of 3D US and MR arthrography with surgical correlation. *Skeletal Radiol.* 2009;38:1063–1069.

10. Lee KS, Rosas HG, Craig JG. Musculoskeletal ultrasound: elbow imaging and procedures. *Semin Musculoskelet Radiol.* 2010;14:449–460.

11. Hashefi M. Ultrasound in the diagnosis of noninflammatory musculoskeletal conditions. *Ann N Y Acad Sci.* 2009;1154:171–203.

12. Fornage BD, Touche DH, Edeiken-Monroe BS. The tendons. In: Rumack CM, Wilson SR, Charbonneau JW, et al., eds. *Diagnostic Ultrasound.* 4th ed. Vol 1. Philadelphia, PA: Elsevier Mosby; 2011:902–934.

13. Silvestri E, Martinoli C, Derchi LE, et al. Echotexture of peripheral nerves: correlation between US and histologic findings and criteria to differentiate tendons. *Radiology.* 1995;197:291–296.

14. Patten RM, Mack LA, Wang KY, et al. Nondisplaced fractures of the greater tuberosity of the humerus: sonographic detection. *Radiology.* 1992;182:201–204.

15. Cross KP, Warkentine FH, Kim IK, et al. Bedside ultrasound diagnosis of clavicle fractures in the pediatric emergency department. *Acad Emerg Med.* 2010;17:687–693.

16. Vasios WN, Hubler DA, Lopez RA, et al. Fracture detection in a combat theater: four cases comparing ultrasound to conventional radiography. *J Spec Oper Med.* 2010;10:11–15.

17. Patton KT, Thibodeau GA. *Anatomy and Physiology.* 7th ed. St. Louis, MO: Mosby; 2010.

18. Moore K, Dalley A, Agur A. *Clinically Oriented Anatomy.* 6th ed. Philadelphia, PA: Lippincott Williams & Wilkins; 2010.

19. American Institute of Ultrasound in Medicine. AIUM practice guidelines for the performance of the musculoskeletal ultrasound examination. October 2007. Available at: http://www.aium.org/publications/guidelines/musculoskeletal.pdf. Accessed March 14, 2010.

20. European Society of MusculoSkeletal Radiology. Musculoskeletal ultrasound technical guidelines: I. Shoulder. Available at: http://www.essr.org/html/img/pool/shoulder.pdf. Accessed March 14, 2011.

21. Tracy MR, Trella TA, Nazarrian LN. Sonography of coracohumeral interval: a potential technique for diagnosing coracoid impingement. *J Ultrasound Med.* 2010;29:337–341.

22. Bouffard JA, Lee SM, Dhanju J. Ultrasound of the shoulder. *Semin in Ultrasound CT MR.* 2000;21:164–191.

23. Jacobson JA, Lancaster S, Prasad A, et al. Full-thickness and partial thickness supraspinatus tendon tears: value of US signs in diagnosis. *Radiology.* 2004;230:234–242.

24. van Holsbeeck M, Introcaso JH, Kolowich PA. Sonography of tendons: patterns of disease. *Instr Course Lect.* 1994;43:475–481.

25. Wohlwend JR, van Holsbeeck M, Craig J, et al. The association between irregular greater tuberosities and rotator cuff tears: a sonographic study. *AJR Am J Roentgenol.* 1998;171:229–233.

26. Tirman PF, Bost FW, Garvin GJ, et al. Posterosuperior glenoid impingement of the shoulder: findings at MR imaging and MR arthrography with arthroscopic correlation. *Radiology.* 1994;193:431–436.

27. van Holsbeeck M, Strouse PJ. Sonography of the shoulder: evaluation of the subacromial-subdeltoid bursa. *AJR Am J Roentgenol.* 1993;160:561–564.

28. Middleton WD, Edelstein G, Reinus WR, et al. Sonographic detection of rotator cuff tears. *AJR Am J Roentgenol.* 1985;144:349–353.

29. Smith J, Finnoff JT, O'Driscoll SW, et al. Sonographic evaluation of the distal biceps tendon using a medial approach: the pronator window. *J Ultrasound Med.* 2010;29:861–865.

30. Tagliafico A, Michaud J, Capaccio E, et al. Ultrasound demonstration of distal biceps tendon bifurcation: normal and abnormal findings. *Eur Radiol.* 2010;20:202–208.

31. Connell D, Burke F, Coombes P, et al. Sonographic examination of lateral epicondylitis. *AJR Am J Roentgenol.* 2001;176:777–782.

32. European Society of MusculoSkeletal Radiology. Musculoskeletal ultrasound technical guidelines: II. Elbow. Available at: http://www.essr.org/html/img/pool/elbow.pdf. Accessed March 14, 2011.

33. European Society of MusculoSkeletal Radiology. Musculoskeletal ultrasound technical guidelines: III. Wrist. Available at: http://www.essr.org/html/img/pool/wrist.pdf. Accessed March 14, 2011.

34. Klauser AS, Halpern EJ, De Zordo T, et al. Carpal tunnel syndrome assessment with US: value of additional cross-sectional area measurements of the median nerve in patients versus healthy volunteers. *Radiology.* 2009;250:171–177.

35. van Holsbeeck M, Introcaso JH. *Musculoskeletal Ultrasound.* St. Louis, MO: Mosby; 1991.

36. Delgado GJ, Chung CB, Lektrakul N, et al. Tennis leg: clinical US study of 141 patients and anatomic investigation of four cadavers with MR imaging and US. *Radiology.* 2002;224:112–119.

37. O'Loughlin PF, Murawski CD, Egan C, et al. Ankle instability in sports. *Phys Sportsmed*. 2009;37:93–103.
38. Lynch SA. Assessment of the injured ankle in the athlete. *J Athl Train*. 2002;37:406–412.
39. Guillodo Y, Riban P, Guennoc X, et al. Usefulness of ultrasonographic detection of talocrural effusion in ankle sprains. *J Ultrasound Med*. 2007;26:831–836.
40. Narváez J, Narváez JA, Sánchez-Márquez A, et al. Posterior tibial tendon dysfunction as a cause of acquired flatfoot in the adult: value of magnetic resonance imaging. *Br J Rheumatol*. 1997;36:136–139.
41. Leung JL, Griffith JF. Sonography of chronic Achilles tendinopathy: a case-control study. *J Clin Ultrasound*. 2008;36:27–32.

# 19 The Pediatric Abdomen

Bridgette M. Lunsford and Regina K. Swearengin

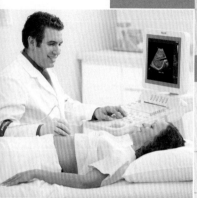

## OBJECTIVES

Demonstrate the sonographic scanning techniques, technical considerations, and routine examination for the neonatal and pediatric abdomen to include the prevertebral vessel evaluation, liver, gallbladder and biliary system, pancreas, gastrointestinal tract, and retroperitoneum.

Describe the pathology, etiology, and clinical signs and symptoms for anomalies and pathology of the aorta and inferior vena cava in the neonate and pediatric patient.

Differentiate between the sonographic appearance of the normal prevertebral vasculature and the sonographic appearance for congenital vascular anomalies and acquired vascular pathology in the neonate and pediatric patient.

Describe the pathology, etiology, and clinical signs and symptoms for hepatic congenital anomalies, cysts, hepatic trauma, infectious and inflammatory disease, diffuse liver disease, hepatic malignant neoplasms, and hepatic vascular disorders in the neonate and pediatric patient.

Differentiate between sonographic appearance of the normal liver and the sonographic appearance for congenital anomalies, cysts, hepatic trauma, infectious and inflammatory disease, diffuse liver disease, hepatic malignant neoplasms, and hepatic vascular disorders in the neonate and pediatric patient.

Describe the pathology, etiology, and clinical signs and symptoms for the gallbladder and biliary congenital anomalies, abnormal size, cholelithiasis, hydrops, biliary obstruction, cholangitis, and biliary neoplasm in the neonate and pediatric patient.

Differentiate between the sonographic appearance of the normal gallbladder and biliary system and the sonographic appearance for normal variants, congenital anomalies, abnormal size, cholelithiasis, hydrops, biliary obstruction, cholangitis, and biliary neoplasm in the neonate and pediatric patient.

Describe the pathology, etiology, and clinical signs and symptoms for pancreatic developmental and congenital anomalies, pancreatic neoplasm, and acute and chronic pancreatitis in the neonate and pediatric patient.

Differentiate between sonographic appearance of the normal pancreas and the sonographic appearance for pancreatic developmental and congenital anomalies, pancreatic neoplasm, and acute and chronic pancreatitis in the neonate and pediatric patient.

Describe the pathology, etiology, and clinical signs and symptoms for pyloric stenosis, small bowel disorders, intussusception, Crohn disease, bowel masses, appendicitis, and Hirschsprung disease in the neonate and pediatric patient.

Differentiate between sonographic appearance of the normal gastrointestinal tract and the sonographic appearance for pyloric stenosis, small bowel disorders, intussusception, Crohn disease, bowel masses, appendicitis, and Hirschsprung disease in the neonate and pediatric patient.

Describe the pathology, etiology, and clinical signs and symptoms for retroperitoneal pathology of the muscles, lymph nodes, neoplasms, and trauma in the neonate and pediatric patient.

Differentiate between sonographic appearance of the normal retroperitoneum and the sonographic appearance of abnormal retroperitoneal muscles, lymph nodes, neoplasms, and trauma in the neonate and pediatric patient.

Identify technically satisfactory and unsatisfactory sonographic examinations of the abdomen on the neonatal and pediatric patient.

## KEY TERMS

appendicitis | biliary atresia | Budd-Chiari syndrome | Caroli disease | cavernous hemangioma | cholecystitis | choledochal cyst | cholelithiasis | cirrhosis | coarctation of the aorta | Crohn disease | cystic fibrosis | echinococcal cyst | hemangioendothelioma | hepatic fibrosis | hepatitis | hepatoblastoma | hepatocellular carcinoma | hepatoma | intussusception | mesenchymal hamartoma | mesenchymal sarcoma | pancreatic carcinoma | pancreatitis | portal hypertension | pseudocyst | pyloric stenosis | sacrococcygeal teratoma | sclerosing cholangitis

## GLOSSARY

**AFP** alpha-fetoprotein; a tumor marker frequently elevated in cases of hepatocellular carcinoma, hepatoblastoma, and certain testicular cancers

**biloma** a walled off collection of bile caused by a disruption of the biliary tree, frequently caused by trauma or surgical procedures

**coarctation** a narrowing or constriction

**hemobilia** hemorrhage or blood in the bile caused by bleeding into the biliary tree

**hemoperitoneum** blood in the peritoneal cavity

**hyperalimentation** the administration of nutrients through intravenous feeding

**hyponatremia** an electrolyte imbalance; low sodium levels in the blood

**ileus** failure of the normal propulsion of the digestive tract

**jaundice** yellowish pigmentation of the skin and whites of the eyes caused by increased levels of bilirubin in the blood

**S**onography is the noninvasive modality of choice to evaluate the neonatal and pediatric abdomen due to the lack of ionizing radiation, the portability of the equipment, and excellent visualization of the abdominal anatomy in this age group. Critically ill patients who are sensitive to stress (i.e., transport, temperature changes) can easily and safely be examined at the bedside. Pediatric sonography presents many opportunities as well as challenges. Childhood obesity is a serious health care problem and obese children may be as challenging to examine sonographically as adults. Obese children may also present with some disease processes previously seen only in adults so the sonographer must have an in-depth knowledge of both pediatric and adult pathology.

## SONOGRAPHIC EXAMINATION TECHNIQUES[1,2]

Scanning the pediatric age group will require sonographic equipment with a wide range of probe frequencies. Depending on the area or organ of interest, when scanning neonates, a high-frequency (7 to 10 MHz) curved or (8 to 15 MHz) linear array transducer is utilized. Lower frequencies will be required to achieve adequate penetration in older pediatric patients. Scanning infants and small children requires the sonographer to be adept at assessing the anatomy and acquiring images quickly. Distraction techniques can be used for this age group rather than sedation. Older children may or may not be able to cooperate fully during the sonogram, so the use of distractions such as appropriate movies or other recordings can be used to ensure the sonographer can complete the examination accurately and in a timely fashion.

The parents will most likely be present for the examination. The sonographer must be prepared to professionally interact with the parents and elicit their assistance with the examination as needed. The sonographer should always explain the examination to the patient using age-appropriate terms and should answer the parent's questions about the examination in accordance with department policies and procedures. Special precautions should be taken to keep infants warm by placing blankets over all but the scanning surface. Warm gel, preferably single packets of gel for infection control, should always be used on children and must be used for neonates and infants. Sterile gel packets should be used whenever a sterile area must be maintained or in cases where infection is of high concern. The sonographer must always follow infection control standards whenever scanning and this can be even more important when examining pediatric patients.

A pediatric abdominal sonogram should include an assessment of all the organs, structures, and vessels of the abdomen. This chapter will discuss the abdominal vessels as well as the liver, gallbladder/biliary system, pancreas, gastrointestinal (GI) tract, and retroperitoneum. Chapter 20 discusses the pediatric urinary system and the adrenal glands. The sonographer should have as much information as possible regarding the reason for the sonogram and should adapt the examination to the patient's condition and any sonographic findings.

## PATIENT PREPARATION

Patient preparation will vary based on the age of the patient and the area or organ of interest. Ideally, the liver and biliary tree are best viewed with the patient in a fasting state. Since infants are fed every 3 to 4 hours, the examination should be performed just before a feeding. Children aged 1 to 3 years are best examined 4 hours after fasting and older children 8 hours after fasting.

# PREVERTEBRAL VESSEL EVALUATION

## SONOGRAPHIC EXAMINATION TECHNIQUE

### Patient Preparation

Although anatomically they are similar to adults, neonates and children require a different scanning approach. Using multiple planes on the neonate, the full length of the great vessels can easily be evaluated from the level of the diaphragm to the bifurcation without any particular patient preparation.

Patients in the neonatal intensive care unit are often intubated, so if it is necessary to turn the patient onto one side or the other, it is advisable to seek the aid of a caregiver. Depending on which great vessel is to be evaluated, it may be necessary to turn the patient to the appropriate side. The left posterior oblique (LPO) or left lateral decubitus (LLD) position is better for evaluating the inferior vena cava (IVC), as the vessel is nearer to the transducer placed on the right lateral abdomen. The LPO position permits use of the liver and right kidney as the sonographic window, thus avoiding bowel gas. In the right posterior oblique (RPO) or right lateral decubitus (RLD) position, the aorta lies nearer the transducer placed on the left lateral abdomen.

### Scan Technique

The sonographic examination of the abdominal vessels should include assessment of the vessels in multiple scan planes and the use of color and/or spectral Doppler to assess blood flow. The sonographer should acquire documentary images that clearly demonstrate the aorta and IVC from proximal to distal (bifurcation), including sonographically visible branches and tributaries. Split screen color Doppler and gray scale imaging can be used to demonstrate the vessels when gray scale alone is insufficient and/or pathology is present. Color Doppler should also be used to evaluate flow in the aorta, IVC, right and left iliac arteries and veins, and right and left renal arteries and veins. Correct presentation of the abdominal aorta and IVC must be documented so that the correct location and course of these vessels is confirmed.

In the neonate, coronal scanning may or may not be effective in demonstrating the aorta and IVC, especially if using a left coronal approach. When present in the neonate, an indwelling catheter in the aorta and its relationship to the renal arteries should be demonstrated. Although an umbilical arterial catheter (UAC) is visible on a radiograph, the location relative to the origin of the renal arteries cannot be reliably determined. Sonographically, the UAC is visualized as hyperechoic parallel lines with an anechoic center. Shadowing from the walls of the UAC may be noted when the beam is perpendicular to the catheter.

## NORMAL ANATOMY

The sonographic appearance of the abdominal vessels in the pediatric patient is the same as in an adult (Fig. 19-1A). The vessels should have anechoic lumens with echogenic or hyperechoic walls. The walls of the abdominal aorta may appear more echogenic than the walls of the IVC. The normal spectral Doppler of the aorta shows a pulsatile vessel with a high-resistance flow pattern (rapid upstroke, sharp systolic peak, and low flow velocity with a small amount of reversed flow possible during diastole) (Fig. 19-1B). The normal spectral Doppler flow pattern of the IVC is monophasic.

## CONGENITAL ANOMALIES

### Coarctation of the Abdominal Aorta[3,4]

Hypoplasia or coarctation of the abdominal aorta is a rare congenital defect. The proximal descending thoracic aorta is affected in 98% of coarctations, only 2% of them actually affect the abdominal aorta (Fig. 19-2A,B) Renal artery stenosis occurs in more than half of abdominal coarctations. Congenital abdominal coarctation can occur at any time in embryonic development. The earlier it occurs, the more obvious the manifestations. Acquired coarctation of the abdominal aorta has been associated with hypercalcemia, neurofibromatosis, tuberous

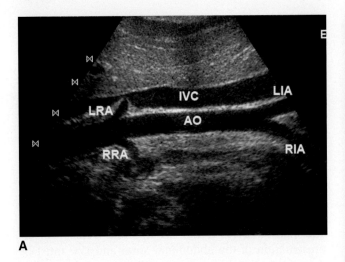

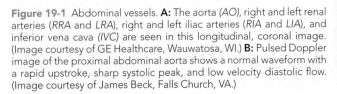

**A**

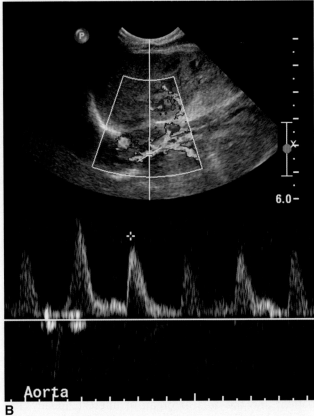

**B**

**Figure 19-1** Abdominal vessels. **A:** The aorta (AO), right and left renal arteries (RRA and LRA), right and left iliac arteries (RIA and LIA), and inferior vena cava (IVC) are seen in this longitudinal, coronal image. (Image courtesy of GE Healthcare, Wauwatosa, WI.) **B:** Pulsed Doppler image of the proximal abdominal aorta shows a normal waveform with a rapid upstroke, sharp systolic peak, and low velocity diastolic flow. (Image courtesy of James Beck, Falls Church, VA.)

sclerosis, rubella, and Turner syndrome. Children present with severe hypertension, headaches, and fatigue, whereas infants exhibit failure to thrive. An interrupted abdominal aorta produces vascular compromise with symptoms such as cyanotic, mottled, and discolored limbs with decreased femoral pulses. The extreme consequences of untreated severe hypertension can be fatal by the age of 30 years.

### Inferior Vena Cava

When scanning the IVC and the aorta, the sonographer must note both the position and relationship of the two vessels. In the normal relationship, the IVC is located on the right side, receiving the hepatic veins as it enters the right atrium. An IVC on the patient's left side is diagnostic of situs inversus. Besides an abnormal relationship of the IVC and aorta, the IVC can also be interrupted, in which case it drains via an azygous continuation, which may lie on either the left or right of the spine. The hemiazygous continuation lies more posterior than the aorta (Fig. 19-3). Another abnormal vessel that may be imaged in the long axis plane is an anomalous venous connection associated with total anomalous pulmonary venous return, which connects to the ductus venosus. It crosses between the aorta and IVC. Displacement or distortion of the IVC or the aorta should alert the sonographer that other anomalies may be present. Sonographers must be cognizant of the fact that unusual presentations of the aorta or IVC and

anomalous vessels in the lower abdomen may indicate complex congenital heart disease.

### ACQUIRED PATHOLOGIES[5,6]

#### Abdominal Aorta in the Neonate

The most common reason for evaluating the aorta in the neonate is for aortic thrombus, a well-recognized complication of indwelling umbilical artery catheters (UACs). Clinical signs of aortic thrombus include: absent femoral pulses, hematuria, cyanosis, hypertension, blanching of the lower extremities, and necrotizing enterocolitis. An overly distended urinary bladder may cause some of the above symptoms.

Suspected aortic thrombus should be evaluated by a thorough scan of the entire aorta and both kidneys in multiple planes. Thrombus typically appears sonographically as echogenic material within the aortic lumen, which may totally or partially fill the vessel. The clot may be long and thick and is termed extensive if it fills 40% of the aorta in a sectional plane, goes to the level of the renal artery or iliac artery, or causes proximal dilatation. As the sonographic appearance of thrombus changes over time, the vessel may appear to contain thin linear structures. Color Doppler should be used to demonstrate any blood flow around the thrombus, normal flow reversal, and the presence of any collateral vessels. Gray scale and color Doppler should be used to follow the progression and/or resolution of the thrombus (Fig. 19-4).

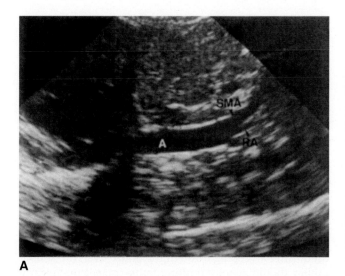

**A**

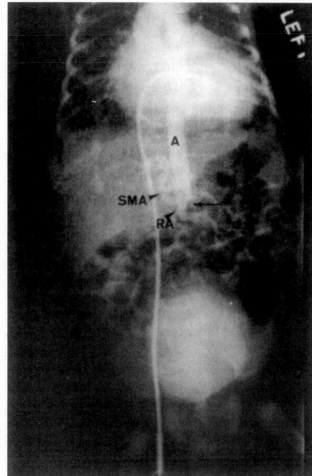

**Figure 19-2** Coarctation of the abdominal aorta. **A:** Coarctation of the abdominal aorta (A) is demonstrated on this longitudinal section with the interruption of the abdominal aorta and collateral circulation of the superior mesenteric artery (SMA) and renal artery (RA). **B:** An aortogram of the same patient shows the interrupted (arrow) abdominal aorta (A) and the collateral circulation of the superior mesenteric artery (SMA) and renal artery (RA).

**B**

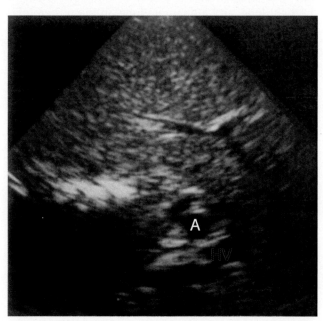

**Figure 19-3** Interruption of the inferior vena cava. In this transverse scan low in the abdomen, the aorta (A) is demonstrated on the left side. The interrupted inferior vena cava is not seen but drains through a hemiazygous vein (HV) with continuation seen posterior to the aorta.

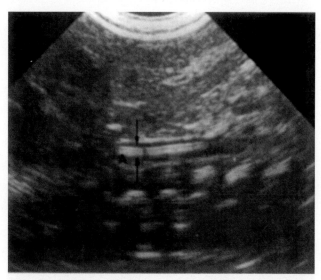

**Figure 19-4** Umbilical artery catheter. An indwelling umbilical artery catheter is visualized as two parallel lines (arrow) with an anechoic center representing the catheter lumen on this longitudinal section of the abdominal aorta (A).

### Inferior Vena Cava[7]

The IVC can be a site of thrombus or calcifications in neonates. Children can have tumor invasion into the IVC, from Wilms tumor (Fig. 19-5).

Extension of renal carcinoma into the IVC has been well documented. Extension can occur from the kidney, adrenal gland (neuroblastoma), retroperitoneum (sarcoma), and from hepatocellular carcinoma (HCC), teratoma, and lymphoma. It is important to evaluate the extension of the tumor into the hepatic veins or right atrium and to seek evidence of tumor invasion into the wall of the IVC. Tumor extension appears similar to the solid texture of the tumor itself. The differential diagnosis includes simple thrombus. Computed tomography (CT) is the modality of choice for evaluating IVC wall invasion; however, sonography is the best modality for evaluating cephalad extension of IVC tumor invasion.

IVC thrombosis can also occur secondary to indwelling catheters, clotting disorders, dehydration, sepsis, nephrotic syndrome, and extension of renal and/or pelvic vein thrombosis.

## LIVER

When imaging the neonatal or pediatric liver, it is important to image all of the "adult" landmarks in an infant's or child's abdomen. Special attention should be paid to the liver parenchyma, the position and size of the gallbladder, portal vein, portal vein bifurcation, hepatic artery, common bile duct, and hepatic veins.

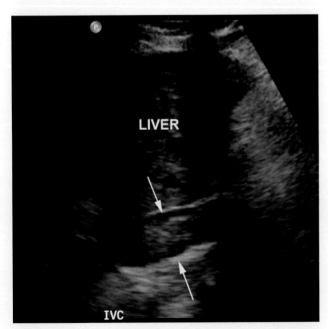

**Figure 19-5** Inferior vena cava thrombus. An echogenic clot (arrow) is visualized within the lumen of the inferior vena cava on this longitudinal section seen posterior to the liver. (Image courtesy of James Beck, Falls Church, VA.)

## SONOGRAPHIC EXAMINATION AND TECHNIQUE

### Scan Technique

Establishing a protocol of longitudinal, coronal, and transverse planes is important to ensure consistency from one patient to the next; however, special attention must be paid to differences such as position of anatomy, pathology, and size. The sonographic examination of the pediatric liver should include assessment of the liver parenchyma, vessels and ligaments in multiple scan planes, and the use of color and/or spectral Doppler to assess blood flow. Patients are most commonly scanned in the supine position but the LPO position may be helpful especially in older and/or obese children. After sweeping through the entire liver, the sonographer should acquire representative images that clearly demonstrate the lobes and segments of the liver including vascular and ligament landmarks. The sonographer should be careful to assess and document the periphery of the liver as well as the bulk of the liver; longitudinal and transverse sweeps should extend past the lateral, superior, and inferior borders of the liver. Normal measurement parameters for the liver have been reported and show correlation with age, height, and weight.

### NORMAL ANATOMY

The normal liver appears as a smooth-outlined, homogeneous organ, usually situated in the right upper quadrant of the abdomen (Fig. 19-6A). The liver is divided into a large right lobe in the right side of the abdomen, a smaller left lobe extending across the midline, a caudate lobe situated on the posterior superior surface of the right lobe, and a quadrate lobe on the posteroinferior surface of the right lobe. The falciform ligament divides the right and left lobes.

The liver receives a dual blood supply. The liver receives oxygenated blood from the hepatic artery, a branch of the celiac artery. Additional blood from the digestive system is carried to the liver via the portal vein, formed by the convergence of the superior mesenteric vein (SMV) and the splenic vein. The portal vein enters the liver at the porta hepatis, where it quickly branches into the right and left portal veins. The hepatic artery also enters the liver at the porta hepatis (Fig. 19-6B). The major vessels of the liver provide important visual and anatomical landmarks.

Applicable laboratory tests include the standard liver function tests and alpha-fetoprotein (AFP), which, if elevated, may indicate the presence of a hepatoblastoma or other malignant tumor.

### CONGENITAL ANOMALIES

Hemangiomas of the liver are rare congenital anomalies arising from an arteriovenous malformation (AVM) forming blood-filled spaces. They are the most common vascular liver tumor in infancy and are either

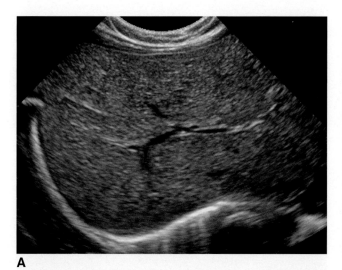
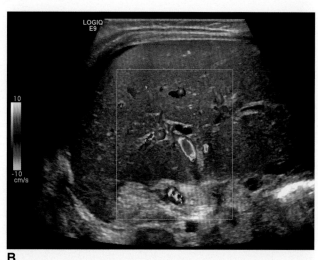

**A**    **B**

**Figure 19-6** Neonatal liver. **A:** Transverse image of the liver in a neonatal patient demonstrates the normal homogeneous echo texture of liver and anechoic vasculature. (Image courtesy of Philips Medical Systems, Bothell, WA.) **B:** Transverse image of the liver in a neonatal patient demonstrating flow in the portal vein. A high-frequency linear transducer is used to image the patient. (Image courtesy of GE Healthcare, Wauwatosa, WI.)

cavernous (blood-filled spaces lined with a single layer of endothelial cells) or hemangioendotheliomas (the lining or endothelium is multilayered or hypertrophic, with primitive or infantile cells).

## Hemangioendothelioma[8–10]

Hemangioendothelioma usually affect infants less than 6 months of age, are typically multiple, and are associated with cutaneous hemangiomas. Patients are typically symptomatic and present clinically with hepatomegaly, congestive heart failure, and hemoperitoneum from rupture. Sonographically, the lesions can appear hypoechoic, isoechoic, or hyperechoic to adjacent liver tissue, homogeneous or complex, and may contain echogenic foci (Fig. 19-7A–D).

Depending on the composition, variable acoustic enhancement may be present.

## Cavernous Hemangioma[8,11]

Hemangiomas are three times more common in girls than in boys. They may or may not be present at birth but usually become evident at about 2 months of age, or they may be found incidentally. Large hemangiomas may cause hepatomegaly, with or without accompanying abdominal distention. Hemangiomas cease to grow and then undergo spontaneous involution.

After the tumor enlarges but before regressing, the infant may experience a number of complications, including fatal rupture of the hemangioma, Kasabach-Merritt syndrome due to platelet trapping, hepatic dysfunction due to portal hypertension, intravascular coagulation, intestinal bleeding, bowel obstruction, obstructive jaundice, and irreversible congestive heart failure, as well as respiratory insufficiency caused by the mass effect.

Typical sonographic findings are of a well-defined, hyperechoic area within the liver (Fig. 19-8A,B). The

hemangioma's hyperechoic appearance results from the multiple interfaces between the walls of the blood-filled sinuses. Less frequently, the mass is hypoechoic and may mimic a collection of simple cysts. It can also appear complex, demonstrating irregular walls and hypoechoic to anechoic areas, possibly due to necrosis (Fig. 19-9A–D).

The presence of calcifications or fibrotic changes within the mass produces a hyperechoic pattern with posterior acoustic shadowing. Doppler interrogation may reveal high flow within the lesion. An enlarged hepatic artery, as well as a small distal aorta due to the increased hepatic flow, can also be seen.

Needle biopsy for confirmation of hemangiomas is a dangerous procedure that can result in fatal hemorrhage, so it is usually used as a last resort when a diagnosis cannot be reached by other means. The cytologic diagnostic criteria include the presence of benign epithelial cells, fresh blood from the mass, and no malignant cells.

The treatment of hemangioma varies with the size of the mass. Most hemangiomas undergo spontaneous involution and regression, but when a large hemangioma threatens the patient's health, aggressive procedures are instigated. A lobectomy or resection of the tumor is sometimes performed, but if the patient is experiencing congestive heart failure, hepatic artery ligation or embolization can be performed. In many cases, the lesion is responsive to steroid therapy and radiation therapy.

The differential diagnosis includes angiomatous tumors, hepatoblastoma, hepatoma and metastatic neuroblastoma, cysts, abscesses, and focal nodular hyperplasia.

## Mesenchymal Hamartoma[8,12]

Mesenchymal or fibrous hamartoma is a rare congenital anomaly that arises from the connective tissue or mesenchyme of the portal tracts. It is considered to be

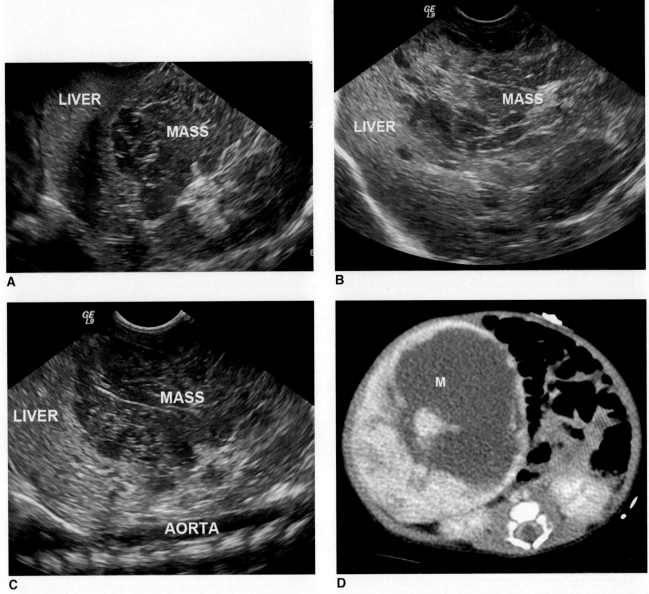

**Figure 19-7** Hemangioendothelioma. This female neonate presents with a distended abdomen and a palpable mass. **A:** The longitudinal image shows a large irregular complex mass, which has both anechoic and hyperechoic areas throughout the mass. **B:** A transverse image demonstrates the irregular borders of the complex mass along with normal liver tissue superior to the mass. **C:** The longitudinal image of the liver demonstrates the size of the mass and the aorta posterior. **D:** On the computed tomography image, the mass (*M*) is seen extending into the midline. The diagnosis was hemangioendothelioma. (Images courtesy of Dr. Nakul Jerath, Falls Church, VA.)

the second most common benign hepatic mass seen in children, and is more common in males.

The lesion usually presents within the first 2 years of life, with painless abdominal swelling and anorexia as the first clinical symptoms. Congestive heart failure has also been noted in patients with mesenchymal hamartoma due to arteriovenous shunting within the tumor. Patients can experience respiratory distress from the large, fluid-filled lesion if fluid accumulation has been rapid. Liver function tests are usually normal.

Sonographically, mesenchymal hamartoma is sometimes mistaken for hemangioma; however, although it frequently reveals internal septations demonstrating a complex appearance, it is avascular. These septations

are strands of hepatocytes, bile duct elements, or mesenchyme separating multiple cysts. The hamartoma is usually situated in the right lobe.

The prognosis of mesenchymal hamartoma is excellent. Resection is usually all that is required, although in patients with respiratory distress, percutaneous drainage of the mass is performed prior to surgery.

The differential diagnosis of mesenchymal hamartoma includes mesenchymoma, hemangioma, parasitic or congenital cyst, teratoma, biliary cystadenoma, and choledochal cyst.

Rare benign lesions include focal nodular hyperplasia, hepatic adenoma, nodular regenerative hyperplasia, and fatty tumors; all of these tumors have the same

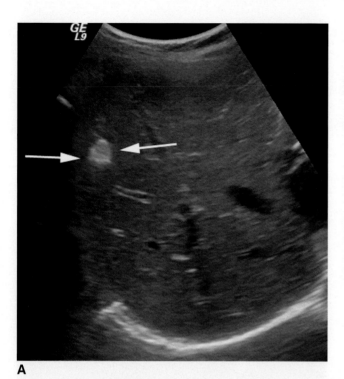

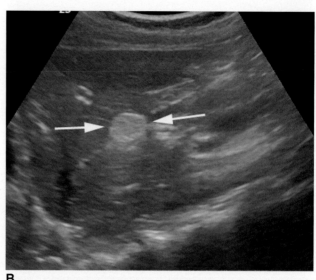

**B**

**A**

**Figure 19-8** Cavernous hemangioma. This pediatric patient has a history of tuberous sclerosis. **A:** The transverse image of the liver demonstrates a well-circumscribed hyperechoic mass *(arrows)* in the right liver lobe and **(B)** the longitudinal image of the left liver lobe shows a second similar mass *(arrows)*. Both masses were diagnosed as cavernous hemangiomas. (Images courtesy of Jillian Platt, Falls Church, VA.)

clinical presentation, sonographic appearance, and complications in adults and children.

## CYSTS[13]

Congenital liver cysts are relatively rare. They range in size from small to large. Multicystic disease of the liver is seen with multicystic kidney disease and von Hippel-Lindau disease. Acquired cysts include hydatid cysts and traumatic cysts caused by blunt trauma. Hemobilia can be detected if there is communication with the biliary tree. The patient is generally asymptomatic unless the lesion is large enough to impair function and cause abdominal distention. The cyst may be palpated on physical examination or found incidentally on an imaging examination.

Sonographically, simple congenital liver cysts appear as smooth-walled, anechoic lesions demonstrating good posterior enhancement (Fig. 19-10A–D). They may be completely intrahepatic, partly intrahepatic, or completely extrahepatic and attached by a stalk.

Hydatid echinococcal cysts or parasitic cysts are usually associated with exposure to livestock, farming, and dogs. After the eggs have been ingested, the gastric juices dissolve the covering of the embryo, allowing the organism to move spontaneously and attach itself to the intestinal wall. From there, it travels through the portal system to the liver, where it lodges and creates a cyst. The sonographic appearances include simple cyst, complex cysts (daughter cysts, echogenic septa, echogenic debris, or floating membranes), and simple or complex cysts with calcifications. The peak incidence occurs in patients 5 to

15 years of age. In this population, 25% are asymptomatic and 60% present with symptoms including urticaria, right upper quadrant pain, and abdominal swelling due to hepatomegaly. Since the lung is the second most common site affected, the right more often than the left, patients with pulmonary hydatid cyst present with pain on the affected side, coughing, high fever, and dyspnea. Forty percent develop complications including rupture into the peritoneal and pleural spaces, resulting in anaphylactic shock and pneumonia. Sometimes, the organism passes through the liver and lodges in the lungs, brain, kidneys, or elsewhere. Depending on the size and location of the lesions, the patient may experience infection, impaired liver function due to biliary obstruction, or other complications due to obstruction or compression of abdominal vasculature.

Treatment usually consists of aspiration, capitonnage, or omentopexy, or a combination of two or more surgical procedures.

Differential diagnosis of extrahepatic cysts includes ovarian or mesenteric cysts, whereas the differential diagnosis of an intrahepatic cyst includes teratoma, mesenchymoma, and tuberculin hepatic granuloma.

## HEPATIC TRAUMA[14]

The most commonly injured abdominal organ in blunt abdominal trauma in children is the liver with the right lobe involved more often than the left lobe. The types of injuries to the liver include subcapsular and parenchymal hematomas, lacerations, and fractures. Hemoperitoneum is often noted in liver trauma injuries (Fig. 19-11A,B).

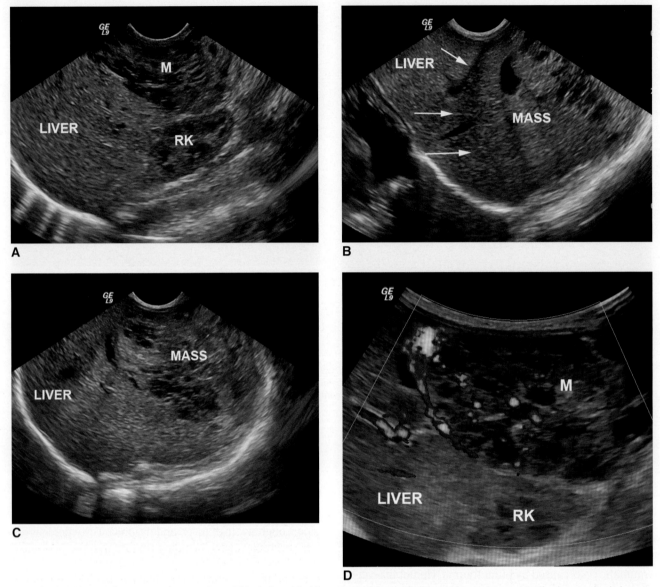

**Figure 19-9** Neonatal cavernous hemangioma. This 1-day-old girl presents with a palpable abdominal mass. **A:** The longitudinal shows a complex mass *(M)* in the anterior right lobe. The right kidney *(RK)* is also seen **B:** A transverse image demonstrates the irregular borders of the mass *(arrows)* and multiple anechoic spaces within the large mass. **C:** This transverse image in the superior portion of the liver demonstrates the mass as well as normal liver tissue. **D:** A power Doppler image demonstrates flow within the mass *(M). RK,* right kidney. (Images courtesy of Dr. Nakul Jerath, Falls Church, VA.)

Hematomas of the liver demonstrate a change in echogenicity over time, progressing from anechoic, to complex, to anechoic with possible development of calcification. Gas or air secondary to tissue ischemia and necrosis may be noted. Biloma (walled-off collections of bile) and pseudoaneurysms may be later complications of liver trauma.

## INFECTIOUS AND INFLAMMATORY DISEASE

### Hepatitis[15]

Hepatitis is a diffuse infection of the liver characterized by inflammation and hepatic cell necrosis. Nearly all cases are viral in origin (hepatitis A, B, C, D, or E; cytomegalovirus, herpes, and Epstein-Barr). Noninfectious causes include toxin exposure, drugs, sclerosing cholangitis, and autoimmune disease. Type A is transmitted by a fecal–oral route of contaminated material. Children and young adults are most often infected by the hepatitis A virus. The extent of liver damage ranges from mild involvement to widespread necrosis and hepatic failure.

The clinical symptoms vary depending on the stage of the disease. The patient can experience abdominal swelling (hepatomegaly) with pain, nausea, fever, chills, jaundice, fatigue, or loss of appetite. An important point to remember is that the clinical symptoms of infectious mononucleosis (IM), jaundice, hepatosplenomegaly, fever, fatigue, sore throat, and lymphadenopathy closely resemble those of acute viral hepatitis (AVH). An important difference with IM is that the spleen is usually larger than in AVH.

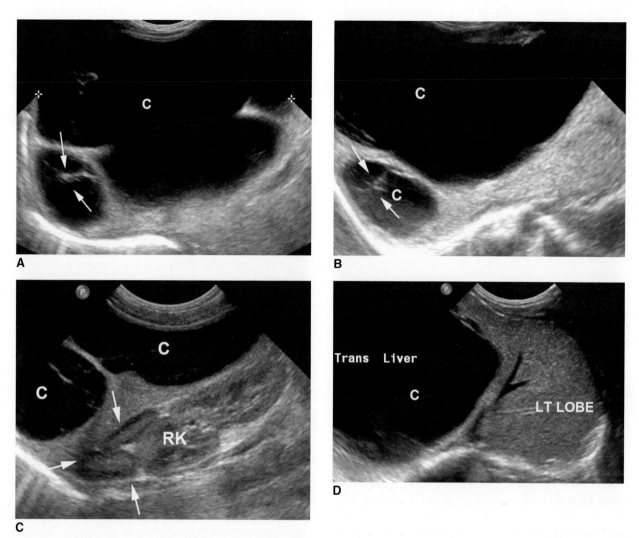

**Figure 19-10** Congenital liver cysts. A female neonate was born with a large abdominal mass. **A,B:** Transverse images of the right lobe demonstrate a large anechoic cyst measuring at least 8.5 cm and a smaller posterior cyst with septations *(arrows)*. **C:** The longitudinal image of the right liver lobe demonstrates two cysts as well as the right kidney (*RK*) and normal neonatal adrenal gland *(arrows)* seen superior to the kidney. **D:** A transverse image of the liver shows the cyst occupying much of the right lobe (*C*). The left lobe appears normal. The diagnosis was congenital liver cysts. No other abnormalities were found. (Images courtesy of Dr. Nakul Jerath, Falls Church, VA.)

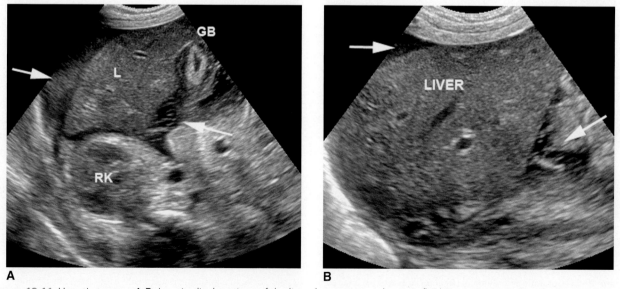

**Figure 19-11** Hepatic trauma. **A,B:** Longitudinal sections of the liver demonstrate echogenic fluid *(arrows)* surrounding the liver in a patient with recent blunt abdominal trauma. The diagnosis was hemoperitoneum. A thickened gallbladder wall is demonstrated in (**B**). *GB*, gallbladder; *L*, liver; *RK*, right kidney. (Images courtesy of Philips Medical Systems, Bothell, WA.)

Depending on the stage of the disease, the sonographic appearance of the liver can range from normal to increasingly hyperechoic. In acute hepatitis, hepatomegaly with decreased parenchymal echogenicity and increased echogenicity of the portal walls may be present. As the patient recovers, the size and echogenicity of the liver return to normal; however, with chronic hepatitis, the size of the liver may decrease but echogenicity and attenuation increase as normal liver tissue is destroyed and replaced by fibrosis and nodular regeneration. Chronic hepatitis may lead to cirrhosis. Liver biopsy is helpful in diagnosing cirrhosis. Thickening of the gallbladder wall, small gallbladder filled with sludge, and enlarged nodes in the porta hepatitis can be found in cases of severe hepatitis (Fig. 19-12A,B).

### Abscess[16,17]

An abscess in the liver of infants usually results from neonatal infection from the umbilicus or mesentery or from surgery and are seeded into the liver via a contaminated portal or umbilical vein. With a neonatal infection, an abscess can form in the ductus venosus as well. Mortality can be high. Vigorous antibiotic therapy is generally the treatment of choice, as surgery or drainage is not always possible. It has also been noted that transplacental (in utero) infections can cause calcifications of the fetal liver. These patients usually present with hepatic dysfunction as well as hepatomegaly.

### Amebic Abscess[16,17]

Amebic liver abscess, although an adult disease, also affects children in areas where drinking water is contaminated and sanitation is poor. Hepatic abscess is the main complication of the organism *Entamoeba histolytica*, forming in 1% of the population that is infected.

*E. histolytica* enters the liver from the colon via the portal system and forms a cavity that becomes the abscess. The organism resides in the wall of the abscess. The abscess is filled with liquified necrotic liver tissue that is reddish brown in color. The right lobe is more commonly affected.

Patients present with abdominal distention, hepatomegaly, fever, and right upper quadrant tenderness. Respiratory distress can also be noted if the abscess has crossed the diaphragm into the right pleural space. This condition is intensified if the right diaphragm is also raised due to a large hepatic abscess. Jaundice is rarely seen.

Laboratory tests show mildly abnormal liver function values, anemia, leukocytosis, and hyponatremia.

Sonographically, the abscess can be readily identified as a hypoechoic, spherical lesion. After treatment, it can be followed with serial sonography.

### Pyogenic Liver Abscess[16,17]

Pyogenic liver abscess (PLA) is rare in children and can be fatal. Pyogenic abscess in children is secondary to generalized infections from the bowel (appendicitis or inflammatory bowel disease), trauma, or surgery. Immunosuppression is an important predisposing condition. The most common causative agents are *Escherichia coli* and *Klebsiella pneumoniae*. PLA can also be seen in Crohn disease, chronic granulomatous disease, intestinal infection or bacteremia of any source, cholecystitis, biliary atresia, polycythemia, perforated viscus, *Candida* organisms, and hematopoietic malignancies.

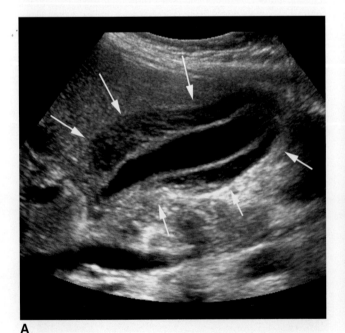

**A**

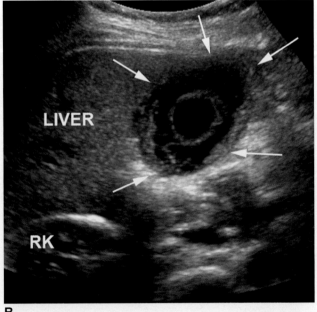

**B**

**Figure 19-12** Hepatitis. Longitudinal **(A)** and transverse **(B)** images of the gallbladder in a pediatric patient with acute hepatitis demonstrate gallbladder wall thickening *(arrows)*. The liver had a normal sonographic appearance. *RK*, right kidney. (Images courtesy of Dr. Nakul Jerath, Falls Church, VA.)

The etiology of abscess is related to the source of the infection and can be introduced to the liver by various routes. These include trauma, direct invasion of adjacent structures, the hepatic artery, the portal vein, or the bile ducts.

Laboratory values vary. The liver enzyme levels may be normal or elevated. Patients are not usually jaundiced. Blood cultures are generally negative. Leukocytosis is common but varies among patients. In neonatal abscesses, the organism is usually gram-negative rather than gram-positive.

Intrahepatic abscesses in infants present sonographically as in older patients and vary from discretely marginated hypoechoic structures with good sound transmission to complex hyperechoic masses with poorly defined margins. Lesions that contain gas (air) are hyperechoic with acoustic shadowing and reverberation artifacts. The mass may also present with a bull's-eye appearance (a central hyperechoic area surrounded by a more anechoic one). In transplacental infection with calcifications, a bright, hyperechoic lesion with posterior shadowing can be seen.

### Fungal Abscess[16,17]

Fungal abscess occurs most often in the immunocompromised patient and is usually due to *Candida albicans*. This type of abscess is most commonly seen as multiple small lesions with irregular walls throughout the liver and may also be seen in the spleen and kidneys. Sonographically, the lesions can appear round and hypoechoic, hyperechoic, or have a target or wheel-within-wheel appearance.

## DIFFUSE LIVER DISEASE

Diffuse parenchymal diseases include fatty infiltration, hepatic fibrosis, cirrhosis, hemosiderosis, and metabolic diseases.

### Fatty Infiltration[14,18,19]

Fatty infiltration of the liver is caused by chronic hepatic injury and results from an accumulation of abnormal amounts of triglycerides and lipids in the hepatocytes. Fatty infiltration may be diffuse or focal, and in children, it is caused by malnutrition, malignancies, tyrosinemia, hyperalimentation, cystic fibrosis, Reye syndrome, glycogen storage disease, malabsorption syndrome, high-dose steroid therapy, acute hepatitis, general obesity, kwashiorkor, Cushing syndrome, galactosemia, fructose intolerance, familial hyperlipidemia, abetalipoproteinemia, diabetic ketoacidosis, exposure to liver toxins, and chronic granulomatous disease. As childhood obesity has emerged as a significant health problem worldwide, the prevalence of fatty infiltration of the liver has increased in children. Fatty infiltration is being seen at a younger age and without the presence of other underlying risk factors.

Depending on the underlying etiology of the steatosis, the fatty infiltration may be reversible. Reversible steatosis is generally asymptomatic. Irreversible steatosis is associated with Reye syndrome, hepatitis D, and certain drugs. Reversible steatosis is associated with nutritional disorders (starvation, obesity), metabolic disorders (diabetes mellitus, hyperlipidemia, galactosemia), steroids, viral infections, and cystic fibrosis (Fig. 19-13A–C).

Diffuse fatty infiltration results in hepatomegaly and sonographic findings of increased parenchymal echogenicity and attenuation of the sound beam. The resulting sonographic appearance is a large echogenic liver with decreased visualization of the intrahepatic vessels, posterior portions of the liver, and the diaphragm. Focal areas of "spared" liver may be found and will appear hypoechoic to the remainder of the liver parenchyma. Focal sparing is most common near the gallbladder fossa, adjacent to the main lobar fissure, in the medial segment of the left lobe near the porta hepatis, and in subcapsular locations.

Focal fatty infiltration is usually noted sonographically as an area of increased echogenicity anterior to the portal vein bifurcation, the gallbladder neck, and in the medial segment of the left lobe. The borders are usually well defined and may appear as finger-like projections. In some cases, the focal infiltration can appear more rounded and will mimic a mass; however, areas of focal infiltration will not produce a "mass effect" within the liver or change the liver contour.

Metabolic disorders of the liver include glycogen story disease (type I von Gierke disease is the most common), lipodystrophy, cystic fibrosis, Gaucher disease, and Wilson disease, all of which have the sonographic appearance of fatty infiltration of the liver.

### Cirrhosis[14,19]

Cirrhosis (parenchymal destruction, scarring, fibrosis, and nodular regeneration) in infants and children is due to biliary atresia, cystic fibrosis, chronic hepatitis, metabolic disease (Wilson disease, glycogen storage disease, tyrosinemia, galactosemia, and $\alpha_1$-antitrypsin deficiency), prolonged parenteral nutrition, Budd-Chiari syndrome, and medications. The clinical presentation is the same as in adults: hepatomegaly (in the earlier stages), jaundice, and ascites.

Laboratory tests show elevations of aspartate aminotransferase (AST), alanine aminotransferase (ALT), lactic dehydrogenase (LDH), and increased direct and indirect bilirubin values if the patient is jaundiced.

Sonographically, the liver is smaller than normal with surface nodularity, a heterogeneous or coarse parenchymal echotexture, increased parenchymal echogenicity with decreased penetration of the sound beam (not as great as fatty liver), regenerative nodules which may be hypoechoic or hyperechoic, and a small or nonvisualized gallbladder. Secondary signs of ascites, splenomegaly, and portal hypertension may be present.

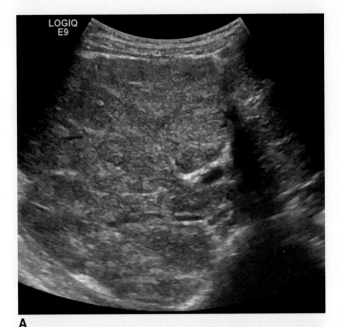

A

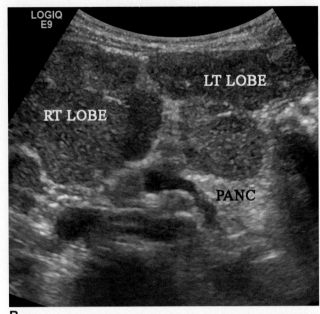

B

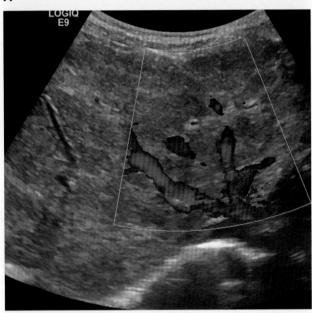

C

**Figure 19-13** Cystic fibrosis. The transverse liver images are on a 10-year-old patient with cystic fibrosis. **A:** The liver is echogenic and has a nodular, patchy appearance with a decreased visualization of the vascular structures. **B:** The pancreas appears echogenic. **C:** A color Doppler demonstrates normal flow within the hepatic veins.

### Hepatic Fibrosis[20]

Hepatic fibrosis is a rare condition and has been associated with autosomal recessive polycystic disease. Hepatomegaly and portal hypertension are common symptoms. Sonographically, the liver demonstrates increased echogenicity and biliary dilatation due to the presence of dense fibrous bands surrounding the liver lobules (Fig. 19-14A,B).

Increased echogenicity of the kidneys may also be noted.

### Hemosiderosis[21]

Hemosiderosis is related to excessive iron storage in the liver usually due to repeated blood transfusions. The liver may demonstrate a decrease in echogenicity.

Magnetic resonance imaging (MRI) is the best imaging test for detecting hemosiderosis.

### MALIGNANT NEOPLASMS[8,9,22]

Primary malignant tumors of the liver are more common in children than in adults and two-thirds of all pediatric hepatic tumors are malignant. These tumors include hepatoblastoma, HCC (hepatoma), mesenchymal (embryonal) sarcoma, and congenital neuroblastoma. Other rare liver tumors include rhabdomyosarcoma, angiosarcoma, germ cell tumors, and undifferentiated sarcomas. Primary liver tumors account for 2% to 5% of all malignant pediatric tumors. The AFP level is usually elevated in the presence of malignant hepatic tumors and invasion of surrounding vessels is commonly noted. Vessel

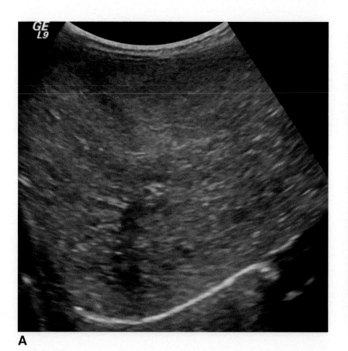

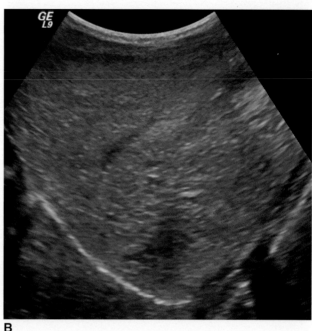

**A**    **B**

Figure 19-14 Hepatic fibrosis. The transverse **(A)** and longitudinal **(B)** liver images were obtained on a 5-year-old male patient with a history of autosomal recessive polycystic kidney disease. The patient presents with worsening renal function and failure to thrive. The sonogram reveals an echogenic heterogeneous liver consistent with hepatic fibrosis. (Images courtesy of Dr. Nakul Jerath, Falls Church, VA.)

involvement generally denotes primary hepatic disease rather than metastases. Since surgical resection is elemental in the treatment of hepatic malignancies, it is of vital importance that imaging modalities accurately assess and identify the location of the tumor, its appearance, its extension into surrounding structures, and its relationship to surrounding major blood vessels.

Sonographically, malignancies usually demonstrate as a solitary, solid, homogeneous, hyperechoic mass, and less frequently as multiple hyperechoic lesions. In some cases, a hypoechoic halo or rim may be seen and infrequently the malignancy may be isoechoic to normal liver tissue.

### Hepatoblastoma[8,9,22,23]

Hepatoblastoma is the most common pediatric liver mass, occurring most commonly in boys younger than 5 years of age. Hepatoblastoma is associated with Beckwith-Wiedemann syndrome (hemihypertrophy, macroglossia, hypoglycemia, organomegaly, omphalocele), fetal alcohol syndrome, the development of Wilms tumor, dysplastic kidney, and Meckel diverticulum.

A tumor should be considered resectable if it does not occupy more than one lobe, has no extrahepatic extension, and does not invade the portal vein. Unresectable tumors can be biopsied and converted to resectable tumors by chemotherapy. Since hepatoblastomas are usually detected in advanced stages, tumor extension outside of the liver or into more than one lobe, as well as being multifocal in origin, makes it unresectable. Chemotherapy is applied before surgery to shrink the tumor, resulting in improved operability.

Clinically, patients usually present with hepatomegaly or a painless, palpable abdominal mass in 90% of cases. In advanced cases, there can be accompanying fever, weight loss, pain, nausea, vomiting, jaundice, anemia, leukocytosis, adenopathy, and fractures due to bone metastases. Laboratory values include an elevation of AFP in 84% to 91% of cases, with a decrease after resection. There may also be a transaminase elevation, as well as anemia and thrombocytosis.

Sonographically, a hepatoblastoma appears as a solitary multinodular mass with a heterogeneous, hyperechoic pattern and indistinct borders (Fig. 19-15A,B).

Anechoic foci may also be present, representing necrosis or hemorrhage. Dense or coarse calcifications with posterior shadowing are also common. The differential diagnosis includes HCC, infantile hemangioendothelioma, and mesenchymal hamartoma.

### Hepatocellular Carcinoma[8,9,22]

HCC, which is also known as hepatoma, affects children older than 3 years of age and has been associated with chronic liver diseases such as type I glycogen storage disease, Wilson disease, extrahepatic biliary atresia, and hepatitis. Pathologically, these lesions have characteristics that differentiate them from other hepatic lesions: daughter nodules, hepatic or portal tumor thrombosis, septa, and pseudocapsules. This tumor can either be well encapsulated or nonencapsulated and is commonly multicentric.

Clinically, the patient presents with sudden liver failure due to invasion of the tumor or thrombosis in the portal or hepatic veins, hepatomegaly, pain, GI bleeding,

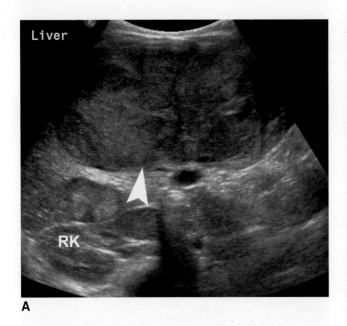

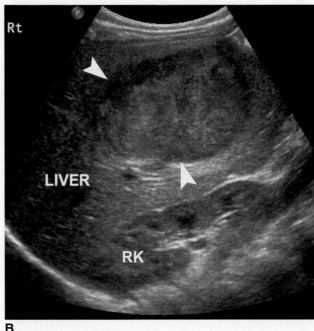

**Figure 19-15** Hepatoblastoma. This 2-year-old has abdominal distention and acholic stool. **A:** The transverse liver scan shows a large, solid, multifocal, heterogeneous mass (*arrowhead*) involving the right liver lobe and the left medial liver segment. **B:** The longitudinal image shows the mass (*arrowheads*) in the right liver lobe. *RK*, right kidney. (Images courtesy of Monica Bacani, Columbus, OH.)

ascites, anorexia, hypoglycemia, anemia, weakness, and fever. Laboratory values include elevated AFP in 60% to 80% of cases.

Sonographically, the tumor may appear similar to a hepatoblastoma. It generally presents as a solid, hyperechoic mass and usually involves the entire liver. It can have well-defined or ill-defined borders. There may be anechoic areas within the mass representing necrosis or hemorrhage, usually as a result of chemotherapy or radiation therapy. An anechoic or hypoechoic halo or rim may also be seen. Tumor thrombi are frequently seen in the portal and hepatic veins and IVC and should be documented if present.

The prognosis of HCC depends on its features and on the general condition of the patient, as well as the possibility of complete resectability. A well-encapsulated mass is easier to resect than a poorly encapsulated hepatoma. The outcome for cirrhotic patients who develop HCC is poor. The differential diagnosis includes hepatoblastoma, abscess, focal nodular hyperplasia, adenoma, hemangiosarcoma, hemangioendothelioma, and biliary rhabdomyosarcoma.

### Fibrolamellar Hepatocellular Carcinoma[8]

Fibrolamellar HCC is histologic subtype of HCC, which most commonly affects teenagers and young adults. Clinical findings include abdominal pain, mass, fever, weight loss, diarrhea, and vomiting. AFP levels are typically normal or mildly elevated. The tumor is usually solitary and well-marginated with variable echogenicity. Some tumors demonstrate a central scar and/or focal calcifications. The sonographic appearance is so similar to other solid hepatic neoplasms that biopsy is needed to differentiate these tumors.

### Mesenchymal Sarcoma[8,9]

Mesenchymal (embryonal) sarcoma is a rare malignant liver tumor that typically presents in patients 5 to 10 years of age, with no gender predisposition as a large fast-growing, round, singular mass with well-defined borders and a thick, fibrous pseudocapsule usually within the right hepatic lobe. It can contain multiple cystic spaces, hemorrhage, necrosis, and brown viscous material, as well as fibrous bands. It can easily spread to the abdominal cavity or to the diaphragm, with metastases to the lungs. These tumors should be resected and respond readily to chemotherapy. Mesenchymal sarcoma is the fourth most common primary pediatric liver tumor following hepatoblastoma, infantile hemangioendothelioma, and HCC. Subtypes of mesenchymal sarcoma include embryonal sarcoma, rhabdomyosarcoma, angiosarcoma, and malignant mesenchymoma.

The clinical findings include abdominal pain and swelling, with a palpable mass. Jaundice is usually not present, and the AFP level is not increased.

Sonographically, mesenchymal sarcoma usually presents as a single hyperechoic mass containing anechoic areas, which represent the cystic spaces. It can also appear homogeneous and hyperechoic or as a complex lesion with anechoic areas as well as calcifications producing posterior shadowing.

## Metastases[8]

Metastatic hepatic neoplasms in children are frequently associated with Wilms tumor, neuroblastoma, leukemia, and lymphoma; the most common cause is neuroblastoma. As in adults, the echogenicity and echotexture of metastases is variable: hypoechoic, isoechoic, hyperechoic and homogeneous, and heterogeneous or complex. Calcifications may be noted. Rarely are pediatric metastases diffuse, with diffuse disease most commonly associated with stage IV-S neuroblastoma.

Lymphoproliferative disorder can be a complication of solid organ transplant. Single or multiple hypoechoic masses in the liver may be noted sonographically; occasionally diffusely infiltrating disease is found.

Lymphoma of the liver is more commonly secondary to non-Hodgkin lymphoma. Sonographically discrete hypoechoic nodules are noted; hepatosplenomegaly may be present.

## HEPATIC VASCULAR DISORDERS

Vascular disorders of the liver include portal hypertension, Budd-Chiari syndrome, portal vein thrombosis, hepatic infarction, peliosis hepatis, and portal venous gas.

### Portal Hypertension[14,24,25]

Portal hypertension is due to increased resistance to normal portal venous flow. The clinical presentation includes splenomegaly, ascites, caput medusa, and, in severe cases, hematemesis, hepatic encephalopathy, and hypersplenism. The obstruction to flow can be prehepatic (portal or splenic vein thrombosis), intrahepatic (secondary to cirrhosis and less commonly hepatic vein obstruction), or posthepatic (secondary to congestive heart failure or constrictive pericarditis).

Sonographic findings include bidirectional or hepatofugal portal vein flow, development of varices, splenomegaly, a thicken lesser omentum, ascites, and evidence of cirrhosis. The portal vein may be dilated, but the size and number of varices or collaterals that develop as the disease progresses can reduce the diameter of the main portal vein. Respiratory variation in portal venous flow may be absent or reduced. Flow in the hepatic artery may increase to compensate for the decrease in blood to the liver via the main portal vein. The hepatic veins may demonstrate a loss of pulsatility and a monophasic flow pattern.

### Portal Vein Thrombosis[14,24,25]

Portal vein thrombosis can be caused by thrombosis or tumor invasion, which most often occurs with hepatoblastoma and HCC. Nonmalignant thrombosis is associated with umbilical vein catheterization, dehydration, shock, hypercoagulable states, and portal hypertension. Clinical presentation includes acute abdominal pain and, in some cases, splenomegaly. Portal vein thrombosis can be acute (enlarged, echogenic vein, absent flow with color Doppler or in cases of tumor invasion, flow within the thrombus) or chronic (cavernous transformation of the portal vein, which is described as multiple tortuous vessels in the porta hepatis and nonvisualization of the portal vein).

Acute portal vein thrombosis may be anechoic and mimic a patent portal vein on gray scale imaging; color Doppler, however, will confirm the finding of thrombosis. Additional sonographic findings in chronic portal vein thrombosis include development of collaterals with the addition of pericholecystic collaterals in some cases (Fig. 19-16A,B).

### Budd-Chiari Syndrome[14,24,25]

Budd-Chiari syndrome may be due to idiopathic occlusion or neoplastic invasion of the hepatic veins, usually secondary to hepatoblastoma, HCC, Wilms tumor, or thrombosis. Idiopathic causes of occlusion include hypercoagulable states, trauma, Gaucher disease, and cirrhosis. The primary sonographic findings include hepatomegaly, echogenic intraluminal clot, and absence of hepatic vein flow using color and pulse-wave Doppler (Fig. 19-17A–D).

Secondary findings include ascites, pleural effusion, and gallbladder wall edema.

Nonvisualization of the hepatic veins is not specific evidence of hepatic vein occlusion as patent veins can be difficult to identify in the presence of hepatomegaly or cirrhosis. In the chronic stages, additional collateral pathways for hepatic vein flow can develop.

Occlusion of the vena cava may be due to a congenital membrane within the IVC (noted sonographically as a thin, hyperechoic band inside the IVC), neoplastic invasion, extrinsic tumor compression, enlarged caudate lobe, and thrombosis. Obstruction of the IVC can cause hepatic venous congestion and development of thrombus in the hepatic veins. Color and pulse-wave Doppler confirms the absence of flow in the obstructed portion of the IVC and abnormal flow in the hepatic veins. The IVC may be dilated inferior to the obstruction.

### Hepatic Infarction

Hepatic infarction is rare due to the liver's dual blood supply but can occur with hepatic artery occlusion. Sonographically, the infarct appears as wedge-shaped, round, or oval area of decreased echogenicity with indistinct margins. Infarcts are usually located at the periphery of the liver but may occur in the middle of the liver as well. Over time, the sonographic appearance of the infarct will change from hypoechoic to hyperechoic and calcification may be noted.

### Peliosis Hepatitis

Peliosis hepatitis is a rare disorder associated with hematologic disorders, HIV infection, and long-term steroid therapy. Sonographically, the liver is heterogeneous

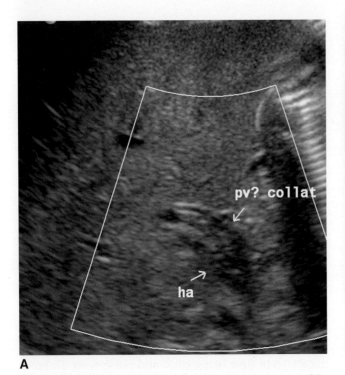

**A**

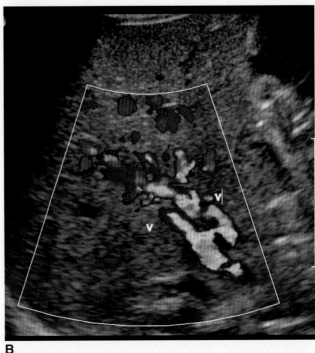

**B**

**Figure 19-16** Portal vein thrombosis. **A:** A longitudinal image of the porta hepatis demonstrates multiple small anechoic structures. The normal portal vein is not visualized. **B:** The color Doppler image demonstrates flow within the small, tortuous vessels consistent with cavernous transformation following portal vein thrombosis. (Image courtesy of James Beck, Falls Church, VA.)

and demonstrates multiple hypoechoic areas, which correlate to blood-filled cystic spaces within the liver.

### Air in the Portal Venous System

Necrotizing enterocolitis occurs in neonates and children with infarcted bowel and can demonstrate air (gas) within the portal venous system and around the gallbladder. Multiple echogenic foci can be seen moving within the vessels in the direction of blood flow, but acoustic shadowing and reverberation are not usually noted.

## GALLBLADDER AND BILIARY SYSTEM[26]

Although gallbladder disease is rare in children, it does occur. The sonographic appearance of the gallbladder is the same as in the adult patient: thin-walled, well-defined structure, with an anechoic lumen and echogenic walls.

### SONOGRAPHIC EXAMINATION TECHNIQUE

#### Scan Technique

Patients are most commonly scanned in the supine and LPO positions. Additional patient positions, such as prone (especially in obese children), semi-erect, erect, and RPO may be helpful.

The sonographer should acquire documentary images that clearly demonstrate the gallbladder and bile ducts in longitudinal and transverse planes. Evaluation, assessment, and documentation should include

the gallbladder periphery; longitudinal and transverse sweeps extending past the medial, lateral, superior, and inferior borders of the gallbladder; and the total length of the bile duct should be evaluated.

### NORMAL VARIANTS AND CONGENITAL ANOMALIES[7,27,28]

Anatomic variations of the gallbladder are common and in some cases can mimic disease states. Careful scanning and use of multiple patient positions can assist in determining if the sonographic appearance is related to a normal variant or an abnormality. The most common normal variants include a gallbladder fold (should elongate in other patient positions), Phrygian cap (fold at fundus), Hartmann pouch (widening at the neck of the gallbladder), and prominent spiral valves of Heister. Congenital anomalies include gallbladder ectopia, agenesis, duplication (division of the gallbladder longitudinally with each compartment having its own cystic duct), biliary atresia, choledochal cyst, and multiseptate gallbladder (Fig. 19-18A–C).

A multiseptate gallbladder has thin septations that give the gallbladder a divided appearance; the septa can lead to bile stasis and the formation of gallstones. Intrahepatic gallbladder is a rare anomaly.

### Biliary Atresia[14,15,27,29–31]

Conjugated hyperbilirubinemia in the newborn has two major causes: diseases of the liver such as hepatitis and biliary tract abnormalities such as atresia.

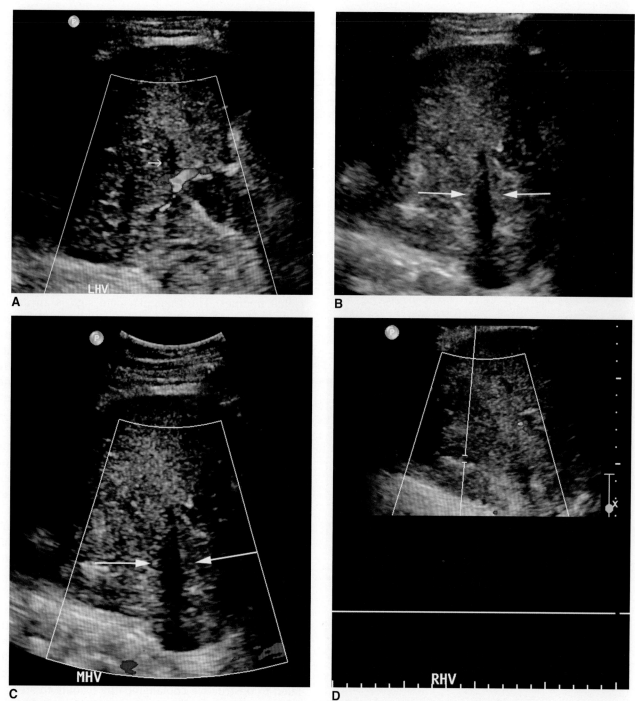

**Figure 19-17** Budd-Chiari syndrome. **A:** The color Doppler image of the left hepatic vein *(arrow)* demonstrates no flow within the vessel. **B,C:** The transverse images show the middle hepatic vein *(arrows)* which also demonstrates no flow with color Doppler. **D:** A pulsed wave image demonstrates a lack of flow in the right hepatic vein. No flow was demonstrated in the right, middle, or left hepatic veins and the liver was echogenic. (Image courtesy of James Beck, Falls Church, VA.)

The manifestations of biliary atresia range from total absence of the biliary tree to a rudimentary gallbladder and cystic duct or a visibly patent gallbladder, cystic duct, and common bile duct. In the most common form, the usual intrahepatic and extrahepatic ducts near the porta hepatis are absent. The cause of biliary atresia is unknown but should be suspected when there is persistent neonatal jaundice and infectious causes have been excluded.

It is extremely important to differentiate extrahepatic biliary atresia from intrahepatic disorders, as early identification improves the clinical outcome of the patient. Biliary atresia requires surgical intervention, whereas neonatal hepatitis syndrome is treated medically. Signs and symptoms of neonatal cholestasis and neonatal hepatitis are similar to those of biliary atresia. In both of these conditions, patients present with jaundice at about 3 to 4 weeks of age. Sonography can demonstrate dilated intrahepatic ducts, which are found in patients with choledochal cyst but not in those with extrahepatic biliary atresia. A gallbladder is usually seen in patients with neonatal hepatitis, whereas in those with atresia, depending on the degree, a gallbladder may not be seen at all or may be partially identified.

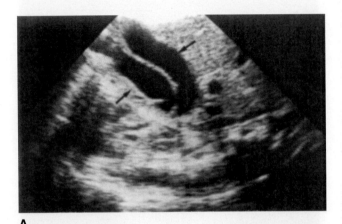

**A**

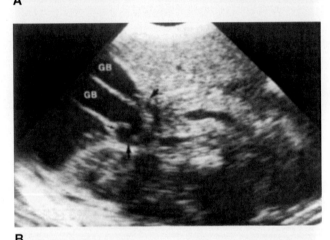

**B**

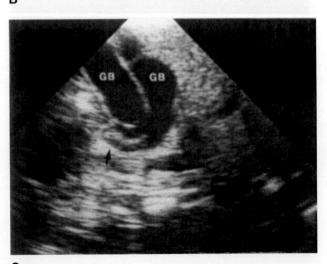

**C**

**Figure 19-18** Duplicated gallbladder. **A:** Two separate gallbladders (*arrows*) are visualized. **B,C:** On longitudinal sections, two separate cystic ducts (*large arrows*) are also visualized, arising from each gallbladder (*GB*) and converging at a distal point (*small arrow*).

Some patients with biliary atresia also have other congenital anomalies, such as anomalous origin of the hepatic artery, azygous continuation of the IVC, polysplenia, bilaterally bilobed lungs, preduodenal portal veins, abdominal malrotation, and visceral situs anomalies.

It is important to make sure that the patient is fasting appropriately for their age to ensure visualization of the gallbladder. If an atretic gallbladder is seen prior to feeding, it should also be checked postprandial to see if the size has changed. If it is not connected to the biliary system, there should be no change in its size.

Sonographically, the gallbladder, cystic duct, common bile ducts, and intrahepatic bile ducts may be seen incompletely, depending on the degree of atresia. If a rudimentary gallbladder is seen, a fasting measurement of less than 1.5 cm suggests atresia. The liver is enlarged and diffusely hyperechoic with increased attenuation, as in cirrhosis. Splenomegaly and ascites may be associated findings. The triangular cord sign is an important sonographic finding in biliary atresia and is seen as an echogenic triangular or tubular focus in the porta hepatis. The cord will follow the portal veins and should measure >4 mm in thickness. Some cases of biliary atresia also involve intrahepatic stone formation. Sonographically, these stones appear tubular or rounded and echogenic, with posterior acoustic shadowing.

Surgical interventions include the Kasai procedure to develop a communication between the duodenum and the gallbladder, common bile duct, or liver to promote drainage of bile into the duodenum and liver transplantation. The success rate of these procedures is greatest when the intervention is performed before 10 weeks of age. One complication of the Kasai procedure is ascending cholangitis probably related to bile stasis. Clinical symptoms include fever and obstructive jaundice, as well as an elevated C-reactive protein level or leukocytosis.

### Choledochal Cyst[9,14,15,27,28,32]

Choledochal cyst is a rare congenital dilatation of the common bile duct that usually presents as abdominal pain, mass, and jaundice. The exact cause of choledochal cyst is not known at this time but may be related to obstructive cholangiopathy leading to stenosis or atresia of the distal common bile duct. Another possible cause is the anomalous insertion of the common bile duct into the main pancreatic duct, which allows pancreatic juice to reflux into the biliary tree causing cholangitis and weakening of the bile duct wall. Both sonography and hepatobiliary scintigraphy are used to establish the diagnosis of this disease with CT and MRI providing additional information.

There are five main types of choledochal cyst. Type I is the fusiform dilatation of the common bile duct and is the most common form found in infants and children (Fig. 19-19A).

If the intrahepatic ducts are also dilated, usually only the distal third of the duct is involved and the peripheral

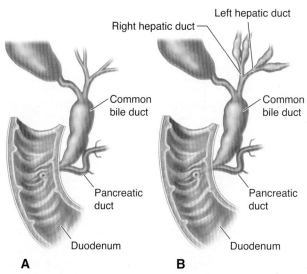

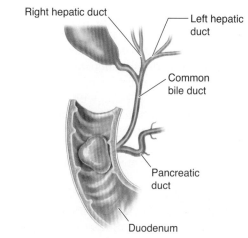

**Figure 19-21** Choledochal cyst. Type III: congenital choledochocele.

**Figure 19-19** Choledochal cyst. **A:** Type I: concentric dilatation and **(B)** type IV: fusiform dilatation, concentric dilatation, with intrahepatic involvement.

intrahepatic ducts are not necessarily affected, as they are in Caroli disease. Type II presents as a diverticulum of the common bile duct and is the second most common (Fig. 19-20A).

Type III is a congenital choledochocele, which is a cystic dilatation of the intraduodenal portion of the common bile duct. Although the cause is not known for certain, it is believed to be the result of a stricture at the ampulla of Vater. This lesion is not considered to be a true choledochal cyst and is generally asymptomatic (Fig. 19-21). Type IV choledochal cysts are concentric dilatations of the common bile duct with intrahepatic ductal dilatation (Figs. 19-19B and 19-20B). Type V is Caroli disease in which the peripheral intrahepatic ducts are affected either diffusely or focally.

Sonographically, a type I choledochal cyst appears as fluid-filled, well-defined mass in the porta hepatis adjacent to the gallbladder (Fig. 19-22). The right, left, and common bile ducts may be seen entering the cyst, and the gallbladder is demonstrated as a separate cystic structure. If the cyst is large, it may contain sludge. A type II choledochal cyst demonstrates one or more diverticula or fluid-filled structures near or coming off of the common bile duct. If there is intrahepatic ductal dilatation, type IV should be considered, and if peripheral ductal dilatation is identified, Caroli disease (type V) cannot be ruled out. In types III and IV intrahepatic ductal dilatation is noted. If biliary atresia is concurrent, the choledochal cyst will be smaller, and the intrahepatic ductal dilatation is absent.

Complications of untreated choledochal cyst include stone formation within the cyst, gallbladder or pancreatic duct, chronic biliary obstruction, chronic cholangitis, cirrhosis, biliary rupture with resulting biliary peritonitis, neoplasia (risk of adenocarcinoma increases with age), and pancreatitis.

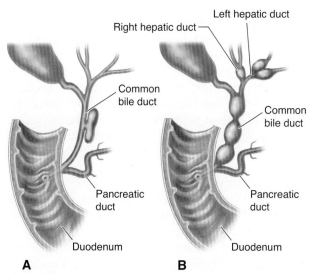

**Figure 19-20** Choledochal cyst. **A:** Type II: eccentric common bile duct diverticulum and a **(B)** type IV: rosary common bile duct diverticulum.

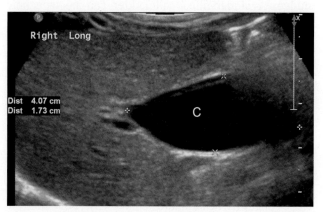

**Figure 19-22** Choledochal cyst. Three-day-old infant presents with jaundice and right upper quadrant cystic mass seen on a prenatal sonogram. A longitudinal scan of the right upper quadrant shows fusiform dilation of the common bile duct (between electronic calipers). This is compatible with a type I choledochal cyst. (Image courtesy of Rechelle Nguyen, Columbus, OH.)

## Caroli Disease[14,15,27,28]

Caroli disease is classified as type V choledochal cyst and occurs in two forms. The first type demonstrates saccular dilatation of the intrahepatic bile ducts with calculus formation and recurrent bacterial cholangitis. These patients typically present with fever, jaundice, and abdominal pain. The second type is associated with hepatic fibrosis and portal hypertension with minimal dilatation of the intrahepatic ducts. Both presentations of Caroli disease are associated with renal tubular ectasia or renal parenchymal cysts.

The sonographic appearance of the first type of Caroli disease demonstrates as multiple dilated tubular structures that extend to the periphery of the liver. Some of these structures may communicate with larger cystic areas (focally ectatic portions of biliary tree). The portal vein appears as a central dot surrounded by the fluid-filled structure; color Doppler should demonstrate blood flow within the area confirming the presence of the portal vein.

## ABNORMAL GALLBLADDER SIZE

If the patient is nonfasting, the gallbladder should be contracted (nondistended). In a fasting patient (4 to 6 hours), a small or nondistended gallbladder may indicate congenital hypoplasia, AVH, cystic fibrosis, or chronic cholecystitis (uncommon in children). A large gallbladder may indicate prolonged fasting, hydrops, or obstruction of the cystic or common bile ducts. Administration of a fatty meal can be used in cases of gallbladder enlargement to determine if the cystic duct is patent. The gallbladder is scanned prior to the fatty meal and should show emptying 45 minutes to 1 hour after the fatty meal if the cystic duct is patent.

Nonvisualization of the gallbladder is most commonly associated with biliary atresia or viral hepatitis. Less common etiologies include agenesis, ectopia, normal contraction after a meal, and the presence of sludge. A sludge-filled gallbladder can be isoechoic with the liver making sonographic detection difficult.

## GALLBLADDER WALL THICKENING[15,17]

Diffuse gallbladder wall thickening is a nonspecific finding associated with numerous inflammatory and noninflammatory causes. In children, as in adults, a gallbladder wall thickness of 2 to 5 mm suggests disease, and thickness of 5 mm or more is considered indicative of disease. Inflammatory causes include acute and chronic cholecystitis. Noninflammatory causes include viral hepatitis, hepatic dysfunction, cirrhosis, hypoalbuminemia, pancreatitis, congestive heart failure, renal disease, bone marrow transplant, sepsis, and AIDS. Diffuse wall thickening may have several sonographic appearances including uniformly echogenic, hypoechoic, or striated (hypoechoic and hyperechoic layers). In patients who are nonfasting, the gallbladder wall will demonstrate thickening due to the lack of distention of the gallbladder. Focal wall thickening is associated with cholecystitis or adenomyomatosis.

## CHOLELITHIASIS[14,15,33–35]

Cholelithiasis is the presence of one or more calculi (stones) in the gallbladder, cystic duct, or common bile duct. Biliary obstruction occurs if calculi are situated in the cystic or common bile ducts. Since bile salt secretion in infants is 50% of that in adults, it is assumed that any treatment that suppresses bile acid formation greatly increases the risk of gallstones. The incidence of gallstones is rising in children due to the increase in childhood obesity and pigmented stones are more common in children than cholesterol stones. Children with sickle cell disease have an increased incidence of cholelithiasis that is nearly double the general population.

Neonatal cholelithiasis is associated with congenital anomalies of the biliary system, total parenteral nutrition (produces bile stasis), dehydration, infection, hemolytic anemia, extracorporeal membranous oxygenation (ECMO), and short-gut syndrome. Common causes of gallstones in older children and teenagers include cystic fibrosis, malabsorption, total parenteral nutrition, liver disease, Crohn disease, bowel resection, sickle cell disease, medication use by pediatric patients for congenital heart disease, and hemolytic anemia. Most children with gallstones are predisposed due to the presence of an underlying disease process; however, some gallstones are idiopathic.

The clinical presentation in younger children with gallstones includes nonspecific symptoms (jaundice, irritability), whereas older children and teens present with more classic symptoms of right upper quadrant pain, intolerance to fatty foods, nausea, and vomiting. The most common complication of gallstones in children is pancreatitis. Often, the gallstones resolve without treatment.

Sonographic findings include a mobile echogenic intraluminal structure with acoustic shadowing, which moves to the dependent portion of the gallbladder with changes in patient position. Small stones may demonstrate little, if any, acoustic shadowing but may exhibit a "twinkle" artifact with color Doppler. Impacted stones may be found in the neck of the gallbladder. Use of multiple patient positions is recommended in cases where small and/or impacted stones are suspected.

A neonate may be examined because gallstones were noted on a fetal sonogram; most resolve spontaneously within the first year of life.

Low-level echoes within the gallbladder may be due to sludge (particulate matter within the bile), slice-thickness artifacts, hemobilia, pus, or inflammatory debris. The formation of sludge within the gallbladder is associated with prolonged fasting, hyperalimentation, and extrahepatic bile duct obstruction. Patients with sickle cell disease and cystic fibrosis are predisposed to the formation of sludge. Sludge may layer within the gallbladder, form "balls," or completely fill the gallbladder. A sludge-filled gallbladder may mimic the echogenicity and echotexture of the liver. Sludge should not exhibit acoustic shadowing.

Cystic duct stones are very difficult to demonstrate if the duct is not dilated. An impacted cystic duct stone can compress the adjacent common bile duct (Mirizzi syndrome) causing extrinsic bile duct dilatation and obstructive jaundice. However, distinguishing a stone in the cystic duct from a stone in the common bile duct is difficult.

## CHOLECYSTITIS[35–37]

Acute or chronic cholecystitis in children has a number of causes: hypoalbuminemia, AVH, heart failure, renal failure, gallbladder carcinoma, ascites, multiple myeloma, congenital obstruction of the cystic duct or obstruction from an external source, biliary stasis, and portal node lymphatic obstruction.

Clinically, the patient can present with right upper quadrant pain, fever, vomiting, and a palpable right upper quadrant lump. The differential diagnosis includes cholecystitis, abdominal abscesses of the right upper quadrant, pancreatitis, appendicitis, peptic ulcer disease, and gallbladder torsion.

In a diseased state, the gallbladder wall presents sonographically as thickened, irregular, and highly reflective. A hypoechoic to anechoic halo seen surrounding the gallbladder wall is usually due to either infection of the wall itself or a disease process in the surrounding liver tissue (Fig. 19-23A,B). At times, sludge can be seen in the gallbladder owing to stasis.

## HYDROPIC GALLBLADDER[38]

Hydropic gallbladder develops in acutely ill children who receive TPN or hyperalimentation therapy and in association with diseases such as Kawasaki (mucocutaneous lymph node) syndrome, leptospirosis, typhoid fever, ascariasis, *Salmonella, Pseudomonas,* or group B streptococcal sepsis, congestive heart failure, shock, chronic biliary tract obstruction, upper respiratory tract infection, gastroenteritis, and Epstein-Barr virus infection. Clinically, patients present with right upper quadrant pain, fever, dehydration, and abdominal distention. The reasons for hydropic gallbladder are unclear. Some suggest that it is due to noncalculous blockage of the cystic duct, resulting in bile stasis. This blockage may be caused by reactive inflammation of the cystic duct, atresia of the cystic duct, lymph node impingement, or cholangitis near the cystic duct. Dehydration can cause bile stasis, and the enlarged gallbladder can further obstruct bile flow by impinging on the cystic duct. Most of the time, a hydropic gallbladder resolves spontaneously.

Sonographically, the gallbladder is dramatically enlarged and completely anechoic with thin walls. Gallstones or sludge may be present. Such a gallbladder generally does not contract well following a fatty meal.

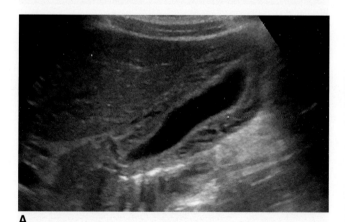

**A**

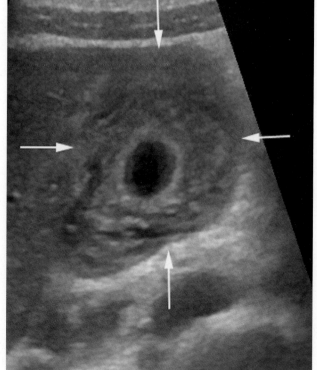

**B**

**Figure 19-23** Cholecystitis. The longitudinal **(A)** and transverse **(B)** images of the gallbladder are on a pediatric patient with acalculous cholecystitis. Note the markedly thickened irregular gallbladder wall. (Image courtesy of GE Healthcare, Wauwatosa, WI.)

## BILIARY OBSTRUCTION[15,39,40]

Intrahepatic and extrahepatic bile duct obstruction may be due to the presence of neoplasm (rhabdomyosarcoma is the most common), enlarged lymph nodes in the porta hepatis compressing the bile duct, acute pancreatitis, biliary calculi, and biliary stricture (uncommon). Patients with biliary obstruction present with jaundice. Sonographically, the dilated intrahepatic bile ducts demonstrate as multiple anechoic irregularly branching structures, which are larger at the porta hepatis. The extrahepatic bile ducts demonstrate as round or tubular anechoic structures near the porta hepatis and/or head of the pancreas. The sonographer should search for the point of obstruction and demonstrate the presence of a mass or calculus that is causing the obstruction. Pancreatitis usually causes the duct to taper significantly

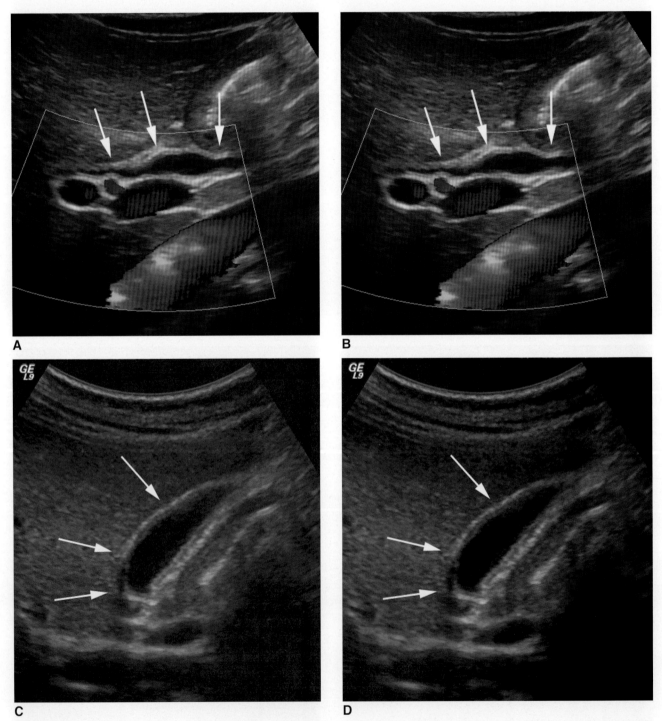

**Figure 19-24** Sclerosing cholangitis. **A,B:** Color Doppler images of the porta hepatis reveal a common bile duct with thickened irregular walls *(arrows)*. The longitudinal **(C)** and transverse **(D)** images of the gallbladder in the same patient demonstrate mild wall thickening. This 16-year-old patient with ulcerative colitis was diagnosed with subsequent sclerosing cholangitis. *(continued)*

at the pancreatic head while a mass, calculus, or stricture demonstrates as an abrupt change from a dilated to a narrowed or absent duct. Calculi in the duct may demonstrate acoustic shadowing or "twinkle" sign with color Doppler.

Dilated bile ducts may spontaneously rupture causing neonatal jaundice and bile ascites or a biloma. The most common location for perforation is at the junction of the cystic and common bile ducts. Affected patients usually present in the first 3 months of life with ascites, mild jaundice, failure to thrive, and abdominal distention. Bilirubin values are elevated but all of the other liver function tests are normal; this distinguishes biliary obstruction from neonatal hepatis syndrome and biliary atresia.

Bile plug syndrome (inspissated bile syndrome) can cause obstruction of the bile ducts. Liver abnormalities are not present in this syndrome, which primarily affects full-term infants. Risk factors include massive hemolysis, total parenteral nutrition, Hirschsprung disease, cystic fibrosis, and intestinal atresias. Echogenic material may be found within dilated ducts and sludge may be noted in the gallbladder. Bleeding into the ducts from trauma, surgery, or biopsy can mimic the sonographic appearance of bile plug syndrome.

## SCLEROSING CHOLANGITIS[14,15,27]

Sclerosing cholangitis is a chronic disease in which there is inflammatory fibrosis that obliterates the intrahepatic and extrahepatic bile ducts. This leads to the development of biliary cirrhosis, portal hypertension, and liver failure. Approximately 70% to 80% of children with sclerosing cholangitis have concurrent inflammatory bowel disease (Fig. 19-24A–D). The clinical presentation of sclerosing cholangitis is right upper quadrant pain and jaundice with abnormal liver function tests and elevated bilirubin.

Sonographic findings include thickening of the walls of the bile ducts, choledocholithiasis (intrahepatic and extrahepatic), cholelithiasis, and ductal strictures (Fig. 19-24E,F).

## AIDS-RELATED CHOLANGITIS[15]

In children with AIDS, the most common biliary tract findings are calculus cholecystitis and cholangitis. The sonographic findings are similar to sclerosing cholangitis with ductal dilatation and gallbladder enlargement with wall thickening. Edema of the ampulla of Vater may demonstrate as a hyperechoic nodule at the distal end of the common bile duct.

## BILIARY NEOPLASM

### Rhabdomyosarcoma[27,41,42]

Biliary rhabdomyosarcoma is a rare soft tissue tumor occurring in children, usually between the ages of 1 and 5 years. It arises in the biliary tract and produces obstruction. It is the second most common cause of obstructive jaundice in older children after choledochal cyst and in neonates after biliary atresia. The tumor appears lobulated and is usually situated in the hilus of the liver. It invades the intrahepatic or extrahepatic ducts, with lacunar polypoid projections causing obstruction. Occasionally, the tumor is discovered in the right lobe of the liver.

Clinical signs are increasing abdominal girth, jaundice, pain, and weight loss. Usually, these clinical

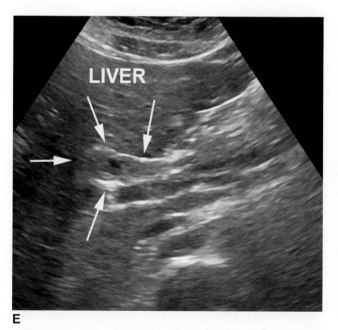

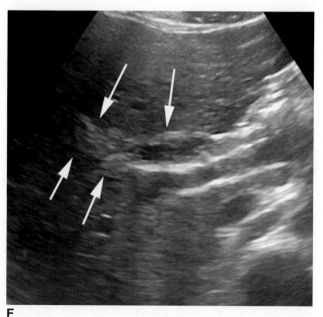

**E**    **F**

Figure 19-24 *(continued)* **E,F:** Images of the common bile duct in a different patient with Crohn disease reveal a thickened irregular wall consistent with sclerosing cholangitis. (Images courtesy of Jillian Platt, Falls Church, VA.)

symptoms are confused with those of infectious hepatitis. Laboratory values may include elevated total serum bilirubin, a marked increase in alkaline phosphatase, and normal or mildly elevated AST. There may also be a moderate increase in the white blood cell count owing to subsequent cholangitis. Unlike hepatoblastoma or HCC, biliary rhabdomyosarcoma may not cause an increase in the AFP level. Biopsy and histologic examination are definitive for diagnosis.

Sonographically, rhabdomyosarcoma is predominantly solid, with hyperechoic formations in the bile duct. With biliary rhabdomyosarcoma, there is no posterior shadowing, as is commonly seen with stones. There may be cystic spaces representing intrahepatic radicles of the bile ducts. There may also be focal areas of necrosis and hemorrhage in the mass. Usually, dilated bile ducts surround the mass.

Surgical excision is a must, although complete excision is almost impossible. Since these tumors are very chemosensitive, the favored method of treatment is surgery with adjuvant chemotherapy and radiation therapy. Rhabdomyosarcomas tend to recur quickly, so the prognosis is poor.

The differential diagnosis includes benign and malignant lesions: choledochal cyst, infectious hepatitis, recurrent cholestasis, gallstones, lymphoma, neuroblastoma, pancreatic pseudocysts, hepatic hemangioma, enteric duplication cysts, hepatoblastoma, HCC, hemangioendothelioma, focal nodular hypoplasia, hepatic adenoma, mixed mesenchymal sarcomas, and gallbladder torsion.

# PANCREAS

Sonography is currently the diagnostic procedure of choice for the examination of children with symptoms of pancreatic disease. Real-time sonography of the pancreas in infants and children is easily performed. Compared to adults, the pancreas is more easily seen in children because most are lean and have a large left hepatic lobe, which serves as an excellent window for visualizing the pancreas. The drawbacks of pancreatic sonography include technically unsatisfactory studies due to obesity or excessive bowel gas, and limited scanning surfaces when surgical dressings or ostomy sites are present.

## SONOGRAPHIC EXAMINATION TECHNIQUE

### Scan Technique

A standard examination of the pancreas includes transverse and longitudinal scans of the supine patient. The transverse scans may require some initial survey to determine the exact position of the gland, as it generally lies oblique in the middle portion of the body, with the head lower than the body and tail. Longitudinal scans should be oriented to the true longitudinal axis of the

pancreas, as determined by the transverse scans. It is not uncommon to examine the patient in different positions (i.e., prone, upright, decubitus) to adequately visualize the pancreas. This is particularly important in the presence of disease, as the scan must demonstrate the lesion's relationship to surrounding pancreatic structure and adjacent organs. Another helpful technique is to use the water-filled duodenum to outline the pancreas. The patient is given ~16 oz of water, and the progress of the water into the duodenum is checked periodically by the sonographer. When the duodenum is appropriately distended, the patient is repositioned until the water-filled duodenum outlines the area of the pancreas that is of interest. A fluid-filled stomach may also be helpful to outline the pancreatic tail. This technique, however, has several drawbacks: (1) many patients suffer severe nausea, and large amounts of water may induce vomiting; (2) fluid filling is contraindicated for fasting patients receiving intravenous fluid; and (3) the method can be time consuming.

### Technical Considerations

During pancreatic sonography, the gain control is usually at settings comparable to those used for scanning the liver. Determination of the normal pancreatic sonographic pattern is based on a comparison to the liver parenchymal pattern. In children, the normal pancreatic parenchyma is relatively homogeneous, with even, high-, and medium-level echo distribution. This is in contrast to the irregular echo texture, or "cobblestone" appearance, considered normal for adults. The normal pancreas is similar to or more echogenic than the liver parenchyma. Vascular structures abound in this area and should have a clearly echo-free pattern and not filled in by too high a gain setting. The transducer frequency selections should be made to obtain the highest resolution with adequate penetration.

### NORMAL ANATOMY

During a sonographic pancreatic study, the sonographer should pay particular attention to surrounding vascular landmarks, to the gland's shape and size, and to delineation of the pancreatic duct.

Attention to the surrounding vascular landmarks may be necessary to identify this rather small structure. Primary vascular landmarks include the following: (1) the splenic vein, which can be seen lying inferior and posterior to the tail of the pancreas (transverse scans) and running left to right from the splenic hilus to the portal vein confluence; (2) the SMV, located posterior to the junction of the head and the body of the pancreas and best seen on the longitudinal scans; (3) the IVC, which passes posterior and slightly to the right of the pancreatic head; and (4) the superior mesenteric artery (SMA), which travels inferiorly along the posterior aspect at the junction of the head and body of the pancreas and anterior to the uncinate process.

Sonographic studies should also give specific attention to the size of the pancreas. The maximum anteroposterior (AP) diameters of the head, body, and tail are measured on transverse images obtained by angling the transducer to visualize more parenchyma. The entire gland can usually be seen in one image if it is oriented transversely across the abdomen, but often it lies oblique to some degree, with the tail more cephalad than the head and body, in which case it may be necessary to obtain several images to demonstrate the entire gland.

The pancreatic duct is not always seen in normal patients. Usually appearing as a single echogenic line <1 mm, it can be located in the pancreatic body in a plane cephalad to the splenic vein.

## DEVELOPMENTAL AND CONGENITAL ANOMALIES

A very small pancreas (head only) is due to agenesis of the dorsal pancreas during the embryonic stage and is associated with polysplenia. Annular pancreas is the result of a bifid pancreatic head, which encases the duodenum. This anomaly is associated with duodenal atresia or stenosis.

### Cystic Fibrosis[43–45]

Cystic fibrosis is a recessively inherited disease with a prevalence of 1 in 3,500 in Caucasians and 1 in 17,000 in African Americans in the United States. Cystic fibrosis affects the exocrine glands in the lungs and GI tract, which produce abnormal highly viscous mucus. Those affected with cystic fibrosis have pancreatic exocrine dysfunction due to obstruction of the small ductules by mucoid secretions. The obstruction of the small ductules leads to subsequent tissue destruction and atrophy and eventual replacement of the pancreatic tissue with fibrosis and fat. Eventually, normal function is compromised and pancreatic insufficiency results. Intraluminal calcifications can be found but inflammatory changes are not common.

The pancreas is hyperechoic due to the replacement of normal pancreatic tissue by fibrosis and fatty tissue. Sonographically apparent cysts may be found. The gallbladder is usually small and gallstones may be present. Pancreatitis may occur but is not common and the sonographic appearance is not affected. Other causes of a hyperechoic pancreas in childhood include steroid therapy, chronic pancreatitis, Cushing syndrome, Shwachman-Diamond syndrome, Johanson-Blizzard syndrome, and obstruction of the main pancreatic duct. Clinical and biochemical tests can distinguish these diseases from cystic fibrosis.

### Congenital Cysts[44]

von Hippel-Lindau disease and autosomal polycystic disease are autosomal dominant disorders that can cause cysts in the pancreas as well as other organs (liver, kidney, adrenal glands, and spleen). Patients with von Hippel-Lindau disease also present with cerebellar, medullary, and spinal hemangioblastomas and pheochromocytomas.

## PANCREATIC NEOPLASMS[45–47]

Pancreatic neoplasms are uncommon in childhood but their clinical appearance is similar to that in adults.

### Pancreatic Carcinoma

Pancreatic carcinoma is a nonfunctioning tumor. Early diagnosis is difficult because of the variety and nonspecificity of early signs and symptoms. Because of this, the tumor is often large by the time it is discovered and metastases to the liver, lymph nodes, and lung have already occurred.

Sonographically, pancreatic carcinoma usually appears as a localized, hypoechoic mass in comparison to the homogeneous texture of the normal pancreas. Focal enlargement is also an important sonographic clue. Lesions <2 cm are often difficult to detect, especially if they create only minor acoustic alterations.

### Islet Cell Tumors

Approximately two-thirds of islet cell tumors are functional, producing a hormone that provokes the clinical suspicion of tumor early in the course of disease. Because of this, most islet cell tumors are small when first detected. The diagnosis is usually made by analyzing serum hormone levels. Therefore, in these cases, diagnostic imaging is used to localize rather than to diagnose.

The remaining third of islet cell tumors are nonfunctional. Owing to a lack of hormone secretion, they remain silent until they grow large enough to produce a palpable mass that obstructs the biliary system or the GI tract.

Sonographically, an islet cell tumor is a well-circumscribed, anechoic mass. It is important to search for metastatic disease, which may be the only reliable sign of malignancy. Sonography can be uniquely helpful in identifying the islet cell tumors in the operating room when all other modalities have failed. Direct pancreatic scanning can aid in tumor localization.

### Insulinoma

Insulinoma, another tumor that occurs in childhood, is round, firm, and encapsulated, and 75% of the time is located in the body or tail of the pancreas. Clinically, patients present with hypoglycemia, which is often manifested in children by erratic behavior and seizures. Ectopic adenomas are rare, and most are benign.

Insulinomas sonographically appear as relatively small hypoechoic well-circumscribed masses. Insulinomas are sometimes difficult to accurately identify and isolate preoperatively. At surgery, palpation is used to aid in detection but is not always reliable. Intraoperative sonography is a more accurate method for detection.

It provides better resolution, the field of view is such that access to the pancreas is improved, and the whole area of interest can be visualized and interrogated, unobscured by bowel gas and overlying structures.

### Lymphoma

Lymphoma of the pancreas is a rare neoplasm that accounts for only 0.16% of pancreatic malignancies. The involvement of the pancreas in a lymphatic process is usually secondary to primary lymph node disease. The neoplasm can be located anywhere in the pancreas, and symptoms depend on anatomic location.

The diagnosis of pancreatic lymphoma should be considered in several clinical situations: when a pancreatic mass develops in a patient known to have disseminated lymphoma, when fine-needle aspiration biopsy of a pancreatic mass reveals lymphocytes without evidence of carcinoma, and when a pancreatic mass is associated with chylous ascites.

Focal infiltration of the pancreas in lymphoma appears sonographically as a large, solitary, hypoechoic lesion. Differential diagnosis is facilitated by the presence of para-aortic lymphomas and the fact that the underlying disease is usually obvious at the time the pancreatic lesions are demonstrated.

### PANCREATITIS[7,43–45,48]

Pancreatitis is significantly less common in children than in adults but is not all that rare. Pediatric pancreatitis may have a variety of causes: (1) trauma (blunt abdominal trauma secondary to childhood accident, motor vehicle accidents, and child abuse); (2) infection (usually viral, such as mumps or mononucleosis); (3) toxicity (secondary to such drugs as prednisone and L-asparaginase); (4) heredity (an autosomal dominant disorder beginning in childhood); and (5) idiopathic. The most common of these is blunt abdominal trauma (Fig. 19-25). To distinguish between the possible causes of pancreatitis, it is important to obtain a detailed patient history.

### Acute Pancreatitis[14,44,45,48]

Acute pancreatic inflammation causes the escape of pancreatic enzymes from the acinar cells into surrounding tissues. Acute pancreatitis can usually be diagnosed with combined clinical and laboratory information without requiring pancreatic imaging. However, diagnostic imaging may be necessary when a wide variety of clinical symptoms, possible causes, and complications cause confusion. Nausea and vomiting are common and may precede or follow the onset of abdominal pain. Other frequent physical findings include fever, tachycardia, abdominal distention due to ileus, and abdominal tenderness. The use of sonography enables earlier diagnosis of acute pancreatitis in children with acute or chronic pain. Diagnostic imaging is also useful in defining the extent of the disease in the patient with suspected complications

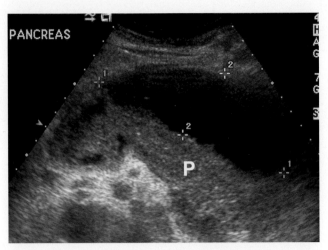

**Figure 19-25** Pancreatic trauma. This transverse pancreas image on an 8-year-old patient with a history of blunt abdominal trauma due to a bicycle accident demonstrates fluid around the pancreas (*electronic calipers*). The pancreas was enlarged and irregular. (Image courtesy of Monica Bacani, Columbus, OH.)

such as necrotizing pancreatitis, hemorrhagic pancreatitis, pseudocyst formation, and superimposed infection.

The primary sonographic appearance in acute pancreatitis is of an enlarged, edematous gland that is less echogenic than the liver parenchyma. These characteristics are most obvious during the first hours after an acute attack. A dilated pancreatic duct is another indication of pancreatitis. A pancreatic ductal diameter of 1.5 mm should be considered abnormal. The pancreas' size and echo pattern usually return to normal as the disease resolves. The entire pancreas is usually involved, but sometimes only portions are affected, particularly in pancreatitis by trauma. Follow-up examinations may help to establish the diagnosis of pancreatitis by showing a decrease in the size of the pancreas. Sonography is also useful in the early detection of complications and the identification of associated biliary disease.

### Complications of Acute Pancreatitis

After an episode of acute pancreatitis, a range of pathologic changes may develop in the gland and peripancreatic region.

### Pseudocysts[9]

The best-known complication of pancreatitis is pseudocyst formation. Pseudocysts can cause pain or bowel or biliary obstruction and can become infected. Pseudocysts are usually located in or adjacent to the pancreas but can occur anywhere in the abdomen or pelvis. Occasionally, pseudocysts may even extend into the mediastinum. Serial examinations are useful for monitoring enlargement and regression of pseudocysts. The majority of pseudocysts resolve spontaneously within 4 to 12 weeks, but those that develop mature, fibrous capsules are unlikely to be reabsorbed spontaneously. Recurrent abdominal pain, elevated serum amylase, and intermittent nausea and vomiting are common clinical symptoms consistent with this complication. When percutaneous drainage of the pseudocyst is indicated, sonographic guidance may be used.

Because children's pseudocysts often have a different pathogenesis, they may resolve more rapidly than the more common adult pancreatitis of biliary or alcoholic origin. Children's pseudocysts are less likely to recur following drainage.

Pseudocysts are usually anechoic masses, with a sharp back wall and increased through transmission. They may be single or multiple (Fig. 19-26A,B). Pseudocysts sometimes contain internal echoes emanating from pus and cellular debris.

### Hemorrhage

Intrapancreatic hemorrhage with acute pancreatitis results from disruption of one or more pancreatic blood vessels. This is uncommon but is a potentially lethal complication that may produce a large pancreatic hematoma.

Sonographically, hemorrhagic pancreatitis appears as an inhomogeneous mass. Initially, acute hemorrhage into the pancreas may appear anechoic, but it becomes moderately echogenic as organization occurs.

### Phlegmon

A phlegmon is a solid inflammatory mass that may develop following acute pancreatitis. Comprised of necrotic tissue mixed with inflammatory exudate and tissue edema, phlegmon may resolve spontaneously whenever the necrotic process is not progressive. With more severe episodes of acute pancreatitis, a necrotizing process may predominate and provoke further complications. The patient is also at risk for developing a pancreatic abscess by bacterial seeding into necrotic tissue.

A phlegmon appears as an anechoic mass in the pancreatic bed. Clinical history plus sonographic findings usually lead to the correct diagnosis.

### Abscess

Abscess formation is more likely to occur in severe cases of pancreatitis with extensive necrosis. Marked by spiking fevers, chills, and a recurrence of abdominal pain 10 to 14 days after the initial episode, drainage is required in all cases because, untreated, mortality is usually 100%. Percutaneous aspiration during drainage provides important material for laboratory studies, assisting in identifying offending organisms for effective antibiotic treatment.

A pancreatic abscess can arise from different sources. A pancreatic phlegmon may develop into an abscess when the necrotic pancreatic and peripancreatic tissues are invaded by infection. An abscess can also occur in a pseudocyst in much the same way. Terminology can be confusing here because the infected pseudocyst is sometimes considered a different entity and not called an abscess. An abscess is present in ~3% of pseudocysts.

Air can be a notable diagnostic criterion for pancreatic inflammation. Air appears within abscesses in 30% to 60% of cases. Air within the pancreatic bed can be produced by a pancreatic abscess with gas-forming organisms or from a fistulous communication with a hollow viscus. The most common site for pancreaticoenteric fistula is the transverse colon at the splenic flexure. Fistulization is considered an ominous finding because it can facilitate seeding and may contribute to a secondary abscess.

Pancreatic abscess usually appears as a large anechoic mass in the pancreatic bed. Because pancreatic abscesses cannot be differentiated sonographically from other anechoic pancreatic masses, it is important to combine the clinical history with the sonographic findings to make the correct diagnosis. The sonographic appearance of the abscess varies with the amount of suppurative material and debris. Abscess walls are usually thick, irregular, and echogenic. When air bubbles are present, the pancreatic area appears highly echogenic

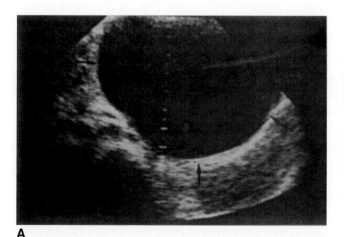

**A**

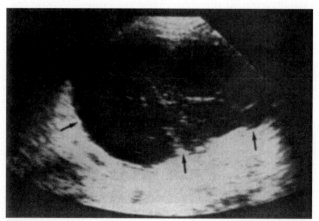

**B**

**Figure 19-26** Pancreatic pseudocyst. The **(A)** transverse image reveals a large single pseudocyst and a **(B)** longitudinal sonogram demonstrates a large septated pseudocyst.

with occasional shadowing. The air may obscure visualization on sonograms.

### Chronic Pancreatitis[43–45]

Chronic pancreatitis, or chronic relapsing pancreatitis, is a clinical condition caused by repeated attacks of acute pancreatitis, which causes fibrosis and destruction of pancreatic cells. In the late stages of the disease, pancreatic tissue fibrosis causes alternating areas of stricture and dilatation in the main pancreatic duct. In very late stages, calcifications can occur within the duct.

A majority of the childhood cases of chronic relapsing pancreatitis have a definite familial clustering pattern and represent examples of the disease called hereditary pancreatitis. Familial cases have an autosomal dominant inheritance pattern with complete penetrance but variable expressivity. More than 200 cases of proven or suspected hereditary pancreatitis have been reported. The likelihood that patients with "hereditary pancreatitis" will develop pancreatic carcinoma is increased, particularly for those with pancreatic calcifications.

Sonographically, in early stages of chronic pancreatitis, the pancreas is less echogenic than the normal liver parenchyma. This appearance is similar to that of acute pancreatitis. There may be dilatation of the main pancreatic duct or common bile duct caused by chronic pancreatitis. In advanced stages, the pancreas shrinks, develops irregular borders, and is more echogenic than usual with fibrosis. Calcifications and dilated ducts may also be present. The calcifications may be so pronounced and cause so much acoustic shadowing that pancreatic identification is difficult.

## GASTROINTESTINAL TRACT[49]

Although sonography is not usually the modality of choice for evaluating the adult GI tract, sonography of the GI tract is readily performed in infants and children using a high-frequency linear transducer. Graded compression is utilized to displace bowel gas and permit visualization of the underlying structures. Pyloric stenosis, intussusception, and acute appendicitis are primarily evaluated using sonography.

### STOMACH

The normal gastric wall, including the mucosa and muscularis muscle layer, measures from 2.5 to 3.5 mm. The gastric wall's thickness can be assessed with the patient lying in the supine and RLD positions before and after ingestion of fluid. For such a study, the child should fast (Fig. 19-27A). With abnormalities associated with stomach wall thickening, the measurements and configuration remain unchanged when water is ingested. The stomach has an echogenic submucosa well seen with a fluid-filled stomach and an outer hypoechoic rim of muscle.

A variety of abnormalities (e.g., eosinophilic gastritis, gastric ulcer, lymphoid hyperplasia, gastric hamartoma) have been reported to cause gastric wall thickening of 5 to 15 mm. Ménétrier disease or transient protein losing gastropathy display hypertrophy of the mucosa. The mucosa is thickened and echogenic, especially in the fundus and antrum. Lymphoma, Henoch-Schönlein purpura, and lymphangiectasia may look similar. In children with gastric ulcer disease, the thickening occurs in the antropyloric mucosa. Moderate or generalized thickening up to 5 mm was present with lymphoid hyperplasia, varioliform gastritis, and Crohn disease involving the stomach. The greatest amount of thickening (up to 10 mm) occurred in children with chronic granulomatous disease (Fig. 19-27B,C).

### Pyloric Stenosis[49,50–56]

Hypertrophic pyloric stenosis (HPS) most commonly affects first-born male infants between 2 and 10 weeks of age with most patients presenting at 1 to 2 months of age. This idiopathic condition is caused by abnormal thickening of the antropyloric region of the stomach. Patients present with dehydration and frequent episodes of projectile nonbilious vomiting; failure to thrive may also be noted. Clinically, the enlarged pylorus can be palpated as an olive-shaped epigastric mass. Sonography is highly sensitive and specific for the diagnosis of this condition providing direct visualization of the pyloric muscle and lack of passage of fluid through the pylorus. With pyloric stenosis, the stomach is often filled with fluid even if the patient has been fasting.

The patient should be examined in the supine and RPO positions. The transverse plane demonstrates the long axis of the pylorus and the longitudinal plane demonstrates its transverse axis. To identify the pylorus, scans should be made in the transverse plane, descending along the lesser curvature of the stomach through the left lobe of the liver, just to the right of the midline. The antrum of the stomach appears just medial to the gallbladder in the transverse plane and the pylorus is continuous with the stomach (Fig. 19-28A,B). If the pylorus is not well visualized, the patient may drink some water to display the gastric lumen.

The mass presents as a doughnut sign: an anechoic to hypoechoic muscle mass with a central lumen of increased echogenicity (Fig. 19-28C). Measurements should be made from the antrum of the stomach to the most distal portion of the identifiable channel (Fig. 19-28D). The diagnosis of pyloric stenosis can be made when the pyloric diameter anterior to posterior exceeds 1.5 cm, the length from the antrum to the distal end of the channel exceeds 1.8 cm, and the muscle thickness exceeds 4 mm. The channel and muscle measurements are the most reliable. To differentiate from antritis, the stomach wall is always normal in patients with pyloric stenosis. The enlarged pyloric muscle is an abrupt change from the normal stomach wall (Fig. 19-28E–G).

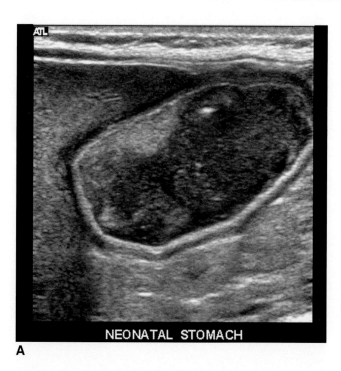

A

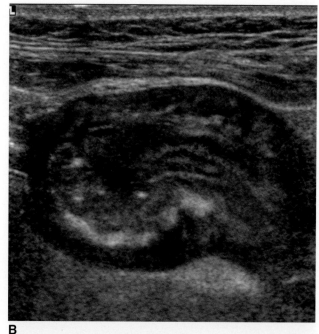

B

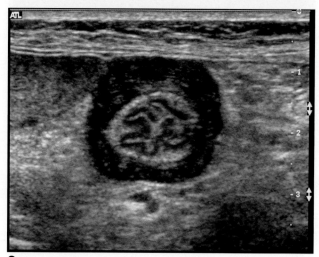

C

**Figure 19-27** Stomach. **A:** In this image of a normal neonatal stomach filled with fluid, the hyperechoic submucosa can be clearly seen surrounded by the hypoechoic muscle layer. **B:** This image of the stomach demonstrates thickened submucosal and muscular layers. **C:** This transverse image of the stomach demonstrates a markedly thickened hypoechoic muscular layer. (Images courtesy of Philips Medical Systems, Bothell, WA.)

## SMALL BOWEL[7,49–52,57,58,59]

Abnormalities of the small bowel include small bowel obstruction (usually congenital anomalies of midgut malrotation, bowel atresia, or meconium ileus in infants), acquired anomalies such as intussusception, incarcerated hernia, and acute appendicitis (older children). Sonography is useful when there is gasless abdominal distention. The normal bowel wall thickness is approximately 5.0 mm when the bowel is contracted. Features of small bowel obstruction include hyperactive, dilated bowel loops with bowel wall thickening in some cases. Graded compression may be used in the sonographic evaluation of the small bowel.

Duodenal atresia, duodenal web, and duodenal stenosis are intrinsic causes of a dilated duodenum and

stomach; the majority of obstructions at this level are intrinsic. Extrinsic causes of an obstruction at this level include malrotation, duodenal duplication cyst, choledochal cyst, and annular pancreas. Sonographically, the duodenum and stomach are seen as large anechoic structures; the esophagus may also be dilated (Fig. 19-29A,B). Duodenal atresia is common in patients with trisomy 21, 30% to 40% of patients with duodenal atresia have trisomy 21. A duodenal web may appear as an echogenic band in the proximal portion of the dilated duodenum.

Jejunal and ileal atresias are the most common causes of obstruction in the small bowel. Neonatal patients present with bilious vomiting, abdominal distention, and failure to pass meconium. Some of these patients will have associated abnormalities of midgut malrotation, gastroschisis, duodenal atresia, or

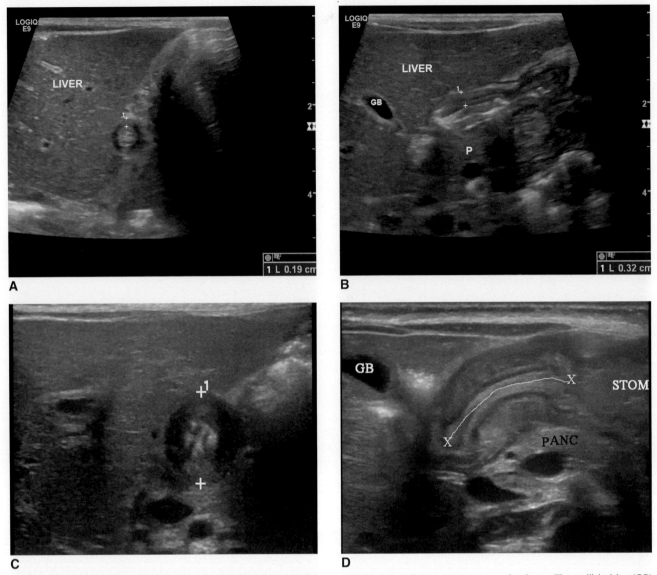

**Figure 19-28** Hypertrophic pyloric stenosis. **A,B:** Transverse and longitudinal images demonstrate a normal pylorus. The gallbladder (*GB*) is seen to the right of the pylorus and the pancreas (*P*) posterior. **C:** This transverse image of the pylorus demonstrates the donut sign with a thickened hypoechoic muscle layer. **D:** A longitudinal image of the pylorus demonstrates an elongated channel with a trace measurement from the antrum of the stomach to the distal end of the channel. A measurement of greater than 1.8 cm is considered abnormal. *(continued)*

tracheoesophageal fistula. The sonographic appearance is of multiple dilated loops of bowel in which active peristalsis can be seen.

Meconium ileus is due to abnormally thick meconium in the distal small bowel and commonly associated with the presence of cystic fibrosis. The sonographic appearance includes echogenic bowel contents, dilated bowel loops, and decreased peristalsis.

A common complication of meconium ileus is antenatal meconium peritonitis and pseudocyst. It is also a complication of bowel atresia and in utero volvulus. Within 12 hours of perforation, calcifications can develop in the fetal abdomen and echogenic ascites may be noted. These calcifications are easily identified in the fetal and neonatal abdomen. Meconium pseudocyst is a walled-off collection of meconium, which commonly

contains calcifications (acoustic shadowing is noted) and may also contain air (shadowing or ring-down artifact may be noted).

Midgut malrotation of the small bowel mesentery is a result of arrested fetal gut development. The mesentery may contain remnant peritoneal folds or shortened mesentery. Other anomalies such as omphalocele, gastroschisis, diaphragmatic hernia, and duodenal atresia or web may be found. Most patients present with bilious vomiting in the first month; abdominal sonography is useful to exclude other reasons for the vomiting.

The sonographer must demonstrate the relative positions of the SMV and SMA, so careful scanning through the transverse axes of these vessels is crucial and should extend as inferiorly in the abdomen as

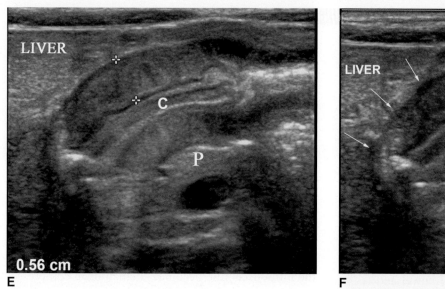

E

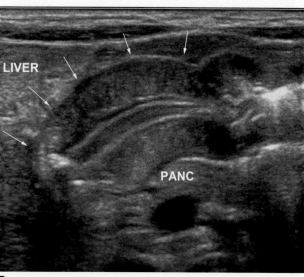

F

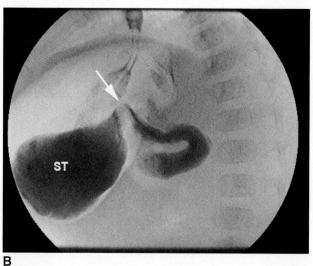

G

Figure 19-28 (continued) E,F: The long axis sections of the pylorus shows a muscle thickness of 0.56 cm and an elongated pyloric channel (C) in a 5-week-old boy with a history of 3 days of projectile vomiting and weight loss. G: Longitudinal image after feeding demonstrates a fluid-filled stomach. During the examination, fluid was not visualized passing through the elongated channel. (Images E and F courtesy of Monica Bacani, Columbus, OH.)

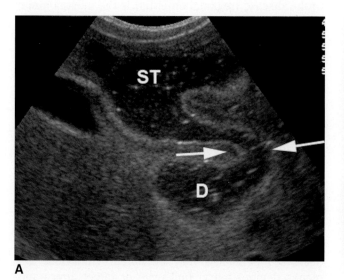

A

B

Figure 19-29 Duodenal atresia. A: Sonogram of the fluid-filled stomach (ST) and duodenum (D) shows a narrowing (arrows) consistent with duodenal atresia. The patient had Down syndrome. B: an upper gastrointestinal (UGI) examination of the same patient again demonstrates the narrowing (arrow). (Images courtesy of Dr. Nakul Jerath, Falls Church, VA.)

possible. In patients with midgut malrotation, the normal positions of the SMV and SMA are reversed with some cases presenting with the SMV directly anterior to the SMA. The SMA, which usually runs inferior to the body of the pancreas, is pulled to the right side to lie anterior to the IVC or to the right of the aorta. If volvulus is present, the whirlpool sign on gray scale and color Doppler has been shown to have 83% to 92% sensitivity and 100% specificity. The whirlpool appearance is a result of the mesentery and SMV wrapped around the SMA.

## INTUSSUSCEPTION[7,9,48,51,55]

Intussusception is the telescoping of bowel and is the most common obstructive bowel disorder of early childhood, found more frequently in males between the ages of 1 to 3. Intussusception occurs when a segment of bowel prolapses into a more distal segment (Fig. 19-30A,B). If the diagnosis is made early, the intussusception can easily be reduced by hydrostatic pressure before complications such as bowel obstruction, perforation, peritonitis, and vascular compromise (which in turn leads to edema of the bowel wall and gangrene) occur.

The most common type is ileocolic, followed by ileoileal and colocolic. The majority of cases are idiopathic but some cases have concurrent Meckel diverticulum, enteric duplication cyst, intestinal polyps, intramural hematoma, or lymphoma. The most common clinical findings are abdominal pain, currant-jelly (dark red in color) stool, and an abdominal mass, which is usually palpable. Sonography is being used more frequently for suspected intussusception and can also identify other abnormalities that might be overlooked when only the enema examination is performed.

Ninety percent of intussusceptions in children are ileocolic and typically occur between the ages of 3 months and 3 years. The child has a history of intermittent colicky abdominal pain, distention, vomiting, and possibly an abdominal mass and rectal bleeding. Intussusception is rare in the first month of life. In children older than 3 years, there is a higher incidence of a lead point for the intussusception, such as a Meckel diverticulum or a small bowel mass or tumor such as lymphoma. Small bowel intussusception has been described postoperatively and may be a cause of early postoperative bowel obstruction in children. The incidence is higher for children who have undergone surgery and for those who have cystic fibrosis, appendicitis, or Henoch-Schönlein purpura.

If intussusception is suspected, a barium enema can be not only diagnostic but also therapeutic. In many pediatric hospitals, intussusceptions are now reduced with either hydrostatic pressure under sonographic or fluoroscopic guidance or retrograde flow of air or barium.

Because sonography is now used as a screening procedure for patients with an abdominal mass as well as for children with vomiting and because the presentation of an intussusception often is not typical, there are sonographic patterns of intussusception that should be recognized. This is the so-called target pattern (multiple concentric anechoic rings surrounding a dense echogenic center) or the doughnut sign (an anechoic ring surrounding an echogenic center), or the pseudokidney appearance in the long axis (a reniform shaped complex mass) (Fig. 19-30C–F). The intussuscipiens (the distal bowel into which the intussusceptum or proximal bowel herniates) does not usually suffer vascular compromise and so is not edematous but normally thin. As the intussusceptum becomes edematous, it compresses the bowel lumen, creating a hypoechoic ring with increased central echogenicity. Depending on the imaging plane, fluid may be present centrally in the obstructed bowel lumen.

Without clinical correlation, the target sign may be nonspecific, as other bowel disease can create this picture; specifically, any process involving the bowel wall, and certainly in adults the target sign is typical of carcinoma. Target patterns have been described in children with Henoch-Schönlein purpura and Burkitt lymphoma. The target pattern has many variations, and the pattern may change in the presence of antegrade or retrograde flow of contrast material.

Patients with ileoileocolic intussusception, or ileum into ileum into colon, show a three-ring sign (target sign). The echogenic center is surrounded by the hyperechoic intussusceptum with intervening mucosa of the more distal ileum, which in turn may be edematous, surrounded again by the intussuscipiens.

## CROHN DISEASE[48,51]

Crohn disease (regional enteritis) is the most common inflammatory disease of the small bowel. The most common bowel segments affected are the terminal ileum and proximal colon. A child with Crohn disease typically present at age 10 years or older and the most common clinical presentation is of abdominal pain, diarrhea, fever, and weight loss. Although contrast radiography examinations and endoscopy are the primary tools for diagnosis of this condition, sonography provides information on complications such as biliary disease, peritoneal abscess, and urinary tract disease.

Sonographic evaluation of Crohn disease utilizes the graded-compression technique. The sonographic findings include symmetrically thickened hypoechoic bowel walls. The bowel may be partially compressible or noncompressible with graded-compression and decreased peristalsis may be noted. Transverse axis planes demonstrate a bull's-eye or target appearance and the longitudinal axis may have a pseudo-kidney appearance. Color Doppler imaging is used to demonstrate

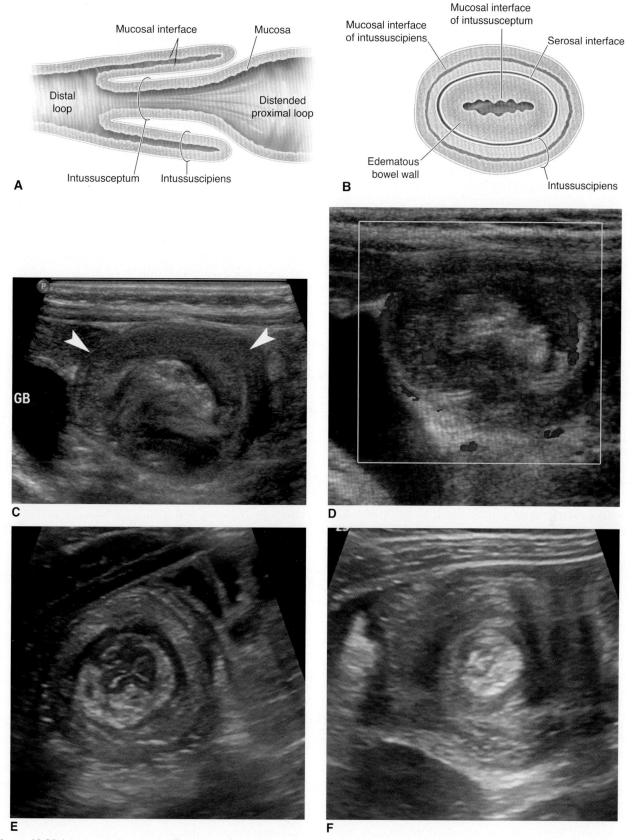

**Figure 19-30** Intussusception. **A:** An illustration of intussusception caused by the proximal bowel loop telescoping into the lumen of the adjacent distal portion. **B:** A cross-sectional illustration of intussusception. **C,D:** The transverse images were obtained on a 14-month-old boy presenting with bloody stool and vomiting. **C:** The gray scale image transverse of the right upper quadrant shows a large donut shaped structure *(arrowhead)* with concentric hypoechoic and hyperechoic rings. **D:** The flow seen on a color Doppler transverse image suggests viable bowel. **E,F:** Transverse images from two different patients demonstrate the donut sign typical of intussusception. (Images C and D courtesy of Rechelle Nguyen, Columbus, OH; images E and F courtesy of Dr. Nakul Jerath, Falls Church, VA.)

the vascularity of the affected segment of bowel and actively inflamed bowel will show increased vascularity. However, this finding is nonspecific for Crohn disease as other bowel inflammations may have the same appearance. Increased flow in the SMA may be noted.

Hypoechoic areas (fibrofatty tissue proliferation in the mesentery) may be noted surrounding the bowel and enlarged lymph nodes may be seen. The appendix may become thickened secondary to the spread of inflammation with findings the same as acute appendicitis. Hypoechoic or complex masses in the right lower quadrant may be related to the presence of abscess or phlegmon. Sonography is useful in the follow-up of treatment for Crohn disease (medical and/ or surgical).

Other inflammatory conditions that cause small bowel wall thickening include cystic fibrosis, malabsorption syndromes, acute enteritis (which may mimic acute appendicitis), tuberculosis, histoplasmosis, *Campylobacter jejuni* infection, and *Salmonella typhosa* infection. Stool cultures and tissue sampling are required to make a definitive diagnosis in most cases of infectious or inflammatory bowel disease.

## BOWEL MASSES[48]

Benign masses of the small bowel include enteric duplication cyst and polyps. Enteric duplication cysts are located along the mesenteric border of the bowel but do not communicate with the bowel. Most of these cysts are found in the ileum. Clinical findings include abdominal pain and distention, vomiting, and rectal bleeding. These cysts can be the lead point of intussusception and may cause pancreatitis if located near the ampulla of Vater.

Sonographically, enteric duplication cysts demonstrate as a well-defined, round, fluid-filled mass that is anechoic to hypoechoic with acoustic enhancement. Duplication cysts have a hypoechoic outer or muscular rim and a hyperechoic inner rim of mucosa. These layers allow differentiation from other cystic masses such as mesenteric or omental cyst, choledochal cyst, ovarian cyst, pancreatic pseudocyst, and abscess which lack a mucosal wall (Fig. 19-31A–C). In some cases, the cyst may appear complex due to hemorrhage or debris.

Polyps may be an isolated finding or associated with multiple polyposis syndromes. Sonographically, the polyps, if seen, appear as nonmobile intraluminal structures.

Malignant masses of the small bowel include lymphoma (the most common small bowel malignancy in children) and, rarely, leiomyosarcoma and adenocarcinoma. Most cases of bowel lymphoma are non-Hodgkin, presenting with palpable abdominal mass or with abdominal pain and vomiting (due to obstruction). The ileum is the most common site within the small bowel for lymphoma involvement, but multiple

areas within the bowel may be affected. Sonographically, lymphoma of the small bowel demonstrates as hypoechoic bowel wall thickening or a focal hypoechoic or complex mass with areas of necrosis. The bowel lumen may be narrowed and intussusception may occur. Other related findings can include splenomegaly and enlargement of the retroperitoneal and mesenteric lymph nodes.

## APPENDICITIS[7,48,51,55,59]

The most common condition requiring emergency surgical intervention in children is acute appendicitis. The incidence in the United States is 1 in 4,000 children under the age of 14. It is almost always associated with obstruction of the appendiceal lumen. The most common clinical presentation is periumbilical abdominal pain that migrates to the right lower quadrant, abdominal tenderness, fever, and leukocytosis, but the presentation may be variable and other conditions, such as gynecologic disorders, can mimic appendicitis.

Sonography is the primary method of imaging for appendicitis in children as the abnormal appendix and surrounding tissues can be evaluated and other conditions, which may be mimicking appendicitis, can be found. The graded-compression technique is used to displace bowel gas and demonstrate the compressibility of the appendix (Fig. 19-32A). The examination is initiated by scanning transversely in the right midabdomen at about the level of the umbilicus, continuing caudad, with gradually increasing compression and then followed by reducing and then increasing the pressure of the transducer. This action allows assessment of the compressibility of normal bowel. Normal cecum and terminal ileum are easily compressed with only moderate pressure. The inflamed appendix is most often visualized at the base of the cecal tip during maximum graded compression (Fig. 19-32B). Scanning at the point of maximum tenderness is useful. Color-flow Doppler demonstrates increased flow to the inflamed appendix (Fig. 19-32C,D). The abnormal appendix is a tubular noncompressible structure with a target appearance of an outer hypoechoic muscular wall with an echogenic submucosa layer surrounding a fluid-filled center. The appendix should not exceed 6 mm in outer diameter (Fig. 19-32E,F).

An appendicolith (echogenic focus with acoustic shadowing) may be noted but is not present in all cases (Fig. 19-32G,H). Enlarged mesenteric lymph nodes, increased echogenicity of the pericecal area, and periappendiceal abscess may be noted as complications of perforation of the appendix (Fig. 19-32I,J). Color Doppler imaging of the appendix demonstrates hyperemia of the wall.

Perforation, which occurs in 80% to 100% of children under the age of 3 years and 10% to 20% in ages

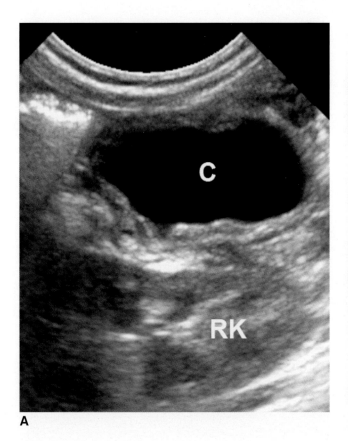

A

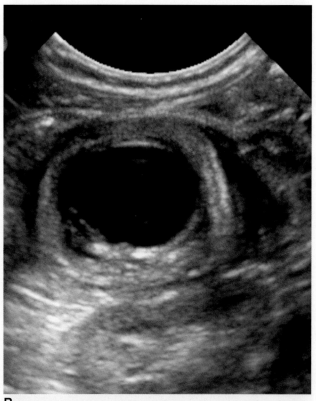

B

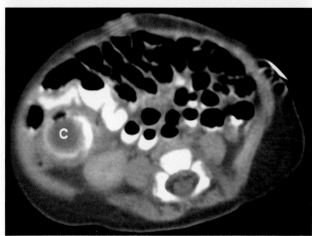

C

**Figure 19-31** Duplication cyst. A 1-month-old patient presents with a history of a fever and bloody stool. The sonograms **(A,B)** of the right lower quadrant reveal a cystic structure with a thick wall. **C:** A computed tomography image on the same patient demonstrates the thick-walled cystic structure filled with simple fluid. A diagnosis of mesenteric duplication cyst was made with Meckel diverticulum as a differential diagnosis. (Images courtesy of Dr. Nakul Jerath, Falls Church, VA.)

10 to 17 years, makes the diagnosis of appendicitis more difficult as the appendix is no longer dilated. Echogenic mucosa, increased periappendiceal echogenicity, and a complex or fluid-filled focal collection (periappendiceal abscess) are the most common features of perforation. Major complications of perforation include abscess formation and peritonitis.

False-negative diagnosis of appendicitis may be due to focal appendicitis, perforation, or retrocecal appendix. False-positive diagnoses are generally related to resolving appendicitis and extension of inflammation from surrounding tissues (Crohn disease, tubo-ovarian abscess, inflamed Meckel diverticulum).

## HIRSCHSPRUNG DISEASE[49,60]

Hirschsprung disease (aganglionic megacolon) is a congenital disorder that is much more frequent in males than in females and is often associated with other anomalies, such as Down syndrome. It is usually manifested in early infancy and has been diagnosed in utero. Hirschsprung disease is caused by congenital absence of parasympathetic ganglion cells in the submucosal and intramuscular plexuses; the bowel becomes enormously dilated and there is no peristaltic action in the aganglionic area. The aganglionic segment remains contracted without reciprocal relaxation and produces

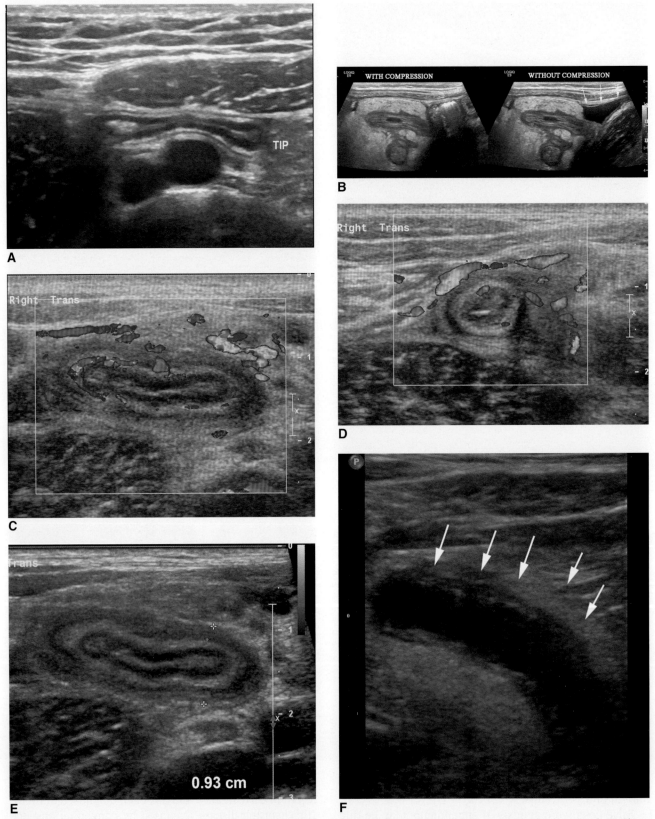

**Figure 19-32** Appendicitis. **A:** The sonogram demonstrates the normal thin-walled appendix seen just anterior to the iliac vessels. **B:** These images with and without compression show no change in the size of the dilated appendix. Fluid is seen in the right lower quadrant when the compression is released. **C:** Longitudinal and transverse (**D**) images of the inflamed appendix demonstrate peripheral hyperemia of the wall. **E:** Longitudinal scan of right lower quadrant shows a dilated blind-ended tubular structure measuring 0.93 cm representing an inflamed appendix. **F:** Longitudinal image of a dilated fluid-filled appendix is seen in the right lower quadrant *(arrows). (continued)*

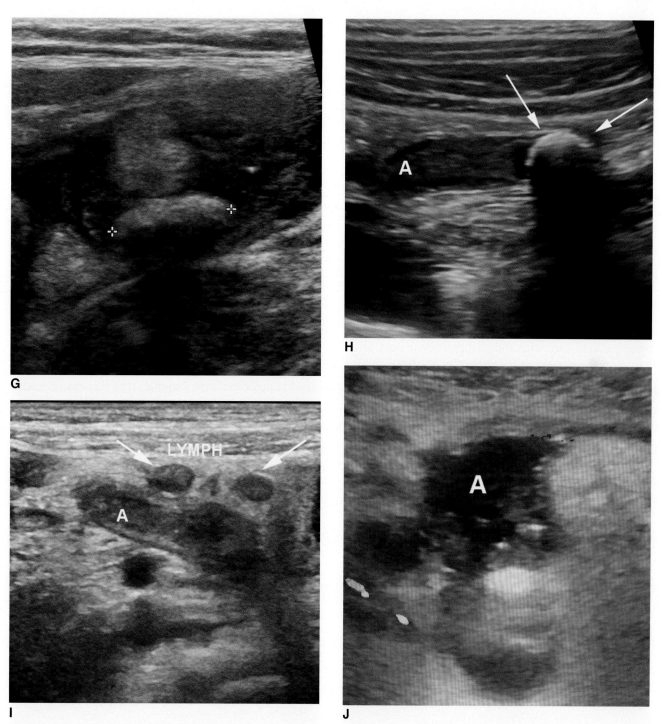

**Figure 19-32** *(continued)* **G:** Sonogram shows a large echogenic appendicolith *(between calipers)* within an irregular dilated appendix. **H:** Echogenic appendicolith *(arrows)* is seen within the appendix (*A*). Note the acoustic shadowing from attenuation distal to the appendicolith. **I:** Enlarged lymph nodes *(arrows)* are seen anterior to an inflamed appendix (*A*). **J:** A complex mass (*A*) seen in the right lower quadrant represents an abscess in a patient with a ruptured appendix. (Images A, F, H, I, and J courtesy of Dr. Nakul Jerath, Falls Church, VA; images C, D, E, and G courtesy of Monica Bacani, Columbus, OH.)

a functional obstruction. The area most frequently affected is the rectosigmoid.

The clinical manifestations depend on the length of aganglionosis or bowel distention. When the disease manifests in early infancy, the patient presents with abdominal distention, constipation, and vomiting and

often appears malnourished and anemic. Hirschsprung disease can be suggested by sonography if the transition zone can be seen high in the sigmoid colon. The findings of distal colon obstruction are dilated distal small bowel and proximal colon, which may be quite echogenic from meconium. The findings of imperforate anus and atresia of the colon cannot be diagnosed by sonography, but by examining the patient from the perineal surface, the distance from the anus to the colon lumen can be measured.

# RETROPERITONEUM[61–63]

The sonographic evaluation of the retroperitoneum includes the muscles (psoas, quadratus lumborum), the crura of the diaphragm, and lymph nodes. Retroperitoneal hemorrhage, retroperitoneal fibrosis (rare in children), and presacral tumors can be evaluated with sonography.

## MUSCLES

The retroperitoneal muscles may become involved in diseases that originate in the lymph nodes, kidneys, pancreas, duodenum, colon, and spinal column. Abscess can occur from bacteremia or adjacent inflammatory conditions; extension of lymphoma, Wilms tumor, Ewing sarcoma; and rhabdomyosarcoma originating in the muscle. A focal mass or a diffuse change may be noted in the psoas muscle. Correlation with clinical history is important.

## LYMPH NODES

When retroperitoneal lymph nodes are found during abdominal sonography of an infant or child, they are abnormal and are generally located near the aorta and IVC. Enlargement of lymph nodes in the retroperitoneum are most commonly associated with lymphoma, Wilms tumor, and neuroblastoma, but can be found in conjunction with other malignancies of the abdomen and pelvis. The sonographic appearance is of one or more hypoechoic homogeneous structures that may combine to appear as one large mass. The enlarged nodes can displace vessels and bowel anteriorly and displace the kidneys laterally (Fig. 19-33A,B).

## NEOPLASMS

Primary retroperitoneal tumors can arise from lymph channels, nerves, and connective tissues. Benign tumors include mature teratoma, hemangiomas, lipomatosis, lymphangioma, and neural tumors. Malignant tumors include rhabdomyosarcoma, fibrosarcoma, neuroblastoma, leiomyosarcoma, malignant germ cell tumor, malignant schwannoma, and Ewing sarcoma. Benign tumors are more likely to be hyperechoic with mature teratomas having a complex appearance due to fat, fluid, and bone contents (Fig. 19-34). Malignant tumors are usually solid with variable echogenicity and a complex appearance due to hemorrhage or necrosis.

Presacral masses in children include sacrococcygeal teratoma (the most common), neuroblastoma, soft tissue sarcomas, lymphoma, lipoma, anterior meningocele, sacral bone tumors, abscess, and rectal duplication. There are four types of sacrococcygeal teratoma: type I is predominately external, type II is external with significant internal components, type III that is predominately internal, and type IV that is entirely presacral without external component or extension. These tumors occur most often in females, are predominately benign, and can be detected prenatally. The sonographic appearance of benign teratoma is of a predominately cystic structure with varied amounts of solid components (fat, calcification, bone, or teeth). Malignant teratomas are mostly solid but may contain cystic areas. Hydronephrosis or urine ascites from bladder rupture may be found. In most cases, CT and/or MRI is needed for a more accurate preoperative assessment.

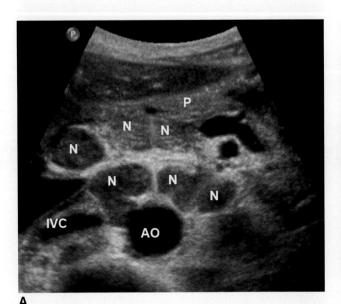

**A**

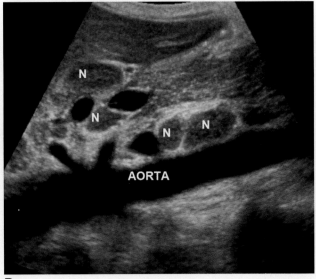

**B**

**Figure 19-33** Lymphadenopathy. Transverse **(A)** and Longitudinal **(B)** images demonstrate multiple hypoechoic lymph nodes (*N*) seen anterior to the aorta (*AO*), adjacent to the pancreatic head (*P*) and porta hepatis. (Images courtesy of Philips Medical Systems, Bothell, WA.)

## TRAUMA

Retroperitoneal hemorrhage in children is associated with blunt abdominal trauma although it can be a complication of renal biopsy or anticoagulant therapy. Hemorrhage associated with renal trauma first surrounds the kidney before extending into the retroperitoneal space. Sonography can detect the presence of fresh hemorrhage (anechoic) and follow the progress of the hemorrhage as it ages and changes in echogenicity.

## RELATED IMAGING PROCEDURES

In 2008, the Alliance for Radiation Safety in Pediatric Imaging launched the image gently campaign to increase awareness of the opportunities to lower radiation dose in pediatric imaging.[64] Children are more sensitive to radiation and the effects last a lifetime. Physicians are encouraged to use sonography and MRI whenever possible.

### MAGNETIC RESONANCE IMAGING

MRI is used in the pediatric abdomen for many different applications including the diagnosis and staging of abdominal masses. Magnetic resonance cholangiopancreatography (MRCP) is used to evaluate congenital biliary anomalies such as choledochal cyst. MRI can also be used to evaluate abnormalities of the GI tract in infants and children.

### COMPUTED TOMOGRAPHY

Although CT is considered to be the largest contributor to medical radiation exposure in the United States, CT does provide useful diagnostic information. The radiation dose should be minimized whenever possible. CT is used in the pediatric abdomen to diagnose and stage abdominal masses and is useful in the evaluation of lymphadenopathy. CT is also used to evaluate the abdomen in cases of trauma and is excellent at detecting lesions of the pancreas.

### RADIONUCLIDE EXAMINATIONS

Hepatobiliary scintigraphy is used to evaluate congenital biliary anomalies such as choledochal cyst.

## SUMMARY

- Sonography is the imaging modality of choice to evaluate the pediatric abdomen because it is portable, has no ionizing radiation, and provides excellent visualization of the abdominal organs and structures.
- Coarctation of the abdominal aorta is a rare congenital defect that causes severe hypertension, headaches, and fatigue in the pediatric population and a failure to thrive in the neonatal patient.
- Aortic thrombus is a complication of indwelling umbilical artery catheters in the neonate and presents clinically as absent femoral pulses, hematuria, cyanosis, hypertension, blanching of the lower extremities, and necrotizing enterocolitis.
- Thrombus in the IVC can be an extension of renal vein or iliac thrombosis.
- Tumor invasion into the IVC can occur from Wilms tumor, neuroblastoma, sarcoma, hepatocellular carcinoma, teratomas, and lymphoma.
- Benign neoplasms of the liver include hemangioendothelioma, cavernous hemangioma, and mesenchymal hamartoma.
- Liver cysts in the neonate and pediatric patient may be due to multicystic kidney disease, von Hippel-Lindau disease, hydatid disease, trauma, or may be simple congenital cysts.
- In patients with acute hepatitis, the liver may sonographically appear normal or may be enlarged and hypoechoic with prominent hyperechoic portal radicles.
- Liver abscesses may be amebic, pyogenic, or fungal.
- Fatty infiltration of the liver may be caused by malnutrition, malignancies, hyperalimentation, cystic fibrosis, Reye syndrome, glycogen storage disease, malabsorption syndrome, acute hepatitis, or obesity.
- With fatty infiltration, the liver appears echogenic with increased attenuation of the sound beam causing decreased visualization of the posterior portions of the liver and the diaphragm.
- Cirrhosis of the liver in infants and children can be caused by biliary atresia, cystic fibrosis, chronic hepatitis, metabolic disorders, and medications.

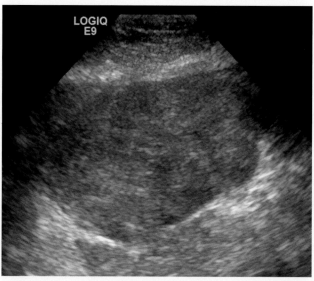

**Figure 19-34** Retroperitoneal tumor. A large solid retroperitoneal tumor was seen in this 4-year-old patient. A diagnosis of fibrosarcoma was made by biopsy.

- Malignant neoplasms of the liver that affect the pediatric population include hepatoblastoma, hepatocellular carcinoma, fibrolamellar hepatocellular carcinoma, and mesenchymal sarcoma.
- AFP is frequently elevated with hepatoblastoma and hepatocellular carcinoma but is typically normal with fibrolamellar hepatocellular carcinoma and mesenchymal sarcoma.
- Portal vein thrombosis can be caused by thrombosis or tumor invasion from hepatoblastoma or hepatocellular carcinoma.
- Conjugated hyperbilirubinemia in the newborn can be caused by neonatal hepatitis or biliary tract abnormalities such as biliary atresia.
- Biliary atresia can range from complete absence of the biliary tree to a rudimentary gallbladder and cystic duct or a visibly patent gallbladder, cystic duct, and common bile duct.
- A fasting gallbladder that measures less than 1.5 cm in the neonate with persistent jaundice is suggestive of biliary atresia.
- Choledochal cyst can present clinically with abdominal pain, palpable mass, and jaundice.
- There are five types of choledochal cysts; type I is the most common type diagnosed in the newborn and is a fusiform dilatation of the common bile duct.
- With sclerosing cholangitis, there is an inflammatory fibrosis that obliterates the intrahepatic and extrahepatic bile ducts, cirrhosis, portal hypertension, and liver failure and usually presents with concurrent inflammatory bowel disease.
- Rhabdomyosarcoma is a rare tumor of the biliary tract occurring between the ages of 1 and 5 that causes biliary obstruction and jaundice.
- In patients with cystic fibrosis, the pancreas is hyperechoic due to fibrosis and the replacement of normal pancreatic tissue with fatty tissue.
- Pancreatitis is less common in children than adults, but can be caused by blunt abdominal trauma, viral infection, drug toxicity, and hereditary disorders.
- Complications of pancreatitis include pseudocyst formation, phlegmon, hemorrhage, and abscess.
- Hypertrophic pyloric stenosis most commonly affects male infants between the ages of 2 and 10 weeks and presents with dehydration, projectile nonbilious vomiting, and possible failure to thrive.
- Pyloric stenosis can be diagnosed when the pyloric anteroposterioer diameter exceeds 1.5 cm, the length of the channel exceeds 1.8 cm, and the muscle thickness exceeds 4 mm.
- Intussusception is found most frequently in males between the ages of 1 and 3 years and occurs when a segment of bowel prolapses into a more distal segment.
- Intussusception appears sonographically as a target pattern, multiple concentric anechoic rings surrounding an echogenic center, doughnut sign, anechoic ring surrounding an echogenic center, or pseudokidney sign, a reniform-shaped complex mass.
- Appendicitis is the most common surgical emergency in children and typically presents with periumbilical pain that radiates to the right lower quadrant, fever, and leukocytosis.

## Critical Thinking Questions

1. A 5-month-old girl presents with a palpable right upper quadrant mass. The sonogram demonstrates a normal liver and gallbladder. A 3-cm cystic mass is seen in the area of the porta hepatis and appears to be separate from the gallbladder. Low-level echoes are seen in the dependent portion of the cyst and appear to change position when the patient is rolled into the left lateral decubitus position. What is the most likely diagnosis?

2. A patient presents with a recent diagnosis of a Wilms tumor for an abdominal sonogram. When scanning the patient, you see an echogenic mass within the lumen of the inferior vena cava and hypoechoic, oval masses surrounding the aorta and inferior vena cava. What is the most likely diagnosis?

3. The sonographer is asked to perform an abdominal sonogram on a 10-year-old patient with cystic fibrosis. What findings might be expected?

4. Which of the following is not true regarding hypertrophic pyloric stenosis? The patient is typically a boy between the ages of 2 and 10 weeks, the patient presents with projectile vomiting and dehydration, the length of the channel is shortened, or the muscle thickness is abnormal if it measures greater than 4 mm.

5. A 7-year-old boy presents for an abdominal sonogram with complaints of abdominal pain and distention. The sonogram of the abdomen demonstrates a large, complex, mass in the right lobe of the liver with a hyperechoic rim. Anechoic areas are seen along with a few calcifications. Laboratory data reveals a normal AFP level. What is the most likely diagnosis?

- The graded compression technique is used to displace bowel gas and evaluate the right lower quadrant for appendicitis.

- The inflamed appendix is most often visualized at the base of the cecal tip as a tubular noncompressible structure with a target appearance in the transverse plane. The appendix should not exceed 6 mm in outer diameter.

## REFERENCES

1. Redmon S. Pediatric sonography: funography for kids. *JDMS*. 2007;23:110–112.
2. Fordham LA. Approach to the pediatric patient. *Ultrasound Clin*. 2009;4:439–443.
3. Saif I, Seriki D, Moore R, et al. Midaortic syndrome in neurofibromatosis type 1 resulting in bilateral renal artery stenosis. *Am J Kidney Dis*. 2010;56:1197–1201.
4. Daghero F, Bueno N, Peirone A, et al. Coarctation of the abdominal aorta: an uncommon cause of arterial hypertension and stroke. *Circ Cardiovasc Imaging*. 2008;1:e4–e6.
5. Nagel K, Tuckuviene R, Paes B, et al. Neonatal aortic thrombosis: a comprehensive review. *Clin Padiatr*. 2010;222:134–139.
6. McAdams RM, Winter VT, McCurnin DC, et al. Complications of umbilical artery catheterization in a model of extreme prematurity. *J Perinatol*. 2009;29:685–692.
7. Miller CR. Ultrasound in the assessment of the acute abdomen in children: its advantages and its limitations. *Ultrasound Clin*. 2007;2:525–540.
8. Varich L. Ultrasound of pediatric liver masses. *Ultrasound Clin*. 2010;5:137–152.
9. Milla SS, Lee EY, Buonomo C, et al. Ultrasound evaluation of pediatric abdominal masses. *Ultrasound Clin*. 2007;2:541–559.
10. Peddu P, Huang D, Kane PA, et al. Vanishing liver tumours. *Clin Radiol*. 2008;63:329–339.
11. Dubois J, Rypens F. Vascular anomalies. *Ultrasound Clin*. 2009;4:471–495.
12. Gow KW, Lee L, Pruthi S, et al. Mesenchymal hamartoma of the liver. *J Pediatr Surg*. 2009;44:468–470.
13. Feleppa C, D'Ambra L, Berti S, et al. Laparoscopic treatment of traumatic rupture of hydatid hepatic cyst—Is it feasible?: A case report. *Surg Laparosc Endosc Percutan Tech*. 2009;19:e140–e142.
14. Nievelstein RAJ, Robben SGF, Blickman JG. Hepatobiliary and pancreatic imaging in children–techniques and an overview of non-neoplastic disease entities. *Pediatr Radiol*. 2011;41:55–75.
15. Siegel MJ. Jaundice in infants and children. *Ultrasound Clin*. 2006;1:431–441.
16. Mishra K, Basu S, Roychoudhury S, et al. Liver abscess in children: an overview. *World J Pediatr*. 2010;6:210–216.
17. Benedetti NJ, Desser TS, Jeffrey RB. Imaging of hepatic infections. *Ultrasound Q*. 2008;24:267–278.
18. Nanda K. Non-alcoholic steatohepatitis in children. *Pediatr Transplant*. 2004;8:613–618.
19. Alfire ME, Treem WR. Nonalcoholic fatty liver disease. *Pediatr Ann*. 2006;35:297–299.
20. Shorbagi A, Bayraktar Y. Experience of a single center with congenital hepatic fibrosis: a review of the literature. *World J Gastroenterol*. 2010;16:683–690.
21. Sirlin CB, Reeder SB. Magnetic resonance imaging quantification of liver iron. *Magn Reson Imaging Clin N Am*. 2010;18:359–381.
22. Tannuri AC, Tannuri U, Gibelli NE, et al. Surgical treatment of hepatic tumors in children: lessons learned from liver transplantation. *J Pediat Surg*. 2009;44:2083–2087.
23. Roebuck DJ, Olsen Ø, Pariente D. Radiological staging in children with hepatoblastoma. *Pediatr Radiol*. 2006;36:176–182.
24. Bittencourt PL, Couto CA, Ribeiro DD. Portal vein thrombosis and Budd-Chiari syndrome. *Clin Liver Dis*. 2009;13:127–144.
25. Harkanyi Z. Pediatric portal hypertension. *Ultrasound Clin*. 2006;1:443–455.
26. Siegel, MJ. *Pediatric Sonography*. Philadelphia, PA: Lippincott Williams & Wilkins; 2002.
27. Rozel C, Garel L, Rypens F, et al. Imaging of biliary disorders in children. *Pediatr Radiol*. 2011;41:208–220.
28. Mesleh M, Deziel DJ. Bile duct cysts. *Surg Clin North Am*. 2008;88:1369–1384.
29. Kanegawa K, Akasaka Y, Kitamura E, et al. Sonographic diagnosis of biliary atresia in pediatric patients using the "triangular cord" sign versus gallbladder length and contraction. *AJR Am J Roentgenol*. 2003;181:1387–1390.
30. Humphrey TM, Stringer MD. Biliary atresia: US diagnosis. *Radiology*. 2007;244:845–851.
31. Lee MS, Kim MJ, Lee MJ, et al. Biliary atresia: color doppler US findings in neonates and infants. *Radiology*. 2009;252:282–289.
32. Souza LR, Pascoal G, Cappellari PF, et al. Giant choledochal cyst as a differential diagnosis for hepatic cyst. *JDMS*. 2010;26:245–248.
33. Attalla BI. Abdominal sonographic findings in children with sickle cell anemia. *JDMS*. 2010;26:281–285.
34. Walker TM, Hambleton IR, Serjeant GR. Gallstones in sickle cell disease: observations from the Jamaican cohort study. *J Pediatr*. 2000;136:80–85.
35. Punia RP, Garg S, Bisht B, et al. Clinico-pathological spectrum of gallbladder disease in children. *Acta Paediatr*. 2010;99:1561–1564.
36. Tsung JW, Raio CC, Ramirez-Schrempp D, et al. Point-of-care ultrasound diagnosis of pediatric cholecystitis in the ED. *Am J Emerg Med*. 2010;28:338–342.
37. Shukla RM, Roy D, Mukherjee PP, et al. Spontaneous gall bladder perforation: a rare condition in the differential diagnosis of acute abdomen in children. *J Pediatr Surg*. 2011;46:241–243.
38. Grisoni E, Fisher R, Izant R. Kawasaki syndrome: report of four cases with acute gallbladder hydrops. *J Pediatr Surg*. 1984;19:9–11.
39. Pryor JP, Volpe CM, Caty MG, et al. Noncalculous biliary obstruction in the child and adolescent. *J Am Coll Surg*. 2000;191:569–578.
40. Karrer FM, Bensard DD. Neonatal cholestasis. *Semin Pediatr Surg*. 2000;9:166–169.
41. Ali S, Russo MA, Margraf L. Biliary rhabdomyosarcoma mimicking choledochal cyst. *J Gastrointestin Liver Dis*. 2009;18:95–97.
42. Kitagawa N, Aida N. Biliary rhabdomyosarcoma. *Pediatr Radiol*. 2007;37:1059.

43. Nijs EL, Callahan MJ. Congenital and developmental pancreatic anomalies: ultrasound, computed tomography, and magnetic resonance imaging features. *Semin ultrasound CT MR*. 2007;28:395–401.

44. Jackson WD. Pancreatitis: etiology, diagnosis, and management. *Curr Opin Pediatr*. 2001;13:447–451.

45. Vaughn DD, Jabra AA, Fishman EK. Pancreatic disease in children and young adults: evaluation with CT. *Radiographics*. 1998;18:1171–1187.

46. Chung E, Travis M, Conran R. Pancreatic tumors in children: radiologic–pathologic correlation. *Radiographics*. 2006;26:1211–1238.

47. Yu DC, Kozakewich HP, Perez-Atayde AR, et al. Childhood pancreatic tumors: a single institution experience. *J Pediatr Surg*. 2009;44:2267–2272.

48. Munden MM, Hill JG. Ultrasound of the acute abdomen in children. *Ultrasound Clin*. 2010;5:113–135.

49. McCarten KM. Ultrasound of the gastrointestinal tract in the neonate and young infant with particular attention to problems in the neonatal intensive care unit. *Ultrasound Clin*. 2010;5:75–95.

50. Hiorns MP. Gastrointestinal tract imaging in children: current techniques. *Pediatr Radiol*. 2011;41:42–54.

51. Sonanvane S, Siegel MJ. Sonography of the surgical abdomen in children. *Ultrasound Clin*. 2008;3:67–82.

52. Cohen HL, Greene EB, Boulden TP. The vomiting neonate or young infant. *Ultrasound Clin*. 2010;5:97–112.

53. Reed AA, Michael K. Hypertrophic pyloric stenosis. *JDMS*. 2010;26:157–160.

54. Forster N, Haddad RL, Choroomi S, et al. Use of ultrasound in 187 infants with suspected infantile hypertrophic pyloric stenosis. *Australas Radio*. 2007;51:560–563.

55. Junewick JJ. Decreasing radiation risks by increasing use of ultrasound in pediatric imaging. *Ultrasound Clin*. 2009;4:273–284.

56. Goldberg BB. *Atlas of Ultrasound Measurements*. St. Louis, MO: Elsevier; 2006.

57. Applegate KE. Evidence-based diagnosis of malrotation and volvulus. *Pediatr Radiol*. 2009;39:S161–S163.

58. Patino MO, Munden MM. Utility of the sonographic whirlpool sign in diagnosing midgut volvulus in patients with atypical clinical presentations. *J Ultrasound Med*. 2004;23:397– S401.

59. Rodriguez DP, Vargas S, Callahan MJ, et al. Appendicitis in young children: imaging experience and clinical outcomes. *AJR Am J Roentgenol*. 2006;186:1158–1164.

60. Baltogiannis N, Mavridis G, Soutis M, et al. Currarino triad associated with Hirschsprung's disease. *J Pediatr Surg*. 2003;38:1086–1089.

61. Heflin D. The two extremes of sacrococcygeal teratomas. *JDMS*. 2008;24:242–245.

62. Wu Y, Song B, Xu J, et al. Retroperitoneal neoplasms within the perirenal space in infants and children: differentiation of renal and non-renal origin in enhanced CT images. *Eur J Radiol*. 2010;75:279–286.

63. Rattan KN, Kadian YS, Nair VJ, et al. Primary retroperitoneal teratomas in children: a single institution experience. *Afr J Paediatr Surg*. 2010;7:5–8.

64. Sidhu M, Coley BD, Goske MJ, et al. Image gently, step lightly: increasing radiation dose awareness in pediatric interventional radiology. *Pediatr Radiol*. 2009;39:1135–1138.

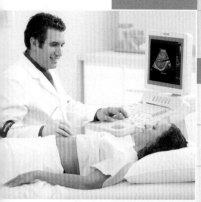

# 20 | The Pediatric Urinary System and Adrenal Glands

Bridgette M. Lunsford and Heidi S. Barrett

## OBJECTIVES

List the indications for the sonographic evaluation of urinary system and adrenal glands in the pediatric patient.

Explain the protocol process for sonographic evaluation of the urinary system and adrenal glands in the pediatric patient.

Identify the normal sonographic appearance of the urinary system and the adrenal glands in the pediatric patient.

Describe the pathology, etiology, clinical signs and symptoms, and sonographic appearance of common congenital abnormalities, tumors, and acquired pathology in the upper and lower urinary system in the pediatric patient.

Discuss three criteria for sonographic documentation of tumors on pediatric patients to include (1) origin of the mass, (2) extent of the mass, and (3) metastases.

Describe the pathology, etiology, clinical signs and symptoms, and sonographic appearance of congenital abnormalities, tumors, hemorrhage, cysts, and abscesses of the adrenal glands in the pediatric patient.

Identify technically satisfactory and unsatisfactory sonographic examinations of the urinary system and adrenal glands on the neonatal and pediatric patient.

## KEY TERMS

adrenal hemorrhage | adrenocortical carcinoma | adult polycystic kidney disease | angiomyolipoma | congenital adrenal hyperplasia | cystitis | duplicated collecting system | glomerular cystic disease | hydronephrosis | infantile polycystic kidney disease | juvenile nephronophthisis | medullary sponge kidney | mesoblastic nephroma | multicystic dysplastic kidney | multilocular cystic nephroma | nephroblastomatosis | nephrocalcinosis | neuroblastoma | pheochromocytoma | posterior urethral valves | renal agenesis | renal cyst | renal dysplasia | renal hypoplasia | rhabdomyosarcoma | urachal cyst | ureterocele | Wilms tumor

## GLOSSARY

**diuresis** increased secretion or production of urine; can result from conditions such as diabetes and acute renal failure or from certain medications or overhydration

**enuresis** involuntary discharge of urine during sleep, or bedwetting

**reflux** occurs when valves at the junction of the ureter and bladder are not working correctly and allow urine from the bladder to back up into the ureter and kidney

**ureteropelvic junction** area where the renal pelvis connects to the ureter

**ureterovesical junction** area where the ureter enters into the urinary bladder

Sonography has become one of the most important means of evaluating the pediatric urinary tract and the adrenal glands, for several reasons. Unlike excretory urography and computed tomography (CT), sonography does not expose the child to ionizing radiation and does not carry the risk of a contrast reaction. Sonography can be performed portably, without sedation, and may be used for serial follow-up examinations. The procedure is also tolerated well by patients and parents.

A common indication for sonographic examination of infants and children is suspected renal anomalies suggested by clinical findings such as vertebral, cardiac, or colon abnormalities. Findings at prenatal sonography may also raise the question of renal anomalies.[1,2] For older infants and young children, the most common reasons for referral are workup for a urinary tract infection, enuresis, diuresis, or, less commonly, a palpable mass. Some of the other current clinical indications for genitourinary sonography include possible obstructive uropathy, ambiguous genitalia, neonatal ascites, anasarca, renal failure, localization for renal biopsy, evaluation of a renal allograft, anomalies of the bladder, assessment of bladder volume, urachal remnant, precocious puberty, pelvic tumors, pelvic abscesses, and pregnancy. Evaluation of the adrenal glands is performed in cases of neonatal hemorrhage and for the evaluation of adrenal masses.

# KIDNEYS

## SONOGRAPHIC TECHNIQUE

For evaluation of the kidneys, no preparation is necessary, although hydration is preferred. Patients need not fast because the kidneys can be imaged from either the posterior surface (prone longitudinal or transverse scan planes) or from the patient's side (coronal planes).

Most pediatric patients are evaluated in the supine or prone position, but scanning children requires a certain amount of flexibility. When necessary, children may be scanned in the sitting position, decubitus positions, or held in a parent's arms, across their shoulders, or on the lap. Because children may be unable or unwilling to hold their breath or obey simple instructions, the sonographer must be prepared to scan from multiple planes or through ribs to visualize all portions of the kidney. As part of the kidney examination, visualizing the ureters is important, particularly if there is evidence of hydronephrosis. The bladder should also be examined as part of the evaluation of the urinary tract.

For neonatal examinations, a 10-MHz transducer affords exquisite resolution and detail of the kidney. Because the kidney is close to the posterior skin surface (0.5 to 3 cm) in young infants, a 10-MHz transducer can easily provide excellent detail. A 7.5-MHz transducer is useful for scanning young children and older, thin children, providing excellent kidney detail. Either a curved-array or a linear-array transducer may be used.

## NORMAL SONOGRAPHIC APPEARANCE

Sonographically, the renal pyramids or medulla of a normal newborn or infant can be identified as hypoechoic, triangular, or rectangular structures.[3] Sonographers unfamiliar with children have mistaken these structures for renal cysts. The renal pyramids show symmetric alignment within the kidney periphery. In 70% of kidneys, a compound renal pyramid or a normal hypoechoic medullary region occurs in the upper pole (50%), lower pole (30%), or middle region (20%). Compound calyces are a conglomerate of calyces that come to one infundibulum and are associated with compound pyramids. Sonographically, these fused medullary pyramids appear as an irregular, hypoechoic area. They are not associated with evidence of renal, pelvic, infundibular, or calyceal dilatation (Fig. 20-1A–E). If obstruction exists or other renal anomalies are present, the renal pyramids may be compressed and poorly visualized.

Renal lobulations are responsible for the irregular renal outlines seen in infants. The lobulations become less pronounced with age and disappear by about 6 years of age, although the normal junctional defects (triangular echogenic indentations in the cortex) on the anterior superior surface and the inferior posterior surface of the kidney may persist. The interrenuncular defect, an echogenic line from the renal cortex to the central sinus, separates the superior and inferior poles of the kidney and is a normal finding (Fig. 20-2A,B). The columns of Bertin are apposing infoldings of cortex, which are not separated by papillae. The cortex is thin compared with the medulla and the renal sinus is less fat filled in infants and young children. The renal pelvis lies within the renal sinus during infancy. In childhood, half the renal pelvis is outside the renal sinus. The renal pelvis should measure <10 mm in the prone and supine positions.[3] The renal pelvic wall should not be visible. A wall may be thickened in cases of chronic infection, reflux, and chronic obstruction (Fig. 20-3).

Table 20-1 summarizes the normal infant and pediatric renal echo patterns. The cortical echogenicity neonates and infants is greater than that in older children, especially in premature infants.[3-5] In older children, however, increased echogenicity in the cortex, although nonspecific, may indicate parenchymal disease. Causes of increased echogenicity are the same as for adults. Specific pediatric conditions include leukemia, progressive glomerulonephritis, nephrotic syndrome, renal artery stenosis, and chronic infection.[5]

Standard measurements of renal size have been published[6] and are related to the length of the kidney for

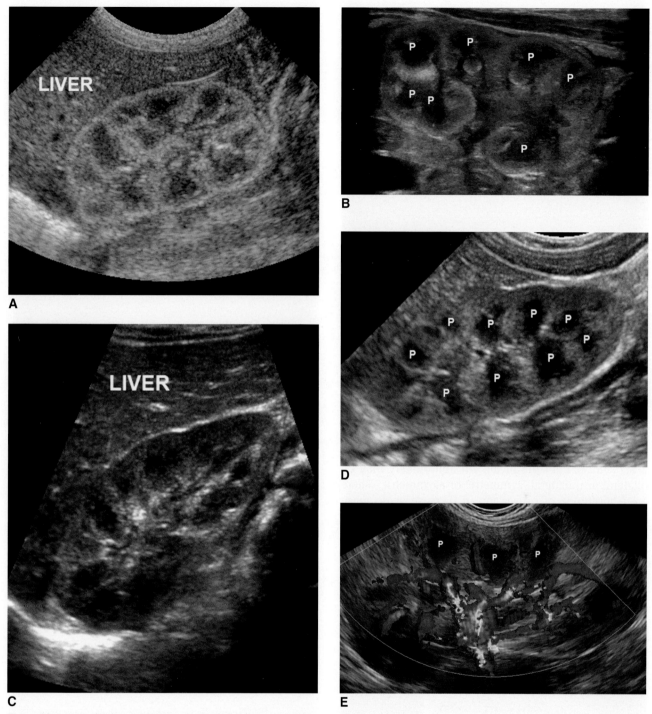

**Figure 20-1** Normal kidneys. **A:** Longitudinal right kidney in a preterm neonate demonstrates the normal sonographic appearance. The pyramids are hypoechoic and the echogenicity of the kidney cortex is greater than that of the adjacent liver. **B:** The normal neonatal kidney is seen in a longitudinal section with the hypoechoic to anechoic pyramids (P) evenly spaced throughout the kidney. **C:** Normal sonographic appearance of the right kidney in an infant. The cortex is isoechoic or slightly hypoechoic to the adjacent liver. **D:** Normal neonatal kidney with hypoechoic to anechoic pyramids (P) seen evenly spaced throughout the kidney. Note the normal mild fetal lobulation and lack of renal sinus fat. **E:** Longitudinal view of the neonatal kidney demonstrates the normal renal vasculature with the interlobar vessels seen coursing between the renal pyramids (P). (Images **A** and **C**, courtesy of Philips Medical Systems, Bothell, WA; Image **B**, courtesy of GE Healthcare, Wauwatosa, WI; Image **D**, courtesy of Monica Bacani, Columbus, OH; E, courtesy of Jillian Platt, Falls Church, VA.)

age and also to the child's weight and body surface area.[7,8] These measurements are particularly useful for examining children who may have a diffuse process such as infection or leukemia.

Comparative measurements should be made to determine appropriate growth in children with chronic infection. Also, in children the renal vein may be unusually prominent, including the intrahilar portion and sinus portion. The renal vein can be distinguished from structures of the collecting system with color and pulsed Doppler. Fetal lobulations are present in most premature infants and in many newborns and infants.[4]

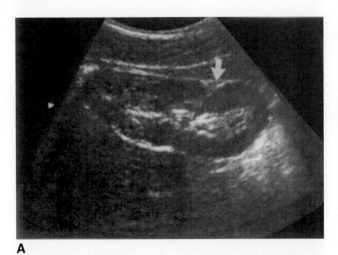

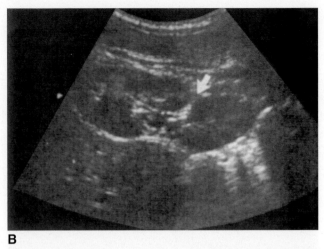

**Figure 20-2** Interrenuncular defect. **A:** This longitudinal sonogram on a 10-year-old boy with enuresis shows a normal kidney. Note the triangular defect in the lower pole *(arrow).* **B:** The hyperechoic defect extends medially to the renal pelvis and represents a normal cleft or interrenuncular defect *(arrow).*

By approximately 1 year of age, fetal lobulations should not be as evident, although in some children they persist as a normal variant. Fetal lobulation may be confused with scarring, but the pyelonephritic scar is usually opposite a clubbed calyx, whereas fetal lobulation is usually seen between the renal pyramids or calyces.

There is a great deal of variation in the size of kidneys. Large kidneys, by definition, are 2 standard deviations (SD) *larger than* the mean. Small kidneys are 2 SD *smaller than* the mean. An abnormality may be bilateral or unilateral, symmetric or asymmetric. There are a multitude of causes for an increase or decrease in the size of the kidneys (Pathology Box 20-1). Compensatory enlargement of a single functioning kidney usually occurs within 6 to 12 months following surgical removal or intrauterine loss.

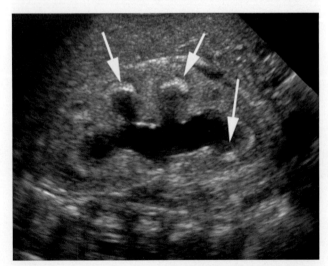

**Figure 20-3** Thickened renal pelvic wall. This longitudinal sonogram of the kidney shows a dilated collecting system with a thick echogenic wall *(arrows)* in an infant with a history of posterior urethral valves and urinary tract infection. (Image courtesy of Dr. Nakul Jerath, Falls Church, VA.)

Duplex Doppler of the renal arteries, as in the adult, demonstrates a sharp systolic peak with a continuous forward diastolic flow (Fig. 20-4A,B). With color flow Doppler, it is easy to identify flow in the interlobar and arcuate arteries. The resistive indices (RIs) obtained in the interlobar and arcuate arteries should be <0.70.[9-11] In the normal neonate, the RI *may exceed* 0.70 but should be <0.70 by 6 weeks of age. The RIs are useful in helping to determine if a dilated system is obstructed. The RI is increased in tubular interstitial disease and vascular disease, whereas frequently normal in glomerular disease.

## CONGENITAL ANOMALIES

### Agenesis

Bilateral renal agenesis is associated with oligohydramnios, an unusually small amount of amniotic fluid. Renal agenesis is associated with Potter syndrome, features of which include abnormal facies with a small mandible and low-set ears. Affected infants also have pulmonary hypoplasia and frequently are stillborn or

| TABLE | 20-1 | |
|---|---|---|
| **Normal Pediatric Renal Echo Pattern** | | |
| **Age** | **Renal Structure** | **Echo Pattern** |
| Newborn | Cortex | More echoic than liver and spleen |
| | Sinus | Poorly defined because of paucity of fat in infants |
| 6–8 weeks | Cortex | Isoechoic to liver and spleen |
| 2–6 months | Cortex | Hypoechoic to liver and spleen |
| >6 months | Cortex | Hypoechoic to renal sinus |

**PATHOLOGY BOX 20-1**

*Causes of Renal Size Variation*

**Enlarged Kidneys**

*Bilateral enlargement*
Congenital: Duplication, cystic disease, storage disease, generalized visceromegaly, systemic infection
Acute: Pyelonephritis, glomerular nephritis
Neoplastic: Nephroblastomatosis, bilateral Wilms tumor, leukemia, lymphoma, tuberous sclerosis, or hamartoma
Vascular: Renal vein thrombosis, acute tubular necrosis, hemolytic uremia, sickle cell anemia
Obstructive: Congenital or acquired
*Unilateral enlargement*
Congenital: Duplication, cystic disease, cross-fused ectopia, horseshoe kidney
Infectious: Acute pyelonephritis, abscess
Neoplastic: Mesoblastic nephroma, Wilms tumor, angiomyolipoma or hamartoma, sarcoma, lymphoma
Vascular: Renal vein thrombosis, transplant complication (rejection or tubular necrosis)
Traumatic: Contusion, hematoma
Obstructive: Congenital, acquired

**Small Kidneys**

*Bilateral*
Congenital: Aplasia, hypoplasia
Acute: Pyelonephritis, glomerular nephritis
Infectious: Chronic pyelonephritis, reflux nephropathy with infarction
Vascular: Renal vein thrombosis, arterial occlusion (intrinsic or extrinsic)
Atrophic: Chronic obstruction, chronic recurrent infarction, chronic failure, dysplasia
Obstructive: Congenital or acquired
*Unilateral*
Congenital: Agenesis, hypoplasia
Infectious: Chronic, chronic reflux with infection
Vascular: Venous thrombosis, arterial obstruction (acquired or congenital)
Atrophic: Chronic obstruction, chronic infection and infarction, dysplasia

survive for only a very short time. They may live longer with ventilatory support, but they die of renal failure. In cases of renal agenesis, the adrenal glands are usually well developed: they can measure up to 3 cm in length and lie in the renal fossa, so they must not be mistaken for the kidneys (Fig. 20-5). It is important to use the highest resolution transducer available to achieve good definition of the adrenal glands and kidneys. With total renal agenesis, the bladder is also absent. Unilateral renal agenesis is more common and may be asymptomatic, in which case it may be detected only incidentally. Renal hypoplasia is probably due to renal infarction, possibly occurring in utero but more likely postpartum. Hypoplasia may result from unsuspected chronic atrophic pyelonephritis, unsuspected reflux nephritis, an anoxic insult, or decreased blood flow due to a vascular problem. Agenesis is associated with multiple anomalies (Pathology Box 20-2).

### Hydronephrosis[1]

Hydronephrosis is a dilatation of the collecting system of the urinary tract, specifically of the renal calyces, the renal pelvis, and the ureters (Fig. 20-6A–C). Congenital hydronephrosis is the most common renal mass in infants and children and is frequently diagnosed in utero.[4,12] In infants, the most frequent site of obstruction is at the ureteropelvic junction (UPJ) (44%).[1,4,12–15] With hydronephrosis, there should be recognizable renal parenchyma surrounding the dilated collecting system. When hydronephrosis is severe, multiple cystic lesions representing the dilated calyces are noted and should be of uniform size and demonstrate communication with the collecting system. Multicystic dysplastic kidney will demonstrate cysts of various sizes that do not communicate with each other or the collecting system[12] (Fig. 20-6D–F). In some cases, no parenchyma is recognizable. Great care must be used to identify the ureter, which may be dilated as well.

Distal ureteral obstructions are the next most common cause of hydronephrosis (21%). Megaureter is an unusual condition of a nonobstructed, nonrefluxing ureter caused by idiopathic dilatation. Usually, there is a distal stenosis or stricture, or the most distal ureter is unable to conduct a peristaltic wave.[1] In cases of bilateral hydronephrosis, the obstruction is going to be located distally, in the bladder or urethra. The bladder

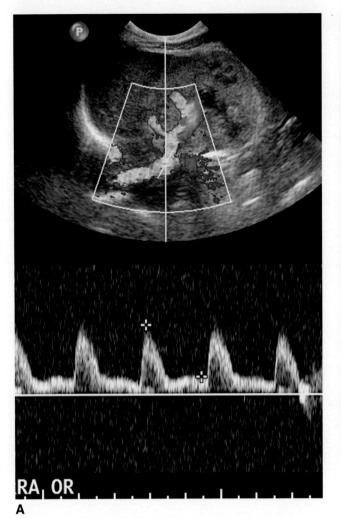

A

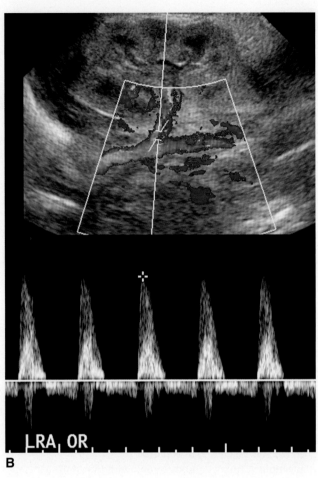

B

**Figure 20-4** Renal artery Doppler. **A:** Pulsed Doppler waveform of the left renal artery in a newborn demonstrates normal flow with a sharp systolic peak and continuous forward diastolic flow. **B:** Pulsed Doppler in a newborn with acute tubular necrosis demonstrates an abnormal waveform with reversed diastolic flow. (Images courtesy of James Beck, Falls Church, VA.)

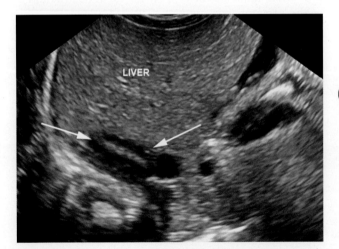

**Figure 20-5** Renal agenesis. Longitudinal sonogram of the right upper quadrant shows an empty renal fossa in a patient with right renal agenesis. In the absence of the right kidney, the normal adrenal gland loses its Y or V shape and is more linear in shape *(arrows)*. Although the shape is different, the neonatal adrenal gland will maintain its normal appearance with the echogenic medulla surrounded by the hypoechoic or anechoic cortex. Care must be taken not to mistake the adrenal gland for the kidney. (Image courtesy of Jillian Platt, Falls Church, VA.)

### PATHOLOGY BOX 20-2

**Associated Anomalies of Renal Agenesis and Hypoplasia**

| | |
|---|---|
| **Cardiovascular** | — |
| Gastrointestinal | Imperforate anus |
| | Esophageal atresia |
| Skeletal | Cervical and thoracic vertebral anomalies |
| | Klippel-Feil syndrome |
| Genital | Duplicated uterus |
| | Duplicated vagina |
| | Hypospadias |
| | Undescended testes |
| | Seminal vesicle cyst |
| | Absent vas deferens |

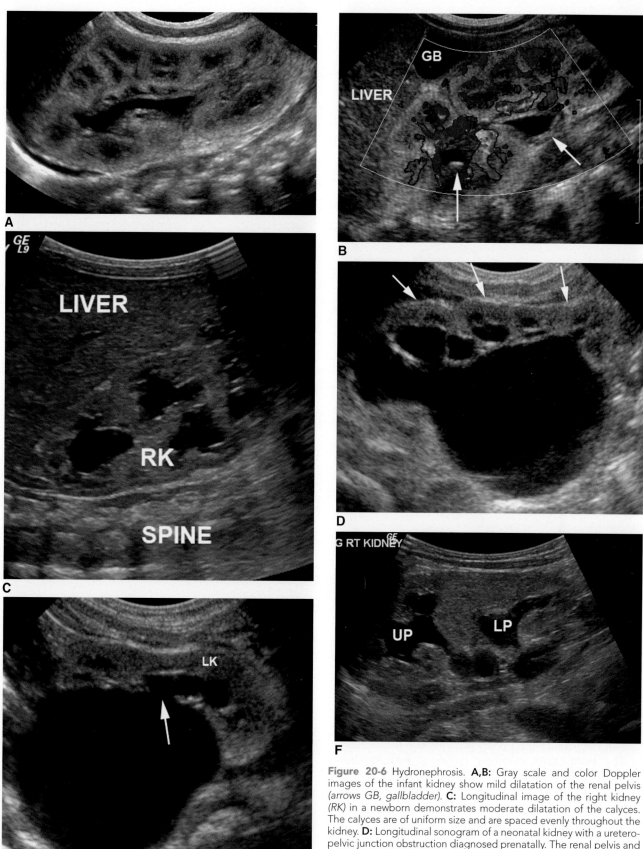

**Figure 20-6** Hydronephrosis. **A,B:** Gray scale and color Doppler images of the infant kidney show mild dilatation of the renal pelvis (arrows *GB, gallbladder*). **C:** Longitudinal image of the right kidney (*RK*) in a newborn demonstrates moderate dilatation of the calyces. The calyces are of uniform size and are spaced evenly throughout the kidney. **D:** Longitudinal sonogram of a neonatal kidney with a uretero-pelvic junction obstruction diagnosed prenatally. The renal pelvis and calyces are massively dilated. Renal parenchyma (*arrows*) is seen surrounding the dilated collecting system. **E:** Transverse image from the same patient in (**D**) shows the communication between a dilated calyx and the dilated renal pelvis (arrow *LK, left kidney*). This can be differentiated from multicystic kidneys, in which the cysts do not communicate. **F:** Longitudinal sonogram of the right kidney in an infant with a history of urinary tract infection demonstrates a duplicated collecting system with a dilated upper (*UP*) and lower (*LP*) pole. *(continued)*

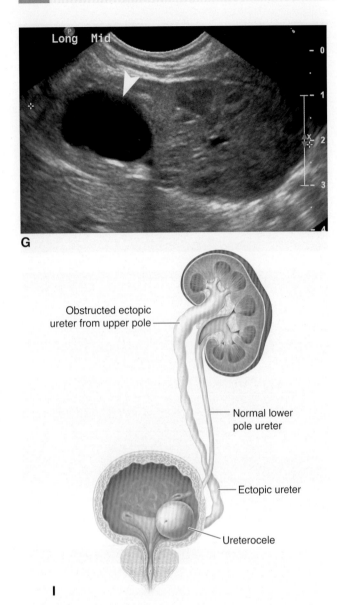

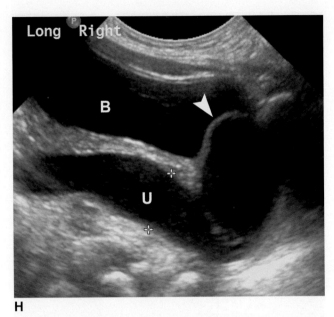

**Figure 20-6** *(continued)* **G–I:** Prenatal sonogram showed right hydronephrosis. **G:** Scan of right kidney shows a duplex kidney with a dilated upper pole collecting system *(arrowhead)* and normal lower pole parenchyma. **H:** Longitudinal scan through the bladder *(B)* in the same patient shows a dilated right ureter *(U)* emptying into an ectopic ureterocele *(arrowhead)*. **I:** A duplicated collecting system is illustrated, with an ectopic ureter from the upper pole ending in an ureterocele in the bladder. (Images **A–B** courtesy of Philips Medical Systems, Bothell, WA; Images **C–F** courtesy of Dr. Nakul Jerath, Falls Church, VA; Images **G–H** courtesy of Rechelle Nguyen, Columbus, OH.)

must be examined for obstructing masses such as dilated distal ureters that obstruct the bladder outlet as is common with ureterocele. A thick-walled small bladder with distention of the posterior urethra, such as has been described in posterior urethral valves, can cause bladder outlet obstruction. A thick-walled bladder indicates chronic obstruction. Children with distal obstruction of the urinary tract often present with infections.

The third most common cause of hydronephrosis is duplication of the collecting system (12%) (Fig. 20-6G,H). These lesions are recognized by dilatation of the upper pole calyx and a separate dilated ureter, which often can be followed to the level of the bladder. The upper pole may be dysplastic or hypoplastic. The upper pole ureter is dilated due to an abnormal ectopic insertion into the bladder with stenosis of the distal ureter.[1,16] It may also be due to an intravesicular obstruction of the distal ureter. When the ureter is obstructed in the area where it enters the bladder, the

anterior wall of the ureter may balloon into the bladder lumen, forming an ureterocele (Fig. 20-6I). There may be dilatation, to a lesser degree in the lower pole, either due to reflux or obstruction by the ectopic ureter. Unobstructed duplicated kidneys may be difficult to image in uncooperative children. The finding of infolding of cortical tissue into the medulla of the kidney and two renal sinuses, as well as a slight discrepancy in the length of the kidneys, should be clues to the existence of duplication. Kidney duplication is often bilateral.

If a dilated collecting system is identified, a voiding cystourethrogram (VCUG) is the examination of choice to determine whether reflux or outlet obstruction is responsible.[1,17] Dilatation does not necessarily mean obstruction. Reflux accounts for up to 14% of cases of hydronephrosis. Reflux may occur with a variety of obstructive bladder lesions, such as prune belly syndrome, posterior urethral valves, or neurogenic bladder with sphincter spasm.[1]

## Posterior Urethral Valves

Posterior urethral valves account for 10% of cases of hydronephrosis and is the most common cause of urethral obstruction in boys occurring in 1 in up to 8,000 boys.[1] A mucosal flap or folds or urethral tissue are responsible for the obstruction. These patients may be identified in utero with hydronephrosis or present with infection, voiding abnormalities, or retention.[18] Sonography demonstrates bilateral hydroureteronephrosis with parenchymal thinning (Fig. 20-7A–H). The kidneys may be

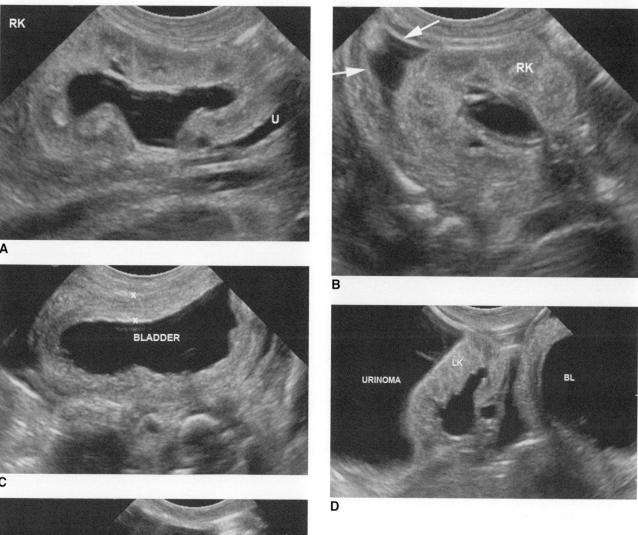

**Figure 20-7** Posterior urethral valves. **A–E:** Sonographic examination of a male neonate with bilateral hydronephrosis diagnosed on a prenatal sonogram. The patient had urinary retention. A diagnosis of posterior urethral valves was made. **A:** Longitudinal image of the right kidney *(RK)* demonstrates hydronephrosis and echogenic renal parenchyma. The dilated ureter *(U)* is seen posterior to the kidney. **B:** Transverse image of the right kidney *(RK)* again demonstrates hydronephrosis and echogenic parenchyma. Free fluid is seen *(arrows)* and is consistent with an urinoma. **C:** The wall of the urinary bladder was markedly thickened *(between calipers)*. **D:** Image of the left side demonstrates a large fluid collection displacing the left kidney *(LK)* inferiorly. The fluid collection is consistent with an urinoma resulting from a ruptured calyx. Hydronephrosis is also present in the left kidney, and the renal parenchyma is echogenic. The urinary bladder *(BL)* is seen inferior to the kidney and again demonstrates a thickened wall. **E:** In this longitudinal image, the urinoma is again seen in the left upper quadrant and is displacing the left kidney *(LK)*. *(continued)*

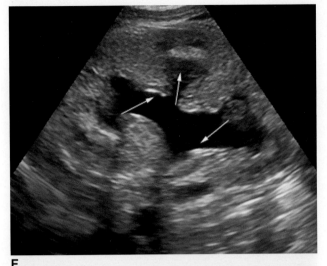

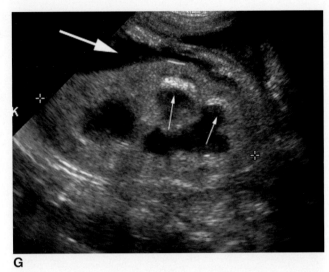

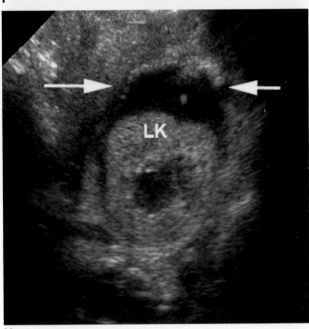

**Figure 20-7** *(continued)* **F–H:** Sonograms on a different male infant with a history of urinary tract infections. Longitudinal images of the right **(F)** and left **(G)** kidneys demonstrate bilateral hydronephrosis. The walls of the collecting system are thickened and echogenic *(small arrows)* consistent with chronic obstruction or infection. A fluid collection is seen anterior to the left kidney *(LK)* *(large arrow)*. **H:** Transverse image of the left kidney again demonstrates the fluid collection *(large arrows)* consistent with a small urinoma. The patient was diagnosed with posterior urethral valves. (Images courtesy of Dr. Nakul Jerath, Falls Church, VA.)

dysplastic with increased parenchymal echogenicity and cysts. They may be small and dysplastic. The ureters are dilated and tortuous. The bladder wall is thickened and a dilated posterior urethra may be seen.[18] Ascites may be present and perirenal or subcapsular fluid can be found.[19] The patient who develops a leak usually through an upper pole calyx has less dysplastic kidneys and better renal function due to decompression of the kidney.

## Prune Belly (Eagle-Barrett) Syndrome

Prune belly syndrome presents with absent abdominal muscles, urinary tract abnormalities, and cryptorchidism.[2,20,21] It occurs in 1 in 50,000 live births and may rarely occur in females.[21] Many infants with prune belly syndrome have small, cystic, dysplastic kidneys, but some have hydronephrotic kidneys. They may also have posterior urethral valves as well as abnormal musculature and lack of contractility of the bladder and ureteral

walls. The flaccid, dilated bladder separates this condition from posterior urethral valves, as well as the clinical observation of the abnormal abdominal wall.

An obstructed kidney, from whatever cause, is an important indication for radionuclide scanning. Even with severely impaired function, radionuclide activity can be detected in an obstructed kidney. Notably, multicystic, dysplastic kidneys exhibit no function on radionuclide scanning and this is a significant finding. Diuretic-augmented radionuclide scanning can in some cases differentiate significant obstruction from insignificant obstruction due to poorly functioning nonobstructed hydronephrotic systems.

## Cystic Dysplastic Kidneys[22,23]

There are several classifications of cystic renal disease based on pathologic or radiographic findings. Sonographically, it may be difficult to differentiate many of the cystic diseases without a family history. Dysplastic kidneys may be small or large without cysts or have small cysts or very large ones. The cysts may involve only a portion of one kidney or both kidneys.

## Multicystic Dysplastic Kidney[1,4]

Multicystic dysplastic kidney, probably the most common cystic dysplasia, is difficult to differentiate from hydronephrosis, but the distinction is important because multicystic dysplasia is a nonsurgical mass, whereas surgical correction of the obstruction may be done to salvage a hydronephrotic kidney. A multicystic kidney develops from a complete ureteral obstruction in utero. Terminal tubules become cysts, and as these cysts develop, they do not communicate and are eventually joined together by small connective tissue cords. There may be multiple cysts of varying sizes or a dominant or single cyst[21] (Fig. 20-8A–F). Multicystic kidneys may be bilateral, but this condition is inconsistent with life and affected infants have a similar presentation to patients with renal aplasia, with Potter syndrome, and respiratory difficulties.

A multicystic kidney may present as a very large mass at birth, as a progressive or decreasing cystic flank mass in utero, or as an unidentifiable kidney at a later age. Multicystic kidneys may enlarge after birth for up to 3 years. Sonography has been useful to document progressive a decrease in the size and number of cysts. A distal ureter is present in multicystic disease, whereas with agenesis no ureter is present. The disorganized cysts do not communicate with the blind ureter, which is otherwise present. Reflux may occur into the blind ureter. Unilateral multicystic kidney disease may be associated with UPJ obstruction in the opposite kidney[1] (Table 20-2).

## Hypoplasia and Dysplasia

Hypoplasia, a small but otherwise normal kidney, most often results from atrophy secondary to infection or from vascular occlusions with infarction. Dysplastic kidneys, however, may be large or small, and all are anatomically abnormal. Dysplasia is associated with urinary tract malformations in 90% of the cases, usually obstruction. Dysplasia occurs with other malformations such as an obstructed ureter, ureterocele with hydroureter, posterior urethral valves, and prune belly syndrome. Ectopic kidneys are often dysplastic. The patient may have urinary ascites. The kidneys are often small and without the corticomedullary junction and pyramids seen in normal neonates. They may or may not have visible cysts. The renal pelvis may be small or dilated, and the ureter may be dilated for some distance. Caliectasis (dilatation of the renal calyx) often is not present. Congenital megacalyces and infundibular stenosis may be the same entity. Affected infants demonstrate asymptomatic hydrocaliectasis without obstruction, which is a radionuclide finding. The calyces are dilated,

but the renal pelvis is of normal size and the kidneys may appear small and hyperechoic.

## Infantile Polycystic Kidney Disease

Infantile polycystic kidney disease or autosomal recessive polycystic kidney disease (ARPKD) is usually present at birth as symmetrically enlarged kidneys.[22] Although this condition is described as a cystic disease, the cysts result from tubular dilatation and are microscopic.[1,4] These cysts cause the pyramids or medulla of the kidney to reflect multiple bright echoes. At birth, the large kidneys are diffusely echogenic with poor differentiation of the renal sinus, medulla, and cortex.[4] Cortical echogenicity is increased, but with time the thin cortex becomes anechoic. It is the medullary portion of the kidney that enlarges and causes stretching of the calyces and renal pelvis (Fig. 20-9A–D).

Congenital hepatic fibrosis is associated with ARPKD.[1,4] All patients who survive with recessive polycystic kidney disease eventually develop congenital hepatic fibrosis, although not all patients with congenital hepatic fibrosis have ARPKD[22] (Fig. 20-9E). Adult polycystic kidney disease and dysplastic kidneys are also associated with hepatic fibrosis. Children with less extensive renal involvement may present with liver disease or portal hypertension.[1] The liver cysts may be visualized without a microscope. Within a given family the presentation may vary, some members developed liver failure, and others developed renal failure.

## Adult Polycystic Kidney Disease

Adult polycystic kidney disease or autosomal dominant polycystic kidney disease (ADPKD) may occur in the neonatal period. ADPKD may affect one or both kidneys. Cysts described in the liver, pancreas, and lung in adults have not been described at this time in neonates. The cysts in neonates may range from 0.1 to 5 mm and can be difficult to visualize with sonography. The most common sonographic finding in the neonate is renal enlargement.[22] Of the cases described in the literature, only 50% had recognizable cysts at presentation. When visible, the cysts appear to be more cortical. Probably, the best way to separate ADPKD from ARPKD is by obtaining a family history or screening the rest of the family. There is a 75% chance that other members of the family have the disease (Table 20-3).

## Glomerular Cystic Disease

Glomerular cystic disease (GKD) is a rare condition. It is hard to separate from ADPKD, ARPKD, and the hamartomas of tuberous sclerosis. At birth, the kidneys may be large and hyperechoic. With age, they become relatively smaller and their echogenicity may decrease. Cortical cysts are present and are usually microscopic, but some may be macroscopic. Although the cortical echogenicity appears to resolve, there is persistent loss

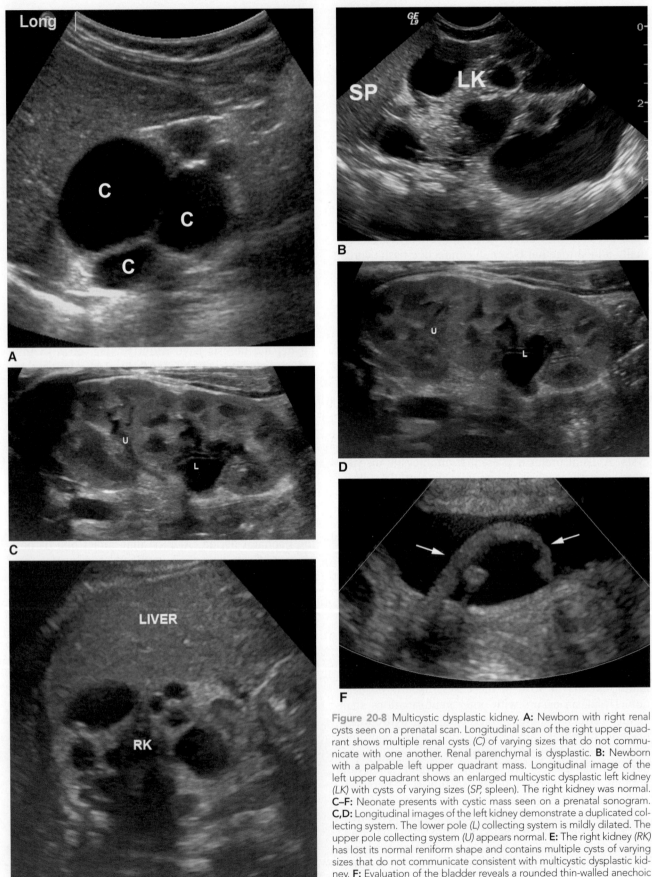

**Figure 20-8** Multicystic dysplastic kidney. **A:** Newborn with right renal cysts seen on a prenatal scan. Longitudinal scan of the right upper quadrant shows multiple renal cysts (*C*) of varying sizes that do not communicate with one another. Renal parenchymal is dysplastic. **B:** Newborn with a palpable left upper quadrant mass. Longitudinal image of the left upper quadrant shows an enlarged multicystic dysplastic left kidney (*LK*) with cysts of varying sizes (*SP,* spleen). The right kidney was normal. **C–F:** Neonate presents with cystic mass seen on a prenatal sonogram. **C,D:** Longitudinal images of the left kidney demonstrate a duplicated collecting system. The lower pole (*L*) collecting system is mildly dilated. The upper pole collecting system (*U*) appears normal. **E:** The right kidney (*RK*) has lost its normal reniform shape and contains multiple cysts of varying sizes that do not communicate consistent with multicystic dysplastic kidney. **F:** Evaluation of the bladder reveals a rounded thin-walled anechoic structure consistent with an ureterocele resulting from an abnormal insertion of the left lower pole ureter into the bladder. (Image **A** courtesy of Monica Bacani, Columbus, OH; Image **B** courtesy of Jillian Platt, Falls Church, VA; Images **C–F** courtesy of Alma Calhoun, Reston, VA.)

**TABLE 20-2**

Sonographic Differentiation of Hydronephrosis and Multicystic Disease[a]

| Feature | Multicystic Kidney | Hydronephrotic Kidney |
|---|---|---|
| Reniform | 2 | 4 |
| Lobular | 4 | 1 |
| Parenchyma present | 1 | 3 |
| Continuity between cysts | 1 | 1 |
| Separated sinus | 1 | 4 |
| Interfaces | 4 | 1 |
| Largest cyst medial | 1 | 4 |
| Largest cyst peripheral | 4 | 0 |
| Single cyst | 2 | 1 |

[a]Reliability of findings 1 (least) to 4 (most).

**TABLE 20-3**

Sonographic Comparison of ARPKD, ADPKD, and GKD

| Disease | Bilateral | Renal Size | Cysts | Inheritance |
|---|---|---|---|---|
| ARPKD | + | Very large | Rare | Autosomal recessive |
| ADPKD | + | Variable | Rare | Autosomal dominant |
| GKD | + | Normal to huge | Variable | Sporadic |

ADPKD, autosomal dominant polycystic kidney disease; ARPKD, autosomal recessive polycystic kidney disease; GKD, glomerulocystic kidney disease.

of the corticomedullary junction. Patients do not develop renal failure but may develop significant hepatic fibrosis and portal hypertension.

### Medullary Cystic Disease

Medullary cystic disease usually presents as metabolic dysfunction in young adults.[24] There are two types.

Medullary sponge kidney or renal collecting tubular ectasia is usually diagnosed in people aged 10 to 30 years of age and on the basis of laboratory and radiologic findings. Neonatal cases of medullary sponge kidney are rarely seen.

Sonographically, medullary sponge kidney demonstrates a normal sonographic pattern except for echogenic pyramids caused by calcium deposits. The findings are similar to renal tubular acidosis.[24]

Juvenile nephronophthisis or uremic medullary kidney disease is familial and may be autosomal dominant or recessive.[22] Patients present in adolescence. The kidneys may be normal or small, with increased parenchymal echogenicity and loss of the corticomedullary junction. There may be sonographically visible cysts at the corticomedullary junction.

### Renal Cysts

Cystic disease may be associated with syndromes such as cerebral hepatorenal or Zellweger syndrome, tuberous sclerosis,[25] short-rib polydactyly, orofacial digital syndrome, renal–retinal dysplasia, Conradi disease, Turner syndrome, von Hippel-Lindau disease, trisomy D or E, and Jeune asphyxiating thoracic dystrophy. Tuberous sclerosis can present initially with bilateral cystic kidneys (Fig. 20-10A,B). Acquired cysts have been described in patients on hemodialysis especially after

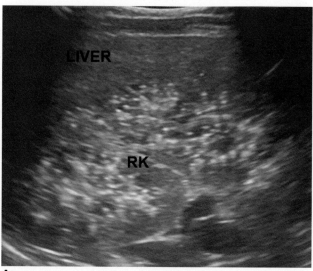

**A**

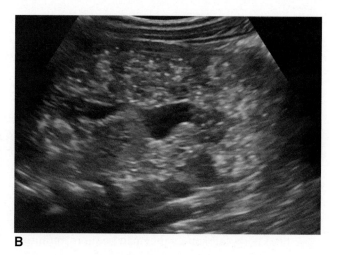

**B**

**Figure 20-9** Infantile polycystic kidney disease. Longitudinal images of the right **(A)** and left **(B)** kidneys in a newborn patient with echogenic kidneys seen on a prenatal sonogram (*RK*, right kidney). Both kidneys are enlarged and contain numerous echogenic foci throughout the kidneys. Normal renal pyramids are not seen. The left kidney demonstrates mild dilatation of the collecting system. *(continued)*

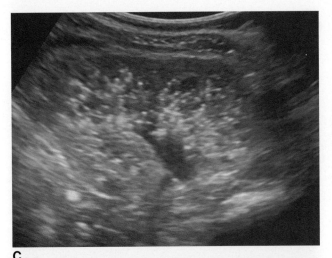

C

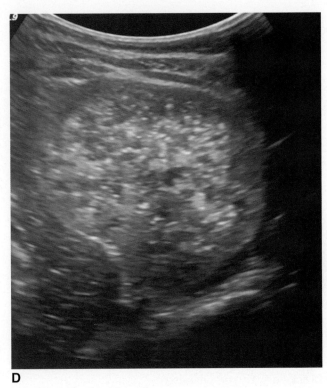

D

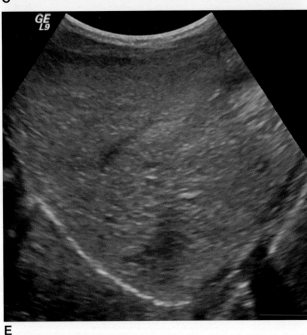

E

**Figure 20-9** *(continued)* **C,D:** Transverse images of the left kidney at the mid pole **(C)** and upper pole **(D)** again demonstrate an enlarged echogenic kidney containing numerous echogenic foci and mild dilatation of the collecting system. The patient was diagnosed with autosomal recessive polycystic kidney disease. **E:** Longitudinal image of the liver in a 5-year-old patient with a history of autosomal recessive polycystic kidney disease demonstrates a heterogeneous liver texture consistent with hepatic fibrosis. (Images courtesy of Dr. Nakul Jerath, Falls Church, VA.)

3 years. Simple cysts are rare in children. Their frequency is <1%. Inflammatory cysts from tuberculosis or other abscesses do occur.

## TUMORS[1]

When a sonographer examines any infant or child with an abdominal mass, there are three important things to determine.

1. The *origin of the mass* if possible. Can the mass be separated from the liver or kidney or other organ? Is the mass intraperitoneal or retroperitoneal? This may be difficult, but in children with little body fat, sonography can be more definitive than CT.

2. The *extent of the mass*. Does the mass extend beyond the organ of origin? Are there adjacent enlarged lymph nodes? Are the adjacent structures such as vessels (inferior vena cava [IVC] or portal vein) displaced or invaded?

3. *Metastases*. Are there metastases to the liver? Of importance to renal tumors, is there involvement of the contralateral kidney?

### Wilms Tumor

Wilms tumor is the most common malignant renal tumor in the pediatric population.[3] There are other malignant renal tumors that may occur, such as clear cell sarcoma and malignant rhabdoid tumor. Many of these tumors cannot be differentiated by any imaging study and are dependent on cytologic and/or histologic examination. The important thing is to determine if the tumor is resectable or if there is bilateral involvement to preclude surgery.

Wilms tumor is the most common solid abdominal tumor in children followed by neuroblastoma. It most often presents as a palpable mass but may cause nonspecific symptoms such as pain, fever, malaise, and weight loss. The patient may also present with hematuria or hypertension. The peak age is 3 to 4 years, but adult and infant cases have been detected. Neonatal Wilms tumor has been

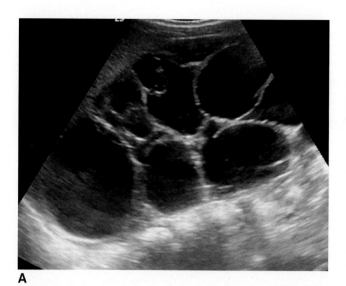
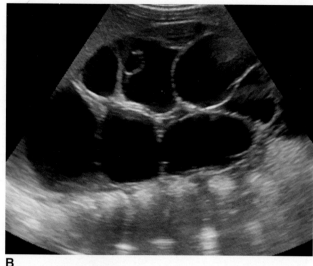

**Figure 20-10** Renal cysts. Longitudinal images of the right **(A)** and left **(B)** kidneys demonstrate multiple cysts of varying sizes in both kidneys. No normal renal parenchyma is identified. The patient was diagnosed with tuberous sclerosis.

described. This may be due to in utero malignant degeneration of nephrogenic rests.[26] Wilms tumor may involve the retroperitoneal nodes and frequently invades the renal vein and IVC and may extend into the heart.[3,27] Distant metastases may occur in the liver and lung. Therefore, these structures should be carefully examined as part of the evaluation of renal tumors. Wilms tumor may be bilateral.

There are congenital malformations associated with Wilms tumors such as aniridia (absent iris), Beckwith-Wiedemann syndrome (omphalocele, macroglossia, and hypoglycemia), Drash syndrome (male pseudohermaphroditism, progressive nephritis, and Wilms tumor), and hemihypertrophy. Children at risk for Wilms tumor should have screening sonography at 3-month intervals up to at least 6 years of age.

Wilms tumors are large, well-circumscribed, smooth masses with a homogeneous echotexture slightly greater than the liver (Fig. 20-11A,B). The tumor has a pseudocapsule that separates it from normal renal parenchyma.[3] The mass may contain hypoechoic or cystic areas and may arise from the renal sinus displacing and distorting the kidney. They may fill the pelvocaliceal system and obstruct the kidney. There is usually a portion of normal kidney that extends over the mass. The tumor may arise on a stalk from a single portion of the renal parenchyma. Anechoic or cystic spaces seen within the mass probably represent necrosis or hemorrhage but could be a remnant of a functioning calyx or infundibulum trapped in the mass. Rhabdoid tumors of the kidney are more likely to have calcification outlining lobulations (best imaged on CT) and subcapsular hematoma (Fig. 20-11C,D).

### Nephroblastomatosis[4]

Nephroblastomatosis is a precursor of Wilms tumor and can be confused with it on histologic examination. Nephroblastomatosis has been found in 25% of patients with Wilms tumor and 100% of patients with

bilateral Wilms tumors.[1] It has also been found in cases of Beckwith-Wiedemann syndrome, aniridia, Denys-Drash syndrome, and hemihypertrophy. There are two patterns. The diffuse form is divided into the pancortical and superficial types. The former replaces the renal parenchyma and the superficial has a subcapsular rind of primitive tissue surrounding normal cortex and medulla. This entity can be identified on sonography as a thick rim of hypoechoic or anechoic subcapsular tissue with irregular central contours and smooth outer margins. The kidneys are large. The sonographic and CT findings are very specific.

In multifocal nephroblastomatosis, there is persistence of primitive tissue along the columns of Bertin. The tissue ranges in size from microscopic rests to large masses in the cortex.[1] The masses may be hypoechoic, anechoic, or isoechoic and only detectable when they alter renal contour or distort the collecting system.

### Multilocular Cystic Nephroma

Also known as benign cystic nephroma, cystic hamartoma, cystic Wilms tumor, cystic lymphangioma, and multicystic nephroblastoma, a multilocular cystic nephroma presents as a mass with multiple thin-walled cysts or as septations within cysts. Normal renal parenchyma may be present elsewhere and is sharply demarcated from the mass. The presence of multiple cysts aids in the diagnosis of a multicystic nephroblastoma. These can occur at any age, and differentiation from a cystic Wilms tumor may be difficult without careful histologic review.

### Mesoblastic Nephroma

Congenital mesoblastic nephroma are the most common abdominal neoplasm seen in the neonate and are sometimes diagnosed prenatally.[1,3,28,29] Solid renal tumors in infants younger than 3 months may represent congenital mesoblastic nephroma.[3,28] Mesoblastic nephroma is a unilateral or bilateral benign tumor composed of connective

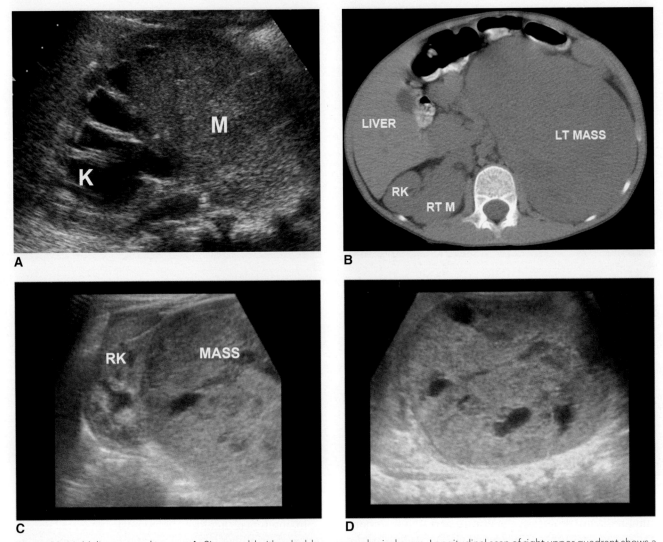

**Figure 20-11** Malignant renal tumors. **A:** Six-year-old with palpable mass on physical exam. Longitudinal scan of right upper quadrant shows a large heterogeneous solid mass arising from the right kidney. There is also dilatation of the calyces of the right kidney *(K)*. **B:** Computed tomography on a 4-year-old patient with a palpable left-sided mass reveals a large solid tumor arising from the left kidney and crossing the midline. A smaller solid mass *(RT M)* is seen arising from the right kidney *(RK)*. A diagnosis of bilateral Wilms tumor was made at biopsy. **C,D:** Longitudinal images of the right kidney in an infant with a clear cell carcinoma. A large solid well-defined mass with anechoic spaces is seen arising from the mid pole of the right kidney *(RK)*. (Image **A** courtesy of Monica Bacani, Columbus, OH; Image **B** courtesy of Dr. Nakul Jerath, Falls Church, VA; Images **C–D** courtesy of Dr. Taco Geertsma, Gelderse Vallei, The Netherlands.)

tissue, which can replace most of the renal parenchyma. Other names are fetal renal hamartoma, mesenchymal hamartoma of infancy, and benign Wilms tumor.[4,29] They present in neonates, whereas Wilms tumors are most common in children older than 2 years.[29] Although the tumor is considered benign there is malignant potential; therefore, if the tumor is unilateral, it may be removed, as Wilms tumor would be; if bilateral, radiation and chemotherapy may be prescribed.[1] Sonographically, they resemble Wilms tumor presenting as a homogeneous mass with slightly increased echogenicity. They may be heterogeneous masses with necrosis or hemorrhage centrally (Fig. 20-12A,B).

### Renal Cell Carcinoma

Renal cell carcinomas have rarely been reported in children.[3] These tumors have been found in association with tuberous sclerosis and von Hippel-Lindau disease. The tumors are isoechoic or slightly hypoechoic compared with the rest of the kidney. On CT, there is marked enhancement. Renal cell carcinoma is highly malignant in children.

### Angiomyolipoma

Angiomyolipomas are hamartomatous masses frequently associated with tuberous sclerosis.[25] Patients with tuberous sclerosis present with seizures due to cortical hamartomas, red papular rash usually over the nose and cheeks, cardiac failure due to rhabdomyomas of the heart, and angiomyolipomas and cysts of the kidneys. Renal cysts and angiomyolipomas can help confirm the diagnosis of tuberous sclerosis. Angiomyolipomas are located within the renal cortex and are homogeneous, markedly hyperechoic, and in cases of tuberous sclerosis, typically bilateral and

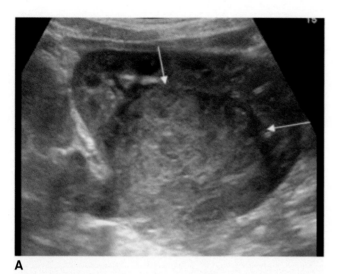
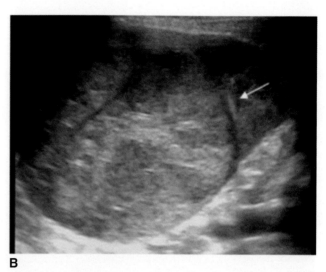

**A**    **B**

**Figure 20-12** Mesoblastic nephroma. **A,B:** Longitudinal images of the left kidney show a large solid heterogeneous central mass (arrows) diagnosed as a mesoblastic nephroma. Renal parenchyma is seen extending over the edges of the tumor indicating origin in the kidney. (Images courtesy of Dr. Taco Geertsma, Gelderse Vallei, The Netherlands.)

multiple[3,25] (Fig. 20-13A–D). There is an increased incidence of renal cell carcinoma associated with tuberous sclerosis.[25]

## ACQUIRED PATHOLOGY

Sonography may be used for evaluating pyelonephritis or infection of the upper urinary tract. Children under the age of 5 with a urinary tract infection typically undergo a sonograph of the urinary tract to evaluate for congenital anomalies.[17,30] The most common sonographic finding in the setting of pyelonephritis is enlargement of the kidneys. Areas of increased cortical echogenicity and less often areas of decreased echogenicity have been described in children with pyelonephritis. The microabscesses described at histologic examination cannot be resolved by sonography and rarely present as renal enlargement. Renal abscesses have been described on sonography. Mild scarring of a kidney due to chronic infection is a difficult sonographic diagnosis to make because the scars may be small and difficult to image and the calyces are not dilated. Sonography is not sensitive for the detection of acute inflammatory changes in the renal cortex.[30] Significant cortical scarring, especially if diffuse, may be easy to identify due to a decrease in overall renal size. Because acute pyelonephritis presents with renal enlargement, baseline measurements for following renal growth should be obtained at least 2 weeks after treatment.[31] In children with continuous lower urinary tract infections, renal measurements may be important to follow over a period of time, to ensure the kidneys are growing properly. Sonography is also a useful screening tool to seek anatomic causes of infection, specifically obstruction.

## Nephrocalcinosis

Nephrocalcinosis is the deposit of calcium in the kidney. It is associated with increased urine calcium from a variety of causes. Both kidneys are usually affected with focal echogenicity, with or without acoustic shadowing. Nephrocalcinosis may present with increased echogenicity of the renal pyramids (Fig. 20-14A–D). Children may present with diffuse cortical nephrocalcinosis. In this situation, the kidneys are normal in size but very echogenic with a loss of the normal corticomedullary junction. Nephrocalcinosis can occur in children with renal tubular acidosis or a defect in tubular reabsorption such as primary hyperoxaluria, cystinosis, and tyrosinemia.[24] Children with hypercalcemia—and particularly those infants receiving long-term furosemide for chronic lung or heart disease, hyperparathyroidism, medullary sponge, and Bartter syndrome—may present with hyperechoic medullary pyramids. Sonography in children at risk for nephrocalcinosis may identify hyperechoic pyramids. This could also represent sloughed papilla, blood clots, fungus balls, cellular debris, or proteinuria. Hyperechoic pyramids with normal urinary calcium have been seen in infancy and are associated with transient oliguria. Children at risk for urolithiasis due to urinary stasis or infection may have echogenic calculi in the ureter or bladder.

## RENAL VASCULAR DISEASE

Renal vascular problems in children are usually the result of trauma or other underlying conditions such as nephrotic syndrome, which predisposes the patient to renal vein thrombosis. Clot formation and emboli can occur in the renal arteries as a complication of umbilical artery catheterization and can result in hypoplasia of the kidneys. In small infants, it can be difficult to

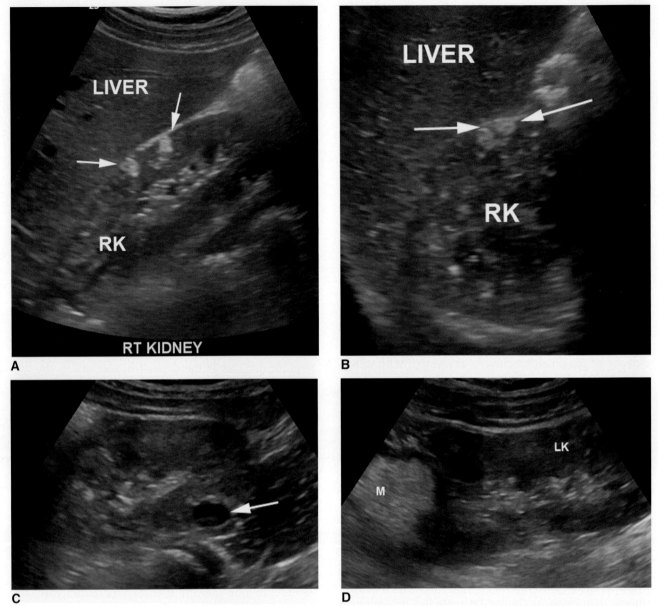

**Figure 20-13** Angiomyolipoma. **A:** Longitudinal image of the right kidney (*RK*) in a pediatric patient diagnosed with tuberous sclerosis. Two hyperechoic, homogeneous, solid masses (*arrows*) are seen in the renal cortex consistent with angiomyolipomas. **B:** Transverse image of the right kidney in a different patient demonstrates multiple echogenic foci seen throughout the renal cortex. The echogenic foci represent angiomyolipomas. A larger angiomyolipoma (*arrows*) is seen at the periphery of the cortex. **C:** Longitudinal image of the left kidney from the same patient as B again shows multiple echogenic foci throughout the cortex as well as a simple cyst (*arrow*) in the lower pole. Both angiomyolipomas and renal cysts are frequently seen in patients with tuberous sclerosis. **D:** Longitudinal image of the left kidney (*LK*) in a pediatric patient with tuberous sclerosis demonstrates an echogenic mass (*M*) arising from the upper pole. The mass was diagnosed as an angiomyolipoma. Patients with tuberous sclerosis must be screened routinely as they are at a higher risk for renal cell carcinoma. (Images courtesy of Dr. Nakul Jerath, Falls Church, VA.)

detect actual renal vein thrombosis, as it often occurs in the small veins, but diffuse enlargement and increased echogenicity of the kidneys can be seen.

### TRAUMA

Renal trauma is unusual in infants but may be related to a birth injury. The cause of a flank mass in a newborn is more often adrenal than renal parenchymal hemorrhage. Sonographically, the appearance of hemorrhage changes over time and may be anechoic to complex. Hemorrhage may be subcapsular or perinephric. For

imaging renal trauma in a child, CT is the modality of choice.

### URINARY BLADDER

In infants, the bladder is an abdominal rather than a pelvic organ, and frequently it is difficult to evaluate because the mere pressure of the transducer on the abdomen causes the bladder to evacuate. When it is necessary for an infant's bladder to be full, a Foley catheter can be used to fill it and the inflated balloon used to keep it full. It is unusual to see a very

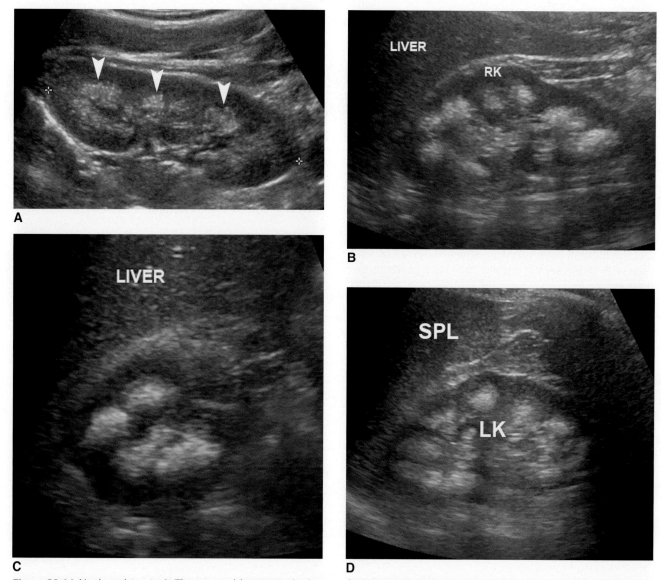

A

B

C

D

**Figure 20-14** Nephrocalcinosis. **A:** Three-year-old patient with a history of William syndrome and hypercalcemia. Longitudinal prone image of the right kidney shows increased echogenicity of the renal pyramids. **B–D:** Longitudinal (**B**) and transverse (**C**) images of the right kidney (*RK*) demonstrate hyperechoic renal pyramids. **D:** Longitudinal image of the left kidney (*LK*) also demonstrates hyperechoic renal pyramids consistent with bilateral nephrocalcinosis (*SP*, spleen). (Image **A** courtesy of Rechelle Nguyen, Columbus, OH; Images **B–D** courtesy of Dr. Nakul Jerath, Falls Church, VA.)

distended bladder in a normal neonate unless the mother received drugs during labor or delivery, which could affect the infant's nervous system for several hours, or the infant is receiving drugs that would inhibit voiding. Bladder distention may be caused by neurogenic disease or a pelvic mass. Cystic pelvic masses can be confused with the bladder, and care must be taken to clearly identify the bladder.

## CONGENITAL ANOMALIES

### Urachal Abnormalities[12]

The urachus is a tubular structure continuous with the anterior dome of the bladder and extending outside the peritoneum to the umbilicus superiorly. Normally, during the fourth and fifth months of gestation, the urachus narrows to a small-caliber tube. The normal urachus is either completely obliterated and fibrotic at or before birth, or it seals off in the neonatal period. Occasionally, the urachus persists. It may persist as a cord from the umbilicus to the superior aspect of the bladder, producing an anterior superior vesical diverticulum, which is usually continuous with the bladder. It may remain as an open structure (patent urachus) between the umbilicus and the bladder, but usually only in cases of bladder outlet obstruction where the urachus decompresses the otherwise obstructed bladder. Such patients may exhibit an abdominal mass after the umbilical cord is clamped at birth. Sometimes the urachus persists in continuity with the umbilicus but not with the bladder; sometimes it is continuous with the bladder but not with the umbilicus. Urachal cysts may present as palpable midline abdominal masses, but more often the patient presents with symptoms of an infection.

Sonography is useful for evaluating urachal cyst. The bladder is tethered anteriorly. Masses are continuous with the bladder, and the echo pattern is cystic or, if infected, complex (Fig. 20-15A–D).

The posterior urethral valve syndrome is another congenital urethral abnormality. The valve is a thin membrane positioned across the membranous portion of the penile urethra in boys. With secondary changes in the bladder, ureters, or kidneys, it can obstruct voiding as previously described. Sonographically, the bladder wall may be thickened, and dilatation of the posterior urethra can be identified. The ureters are tortuous and dilated, and the kidneys have varying degrees of dysplasia. Children with prune belly syndrome may have posterior urethral valves with hydroureteronephrosis and renal dysplasia, but the bladder is usually very large and flaccid.

## BLADDER TUMORS

### Rhabdomyosarcoma

Rhabdomyosarcomas often involve or arise from the bladder, prostate, uterus, or vagina of children. Depending on the point of origin, they may cause various changes in the urinary tract. With rhabdomyosarcoma of the bladder, patients present with hematuria, dysuria, retention, and urinary tract infection.[16] Sonographically, rhabdomyosarcomas are seen as a homogeneous polypoidal mass.[16] Masses within the bladder are often immovable blood clots that are adherent to the thick wall. The bladder may also be obstructed by sacrococcygeal teratoma (see Chapter 19).

## INFECTION

Cystitis, the most common urinary tract infection in children, is 10 times more common in girls than in boys. In children with chronic cystitis, the bladder wall may

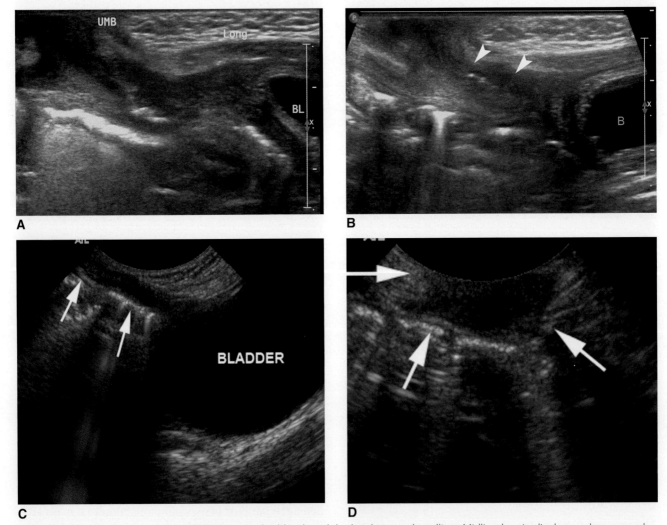

**Figure 20-15** Urachal abnormalities. **A,B:** Two-month-old with umbilical redness and swelling. Midline longitudinal scan shows an echogenic tract from the dome of the urinary bladder *(BL)* to the umbilicus *(UMB)* most likely representing an infected umbilical remnant *(UMB, arrowheads)*. **C,D:** Longitudinal scan of the pelvis demonstrates a hypoechoic tract *(arrows)* arising from the dome of the bladder to the umbilicus. **D:** A hypoechoic mass *(arrows)* is seen just posterior to the umbilicus representing an infected patent urachus. The urachus was found to be patent at the bladder and closed at the umbilicus allowing a cyst to form. (Images **A-B** courtesy of Rechelle Nguyen, Columbus, OH; Images **C–D** courtesy of Dr. Nakul Jerath, Falls Church, VA.)

be thickened, measuring >0.3 cm with a full bladder and 0.5 cm with an empty bladder.[32] Usually, cystitis produces diffuse thickening of the bladder wall, which can be a nonspecific finding. Bladder wall changes may be asymmetrical with marked localized thickening of the wall suggestive of a mass or pseudotumoral cystitis. If there is evidence otherwise of acute infection, this should be treated conservatively and with follow-up sonography in a week to make sure there is no progression of the mass to suggest tumor. Bladder calculi in children are extremely unusual unless there is urinary stasis in the bladder. Children with active urinary tract bleeding may show clots or blood in the bladder. Bladder perforation and trauma are best evaluated by cystography.

# ADRENAL GLANDS

Diagnostic sonography is particularly useful in the examination of the neonatal adrenals. The right adrenal gland can be successfully imaged 97% of the time and the left adrenal gland 83% of the time. The ability to visualize the normal neonatal adrenal glands by sonography is due to several factors: (1) the neonatal adrenals are proportionally larger than adult glands (about one-third the size of the kidney at birth, as opposed to one-thirteenth in adults); (2) newborn infants' sparsity of perirenal fat affords better image resolution than the abundance of areolar fatty tissue surrounding the adult gland; and (3) the neonatal adrenal glands are closer to the skin surface, which permits the use of higher frequency transducers for sharper resolution of small structures.[33] In older infants and children, normal adrenal glands are sometimes difficult to identify, especially the left one. Adrenal sonography provides an opportunity to image from several directions, avoids the negative effects of ionizing radiation, is less expensive than CT, and can be performed at the bedside of a critically ill patient. The drawbacks of adrenal sonography include technically unsatisfactory studies resulting from the small size of the gland in older children, obesity, and overlying bowel gas.[33]

## SONOGRAPHIC TECHNIQUE

### Patient Preparation

Pediatric patients require no preparation for this exam, but should be encouraged to be well hydrated. Adrenal visualization may be limited because the attenuation by bowel gas. Because air is a major culprit, it may be helpful to examine the patient after fasting using an approximate time line of 3 hours for patients younger than 1 year, 6 hours for patients 1 to 5 years of age, and 12 hours for older children.

### Scan Technique

The accuracy of adrenal sonographic visualization varies greatly, depending on what technique is used and on the experience and skill of the operator. The age of

the patient is also an important factor because the adrenal glands of neonates and young infants are larger and more easily identified.[34] It is not uncommon to examine the patient in different positions until the entire gland can be optimally visualized. The adrenal glands may be demonstrated by scanning from the flanks in longitudinal, coronal, and transverse planes. These planes are useful for avoiding overlying bowel.

The use of various decubitus and oblique positions may aid visualization.[33] A combination of transverse and longitudinal oblique scans has been reported to be accurate in identifying adrenal disease. When the patient lies in the decubitus position, the kidney falls forward and the adrenal gland may come into the scanning plane. However, because the gland is a complicated, folded piece of tissue, a single scan may demonstrate only part of it. For a complete adrenal evaluation, the sonographer should scan anterior as well as posterior to the gland until it is imaged in its entirety.

Another helpful technique in left adrenal gland visualization is the cava-suprarenal line (CSL) position, in which the patient lies in a 45-degree left posterior oblique position while transverse scans are made from the right side to localize the left adrenal gland. The patient's position is then adjusted so that the acoustic beam lines up and passes through the IVC and aorta. The left adrenal gland is then visualized. Longitudinal planes are obtained by using the IVC and aorta as a double window for transmission.

The left adrenal gland is more difficult to visualize than the right one because of nearby stomach or bowel gas interference. This difficulty may be overcome by scanning through the intercostal spaces near the posterior axillary line. In difficult cases, it may be helpful to elevate the patient's left side, so that the adrenal area can be scanned through the spleen and kidney and behind the stomach gas bubble.

### Technical Considerations

During adrenal scanning, the gain control setting should be comparable to that used for studying the liver. The normal adrenal glands have about the same echogenicity as the normal liver.

## NORMAL SONOGRAPHIC APPEARANCE

The use of adjacent structural landmarks facilitates accurate localization of the adrenal glands. These paired retroperitoneal structures are located within the perirenal space. The right adrenal gland is pyramid-shaped and lies over the kidney between the right crus of the diaphragm and the liver, posterior to the IVC. Any mass in the right adrenal area must be differentiated from a renal, hepatic, or retrocaval lymph node mass.

Imaging the left adrenal gland may be more difficult because of the numerous structures located in the left upper quadrant. The left adrenal is crescent-shaped and lies anterior to the upper pole of the left kidney but lateral to the left crus of the diaphragm and posterior to the pancreatic tail. The esophagogastric junction is superior to the left gland and the fourth portion of the duodenum, inferior to it. It is important not to mistake the spleen, the splenic vessels, or the left renal vessels for the adrenal gland. These structures are usually distinguishable by their differing sonographic textures and contours, although masses originating in any of these structures can be mistaken for left adrenal masses or vice versa. A collapsed stomach or the duodenum can also be differentiated from the adrenal by the presence of "bright" central mucosal echoes and the real-time demonstration of peristalsis. The patient can drink water to demonstrate the stomach if there is any question. The spleen varies in size and location and may have lobulations (accessory spleens). Such findings can cause confusion and lead to misdiagnosis of an enlarged left adrenal gland.[35] Abdominal vessels can be identified by observing their pulsations and using Doppler instrumentation to detect blood flow.

The typical sonographic appearance of the adrenal gland is a Y- or V-shaped structure on longitudinal scans and a curvilinear structure on transverse scans[33] (Fig. 20-16A,B). The adrenal gland is made up of two parts: the medulla, which is sonographically visualized as a thin, echogenic central area; and the cortex, which appears as a thicker, anechoic zone surrounding the medulla. The newborn's adrenal cortex is relatively thick because it is composed of two layers: a thick fetal zone that occupies ~80% of the gland and a thin peripheral zone that will become the adult cortex. After birth, the fetal zone undergoes involution, gradually shrinking, and taking on a more typical adult appearance as it is replaced by connective tissues by 1 year of age.[33]

Sonographic studies should note the size of the adrenal glands. The normal adrenal length ranges from 0.9 to 3.6 cm and the width between 0.2 and 0.5 cm. Their study found no statistically significant difference in the size of right and left adrenals. It is important to note that with renal agenesis, the adrenal gland is large and occupies the renal fossa. It may lose its typical Y or V shape but should not be mistaken for the kidney or another mass.[34]

## ABNORMAL FINDINGS

### Tumors

Sonography can document the presence of adrenal masses, but it cannot differentiate tumor types.[35] Masses are usually more readily visualized than the normal gland. The sonographic appearance must be correlated with clinical and laboratory data to determine the type of lesion.[35] Adrenal masses usually appear as sonographically discrete lesions superior and medial to the upper pole of the kidney. A large mass may compress and deform the kidney, producing the appearance of tumor invasion. The most important

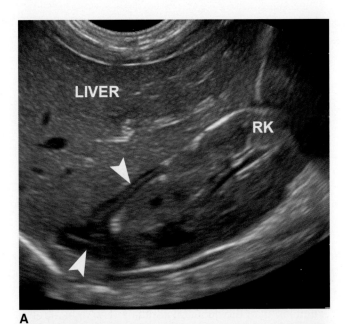

**A**

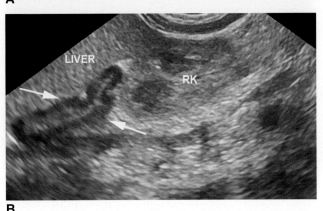

**B**

**Figure 20-16** Normal neonatal adrenal gland. **A:** Longitudinal scan of right upper quadrant in a 35-week neonate shows the normal Y-shaped adrenal gland *(arrowheads)* superior to right kidney *(RK)*. **B:** Longitudinal scan of the right upper quadrant in a term neonate shows the adrenal gland with the normal echogenic medulla surrounded by the hypoechoic cortex. RK, right kidney: (Image **A** courtesy of Monica Bacani, Columbus, OH; Image **B** courtesy of Jillian Platt, Falls Church, VA.)

feature for differentiating adrenal and renal masses is an interface or demarcation between the mass and the kidney. An adrenal mass shows such a demarcation, whereas a renal mass does not.

### Neuroblastoma[1,36]

The most common adrenal tumors of childhood are the complex of neuroblastomas, which include ganglioneuromas, ganglioneuroblastomas, and neuroblastomas. All of the tumors are of neural crest origin, but the ganglioneuroma is considered less malignant and actually is a mature neuroblastoma.[34] Neuroblastoma is a tumor of infancy. Half the reported cases appear in the first year of life. Uncommon after age 8, neuroblastoma almost never occurs in adults.[37] It is important to note that these lesions can also arise from sympathetic ganglia in the lower abdomen, presacral region, chest, and even the neck and nasopharynx.[34] In the first year of life, almost all neuroblastomas involve the adrenal gland. The older the patient, the more likely the tumor is to arise outside the adrenal gland.[38] Children with abdominal neuroblastomas usually present with a palpable mass. It is less common for the presenting signs or symptoms to be caused by metastases. Pelvic tumors can cause urinary or gastrointestinal symptoms. Clinically, systemic signs and symptoms, such as fever, weight loss, abdominal distention, irritability, hypertension, and anemia are sometimes seen.[36,39] The prognosis for neuroblastoma is usually better in neonates and young infants than in older infants or children. Prognosis is also dependent on the site of origin of the tumor and the extent of disease at the time of diagnosis.[40] Early detection of the tumor is crucial to improve outcome.

Neuroblastoma is well known to have an unpredictable course.[37,41] Ordinarily, staging is based on the local extent of the lesion and the presence or absence of metastases. In most cases, patients with neuroblastoma present with advanced disease, having a large abdominal mass, or signs of metastases. Unlike Wilms tumor, most neuroblastomas are not "clean" lesions; usually, they spread rapidly beyond the confines of the adrenal glands, often crossing the midline in the abdomen and sometimes extending into the chest.[27] Calcification is a common finding in neuroblastoma, and calcifications frequently are irregular and visible in the primary tumor or its metastases.[34,38]

Sonographically, neuroblastoma is predominately echogenic, with poorly defined borders[36] (Fig. 20-17). When tumor calcification is present, focal echogenic areas can be seen producing acoustic shadowing. Hypoechoic areas within the neoplasm may result from necrosis. In the classic case of neuroblastoma arising from the adrenal gland, sonography clearly demonstrates the relationship of the tumor to the kidney, with its typical downward and outward displacement. Sonography is also useful for identifying urinary obstruction, vascular displacement and compression, nodal involvement, tumor extent, and liver involvement.[40] Extra-adrenal lesions exhibit a variety of configurations and relationships between the kidney and other organs.[34]

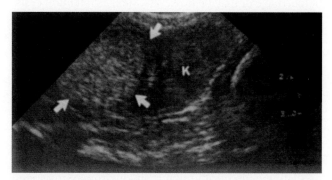

**Figure 20-17** Neuroblastoma. Longitudinal sonogram of a neuroblastoma *(arrows)*, displacing the right kidney *(K)* downwardly.

Sonographic evaluation of neuroblastoma occurring in the chest and paraspinal area has obvious limitations. In these and other cases, CT more clearly demonstrates the extent and borders of the mass. Thus, even though sonography may originally make the diagnosis, CT is generally necessary to provide precise tumor mapping.[27] Magnetic resonance imaging (MRI) also provides similar information important to both the initial diagnosis and posttreatment follow-up.[34]

The sonographer must attempt to differentiate the neuroblastoma from other abdominal masses, define the margins of the tumor, and identify any signs of metastatic disease. It may not be possible on the basis of the sonographic study alone to differentiate neuroblastoma from other solid tumors. Like Wilms tumor, neuroblastoma can metastasize to almost any organ.[41] In a neonate with a suprarenal mass, adrenal hemorrhage should be distinguished from necrotic neuroblastoma. An adrenal hemorrhage should show a characteristic pattern of resolution over a short time.

### Adrenocortical Carcinoma

In children, adrenal gland tumors other than neuroblastomas are rare. The most common of these is the congenital adrenocortical carcinoma, which can produce virilizing symptoms or be linked with fetal alcohol syndrome or congenital hemihypertrophy and Beckwith-Wiedemann syndrome. Other clinical signs include abdominal mass, deepened voice, hypertension, seizures, and, rarely, weight loss. These lesions tend to be highly malignant and locally invasive[34] with frequent venous extension, regional lymph node involvement, and distant metastases to liver, lung, bone, and brain. Adrenocortical carcinoma is more common in adults than in children.[34]

Sonographically, adrenocortical carcinoma has a moderately echogenic complex pattern. The heterogeneous pattern probably represents areas of hemorrhage and necrosis dispersed throughout the tumor.[34] Calcification is seen in approximately one-fifth of the tumors. A thick, echogenic capsule-like rim may also be visualized in adrenocortical carcinoma.[40] Diagnostic imaging is an important tool for defining the extent of the primary tumor and determining the presence or absence of metastatic disease. Vascular extension is characteristic of adrenocortical carcinoma, and sonography can clearly demonstrate tumor extension into the IVC, hepatic veins, and right atrium. Metastasis in the retroperitoneum can also be visualized.

### Pheochromocytoma

Pheochromocytomas are rare, functioning tumors that originate in chromaffin tissue. Fewer than 5% of all pheochromocytomas affect children, but most of those occur in the adrenal medulla. Pheochromocytomas may also be found in aberrant tissue along the sympathetic chain, the thorax, the para-aortic area, the aortic bifurcation, the retroperitoneum, and the bladder. Multiple pheochromocytomas are sometimes found in children, so it is important to search for a second and even a third lesion. In ~10% of pediatric cases, other family members are similarly affected, so careful examination of the child's immediate family is in order. Clinically, the diagnosis of pheochromocytoma is made by determination of urinary catecholamine excretion. Clinical symptoms include hypertension, headaches, palpitations, and diaphoresis.[37]

Sonographically, pheochromocytomas have a broad spectrum of appearance. A variety of internal echo patterns can be observed, including purely solid tumors, mixed solid and cystic masses, and cyst-like lesions. When lesions are large, they often contain areas of hemorrhage and necrosis, which result in a heterogeneous sonographic appearance.[35] Pheochromocytomas are almost always sharply encapsulated, producing a sharp, echogenic wall. Extra-adrenal masses are difficult to image sonographically and are often obscured by bowel gas.[35]

### Metastases

Adrenal metastases often occur in a variety of adult malignancies but are rare in children.[39] Although metastases to the adrenal gland infrequently cause clinical symptoms, sonography is helpful for examining patients with known primary tumors for the progression of metastatic adrenal disease.[35] Such tumors are often bilateral and large.

Given the increased proportion of malignant lesions, adrenal masses in children and adolescents probably warrant resection unless they are seen in conjunction with a specific disorder such as congenital adrenal hyperplasia.[42]

Sonographically, adrenal metastasis is nonspecific and may look identical to a primary adrenal tumor. Metastases appear solid, with varying degrees of echogenicity. Bilateral masses heighten the suspicion of adrenal origin.

### HEMORRHAGE[43]

Adrenal hemorrhage in the newborn may result from prematurity, neonatal sepsis or hypoxia, or birth trauma inflicted on the rapidly involuting adrenal gland, particularly in large infants of diabetic mothers.[43,44] Often more than one factor is responsible. Neonatal adrenal glands are susceptible to hemorrhage due to their large size and high vascularity.[43,44] Adrenal hemorrhage is most frequently identified between the second and seventh days of life. Clinically, there may be a palpable mass, anemia, hypotension, hyponatremia, jaundice, and scrotal discoloration in males.[43,44] Jaundice may occur because of the resorption of excessive hemoglobin from massive hemorrhage, but with massive hemorrhage complete exsanguination of the infant can

result.[34] Adrenal hemorrhage can also be identified after accidental blunt abdominal trauma[45] or child abuse in children. The hemorrhage is usually small, unilateral, in the right gland, and associated with ipsilateral intra-abdominal and intrathoracic injuries. Care should be taken not to incorrectly identify the hemorrhage as adrenal neoplasm, retroperitoneal blood, or hepatic or renal injury. An uncommon complication of adrenal hemorrhage is adrenal insufficiency.

Sonographically, the appearance of adrenal hemorrhage depends on the age of the hemorrhage. Initially, hemorrhage appears as an echogenic mass in the suprarenal area. As it liquefies, the mass becomes progressively more anechoic, so that eventually a suprarenal anechoic, cyst-like structure is visualized[34] (Fig. 20-18A–C). The diagnosis of adrenal hemorrhage may be established if sonography is repeated at 3- to 5-day intervals to observe the appearance of the mass as it changes from solid to cystic (Fig. 20-18D,E). Follow-up is appropriate at intervals of several weeks for 2 to 3 months because neuroblastoma may mimic the appearance of adrenal hemorrhage. Neuroblastoma will increase in size over time, whereas hemorrhage will resolve.[40] Elevated urinary catecholamines also can be indicative of neuroblastomas assisting with the differential diagnosis.

In most cases, the enlarged, hemorrhagic adrenal gland shrinks rapidly and calcifications may become visible within a few weeks or months. Initially, the calcifications outline the enlarged anechoic adrenal gland in a rim-like fashion. With time, as the adrenal becomes progressively smaller, the calcifications become more compact and eventually conform to the triangular configuration of the normal gland. Calcifications may be found incidentally on abdominal radiography or sonography. Documentation or adrenal hemorrhage is uncommon in these cases, but calcifications are assumed to be evidence of this. The calcified glands are echogenic.[34]

### CYSTS

Adrenal cysts are rare.[35] They are usually unilateral, asymptomatic lesions that may be large and may cause hypertension. Adrenal cysts may occur secondary to hemorrhage or may be true cysts, such as retention cysts, cystic adenomas, or angiomatous cysts. Malignancies associated with adrenal cysts have not been reported.[35]

Sonographically, adrenal cysts usually appear as anechoic structures in the adrenal area that demonstrate well-defined walls and posterior acoustic enhancement. Typically, they displace the kidney inferiorly and present a definite interface with the upper pole of the kidney. Some adrenal cysts contain debris and have irregular borders; for example, adrenal pseudocysts and hemorrhagic cysts. Adrenal cysts can simulate and must be distinguished from renal cysts, hydronephrosis, and splenic or pancreatic pseudocysts.[35]

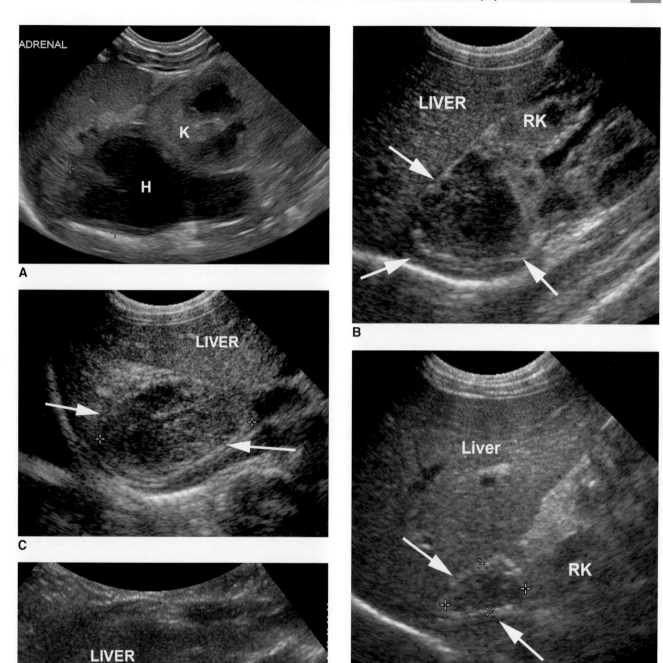

**Figure 20-18** Adrenal hemorrhage. **A:** Prenatal sonogram showed a mass in left upper quadrant. Longitudinal scan of the left kidney *(K)* in the neonate shows a cystic mass *(H)* superior to kidney consistent with adrenal hemorrhage. **B–E:** Serial sonographic evaluations in a patient with adrenal hemorrhage following a traumatic delivery. Longitudinal **(B)** and transverse **(C)** images of the right upper quadrant 2 days after delivery demonstrate a heterogeneous mass *(arrows)* superior to the right kidney *(RK)*. **D:** Follow-up examination 3 weeks later demonstrates a much smaller more echogenic mass *(arrows)* again seen superior to the right kidney *(RK)*. **E:** A second follow-up examination 6 weeks after delivery demonstrates complete resolution of the mass with only small residual calcifications *(arrow, RK, right kidney)*. Follow-up examination will help distinguish an adrenal hemorrhage from an adrenal tumor as an adrenal tumor should decrease in size over time. (Image **A** courtesy of Monica Bacani, Columbus, OH; Images **B–E** courtesy of Dr. Nakul Jerath, Falls Church, VA.)

## ABSCESS

Adrenal abscesses are rare in children but have been documented in the neonatal period, probably the result of neonatal sepsis.[34] Bacterial seeding of adrenal hemorrhage is probably the cause of many adrenal abscesses.[39] The adrenals are relatively resistant to ordinary bacterial infection; although pyogenic abscesses can develop in the cortex with bacteremia, staphylococcal infections are the most common. The adrenal gland may also be involved by disseminated granulomatous disease. Adrenal abscesses are usually unilateral, but bilateral abscesses have been documented. Before 1946, adrenal tuberculosis accounted for nearly 90% of reported Addison disease cases in childhood. Since that time, histoplasmosis has become the most common childhood granulomatous disease of the adrenal gland. Infection of the adrenal gland by other fungi, particularly *Candida* (*Monilia*) or *Aspergillus*, may occur in terminal stages of leukemia or other hematopoietic diseases. Antibiotics alone are inadequate in treating a walled-off abscess and percutaneous drainage is necessary.[40] Clinically, abscesses are characterized by fever, chills, and abdominal pain.

Sonographically, an adrenal abscess is identified as a relatively anechoic suprarenal mass, sometimes containing echogenic debris,[34] or a fluid-debris level with layering of debris altering with changes in position.[40] Abscesses are usually unilateral, although bilateral ones have been documented.[34] It can be difficult to sonographically distinguish between adrenal abscess and adrenal hemorrhage or neuroblastoma with central hemorrhage and necrosis. The failure of an adrenal hemorrhage to resolve or an increase in the size of a mass in an infant with fever should raise the suspicion of an abscess.[39] It is important to correlate the clinical history with the sonographic findings to make the correct diagnosis.[35]

## RENAL AGENESIS

In patients with renal agenesis or severe renal hypoplasia (Potter syndrome) or ectopia of the kidney, the adrenal glands may become elongated and increase in thickness or may assume an unusual flattened or discoid shape.[39] Although this condition has been described as "hypertrophied," the adrenal gland is actually of normal weight and is normal in all other respects, except for shape.

In cases of renal agenesis, ectopia, or hypoplasia, it is important to recognize the characteristic sonographic appearance of the neonatal adrenals.[33] When normal renal tissue is absent, the adrenal gland preserves its typical echogenic medulla and hypoechoic cortex but enlarges, losing its characteristic Y or V shape and assuming a more elliptic, flattened shape. The distinctive appearance of the adrenal medulla and cortex should not be mistaken for the kidney.[33]

An enlarged adrenal gland without an adjacent kidney does not necessarily indicate renal agenesis, as the kidney may merely be ectopic. Whenever enlarged adrenal glands are identified, a careful search should be made for renal tissue elsewhere in the abdomen or pelvis. Because renal agenesis is accompanied by Potter syndrome and pulmonary hypoplasia, it is important to identify affected fetuses and neonates because of direct therapeutic implications. The sonographic appearance of an elongated and thickened adrenal is probably the result of lack of pressure from the kidney against the developing adrenal.

## CONGENITAL ADRENAL HYPERPLASIA

Congenital adrenal hyperplasia (CAH) is an inborn error of the metabolism involving a deficiency of one of several enzymes necessary for normal steroid biosynthesis. It is transmitted as an autosomal recessive trait; the incidence is ~1 in 50 births in the United States.[41] The diagnosis of CAH depends on specific biochemical tests. The clinical signs include virilism in newborn females, premature masculinization in males, and advanced somatic development in both sexes.[39] Adrenocortical adenomas can develop in patients afflicted with CAH from hyperplastic tissue when the adrenal cortex undergoes increased hyperstimulation. Most cases of incidentally discovered adrenocortical adenomas (incidentalomas) have been reported in adults due to increased CT and MRI scans being done for other diagnostic reasons. Lho et al. reported a case of a 12-year-old girl with CAH, who developed an adrenocortical adenoma tumor despite being treated with steroids after birth.[46]

Sonographically, CAH is demonstrated by increased adrenal size. The adrenal glands become markedly enlarged, with preservation of the characteristic anechoic cortex and echogenic medulla. The enlargement involves the cortex predominantly, without obvious medullary enlargement except in length. Sonographic adrenal measurements of ≥20 mm and a mean width of ≥4 mm are suggestive of the presence of adrenal hyperplasia. Sonography is used in CAH to measure the size of the adrenal glands to monitor the response to treatment, to reduce the likelihood of overtreatment and oversuppression, and their effects on growth and maturation. Some neonates with biochemically proved CAH may have normal sonograms. Therefore, identification of sonographically normal-sized adrenal glands does not exclude CAH.

# RELATED IMAGING PROCEDURES

Because no single procedure always provides all the necessary diagnostic information, the appropriate use of each modality requires an understanding of its strengths and weaknesses.

## RADIOGRAPHIC EXAMINATIONS

Intravenous pyelography (IVP) and the VCUG are used to evaluate the urinary tract in children and infants. Both examinations can provide information regarding congenital anomalies and the functionality of the urinary tract. VCUG is used to evaluate for reflux in cases of urinary tract infection. An IVP provides limited diagnostic information, and its importance has decreased with the introduction of sonography and CT. Both examinations have the disadvantage of using ionizing radiation and injected radiopaque contrast medium.

## COMPUTED TOMOGRAPHY

High-resolution CT can accurately image the normal kidneys and adrenal glands as well as tumors or masses, particularly in obese patients. It has been suggested that CT is the most important modality for assessment of primary and metastatic disease at the time of diagnosis and for follow-up. The advantages of CT are that it provides a more complete abdominal examination that is not limited by bowel gas, clearer definition of anatomic relationships, and very few unsatisfactory examinations. Disadvantages of CT include its ionizing radiation, opaque contrast material, relative expense, and limitation to imaging suite.

## MAGNETIC RESONANCE IMAGING

MRI demonstrates excellent soft tissue contrast and is very helpful in differentiating among several diagnostic possibilities. MRI offers a combination of good anatomic information and tissue-specific information based on signal intensity. It is effective in diagnosing renal masses, adrenal hemorrhage, adrenal cortical carcinoma, metastases, pheochromocytoma (particularly ectopic lesions), and neuroblastoma, including staging (in children beyond the neonatal period). Magnetic resonance urography (MRU) has become more widely used and provides anatomic and functional information without the use of ionizing radiation.[15] MRU provides useful information in cases of complex congenital anomalies, urinary tract obstruction, and urinary tract infections.[15]

## NUCLEAR MEDICINE SCINTIGRAPHY

Renal scintigraphy provides functional information about the urinary system and can provide valuable information in cases of congenital renal anomalies, obstruction, and reflux. Specifically, a metaiodobenzylguanidine (MIBG) scan can be used for detecting recurrent or metastatic adrenal tumors with fibrosis, distorted anatomy, or masses in an unusual location. Disadvantages include an increased dose of radiation and the patient's thyroid gland must be blocked or protected during the scan.[47,48]

## POSITRON EMISSION TOMOGRAPHY

Positron emission tomography (PET) can be utilized to target specific processes unique to certain types of tumors. Advantages are low radiation and no blocking of the thyroid needed (as in the MIBG scan). Disadvantages include an increased cost of the exams.[47,48]

## SUMMARY

- Sonography is widely used to evaluate the urinary tract and adrenal glands in the pediatric patient population as it can be performed portably; does not employ ionizing radiation, contrast, or sedation; and it can be used for follow-up examinations.

- A 10-MHz transducer is used for neonatal examinations, whereas a 7.5-MHz transducer is more appropriate for older children.

- The medulla or renal pyramids are more prominent in infants and should not be mistaken for renal cysts.

- The renal pelvis should measure <10 mm in a normal kidney and the wall should not be visible; a thickened wall may indicate chronic infection, reflux, or chronic obstruction.

- The cortex of the kidneys in newborns, especially premature infants, is more echogenic than the liver and spleen.

- Bilateral renal agenesis is incompatible with life and is associated with oligohydramnios and Potter syndrome; unilateral renal agenesis is more common and may be asymptomatic.

- In cases of renal agenesis, the adrenal gland may fill the renal fossa and should not be mistaken for the kidney.

- Congenital hydronephrosis is the most common renal mass in infants and children and most commonly results from an obstruction at the ureteropelvic junction.

- Duplication of the collecting system is a common cause of hydronephrosis due to the anomalous insertion of the ectopic ureter into the bladder; the upper pole collecting system is typically dilated.

- A ureterocele occurs when the ureter is narrowed at its distal insertion into the bladder; the anterior wall of the ureter projects into the bladder lumen forming a ureterocele.

- Posterior urethral valves cause bilateral hydronephrosis, a thickened bladder wall, and dilated ureters.

- Multicystic dysplastic kidney may be hard to differentiate from hydronephrosis and is the result of a complete ureteral obstruction in utero.

- Hypoplastic kidney is a result of atrophy secondary to infection or vascular infarction.

- Infantile polycystic kidney disease presents at birth as symmetrically enlarged kidneys that are diffusely echogenic; the condition is associated with hepatic fibrosis.

## Critical Thinking Questions

1. A 3-year-old boy presents with hematuria, a mild fever, and a left upper quadrant palpable mass. The sonogram demonstrates a well-defined, homogeneously solid, 3-cm mass in the lower pole of the left kidney. What is the most likely diagnosis and where else should the sonographer include in the examination?

2. The sonographer receives a requisition to perform an abdominal sonogram on a 2-day-old infant with a right upper quadrant abdominal mass following a difficult delivery. The examination reveals a large echogenic mass superior to the right kidney and appears separate from the right kidney. What is the most likely diagnosis and what would help to confirm the diagnosis?

3. A 6-month-old girl presents with a palpable mass just inferior to the umbilicus. The area appears red and inflamed. The sonogram reveals a cystic mass that contains some debris. With further evaluation, a small tract is seen connecting the cystic area to the superior urinary bladder. What is the most likely diagnosis?

4. What is the most common cause of hydronephrosis in infants?

5. While scanning a newborn patient for a renal examination, the sonographer notices both kidneys are enlarged and echogenic with hyperechoic foci scattered throughout both kidneys. What is the most likely diagnosis?

---

- Simple renal cysts are rare in children and are usually associated with a syndrome such as tuberous sclerosis or von Hippel-Lindau disease.

- Wilms tumor is the most common malignant renal tumor in children and frequently presents before the age of 4 with pain, fever, malaise, weight loss, and a palpable abdominal mass.

- Wilms tumors are typically large, well-circumscribed, homogeneous masses that may contain cystic spaces within the mass representing necrosis or hemorrhage.

- Mesoblastic nephroma occur in infants younger than 3 months of age and may be unilateral or bilateral; sonographically, they resemble a Wilms tumor.

- Angiomyolipoma are echogenic, well-defined masses that are rare in children except in cases of tuberous sclerosis where they are typically bilateral and multiple.

- Cystitis is the most common urinary tract infection in children, occurs 10 times more often in females than males, and may cause thickening of the bladder wall.

- The most common adrenal tumor of childhood is the neuroblastoma, which most commonly occurs in the first year of life.

- Sonographically, neuroblastoma are poorly defined, echogenic, solid masses that frequently have internal calcifications.

- Pheochromocytomas are rare, functioning adrenal gland medullary tumors that can occur in children and sonographically may appear solid, complex, or cystic.

- Adrenal hemorrhage may occur in the newborn as a result of prematurity, neonatal sepsis, birth trauma, or hypoxia; is most frequently identified between the second and seventh days of life; and may result in a palpable mass and anemia.

- Sonographically, the appearance of adrenal hemorrhage varies from echogenic to anechoic depending on the age of the hemorrhage.

## REFERENCES

1. Milla SS, Lee EY, Buonoma C, et al. Ultrasound evaluation of pediatric abdominal masses. *Ultrasound Clin.* 2007;2:541–559.
2. Becker AM. Postnatal evaluation of infants with an abnormal antenatal renal sonogram. *Curr Opin Pediatr.* 2009;21:207–213.
3. Paltiel HJ. Sonography of pediatric renal tumors. *Ultrasound Clin.* 2007;2:89–104.
4. Lawande A. Ultrasonography in pediatric renal masses. *Ultrasound Clin.* 2010;5:433–441.
5. Kasap B, Soylu A, Türkmen M, et al. Relationship of increased renal cortical echogenicity with clinical and laboratory findings in pediatric renal disease. *J Clin Ultrasound.* 2006;34:339–342.
6. Michel SC, Forster I, Seifert B, et al. Renal dimensions measured by ultrasonography in children: variations as a function of the imaging plane and patient position. *Eur Radiol.* 2004;14:1508–1512.
7. Creel SA, Anderson J, Michael K, et al. Evaluation of pediatric renal size by sonography. *JDMS.* 1999;15:1–6.
8. Pantoja Zuzuárregui JR, Mallios R, Murphy J. The effect of obesity on kidney length in a healthy pediatric population. *Pediatr Nephrol.* 2009;24:2023–2027.
9. Ozçelik G, Polat TB, Aktaş S, et al. Resistive index in febrile urinary tract infections: predictive value of renal outcome. *Pediatr Nephrol.* 2004;19:148–152.
10. Okada T, Yoshida H, Iwai J, et al. Pulsed Doppler sonography of the hilar renal artery: differentiation of obstructive from nonobstructive hydronephrosis in children. *J Pediatr Surg.* 2001;36:416–420.
11. Yildirim H, Gungor S, Cihangiroglu MM, et al. Doppler studies in normal kidneys of preterm and term neonates: changes in relation to gestational age and birth weight. *J Ultrasound Med.* 2005;24:623–627.

12. Sivit CJ. Sonography of pediatric urinary tract emergencies. *Ultrasound Clin*. 2006;1:67–75.

13. Vorvick L. Medline Plus. Ureteropelvic junction obstruction. 2009. Available at http://nlmnih.gov/medlineplus/ency/article/001267.htm. Accessed May 13, 2010.

14. Singh H, Ganpule A, Malhotra V, et al. Transperitoneal laparoscopic pyeloplasty in children. *J Endourol*. 2007;21:1461–1466.

15. Renjen P, Bellah R, Hellinger JC, et al. Pediatric urologic advanced imaging: techniques and applications. *Urol Clin North Am*. 2010;37:307–318.

16. Sidhu R, Bhatt S, Dogra VS. Ultrasonography of the urinary bladder. *Ultrasound Clin*. 2010;5:457–474.

17. Zamir G, Sakran W, Horowitz Y, et al. Urinary tract infection: is there a need for routine renal ultrasonography? *Arch Dis Child*. 2004;89:466–468.

18. Bernardes LS, Aksnes G, Saada J, et al. Keyhole sign: how specific is it for the diagnosis of posterior urethral valves? *Ultrasound Obstet Gynecol*. 2009;34:419–423.

19. Heikkilä J, Taskinen S, Rintala R. Urinomas associated with posterior urethral valves. *J Urol*. 2008;180:1476–1478.

20. Metwalley KA, Farghalley HS, Abd-Elsayed AA. Prune belly syndrome in an Egyptian infant with Down syndrome: a case report. *J Med Case Reports*. 2008;2;322.

21. Lin CC, Tsai JD, Sheu JC, et al. Segmental multicystic dysplastic kidney in children: clinical presentation, imaging finding, management, and outcome. *J Pediatr Surg*. 2010;45:1856–1862.

22. Garel L. Renal cystic disease. *Ultrasound Clin*. 2010;5:15–59.

23. Sweeney WE Jr, Avner ED. Diagnosis and management of childhood polycystic kidney disease. *Pediatr Nephrol*. 2011;26:675–692.

24. El-Sawi M, Shahein AR. Medullary sponge kidney presenting in a neonate with distal renal tubular acidosis and failure to thrive: a case report. *J Med Case Reports*. 2009;3:6656.

25. Letourneau K, Harrington C, Reed M, et al. Tuberous sclerosis complex: typical and atypical sonographic findings. *JDMS*. 2005;21:491–496.

26. Ritchey ML, Azizkhan RG, Beckwith JB, et al. Neonatal Wilms tumor. *J Pediatr Surg*. 1995;30:856–859.

27. Mehta SV, Lim-Dunham JE. Ultrasonographic appearance of pediatric abdominal neuroblastoma with inferior vena cava extension. *J Ultrasound Med*. 2003;22:1091–1095.

28. Celik H, Kefeli M, Tosun M, et al. Congenital mesoblastic nephroma: prenatal diagnosis by sonography. *JDMS*. 2009;25:112–115.

29. Fuchs IB, Henrich W, Brauer M, et al. Prenatal diagnosis of congenital mesoblastic nephroma in 2 siblings. *J Ultrasound Med*. 2003;22:823–827.

30. Bauer R, Kogan BA. New developments in the diagnosis and management of pediatric UTIs. *Urol Clin North Am*. 2008;35:47–58.

31. Pickworth FE, Carlin JB, Ditchfield MR, et al. Sonographic measurement of renal enlargement in children with acute pyelonephritis and time needed for resolution: implications for renal growth assessment. *AJR Am J Roentgenol*. 1995;165:405–408.

32. Bellah RD, Epelman MS, Darge K. Sonography in the evaluation of pediatric urinary tract infection. *Ultrasound Clin*. 2010;5:1–13.

33. Oppenheimer DA, Carroll BA, Yousem S. Sonography of the normal neonatal adrenal gland. *Radiology*. 1983;146:157–160.

34. Hayden KC Jr, Swischuk LE. *Pediatric Ultrasonography*. Baltimore, MD: Lippincott Williams & Wilkins; 1987.

35. Worthen NJ. Adrenal sonography. In: Sarti D, ed. *Diagnostic Ultrasound: Text and Cases*. 2nd ed. Chicago, IL: Year Book Medical Publishers; 1987.

36. Perry CL. Sonographic evaluation of neuroblastoma. *JDMS*. 2009;25:101–107.

37. Dunnick NR, Korobkin M. Imaging of adrenal incidentalomas: current status. *AJR Am J Roentgenol*. 2002;179:559–568.

38. Arce GJ, Arce TY, Angerri FO, et al. Retroperitoneal ganglioneuroma in the infancy. *Actas Urol Esp*. 2008;32:567–570.

39. Shackelford GD. Adrenal glands, pancreas and other retroperitoneal structures. In: Siegel MJ, ed. *Pediatric Sonography*. 2nd ed. New York, NY: Raven Press; 1995.

40. Silverman FN, Kuhn JP. *Caffey's Pediatric X-Ray Diagnosis: An Integrated Imaging Approach*. Vol 2. St. Louis, MO: CV Mosby; 1993.

41. Filiatrault D, Hoyoux C, Benoit P, et al. Renal metastases from neuroblastoma. Report of two cases. *Pediatr Radiol*. 1987;17:137–138.

42. Pescovitz OH, Eugster EA. *Pediatric Endocrinology: Mechanisms, Manifestations, and Management*. Philadelphia, PA: Lippincott Williams & Wilkins; 2004.

43. Valdespino RS. The importance of sonography in the evaluation of neonatal adrenal hemorrhage. *JDMS*. 2009;25:221–225.

44. Abdu AT, Kriss VM, Bada HS, et al. Adrenal hemorrhage in a newborn. *Am J Perinatol*. 2009;26:553–557.

45. Soundappan SV, Lam AH, Cass DT. Traumatic adrenal haemorrhage in children. *ANZ J Surg*. 2006;76:729–731.

46. Lho SR, Park SH, Jung MH, et al. A case of adrenocortical adenoma following long-term treatment in a patient with congenital adrenal hyperplasia. *Korean J Pediatr*. 2007;50:302–305.

47. Willatt JM, Francis IR. Radiologic evaluation of incidentally discovered adrenal masses. *Am Fam Physician*. 2010;81:1361–1366.

48. Sahdev A, Willatt J, Francis IR, et al. The indeterminate lesion. *Cancer Imaging*. 2010;10:102–113.

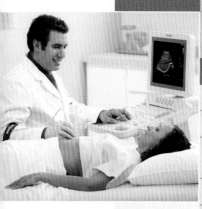

# 21 The Neonatal Brain

Monica M. Bacani

## OBJECTIVES

Identify the sonographic appearance of the normal neonatal brain.

Demonstrate the process for sonographic evaluation of the neonatal brain.

Describe the differences in sonographic appearance of the mature and immature neonatal brain.

Identify the risk factors for development of an intracranial hemorrhage.

Illustrate the sonographic appearance of the four grades of intracranial hemorrhage.

Describe the mechanism and sonographic appearance of hydrocephalus.

List common intracranial pathologies that can be visualized sonographically.

## KEY TERMS

agenesis of the corpus callosum | cerebellar hemorrhage | Chiari malformation | coarctation of the lateral ventricle | cytomegalovirus | Dandy-Walker complex | germinal matrix intraventricular hemorrhage | holoprosencephaly | hydrocephalus | intracranial hemorrhage | periventricular leukomalacia | porencephaly | prominent periventricular blush | subarachnoid space | TORCH complex | vein of Galen malformation

## GLOSSARY

**cerebellum** posterior portion of the brain composed of two hemispheres; lies below the tentorium

**cerebrum** largest section of the brain; divided into two hemispheres joined by the corpus callosum

**choroid plexus** echogenic cluster of cells located within the lateral ventricles responsible for the production of cerebral spinal fluid

**corpus callosum** largest white matter structure in the brain; contains nerve tracts that allow communication between the right and left hemispheres of the brain

**falx cerebri** fold of dura matter that divides the two hemispheres of the brain

**fontanelle** soft spot between the cranial bones; anterior, posterior, and mastoid fontanelles are used as acoustic windows during sonographic examination of the neonatal brain

**hypoxia** lack of oxygen

**porencephaly** cyst or cavity in the brain usually the result of a destructive lesion

**thalamus** paired ovoid structures in the central brain responsible for relaying nerve impulses and carrying sensory information into the cerebral cortex

**C**ranial sonography has evolved into a vital clinical tool and is the primary modality for both screening and follow-up of intracranial hemorrhage (ICH), hydrocephalus, and congenital anomalies of the neonatal brain. Widespread utilization is the result of its proven diagnostic value, bedside availability, nonionizing nature, and its cost-effectiveness compared to other imaging modalities.

Unlike other sonographic examinations, cranial sonography is not a common procedure performed in hospitals or institutions without a level II or III neonatal intensive care unit. The overall aim of this chapter is to provide the sonographer or sonography student with an introduction to neonatal cranial sonography. The focus is on normal sonographic anatomy of the neonatal brain, scanning protocols, normal variants, and some of the more common intracranial pathology and anomalies. For a more comprehensive study of intracranial anomalies, there are several texts the reader should reference.[1,2]

## TECHNIQUE

The current standard of practice utilizes the anterior fontanelle as the primary acoustic window to image the neonatal brain. Closure of the anterior fontanelle begins at about 9 months of age and is usually complete by 15 months of age. However, rarely is it suitable to scan an infant older than 9 months except in cases of increased intracranial pressure (ICP) or prematurity. Routine images are obtained in the coronal and sagittal planes. Two alternate acoustic windows, the posterior fontanelle (PF) and the mastoid (posterolateral) fontanelle (MF) have shown considerable diagnostic benefits as supplemental imaging sections to the routine anterior fontanelle approach. Illustration of their clinical utility will be discussed further in this chapter.

A small footprint high-frequency 7- to 10-MHz phased curved array or sector transducer is typically used to image the neonatal brain. A lower frequency (5 to 7 MHz) transducer may be needed for older infants with closing fontanelles or infants with a large amount of hair. A small footprint, high-frequency linear transducer (10 to 15 MHz) is useful for imaging superficial structures such as the superficial cortex or the extracranial space around the convexity of the brain.

Preterm infants in the intensive care nurseries are at high risk for infections due to their immature immune systems. Transducers and cables must be cleaned thoroughly between each patient. Proper hand washing technique, adherence to isolation protocols, and the use of single-use gel packets will help minimize the spread of infection. Before proceeding with the scan, the examiner needs to communicate with the nurse in charge of the infant to discuss any potential complications that may arise during scanning and to solicit help with ventilator tubes or other equipment that may need to be rearranged in order to access the fontanelles. There are also some procedural precautions that need to be observed in order to prevent additional stress on the preterm infant. These precautions include limiting head and neck movement on babies that have endotracheal tubes in place, thus minimizing the risk of dislodging critical airway support; applying too much pressure to the anterior fontanelle with the transducer causing the onset of bradycardia; and thermal regulation. Opening the isolette doors should be avoided when possible. Scanning through the portholes of the isolette and the use of prewarmed gel can help the infant maintain thermal stability during the sonography examination.

## NORMAL BRAIN ANATOMY

The brain and spinal cord comprise the central nervous system (CNS). Three protective membranes called meninges cover and protect the brain and spinal cord. They consist of the pia mater, dura mater, and the arachnoid. The dura mater is the outer layer and the most resilient of the three. It attaches to the inside of the cranial vault. The pia mater surrounds the surface of the cerebral cortex, and the arachnoid is interposed between the pia and dura mater.

### CEREBROSPINAL FLUID

Cerebrospinal fluid (CSF) surrounds the brain and the spinal cord. This fluid acts like a buffer to help cushion the brain and spinal cord from injury. The brain maintains a balance between the amount of CSF that is produced and the amount that is absorbed.

### FONTANELLES

The anterior fontanelle is formed at the junction of the coronal, sagittal, and frontal sutures. The posterior fontanelle is formed by the junction of the lambdoid and sagittal sutures. The mastoid (posterolateral) fontanelle is located at the junction of the squamosal, lambdoidal, and occipital sutures (Fig. 21-1).

### DIVISIONS OF THE BRAIN

The brain can be divided into the cerebrum, the cerebellum, and the brain stem. The cerebrum is the largest section and is divided into right and left cerebral hemispheres and is separated by a fissure or groove called the *interhemispheric (longitudinal) fissure.* The falx cerebri is a section of dura that lies within this fissure.

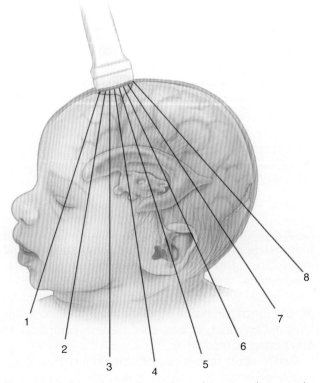

**Figure 21-1** Coronal scan planes. Coronal imaging planes via the anterior fontanelle approach.

The cerebrum is composed of both gray and white matter. The outer portion called the *cortex* is composed of gray matter, whereas the white matter is found deeper within the cerebrum.

The cortex is divided into four lobes: frontal, parietal, occipital, and temporal. The brain stem is a stalk-like structure connecting the cerebral hemispheres with the spinal cord. It consists of three parts: the midbrain, pons, and medulla oblongata. The cerebellum is located at the back of the brain beneath the occipital lobes and is separated from the cerebrum by the tentorium (a fold of dura). The cerebellum is composed of two hemispheres with a median structure called the *vermis* that connects the two hemispheres. The cavity containing the cerebellum, fourth ventricle, brain stem, and cranial nerves is called the *posterior fossa*.

## VENTRICLES

The purpose of the ventricular system is to provide a pathway for the circulation of CSF. The ventricular system is composed of four ventricles: the paired lateral ventricles and the midline third and fourth ventricles. The paired lateral ventricles are the largest of the ventricles and are located on either side within the cerebrum of the brain. They are divided into four segments: the frontal (anterior) horn, body, temporal, and occipital (posterior) horn. The trigone (atrium) of the lateral ventricle is the region where the anterior, occipital, and temporal horns join.

The paired lateral ventricles drain into the third ventricle through the foramina of Monro, and the third ventricle drains into the fourth through the aqueduct of Sylvius. The fourth ventricle drains into the subarachnoid space through the foramina of Luschka and Magendie and then into the basal cistern. CSF flows upward around the brain to the vertex, where it is resorbed by the arachnoid granulations into the superior sinuses. CSF also flows around and down the spinal subarachnoid space.

## CHOROID PLEXUS

The choroid plexus is responsible for the production and regulation of CSF. The largest part of the choroid plexus, which is known as the *glomus,* lies within the lateral ventricles at the level of the trigone. It tapers to a point as it courses anteriorly and ends at the caudothalamic groove. The choroid plexus never extends anterior to the foramen of Monro into the frontal horns or posterior into the occipital horns. Choroid plexus is also present in the roof of the third and fourth ventricles.

## CORPUS CALLOSUM

The two sides of the cerebrum are joined by the corpus callosum. The corpus callosum is the largest white matter structure in the brain and contains nerve tracts that allow communication between the right and left hemispheres of the brain. It is divided into the rostrum, genu, body, and splenium (posterior part) and forms the roof of the lateral and third ventricle.

## CAUDATE NUCLEUS

Located in each hemisphere of the brain, the caudate nucleus is the most medial of the four basal ganglia. An elongated, curved mass of gray matter its consists of head, body, and tail. The head and body form part of the floor of the anterior horn of the lateral ventricle and the tail curves back toward the anterior forming the roof of the inferior horn of the lateral ventricle.

## THALAMUS

The thalami are paired structures of gray matter situated between the cerebral cortex and the midbrain. They are located in the center of the brain, one beneath each cerebral hemisphere, next to the third ventricle. The thalami can be thought of as relay stations for nerve impulses carrying sensory information into the cerebral cortex.

## CISTERNA MAGNA

The cisterna magna is a fluid-filled structure that communicates with the fourth ventricle. It lies between the cerebellum and the dorsal surface of the medulla.

# SCANNING PROTOCOL

Scanning of the neonatal head should be performed in a standardized manner with a specific sequence of images and key anatomical structures identified on each scan. Most premature infants will have serial scans over the course of their hospital stay and a standard approach will ensure that consistency will be maintained from examiner to examiner. The examiner should also know the approximate gestational age of the infant. This will aid in differentiating age-related features from pathology.

## CORONAL SCANNING PROTOCOL

Scanning in the coronal plane via the anterior fontanelle should minimally include six to eight images. Magnified image planes should be incorporated to draw attention to suspicious areas or to enhance visualization of abnormal areas. Maintaining side-to-side symmetry while scanning in the coronal plane is a technique that will require some practice; however, doing so is essential to obtaining a good study. Representative coronal sections are obtained by systematically angling the transducer from the frontal lobe of the infant brain to the occipital cortex. The scanning planes are depicted in Figure 21-1. In the coronal plane, by convention, image labeling should have the right side of the brain projected on the left side of the image.

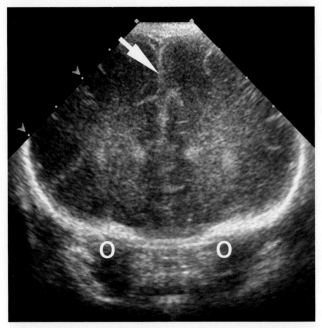

**Figure 21-2** Frontal lobes. Coronal image at the level of the frontal lobes shows interhemispheric fissure *(arrow)*, normal echogenicity of the frontal lobes, and orbital ridges *(O)*. This image is just anterior to the frontal horns of the lateral ventricles.

The most anterior coronal image is obtained through the frontal lobes of the cerebral cortex at the level of the orbital rims and the interhemispheric fissure (Fig. 21-2). This scan is anterior to the frontal horns. The next scan should include the triangular-shaped, fluid-filled frontal horns and the head of the caudate nuclei adjacent to the lateral walls of the ventricles. The fluid-filled cavum septi pellucidi can be seen between the frontal horns of the lateral ventricles. Anterior to the cavum is the corpus callosum (Fig. 21-3). The next scan is slightly more posterior and is obtained at the level of the foramen of Monro. This is where the lateral ventricles and the third ventricle communicate. The normal slit-like third ventricle is often difficult to visualize due to the fact that its transverse diameter often falls within the beam width. Slight off axis angulation will offset the beam thickness effect and will often allow visualization of the normal third ventricle. When dilated, it can be imaged quite easily (Fig. 21-4). Continuing with further posterior angulation, the echogenic choroid plexus can be seen in the floor of the lateral ventricle and in the roof of the third ventricle. This scan is slightly posterior to the third ventricle. The echogenic V-shaped tentorium can be seen in this scan anterior to the cerebellum. Posterior to the vermis of the cerebellum is the cisterna magna. The Y-shaped sylvian fissure can also be seen in this plane (Fig. 21-5). With more posterior angulation, the next scan demonstrates the echogenic star-shaped quadrigeminal cistern posterior to the thalami. Posterior to the tentorium is the posterior fossa containing the echogenic cerebellum (Fig. 21-6).

Angling slightly more posterior, the trigones of the lateral ventricles dominate this section. The glomi of the choroid plexus fills most of the lateral ventricles at this level. The periventricular parenchyma lateral to the ventricles should be evaluated carefully. These

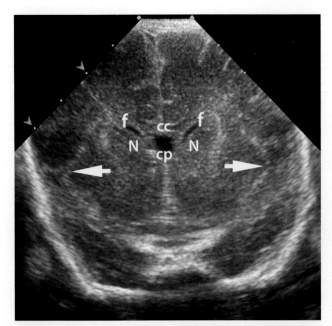

**Figure 21-3** Frontal horns. In this coronal image, the frontal horns *(f)* appear as triangular-shaped, fluid-filled spaces separated by the cavum septum pellucidum *(cp)*. The head of the caudate nuclei *(N)* lie adjacent to the lateral walls of the ventricles. The hypoechoic corpus callosum *(cc)* forms the roof of the cavum. The echogenic Y-shaped sylvian fissures *(arrows)* are seen laterally.

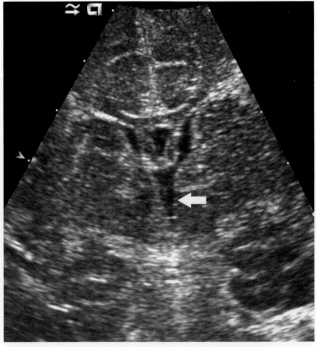

**Figure 21-4** Third ventricle. Magnified coronal image at the level of the normal third ventricle. Slight off-axis scan shows the normal size third ventricle *(arrow)* at the level of the foramen of Monro.

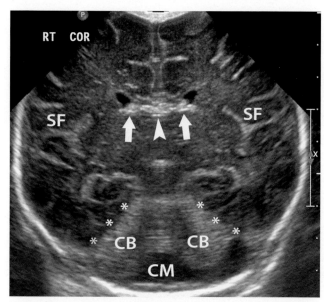

**Figure 21-5** Coronal scan posterior to the third ventricle. The echogenic choroid plexus is seen in the floor of the lateral ventricles *(arrows)* and the roof of the third ventricle *(arrowhead)*. The Y-shaped sylvian fissures *(SF)* are seen laterally. Also visible are the echogenic tentorium *(\*)*, the cerebellar hemispheres *(CB)*, and the cisterna magna *(CM)*.

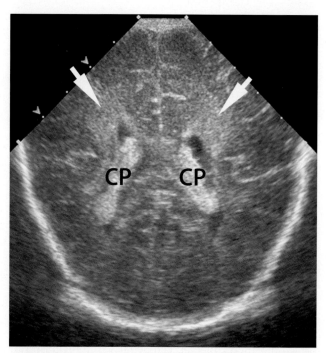

**Figure 21-7** Choroid plexus. Coronal scan at the level of the trigones of the lateral ventricles. The largest part of the choroid plexus *(CP)*, the glomus, can be seen occupying most of the lateral ventricles. The periventricular matter is located lateral to the ventricles *(arrows)*.

areas represent the periventricular white matter and the echogenicity of this area should not be brighter than the choroid plexus. (See section on periventricular halo or blush). A benefit of the coronal plane is that it allows contralateral comparison of the echogenicity between the choroid plexus and the periventricular parenchyma. Increased echogenicity of this area should arouse

suspicion for hemorrhage/infarction and requires follow-up evaluation (Fig. 21-7). The final and most posterior scan visualizes predominantly the gyri and sulci of the occipital lobe, the periventricular white matter, and the posterior interhemispheric fissure (Fig. 21-8).

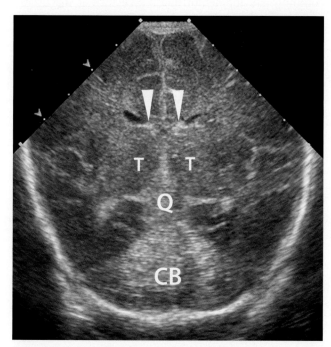

**Figure 21-6** Quadrigeminal cistern. Coronal image taken at the level of the quadrigeminal cistern. The star-shaped echogenic quadrigeminal cistern *(Q)* is seen inferior to the thalami *(T)*. The cerebellum *(CB)* and the echogenic choroid plexus *(arrowhead)* in the floor of the lateral ventricles are also visualized on this image.

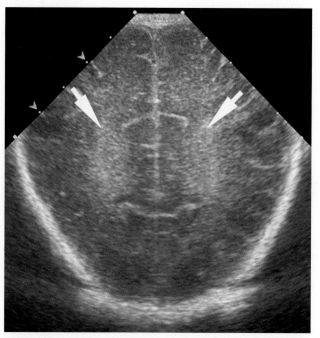

**Figure 21-8** Occipital lobe. Coronal image taken posterior to the occipital horns of lateral ventricles shows the normal echogenic periventricular white matter *(arrows)* and the occipital cortex.

## SAGITTAL/PARASAGITTAL SCANNING PROTOCOL

The transducer is rotated 90 degrees from the coronal plane and, starting at the midline, is angled medial to lateral sequentially through each cerebral hemisphere via the anterior fontanelle. Scanning planes are depicted in Figure 21-9. Image labeling, by convention, places the anterior aspect of the brain on the left side of the image. The midline, right, and left side need to be annotated, respectively. In the midline, the crescentic hypoechoic corpus callosum is visualized just above the cavum septum pellucidum and vergae (seen in premature infants only). Superiorly, the corpus callosum is surrounded by the hyperechoic pericallosal sulci, which contains the pericallosal artery. The vascular pulsations from these vessels can be appreciated on real-time imaging. Inferior to the corpus callosum is the third ventricle. Anterior to the echogenic vermis of the cerebellum is the triangular-shaped fourth ventricle. The moderately echogenic midbrain is anterior to the fourth ventricle, and the echogenic cerebellar vermis is posterior to the fourth ventricle (Fig. 21-10). The cisterna magna is seen inferior to the vermis and should always be visualized. Absence of the cisterna magna is indicative of pathology. Parasagittal images are obtained by angling the transducer from the midline through the right and left cerebral hemispheres from medial to lateral (or lateral to medial). The main anatomic landmark in the next image is the caudothalamic groove. The anterior

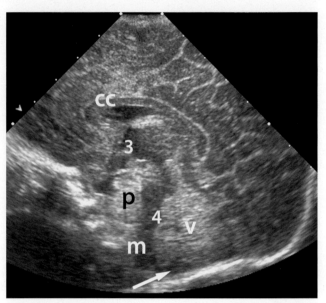

**Figure 21-10** Sagittal midline. Normal midline sagittal image on a term infant. The hypoechoic corpus callosum *(cc)* is seen anterior to the cavum septum pellucidum. The third *(3)* and fourth *(4)* ventricles are visible in this plane. Posterior to the fourth ventricle is the echogenic vermis of the cerebellum *(v)* and the cisterna magna *(arrow)*. Anterior to the fourth ventricle is the pons *(p)* and medulla *(m)*.

extent of the choroid plexus tapers to a point into this groove, which is formed by the head of the caudate nucleus anteriorly and the thalamus posteriorly. The head of the caudate nucleus is slightly more echogenic than the thalamus. In the premature neonate, the fragile germinal matrix is located in these areas and is a common site for hemorrhage. (See further discussion under Intracranial Hemorrhage.) This is an area where a magnified image plane is recommended (Fig. 21-11). With continued angulation laterally, the next image is through the lateral ventricle. The frontal horn of the lateral ventricle is more medial than the occipital horn, so to visualize the entire ventricle, the anterior part of the transducer needs to be angled obliquely with the front end of the transducer angled medially and the posterior part angled slightly more lateral. This parasagittal section will visualize a good portion of the frontal horn and body of the lateral ventricle. The thalamus is seen inferior to the head of the caudate nucleus, and the choroid plexus should taper into the caudothalamic groove (Fig. 21-12). Angling more laterally, the highly echogenic glomus of the choroid plexus is seen filling the trigone of the lateral ventricle and has a comma-shaped configuration as it courses posterior toward the temporal horn (Fig. 21-13). There should be no choroid plexus extending anterior to the third ventricle or into the occipital horn. Several images may be needed to image the complete ventricular system. The temporal horn or occipital horn will need to be imaged separately as it is not always possible to line up the entire ventricle system in one plane. In a nondilated ventricular system, the temporal and occipital horn may be difficult to

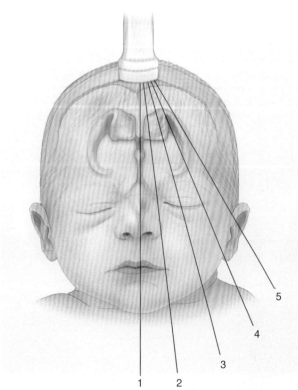

**Figure 21-9** Sagittal scan planes. Sagittal/parasagittal imaging planes via the anterior fontanelle approach.

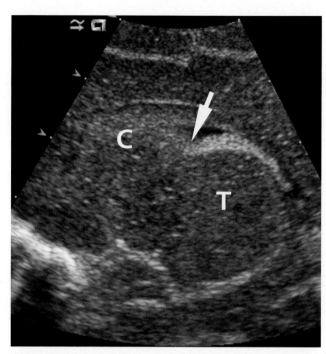

**Figure 21-11** Caudothalamic groove. Magnified parasagittal scan at the level of the caudothalamic groove. Head of the caudate nucleus *(C)* is seen anterior to the thalamus *(T)*. Between these two structures is the caudothalamic groove *(arrow)*, which contains the anterior extent of the choroid plexus.

visualize. As on the coronal section, the periventricular white matter lateral and posterior to the trigones of the lateral ventricles requires careful evaluation. This area should not be brighter than the choroid plexus. Angling more lateral to the ventricle, the next scan demonstrates the far lateral periventricular white matter tracts and

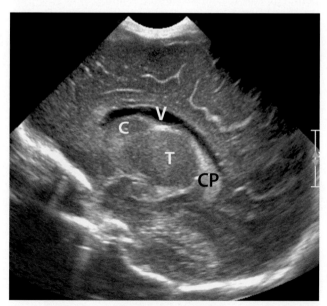

**Figure 21-12** Lateral ventricle. Nonmagnified parasagittal scan through the area of the lateral ventricle. The highly echogenic choroid plexus *(CP)* is seen within the body of the lateral ventricle *(V)* and tapers to a point at the caudothalamic groove. The caudate nucleus *(C)* anterior to the thalamus *(T)* is again noted. This is the location of the germinal matrix in premature infants.

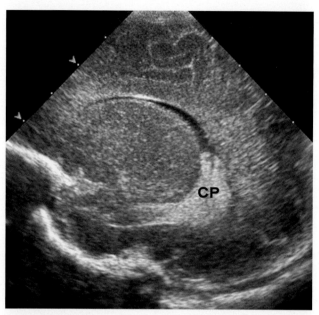

**Figure 21-13** Parasagittal choroid plexus. Parasagittal scan through the body of the lateral ventricle. The echogenic choroid plexus *(CP)* is seen within the trigone of the ventricle.

the echogenic sylvian fissure. On real-time scanning, the middle cerebral artery branches can be seen pulsating within this fissure (Fig. 21-14).

# NORMAL VARIANTS

## SONOGRAPHIC FEATURES OF THE MATURE VERSUS IMMATURE BRAIN

Sonographically, certain features are markers of prematurity and should not be misinterpreted as abnormal. The premature brain changes significantly in appearance from 26 weeks until term. Knowing the

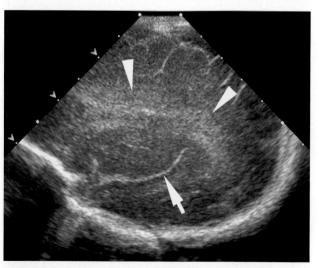

**Figure 21-14** Sylvian fissure. Parasagittal scan lateral to the ventricle. The sylvian fissure is seen in this scan and on real-time scanning, the branches of the middle cerebral arteries can be seen pulsating within this fissure. Normal periventricular white matter *(arrowheads)* lateral to the ventricle.

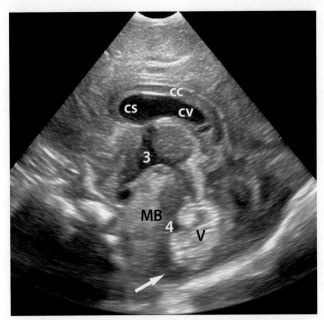

**Figure 21-15** Cavum vergae. Sagittal midline scan of an immature brain. The midline cystic cavum septum pellucidum *(CS)* and cavum vergae *(CV)* are prominent in the premature infant. Superior to the cavum is the hypoechoic corpus callosum *(CC)*. The third *(3)* and fourth *(4)* ventricles are seen in this plane with the fourth ventricle seen as a triangular lucency indenting the vermis *(V)*. The cisterna magna *(arrow)* is visible posterior to the vermis and the midbrain *(MB)* is seen anterior to the fourth ventricle.

approximate gestational age of the infant will aid in differentiating age-related features from pathology.

## Cavum Septum Pellucidi and Cavum Vergae

The cavum septum pellucidum is a CSF-filled space lying between the frontal horns of the lateral ventricles. In very premature infants, a posterior extension of the cavum septum pellucidum called the *cavum vergae* is often seen. On the coronal scan, it can be seen lying between the bodies of the lateral ventricles, and on the midline sagittal scan, posterior to the corpus callosum (Fig. 21-15). Closure of this space starts at approximately 6 months of gestation and progresses from the posterior to the anterior. In late gestation infants, only the anterior cavum septum pellucidum may be appreciated. This fetal structure is completely closed by 3 to 6 months after birth.

## Brain Parenchyma

In the very premature infant, the sulci and gyri are not fully developed and the brain appears quite smooth and featureless (Fig. 21-16A,B). Sulci development begins to appear during the fifth month of gestation. Generally, the sulci are not seen sonographically until about 26 weeks gestation (Fig. 21-16C,D). Before the age of 24 to 26 weeks gestation, the area of the insula is exposed and the sylvian fissure is wide open. The sonographic appearance of widely separated sylvian fissures on the coronal/parasagittal section is a marker of extreme prematurity (Fig. 21-16E). As the brain continues to mature, specific sulci become visible. The sulci branch and bend further in the eighth and ninth month with the development of secondary and tertiary sulci.[3]

## Prominent Periventricular Blush

Nearly all premature and some term infants show an increased echogenicity in the parenchymal region around the peritrigonal area of the ventricles. This appearance has been termed the "peritrigonal blush"[4] or the "periventricular halo."[5] When scanning through the anterior fontanelle, the orientation of the normal fiber tracts superior and posterior to the peritrigonal area are perpendicular to the interrogating sound beam, thus producing this increased echogenicity. Scanning through the posterior fontanelle (Fig. 21-17) places these fiber tracts more parallel to the beam, and in most cases,

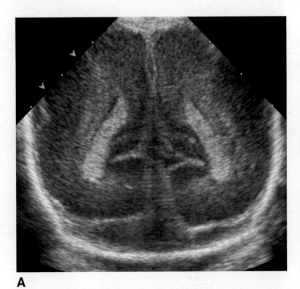

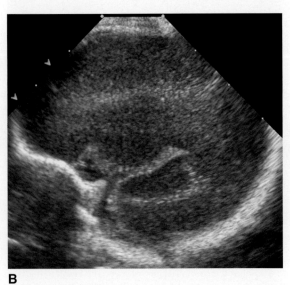

**A**    **B**

**Figure 21-16** Mature verses immature patterns of brain parenchyma. Coronal **(A)** and sagittal **(B)** scans of a 26-week premature infant. The brain parenchyma is smooth due to underdeveloped gyri and sulci. *(continued)*

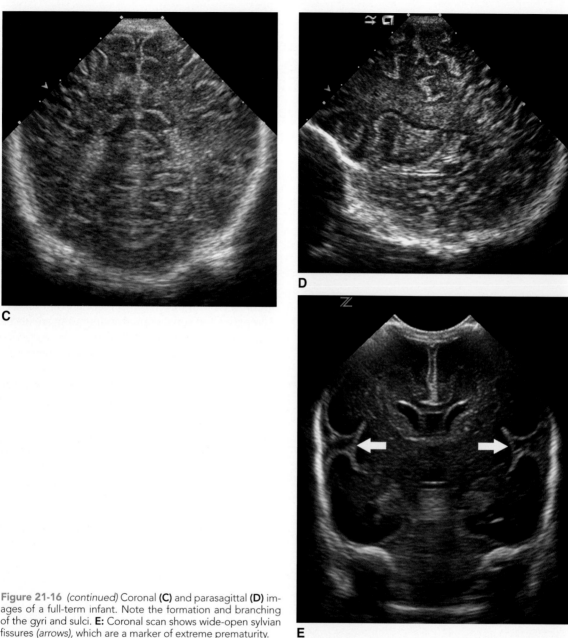

**Figure 21-16** *(continued)* Coronal **(C)** and parasagittal **(D)** images of a full-term infant. Note the formation and branching of the gyri and sulci. **E:** Coronal scan shows wide-open sylvian fissures *(arrows)*, which are a marker of extreme prematurity.

the blush disappears (Fig. 21-18A,B). The change in echogenicity of this area from the anterior fontanelle approach to the posterior fontanelle approach is due to the anisotropic effect of scanning. *Anisotropy* refers to the difference in echogenicity of an organ based on its orientation to the sound beam. This normal finding must be differentiated from the abnormal increased echogenicity caused by periventricular leukomalacia (PVL). If the increased peritrigonal echogenicity persists on the posterior fontanelle section, follow-up scans are needed to check for the evolution of PVL.

### Ventricular Size

Ventricular size also varies with maturity. The ventricles in the preterm infant appear relatively larger than those of a term infant. Narrow slit-like ventricles,

particularly in the frontal horn, can be seen in most normal full-term infants. Slit-like ventricles can also be seen in infants with cerebral edema; however, there are often other associated findings. Some degree of ventricular asymmetry can be seen in 20% to 40% of infants with the left ventricle often larger than the right[6] (Fig. 21-19).

### COARCTATION OF THE LATERAL VENTRICLE

Cranial sonograms will occasionally demonstrate cystic areas adjacent to the superolateral angles of the lateral ventricles. Coarctation of the lateral ventricle is an unusual variant that consists of a focal approximation of the ventricle wall at the external angle of the lateral ventricle at the level of the foramen of

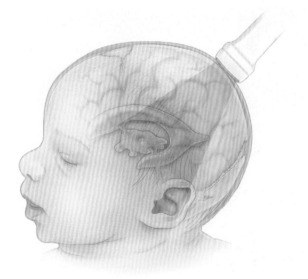

Figure 21-17 Posterior approach. Sagittal imaging plane through the posterior fontanelle. Coronal plane is obtained by rotating the transducer 90 degrees.

Monro. Unilateral or bilateral cystic areas located adjacent to the superolateral margins at the external angle of the lateral ventricle are a normal variant and should not be confused with hemorrhage or ischemia (Fig. 21-20). Position of these cystic areas as related to the external angle of the frontal horn of the lateral ventricle is the key in differentiating them from other cystic lesions. Lesions such as cystic PVL are located above the external angle and germinal matrix cysts are located below.[7]

## INTRACRANIAL PATHOLOGIES

### INTRACRANIAL HEMORRHAGE

One of the main indications for cranial sonography is to evaluate the premature neonate for ICH. ICH is a major cause of neonatal morbidity and mortality in the premature infant. Prognosis varies with the extent and severity of the hemorrhage.

#### Germinal Matrix Intraventricular Hemorrhage

Germinal matrix intraventricular hemorrhage (GM-IVH) is a complication occurring in the first weeks of life of the premature infant. The majority of ICH usually occurs within the first 3 days of life, with about 50% occurring on day 1, 25% on day 2, and 15% on days 3 to 4. By 72 to 96 hours, 80% to 90% of ICH has occurred.[2,8]

Preterm neonates with a birth weight less than 1,500 g and a gestational age of less than 32 weeks have the greatest risk for developing cerebral events such as ICH. Screening and serial cranial sonography are necessary in this group because ICH can occur without clinical signs. Most bleeds originate in the germinal matrix, which is a fetal structure located in the subependymal region of the lateral ventricles. The most prominent portion lies between the head of the caudate nucleus and the thalamus at the caudothalamic groove. The germinal matrix is not seen sonographically as a discrete structure; however, it is important to understand its location, development, and the effects of certain physiologic stressors that make it predisposed to hemorrhage.

The germinal matrix is a metabolically active, highly vascular network composed of immature fragile blood vessels with poor supporting connective tissues.

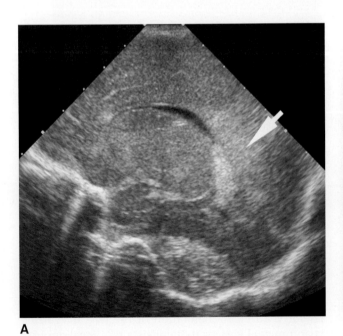

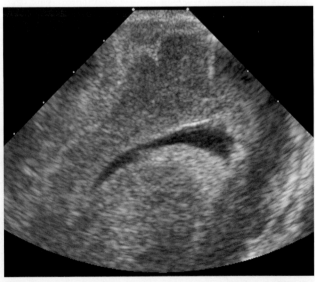

**A**

**B**

Figure 21-18 Prominent periventricular blush. **A:** Parasagittal scan on a premature infant shows prominent echogenicity in the periventricular region *(arrow).* **B:** Sagittal scan performed through the posterior fontanelle shows blush has disappeared.

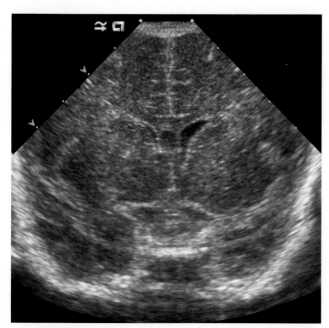

**Figure 21-19** Ventricular asymmetry. Coronal scan shows the left lateral ventricle larger than the right. This is a normal variant.

Between 8 and 28 weeks gestation, the germinal matrix produces neurons and glial cells, which migrate to populate the cerebral cortex during embryologic development. The germinal matrix reaches its greatest size at approximately 23 to 24 weeks gestation. It continues to regress, and involution is usually complete by the 36th week of gestation; therefore, the incidence of GM-IVH is low in the term infant. Hypoxia (decreased oxygen) predisposes the premature infant to the loss of autoregulation of the cerebral circulation. Loss of autoregulation allows fluctuations in blood pressure to

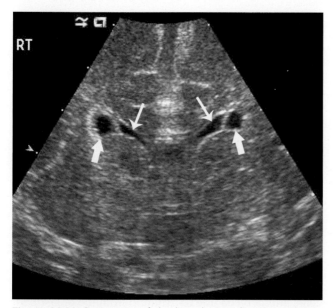

**Figure 21-20** Coarctation of the lateral ventricles. Coronal scan shows bilateral cysts (*large arrows*) at the external angle of the lateral ventricles (*small arrows*).

be transmitted to the cerebral circulation, which leads to hypotension and vascular dilatation. These factors along with the structurally fragile nature of the germinal matrix vasculature predispose it to hemorrhage.[8]

## CLASSIFICATION OF INTRACRANIAL HEMORRHAGE

The most widely used classification to grade the severity of ICH is that of Papile and colleagues.[9] ICH is divided into four grades (Pathology Box 21-1).

### Grade I Hemorrhage

The area of the caudothalamic groove is the primary site for hemorrhage in the preterm infant. On the parasagittal scan, the choroid plexus should taper to a point at the caudothalamic groove. The choroid plexus does not extend anterior to the third ventricle into the frontal horns of the lateral ventricles. Germinal matrix hemorrhage, subependymal hemorrhage (SEH), or grade I hemorrhage appear as a bulbous focal area of increased echogenicity at the inferolateral area of the floor of the frontal horn on the coronal section and anterior to the caudothalamic grove on the parasagittal section. The hemorrhage can be unilateral or bilateral. Over time, the clot evolves and liquefies creating a cystic center (Fig. 21-21A–C). This grade of hemorrhage is the mildest form of GM-IVH and carries no long-term neurologic sequelae.

### Grade II Hemorrhage

When germinal matrix hemorrhage ruptures through the ependymal lining and enters the ventricular cavity, it is classified as a grade II GM-IVH. Ventricular dilatation is not present in a grade II hemorrhage. Distinguishing hemorrhage from the normal echogenic choroid plexus can be quite difficult in a nondilated ventricle. Clot can adhere to the normal choroid, causing it to appear irregular and thickened. Doppler imaging may help in differentiating blood flow in the normal choroid plexus from nonvascular clot. Most often, the blood accumulates and migrates to the most dependant part of the ventricle, the occipital horn. Intraventricular echogenicity anterior to the foramina of Monro or in the occipital horn may be the only sign of a grade II GM-IVH. Scanning through the posterior fontanelle

**PATHOLOGY BOX 21-1**

*Intracranial Hemorrhage*[9]

| | |
|---|---|
| Grade I: | Germinal matrix (subependymal hemorrhage) |
| Grade II: | Intraventricular hemorrhage without ventricular dilatation |
| Grade III: | Intraventricular hemorrhage with ventricular dilatation |
| Grade IV: | Intraparenchymal hemorrhage with or without ventricular dilatation |

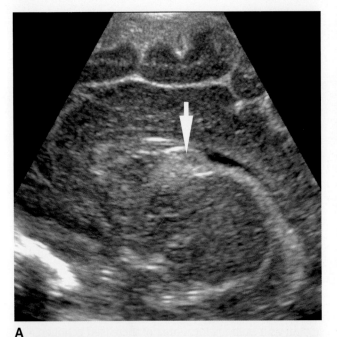

**A**

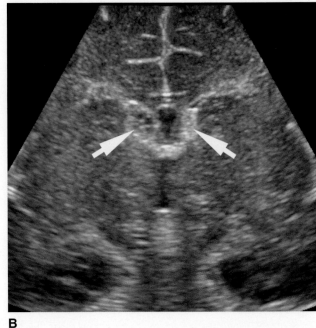

**B**

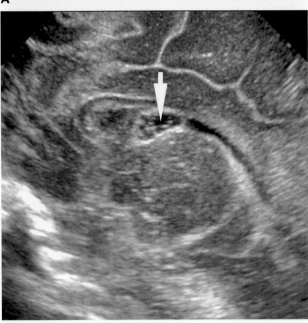

**C**

**Figure 21-21** Germinal matrix hemorrhage, grade I. **A:** Parasagittal scan through the area of the caudothalamic groove shows a focal area of increased echogenicity *(arrow)*. **B:** Coronal scan reveals bilateral echogenic foci at the caudothalamic grove *(arrows)*. **C:** Resolving grade I hemorrhage. Parasagittal image same infant several weeks later shows clot has undergone cystic liquefaction *(arrow)*.

(PF) can aid in determining the presence or absence of blood in the occipital horns.[10,11] Echogenic material in the occipital horn utilizing the PF section should be suspicious for a grade II GM-IVH (Fig. 21-22A–C).

### Grade III Hemorrhage

Grade III GM-IVH consists of intraventricular hemorrhage with ventricular dilatation. Initially, hemorrhage may completely fill the lateral ventricular cavity forming a cast of the ventricle with the contour of the ventricles becoming rounded (Fig. 21-23A,B). Over a period of weeks, the clot begins to resolve and becomes less echogenic owing to internal liquefaction (Fig. 21-23C).

The clot gradually retracts and fragmentation may occur, resulting in small segments of clot moving freely within the ventricle. With real-time scanning, the movement of these low-level echoes can be appreciated (Fig. 21-23D).

When the third ventricle is dilated, a structure called the *massa intermedia* can be seen (Fig. 21-23E). It connects the two thalami and crosses the third ventricle and should not be mistaken for a clot (bleed). Often, the lining of the ventricles become thickened and echogenic after a bleed due to irritation from the breakdown of blood products. Posthemorrhagic hydrocephalus is often a complication. (See section on Hydrocephalus.)

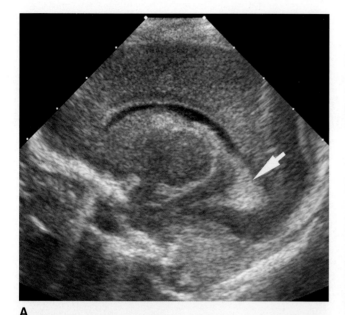

**A**

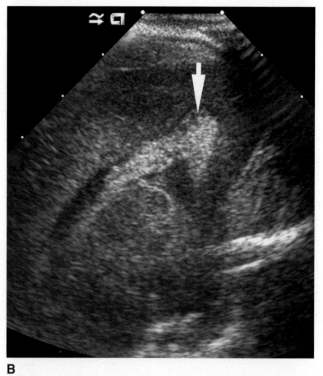

**B**

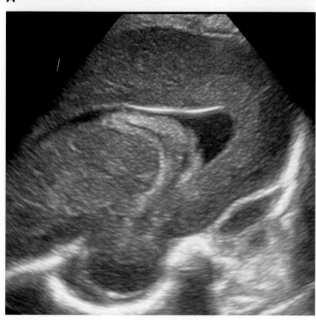

**C**

**Figure 21-22** Germinal matrix hemorrhage, grade II. **A:** Sagittal scan through anterior fontanelle is suggestive for clot in the occipital horn. **B:** Scanning through the posterior fontanelle confirms clot in the occipital horn *(arrow)*. **C:** Posterior fontanelle scan on another patient shows the occipital horn free of clot.

## Grade IV Hemorrhage

Grade IV GM-IVH is parenchymal involvement with or without ventricular dilatation. Traditionally, this was considered to be due to an extension from a ventricular bleed; however, it is now considered to be the result of a venous infarction secondary to obstruction of the terminal veins by germinal matrix hemorrhage.[8,12] When draining veins become obstructed, the area they drain becomes congested, and this leads to venous infarction and subsequent hemorrhagic necrosis of the periventricular white matter. Intraparenchymal hemorrhage (IPH) is most common in the frontal and parietal lobes (Fig. 21-24A,B). Over time, the clot demonstrates characteristic evolution with retraction from the surrounding brain parenchyma. An area of porencephaly can develop, which represents the resorption of the infarcted area of brain parenchyma. *Porencephaly* is defined as fluid-filled spaces that have replaced normal brain parenchyma due to the result of a destructive process. These areas may or may not communicate with the ventricular system (Fig. 21-24C,D). These cysts rarely resolve. Long-term neurologic sequelae include deficits such as cerebral palsy, developmental delays, and seizures.

## HYDROCEPHALUS

Hydrocephalus is a progressive dilatation of the ventricular system that is a result of impairment of CSF dynamics or brain parenchymal loss. Posthemorrhagic hydrocephalus (PHH) is a common complication of IVH

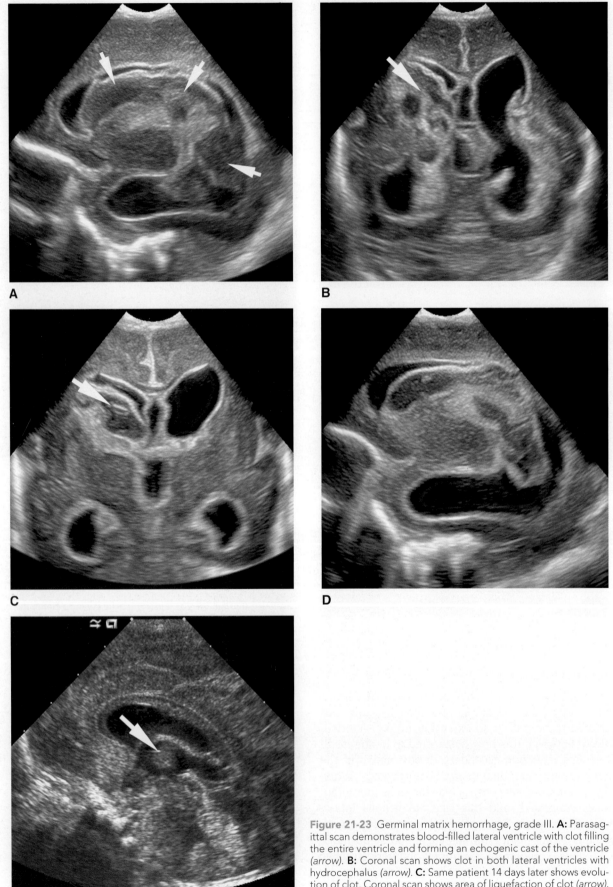

**Figure 21-23** Germinal matrix hemorrhage, grade III. **A:** Parasagittal scan demonstrates blood-filled lateral ventricle with clot filling the entire ventricle and forming an echogenic cast of the ventricle *(arrow)*. **B:** Coronal scan shows clot in both lateral ventricles with hydrocephalus *(arrow)*. **C:** Same patient 14 days later shows evolution of clot. Coronal scan shows area of liquefaction of clot *(arrow)*. **D:** Parasagittal scan shows some retraction of the intraventricular clot. **E:** Parasagittal scan show the massa intermedia *(arrow)*.

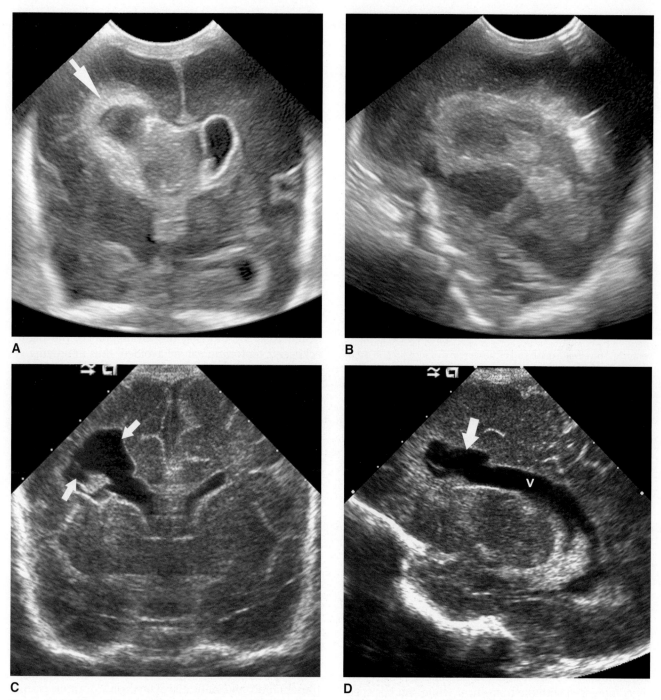

**Figure 21-24** Germinal matrix hemorrhage, grade IV. **A:** Coronal scan shows a right germinal hemorrhage with intraventricular blood and extension of the hemorrhage into the right frontoparietal area. **B:** Right parasagittal scan shows the lateral extension of the parenchymal hemorrhage. Same infant 4 weeks later. Coronal **(C)** and parasagittal **(D)** scan shows a large area of porencephaly in the area of the brain involved by the hemorrhagic infarction *(arrows)*. This cystic cavity communicates with the adjacent ventricle *(v)*.

and may initially result from an acute increase in ventricular size due to hemorrhage, later by obstruction of the outflow tracts of the ventricles, or occlusion of the arachnoid granulations with blood. When these membranes swell, the normally small channels (e.g., foramina of Monro, aqueduct of Sylvius) become blocked.

If the obstruction occurs within the ventricular system, it is referred to as *noncommunicating hydrocephalus,* whereas if it occurs outside the ventricular system,

(extraventricular) the term *communicating hydrocephalus* is applied.[13] The trigones and the occipital horns of the lateral ventricles are initially the first parts of the ventricular system to dilate. A chemical ventriculitis resulting from blood products within the CSF causes thickening and increased echogenicity of the ependymal lining of the ventricular system (Fig. 21-25).

The classic clinical signs of hydrocephalus; increasing head size; bulging of the anterior fontanelle; and

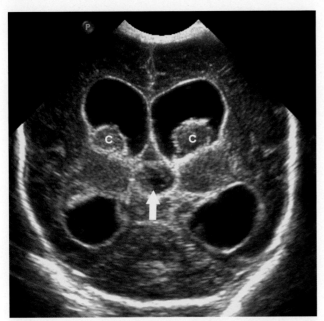

**Figure 21-25** Post hemorrhagic hydrocephalus. Coronal scan shows grade III hemorrhage, hydrocephalus with clot in lateral and third ventricle. The ependymal lining of the ventricles is increased in echogenicity consistent with ependymitis.

separation of the cranial sutures, bradycardia, apnea, and increased ICP often lag behind the onset of ventricular dilatation by days or weeks. For this reason, serial sonograms are often required to monitor the progression of hydrocephalus.

Infants with progressive hydrocephalus and elevated ICP may require the placement of a shunt or ventricular reservoir. Hemodynamic changes in response to fontanelle compression during Doppler sonography can be a useful technique in identifying infants with elevated ICP and in determining optimal timing for shunt placement. This method involves compression of the anterior fontanelle with the transducer while obtaining a spectral Doppler tracing from the pericallosal branches of the anterior cerebral artery, easily located in the midline sagittal section. The Doppler gate is positioned in the artery, and a spectral tracing is obtained without any fontanelle compression. The fontanelle is then gently compressed with the transducer while another spectral Doppler tracing is obtained. The duration of the pressure should not exceed 3 to 5 seconds. Prolonged or continuous compression should be avoided, and pressure should be discontinued if the infant's heart rate decreases. A resistive index is obtained from both spectral Doppler tracings. An RI increase of >0.1 above a baseline measurement or reversal of flow in diastole is an indication of elevated ICP (Fig. 21-26A–C). If reversal of flow is present without compression, this is suggestive of an increase in ICP and fontanelle compression is not recommended.[14]

Shunt tubes are highly echogenic on the sonogram and can be seen as bright parallel lines if imaged perpendicularly to their long axis. Otherwise, they will appear as echogenic foci with distal shadowing. Sonography is useful in monitoring ventricular size after shunt placement.

## CEREBELLAR HEMORRHAGE

Detection of hemorrhage within the cerebellum is difficult to visualize from the traditional anterior fontanelle approach. This is primary due to the poor delineation of the posterior fossa structures from the anterior fontanelle approach. Recent utilization of the MF, as an alternate acoustic window has improved visualization of the infratentorial structures of the posterior fossa, especially the cerebellum, and should routinely be incorporated as part of the protocol when performing sonography of the neonatal brain. From the anterior fontanelle approach, the posterior fossa structures lie in the far field of the transducer beam, and many of these structures lie parallel to the sound beam. Utilizing the MF places these structures in a more optimal focal zone of the transducer and at a more perpendicular orientation to the sound beam. Also, by utilizing the MF approach, the highly echogenic tentorium can be avoided, thus improving visualization of the cerebellum.[10,15,16]

Mastoid scanning is best performed with the infant's head on the side. The most accessible side should be used, with care taken to indicate on the images which side of the brain is nearest the transducer. Axial and coronal scanning can be performed depending on the desired anatomical information. For the coronal section, the transducer is placed over the MF just behind the pinna of the ear and rotated until the desired structures of the posterior fossa are seen. Orientation of the transducer places the notch up toward the top of skull for a coronal section (Fig. 21-27). Four to five images are obtained in this plane, angling from superior to inferior. Images are obtained from the tentorii cerebelli superiorly through the fourth ventricle, the cerebellar hemispheres, vermis, and cistern magna inferiorly (Fig. 21-28). For an axial section, the transducer is positioned above the tragus of the ear with the notch of the transducer toward the infant's face.

Cerebellar hemorrhage may be clinically silent in presentation and only discovered on a routine cranial sonogram. Cerebellar hemorrhages may or may not be associated with supratentorial hemorrhage (Fig. 21-29). Posterior fossa hemorrhages have also been associated with traumatic delivery and infants on extracorporeal membrane oxygenation (ECMO).[17,18] The MF approach permits a more comprehensive evaluation of the third and fourth ventricles in the presence of hydrocephalus (Fig. 21-30).

### Periventricular Leukomalacia

PVL is the most common hypoxic–ischemic brain injury in the premature infant. Hypoxia is the lack of adequate oxygen, and ischemia is the lack of adequate blood flow to a region.

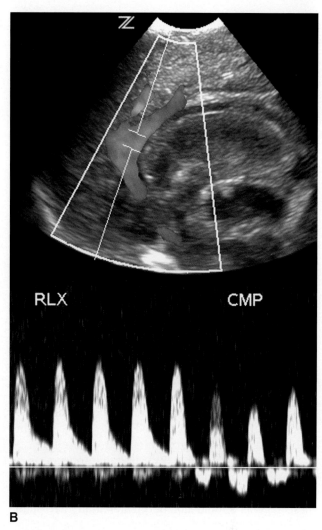

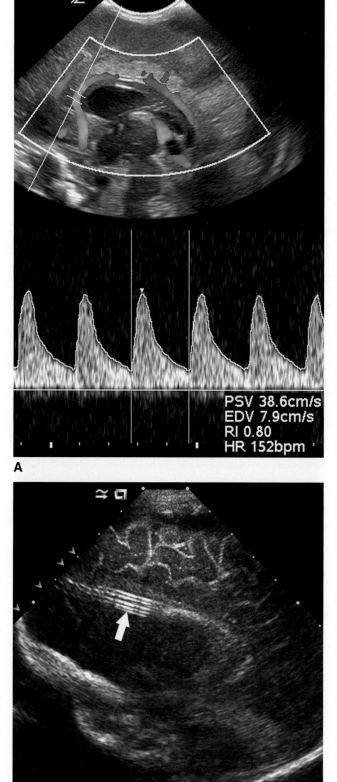

**Figure 21-26** Spectral Doppler with fontanelle compression. **A:** Sagittal midline of a normal spectral Doppler signal from a branch of the pericallosal artery demonstrating normal resistive index. **B:** Sagittal midline with fontanelle compression shows reversal of flow in diastole, indicating elevated intracranial pressure. **C:** Shunt tube. Parasagittal scan shows bright parallel lines from a shunt tube *(arrow)* in the decompressed ventricle.

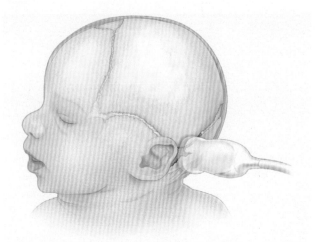

**Figure 21-27** Mastoid fontanelle. Image shows placement of transducer over mastoid fontanelle.

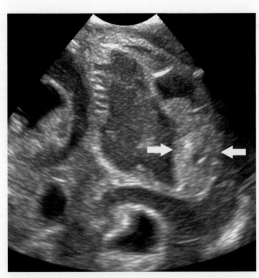

**Figure 21-29** Cerebellar hemorrhage. Coronal image shows large echogenic hemorrhage in the right cerebellar hemisphere *(arrows)*.

The white matter most affected is the parenchyma adjacent to the region of the peritrigonal area of the posterior lateral ventricles and the frontal cerebral white matter just anterolateral to the frontal horns. In the premature infant, the blood flow watershed area is located in the periventricular area and is a zone of end arteries that lack collateral circulation. When blood supply to this area is decreased, ischemia occurs and leukomalacia (softening of white matter) results.[13]

Sonographically, acute PVL initially appears as an increase in echogenicity in these areas. PVL is almost always bilateral and symmetric. The echogenicity of these regions should not be greater than that of the choroid plexus (Fig. 21-31A,B). Sonography has limited sensitivity in detecting acute PVL due to the difficulty in differentiating it from the normal periventricular blush that is seen in most premature infants. (See section on variants.) The later changes of PVL are the formation of cysts in the periventricular area. These findings may only become apparent over a period of weeks after the initial insult. The cystic spaces represent areas of necrosis and cavitation (Fig. 21-32A,B). Neurologic sequelae associated with PVL include cerebral palsy, developmental abnormalities, intellectual impairment, and visual disturbances.

## SUBARACHNOID VERSUS SUBDURAL COLLECTIONS

Extra-axial fluid collections are a relatively common finding on cranial sonograms and are easily demonstrated as anechoic areas on gray scale imaging. This fluid is usually seen within the interhemispheric fissure and over the convexities of the brain.

Color flow or power Doppler and a high-frequency linear array transducer are used to differentiate subarachnoid from subdural fluid collections. Fluid in the subarachnoid space produces a cortical vein sign while subdural fluid does not. Superficial cortical blood vessels lie between the pia and arachnoid. Fluid in the subarachnoid space displaces cortical vessels away from the brain surface toward the cranial vault. The cortical veins can be seen bridging the fluid collection (Fig. 21-33A,B). Fluid in the subdural space displaces cortical vessels toward the brain surface and contains no crossing vessels[19] (Fig. 21-33C).

Subarachnoid fluid is commonly seen with benign macrocrania and in former premature infants. Subdural fluid is usually blood and related to infection, traumatic delivery, or should be considered in cases of child abuse in the appropriate setting.

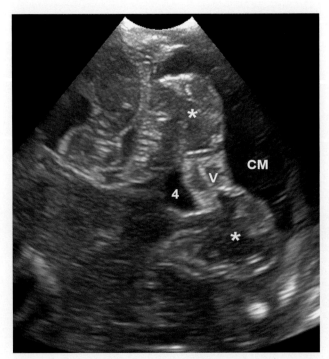

**Figure 21-28** Posterior fossa. Normal posterior fossa structures obtained via the mastoid fontanelle. Coronal sonogram shows a normal fourth ventricle *(4)*, cerebellar hemispheres *(*)*, midline vermis *(V)*, and cisterna magna *(CM)*.

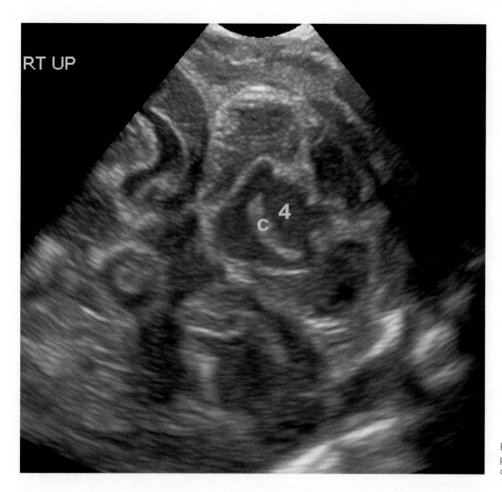

RT UP

**Figure 21-30** Mastoid section on preterm neonate. Coronal scan shows clot *(c)* in dilated fourth ventricle *(4)*.

## AGENESIS OF THE CORPUS CALLOSUM

The corpus callosum forms during the third and fourth months of fetal life. Complete or partial agenesis, is possible and depends on the stage of callosal development when the intrauterine insult occurs. Complete agenesis usually occurs before 12 weeks of gestation. The direction of embryonic development is from anterior to posterior; therefore, in partial agenesis, the posterior portion is absent. Agenesis of the corpus callosum can occur as an isolated condition or in combination with

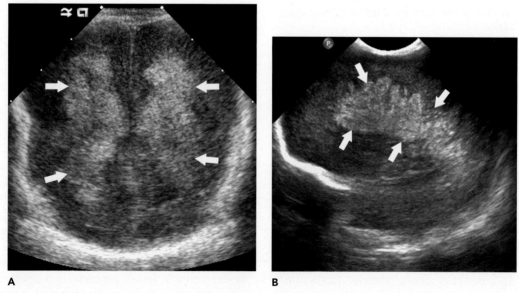

**A**                                                **B**

**Figure 21-31** Periventricular leukomalacia in premature infant. **A:** Posterior coronal scan shows symmetrically increased echogenicity *(arrows)* in the periventricular areas bilaterally. **B:** Right parasagittal scan shows increased echogenicity at the lateral angles of the ventricle *(arrow)*.

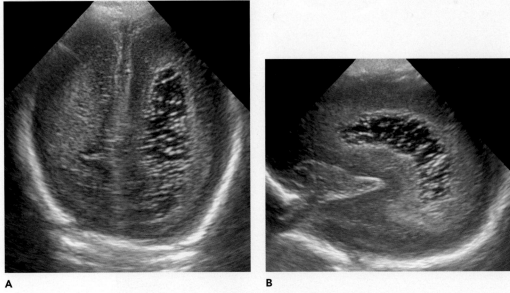

**A**                                          **B**

**Figure 21-32** Evolving periventricular leukomalacia. Coronal **(A)** and left parasagittal **(B)** follow-up scan 4 weeks after initial insult in a premature infant shows development of cystic areas adjacent to the occipital and frontal horns of the lateral ventricles.

other cerebral abnormalities, including Chiari II malformation, Dandy-Walker syndrome, holoprosencephaly, and septo-optic dysplasia.[2]

Sonographically, agenesis of the corpus callosum presents as the complete or partial absence of the hypoechoic band usually seen in the midline superior to the third ventricle. The third ventricle may be displaced upward between the separated frontal horns. On the coronal scan, the frontal horns of the lateral ventricles are widely separated and sharply angled laterally, and the occipital horns have a parallel orientation and a teardrop shape. There is relative enlargement of the posterior horns (colpocephaly). Best seen on the midline sagittal image is the radial arrangement of the medial sulci and gyri above the third ventricle, also known as the "sunburst sign" rather than the normal parallel orientation when the corpus callosum is present (Fig. 21-34A–D).

## DANDY-WALKER COMPLEX

The *Dandy-Walker complex* is a term used to indicate a spectrum of anomalies of the posterior fossa that include the Dandy-Walker malformation and Dandy-Walker variant. The classic Dandy-Walker malformation is characterized by cystic dilatation of the fourth ventricle, superior elevation of the tentorium, partial or complete absence of the vermis, and small cerebellar hemispheres (Fig. 21-35A–C). Hydrocephalus is present in 80% of cases.[2,20]

Dandy-Walker malformation is frequently associated with other intracranial anomalies. These include partial or complete agenesis of the corpus callosum, holoprosencephaly, and occipital encephalocele. Extracranial anomalies include cystic renal disease, chromosomal, and cardiac abnormalities. Dandy-Walker variant refers

to a milder form of the Dandy-Walker malformation. The fourth ventricle is slightly to moderately enlarged, the cerebellar hemispheres are normal, and there is variable hypoplasia of the cerebellar vermis. Hydrocephalus is usually not present.[2]

A mega cisterna magna and arachnoid cyst can be confused with a Dandy-Walker cyst. Arachnoid cysts do not communicate with the fourth ventricle, and a mega cisterna magna is a normal variant and is associated with a normal fourth ventricle and isolated enlargement of the cisterna magna.[1]

## CHIARI MALFORMATION

The Chiari malformation is a complex congenital malformation of the brain involving the hindbrain and has been classified into three main types. Type I is a downward displacement of the cerebellar tonsils without displacement of the fourth ventricle. Chiari II malformation is the most common type seen in infants and neonates and is nearly always associated with myelomeningocele. It is characterized by a relatively small posterior fossa, downward displacement of the cerebellum, medulla, and fourth ventricle into the upper spinal canal, and elongation of the pons and fourth ventricle. Hydrocephalus is present in varying degrees and tends to worsen after repair of the myelomeningocele because CSF can no longer decompress into the spinal defect. These patients are treated with the placement of a ventriculoperitoneal shunt in which the proximal end is placed in the lateral ventricles and the distal end is placed in the peritoneal cavity. Chiari III malformation is rare and is characterized by a high cervical encephalomeningocele containing the medulla, fourth ventricle, and cerebellum.[1,2]

Sonographic findings in Chiari II include hydrocephalus with a prominent massa intermedia, inferior

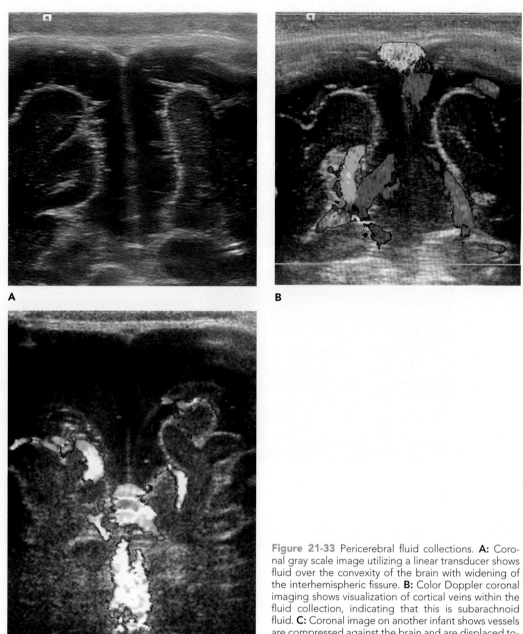

A

B

C

**Figure 21-33** Pericerebral fluid collections. **A:** Coronal gray scale image utilizing a linear transducer shows fluid over the convexity of the brain with widening of the interhemispheric fissure. **B:** Color Doppler coronal imaging shows visualization of cortical veins within the fluid collection, indicating that this is subarachnoid fluid. **C:** Coronal image on another infant shows vessels are compressed against the brain and are displaced toward the parenchyma of the brain, indicating a subdural fluid collection.

pointing of the frontal horns of the lateral ventricles referred to as the "bat-wing" appearance and downward displacement and elongation of the cerebellum, fourth ventricle with loss of visualization of the cisterna magna (Fig. 21-36A). The posterior fossa is small and the tentorium appears low and dysplastic (Fig. 21-36B). The occipital horns of the lateral ventricles are larger than the frontal horns (colpocephaly) and there is usually a partial or complete absence of the corpus callosum.

## VEIN OF GALEN MALFORMATION

The vein of Galen malformation (VGM) is the most common intracranial vascular anomaly presenting in the neonatal period. The VGM is a midline cerebral

arteriovenous malformation, which causes dilatation of the vein of Galen. Large arteries from the anterior and posterior cerebral artery circulation feed the malformation. These abnormal feeding vessels drain in to the vein of Galen, causing it to become markedly enlarged. Most VGMs present during the neonatal period.

Neonates classically present with congestive heart failure and a cranial bruit. Due to shunting of blood into the lower resistive vein of Galen, perfusion of blood to the periphery of the brain can be decreased, causing brain atrophy and calcifications.

Sonographic features include a well-circumscribed anechoic or hypoechoic mass in the midline posterior to the third ventricle. Hydrocephalus may be present. Color Doppler demonstrates turbulent flow within the

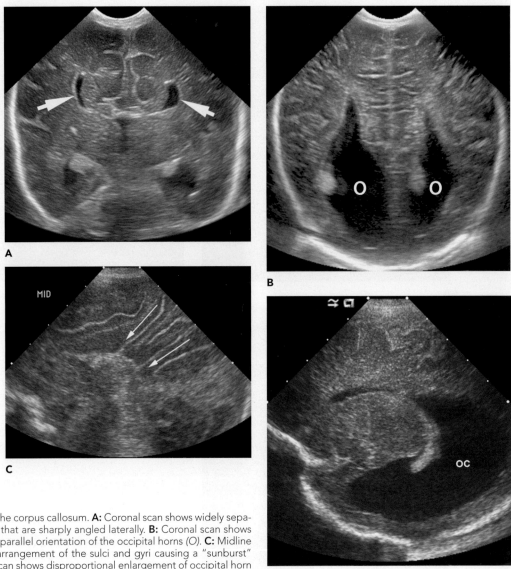

**Figure 21-34** Agenesis of the corpus callosum. **A:** Coronal scan shows widely separated frontal horns *(arrows)* that are sharply angled laterally. **B:** Coronal scan shows teardrop configuration and parallel orientation of the occipital horns *(O)*. **C:** Midline sagittal scan shows radial arrangement of the sulci and gyri causing a "sunburst" effect *(arrows)*. **D:** Sagittal scan shows disproportional enlargement of occipital horn *(OC)* compared with the rest of the ventricle (colpocephaly).

vein of Galen. Spectral Doppler shows elevated systolic and diastolic flow velocities and damped pulsatility (Fig. 21-37A–C).

Although sonography can identify the VGM, magnetic resource imaging (MRI) is required to more accurately identify the feeding arteries and draining veins. Angiography remains the definitive examination to identify vascular anatomy prior to embolization therapy.

## HOLOPROSENCEPHALY

Holoprosencephaly represents a spectrum of congenital malformations that result from a disorder of diverticulation in which the primitive forebrain (prosencephalon) fails to divide into two separate cerebral hemispheres. There are three distinct forms of holoprosencephaly depending on the degree of diverticulation: alobar, semilobar, and lobar. A wide variety of midline craniofacial anomalies are associated with these malformations.

Alobar holoprosencephaly is the most severe form. There is a thin pancake-like primitive cerebrum covering a horseshoe-shaped midline monoventricle. The corpus callosum, third ventricle, and interhemispheric fissures are absent and the thalami are fused (Fig. 21-38). The optic tracts and olfactory bulbs are also absent. Infants born with this form are usually stillborn or die shortly after birth. Facial anomalies are severe and can include close-set eyes (hypotelorism), cleft lip and/or palate, single central eye (cyclopia), a nose located on the forehead (proboscis), or missing facial features.[2]

Semilobar holoprosencephaly or incomplete forebrain division results in partial separation of the cerebral hemispheres posteriorly; however, a single ventricle persists. The occipital and temporal horns may be formed. A small portion of the falx may be present, along with variable degrees of fusion of the thalami. The third ventricle is small or absent.

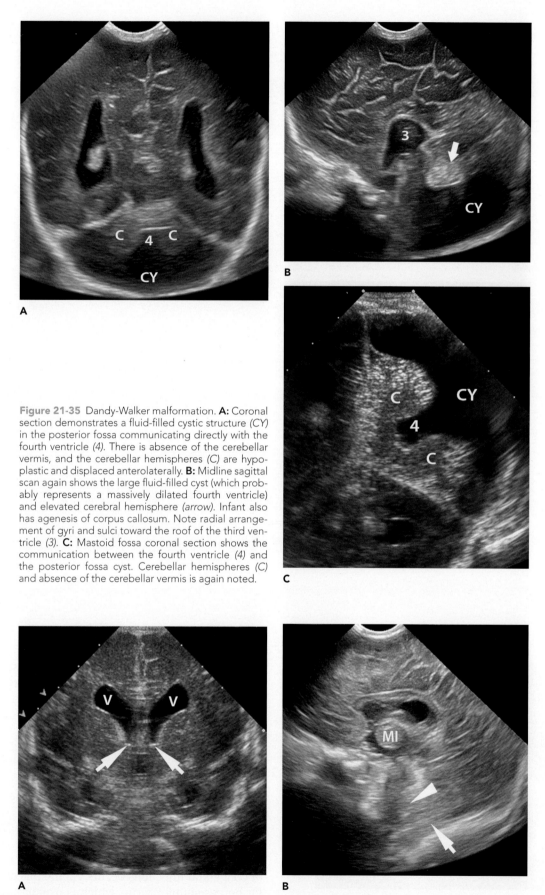

**Figure 21-35** Dandy-Walker malformation. **A:** Coronal section demonstrates a fluid-filled cystic structure *(CY)* in the posterior fossa communicating directly with the fourth ventricle *(4)*. There is absence of the cerebellar vermis, and the cerebellar hemispheres *(C)* are hypoplastic and displaced anterolaterally. **B:** Midline sagittal scan again shows the large fluid-filled cyst (which probably represents a massively dilated fourth ventricle) and elevated cerebral hemisphere *(arrow)*. Infant also has agenesis of corpus callosum. Note radial arrangement of gyri and sulci toward the roof of the third ventricle *(3)*. **C:** Mastoid fossa coronal section shows the communication between the fourth ventricle *(4)* and the posterior fossa cyst. Cerebellar hemispheres *(C)* and absence of the cerebellar vermis is again noted.

**Figure 21-36** Chiari malformation. **A:** Coronal sonogram through the anterior fontanelle shows "bat-wing" appearance of the frontal horns of the lateral ventricles *(v)* and inferior pointing of the frontal horns *(arrows)*. **B:** Sagittal scan shows prominent massa intermedia *(MI)*; posterior fossa is small and low lying and cisterna magna is obliterated *(arrow)*. The fourth ventricle is flattened and displaced caudally *(arrowhead)*.

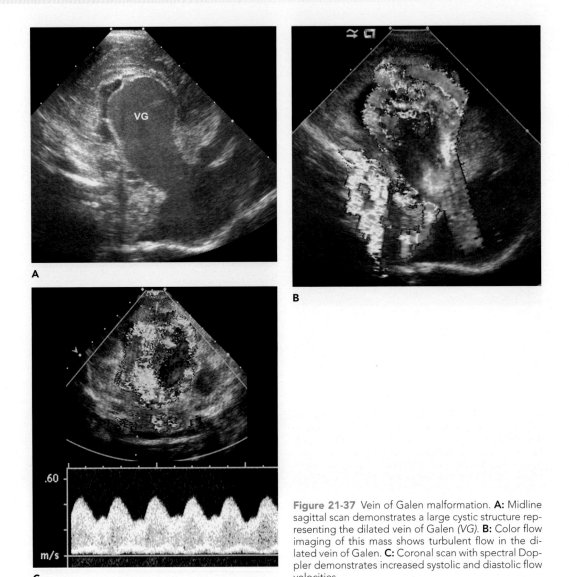

**Figure 21-37** Vein of Galen malformation. **A:** Midline sagittal scan demonstrates a large cystic structure representing the dilated vein of Galen *(VG)*. **B:** Color flow imaging of this mass shows turbulent flow in the dilated vein of Galen. **C:** Coronal scan with spectral Doppler demonstrates increased systolic and diastolic flow velocities.

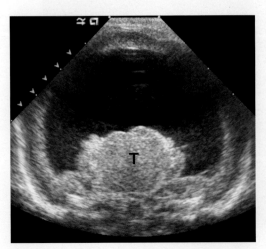

**Figure 21-38** Alobar holoprosencephaly. Coronal scan shows a single horseshoe-shaped ventricle with fused thalami *(T)* and a thin primitive cerebral cortex.

The least severe form is lobar holoprosencephaly. Facial anomalies are much milder and there is nearly complete separation of the hemispheres with formation of the falx, interhemispheric fissure, third ventricle, and normal posterior fossa.

## INTRACRANIAL INFECTION

The most common neonatal congenital infections are those referred to as the TORCH complex (toxoplasmosis, others, rubella, cytomegalovirus [CMV] and herpes simplex). CMV is the most common with toxoplasmosis as the second most common. Transmission of congenital infections occurs via the placenta except for herpes simplex virus, which is usually transmitted at the time of birth as a result of contact with lesions in the vagina.

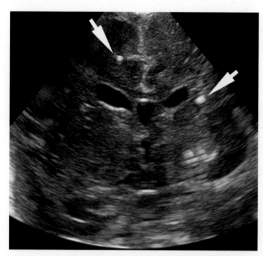

**Figure 21-39** Intracranial infection. Coronal scan shows nonshadowing echogenic foci, which represent parenchymal calcifications in and infant with cytomegalovirus infection (*arrows*).

The diagnosis of CNS infections is made clinically, and the role of sonography is to diagnose complications resulting from infections. Parenchymal calcifications and lenticulostriate vasculopathy are sonographic findings that can be seen with neonatal infections. Parenchymal calcifications are the classic sonographic finding and can be seen with or without distal acoustic shadowing and can vary in number and location (Fig. 21-39). Other complications include abscess, infarction, encephalomalacia, and hydrocephalus.

Lenticulostriate vasculopathy is characterized by linear branching of echogenic foci within the basal ganglia and thalamus. These echogenic foci may be unilateral or bilateral and follow the distribution of the lenticulostriate vessels (Fig. 21-40A,B). This finding, however, is not specific for the TORCH infections and can be seen in a wide range of nonspecific clinical conditions: fetal alcohol syndrome, intrauterine cocaine exposure, hypoxic/ischemic conditions, cardiac disease, and chromosomal abnormalities.[21,22]

## THREE-DIMENSIONAL SONOGRAPHY

Three-dimensional (3D) sonography has gained acceptance as a component of clinical imaging. Although the early applications of 3D sonography have focused on obstetrical, gynecologic, and cardiac applications, 3D sonography is showing promise as an emerging technique in imaging the neonatal brain.[23] Recent advances in computer technology and improvements in reconstruction software and transducer technology have driven the expansion. 3D imaging capabilities are available on most sonography systems.

Some of the advantages of 3D over two-dimensional (2D) are a decrease in the examination time, less variability among operators, and the capability of viewing anatomy and pathology in an infinite number of scanning planes unattainable through 2D scanning. 3D sonography also provides additional benefits for education and training, as the data can be virtually rescanned and manipulated at a workstation long after the exam is completed. A typical 2D neonatal head scan takes approximately 10 to 15 minutes to perform. The time needed for 3D image acquisition is only a few minutes. Rapid acquisition of data reduces the duration of stimulation to the infant and may have the potential of reducing some musculoskeletal injuries suffered by sonographers. The digital data sets are saved and recalled for reconstruction and interpretation at an offline computer. Recent advances in volumetric sonography have enabled the volumetric data to be viewed in tomographic slices and in the axial plane much like computed tomography (CT) and MRI. With this technique, a volumetric transducer sweeps through the

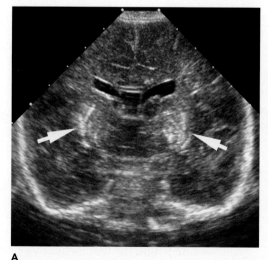

A

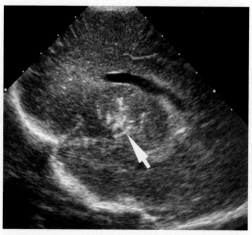

B

**Figure 21-40** Lenticulostriate vasculopathy. **A:** Coronal section shows bilateral branching of echogenic foci in the basal ganglia representing mineralized deposits along the lenticulostriate vessels (*arrows*). **B:** Parasagittal section shows linear location of deposits within the basal ganglia (*arrow*).

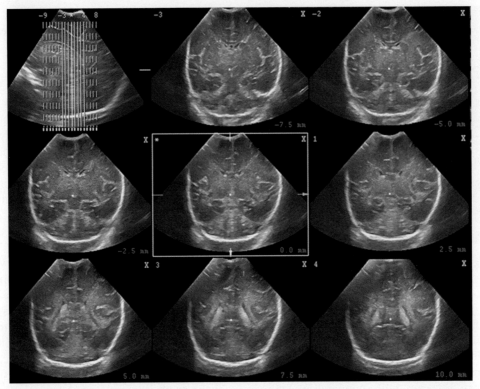

**Figure 21-41** Volume imaging. Three-dimensional data set was acquired in a single sweep using a volumetric transducer. Volumetric acquisition is reformatted into tomographic coronal slices of the neonatal brain.

brain acquiring a volume of images. After capturing the volume data set, the images are sliced into axial, coronal, and sagittal planes (Fig. 21-41). Research is still needed to evaluate the ultimate clinical utility that 3D sonography will have on patient management and quality of care.

## SUMMARY

- The anterior fontanelle is the primary acoustic window used to image the neonatal brain; the posterior and mastoid fontanelles can also be utilized.
- Closure of the anterior fontanelle begins at about 9 months, making imaging after this time difficult.
- A small footprint, high-frequency 7- to 10-MHz phased curved array or sector transducer is used to image the neonatal brain; a linear transducer may be used to image the subarachnoid and subdural spaces.
- The brain is divided into the cerebrum, cerebellum, and brain stem.
- The ventricular system provides a pathway for circulation of CSF and is made up of the paired lateral ventricles and the midline third and fourth ventricles.
- The corpus callosum lies in the midline and contains nerve tracts that allow communication between the right and left hemispheres of the brain.

- A standardized protocol, including coronal and sagittal images should be used when evaluating the neonatal brain.
- Coronal evaluation should include images from the frontal lobe of the brain to the occipital cortex with the right side of the brain displayed on the left side of the image.
- Sagittal evaluation should include images from the right and left hemispheres and the midline with the anterior aspect of the brain on the left side of the image.
- The sonographic appearance of the premature brain differs from that of the mature brain and these differences should not be mistaken for pathology.
- Sulci are not seen sonographically until 26 weeks gestation; therefore, the very premature brain appears smooth.
- An increased area of echogenicity, termed *peritrigonal blush*, is seen in the parenchymal region around the peritrigonal area of the ventricles in most premature infants.
- Scanning through the posterior fontanelle should cause the blush to disappear; however, if it persists, follow-up scans are needed to check for the evolution of PVL.
- Germinal matrix intraventricular hemorrhage typically occurs within the first 3 days of a premature infant's life and neonates with a birth weight less than 1,500 g and a gestational age of less than 32 weeks are at the greatest risk.

# Critical Thinking Questions

1. Where do the majority of intracranial hemorrhages originate and why is the risk lower in term infants?

2. How would the sonographer distinguish a peritrigonal blush from early periventricular leukomalacia?

3. What differences would a sonographer expect to see in the sonographic appearance of the brain in an infant born at 24 weeks gestation compared to an infant born at term?

4. You are asked to perform a sonographic examination of the brain in a 26-week gestational age neonate.

The examination reveals a dilated left ventricle that is filled with echogenic material. The lining of the ventricle is echogenic and slightly thickened. The right side of the brain appears normal. What is the most likely diagnosis?

5. The examination of the brain in a 29-week gestational age neonate demonstrates multiple echogenic foci throughout the cortex. The remainder of the examination is unremarkable. What is the most likely diagnosis?

---

- Intracranial hemorrhages are classified as grades I to IV based on the severity.

- Grade I intracranial hemorrhages include germinal matrix or subependymal hemorrhage.

- Grade II intracranial hemorrhages are intraventricular hemorrhages that occur without ventricular dilatation.

- Grade III intracranial hemorrhages are intraventricular hemorrhages with ventricular dilation.

- Grade IV are the most severe and consist of intraparenchymal hemorrhage with or without ventricular dilatation.

- Hydrocephalus is a dilatation of the ventricular system and can be classified as communicating or noncommunicating.

- PVL is the most common hypoxic–ischemic brain injury in the premature infant and affects the parenchyma adjacent to the region of the peritrigonal area of the posterior lateral ventricles and the frontal cerebral white matter just anterolateral to the frontal horns.

- Initially, PVL appears sonographically as an increased area of echogenicity; over time, cystic spaces form as a result of necrosis.

- Fluid in the subarachnoid space will displace cortical vessels away from the brain surface toward the cranial vault, and the cortical veins will be seen bridging the fluid collection.

- Fluid in the subdural space displaces cortical vessels toward the brain surface and contains crossing vessels will not be seen.

- Agenesis of the corpus callosum presents sonographically as an absence of the hypoechoic band seen in the midline superior to the third ventricle, which may be displaced upward between the separated frontal horns.

- With agenesis of the corpus callosum, a radial arrangement of the medial sulci and gyri above the third ventricle is seen and referred to as the "sunburst sign."

- The Dandy-Walker complex is a term used to indicate a spectrum of anomalies of the posterior fossa that include the Dandy-Walker malformation and the less severe Dandy-Walker variant.

- The Chiari malformation is a complex congenital malformation of the brain involving the hindbrain.

- The vein of Galen malformation (VGM) is a midline cerebral arteriovenous malformation, which causes dilatation of the vein of Galen.

- Holoprosencephaly represents a spectrum of congenital malformations in which the primitive forebrain (prosencephalon) fails to divide into two separate cerebral hemispheres.

- Depending on the degree of diverticulation, holoprosencephaly is divided into alobar, semilobar, and lobar varieties.

- TORCH complex (toxoplasmosis, others, rubella, cytomegalovirus [CMV] and herpes simplex) are the most common neonatal congenital infections and present sonographically as parenchymal calcifications.

- Three-dimensional sonography continues to evolve and has the potential to decrease examination time, improve consistency among sonographers, and provide an infinite number of scan planes from one volume data set.

- With the increasing survival rate of very low birth weight neonates, sonography will continue to play a major role in the diagnosis, follow-up, and management of intracranial problems in the sick neonate.

## REFERENCES

1. Rumack CM, Drose JA. Neonatal and infant imaging. In: Rumack CM, Wilson SR, Charboneau JW, et al. *Diagnostic Ultrasound*. Vol. 2, 3rd ed. St. Louis, MO: Elsevier Mosby; 2005:1623–1702.

2. Siegel MJ. *Pediatric Sonography*. 3rd ed. Philadelphia, PA: Lippincott Williams & Wilkins; 2002:43–141.

3. Worthen NJ, Gilbertson V, Lau C. Cortical sulcal development seen on sonography: relationship to gestational parameters. *Ultrasound Med*. 1986;5:153–156.

4. DiPietro MA, Brody BA, Teele RL. Peritrigonal echogenic "blush" on cranial sonography: pathologic correlates. *AJR Am J Roentgenol.* 1986;146:1067–1072.

5. Grant EG, Schellinger D, et al. Echogenic preventricular halo: normal sonographic or neonatal cerebral hemorrhage. *Am J Roentgenol.* 1983;140:793–796.

6. Hobar JD, Leahy KA, Lucey JF. Ultrasound identification of lateral ventricular asymmetry in premature infants. *Clin Radiol.* 1983;35:29–31.

7. Rosenfeld DL, Schonfeld SM, Underberg-Davis S. Co-arctation of lateral ventricles: an alternative explanation for subependymal pseudocyst. *Pediatr Radiol.* 1997;27:859–897.

8. Bassen H. Intracranial hemorrhage in the preterm infant: understanding it, preventing it. *Clin Perinatol.* 2009;36:737–762.

9. Papile LA, Burstein J, Burstein R, et al. Incidence and evolution of subependymal and intraventricular hemorrhage: a study of infants with birth weights less than 1500 g. *J Pediatr.* 1978;92:529–534.

10. DiSalvo DN. A new view of the neonatal brain: clinical utility of supplemental neurologic US imaging windows. *Radiographics.* 2001;21:943–955.

11. Flavia C, Goya E, Rosselló J, et al. Posterior fontanelle sonography: an acoustic window into the neonatal brain. *AJNR.* 2004;25:1274–1282.

12. Ghazi-Birry HS, Brown WR, Moody DM, et al. Human germinal matrix: venous origin of hemorrhage and vascular characteristics. *AJNR Am J Neuroradiol.* 1997;18:219.

13. Benson JE, Bishop MR, Cohen HL. Intracranial neonatal neurosonography: an Update. *Ultrasound Q.* 2002:178:89–114.

14. Taylor GA, Madsen JR. Neonatal hydrocephalus: hemodynamic response to fontanelle compression: correlation with intracranial pressure and need for shunt placement. *Pediatr Radiol.* 1996;201:685–689.

15. Enriquez G, Correa F, Enriquez G, et al. Mastoid fontanelle approach for sonographic imaging of the neonatal brain. *Pediatr Radio.* 2006;36:532–540.

16. Luna JA, Goldstein RB. Sonographic visualization of the neonatal posterior fossa abnormalities through the posteriolateral fontanelle. *AJR Am J Roentgenol.* 2000;174:561–567.

17. Bulas DI, Taylor GA, Fitz CR, et al. Posterior fossa intracranial hemorrhage in infants treated with extracorporeal membrane oxygenation: sonographic findings. *AJR Am J Roentgenol.* 1991;156:571–575.

18. Merrill JD, Piecuch RE, Fell SC, et al. A new pattern of cerebellar hemorrhages in preterm infants. *Pediatrics.* 1998;102:62–66.

19. Chen CY, Chou TY, Zimmerman RA, et al. Pericerebral fluid collection: differentiation of enlarged subarachnoid spaces from subdural collections with color Doppler US. *Radiology.* 1996;201:389–92.

20. Epelman M, Daneman A, Blaser Sl, et al. Differential diagnosis of intracranial cystic lesions at head US: correlation with CT and MR imaging. *Radiographics.* 2006;26:173–196.

21. Coley BD, Rusin JR, Boune DR. Importance of hypoxic/ischemic conditions in the development of cerebral lenticulostriate vasculopathy. *Pediatr Radiol.* 2000;30:846–855.

22. Malhoul IR, Eisenstein I, Sujov P, et al. Neonatal lenticulostriate vasculophy: further characterization. *Arch Dis Child Fetal Neonatal Ed.* 2003;88:F410–F414.

23. Riccabona M, Nelson TR, Weitzer C, et al. Potential of three-dimensional ultrasound in neonatal and paediatric sonography. *Eur Radiol.* 2003;13:2082–2093.

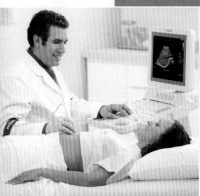

# 22 The Infant Spine

Rechelle A. Nguyen

## OBJECTIVES

Describe the embryological development of the spine.

Define the process for sonographic evaluation of the spine.

List the clinical indications for sonographic evaluation of the spine.

Describe the normal sonographic appearance of the neonatal spinal canal and cord.

Define open and closed spinal dysraphism.

Identify the sonographic appearance of congenital anomalies of the spine.

## KEY TERMS

Ventriculus terminalis | filar cyst | myelocele | myelomeningocele | tethered cord | diastomyelia | dorsal dermal sinus | sacral dimple | pilonidal sinus | spinal lipoma | lipomyelocele | lipomyelomeningocele | terminal myelocystocele.

## GLOSSARY

**cauda equina** collection of nerve roots at the end of the spinal column; includes lower lumbar and sacral nerve roots; Latin for horse's tail due to its appearance

**conus medullaris** the most caudal portion of the spinal cord

**dura** outmost layer of the covering of the spinal cord

**dysraphism** anomalies associated with an incomplete fusion of the neural tube during embryological development

**epidural space** space between the outermost layer of the spinal cord, the dura, and the spinal column

**filum terminale** tapering end of the spinal cord, caudal to the conus medullaris

**hydromyelia** dilatation of the central canal of the spinal cord

**myelomalacia** softening of the spinal cord frequently caused by a lack of blood supply

**syrinx** fluid filled cavity in the spinal cord

Sonography is a useful imaging tool when evaluating the spinal canal and cord in specific settings. It is expedient, cost effective, and has no known side effects or harmful exposure to radiation. However, due to the obvious bony nature of the spine, the usefulness of sonography is limited to infants under the age of 6 months, surgical procedures, interventional radiology, and settings in which there is an acoustic window.

Sonography is possible in the infant because the posterior spinous processes are not yet ossified, thus providing an acoustic window. Sonography of the spine becomes increasingly difficult as these bones begin to ossify. The diagnostic value of sonography decreases at 3 months and is nearly nondiagnostic after 5 to 6 months.[1] Sonography can be utilized in the surgical setting using a surgically created acoustic window. Known spinal defects where the posterior spinal elements are missing can also be used as an acoustic window to image the spinal canal.

Clinical indications for spinal sonography include evaluation of spinal dysraphism and any associated mass, including meningoceles, myelomeningoceles (MMCs), lipomyelomeningoceles, and lipomas.[2] Patients with lumbosacral skin anomalies, including pigmented spots, hairy nevus, dermal sinuses, dimples, and hemangiomas, may be evaluated for an associated tethered spinal cord.[3-5] Sonographic evaluation readily detects spinal tumors, masses, cysts, and syrinx. Acquired lesions, such as cord birth trauma, subarachnoid and epidural hemorrhage, and epidural abscess, can also be detected in the infant.[6] Intraoperative use of spinal sonography is helpful to localize intramedullary lesions, including tumors, cysts, hydrosyrinx, and vascular malformations, which may otherwise be difficult to locate by direct visualization of the cord.

## SONOGRAPHIC TECHNIQUE

High-frequency transducers are used to optimally evaluate the spinal cord due to its superficial location. Linear or sector transducers with frequencies between 8 to 15 MHz are used routinely.[1,7] Sector transducers may be useful in the older patient where the acoustic window is small. High-frequency linear transducers are the best choice for the neonatal spine. The high-resolution images provide detailed evaluation of the spinal cord and the nerve roots. Dual screen images can extend the field of view to image longer sections of the spine. Panoramic views, which are now readily available on many machines, provide extended images to encompass the length of the spine.[7] Panoramic imaging is especially helpful when determining the level of the conus (Fig. 22-1).

To evaluate the spine, the patient should be placed in a position to optimize the acoustic window. For the infant, place the patient prone over a towel or pillow. This will round out the back, creating a slight kyphosis.[7] A decubitus position can also be helpful as the legs can be tucked up in front of the body, increasing the splaying of the spinous processes.[7] A bottle or pacifier can be helpful during this examination as it will help to keep the patient still.

The examination should include longitudinal and transverse images from the craniocervical junction to the coccyx. The rounded surface of a curvilinear transducer will optimize imaging of the craniocervical junction.[7] For the remainder of the exam, a linear transducer is placed midline, directly over the spine. An exception is made for the older child, where a parasagittal approach may diminish shadowing from the ossified spinous process.[7] The level of the conus medullaris, as well as the position of the spinal cord in the spinal canal, is documented. During the examination, cord and nerve root motion should be detected and noted. Any cutaneous lesions should be documented and evaluated for associated tracts or masses.

## NORMAL ANATOMY

The spinal canal and cord can be observed from the base of the skull to the tip of the coccyx. Scanning from a posterior approach, in the sagittal plane, the canal

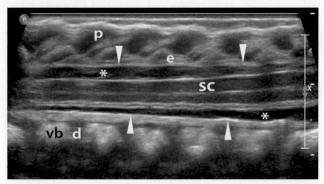

**Figure 22-2** Spinal canal. The canal is bordered anteriorly by the echogenic vertebral bodies (vb) with hypoechoic intervertebral disks (d) and posteriorly by the hypoechoic spinous processes (p). The canal is surrounded by a thin brightly echogenic layer which represents the arachnoid/dural layer (arrowheads). Just posterior to the arachnoid/dural layer and anterior to the spinous process is the epidural space (e). Anechoic cerebrospinal (*) encompasses the hypoechoic spinal cord (sc) and occupies the subarachnoid space.

will be anechoic. The echogenic vertebral bodies and hypoechoic intervertebral disks border the length of the spinal canal anteriorly.[7] Posteriorly, the canal is bordered by the hypoechoic spinous processes and the narrow echogenic epidural space. An intense linear echo, representing the arachnoid-dural layer, is seen lining the canal both anteriorly and posteriorly. Between the echogenic dura, the hypoechoic spinal cord is situated centrally to slightly anterior and is surrounded by anechoic cerebrospinal fluid (CSF) of the subarachnoid space[8] (Fig. 22-2). The subarachnoid space or thecal sac extends into the sacral region.

In the sagittal plane, the cord is a hypoechoic, tubular structure bordered by two echogenic nearly parallel lines anteriorly and posteriorly and a linear echogenic central canal[8] (Fig. 22-3). Between 1 to 3 months of age, the cervical, thoracic, and lumbar segments of the spine are 5.3 ± 0.29, 4.4 ± 0.42, and 5.8 ± 0.66, respectively.[8] The spine is larger in the cervical and lumbar regions due to the amount of nerves in these areas. The spinal cord tapers to a point and terminates with the conus medullaris between L1 and L2. The conus gives way to the filum terminale, which is surrounded by the echogenic strands of the cauda equina[8] (Fig. 22-3B). The filum terminale can be slightly more echogenic and thicker (≤2mm) than the surrounding nerve roots.[8,9] The roots of the cauda equina form a collection of less echogenic linear strands that move freely with changes in patient positioning and with crying. The filum terminale and nerve roots extend into the distal portion of the thecal sac. Inferior to the thecal sac, the echogenic sacral vertebral bodies are noted coursing posteriorly toward the skin surface (Fig. 22-3C). Caudal to the sacrum are the two to three hypoechoic coccygeal segments. The coccyx is hypoechoic due to its cartilaginous nature (Fig. 22-3D).

In the axial plane, the spinal cord appears as an oval to round hypoechoic structure located within

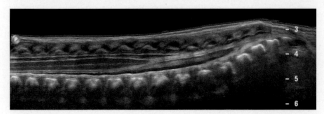

**Figure 22-1** Extended field-of-view image. This feature enables the sonographer to display the full length of the spine in one image. This image displays the thoracic spine to the sacrum.

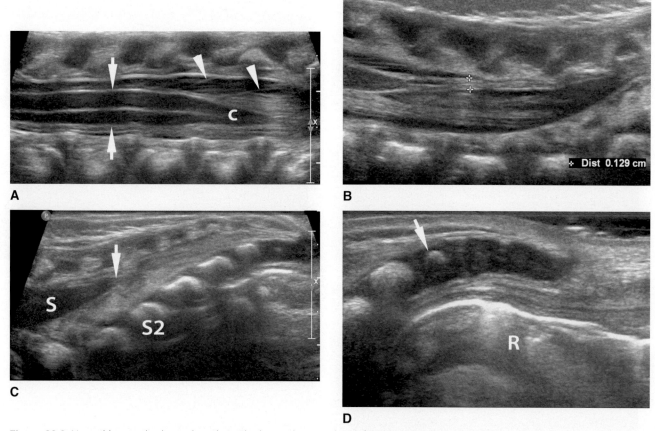

**Figure 22-3** Normal longitudinal spinal cord. **A:** The hypoechoic cord is defined by two parallel echogenic lines anteriorly and posteriorly *(arrows)* with an echogenic central canal. The cord tapers to the conus medullaris *(c)* and echogenic nerve roots are observed extending distally *(arrowheads)*. **B:** The echogenic filum terminale *(cursors)* extends from the conus and floats among the echogenic nerve roots in the anechoic cerebrospinal fluid. **C:** The hypoechoic thecal sac *(S)* comes to a point *(arrow)* and terminates at S2. The echogenic sacral vertebral bodies are coursing posterior toward the skin. **D:** The hypoechoic coccyx contains two to three cartilaginous segments one of which is partially calcified *(arrow)*. The air-filled rectum *(R)* is seen anterior to the coccyx.

the spinal canal with an echogenic circumferential border and echogenic dot centrally. The cord is surrounded by CSF, which is contained by the echogenic dura surrounding the canal (Fig. 22-4A). Posteriorly, the spinous process is noted centrally as a small hypoechoic circle. The echogenic vertebral arches are seen posterior and lateral on both sides of the canal. Again, the cord diameter is larger in the cervical region, narrows through the thoracic segment, and then enlarges again near the conus. As the spinal cord tapers to the conus, the cord diameter diminishes to a small hypoechoic circle. The filum terminale appears as a slightly thicker, round, echogenic, centrally located nerve arising from the tip of the conus (Fig. 22-4B). The nerves of the cauda equina appear as smaller echogenic dots surrounding the conus and filum (Fig. 22-4C). Because of these surrounding nerves, it can be difficult to differentiate the filum from the cauda equina.[8] As the thecal sac tapers distally, the sacral vertebral bodies appear as round, echogenic structures in the far field, which gives way to the round hypoechoic cartilaginous bones of the coccyx just below the skin surface.

Determining the exact level of the vertebral column allows determination of normal or abnormal levels of the position of the conus medullaris and exact localization of intraspinal abnormalities. As stated previously, the spinal cord should terminate between L1 and L2. Determination, however, can be difficult.[10] In the earlier reports of sonography use in the spine, methods used to determine the exact level in the spinal cord included palpation of the end of the lower ribs (said to indicate the level of L2). Another method involves determining the supracristal line by connecting the top of the palpated iliac crest (supposed to transect the L3–L4 space). A more objective method of determining the level of the conus is to count vertebrae up from the sacrum or down from the thoracolumbar junction. Generally, there are five sacral vertebrae and five lumbar vertebrae. Starting at S5 (the last echogenic structure in the sacrum), count cephalad five vertebrae to the lumbosacral junction (LSJ) (S1/L5) and then five more vertebrae to the thoracolumbar junction (T12/L1) (Fig. 22-5). The count could be confirmed by locating T12 by following the last rib to the junction with the spine and counting the lumbar

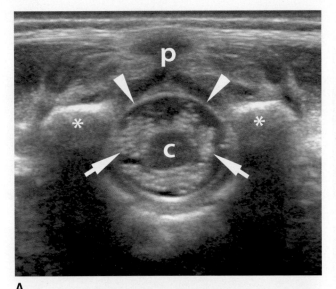

**A**

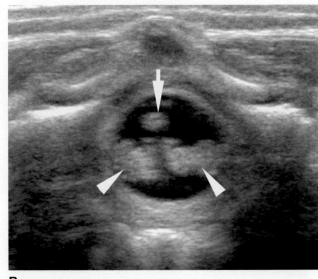

**B**

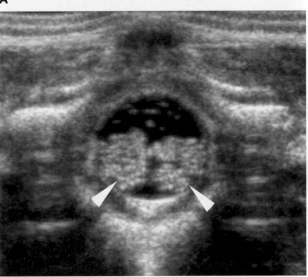

**C**

**Figure 22-4** Normal transverse spinal cord. **A:** The hypoechoic spinal cord *(c)* is surrounded by the echogenic nerve roots of the cauda equina *(arrows)*. Cerebrospinal fluid surrounds the cord that is contained by the echogenic dura *(arrowheads)* encompassing the canal. Echogenic vertebral arches *(\*)* are noted posterior and laterally joining with the hypoechoic spinous process *(p)* posteriorly. **B:** A slightly more prominent echogenic round filum terminale *(arrow)* floats among echogenic nerve roots *(arrowheads)*. **C:** Nerve roots can appear as small echogenic dots *(arrowheads)* or clump together, sometimes obscuring the filum terminale.

vertebrae caudally. Another way to confirm the level of the conus is to visually identify the LSJ and count upward.[7] The LSJ is identified by the transition from the relatively straight line of the lumbar vertebral bodies to the gentle kyphosis of the sacrum.[10] Because

there can be variants in the bony anatomy, if the level of the conus is uncertain, an X-ray may be needed to confirm the level. Using sonographic guidance, a radiopaque marker can be placed on the skin, over the tip of the conus, and an X-ray of the spine can be obtained.[11] The X-ray will confirm any variant in the bony anatomy and the level of the conus.

## NORMAL VARIANTS

There are a few normal variants that can be discovered during sonography of the spine. These variants are incidental findings and have no significant clinical implications. They should be identified and documented to prevent further unnecessary testing.[11]

### Ventriculus Terminalis

The *ventriculus terminalis* is a slight widening of the distal central canal. The dilated area is linear to slightly irregular and is anechoic. The widening is thought to

**Figure 22-5** Counting vertebrae. Utilizing an extended field-of-view image, starting with the fifth sacral vertebral body, count cephalad and backward five vertebrae ending at the first sacral vertebrae. Continue counting five more lumbar vertebrae ending at the first lumbar vertebrae. Note the gentle curve of the sacral vertebral bodies as it meets the more straight lumbar vertebrae at the lumbosacral junction.

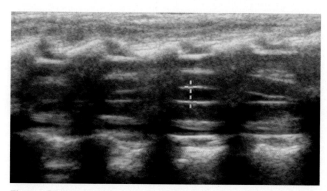

**Figure 22-6** Ventriculus terminalis. Longitudinal image shows the echogenic walls of the central canal are slightly separated by anechoic fluid near the conus (cursors). Note that the central canal widening is confined to the distal cord and does not extend cranially into the thoracic spinal cord.

be the incomplete resolution of the embryonic terminal ventricle and is sometimes referred to as *the fifth ventricle.*[11,12] Typically, it disappears after the first few months of life[7] (Fig. 22-6).

### Filar Cyst

A *filar cyst* is an ovoid midline anechoic structure just inferior to the tip of the conus medullaris. It is thought to be an ependyma-lined cyst that develops during embryogenesis. Some consider this the ventriculus terminalis, whereas others define it as the fifth ventricle. This structure is 8 to 10 mm long and 2 top 4 mm in the transverse diameter[7,8,11] (Fig. 22-7).

## CONGENITAL ANOMALIES

*Spinal dysraphism* refers to an array of spinal abnormalities caused by inadequate or improper fusion of the neural tube (NT) early in fetal life.[13] The incidence of spinal dysraphisms is 0.5 to 0.8 per cases per 1,000 births.[13] Most commonly, the defect occurs in the lower spine, although

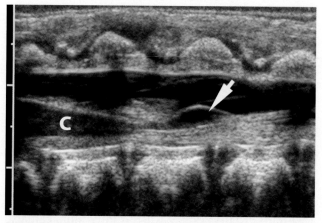

**Figure 22-7** Filar cyst. A longitudinal view of the conus and nerve roots demonstrates a small anechoic fluid collection (arrow) among the nerve roots just inferior to the conus medullaris (c).

any part of the spine may be affected. The spectrum of spinal dysraphism can be categorized into two major groups. *Open spinal dysraphism* (OSD) is characterized by neural tissue exposed without skin covering. A *closed spinal dysraphism* (CSD) is a skin-covered spinal abnormality. Due to the obvious defect, open dysraphisms like myeloceles and MMCs are easily classified.

The second group, closed dysraphisms, can present with a skin covered subcutaneous mass or various cutaneous markers. CSDs presenting with a subcutaneous mass include lipomyelocele/lipomyelomeningocele and myelocystocele. Closed dysraphisms without a subcutaneous mass like tethered cord, spinal lipoma, diastematomyelia, or a dorsal dermal sinus (DDS) can present with various cutaneous markers that can indicate an underlying abnormality. These cutaneous markers are typically located in the midline lumbosacral region and include hair tufts, sacral dimples or pits, pigment changes, hemangiomas, and skin tags.[14–17] Nearly all of the previously mentioned anomalies are associated with a tethered cord.

### EMBRYOLOGY

A brief summary of embryogenesis can provide some understanding as to why these anomalies occur. Development of the NT begins early in fetal life and is completed around the eighth week of gestation.[1,7] Initially, the NT (which becomes the spinal cord) starts as a flat plate comprised of a single layer of ectodermal cells.[7,18] Skin and nerve tissue will differentiate from the single ectodermal layer.[18] The neural plate begins to fold in the center, creating two opposing ridges. As the fold deepens, the ridges come together and fuse, forming a tube starting in the middle and extending superiorly and inferiorly.[7] During the fusion of the NT, the ectoderm separates from the NT. Mesenchymal cells separate from the ectoderm and will become the bony spine, meninges, and muscle.[1] Because the fusion of the NT and separation of the ectodermal and mesenchymal layers occur simultaneously, any disruption in the process can lead to spinal abnormalities.[7]

### OPEN SPINAL DYSRAPHISM

#### Myelocele/Myelomeningocele

Myelocele and myelomeningocele (MMC) represent two forms of spinal dysraphism in which there is a failure of the spinal cord to fold into an NT with a herniation of the leptomeninges through a defect in the dura matter. The NT persists as a flat plate. This occurs in 2 out of every 1,000 births.[8] A myelocele presents as a flat plate of neural tissue flush with the skin surface. The neural plate, of the more common MMC, is elevated above the skin surface due to an enlarged underlying subarachnoid space.[16] The developmental process stopped in the area of the defect because the NT did not fuse.[8] The ectoderm failed to separate from the NT and the mesenchymal cells did not migrate to form the bones. The skin, paraspinal musculature, and bony vertebral arches overlying the defect are attached and splayed lateral to the defect. The spinal cord is tethered at the level of the abnormality. Because the pathology is visible and the risk of infection is high, preoperative evaluation is not necessary.[16] Some of the problems these patients will encounter are decreased lower limb function to paralysis, bladder and bowel dysfunction, and hydrocephalus.[16]

In patients with MMC and myelocele, sonography displays absent spinous processes in the midline, the laminae are everted anteriorly, and the paraspinal musculature rotates anteriorly with the laminae.[19] The *myelocele* or *MMC* is a fluid-containing anechoic mass that is continuous with the spinal canal through the defect in the spine (Fig. 22-8). The spinal cord is low in position and may extend the entire length of the canal, never tapering into the conus, and terminating into the dorsal plate of neural tissue. The fluid-filled sac may contain fibrous septa that may be difficult to distinguish from nerve roots. Real-time evaluation will be helpful in that nerve roots demonstrate arterial-like pulsations, provided that the tension from the tethered cord is not so great as to completely dampen these pulsations. Postoperatively, a sac-like enlargement of the subarachnoid space is often seen (Fig. 22-9). Due to the bony defect, sonographic evaluation may be useful to diagnose any associated abnormality such as lipoma, hydromyelia, and retethering. Associated lipomas will appear as echogenic masses that may be situated between the cord and the posterior defect or into which

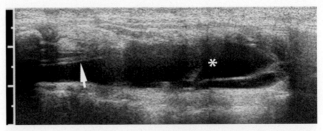

**Figure 22-9** Myelomeningocele repair. Scanning sagittal over the repaired defect, the missing posterior elements allow for an unobstructed view of the enlarged fluid-filled subarachnoid space (*). Note the thinned distal spinal cord terminating in the posterior placode *(arrow)*.

the cord may insert. Concurrent hydromyelia will be manifested by a centrally positioned anechoic collection within the spinal cord that will displace the cord peripherally. The hydromyelia may be focal or extend the entire length of the cord.

## CLOSED SPINAL DYSRAPHISM

### Tethered Cord

A *tethered cord* is a low-lying cord with a thickened filum terminale. It is almost always associated with dysraphic spinal anomalies. Physically, a tethered cord as well as dysraphic states can present with a wide range of symptoms. OSDs and CSDs can cause decreased lower limb, bowel, and urinary function.[20,21] Tethered cord symptoms are similar but may present later as a child grows and the spinal cord is pulled tight, causing neurological symptoms.[8,20] For this reason, early detection can decrease nerve damage, as the cord is surgically released before the cord is pulled tight and damaged. Clinically, aside from obvious lumbar masses, any abnormal markings over the midline spine should be investigated for possible spinal anomalies. As mentioned previously, hair tufts, vascular malformations, deep dimples, skin tags, and deep clefts, especially in the lumbar region or higher, are highly suspicious for a spinal abnormality. Also, patients with anal or urogenital malformations or VACTERL (vertebral defects, anal or duodenal atresia, cardiac defects, tracheoesophageal fistula, renal anomalies, and limb malformations) syndrome have a high association with tethered cord.[17,20,21]

Sonographically, the spinal cord is low in position. The conus is considered abnormally low at or below the level of the L3 vertebral.[5,11] The spinal cord will be pulled dorsally. The conus will be abnormally elongated and may lack the normal tapering.[1,11] The cord and nerve roots will also have decreased motion. Instead of floating freely in the CSF, the nerve roots will be floating more dorsally and lack normal movement. The filum terminale, if not associated with a dysraphic mass, may be abnormally thick (>2 mm) or fatty[5] (Fig. 22-10). A fatty filum can also be an incidental finding and is known as *tight filum terminale syndrome*. The abnormally thick filum gets

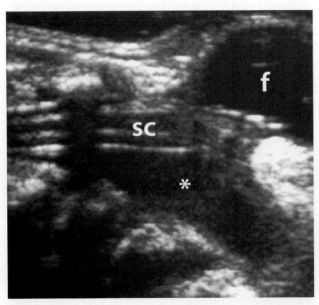

**Figure 22-8** Myelomeningocele. This sagittal image shows the spinal cord *(sc)* terminating in an enlarged fluid-filled area *(f)* that extends above the skin surface. A normal conus is not identified. Note the dilated subarachnoid space (*) anterior to the defect.

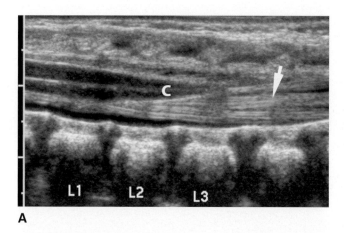

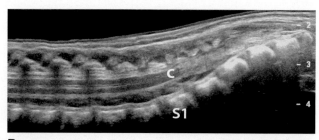

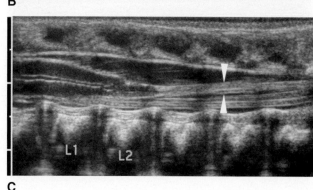

**Figure 22-10** Tethered cord. **A:** Sagittal image of the lumbar spinal cord indicates tethered cord. The conus is low, elongated, and pulled posteriorly. The nerve roots are also pulled more posteriorly *(arrow)*. **B:** The extended field-of-view image of the lumbosacral spine demonstrates an extremely low conus and dorsally displaced spinal cord. The conus *(c)* ends at S1. **C:** Longitudinal image of a fatty filum *(arrowheads)* with a conus ending at L2–L3.

tethered in the distal canal, which may or may not cause symptoms.[9]

### Diastomyelia

*Diastomyelia* is the separation of the spinal cord into two hemicords.[4,16] The split cord can be separated by a bony or fibrous septum, which can make imaging difficult.[16] This defect most commonly occurs in the thoracolumbar region and is usually associated with a cutaneous marker in the region of the defect.[4,9] The two hemicords reunite to form a single distal cord in the majority of cases. It is associated with tethered cord, scoliosis, clubfoot, vertebral anomalies, and dilation of the central canal (hydromelia).[4,8,9]

Sonographic diagnosis is made in the axial plane with demonstration of two hemicords, each with their own central echo complex[4,8] (Fig. 22-11). Evaluation in the sagittal plane will fail to detect its presence because the hemicords will not be visible simultaneously. The septum separating the hemicords may cause an acoustic barrier making diagnosis difficult. Associated severe scoliosis can also limit the sonographic window.

### Dorsal Dermal Sinus

The *dorsal dermal sinus* (DDS) is a thin, epithelial lined tract that passes from the skin toward the spinal canal.[16,19,22] They represent a very focal disruption in the development or fusion of the spinal canal. Dermal sinuses are most common in the lumbosacral region; however, they can occur in any region of the spine. Clinically, they manifest as deep midline dimples or pits. They should not be confused with a sacral dimple located in the gluteal fold.[16] Patients are at risk for meningitis because of the open tract to the spinal canal.[14,23]

Sonographically, a dermal sinus appears as a midline opening/defect that leads to the deep tract of the sinus. Appearance may vary depending on the width of the lumen. The sinus tract may appear as a single echogenic band if the lumen is very narrow or as a triple tract with two parallel lines of echogenicity with a central hypoechoic space if the lumen is large enough to visualize (Fig. 22-12A). It is frequently difficult, if not impossible, to trace the sinus into the canal

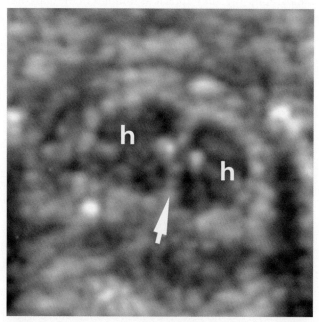

**Figure 22-11** Diastomyelia. The transverse spinal cord image demonstrates two hemicords *(h)*, each with its own central echo complex, separated by a fibrous septum *(arrow)*.

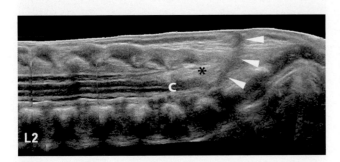

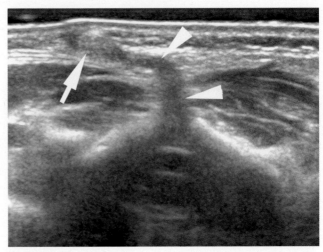

**A**

**B**

**Figure 22-12** Dorsal dermal sinus. **A:** The longitudinal extended field-of-view image displays a hypoechoic tract (*arrowheads*) extending from the skin to the spinal canal terminating in diffusely echogenic tissue (*\**) surrounding a low conus (*c*). **B:** In the axial plane, a hypoechoic tract (*arrowheads*) with an echogenic component representing a dermoid (*arrow*) is noted in the thoracic spine.

itself. If the spinal cord is low in position, tethering from an intraspinal extension of the sinus can be suspected. In addition, an abnormal focus of echogenicity within the canal suggests an associated dermoid (Fig. 22-12B).

## Sacral Dimple/Pilonidal Sinus

The *sacral dimple* or *pit* is the most common reason an infant is referred for spinal sonography. This skin anomaly, which quite possibly is a normal variant, is located within the gluteal fold <2.5 mm from the anus.[5,7,14] The dimple can be blind ending or associated with a pilonidal sinus/tract that extends to the coccyx. Sonographically, they appear as dimples in the skin that lead to a hyperechoic or hypoechoic tract (Fig. 22-13). If there is an associated pilonidal cyst, the sinus will

widen deeply into a fluid collection. Again, the pilonidal sinus should not be confused with a DDS as it has no connection to the normal spine.

## Spinal Lipoma

*Spinal lipomas* are collections of fat and connective tissue that appear at least partially encapsulated and have definite connection with the spinal cord.[19] There are three major types: (1) lipomyeloceles/lipomyelomeningoceles (most common), (2) intradural lipomas, and (3) lipomas of the filum terminale. These defects make up 20% to 50% of closed spinal defects.[9] Lipomas are caused when mesenchymal cells separate and migrate too early and end up in the not yet closed NT. The cells develop into fat thus causing the fatty masses.[8] They will appear hyperechoic or mixed in echogenicity.

The most common of the three, lipomyelocele/lipomyelomeningocele, presents with a skin covered back mass typically located in the lumbar region.[8] Both abnormalities are associated with a midline bony defect and an echogenic fatty mass that distorts and tethers the spinal cord.[22] The difference between the lipomyelocele and lipomyelomeningocele is similar to the difference between a myelocele and MMC. The lipomyelocele stays within the spinal canal whereas the lipomyelomeningocele has an enlarged subarachnoid space and the fatty mass extends through the posterior bony defect[16] (Fig 22-14).

The last two spinal lipomas, intradural lipoma and lipoma of the filum terminale, are different from the lipomyelocele/lipomyelomeningocele because they are not associated with a subcutaneous mass. They also differ in that they may or may not be associated with a tethered cord.[19] An intradural lipoma lies within the spinal cord and is completely confined by the dura.

**Figure 22-13** Pilonidal sinus. The patient presented with a simple sacral dimple. Longitudinal image over the dimple (*\**) shows a hypoechoic tract (*arrowheads*) coursing toward the coccyx (*c*) in this longitudinal image.

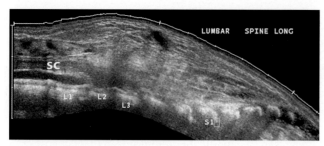

**Figure 22-14** Lipomyelomeningocele. This infant presented with a skin covered lumbar mass. In this longitudinal image, the spinal cord *(sc)* is low and tethered by a diffuse echogenic mass. The distal cord is displaced anteriorly and disappears into the echogenic mass.

The echogenic mass can be located in the lumbosacral region and sometimes higher in the cervicothoracic area.[16] Lipomas of the filum terminale can present as a thickened filum (>2 mm) or a small echogenic fatty mass associated with the filum (Fig. 22-15). A fatty filum can be an incidental finding (Fig. 22-16).

### Terminal Myelocystocele

A *terminal myelocystocele* is a skin covered, fluid-filled lumbar mass protruding through a dysraphic defect.[9] The fluid-filled cyst is an abnormal dilation of the terminal ventricle which communicates with the central spinal cord canal. The cyst does not communicate with the subarachnoid space.[16] Although the etiology is unclear, it is suggested that an abnormal circulation of CSF results in a massively dilated terminal ventricle.[8]

Sonographically, a large skin-covered fluid-filled mass is identified in the lumbar region. The central

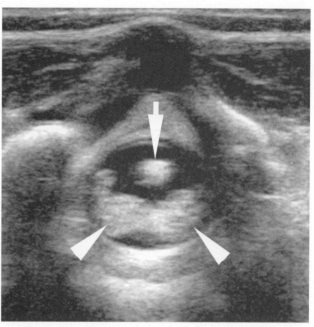

**Figure 22-16** Fatty filum. The transverse image of the lumbar spine documents an incidental prominent fatty filum in an otherwise normal exam. The prominent filum *(arrow)* floats posterior to the more anterior group of nerve roots *(arrowheads)*.

canal widens and directly communicates with the fluid-filled sac. The large sac herniates through the dysraphic defect creating a large lumbar mass[9] (Fig. 22-17). Hydromelia (dilated central canal) can be seen extending superiorly in some cases.

Myelocystocele is associated with omphalocele, bladder exstrophy, and imperforate anus. As with other

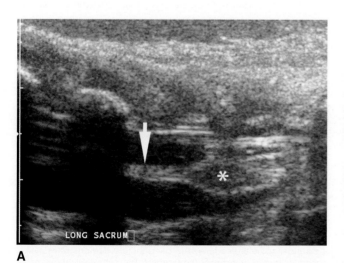

A

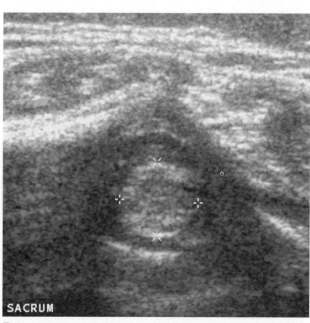

B

**Figure 22-15** Filum lipoma. **A:** The longitudinal image shows the filum terminale *(arrow)* expanded by a focal echogenic mass *(\*)*. The lipoma is confined to the filum. **B:** Transversely, the echogenic lipoma is obvious *(cursors)*, surrounded by cerebrospinal fluid, and located posterior to echogenic nerve roots.

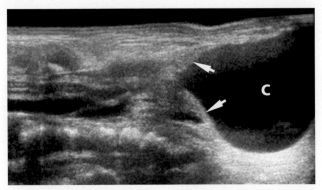

**Figure 22-17** Myelocystocele. The longitudinal image of the spinal cord shows the spinal cord splitting *(arrowheads)* and the central canal balloons into the large lumbar cystic *(c)* mass.

spinal dysraphisms, patients suffer from decreased lower extremity and poor bladder/bowel function.[16]

## MISCELLANEOUS SPINAL ABNORMALITIES

### Spinal Cord Injuries

Sonography can be useful in the evaluation of birth trauma to the spinal cord, especially because it can be done portably. Although the majority of cases will be evaluated by MRI, because of sedation issues as well as portability, sonography may be used. Sonography can also be utilized after failed lumbar puncture (LP) to evaluate for epidural hematoma.

Typically, spinal cord injury resulting from birth trauma occurs during a difficult breech delivery. Severe spinal cord injury is infrequent but may manifest sonographically as cord edema, hematomyelia, and hemorrhage outside the cord. Subacute or serial follow-up evaluation may identify a focal area of cord narrowing from myelomalacia, which will appear as focal increased echogenicity of the cord with obliteration of the central echo complex. Extramedullary hematomas resulting from trauma displace and compress the

spinal cord. They can appear echogenic or anechoic depending on their chronicity. The older the hematoma, the more anechoic it becomes. Acute hemorrhage is more echogenic.

LPs are performed routinely for sepsis in infants to obtain CSF for culture.[24] Unfortunately, approximately 50% of LPs in neonates are unsuccessful.[24] Because there is a network of vessels in the epidural space and thecal sac, a significant hematoma can occur after a failed or traumatic LP.[25] Sonography is utilized after a failed LP to confirm the presence of CSF to avoid another failed attempt.[26]

Following a failed LP, the lumbar region of the epidural space and thecal sac should be evaluated for blood products. Sonographically, as mentioned previously, hematomas vary in echogenicity depending on the age. Acutely, the epidural space will be enlarged and filled with echogenic blood compressing the thecal sac. As the thecal sac is compressed, the CSF is displaced cephalad[25] (Fig. 22-18A). As the hematoma resolves, it will become more anechoic (Fig. 22-18B). The compression will become less severe, and the CSF will return slowly. Blood in the thecal sac appears as debris filled CSF. Once reaccumulation of CSF is confirmed, an sonography-guided LP can be performed to assure a successful outcome.

### Tumor/Intraoperative Sonography

The use of sonography in the evaluation of spinal cord tumors is not routine in the initial evaluation and diagnosis but is used in the operating room and following therapy or treatment. Evaluation can be performed through the laminectomy defect to localize tumor, follow postoperative associated complications (syrinx or cyst formation, recurrent disease, or myelomalacia), or evaluate response to therapy.

Sonographic characteristics of intramedullary tumors include expansion of the spinal cord with the tumor itself usually demonstrating homogeneous or

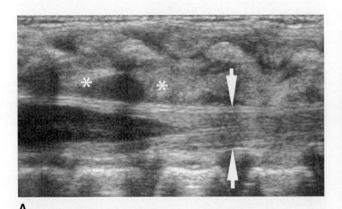

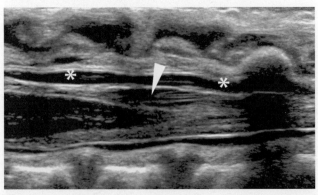

A                                    B

**Figure 22-18** Bleeding after lumbar puncture. **A:** Longitudinal image of the lumbar spine after a failed lumbar puncture demonstrates mixed echogenicity blood *(*)* in the epidural space. The enlarged epidural space is compressing the thecal sac *(arrows)*. The echogenic nerve roots are compressed together. No cerebrospinal fluid is identified. **B:** After several days, the hematoma resolves, becoming less echogenic and more anechoic *(*)*. The nerve roots continue to be compressed together with a minimal amount of cerebrospinal fluid *(arrowhead)* noted distal to the conus.

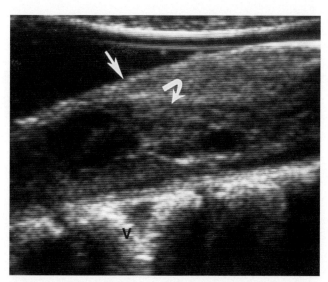

**Figure 22-19** Intraoperative sonography. Intraoperative sonogram in the longitudinal section through a laminectomy defect in a 9-year-old boy, who 3 years earlier had resection of brain tumor. The spinal cord *(arrow)* is expanded by a heterogeneously echogenic mass *(curved arrow)*, which was a metastatic pilocytic astrocytoma of the cord at pathology *(v, vertebrae).*

heterogeneous increased echogenicity (Fig. 22-19). Some tumors, however, may have an echo texture that is indistinguishable from the normal cord and are apparent only because of the change in the caliber or margins of the cord itself. The central echo complex is either partially or totally obliterated by the tumor. There may or may not be associated cystic structures present. Extramedullary tumors are most frequently echogenic with respect to the spinal cord and displace the spinal cord. Whereas the central echo complex is at least partially obliterated by intramedullary tumors, the central echo complex is usually preserved when extramedullary tumors are present.

Intraoperative sonography during neurosurgical procedures allows for localization of intramedullary

tumor,[27,28] differentiates cystic from solid components,[27,29] identifies and localizes spinal arteriovenous malformations, and provides guidance for placement of shunts in the treatment of syrinx (Fig. 22-20).

The technique used for intraoperative sonography evaluation involves scanning with the patient in a prone position through the laminectomy defect. Before the dura is opened, sterile saline is used to fill the defect. Gel should be applied to a high-frequency transducer and enclosed in a sterile probe cover. The neurosurgeon or radiologist will perform the scanning while the technologist operates the machine.

## SUMMARY

- Sonographic evaluation of the spine can be performed in the infant up to 6 months of age as well as in the patient with a congenital or postsurgical defect in the posterior arch of the vertebrae.

- The most frequent use will be in the infant with a sacral dimple or other midline cutaneous abnormalities in which evaluation of the cord and the level of the conus medullaris is desired to exclude the presence of a tethered cord.

- Intraoperative use in cooperation with the neurosurgeon for localization of tumor, cysts, and other lesions as well as in the setting of trauma has become widely accepted.

- Clinical indications for sonographic evaluation of the neonatal spine include patients with lumbosacral skin anomalies including pigmented spots, hairy nevus, dermal sinuses, dimples, and hemangiomas.

- A high-frequency (8 to 15 MHz) linear transducer is routinely used to evaluate the neonatal spine.

- The infant should be placed prone on a towel or pillow to provide an optimal acoustic window.

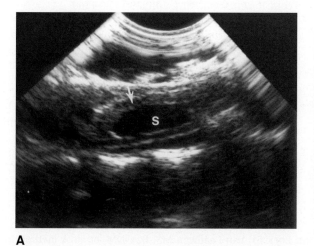

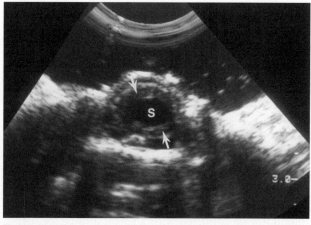

**A**    **B**

**Figure 22-20** Sonography guided drainage. Intraoperative sonography was performed for guidance in drainage of a syrinx in the cervical spinal cord in a 7-year-old boy. Both a longitudinal section **(A)** and an axial section **(B)** were obtained via a laminectomy defect. The spinal cord *(arrow)* is displaced peripherally by an anechoic fluid collection, which is the syrinx (s) in the center of the spinal cord.

- The level of the conus medullaris, as well as the position of the spinal cord in the spinal canal, is documented along with visualization of normal cord and nerve root motion.

- Between the echogenic dura, the hypoechoic spinal cord is situated centrally to slightly anterior and is surrounded by anechoic cerebrospinal fluid (CSF).

- The spinal cord tapers to a point and terminates with the conus medullaris between L1 and L2.

- The conus gives way to the filum terminale which is surrounded by the echogenic strands of the cauda equina.

- The roots of the cauda equina form a collection of less echogenic linear strands that move freely with changes in patient positioning and with crying.

- Spinal dysraphism refers to an array of spinal abnormalities caused by inadequate or improper fusion of the neural tube (NT) early in fetal life.

- Most defects occur in the lower spine, although any part of the spine may be affected.

- Spinal dysraphisms are classified as open or closed depending on whether or not the lesions are covered by skin.

- Myelocele and the more common myelomeningocele (MMC) are two forms of spinal dysraphism in which there is a herniation of the leptomeninges through a defect in the dura matter.

- With myelocele and MMC, the skin, paraspinal musculature, and bony vertebral arches overlying the defect are attached and splayed lateral to the defect, and the spinal cord is tethered at the level of the abnormality.

- The myelocele or MMC is a fluid-containing anechoic mass that is continuous with the spinal canal through the defect in the spine.

- A tethered cord is a low-lying cord with a thickened filum terminale, almost always associated with dysraphic spinal anomalies.

- The conus is considered abnormally low at or below the level of the L3 vertebral.

- With a tethered cord, the cord and nerve roots will have decreased motion.

- Diastomyelia is the separation of the spinal cord into two hemicords.

- The dorsal dermal sinus (DDS) is a thin, epithelial lined tract that passes from the skin toward the spinal canal as a result of a very focal disruption in the fusion of the spinal canal.

- DDS manifest as deep midline dimples or pits, but should not be confused with a sacral dimple located in the gluteal fold.

- The sacral dimple or pit is the most common reason an infant is referred for spinal sonography.

- The sacral dimple can be blind ending or associated with a pilonidal cyst that extends to the coccyx; however, the pilonidal sinus has no connection to the normal spine.

- Spinal lipomas, which make up 20% to 50% of closed spinal defects, are collections of fat and connective tissue that appear at least partially encapsulated and have definite connection with the spinal cord.

- Trauma to the spinal cord during birth can present sonographically as cord edema, hematomyelia, and hemorrhage outside the cord.

## Critical Thinking Questions

1. What clinical signs would lead a clinician to order a sonography evaluation of the neonatal spine?

2. What is the importance of detecting a tethered cord as early as possible?

3. How would a dorsal dermal sinus be differentiated from a sacral dimple?

4. How is a tethered cord diagnosed sonographically?

## REFERENCES

1. Dick EA, Patel K, Owens CM, et al. Spinal ultrasound in infants. *Br J Radiol.* 2002;75:384–392.
2. Siegel MJ, McAlister WH. Musculoskeletal system and spine. In: Siegel MJ, ed. *Pediatric Sonography.* 2nd Edition. New York: Raven Press; 1995:532–540.
3. Bates D, Ruggieri P. Imaging modalities for evaluation of spine. *Radiol Clin North Am.* 1991;29:675–690.
4. Hung PC, Wang HS, Lui TN, et al. Sonographic findings in a neonate with diastematomyelia and a tethered spinal cord. *J Ultrasound Med.* 2010;29:1357–1360.
5. Ben-Sira L, Ponger P, Miller E, et al. Low-risk lumbar skin stigmata in infants: the role of ultrasound screening. *J Pediatr.* 2009;155:864–869.
6. Gudinchet E, Chapuis L, Berger D. Diagnosis of anterior cervical spinal epidural abscess by US and MRI in a newborn. *Pediatr Radiol.* 1991;21:515–517.
7. Deeg KH, Lode HM, Gassner I. Spinal sonography in newborns and infants—Part I: method, normal anatomy and indications. *Ultraschall in Med.* 2007;28:507–517.
8. Unsinn KM, Geley T, Freund MC, et al. US of the spinal cord in newborns: spectrum of normal findings, variants, congenital anomalies, and acquired diseases. *Radiographics.* 2000;20:923–938.
9. Dick EA, de Bruyn R. Ultrasound of the spinal cord in children: its role. *Eur Radiol.* 2003;13:552–562.
10. Beek FJ, van Leeuwen MS, Bax NM, et al. A method for sonographic counting of the lower vertebral bodies in newborns and infants. *AJNR Am J Neuroradiol.* 1994; 15:445–449.

11. Lowe LH, Johanek AJ, Moore CW. Sonography of the neonatal spine: part I, normal anatomy, imaging pitfalls, and variations that may simulate disorders. *AJR Am J Roentgenol.* 2007;188:733–738.

12. Kriss VM, Kriss TC, Coleman RC. Sonographic appearance of the ventriculus terminalis cyst in the neonatal spinal cord. *J Ultrasound Med.* 2000;19:207–209.

13. Drolet BA, Chamlin SL, Garzon MC, et al. Prospective study of spinal anomalies in children with infantile hemangiomas of the lumbosacral skin. *J Pediatr.* 2010; 157:789–794.

14. Schenk JP, Herweh C, Günther P, et al. Imaging of congenital anomalies and variations of the caudal spine and back in neonates and small infants. *Eur J Radiol.* 2006;58:3–14.

15. Robinson AJ, Russell S, Rimmer S. The value of ultrasonic examination of the lumbar spine in infants with specific reference to cutaneous markers of occult spinal dysraphism. *Clin Radiol.* 2005;60:72–77.

16. Rossi A, Biancheri R, Cama A, et al. Imaging in spine and spinal cord malformations. *Eur J Radiol.* 2004;50: 177–200.

17. Cornette L, Verpoorten C, Lagae L, et al. Closed spinal dysraphism: a review on diagnosis and treatment in infancy. *Eur J Paediatr Neurol.* 1998;2:179–185.

18. Sneineh AK, Gabos PG, Keller MS, et al. Ultrasonography of the spine in neonates and young infants with a sacral skin dimple. *J Pediatr Orthop.* 2002;22: 761–762.

19. Naidich TP, Radkowski MA, Britton J. Real-time sonographic display of caudal spinal anomalies. *Neuroradiology.* 1986;28:512–527.

20. O'Neill BR, Yu AK, Tyler-Kabara EC. Prevalence of tethered spinal cord in infants with VACTERL. *J Neurosurg Pediatr.* 2010;6:177–182.

21. Kim SM, Chang HK, Lee MJ, et al. Spinal dysraphism with anorectal malformation: lumbosacral magnetic resonance imaging evaluation of 120 patients. *J Pediatr Surg.* 2010;45:769–776.

22. Sorantin E, Robl T, Lindbichler F, et al. MRI of the neonatal and paediatric spine and spinal canal. *Eur J Radiol.* 2008;68:227–234.

23. Lin KL, Wang HS, Chou ML, et al. Sonography for detection of spinal dermal sinus tracts. *J Ultrasound Med.* 2002;21:903–907.

24. Baxter AL, Fisher RG, Burke BL, et al. Local anesthetic and stylet styles: factors associated with resident lumbar puncture success. *Pediatrics.* 2006;117:876–881.

25. Coley BD, Shiels WE ll, Hogan MJ. Diagnostic and interventional ultrasonography in neonatal and infant lumbar puncture. *Pediatr Radiol.* 2001;31:399–402.

26. Molina A, Fons J. Factors associated with lumbar puncture success. *Pediatrics.* 2006;118:842–844.

27. Brunberg JA, DiPeitro MA, Venes JL, et al. Intramedullary lesions of the pediatric spinal cord: correlation of findings from MR imaging, intraoperative sonography, surgery and histologic study. *Radiology.* 1991;181:573–579.

28. Kawakami N, Mimatsu K, Kato F. Intraoperative sonography of intramedullary spinal cord tumours. *Neuroradiology.* 1992;34:436–439.

29. Kochan JP, Quencer RM. Imaging of cystic and cavitary lesions of the spinal cord and canal. The value of MR and intraoperative sonography. *Radiol Clin North Am.* 1991;29:867–911.

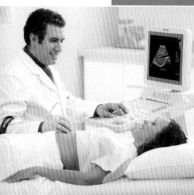

# 23 The Infant Hip Joint

Charlotte Henningsen

## OBJECTIVES

Describe the embryologic development of the hip joint.

Illustrate the bones and joints of the hip.

List the risk factors associated with developmental dysplasia of the hip.

Define the process for sonographic evaluation of the hip.

Describe the etiologies of hip effusion.

Identify the sonographic appearance of hip effusion.

Define proximal femoral focal deficiency.

## KEY TERMS

developmental dysplasia of the hip | hip effusion | proximal focal femoral deficiency | septic arthritis | transient synovitis

## GLOSSARY

**abduct** to move toward the midline

**adduct** to move away from the midline

**arthrocentesis** to remove fluid from a joint through a needle

**erythrocyte sedimentation rate** a nonspecific indicator for inflammation; a measurement of the time it takes for red blood cells to settle in a tube of unclotted blood

**mesoderm** the middle germ cell layer that contributes to the embryologic development of connective tissue, bone, blood, muscle, vessels, and lymphatics

**oligohydramnios** a decreased amount of amniotic fluid around the fetus

**osteomyelitis** infection of the bone marrow and bone

**torticollis** a head that is held sideways due to a muscle contraction

Developmental dysplasia of the hip (DDH) describes a range of dysplasia that includes instability, subluxation, and frank dislocation. DDH was previously known as *congenital dysplasia of the hip*, but most dislocations occur after birth. The frequency of DDH is 10 in 1,000 live births.[1] Early diagnosis and treatment is important to avoid significant disability. Clinical assessment and sonography are the two most common methods utilized in the detection of DDH.[2] This chapter provides an overview of the development and anatomy of the hip and explore the risk factors associated with DDH. Sonographic evaluation for DDH is explained in addition to other diseases that can affect the hip including hip effusion and focal femoral deficiency.

## EMBRYOLOGY

There are three germ layers from which all body systems form: the ectoderm, the mesoderm, and the endoderm. The bones, connective tissues, and muscles are derived from the mesoderm. The initial development of the mesoderm occurs in the latter part of the third week postconception, which marks the beginning of bone formation. From the mesoderm, mesenchymal cells arise that are concentrated in the cephalic end of the body and, along with cells derived from the neural crest, contribute to the development of the face and head. The ossification of the bones of the arms and legs begins at the end of the third week, which marks the end of the embryonic period, although the development of bones continues into adult life. Initially, the limbs arise as buds with the distal ends developing into paddle-like structures from which the bones continue to develop and fingers and toes arise. Myoblasts differentiate to develop into the muscles of the long bones. The joints of the body begin to develop during the sixth week, and during the seventh week of development, the upper and lower limbs will rotate on their longitudinal axes.[3]

## ANATOMY

The bones of the hip joint are composed of the pelvic girdle and the femur. The hip bone or coxal bone is composed of the ilium, ischium, and pubis (Fig. 23-1). The acetabulum is located at the lateral aspect of these bones and is joined by a growth plate, the triradiate cartilage. This creates an articulation point for the femur.[4] The proximal aspect of the femur, the femoral head, is rounded and sits in the acetabulum. At the rim of the acetabulum sits a lip of cartilage called the *acetabular labrum* (Fig. 23-2A,B). The femoral head is contiguous with the neck, which is contiguous with the diaphysis or shaft of the femur. The femoral head is cartilaginous at birth and the acetabulum is composed of cartilage and bone. The femoral head begins to ossify from the center outward at 2 to 8 months of age (Fig. 23-3).[1] The cartilaginous characteristics allow for sonographic evaluation of the hip in infants. It is also because of the large cartilaginous component of the hip that it is subject to molding with normal development dependant on the femur being in good contact with the acetabulum. Additionally, during fetal development, maternal hormonal influences contribute to the laxity of fetal ligaments, which may in turn create a vulnerable atmosphere for the hip to become subluxable or dislocatable.[5]

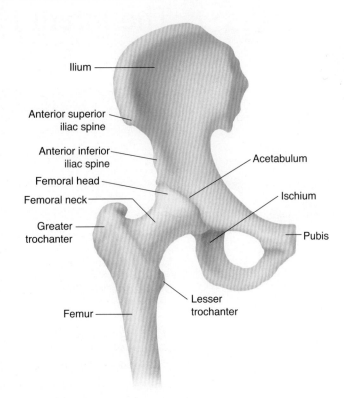

**Figure 23-1** Hip joint anatomy. The illustration of the anterior hip joint shows the ilium, ischium, and pubis forming the hip bone. The acetabulum is located at the lateral aspects and has the triradiate cartilage (growth plate), which creates an articulation point for the femoral head.

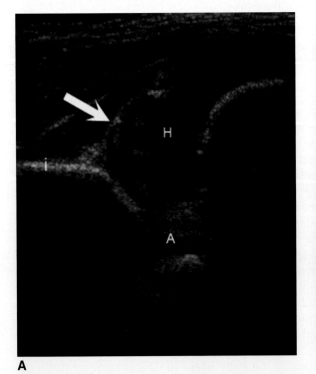

**A**

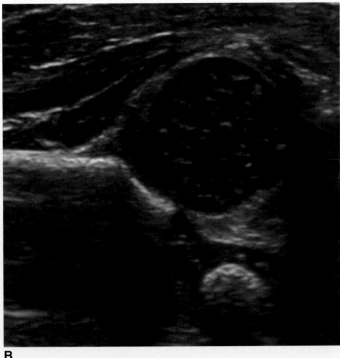

**B**

**Figure 23-2** Coronal sections. **A:** A coronal section of the hip with the leg in the neutral position shows the femoral head (*H*), the iliac line superiorly (*i*), the labrum (*arrow*), and the acetabulum (*A*). **B:** This coronal section in a flexed position demonstrates similar anatomy; however, the femoral neck is not seen.

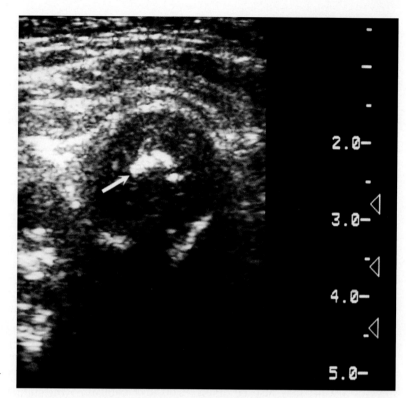

**Figure 23-3** Ossification. The femoral head ossification *(arrow)* is seen on a 7-month-old girl.

## DEVELOPMENTAL DYSPLASIA OF THE HIP

DDH occurs most frequently at birth but may appear through the infant period. The cause may be mechanical as a result of positional influences in utero and after birth or the cause may be physiologic resulting from a response to maternal hormones in utero or physical makeup after birth.

### RISK FACTORS

Those at risk for DDH include those born in the breech position, those with a positive family history, those living in cultures that swaddle infants in the extension and hip adduction, and those with an abnormal physical examination.[6] A pregnancy affected by oligohydramnios can lead to DDH and both metatarsus adductus and torticollis are associated with DDH. DDH is also identified more frequently in the first pregnancy or firstborn, females, whites, infants with high birth weights, and native North American populations.[5]

### CLINICAL ASSESSMENT

A routine neonatal screening typically includes clinical assessment of both hips. The assessment should be completed by experienced hands and when the infant is relaxed. Even in experienced hands, sonographic evaluation may detect instabilities that are undetected by clinical examination[2]; however, research has shown that most of these dysplasias will become normal without treatment.[7] More significant dysplasias can lead to disability and require surgical treatment including hip replacement in adult life.[8] The proper diagnosis which results in the best treatment plan is dependent on the expertise of the individual examining the infant.

### Barlow and Ortolani Maneuvers

The Barlow and Ortolani tests are two maneuvers for assessing hip stability. With the Barlow maneuver, the examiner attempts to push the femoral head posteriorly out of the socket, and with the Ortolani maneuver, the examiner attempts to reduce a recently dislocated hip.

The Barlow provocative maneuver test is performed on a supine infant with legs flexed 90 degrees. The examiner grasps the symphysis pubis and sacrum with one hand while the other hand is placed over the knee area and adducts the leg. Slight outward pressure is then exerted over the knee and distal thigh area in an effort to dislocate the hip. A palpable sensation of movement called a *clunk* is felt as the femoral head exits the acetabulum posteriorly.[5,9]

The Ortolani maneuver is performed on a supine infant and the index and middle finger of the examiner is placed along the greater trochanter with the thumb placed along the inner thigh. The hip is flexed to 90 degrees and held in a neutral position as the hip is gently abducted simultaneously lifting the leg anteriorly. A palpable physical movement called a clunk is felt as the dislocated femoral head reduces into the acetabulum.[5,9]

The palpable and at times audible clunk are strong positive Barlow and Ortolani signs.[5,9]

### Visual Assessment

Other features that arouse suspicion include asymmetry of thigh folds, a positive Allis or Galeazzi sign (relative shortness of the femur with the hips and knees flexed), and discrepancy of leg lengths. These physical findings alert the examiner that abnormal relationships of the femoral head to the acetabulum (dislocation and subluxation) may be present.

A visual assessment should be performed for signs that would raise suspicion of DDH. Dislocation can be observed using the Allis or Galeazzi sign of the relative shortness of the femur by noting that when the knees are flexed, one knee will appear lower than the other.[5] For unilateral hip dysplasia, the Allis or Galeazzi sign can be assessed with the patient in the supine position with the knees flexed noting limb-length discrepancy. Other visual signs include a shortening of the thigh, redundant and asymmetric skin folds on the thigh of the affected leg, and asymmetry of gluteal folds.[9] A female profile with an increased pelvic width and the appearance of a waist may also be noted. A positive clinical examination may prompt a follow-up sonographic examination. To reduce the likelihood of a false-positive examination due to laxity of the muscles in response to maternal hormones, sonographic examination of the hip should be performed at 4 to 6 weeks of age.[2]

## SONOGRAPHIC EVALUATION

### Preparation

The literature describes a variety of techniques to examine infants for DDH with sonography. Most authors agree that to gain the best results, it is important for the infant to be relaxed and cooperative. The best time to examine the infant will be immediately following or during feeding. Additionally, it may be helpful to have distractions such as toys available during the examination. It is beneficial to position bolsters of foam or rolled bedding on both sides of the body to aid in stabilizing the infant when scanning in a decubitus position. Parents can be valuable during the examination by helping to hold the infant and by calming the infant with soothing conversation.

Preparation for the examination includes removing clothing below the waist that might impede making contact with the infant's hip. Clothing above the waist should not be removed and care must be taken to maintain the infant's warmth. It is recommended that the diaper be left in place exposing each side as it is being examined. A warm room and warm gel are a must to maintain as much cooperation as possible.

A linear transducer is preferred over a sector transducer due to the larger footprint and better near field resolution. The highest frequency that allows adequate

penetration should always be utilized.[10] Generally, a 7.5-MHz transducer may be used for infants from birth to 3 months of age, and a 5-MHz transducer may be needed for older infants. On rare occasions, a 3-MHz transducer may be needed for adequate penetration. Sonography of the hip is best performed up to 6 months of age but between 6 months and 1 year of age, radiography is more reliable due to the increasing bony ossification that will eventually preclude adequate sonographic imaging.[10]

### Technique

In the 1980s, sonography of the hip was introduced by Graf, an Austrian orthopedic surgeon. Graf used static images with a coronal approach measuring the acetabular depth. A dynamic technique was then developed by Harcke and others, which evaluated femoral head coverage.[11] Current guidelines recommend imaging with and without stress utilizing either the measurement technique or assessing for femoral head coverage. Imaging planes include the coronal plane without stress and the transverse plane with and without stress maneuvers.[10] To assess for asymmetry, both hips must be included in the protocol. The infant can be imaged in the supine or decubitus position. It is easiest to assess if the sonographer holds the transducer in one hand and the infant's leg in the other hand.[12]

Reproducibility and accuracy are important aspects of the sonographic examination. There is a learning curve for the sonographer during which time experience with normal and abnormal hips should be obtained. Harke suggested that at least 100 examinations should be performed to gain adequate experience.[13]

### Coronal Scan Plane

The coronal scanning plane may be obtained with the hip in a neutral or flexed position and the infant may be either in a decubitus or a supine position (Fig. 23-2A,B). The transducer is placed at the lateral aspect of the hip providing a longitudinal image of the hip from the coronal plane.[1,10,12] In this scan plane, the femoral head can be identified sitting in the acetabulum. The iliac line will be identified superiorly, and the bony shaft of the femoral neck will be identified inferiorly. The iliac line should appear as a straight line, which is important in making an accurate assessment. If the iliac appears concave, the transducer should be positioned slightly more anteriorly, and if the iliac line appears to incline laterally, then the transducer should be positioned slightly more posteriorly. In the coronal/neutral scan plane, the leg can either be extended or remain in a neutral position. Care should be taken to guard against forcing the leg beyond what would be a natural extension. In an infant, the physiologically neutral state maintains an approximate 15 to 20 degrees of flexion.[13]

Both the alpha and beta angles can be obtained using the coronal scan plane. To obtain the angles, a sonography hip applications package may be used or lines

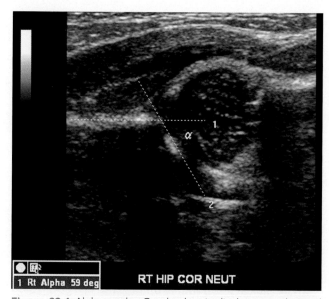

**Figure 23-4** Alpha angle. On the longitudinal image obtained with a coronal scan plane, there is an alpha angle of 59 degrees in a 3-month-old girl with an abnormal physical exam. No subluxation was noted with stress maneuvers.

| TABLE 23-1 | |
|---|---|
| **Graff Classification** | |
| **Classification** | **Criteria** |
| Type I hip | Normal, alpha angle >60 degrees |
| Type II hip | Normal if newborn, up to 3 months of age; indicates slowed development, alpha angle 44–60 degrees |
| Type III hip | Dislocated hip, alpha angle <43 degrees |
| Type IV hip | Gross dislocation, alpha angle not measurable |

may be drawn on the image. The first line is aligned with the ilium and extends through the head of the femur. The second line extends from the ilium along the labrum. The third line extends from the bony edge of the acetabulum at the triradiate cartilage to the lowest point of the ilium. The alpha angle is the angle formed between the first and second line (Fig. 23-4). The beta angle is the angle formed between the first and third line. The alpha angle is defined as the bony or osseous roof of the acetabulum and the beta angle is defined as the cartilaginous roof of the acetabulum. The angles can be used to measure the depth of the acetabulum and the position of the acetabular labrum. The alpha angle has been used as the primary measure for hip dysplasia. When the alpha angle is ≥60 degrees, it is considered normal.[14] Furthermore, utilizing the Graf classification,[15] the hip can be classified using the criteria presented in (Table 23-1).

The beta angle is not addressed as frequently in the literature and is not relied on as often as a determinate for DDH. It should be noted that a beta angle of <55 degrees is considered normal.[14] It should be noted that both premature and newborn infants may present with type II hips and may only require follow-up to determine if treatment is necessary, as many of these hips may appear normal at 4 to 6 weeks of age without medical intervention.

The coronal scan plane also allows for an assessment of femoral head coverage with respect to how well it is contained in the acetabulum and whether or not the femoral head is in contact with the acetabular floor. The mean femoral head coverage is 54% in females and 56% in males with the lower limit of normal at approximately 45% (Fig. 23-5A). Hip instability will

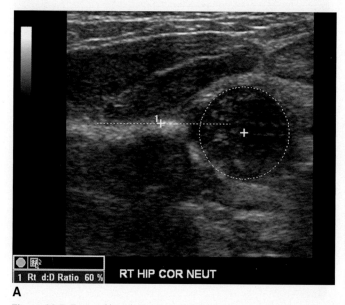

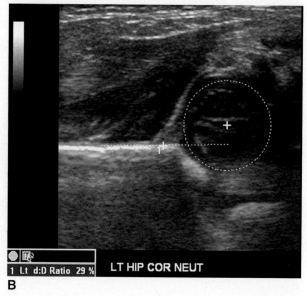

**A**      **B**

**Figure 23-5** Femoral head coverage. **A:** On the coronal image of the right hip with the patient in a neutral position, the femoral head coverage of 60% is consistent with a normal examination. **B:** On the coronal image of the left hip, the femoral head coverage of 29% is seen in a 2-month-old in a neutral position with a positive clunk on physical exam. The interpretation report stated the presence of shallow coverage of the femoral head.

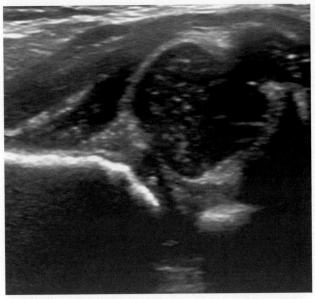

**Figure 23-6** Hip dislocation. The femoral head is completely out of the acetabulum which is consistent with dislocation in this 10-week-old girl.

present with femoral head coverage of approximately 36% to 37% defining subluxation.[12] A dislocated hip will sit completely out of the acetabulum. Although indexes and application's software have been developed to quantify the percentage of coverage, a qualitative assessment is commonly thought to be sufficient and can be classified as shallow, intermediate, or deep

(Fig. 23-5B). Assessing hip dysplasia using the alpha angle has shown to be more reproducible than assessing femoral head coverage.[11]

A coronal/flexion image is made in the coronal scan plane with the hip held at a 90-degree angle. The transducer should be positioned at the lateral aspect of the hip and in a coronal plane with respect to the acetabulum similar to the coronal/neutral scan/position. When viewing a coronal/flexion sonogram, the normal hip will have a "ball on a spoon" appearance. The ball is the femoral head, the iliac line represents the handle of the spoon, and the scoop of the spoon is the acetabulum.[1] When the hip is subluxable, posterior, superior, and lateral displacement of the femoral head will be identified. With hip dislocation, the femoral head will appear completely out of the acetabulum (Fig. 23-6).

In the flexed position, the infant's hip can be stressed when scanning by exerting downward pressure and simultaneously adducting and abducting the hip slightly. A stress maneuver utilizing a push–pull method can also be used to test for instability. Additionally, utilizing an abduction maneuver, similar to the Ortolani maneuver, can demonstrate whether or not a subluxed or dislocated hip is reducible.[12] Images are then obtained noting any movement of the femoral head (Fig. 23-7A,B). The sonogram should be labeled with the scan plane, the flexed position, and whether the hip is stressed or unstressed.

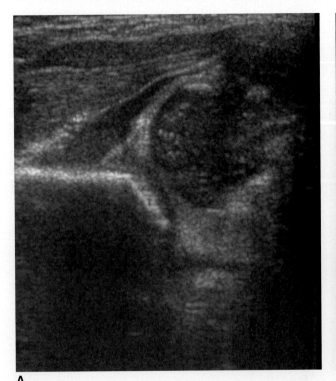

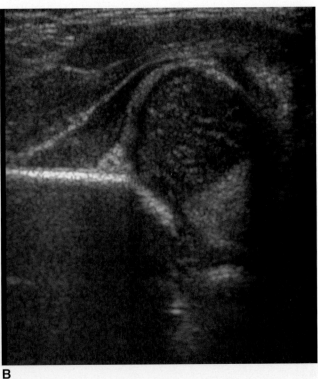

**A**      **B**

**Figure 23-7** Subluxation. Stress maneuvers demonstrate subluxation in this 3-month-old with bilateral developmental dysplasia of the hip. Compare the image made **(A)** without stress to the image made **(B)** with stress and note the movement of the femoral head.

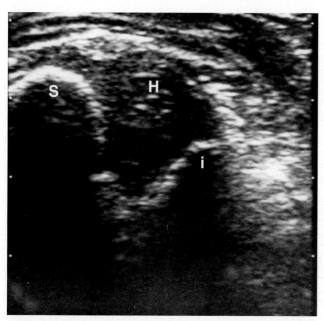

**Figure 23-8** Transverse image/flexion position. On a transverse image made with the patient in the femur flexed 90 degrees, U configuration formed by the femoral shaft (S) and the ischium (i) can be identified (H, femoral head).

## Transverse Scan Plane

In the transverse scan plane, the transducer is rotated 90 degrees from the coronal orientation. The transverse image may also be obtained in a neutral or flexed position; however, current guidelines suggest that the flexion position is adequate.[10] In the transverse/flexion, the image is made from a transverse scan plane with the femur flexed 90 degrees. The transducer may need to be shifted slightly posterolaterally on the infant's hip to obtain the image plane of the femoral shaft and the ischium as they form a U or V configuration around the femoral head (Fig. 23-8).[1] The relationship of the femoral head to the acetabulum should then be observed by performing stress maneuvers, which may include a piston maneuver and/or abduction and adduction. If the hip is abnormal, the femoral head will be positioned away from the ischium and soft tissue echoes will be identified in between. If the hip is dislocated, the U configuration will not be identified. Additionally, the sonographer may be able to observe reduction of the dislocation by abducting the hip. Images should be made of each scan plane with the proper annotation of each stress maneuver. Measurements are not taken in this imaging plane.

## HIP EFFUSION

When young children present with hip pain, the diagnosis can be variable with a range in severity to innocuous to a true emergency. Clinically, patients can present with localized pain, limping or refusal to bear weight, limited movement, and fever.[16] Sonography can evaluate for the presence of a hip effusion and the evaluation of the aspirate of that effusion can differentiate between transient synovitis versus septic arthritis.

Transient synovitis is a relatively common cause of a painful hip in children. It is a self-limiting disease that can be treated with anti-inflammatory medication and rest.[16] Patients may present with a history of a recent upper respiratory infection, although most patients will be afebrile at the time of the onset of hip pain. Once symptoms abate, there are no long-term effects.

Septic arthritis is a serious bacterial infection that can present with more severe clinical symptoms than transient synovitis, but differentiation clinically may be difficult, although children will usually present with a fever. In addition, the patient may have an elevated erythrocyte sedimentation rate and elevated serum white blood cell count. Septic arthritis is considered a medical emergency requiring rapid treatment in order to avoid long-term sequelae including avascular necrosis of the femoral head, osteomyelitis, systemic sepsis, limb-length discrepancy, and osteoarthritis of the hip joint.[17,18] Sonography-guided arthrocentesis is utilized to aspirate the fluid for laboratory evaluation. When septic arthritis is confirmed, it usually leads to hospitalization for intravenous antibiotics. The arthrocentesis can also have the added benefit of providing some pain relief to the child.

## SONOGRAPHIC TECHNIQUE

Patients presenting for sonography-guided arthrocentesis may be placed under general anesthesia or given local anesthesia with sedation. The patient is placed in the supine position with the legs placed in a neutral position. A linear transducer should be utilized and the highest frequency possible. Imaging is performed from the anterior aspect of the leg with the transducer oriented oblique, parallel to the long axis of the femoral neck. A normal hip capsule will usually have a concave appearance and with the presence of an effusion, it bulges outward (Fig. 23-9A,B). The hip capsule is usually 2 to 5 mm in thickness and should be symmetric, so both hips should be imaged for comparison.[19] An abnormal appearance is defined as a capsular thickness of greater than 5 mm or a 2-mm difference between both hips, assuming it is not a bilateral process.[19,20] Once an effusion is identified, sonographic guidance for aspiration may be performed.

## FEMORAL FOCAL DEFICIENCY

Proximal femoral focal deficiency (PFFD) is a rare congenital anomaly involving the proximal femur and the acetabulum. The range of severity of PFFD greatly varies from decreased ossification to absence of the hip joint with significant shortening or absence of the femur. PFFD has been associated with numerous

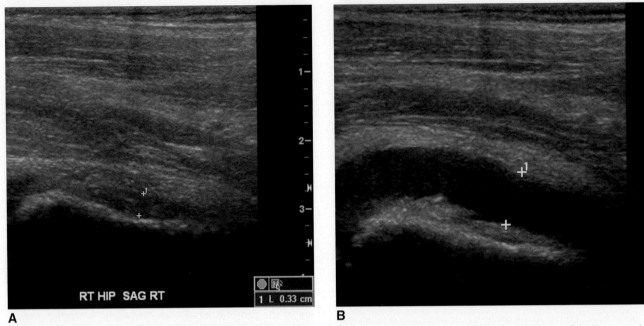

RT HIP  SAG RT

1 L  0.33 cm

A

B

**Figure 23-9** Hip joint capsule. **A:** A longitudinal image demonstrates a normal hip capsule. **B:** This longitudinal image on an afebrile 3-year-old with left sided hip pain shows the left joint capsule with an effusion measuring 7.4 mm in diameter. The patient's right hip capsule was normal.

syndromes.[21,22] Radiographic imaging, sonography, and magnetic resonance imaging (MRI) may be utilized in the evaluation of PFFD. Sonographic evaluation is not definitive but may be able to identify the presence or absence of the femoral head and if the head and shaft are connected.[1]

## DIAGNOSIS AND TREATMENT

### SCREENING

Sonography has become an excellent screening modality for identification of hip dysplasias and other hip joint pathology in infants. There is, however, controversy as to when infants should be screened and which infants should be screened. Clinical screening is available to most newborns, but it does not identify all abnormalities. A sonography screening program appears to identify a number of the abnormalities that may be missed by clinical assessment; however, the cost-effectiveness of a sonography screening program is questioned. The current recommendation is to screen all newborns with physical examination and utilize sonographic assessment for those infants with an abnormal clinical examination and those with a compelling risk factor that would place the infant at increased risk for the development of hip abnormalities.[9] If the sonography examination is scheduled when the infant is 4 to 6 weeks of age, the time lapse provides the opportunity for physiologic laxity to resolve which diminishes the need to require follow-up treatment; however, if the newborn is screened earlier due to an abnormal physical examination, follow up may be required before determining if treatment is necessary.

### FOLLOW-UP

Once an infant has been diagnosed with a hip abnormality of mild instability, subluxation, a dislocatable hip, or frank dislocation, various treatment methods may be utilized depending on the severity of the abnormality. Sonography of the hip may be utilized to follow a borderline hip that will typically become normal within a few weeks without treatment. Treatment plans may include placing the infant in a Pavlik harness, bracing the lower extremities, casting, or surgical reduction. The Pavlik harness, developed by Arnold Pavlik in 1946, is an effective method for treating hip dysplasia in the first 4 months. The Pavlik harness is designed to brace the hip in abduction and flexions so the acetabulum will remodel as the femoral head is placed to rest centered in the acetabular socket. Sonographic evaluation of the treatment progress can be performed with the infant in the harness, it can assist in determining when the harness can be removed, and as follow-up once harness use has been discontinued.[23]

Once the treatment plan is operational, sonography follow-up can be used to confirm the presence of the correct location of the femoral head in the acetabulum. If the infant is in a harness, stress maneuvers should not be performed until the treatment has been completed or unless directed by the referring physician. An infant in a cast can also be monitored in the cast by cutting a window over the lateral aspect of the hip. Sonographic evaluation of an infant in a cast may be unsatisfactory, but when successful can prevent unnecessary radiation.[24] A computed tomography (CT) hip examination may be more accurate and will diminish the chance of increasing mobility by cutting the cast for the sonographic scanning window.

## *Critical Thinking Questions*

1. The 4-month-old infant is referred for sonography examination with a positive Galeazzi sign on the left side. The patient's mother wants to know why sonography rather than radiography of the hip joint was ordered, what the sonographer will be looking for, and if can she stay with her baby during the examination.

2. If an infant is less than 4 months of age is diagnosed with mild–moderate DDH, what is the treatment of choice and follow-up procedure?

3. A 2-year-old boy presents with an elevated temperature. His father said the boy refuses to walk the past day with right-sided hip pain. The sonographer scans both hips and the joint capsule appear to both have a concave appearance. The left hip capsule thickness is 2.4 mm and the right hip capsule thickness is 4.5 mm. Based on the patient's clinical presentation and sonographic appearance, what is the most likely diagnosis?

4. A patient presents with asymmetry of the gluteal folds, leg length discrepancy, and pain. Which of these is considered a late sign or symptom of DDH?

5. When scanning an infant, the sonographer documents a femoral head, which maintain contact with the acetabulum but is not well seated within the hip joint. The acetabulum appears shallow but the femur appears normal. What is the likely diagnosis?

## OTHER IMAGING MODALITIES

In the past, radiographic imaging of the infant hip was widely used. Because the newborn hip is primarily composed of cartilage, the radiograph may fail to identify marginal abnormalities. The radiographic examination is less costly to perform and may be more effective at 6 months and older when the ossification centers are more likely to be evident. Using CT for infant hip imaging is primarily indicated for follow-up rather than screening. It is especially useful, as previously noted, when imaging casted patients.[24] The advantages of using MRI for screening and follow-up includes the fact that it is an excellent modality for identifying musculoskeletal abnormalities and, like sonography, does not use ionizing radiation. The major disadvantages of MRI for screening are that it is expensive and the long examination time requires sedation.

## SUMMARY

- The bones of the hip joint are composed of the pelvic girdle (ilium, ischium, and pubis), the acetabulum, the triradiate cartilage (growth plate), and the femoral head.

- Developmental dysplasia of the hip (DDH), previously known as congenital dysplasia of the hip, describes a range of dysplasia that includes instability, subluxation, and frank dislocation.

- The risk factors of DDH include breech position and delivery position, positive family history, and being swaddled.

- There is a higher incidence of DDH in the first born, females, whites, infants with high birth weights, and native North American populations.

- The Barlow test, Ortolani test, and visual assessment are used to screen for DDH.

- The sonography procedure should include an evaluation of both hips in coronal and transverse scan planes with neutral and flexed patient positions.

- Both the alpha and beta angle can be obtained in the coronal scan plane with a higher reliance on the alpha angle for diagnosis.

- There are four types of hip joint classifications using criteria developed by Graf.

- Sonography assessment of the hip is best performed up to 6 months of age after which time radiography is more reliable due to increasing bony ossification

- Evaluation of both hips is included in the protocol.

- The reproducibility and accuracy of the sonography examination relies on the skill, knowledge, and experience of the sonographer who has performed multiple examinations on both normal and abnormal hips.

## ACKNOWLEDGMENT

The author would like to acknowledge Kelli Gohrs, RDMS, Florida Hospital, Orlando, Florida, for her valuable assistance in gathering images for this chapter.

### REFERENCES

1. Harcke HT, Grissom LE. Pediatric musculoskeletal ultrasound. In: Rumack C, Wilson S, Charboneau J, eds. *Diagnostic Ultrasound.* 3rd ed. Vol II. St. Louis, MO: Elsevier Mosby; 2005:2035–2060.
2. Dogruel H, Atalar H, Yavuz Y, et al. Clinical examination versus ultrasonography in detecting developmental dysplasia of the hip. *Int Orthop.* 2008;32:415–419.
3. Moore KL, Persaud TVN. *Before We Are Born: Essentials of Embryology and Birth Defects.* 6th ed. Philadelphia, PA: Saunders; 2003.
4. Seeley RR, Stephens TD, Tate P. *Anatomy & Physiology.* 8th ed. New York, NY: McGraw-Hill; 2008.
5. Henningsen C. *Clinical Guide to Ultrasonography.* St. Louis, MO: Mosby; 2004.

6. von Kries R, Ihme N, Oberle D, et al. Effect of ultrasound screening on the rate of first operative procedures for developmental hip dysplasia in Germany. *Lancet*. 2003;362:1883–1887.

7. Tegnander A, Holen KJ, Terjesen T. The natural history of hip abnormalities detected by ultrasound in clinically normal newborns: A 6–8 year radiographic follow-up study of 93 children. *Acta Orthop Scand*. 1999;70:335–337.

8. Paton RW, Hinduja K, Thomas CD. The significance of at-risk factors in ultrasound surveillance of developmental dysplasia of the hip. A ten-year prospective study. *J Bone Joint Surg Br*. 2005;87:1264–1266.

9. Committee on Quality Improvement and Subcommittee on Developmental Dysplasia of the Hip. Clinical practice guideline: early detection of developmental dysplasia of the hip. *Pediatrics*. 2000;105:896–905.

10. American Institute of Ultrasound Medicine; American College of Radiology. AIUM practice guideline for the performance of an ultrasound examination for detection and assessment of developmental dysplasia of the hip. *J Ultrasound Med*. 2009;28(1):114–119.

11. Falliner A, Schwinzer D, Hahne HJ, et al. Comparing ultrasound measurements of neonatal hips using the methods of Graf and Terjesen. *J Bone Joint Surg*. 2006;88:104–106.

12. Terjesen T. Ultrasonography for evaluation of hip dysplasia. Methods and policy in neonates, infants, and older children. *Acta Orthop Scand*. 2008;69:653–662.

13. Harcke HT, Grissom LE. Infant hip sonography: current concepts. *Semin Ultrasound*. 1994;15:256–263.

14. Phillips WE II, Burton EM. Ultrasonography of developmental displacement of the infant hip. *Appl Radiol*. 1995;24:25–31.

15. Haggstrom JA, Brown JC, Schroeder BA, et al. Ultrasound in congenital hip disease. Part I—Review of technique. *Nebr Med J*. 1990;75:134–141.

16. Eich GF, Superti-Furga A, Umbricht FS, et al. The painful hip: evaluation of criteria for clinical decision-making. *Eur J Pediatr*. 1999;158:923–928.

17. Givon U, Liberman B, Schindler A, et al. Treatment of septic arthritis of the hip joint by repeated ultrasound-guided aspirations. *J Pediatr Orthop*. 2004;24:266–270.

18. Caird MS, Flynn JM, Leung YL, et al. Factor distinguishing septic arthritis from transient synovitis of the hip in children. *J Bone Joint Surg Am*. 2006;88:1251–1257.

19. Zabala VA. The role of ultrasound in the diagnosis of joint hip effusions in small children. *JDMS*. 2000;16:73–75.

20. Tsung JW, Blaivas M. Emergency department diagnosis of pediatric hip effusion and guided arthrocentesis using point-of-care ultrasound. *J Emerg Med*. 2008;35:393–399.

21. Filly AL, Robnett-Filly B, Filly RA. Syndromes with focal femoral deficiency: strengths and weaknesses of prenatal sonography. *J Ultrasound Med*. 2004;23:1511–1516.

22. Bernaerts A, Pouillon M, De Ridder K, et al. Value of magnetic resonance imaging in early assessment of proximal femoral focal deficiency (PFFD). *JBR-BTR*. 2006;89:325–327.

23. Carmichael KD, Longo A, Yngve D, et al. The use of ultrasound to determine timing of Pavlik harness discontinuation in treatment of developmental dysplasia of the hip. *Orthopedics*. 2008;31:1–5.

24. van Douveren FQ, Pruijs HE, Sakkers RJ, et al. Ultrasound in the management of the position of the femoral head during treatment in a spica cast after reduction of hip dislocation in developmental dysplasia of the hip. *J Bone Joint Surg*. 2003;85:117–120.

## 24 Organ Transplantation

Kevin D. Evans

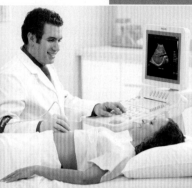

### OBJECTIVES

Describe each part of the comprehensive patient history including laboratory values and medications and its importance in evaluating the patient with an organ transplantation.

Describe the clinical presentations, pathologies, and sequelae leading to the need for an organ transplantation.

Differentiate between organ donations from a living donor or one harvested from a cadaver.

Illustrate the most common surgical placements for the renal, pancreas, and liver allografts with a rationale for each location.

Correlate the sonography evaluation of a transplant patient to include the gray scale parenchymal echogenicity, Doppler data, and medical complications associated with pathology or rejection.

Demonstrate completing a diagnostic sonography examination on patients with a renal, pancreas, and/or liver transplant.

Discuss other procedures used to evaluate patients with organ transplants.

### KEY TERMS

allograft | Doppler | heterotopically | histocompatibility | perfusion

### GLOSSARY

**allograft** graft transplanted between genetically non-identical individuals of the same species

**histocompatibility** the state of a donor and recipient sharing a sufficient number of histocompatibility

antigens so an allograft is accepted and remains functional

**immunosuppressive medication** pharmaceutical agents prescribed to prevent or decrease the immune response

**A**lthough the sonographic evaluation of transplanted organs may have become a common sonography examination, truly understanding the diagnostic information is still evolving. As with many sonography examinations, a holistic approach is needed to ensure that the data acquired is placed in context with the many other pieces of diagnostic information obtained on these patients.

## COMPREHENSIVE PATIENT HISTORY

A paramount activity, prior to conducting a sonographic examination on a patient with a transplanted organ, is to obtain a very comprehensive patient history. In order to accomplish this activity on a hospitalized patient, it will require access to the patient's electronic medical record so that a thorough search can be conducted to gather information, such as the origin of the native organ disease, site of transplantation, preexisting malignancy or infections, and any other medical issues that could impact the activity of the organ.[1] This is a similar activity for a patient who has already been discharged from the hospital and is returning with a change in their health. Typically, these patients provide an extensive oral history, which needs to be checked against the medical record for accuracy.

An additional piece needed in the diagnostic puzzle is the review of current clinical laboratory values with a focus on the typically most sensitive tests[2] (Table 24-1). It is also advised to consult the record for information on the patient's immune status and any pathology reports that might be available.

As with conducting any sonography examination, it is imperative to spend time evaluating the previous imaging studies in order to form a diagnostic baseline for the current study to be performed. Often, Doppler information and the gray scale dimensions of the transplanted organ can provide important formative information while new information is being gathered. The interpreting physician's reports, the postoperative notes, and the transplant surgeon's diagrams cumulatively provide the background material that can prove to be invaluable during the sonographic examination as it will expedite the time spent in examination.

Patients are usually very good about self-reporting their medications, and although valuable to the interpreting physician, this information needs to be verified against the medical record. Most patients will be taking some amount of immunosuppressive medication, with the most common being cyclosporine A (CsA), sirolimus (Rapamycin), or tacrolimus (Prograf), and patients are often taking some accompanying levels of steroids.[2] These drugs must be closely monitored to ensure that they are providing the proper protection since lower levels lead to rejection and higher levels can contribute to toxicity. High-pressure liquid chromatography is considered to be the current gold standard for obtaining quantitative levels for the drugs.[2] Certainly, these values can be important to the referring physician who has to assemble all the diagnostic information to adjust the patient's treatment plan.

The comprehensive patient history can assist the sonographer in obtaining and in evaluating the images and Doppler data. Sonography of the transplanted organ is a key part of the diagnostic workup and is a vital part of a holistic plan of action in determining the proper medical course of action.

## CLINICAL PRESENTATION

The patient diagnosed with chronic renal failure is likely undergoing some form of dialysis to reduce nitrogen-containing wastes that have accumulated in the blood stream. A failure to clear nitrogen-containing wastes from the body results in increased blood urea and creatinine. This condition is referred to as *uremia*. Uremia has a toxic effect on many different body systems such as the gastrointestinal and nervous systems and causes the skin to take on a yellow color and causes itching. These physical manifestations are a combination of uremia and developing anemia in the patient. The inability to synthesize erythropoietin, which governs the production of red blood cells, results in the development of anemia.[3] Either hemodialysis three times a week or peritoneal dialysis, which is often done at home at night, should assist the patient in reducing uremia and anemia; however, the process is very hard on the cardiovascular system.[4]

A patient suffering from cirrhosis, and its poor prognosis, is one condition that leads to liver transplantation.[5] A patient is deemed a candidate for liver transplantation when their underlying disease becomes so threatening that the risk of surgery is less than the continued life expectancy with the native liver. The 1-year survival rate for a liver transplant patient is 87% and the 1-year graft survival rate is 80.3%.[1] The causes for liver failure and ultimate transplantation are hepatitis C, alcoholic liver disease, and cryptogenic cirrhosis.[1] Those patients with metastatic cancer, active substance abuse, sepsis, and compromised cardiac function are not typical candidates for a liver allograft.[1] Patients with portal vein thrombosis are considered high risk because it complicates the surgical procedure and results in lower survival rates.

Uncontrolled diabetes manifests in a variety of pathologies, and many type I diabetics are more likely to seek pancreatic allografts. Since diabetics are at risk for chronic renal failure, there is a tendency to advocate for a dual transplant of a kidney and pancreas. A simultaneous pancreas and kidney transplant (SPK) is reportedly 85% successful, whereas a pancreas following a renal transplant (PAK) diminishes to only 78% effective, and a pancreas transplant alone (PTA) is only 77% effective.[2]

## SURGICAL PLACEMENT

The orientation of the transplanted organ anatomy or allograft is very often dictated by the medical condition of the patient at the time of surgical implantation. The term *allograft* is defined as graft transplanted between genetically nonidentical individuals of the same species.[6] The medical condition of the allograft recipient can vary according to the severity of their underlying disease.

There are two types of organ donations: either a living donor or one harvested from a cadaver. The benefits of matching donor and recipient are that both the

| TABLE | 24-1 |
| --- | --- |

**Sensitive Clinical Laboratory Tests[2]**

| Entity | Laboratory Test |
| --- | --- |
| Kidney | Creatinine |
| Liver | Gamma-glutamyl transferase (GGT) |
| | Alanine aminotransferase (ALT) |
| | Aspartate aminotransferase (AST) |
| Pancreas | Amylase |
| | Lipase |
| | Blood glucose |
| Inflammation | Cytokines |
| | Chemokines |

cellular and humoral rejection pathways can be suppressed. The use of immunosuppression drugs is necessary to avoid these cellular pathways; however, they do not protect the recipient from fungal, viral, and other infections.[2] The postsurgical risks for infection is coupled with the challenge to regulate the immunosuppressive drugs to achieve an optimal balance for the patient.

## RENAL ALLOGRAFT

The renal allograft is surgically implanted in a superficial placement in either the right or left lower abdomen.[4] Although the renal allograft can be placed transperitoneal or intraperitoneal, the surgical preference is an extraperitoneal placement, which is usually in the right iliac fossa.[7] Compared to the left iliac fossa, the right iliac fossa is nearer to major vessels and the urinary bladder. If the transplanted kidney is placed heterotopically, it means a right kidney is transplanted in the left iliac fossa or a left kidney is transplanted in the right iliac fossa.[7]

En block is a type of harvesting that preserves cadaveric ureters, main renal arteries and veins, segments of the suprarenal and infrarenal arteries and veins, as well as segments of the aorta and inferior vena cava (IVC).[1] In the case of a cadaveric transplant with a donor renal artery and a portion of the aorta, the multiple donor arteries are anastomosed end-to-side to the external iliac artery using a Carrel patch.[1,7,8] In the case of a living donor transplant harvested with only the main renal artery, the artery is anastomosed either end-to-end to the internal iliac artery or end-to-side to the recipient external iliac artery[7] (Fig. 24-1). Hilar fat and adventitia surrounding the ureter is harvested to maximize the blood supply to these areas.[1] The ureter is implanted directly into the superolateral wall of the bladder via ureteroneocystostomy.[1] The ureter can also be joined to the native ipsilateral ureter, otherwise known as an *ureteroureterostomy*.[8] Although the health of the recipient is of primary concern, it is also important to be aware of any intrinsic pathology that might be passed on from the donor and donated tissue.

## PANCREATIC ALLOGRAFT

The pancreatic allograft is implanted as a whole organ and placed either in the pelvis or the upper abdomen. In the pelvis, the pancreatic allograft is oriented vertically and the arterial anastomosis is made with the iliac artery. The donor's portal vein is sewn into the external iliac vein and a stump of the donor's duodenum is inserted so that it empties into the recipient's urinary bladder.[1] In the upper abdomen, the pancreatic allograft is oriented diagonally and this placement puts donor's portal vein attached to the recipient's superior mesenteric vein (SMV). The donor's duodenal stump is sutured into the recipient's jejunum, which is much like a Roux-en-Y gastric bypass procedure.[1]

## LIVER ALLOGRAFT

The surgery for a liver allograft is quite complex as it requires that four vascular connections be made as well as a biliary anastomosis for proper perfusion and drainage. The hepatic artery is typically anastomosed by either suturing in the donor's celiac artery to the recipient's split right and left hepatic or at the branch point of the gastroduodenal and proper hepatic arteries.[1] In some cases, an interposition graft must be used to hook the donated celiac axis directly into the recipient's aorta.

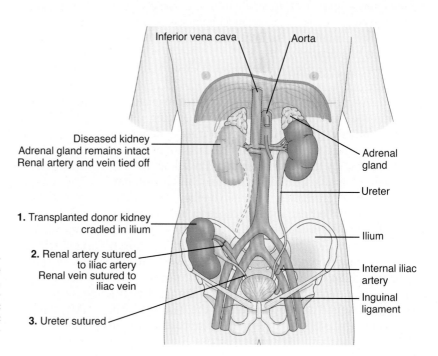

**Figure 24-1** Renal transplantation. The illustration shows the diseased kidney, which may be removed with the renal artery and vein tied off. The transplanted kidney is placed in the iliac fossa. The donor renal artery is sutured to the iliac artery, the donor renal vein is sutured to the iliac vein, and the donor ureter is sutured to the superolateral urinary bladder wall of the recipient.

Inferior vena cava

Aorta

Diseased kidney
Adrenal gland remains intact
Renal artery and vein tied off

Adrenal gland

Ureter

1. Transplanted donor kidney cradled in ilium

2. Renal artery sutured to iliac artery
Renal vein sutured to iliac vein

Ilium

Internal iliac artery

Inguinal ligament

3. Ureter sutured

The donated portal vein is end-to-end anastomosed to the recipient's portal vein. In the situation of a portal vein thrombosis, a jump graft may be needed in order to unite the vessels around the area of thrombosis.

The IVC is transected above and below the donated liver so that these vascular connections can be made with an end-to-end anastomosis with the native IVC. Additional surgical techniques, such as a side-to-side or an end-to-side connection between the donor IVC and the recipient's IVC, are connections that are likely made between the donor's IVC and the stump of the recipient's hepatic veins.

The donor's bile duct can be united with the recipient's biliary system by an end-to-end anastomosis after the gallbladder has been removed. A T tube can be left in place for those patients that have a diseased biliary tree. Those with advanced biliary disease may need a choledochojejunostomy.

This type of allograft is typically provided as a result of a cadaver donation; however, living donations are sometimes made. These partial donations involve a right hepatectomy for segments V, VI, VII, and VIII along with the right hepatic vein.[1] But, regardless of the donation source, the anastomotic connections must be carefully interrogated to ensure that the vascular connections are not stenotic and provide adequate perfusion to the allograft.

## ALLOGRAFT PHYSIOLOGY

The renal allograft has an average life span of 7 to 10 years; however, this is increased for those who receive a living donor organ to a life span expectancy between 15 and 20 years of function.[1,8] Upon transplantation, the renal allograft experiences a margin of hypertrophy of up to 15% in size within the first 2 weeks postsurgically. It also is expected to increase in volume by 40% and maintain its final size and shape about 6 months postoperatively.[1]

Pancreatic allografts have a reported survival of 95% at 1 year and have decreasing percentages of acute rejection. As many as 80% of pancreatic transplant recipients are freed from insulin injections after 1 year postoperatively.[1] Postoperative monitoring of active rejection is necessary along with increased immunosuppressive therapy to avert ischemia of the allograft.[9]

Liver allografts should begin functioning immediately and the normal flow anticipated in the hepatic artery is a rapid acceleration of less than 100 msec. The flow should be continuous throughout diastole with a resistive index (RI) between 0.5 and 0.7.[10] The portal vein will have hepatopetal flow into the liver and may appear turbulent. Additionally, the hepatic veins should demonstrate their expected phasic flow that crosses the Doppler baseline due to changes in the cardiac cycle. Assessing perfusion and determining the patency of the IVC is an important factor in predicting the success of the liver transplant procedure.

## LABORATORY TEST RESULTS

Renal allografts can be monitored in conjunction with imaging by analyzing biomarkers. The two most often monitored during acute rejection are increased levels of blood urea nitrogen (BUN) and creatinine. Alongside these lab tests, the electrolytes for the patient need to be closely monitored for changes. If the rejection episode progresses, the laboratory values for BUN and creatinine will also continue to escalate.[11] A glomerular filtration rate (GRF) can be derived for a kidney transplant, and careful evaluation is needed when the values drop below 10 rnl/rnin.[12] A successful renal allograft should have a GFR value of between 50 and 60 mL/hr.[12]

The pancreatic allograft provides exocrine secretions of amylase, lipase, and anodal trypsinogen into the bladder, which help to provide biomarkers of acute acinar cellular injury. Elevated levels of amylase and lipase are indicative of inflammation.[11] An increase in parenchymal water content is associated with rejection and is thought to be related to a swelling in overall allograft size.[13] Blood glucose also provides a measure of endocrine function.

The liver allograft should be monitored for function with biomarkers that are typically used for a native liver. The allograft is expected to function at an optimal level and any decrease in function may be an indicator of tissue ischemia. Sonographic evaluation of the vascular patency of the liver allograft is indicated due to abnormal liver function biomarkers.

## SONOGRAPHIC ANATOMY

### RENAL ALLOGRAFT

The renal allograft must be evaluated sonographically for its size and overall echogenicity. The gray scale images that are chosen for inclusion in the patient's record should demonstrate the echogenicity of the cortex as well as the renal sinus. The normal sonographic appearance of the renal cortex is hypoechoic with prominent medullary pyramids that are anechoic. The thickness and the qualitative assessment of the renal allograft cortex will be highly relevant for gauging the potential for rejection and possible ischemia of the tissue. Because the cortex is the primary site for urine production, close attention needs to be paid to this area of the allograft. The renal allograft sinus is normally hyperechoic and contains the hilum for vascular insertion as well as the pelvis for urine excretion. Depending on the stage of transplantation, small amounts of fluid can be visualized within the renal pelvis, especially immediately after the postoperative period. If there is confusion when identifying vessels versus the ureteropelvic junction, power Doppler is a good tool to clarify the anatomic difference. Color and power Doppler are the primary tools for the evaluation of the renal transplant and facilitate a rapid assessment of global renal artery perfusion and venous patency.[10] Current technology allows for

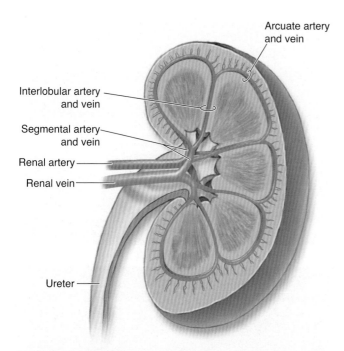

Arcuate artery and vein

Interlobular artery and vein

Segmental artery and vein

Renal artery

Renal vein

Ureter

**Figure 24-2** Vascular assessment. Doppler evaluation of the renal allograft includes the renal sinus and renal cortex as well as the segmental, interlobar, and arcuate arteries with the corresponding veins.

definitive visualization of the main, anterior, and posterior divisions of the renal artery and vein. Additionally, within the renal sinus and cortex, Doppler allows for the assessment of the segmental, interlobar, and arcuate arteries with the corresponding veins (Fig. 24-2).

The normal renal allograft has a low-resistance vascular bed, which is characterized by streamlined systolic flow and continuous forward flow during diastole. The normal main renal artery has a velocity that ranges between 80 and 118 cm/sec.[10] As mentioned earlier, the renal allograft will be expected to increase in size during the postsurgical period. Resolution of any fluid collections adjacent to the renal allograft should be carefully documented as these have the potential to compress vital arterial flow to the allograft or venous drainage from the allograft.

## PANCREATIC ALLOGRAFT

The sonographic appearance of the pancreatic allograft is very similar in echogenicity to the native pancreas (Fig. 24-3A). The transplant is surgically placed either vertically in the right lower quadrant or diagonally in the

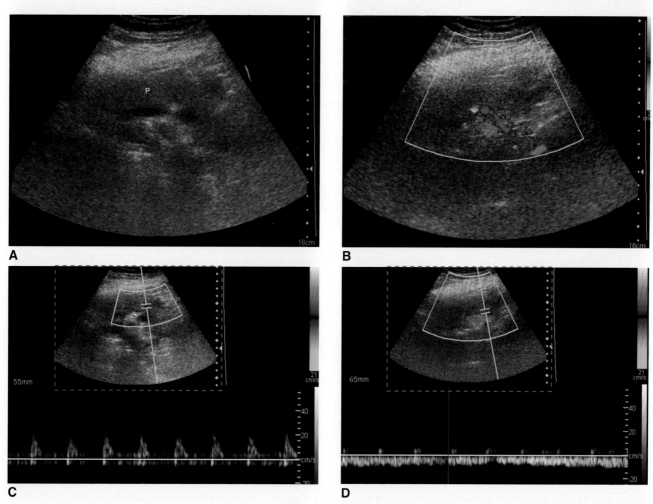

**Figure 24-3 A:** Gray scale evaluation. The longitudinal image of the normal pancreas (P) transplant located in the pelvis shows normal echogenicity similar to a native pancreas. **B:** Color Doppler evaluation. The longitudinal section of the pancreas demonstrates vascular patency and perfusion of the allograft. **C,D:** Spectral Doppler evaluation. The images of the transplanted pancreas sonograms documents both **(C)** the presence of arterial flow and **(D)** venous patency.

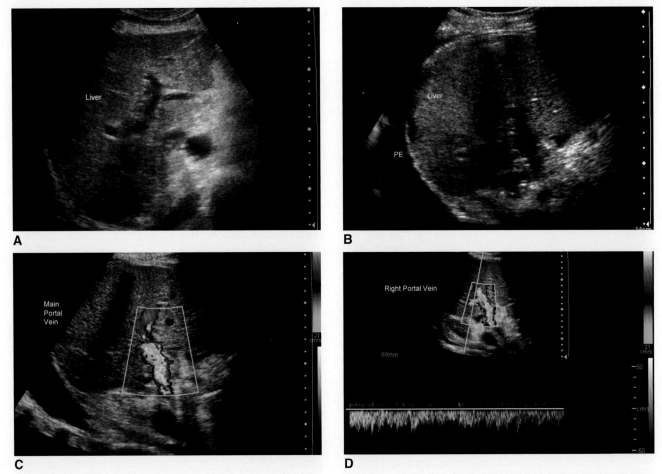

**Figure 24-4 A,B:** Gray scale liver allograft. The echogenicity of the transplanted liver is similar to the native liver. **A:** The longitudinal image is obtained on a liver allograft transplanted 8 days previously. **B:** The transverse image of the liver allograft demonstrates normal echogenicity on a patient with an associated right pleural effusion *(PE)*. **C–F:** Evaluation of portal triad vessels. **C:** Color Doppler images of turbulent main portal vein of a liver allograft. **D:** Spectral Doppler tracing of the forward flow into the right branch of the portal vein. *(continued)*

upper abdomen for enteric drainage into the portal vein. Regardless of placement, patency of the vasculature associated with the transplanted pancreas is important to assure proper perfusion of the tissue (Fig. 24-3B). The arterial and venous flow should be carefully documented to determine the potential for resistance. Spectral Doppler should document monophasic venous flow and low-resistant arterial waveforms (Fig. 24-3C,D). The pancreatic duct should also be visualized to ensure that pancreatic digestive enzymes and juices are being generated and are flowing out of the allograft. Extra pancreatic fluid collections should be carefully monitored. Again, documentation of fluid collections adjacent to the pancreatic allograft has the potential to compress the vascular flow directed into and out of the organ. Bowel gas in the abdomen or pelvis limits the evaluation of the area around the pancreatic allograft.

## LIVER ALLOGRAFT

The transplanted liver is in many ways similar in echogenicity to the normal healthy liver (Fig. 24-4A,B). The portal triad of the portal vein, hepatic artery, and bile duct must be carefully documented to ensure that the surgical anastomosis between the allograft and the native vasculature is patent (Fig. 24-4C–F). Additionally, the hepatic veins must also be evaluated to ensure that they are patent and flowing in the correct direction and draining into the IVC (Fig. 24-4G,H). Doppler tracings of the hepatic artery, portal vein, and hepatic veins are necessary to ensure that proper perfusion of the allograft is accomplished. Angle correction of the Doppler cursor to ≤60 degrees is necessary in order to capture accurate and reproducible spectral tracings of the flow in the segments of vessels interrogated. The sonographic evaluation of the liver allograft is very dependent on the documentation of flow in the intrahepatic and extrahepatic vessels. Often, if patency and correct direction of flow is not demonstrated, the patient will have more invasive vascular studies and/or will return to the surgical suite. Since narrowing or occlusions within the vasculature are a risk, careful interrogation at points both inside and outside of the liver allograft need to be made. The portal vein should be sampled in both the main, right, and left branches to ensure hepatopetal flow. Due to the importance of these measurements,

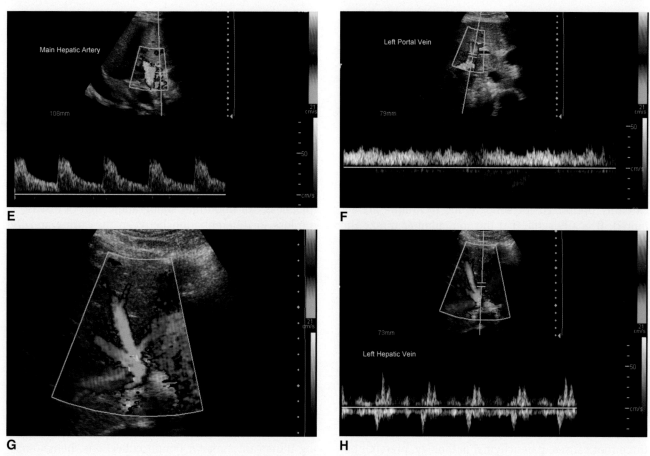

**Figure 24-4** *(continued)* **E:** Spectral Doppler tracing of the main hepatic artery perfusing the liver allograft. **F:** Spectral Doppler tracing of the left portal vein with forward flow into the left lobe of the allograft. Evaluation of hepatic veins. **G:** Color Doppler evaluation of the hepatic veins within the liver allograft. **H:** Spectral tracing of the turbulent flow within the left hepatic vein in the liver allograft.

careful use of the sonographic equipment is required to provide quick and accurate results.

## SONOGRAPHIC TECHNIQUE AND ASSESSMENT

Since the placement of the renal/pancreatic allograft is in the iliac fossa of the lower abdominal quadrant, a 3- to 6-MHz curvilinear transducer with an adjustable bandwidth frequency will provide high-resolution images. The liver transplant is a much more difficult investigation on those patients who are at a fresh stage, postoperatively. These patients are heavily bandaged, and many times the only area for contact scanning with a transducer is below the rib cage. On occasion, bandages can be adjusted to provide an intercostal space for sonographic investigation of the liver and associate vessels.

All three primary transplanted organs (renal, pancreas, and liver) will require the use of Doppler to generate both quantitative and qualitative information on the perfusion of the allograft. Again, a 3- to 6-MHz transducer that can provide duplex scanning will facilitate the interrogation of vessels at specific locations throughout the transplanted tissue. All Doppler interrogation needs to be angle corrected to ≤60 degrees

so that the quantitative values can be compared and reproduced. Attention to detail for each gray scale image and Doppler waveform is required, such that image optimization needs to be a primary concern. At the end of scanning, most sonographic equipment allows the sonographer to complete postprocessing of images, which can ensure a quality image or volume clip was acquired. Often, spectral waveforms are set up to be autocalculated, and this needs to be carefully scrutinized to ensure that proper waveforms have been selected by the software for analysis. It is advisable to consider manual calculation for those waveforms that appear to have been neglected or disregarded by the software during autocalculation. The precision demanded by these studies requires that the sonographer and sonologist carefully review all images and data generated for each and every patient in the laboratory.

Each selected sonographic image needs to be carefully labeled for the anatomy and vessel being imaged and the orientation of the transducer. The use of Doppler measurements taken at varied segments of the vasculature will require proper annotation such that the sonologist and subsequent sonographers can be assured that the data was taken from discrete locations within the allograft and the supporting vessels. Again, a key component to these studies is accuracy and reproducibility, and this includes proper annotation of the images selected by the sonographer. Ultimately, these images and Doppler tracings will be used as a guide for subsequent follow-up examinations throughout the life of the allograft.

## RENAL ALLOGRAFT

### Gray Scale

Evaluation of the renal allograft is highly dependent on the representative images presented to the sonologist for interpretation. High-quality images that have been carefully optimized for sonographic technique are required. It is advisable that the sonographer utilize the width of the frequency bandwidth to ensure proper penetration of the allograft and surrounding pelvic anatomy. Since the renal allograft has a more superficial position in the lower abdomen/pelvis, it has a more reflective quality than what is normally encountered with the native kidney. This may require postprocessing of the image to achieve a suitable presentation. Allografts tend to have an appearance much like a pediatric renal study with the noted prominence of the renal pyramids within the cortex. This can give an erroneous, false-positive appearance of a dilated collecting system (Fig. 24-5A,B). Sonographic documented abnormities in the renal allograft are associated diagnostically with three root causes: parenchymal pathology, prerenal pathology, and postrenal complications.[1,8]

It is difficult to detect the early stages of parenchymal pathology, within the cortex of the allograft, as acute accelerated rejection (AAR) and acute tubular necrosis (ATN) both appear the same sonographically. Both AAR and ATN cause subtle changes in the dimensions of the allograft. Color Doppler is also not very helpful in the early stages of these two pathologies.[1] What can be noticed at an early stage in the parenchyma is focal regions of cortical hypoechoic spaces that are indicative of edema and possible necrosis of the tissue.[10] The pyramids can appear to be prominent, but this is rather nonspecific and some swelling of the cortex adds to its thickness. An important sonographic sign of disease is the loss in differentiation between the cortex and the medullary sinus. This blending of the echogenicity of these tissues has also been seen as a result of nephrotoxicity from CsA. Chronic rejection is associated with a loss of renal allograft function after 3 months. The kidney begins to atrophy, and interstitial fibrosis becomes noticeable sonographically. This atrophy of the tissue is believed to be a result of recurrent episodes of acute rejection. The allograft can be measured from the sonogram and compared to previous studies; however, a biopsy is needed to confirm the diagnosis.[8]

Prerenal pathologies are most often fluid collections or other entities that cause compression of the vascular flow to the renal allograft. In the early stages following transplant surgery, lymph collections, hematomas, or even urinomas can create a mass effect that occludes

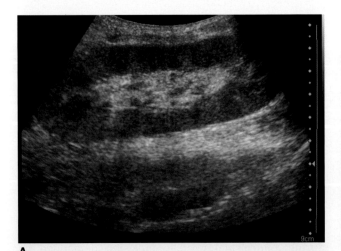

A

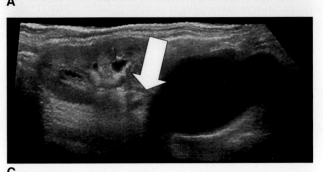

C

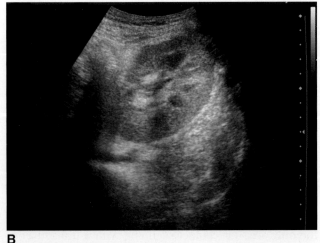

B

**Figure 24-5** Gray scale evaluation. The sonographic evaluation of a renal allograft uses **(A)** a transverse transducer orientation to obtain a longitudinal image and **(B)** a longitudinal transducer orientation to obtain a transverse image. The superficial surgical placement of the renal allograft allows for visualizing prominent renal pyramids within the cortex. **C:** Lymphocele. A large lymphocele poses an obstruction to the vasculature and ureter of the renal allograft. The *white arrow* indicates the "mass effect" compressing the renal artery, vein, and ureter. (Image courtesy of General Electric HealthCare, Inc, Milwaukee, WI.)

blood flow to and from the organ. Fluid collections can either naturally resolve or be drained to relieve the pressure and help to restore vascular perfusion (Fig. 24-5C). More information on these entities is presented in the Allograft Pathology and Rejection section in this chapter.

Postrenal complications are intrinsic or extrinsic lesions that result in the obstruction of the ureter and prevent urine drainage from the allograft. Some of the previously presented fluid collections can also cause compression of the ureter and can cause hydronephrosis within the transplant. Again, the mass effect needs to be removed in order to restore normal urine flow to the bladder.

## Doppler

Color and power Doppler are very helpful in identifying arteries and veins within the renal allograft as well as global perfusion within the cortex[14] (Fig. 24-6A). Likewise, color or power Doppler is extremely helpful in

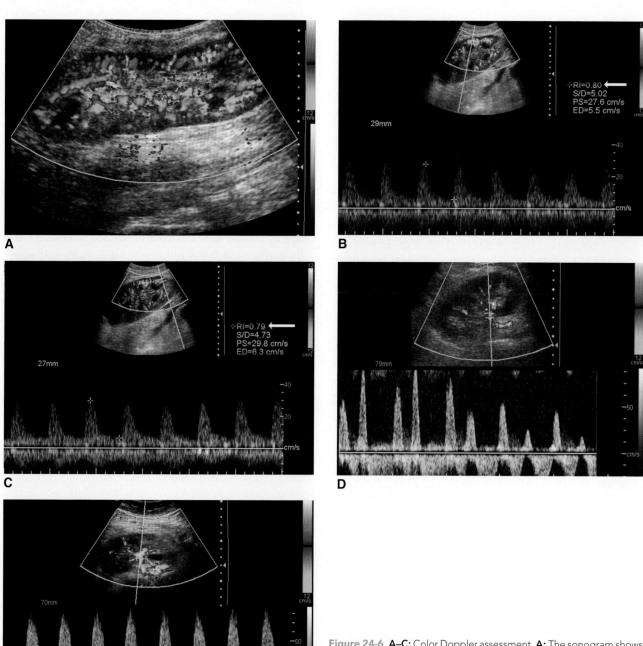

**Figure 24-6  A–C:** Color Doppler assessment. **A:** The sonogram shows the normal vasculature and cortical perfusion within the renal allograft. **B:** A spectral tracing is seen of the midportion of a lobular artery in a renal allograft with the RI ≤0.80 (arrow). **C:** A spectral tracing on this patient in the lower portion of a lobular artery in a renal allograft with the RI ≤0.80 (arrow). **D,E:** Quantitative documentation of rejection. **D:** The spectral Doppler tracing documents a highly resistant renal artery in the hilum of the allograft. **E:** On this patient, the spectral Doppler tracing displays a steep spectral peak and spectral broadening.

detecting areas that lack perfusion and could indicate areas of early ischemia.[1]

Spectral interrogation of the renal allograft has been an evolving diagnostic tool, and benchmarking for spectral data points is strengthened by continued published research. Spectral tracings of the interlobar arteries should be obtained from the upper, mid, and lower portion of the allograft with a low-filter setting, maximum gain, and a small velocity scale to profile the spectral peak. An RI $\leq 0.8$ and/or a pulsatility index (PI) $\leq 1.5$ have been suggested as normal parameter for diagnostic purposes[10] (Fig. 24-6B,C). Published research has posed morphologic indicators for spectral Doppler to document a rejection episode[10] (Pathology Box 24-1, Fig. 24-6D,E). Quantitatively, spectral Doppler information can be compared to published clinical guidelines that can help to suggest that the allograft is undergoing a rejection episode. An RI that is $\geq 0.9$ and/or a PI that is $\geq 1.8$ are regarded as an abnormal finding.[10]

Recent research conducted in Europe with pulse inversion imaging (PII) and contrast media was done to assess the function of the cortical perfusion of an allograft suspected of acute rejection.[15,16] These studies adjusted the overall power to low diagnostic levels and then after bolus injection, assessed the cortex with increased overall power and the shattering of microbubbles in the contrast. This revealed detailed information about the cellular activity of the allograft. Dynamic ability to determine the rate at which contrast clearance was obtained gave functional information about the transplanted organ. The levels of evidence provided by these studies point to the progression of using sonography to document pathology at the level of the glomerulus. It is hoped these techniques could someday be approved for use in the United States.

## PANCREATIC ALLOGRAFT

The pancreas is difficult to evaluate due to its placement in the body and the amount of bowel gas encountered while scanning. Color and power Doppler can be very helpful in identifying the vasculature and obtaining spectral tracings. As with any transplanted organ, it is important to determine whether there is reversal of flow and if all the tissue is adequately perfused. Sonographic

information should be paired with medical laboratory testing to present a complete picture of the health of the allograft. An RI of 0.7 has been published as a clinical guide to suggest possible acute pancreatic allograft rejection.[10] Interestingly, a study conducted by Wong et al.[9] used biopsy specimens to confirm that acute rejection in selected pancreatic allografts were best suggested by using gray scale images that demonstrated a heterogeneous echotexture and an overall increase in graft size.[9] Although rigorous, the research is limited by the number of patients studied so biopsy results on a larger number of pancreatic allografts would assist in establishing these sonographic features as a clinical benchmark.

## LIVER ALLOGRAFT

The liver allograft should have a native liver sonographic appearance with minimal fluid collections surrounding the organ. These fluid collections should resolve within 7 to 10 days postoperatively. The biliary system should have a normal appearance with the measurements following those guidelines established for a postcholecystectomy patient. The anastomosis of the common bile duct should be carefully scrutinized in order to ensure that a stricture has not developed and biliary obstruction will not ensue. Gray scale evaluation of the caliber of the common bile duct and wall thickness can be important diagnostic indicators.

## ALLOGRAFT PATHOLOGY AND REJECTION

Human lymphocytic antigens (HLAs) are broken into three classifications, each located on chromosome 6, which must be matched between donor and recipient in order to prolong allograft survival.[1] This process leads to measuring histocompatibility. The timing for surgery is also important as it allows the donated tissue to be warm and functional, ideally 24 to 48 hours after harvest. Cold transplanted renal tissue will often require dialysis to encourage function of the newly implanted allograft.[10]

### RENAL ALLOGRAFT

#### Parenchymal Pathology

Acute accelerated, acute, and chronic rejection are general terms, which should be considered imprecise as the terms are not well suited to categorize patients for diagnosis and treatment. These terms are best used to represent a continuum of assaults that affect the parenchyma and longevity of a renal allograft.

The condition known as *acute accelerated rejection* (AAR), or hyperacute, should not occur if proper steps have been made to ensure major histocompatibility (MHC) between the donor and the recipient.[17]

Circulating antibodies prior to transplantation are available and can cause an immediate rejection at the vascular level. Graft rejection during surgery in the pre-sensitized patient causes a series of vascular reactions, which are widespread. AAR begins with acute arteritis and arteriolitis and leads to massive vessel thrombosis and ischemic necrosis due to the binding of humoral antibodies. All arteries and arterioles exhibit acute necrosis as a result of binding to humoral antibodies. To minimize the potential for AAR, it is vital to adhere to rigorous preadmission testing, crossmatch, and typing of HLA, thereby avoiding antibodies that can develop against the donor's lymphocytes. AAR has become less of a concern due to the histocompatibility testing, and as a result it occurs in less than 0.4% of transplants.[1,5] Heart and liver transplants become available on a very emergent basis; therefore, the same level of histocompatibility testing cannot be accomplished, which results in a higher percentage of HLA rejection in the emergent types of transplants.

The early necrosis of the cortical filtration system, referred to as *acute tubular necrosis* (ATN), is most often detected within the first few days after transplantation of the allograft. ATN can be reduced by allowing the patient to undergo dialysis to assist the allograft to achieve maximal function. ATN has been noted in 10% to 30% of transplanted patients and is often attributed to the transplantation of cold preserved tissue.[12] The process "delayed graft function," which includes ATN, describes diminished activity and a variety of clinical problems.[17] Distinguishing between an acute rejection episode (AR) and ATN is difficult clinically as symptoms and signs of AR are rare while ATN has been commonly noted in cadaveric grafts[1] (Fig. 24-7A–C).

The next phase of concern has been labeled acute rejection (AR) and it typically occurs in 40% of patients from the first to third week posttransplantation (Fig. 24-7D–F). AR is believed to be manifest due to activity from cellular and humoral/antibody pathways.[1,12] The cellular pathway of AR encompasses rejection that is attributed to tubule-interstitial rejection, transplant endarteritis, and transplant glomerulitis. The humoral/antibody pathway of AR is believed to cause fibrinoid arterial wall necrosis and rare forms of AAR.[17] A transplant biopsy is indicated in order to histologically classify the cause of a suspected rejection episode. The treatment to reverse AR is accomplished by utilizing high doses of steroids or antibody therapy. Flu-like symptoms, fever, and malaise, along with graft tenderness, are some of the reported symptoms by patients who are undergoing an AR episode.[1] In these cases, the patient's symptoms are not specific enough to indicate AR as a potential for renal disease and can be manifest due to an allograft's "previous life."

These two pathways that contribute to AR are not sharply divided and work together to reject the donation of the transplanted organ. The cellular pathway is based on activity that occurs within a period of 10 to 14 days. During this time, mononuclear cells infiltrate and invade, causing edema and parenchymal damage. Further damage is created at the cellular level by these mononuclear cells, which further permeate into the glomerulus and peritubular capillaries, which begins to cause focal tubular necrosis. The antibody pathway is also actively engaged and contributes to rejection more than was previously believed. Humoral antibodies react and cause narrowing of the arterioles, which results in infarction or renal cortical atrophy. These resulting lesions resemble arteriosclerotic thickening.[1,2] Specific antibodies are identified as the instigators of tissue rejection. CD4 and CD8 are two specific antibodies that work in tandem to activate separate processes that result in a rejection of the allograft.[2] The immune complex is activated by requiring T cell activation and that is caused by both CD4 and CD8. A direct recognition of foreign tissue is made by CD8, which unites with T cells to lysis the allograft cells through the vascular membrane. This allows direct attack on the renal parenchyma and is considered an antigen class I process.[2] An indirect recognition of the donated tissue is made by CD4, which unites with B lymphocytes to attack the allograft with an aggressive macrophage. This process increases vascular permeability and allows more mononuclear cells to collect and results in cellular death. This indirect attack through the permeability of mononuclear cells is classified as an antigen class II process.[2]

The life of an allograft is jeopardized by episodes of rejection, and these bouts are conceptualized as a continuum of infiltration that moves from AR to a more chronic condition that results in sclerosed renal cortical tissue. The sclerosing renal cortical tissue ends in a diagnosis of chronic allograft rejection (CR). CR is theorized to culminate in the loss of function in the renal parenchyma due to the aforementioned mononuclear infiltration (Fig. 24-7G,H). This loss of function within the allograft is completed by long-standing arteritis and is termed *interstitial fibrosis*. This fibrotic renal tissue is likely due to the healing and scarring that occurred from earlier inflammatory episodes. CR is diagnostically inferred with sonography due to the reduction in size of the transplanted organ. A change in the echogenicity of the allograft can be noted as well as a change in vascular perfusion. An interesting point to consider is that CsA nephrotoxicity can have a similar sonographic appearance much like rejection.[10,18]

A critical assault on the parenchyma of the renal allograft is a stenosis of the anastomosed renal artery.[12] Renal artery stenosis (RAS) quickly curtails the arterial flow into the allograft and compromises its parenchymal function. RAS occurs at a rate of 10% and occurs within 1 to 3 years after the surgical implantation.[12] The gray scale evaluation of this pathology would cause a decrease in the size of the allograft and, long term, would demonstrate ischemic tissue. The use of spectral

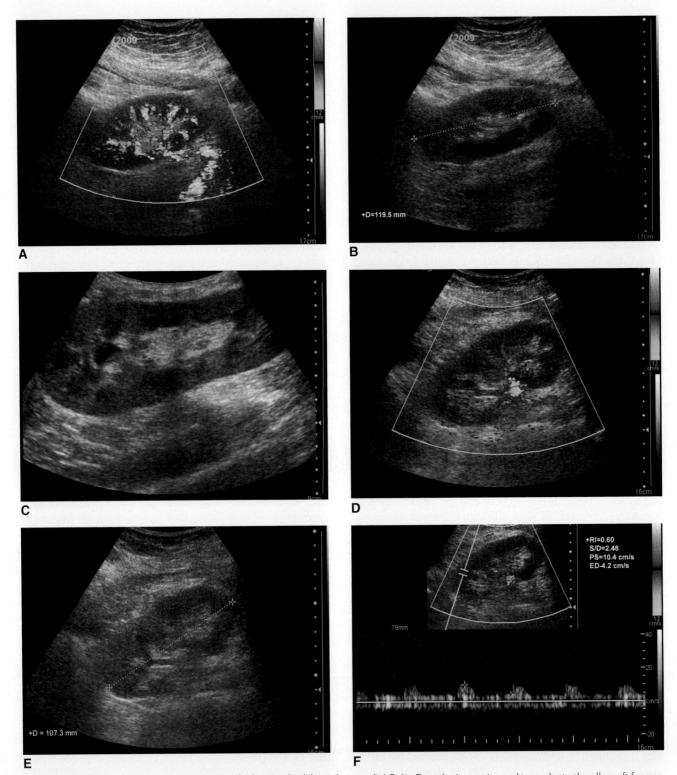

**Figure 24-7** **A–C:** Third day postoperative. **A:** The longitudinal, lateral-to-medial Color Doppler image is used to evaluate the allograft for perfusion. **B:** Gray scale imaging is used to obtain the baseline measurements. This sonogram demonstrates a longitudinal image of the right kidney measuring 119.5 mm in length. **C:** The longitudinal sonogram shows prominent pyramids within the parenchyma of the superficially located renal allograft. **D–F:** Acute rejection. The second day postoperative sonographic evaluation provides evidence to suspect acute rejection of the right renal allograft. The three images are of the renal allograft surgically paced in the right lower quadrant. **D:** The color Doppler sonogram documents lack of perfusion in the allograft parenchyma. **E:** The gray scale sonogram documents swelling of the parenchyma. **F:** The spectral Doppler sonogram documents diminished flow in the lobular arteries in the upper pole of the renal allograft. *(continued)*

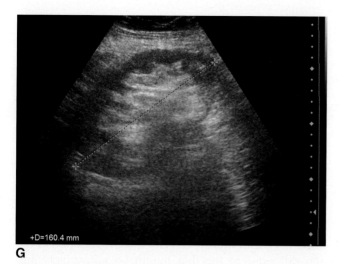

+D=160.4 mm

**G**

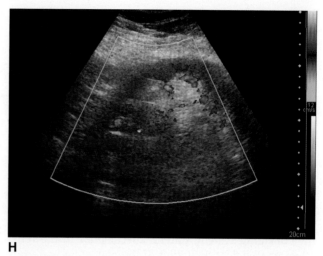

12 cm/s

20cm

**H**

**Figure 24-7** *(continued)* **G,H:** Chronic rejection. **G:** The gray scale image of the right renal allograft is seen in a longitudinal section using a lateral-to-medial transducer orientation. The sonogram shows the documentation of a chronic rejection episode with a noticeable thin cortex compared to the sinus. **H:** The color Doppler sonogram made through the hilum of the right kidney shows documentation of a chronic rejection episode in a renal allograft with diminished cortical flow.

Doppler has been used to document proper arterial flow through the united renal artery. Stenotic areas within the transplant renal artery display a peak systolic velocity >200 cm/s with distant turbulence.[10] Interrogation of vessels within the allograft would demonstrate diminished flow and dampened waveforms.

A thrombosis within the allograft vein or artery is considered to be rare.[10,12] A venous thrombosis in the allograft would demonstrate a reversal of flow in diastole prior to the clot and an absence of venous flow beyond the obstruction. An arterial thrombosis, although rare, would occur in the first month and often is hard to distinguish from AAR or AR.

### Prerenal Pathology

Infection can occur postoperatively, and this can negatively influence the function of the newly transplanted kidney. One of the most difficult infections to treat is polyoma-BK virus nephropathy (PVN), which has been blamed for up to 10% of allograft failures.[17] Unfortunately, potent drugs to treat PVN are not available.[17] Infections can be localized and arise from otherwise sterile fluid collections. An abscess is hallmarked by a patient that presents with fever, leukocytosis, and pain.

Much like the disease of the native kidney, pyelonephritis can attack at the cellular level and is believed to be the result of bacteria that has ascended from the bladder. This infection of the renal parenchyma can be caused by obstruction, stasis, reflux, or the spread of *Escherichia coli*.[11] A renal allograft that has survived an episode of hydronephrosis can be susceptible to attack by bacteria that has communicated upward and contaminated the cortex. Recurrent urinary tract infections (UTIs) are another contributor to the spread of *E. coli* to the allograft.[11] The sonographic appearance is an echogenic cortex, loss of corticomedullary junction, and

inflammatory changes surrounding the allograft. An alternative form of this infection is emphysematous pyelonephritis, which results in air developing in the collecting system. The sonographic appearance is bright echogenic foci with distal dirty shadowing.

An abscess can occur weeks to months after the transplant surgery and sonographically presents as well-defined collection of contents that vary from anechoic to echogenic in appearance. These infectious collections can cause compression of the vasculature as a prerenal pathology.

A prerenal pathology that can result in compression of the vascular structures of an allograft is perinephric fluid collections.[12] A common fluid collection that can be noted in association with a renal transplant is a localized hematoma. A hematoma presents asymptomatically and is often found sonographically immediately after surgery. A hematoma can be either anechoic at an early stage and progress to a more mixed echogenicity. Hematomas are generally absorbed and should decrease in size over time.

Another asymptomatic fluid collection associated with a renal allograft is a lymphocele. The patient with a lymphocele presents asymptomatically and again can have an obstructed ureter due to this postrenal complication (Fig. 24-5C). A lymphocele typically is found postsurgically between the first and second month. It is believed to be caused by an interruption of lymphatics that occurred at the time of surgery. Sonographically, these fluid collections can be multilocular with thin septa and anechoic fluid. Commonly, they are located between the lower pole of the transplant and the urinary bladder.

A urine leak or urinoma is another prerenal pathology that can be discovered sonographically. Urinomas are well defined, appear anechoic, and on rare occasion, can also cause compression of the ureter. A urinoma has been reported in association with 6% of renal allograft and usually discovered in the first month after surgery.[1]

The detection of an arteriovenous malformation (AVM) can be made with color or power Doppler, and these are often created as a result of biopsy trauma.[10,12]

### Postrenal Complication

Hydronephrosis is the most common postrenal complication; however, some slight dilation of the collecting system is common postoperatively.[10] Compression of the ureter or stricture at the site of anastomosis of the ureter to the urinary bladder could result in pressure in the collecting system. Careful surveillance of the renal allograft to detect dilatation of the collecting system is paramount (Fig. 24-8).

### PANCREATIC ALLOGRAFT

The pancreatic allograft is susceptible to many of the same risks for early rejection as a renal allograft. Combining immunosuppressive drugs and histocompatibility testing helps to reduce the incidence of acute rejection in these patients. Acute rejection is commonly suspected when there is an incidence of a 50% drop in timed urine amylase output.[1] This indicates diminished allograft function, which is likely due to humoral/cellular attack and injury to the tissue. The pancreatic tail is usually fixed when implanted in the left lower quadrant because the descending colon can physically hold it in place.[1] The pancreatic tail develops an attachment to the lateral parietal peritoneum. The placement in the lower quadrant makes the pancreatic allograft tail an ideal location for biopsies to determine a true rejection episode.

The second contributor to loss of a pancreatic allograft is vascular thrombosis, which has a 2% to 19% incidence.[1] Thrombosis can cause acute rejection of the allograft prior to the first month postoperatively and chronically afterward. The rationale for this to occur is due to the slower rate of perfusion in the pancreatic allograft. The rate of flow is much lower compared to the renal transplant. Thrombosis can cause pancreatic ischemia and pulmonary embolus, as well as pancreatitis. An arterial malformation is considered to be rare and therefore not commonly considered as a cause for rejection.

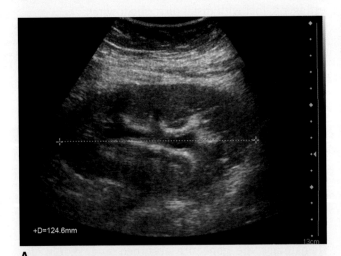

A

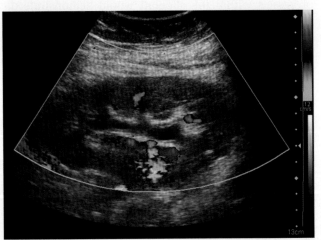

B

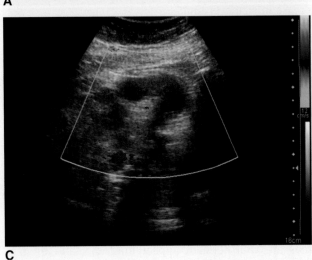

C

**Figure 24-8** Hydronephrosis. **A:** The gray scale longitudinal sonogram shows documentation of a hydronephrotic renal allograft and a baseline measurement. **B:** The color Doppler longitudinal sonogram shows documentation of a hydronephrotic renal allograft and continued perfusion of the tissue. **C:** The gray scale and color Doppler sonogram shows documentation of a hydroureter, which confirms a postrenal complication.

## LIVER ALLOGRAFT

The most significant liver allograft pathology is biliary strictures, which can develop and can result in complications in as many as 25% of patients.[19] The onset of a biliary stricture is complicated by the fact that the nerve supply to the liver allograft is minimal, and patients have no sense of impending obstruction. Often, they present with painless jaundice and abnormal liver function tests. This requires a careful investigation to determine the location of the stricture, which could be either intrahepatic or extrahepatic. The process of transplantation can be the cause of postsurgical scarring, which results in a narrowing of the biliary system. A sonogram can demonstrate a focal area of dilation proximal to the area of stricture. A stricture needs to be surgically corrected to avoid biliary obstruction and subsequent bacteria that can develop due to stasis. Ascending cholangitis develops due to an overgrowth of bacteria that moves through the biliary tree.[1] These pathologic conditions are commonly reviewed and managed with endoscopic retrograde cholangiopancreatography (ERCP).

Recurrent sclerosing cholangitis can occur after 350 days posttransplant and sonographically can present much like acute sclerosing cholangitis.[1] This condition permits bacteria to invade the liver allograft such as enteric flora, cytomegalovirus, and cryptosporidium. Sonographically, this can be noted as thickening of the ducts and diverticulum-appearing outpouchings of the common bile duct.[1]

An additional concern is the development of sludge in the biliary tree, which has been seen in up to 29% of liver allograft patients as late as 8.5 years postoperatively.[1] The development of sludge is not clearly understood; however, it has been linked to bacterial infection, rejection, biliary obstruction, and biliary leaks. Since the presence of sludge in the biliary tree has the ability to promote sclerosing cholangitis, it is important to document the sonographic pathology and amend medical treatment to avert ischemia of the allograft. It is important to also ensure that bile is not leaking from the site of biliary anastomosis.

The sphincter of Oddi must also be closely evaluated to make sure that it is not dysfunctional and the source of biliary stasis. Although this is a more infrequent pathology associated with the liver transplant patient, an ERCP is an appropriate procedure to evaluate the insertion of the common bile duct to the ampulla of Vater. An ERCP can help to decompress the biliary system and ensure that digestive juices are freely flowing into the duodenum.[1]

The potential of hepatic artery thrombosis is a major clinical concern and must be closely monitored as the biliary system is highly dependent on the hepatic artery for its arterial blood supply as well as for overall organ perfusion. Capturing a spectral Doppler tracing that documents forward flow in the hepatic artery is often difficult to obtain but can save the patient from additional imaging studies, such as angiography. The use of Doppler to detect hepatic artery thrombosis is reported to be as high as 92%.[20] As collateral vessels begin to form throughout the liver, diminished flow can be expected as these new vascular connections are forming.

Stenosis of the hepatic artery is also a secondary concern due to narrowing that can occur at the anastomotic site. The incidence of stenosis of the hepatic artery can be caused by the surgical technique, catheters used during surgery, or a rejection episode. The patient will present with abnormal liver function tests and biliary ischemia.[1] Duplex sonography can be used to directly investigate the course of the hepatic artery and detect areas of high flow or turbulence. Spectral waveforms can also be helpful, and a tardus parvus signal, suggests a stenosis proximally.[1] Since the hepatic artery is difficult to directly investigate throughout its entire course, angiography may be the best imaging choice if a stenosis is suspected. Evaluation of the portal vein must also be completed to ensure that hepatopetal flow has been restored and maintained. If recanalizations of varices are noted, then a portal vein thrombosis or stenosis should be suspected. Gray scale images of the portal vein will be helpful in confirming if a portal vein thrombosis has developed; however, an acute thrombosis can be anechoic and easily missed. This makes the use of duplex necessary to record a spectral tracing and to document the direction of flow at several points within the liver.

## OTHER PROCEDURES

### RENAL ALLOGRAFT BIOPSIES

The gold standard for diagnosis is the evaluation of core tissue from the allograft. Biopsies are more accurate when the procedure is sonographically guided. It has been reported that using sonography to guide a biopsy procedure increases the probability of obtaining renal cortex in 75% to 90% of patients.[21] The percentage increases when the core samples can be immediately evaluated with an electron microscope and accuracy approaches 100%.

Besides defining the diagnosis of rejection, a biopsy has a significant impact on the treatment of the patient. Biopsy results have helped modify the treatment of 27% to 46% of patient cases, have revised therapies in 42% to 83% of patient cases, and have helped to avoid the use of additional immunosuppressive therapy in 19% to 30% of patient cases.[17] In order to ensure that the pathologist can provide these important diagnostic results, a proper sample of the allograft is needed. Histology can pinpoint the cause of rejection from a broad spectrum of diseases that can be superimposed on the rejection episode.[17] It is also important to obtain tissue from the allograft during the rejection episode so that a morphologic episode can be diagnosed. Waiting

| TABLE 24-2 |
| --- |
| **Renal Allograft Biopsy Criteria[17]** |
| 1. Obtain at least two biopsy cores for standard light microscopic evaluation. |
| 2. A biopsy sample needs to contain greater than 12 glomeruli (located in the deep cortex). |
| 3. A biopsy sample needs to contain greater than two large interlobular arteries/branches of arcuate arteries (with at least 2–3 layers of medial smooth muscle cells). |
| 4. The sample should contain a portion of the medulla. |

until an episode has concluded will make the diagnosis less definitive and only document sclerosis.[17] A biopsy gun is an important tool, and utilizing sonographic guidance is recommended so criteria can be followed to obtain sufficient tissue and to ensure a diagnostic sample is obtained from the renal allograft[17] (Table 24-2).

The research conducted by Bartlett et al.[13] documents the usefulness of taking a biopsy sample of both the renal and pancreatic allograft to determine the extent of a rejection episode.[13] Securing biopsies of both allografts can be used to ensure that the appropriate medical therapy is used and the overall dosage can be regulated. Sonography guidance is vital and helps with the appropriate diagnosis to tailor treatment for patients with compromised health due to rejection (Fig. 24-9).

## COMPUTED TOMOGRAPHY

Computed tomography (CT) has been described as a central imaging modality, and other imaging options are utilized when a CT is deemed inconclusive. Due to the use of ionizing radiation and patient dose, CT is not a primary imaging tool for transplant patients

because these patients are generally followed through their clinical course for changes in their medical status postoperatively. CT is very helpful as part of the workup of potential donors when screening for compatibility.[22] Three-dimensional (3D) CT and CT angiography (CTA) studies provide preoperative assessment of renal donors and give the surgeon important information about the ureters, number of vessels, and the location of renal arteries.[23] This allows for preplanning of the living allograft surgical procedure and the associated complications that might be encountered.

The CT examination can play a role in the evaluation of the pancreatic allograft since it is usually surgically placed in the lower pelvis and is often partially obscured by bowel gas and other pelvic organs. A CT evaluation can help to define all the margins of the pancreatic allograft and also detect associated fluid collections. CT can also provide added information for those liver allograft patients with extrahepatic biliary duct strictures. A study of 38 patients demonstrated that helical CT provided a volumetric image that predicted the donated right liver lobe volume with 92% of actual graft volume.[24] Detailed CT sectional images of the duodenum and ampulla of Vater would allow the site of obstruction to be located and perhaps avoid the need to undergo an ERCP.

## NUCLEAR MEDICINE

A nuclear medicine allograft study requires the injection of a radioisotope into the transplant recipient's venous system. This allows the radionuclide to circulate back through the arterial system and traces perfusion of the allograft suspected of rejection. Using a camera to collect the radiation emitted by the patient over the site of the allograft provides information regarding

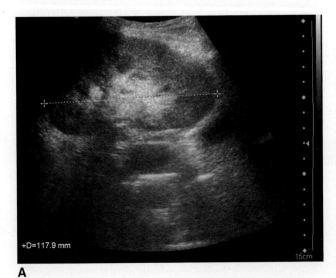

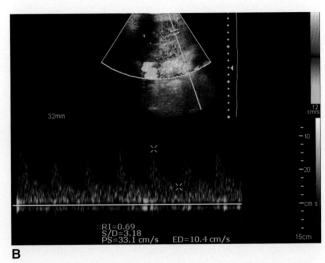

**A**    **B**

**Figure 24-9** Seventeen-year-old renal allograft. **A:** The gray scale longitudinal sonogram of the renal allograft documents parenchymal echogenicity, which aids in tailoring treatment for patients with compromised health due to rejection. **B:** The color and spectral Doppler evaluation shows perfusion within the cortex of the renal allograft.

the function of the organ. A lack of vascular perfusion within the allograft would suggest that the arterial supply is being rejected and is under a state of vasodilatation even though the volume of flow is inadequate. A function study of the allograft is very helpful to determine whether acute or chronic ischemia has occurred. Positron emission tomography (PET) studies coupled with CT have been shown to be helpful in monitoring perfusion in posttransplant patients and also could aid in regulating medical therapy.[25]

## SUMMARY

- Sonography of patients with organ transplantations requires a holistic approach to ensure the data acquired is placed in contexts with all diagnostic information.

- A comprehensive patient history includes a thorough check of the patient's electronic medical record with evaluation of current clinical laboratory values, immunosuppressive drugs, other medications, surgical placement of the organ, immune status, pathology reports, and imaging examinations.

- Patients with clinical presentations, which include chronic renal failure, hepatitis C, alcoholic liver disease, cryptogenic cirrhosis, and/or type I diabetics are the most likely candidates for organ transplantation.

- The two types of organ donations are from a living donor or one harvested from a cadaver.

- Renal allografts can be placed transperitoneal or intraperitoneal, but the surgical preference is an extraperitoneal placement and usually in the right iliac fossa.

- The pancreatic allograft is oriented vertically in the pelvis or diagonally in the upper abdomen.

- The liver allograft is surgically placed in the right upper quadrant and involves complex anastomosis of vasculature and biliary ducts.

- The renal allograft has an average life span of 7 to 10 years for a harvested organ from a cadaver and 15 to 20 years for an organ from a living donor organ.

- One year following transplantation, successful pancreatic allografts free 80% of the recipients from insulin injection.

- With a liver allograft, flow should be continuous throughout diastole with a resistive index between 0.5 and 0.7.

- Postoperatively, the renal, pancreas, and liver transplants should be evaluated with both gray scale for the parenchymal echogenicity and with Doppler to generate both quantitative and qualitative information on the perfusion of the allograft.

- Acute accelerated renal allograft rejection can be greatly diminished with rigorous preadmission testing, crossmatch, and typing of HLA to help avoid antibodies against the donor's lymphocytes.

- Renal allograft pathologies, which increase the incidence of rejection are classified as parenchymal pathology, prerenal pathology, and postrenal complications.

- The primary contributors to the loss of a pancreatic allograft include diminished function likely due to humoral/cellular attach and injury to the tissue or vascular thrombosis.

- Biliary strictures are the most significant liver allograft pathology, and vascular thrombosis, stenosis, and flow direction are also of major clinical concern.

- Other procedures to evaluate the health of an allograft include biopsy, CT, and nuclear medicine.

- Follow-up examination accuracy and reproducibility is possible when each study includes proper annotation of the images, which includes labeling the anatomy, vessels, and the orientation of the transducer.

## DEDICATION

Dedicated to my sister who was the recipient of my kidney donation more than 25 years ago.

## *Critical Thinking Questions*

1. A 48-year-old man with a renal transplant and elevated creatinine and blood urea nitrogren presents with increased lower quadrant pain. The gray scale sonogram shows prominent renal pyramids within the cortex normally identified on the superficially placed renal allograft. There is an anechoic "mass" in the renal pelvis, which appears to be impinging on the vascular structures and the urethra. Color Doppler and spectral tracings were within normal limits. Baseline measurements were within normal limits. Based on the clinical presentation and sonographic findings, what is the most likely diagnosis?

2. The 51-year-old woman is 2 weeks postoperative pancreatic transplantation. Her sonogram report suggests acute rejection of the allograft due to thrombosis. Explain how thrombosis can lead to rejection of the pancreatic transplant.

3. A liver transplant sonography examination is scheduled on a 45-year-old man. He is 6 months postoperative and presents with painless jaundice and abnormal liver function tests. The sonogram demonstrates a focal area of dilatation in the hepatic duct. The Doppler and spectral evaluation were normal. What is the likely diagnosis and treatment for this patient?

## REFERENCES

1. Muradali D, Wilson SR. Organ transplantation. In: Rumack CM, Wilson SR, Charbonneau JW, eds. *Diagnostic Ultrasound.* 3rd ed. Vol 1. St. Louis, MO: Elsevier Mosby; 2005:657–701.

2. Mitchell RN, Kumar V. Diseases of immunity. In: Kumar V, Cotran RS, Robbins SL, eds. *Basic Pathology.* 7th ed. Philadelphia, PA: Elsevier Saunders; 2003:103–164.

3. Eisenberg RL, Johnson NM. Urinary system. In: Eisenberg RL, Johnson NM, eds. *Comprehensive Radiographic Pathology.* 4th ed. St. Louis, MO: Elsevier Mosby; 2007:231–265.

4. Brown ED, Chen MYM, Wolfman NT, et al. Complications of renal transplantation: evaluation with US and radionuclide imaging. *Radiographics.* 2000;20:607–622.

5. Kowalczyk N, Mace JD. Hepatobiliary system. In: Kowalczyk N, Mace JD, eds. *Radiographic Pathology for Technologists.* 5th ed. St. Louis, MO: Elsevier Mosby; 2009:140–160.

6. Stedman TL, Dirckx JH. *Stedman's Concise Medical Dictionary for the Health Professions.* Philadelphia, PA: Lippincott Williams & Wilkins; 2001:50.

7. Kobayashi K, Censullo ML, Rossman LL, et al. Interventional radiologic management of renal transplant dysfunction: indications, limitations, and technical consideration. *Radiographics.* 2007;27:1109–1130.

8. Wise A, Cox LA, Long BW. Renal transplant: a review. *J Diagn Med Sonography.* 1998;14:60–66.

9. Wong JJ, Krebs TL, Klassen DK, et al. Sonographic evaluation of acute pancreatic transplant rejection: morphology-Doppler analysis versus guided percutaneous biopsy. *Am J Roentgenol.* 1996;166:803–807.

10. Zwiebel WJ. Duplex evaluation of native and renal vessels and renal allografts. In: Zwiebel WJ. *Introduction to Vascular Ultrasonography.* 4th ed. Philadelphia, PA: Elsevier Saunders; 2000:455–475.

11. Hall R. *The Ultrasound Handbook.* 3rd ed. Philadelphia, PA: Lippincott Williams & Wilkins; 1999.

12. Baxter GM . Ultrasound of renal transplantation. *Clin Radiol.* 2001;56:802–818.

13. Bartlett ST, Schweitzer EJ, Johnson LB, et al. Equivalent success of simultaneous pancreas kidney and solitary pancreas transplantation: a prospective trial of tacrolimus immunosuppression with percutaneous biopsy. *Ann Surg.* 1996;224:440–452.

14. Schwenger V, Korosoglou G, Hinkel UP, et al. Real-time contrast-enhanced sonography of renal transplant recipients predicts chronic allograft nephropathy. *Am J Transplant.* 2006;6:609–615.

15. Lefevre F, Correas JM, Briancon S, et al. Contrast-enhanced sonography of the renal transplant using triggered pulse-inversion imaging: preliminary results. *Ultrasound Med Biol.* 2002;28:303–314.

16. Lockhart ME, Wells CG, Morgan DE, et al. Reversed diastolic flow in the renal transplant: perioperative implications versus transplants older than 1 month. *Am J Roentgenol.* 2008;190:650–655.

17. Nickeleit V. The pathology of kidney transplantation. In: Ruiz P, ed. *Transplantation Pathology.* New York, NY: Cambridge University Press; 2009:45–110.

18. Weinberg K. The urinary system. In: Hagen-Ansert SL, ed. *Textbook of Diagnostic Ultrasonography.* 6th ed. Vol 1. St. Louis, MO: Elsevier Mosby; 2006:290–356.

19. Demetris AJ, Minervini M, Nalesnik M, et al. Histopathology of liver transplantation. In: Ruiz P, ed. *Transplantation Pathology.* New York, NY: Cambridge University Press; 2009:111–184.

20. Flint EW, Sumkin JH, Zajko AB, et al. Duplex sonography of hepatic artery thrombosis after liver transplant. *Am J Roentgenol.* 1988;151:481–483.

21. Damjanov I. *Pathology for the Health Professional.* 3rd ed. St. Louis, MO: Elsevier Mosby; 2006:301–315.

22. Kamell R, Kruskal JB, Pomfret EA, et al. Impact of multidetector CT on donor selection and surgical planning before living adult right lobe liver transplantation. *Am J Roentgenol.* 2001;176:193–200.

23. Flak B. Computed tomography of the body. In: Seeram E, ed. *Computed Tomography: Physical Principles, Clinical Applications, and Quality Control.* 3rd ed. St. Louis, MO: Elsevier Mosby; 2009:421–449.

24. Pomfret A, Pomposelli JJ, Lewis WD, et al. Live donor adult liver transplantation using right lobe grafts: donor evaluation and surgical outcome. *Arch Surg.* 2001;136:425–433.

25. McCormack L, Hany T, Hubner M, et al. How useful is PET/CT imaging in the management of post-transplant lymphoproliferative disease after liver transplantation? *Am J Transplant.* 2006;6:1731–1736.

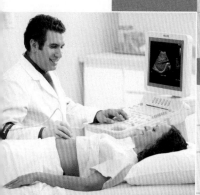

# 25 Emergency Sonography

J. P. Moreland and Michelle Wilson

## OBJECTIVES

Identify what new instrumentation and medical record archiving practices contributed to establishing sonography as an integral part of emergency medicine and acute care.

List the primary applications of emergency cardiac sonography evaluation.

Explain the common acoustic windows, probe placement, and anatomy seen in emergency echocardiography.

Discuss the importance of evaluating pericardial fluid, respiratory variation, and heart wall contraction during emergency echocardiography.

Demonstrate the clinical application and sonographic differentiation for the two different techniques used to exam the parietal pleura to rule out a pneumothorax and examine for hemothorax.

Explain the advantage of using a Trendelenburg patient position versus a supine patient position when evaluating the abdomen and pelvis for free fluid.

Demonstrate the FAST exam protocol for each of the common acoustic windows for the abdomen and pelvis.

Locate the veins included in a three-point evaluation for deep venous thrombosis.

Describe the goal and the protocol of each of the two components of a targeted evaluation of the deep venous system.

## KEY TERMS

cardiac tamponade | deep venous thrombosis | eFAST | FAST | hemoperitoneum | hemothorax | pneumothorax

## GLOSSARY

**cardiac tamponade** the mechanical compression of the heart resulting from large amounts of fluid collecting in the pericardial space and limiting the heart's normal range of motion

**deep vein thrombosis (DVT)** the formation or presence of a thrombus within a vein

**diagnostic peritoneal lavage (DPL)** this is a surgical procedure used to insert a catheter through the abdominal wall and fascia; a syringe is attached to the catheter to aspirate fluid; bleeding is confirmed when gross blood is aspirated; saline solution is injected into the catheter, then it is drained and analyzed; the procedure is performed when computed tomography or sonography is unavailable

**hemoperitoneum** the presence of extravasated blood in the peritoneal cavity

**hemothorax** accumulation of blood in the pleural cavity (the space between the lungs and the walls of the chest)

**laparotomy** an incision is made into the abdomen to insert a camera (laparoscope) into the abdomen to visualize and examine the abdomen and pelvic structures and spaces

**parietal pleura** pleura that lines the inner chest walls and covers the diaphragm

**pericardial effusion** presence of fluid within the pericardium

**pleural effusion** presence of fluid in the pleural cavity

**pneumothorax** the abnormal presence of air between the lung and the wall of the chest (pleural cavity), resulting in collapse of the lung

**pulsatility** pertaining to an activity characterized by rhythmic pulsations

**vein lumen** the central open

**visceral pleura** pleura that covers the lungs

**S**onography continues to establish itself as an indispensible tool in the evaluation of the acute patient. The technology advancements in instrumentation allow for a less complicated user interface, which increases the ease of operating the equipment. The improved medical record archiving practices allows for the movement of sonography from traditional imaging departments to the patient's bedside in the acute setting. Sonographic evaluation has become an integral part of emergency medicine and acute care. It is included in the Advanced Trauma Life Support (ATLS) guidelines as a diagnostic tool in trauma patients.[1] This chapter focuses on some of the primary indications for the sonography examination in the emergency department and discusses how sonography is more readily utilized on acute patients.

## PERFORMANCE STANDARDS

Sonography became a well-established, reliable, and noninvasive diagnostic tool that can rapidly detect free fluid in body cavities without exposing the patient to ionizing radiation. This concept and its implications began spreading in Japan and Europe in the 1970s.[2] It was not until the 1980s and 1990s that physicians in the United States began publishing studies focused on the depiction of free fluid or blood within the peritoneal and pericardial spaces. As the medical profession gained experience and as the technology continued to ascend, trauma sonography was utilized at the bedside, in more applications, and in a broad spectrum of disciplines.[3-6]

The growth of sonographic assessment of trauma and other recent sonographic enhancements led to an evolving standard of care developed from what began as best practice for some emergency department physicians. Professional associations have developed recognized guidelines, recommendations, and standardizations for sonography examinations in the emergency department. Three of these associations with Web sites containing valuable clinical information include the American College of Emergency Physicians (ACEP), the American College of Radiology (ACR), and the American Institute of Ultrasound in Medicine (AIUM).[7-9] A summary of the practice guidelines for emergency sonography published by these organizations are briefly summarized on Table 25-1. Each publication includes standards for personnel, education, protocols, risk management, quality control, quality improvement, and scanning equipment and maintenance.[7-9]

## PROTOCOLS

The focused assessment with sonography for trauma (FAST) exam and the extended FAST (eFAST) exam are two protocols used to detect sequelae of trauma in emergency sonography. Implementing FAST and eFAST for emergency sonography provides a rapid evaluation tool for the everyday practice of trauma patients, which can significantly

| TABLE | 25-1 |
|-------|------|

**Summary of Practice Guidelines for Emergency Sonography[7-9]**

1. Typically, emergency sonography is a goal-directed focused examination that answers brief and important clinical questions in an organ system or for a clinical symptom or sign involving multiple organ systems.

2. Emergency sonography is complimentary to the physical examination but should be considered a separate entity that adds anatomic, functional, and physiologic information to the care of the emergent patient.

3. Emergency sonography is performed, interpreted, and integrated in an immediate and rapid manner dictated by the clinical scenario. It can be applied to any emergency medical condition in any setting with the limitations of time, patient condition, operator ability, and technology limitations.

4. The information gained from the emergency sonography examination is the basis for immediate decisions about further evaluation, clinical management, and therapeutic interventions.

5. Emergency sonography requires emergency physicians to become knowledgeable in the indications for sonography applications, competent in image acquisition and interpretation, and able to integrate the findings appropriately in the clinical management for each patient.

improve patient care and balance the differences between medical and surgical emergencies. The concept behind the FAST exam is based on the fact that many life-threatening injuries cause bleeding in the pericardium, thorax, abdomen, and pelvic regions. The primary purpose of the FAST exam is the methodical search for anechoic or hypoechoic free fluid (blood) in the dependent regions of the pericardium, pleural spaces, intraperitoneal spaces, and the retroperitoneum. The primary purpose of eFAST is to extend the search for a pneumothorax.

Although neither FAST or eFAST exams provides a comprehensive examination, there are major benefits which include that it is a noninvasive bedside examination, which can be performed on pregnant women and children without exposing the patient to ionizing radiation or requiring nephrotoxic contrast agents. Patients who benefit from a FAST exam include those who are hemodynamically unstable and those with penetrating trauma with multiple wounds or unclear trajectory. The limitations include the inability to differentiate blood from other fluids (ascites, urine) and the difficulty examining obese patients. The examination, like all other sonography examinations, is operator dependent.

## CARDIAC

The emergency cardiac sonography examination is a rapid, dynamic method of evaluating in the acute setting patients suspected of having impaired cardiac disease. Its primary applications are directed toward the detection of pericardial fluid, cardiac function, and the detection of cardiac motion in patients with pulseless electrical activity.[10-13] In the trauma setting, cardiac sonography is a defined component of the FAST examination.[7]

The subxiphoid, parasternal, and apical regions provide the three common acoustic windows used in emergency echocardiography (Table 25-2). The subxiphoid window is the most commonly used and convenient method to sonographically visualize cardiac structures including the pericardial sac. With the transducer orientated transversely in the subxiphoid region, the four-chamber cardiac image can be recognized. The liver serves as an acoustic window and often a small segment of the liver can be visualized in the near field. The base of the heart including both atria should be located to the patient's right and is slightly posterior. The apex of the heart is located more to the patient's left and is situated more anteriorly and inferiorly. If any of the four chambers are not fully visualized within this acoustic window, an attempt should be made to adjust the transducer orientation so it is almost parallel to the skin of the anterior torso. In certain patients, especially those with abdominal distention or pain, the subxiphoid window may not be optimal; therefore, familiarity and mastery of all four cardiac scanning planes should be utilized to rule out any pericardial or cardiac pathologies. Whichever scanning plane is used, the same goal remains and that is to observe for pericardial effusion and identify cardiac activity. If an effusion is present, then demonstrating right ventricular collapse will make the diagnosis of pericardial tamponade.

## PERICARDIAL EFFUSION

Sonography of the pericardial space to evaluate for fluid collections is a well-documented practice.[14-16] In the absence of fluid collections, the parietal and visceral pericardium are typically indistinguishable. Sonographically, they should be visualized as a combined white echogenic line surrounding the surface of the heart (Fig. 25-1A). A sonographic finding often noted which can be seen with cardiac imaging is up to 10 mL of normal serous physiologic fluid and sometimes a small amount of pericardial fat.

The detection of pericardial fluid is evident by its hypoechoic presence surrounding the heart (located within the pericardial sac) (Fig. 25-1B,C). In the acute setting, the hypoechoic echogenicity is consistent with blood found within the cardiac chambers. When present, blood collections will most often be noted in the subxiphoid window between the liver and right side of the heart. In the parasternal window, blood will most often be noted superior to the right ventricle, or even posteriorly as it outlines the free wall of the left atria and ventricle. The descending aorta may be used as a landmark for the posterior aspect of the pericardial sac and is often another site for pericardial fluid collections. Hemorrhage has the ability to quickly collect between the visceral and parietal space, which causes hypotension due to the cascade of increasing intrapericardial pressure; which in turn causes a decrease in right heart filling; which then causes decreased left ventricular stroke volume. Even small pericardial effusions can set this cascade in motion, causing tamponade. In the event of a pericardial effusion, it is imperative that patients receive immediate treatment to avoid the life-threatening clinical course with the onset of tamponade physiology.

## CARDIAC TAMPONADE

Pericardial tamponade is a known finding often presents in certain traumatic settings and can be rapidly assessed sonographically. It is demonstrated by visualizing an anechoic space surrounding the heart (pericardial effusion) with the collapse of all or some of its chambers during diastole. Normally, the ventricles contract symmetrically. With tamponade, the outer wall of the ventricle will depress centrally. Often this finding is more difficult to appreciate in the setting of tachycardia. A pathognomonic sonographic finding that distinguishes tamponade is the visualization of the interventricular septum bowing into the left ventricle, known as *paradoxical septal movement*. Another sign of tamponade is the loss of respiratory variation in the inferior vena cava (IVC). This is sonographically noted by the loss of collapse in the anteroposterior plane of the IVC with forceful inhalation or a "sniff" test performed by the patient (Fig. 25-2).

## CARDIAC ACTIVITY

Additional primary applications of emergent cardiac sonography include the evaluation of gross cardiac activity in the setting of cardiopulmonary resuscitation and the assessment of global left ventricular systolic function. One can assess the overall cardiac contractility by observing the relative percentage of change in the movement of ventricular endocardial walls from relaxation during diastole to contraction during systole. A uniformly and circumferentially contracting endocardium is indicative of good function. Poor left ventricular function often coupled with a dilated or plethoric IVC may indicate a fluid overload or congestive heart failure. Again, a visual image of the heart and IVC may quickly establish whether poor perfusion is due to a direct cardiac problem, or a volume problem. In the setting of a pulseless patient, the lack of cardiac activity carries a grave prognosis. Multiple possibilities relating to low flow states can contribute to the presence of electrical activity without a palpable pulse. These conditions may include but are not limited to hypovolemia, peripheral vascular disease, tamponade, and possibly tension pneumothorax.[11,17,18] The sonographic evaluation of cardiac structures allows for the rapid dynamic visualization of heart wall contractions as they occur undetected. Having this immediate diagnostic tool allows for the prompt correction of the low flow state, which may be a potential life-saving event.

**TABLE  25-2**

## Common Acoustic Windows in Emergency Echocardiography

| Acoustic Window | Probe Position | Probe Placement | Anatomy | Sonographic Image |
|---|---|---|---|---|
| Subxiphoid | Just inferior to the xiphoid tip of the sternum; transducer angled superiorly toward left shoulder | | | |
| Parasternal Long Axis | Third to fifth intercostal space, left side of sternum, directly over heart | | | |
| Parasternal Short Axis | Same position as Parasternal long axis; rotate transducer 180 degrees clockwise | | | |
| Apical | Patient in left lateral decubitus position; transducer placed at point of maximum impulse on the lateral chest wall (often just below the nipple) | | | |

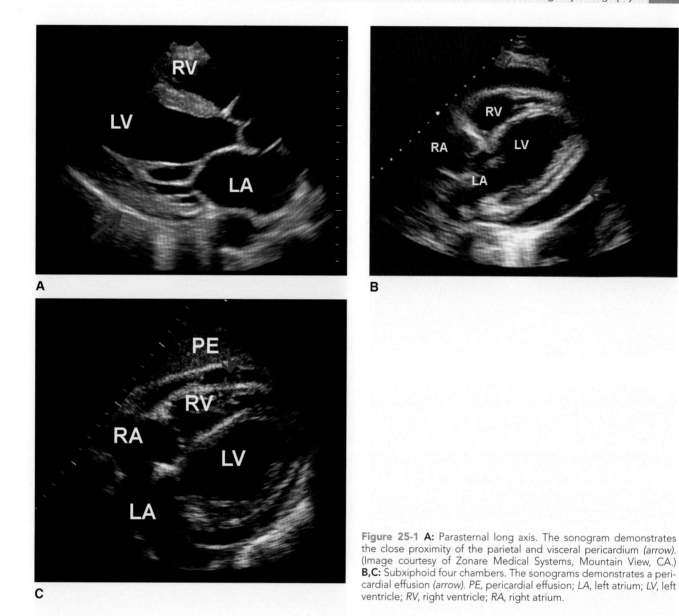

A

B

C

**Figure 25-1 A:** Parasternal long axis. The sonogram demonstrates the close proximity of the parietal and visceral pericardium (arrow). (Image courtesy of Zonare Medical Systems, Mountain View, CA.) **B,C:** Subxiphoid four chambers. The sonograms demonstrates a pericardial effusion (arrow). PE, pericardial effusion; LA, left atrium; LV, left ventricle; RV, right ventricle; RA, right atrium.

## THORAX

Sonography is more sensitive than chest radiography or physical examination for the evaluation of a pneumothorax.[19-22] The eFAST examination is easily mastered by proper identification of the normal anatomy and its appearance during normal respiration. To gain scanning competence, one should be able to identify in normal individuals, a sliding motion caused by the movement of the mobile visceral pleura during respiration along the static parietal pleura. The parietal pleura can be visualized in the near field, distal to the echogenic ribs with distal shadowing, which serves as a sonographic landmark. Air has a high acoustic impedance.

**Figure 25-2** Longitudinal plane of upper abdomen. Normal respiratory variation is seen when comparing the two longitudinal sonograms of the upper abdomen. The left image displays the inferior vena cava (IVC) with expiration and the right image demonstrates the normal 50% collapse of the IVC with inspiration. L, liver

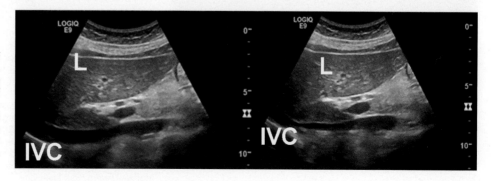

The air-filled lung covered by visceral pleura is a potent reflector of the ultrasound beam, blocking sound penetration deeper into the chest and producing a bright linear interface that moves with respiration. Using a 5- to 7-MHz frequency transducer with a larger footprint, such as a curved linear or a linear probe, allows for proper visualization of the ribs (rounded echogenic interfaces) and of the intercostal spaces located between two ribs (Fig. 25-3A). With the transducer oriented perpendicular to the intercostal space in the parasagittal plane, one or two ribs will be identified and subcutaneous tissue and muscle can be visualized between the

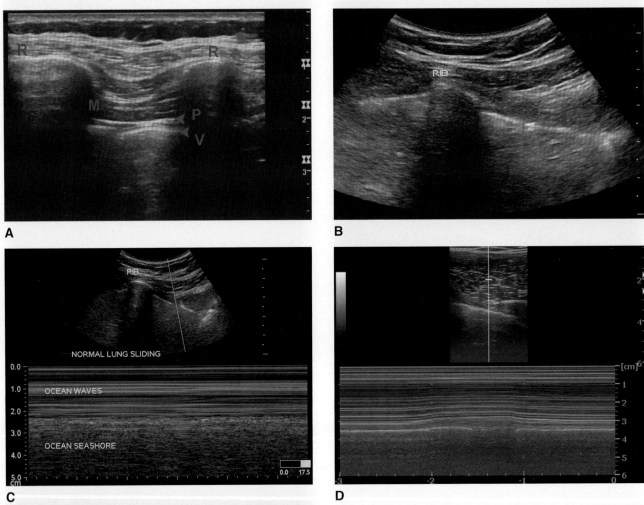

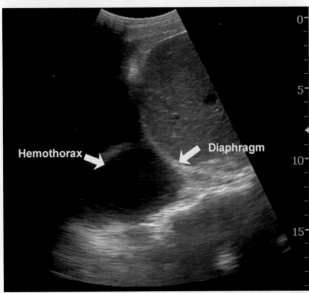

Figure 25-3 **A:** Transverse plane of the upper thorax. The echogenic ribs *(R)* can be seen with normal distal shadowing. The intercostal muscles *(M)* are seen between the ribs. Distal to the ribs, the parietal pleura *(P)* lining the chest wall is seen, and distal to this is the visceral pleura *(V).* The parietal pleura and visceral pleura should be visualized sliding over each other with respiration *(arrowheads).* **B:** Longitudinal plane of the upper thorax. The echogenic rib *(RIB)* can be seen with its normal distal shadowing. The parietal and visceral pleura are noted in close proximity *(red arrows).* On normal individuals, a sliding motion caused by the movement of the mobile visceral pleural during respiration along the static parietal pleura to slide over one another with patient respirations can be observed in real time. **C,D:** M-mode (motion mode) tracing of the upper thorax. The gray scale image corresponds anatomically with the M-mode tracing. The nonmobile superficial structures of the chest, ribs, and muscle above the pleural line correspond to the "ocean waves" on the M-mode display. The moving parietal and visceral pleura are noted in the "ocean seashore" area, with normal air in the lungs corresponding to the in homogeneous M-mode tracing below. **E:** Coronal plane. The sonogram shows a hemothorax in the costophrenic angle and within the pleural cavity as the diaphragm is located inferiorly. Images **B**, **C**, **D** courtesy of Zonare Medical Systems, Mountain View, CA; Images **D**, **E**, courtesy of Mathew Ahern, Salt Lake City, UT.

rib shadows. Finally, the pleura itself is located within 1 cm of depth from the rib space, with the parietal pleura immediately distal to the chest muscle. The pleura is identified by its pronounced superficial echogenic line.

There are two techniques that can be used for the eFAST exam of the parietal and visceral pleura to rule out a pneumothorax. The first is to try to identify the normal back and forth movement of the pleural layers, corresponding to the patient's respirations that is called the "gliding sign" or "sliding sign." The second is to identify comet tail artifacts at the pleural interface.[22] The sliding should be readily appreciated once the echogenic reflectors (parietal pleura and visceral pleura) just distal to the ribs are seen in real time with the visceral pleura sliding back and forth under the parietal pleura with patient respiration (Fig. 25-3B). The sliding sign and moving comet tail artifacts are synchronized with respiratory movement. Absence of the sliding sign indicates there is a pneumothorax. The sliding sign can immediately rule out a pneumothorax at this particular location; however, bilaterally, multiple areas should be evaluated, especially in the absence of the sliding sign.[23] Although this imaging finding should be present along any and all acoustic windows in the upper thorax, with the patient in the supine position, the more superior location is the common site for a pneumothorax.

The second sonographic technique used to identify a pneumothorax is with the application of M-mode (motion mode), which is used to detect motion along a select line of interrogation (line of site). With this technique, motion creates waves or curves and stillness creates straight horizontal lines. A tracing is displayed by placing the M-mode cursor on the pleura between the ribs. The M-mode will reveal parallel lines above the pleural line corresponding to the motionless parietal tissue of the chest wall. In the presence of sliding, a homogeneous granular (sandy) pattern is seen below the pleural line due to the corresponding constant motion of the underlying lung. This normal lung sliding motion has the appearance of a sandy beach intersecting with rolling waves and is known as the "seashore sign" (Fig. 25-3C,D).[24] In the case of pneumothorax with absent normal sliding, the M-mode reveals a series of parallel horizontal lines, suggesting complete lack of movement both over and under the pleural line. This pattern is known as the "barcode sign" or "stratosphere sign."[24,25] Although absent lung sliding suggests pneumothorax, it can occur in the presence of multiple other conditions such as main stem intubation, acute respiratory distress syndrome, or pleural adhesions.[24]

If a pneumothorax is suspected, one should attempt to document the size or extent of the pneumothorax by localizing the point on the chest wall where the normal lung pattern can be seen. The phenomenon of demonstrating absent lung sliding and normal lung sliding occurring between the pneumothorax and the normal lung is known as the "lung point."[25] At the lung point position during expiration, no sliding is seen; but, with inspiration, the lung inflates and the visceral pleura moves up in apposition with the parietal pleura beneath the probe and sliding is again seen.[24] The ability to demonstrate the alternating lung sliding and absence of lung sliding within the same field is diagnostic of pneumothorax with a sensitivity of 66% and specificity of 100%.[24,26,27] Due to the dynamic nature of lung scanning, the concept is not appreciated with individual sonograms.

The incidence of a hemothorax after blunt or penetrating chest injury can be noted sonographically as an anechoic or hypoechoic fluid collection localized to the costophrenic angle.[19] Visualizing an intact diaphragm inferiorly will allow for the certainty that the fluid collection rests within the pleural cavity (Fig. 25-3E). If there is a pleural cavity fluid collection, the lung may sometimes be identified as a triangular structure superior to the diaphragm and should display rhythmic movement corresponding to the patient's respirations.

## ABDOMEN AND PELVIS

When penetrating or blunt abdomen or pelvic trauma occurs, the useful and proven FAST exam protocol can be employed to locate free fluid, intraperitoneal hemorrhage, and other abnormal fluids, such as urine and bile. The FAST exam is about 90% sensitive for detecting any amount of intraperitoneal free fluid,[28] and nearly perfect for the detection of intraperitoneal bleeding significant enough to cause shock and requiring diagnostic peritoneal lavage (DPL) or an emergent laparotomy.[29-31]

Like the FAST and eFAST exam of the pericardium and pleural spaces, learning to perform the FAST exam involves learning how to visualize the abdomen and pelvic structures to include the diaphragm, liver, spleen, kidneys, and urinary bladder. Interpretation of the FAST exam involves learning the spaces where free fluid commonly collects adjacent to these organs, and how to recognize these areas sonographically.

The examination protocol is performed with the patient in a supine position. Placing the patient in the Trendelenburg position shifts the areas of dependency and increases the sensitivity of the FAST exam, especially in the detection of free fluid in the hepatorenal space (Morrison pouch) and the perisplenic space.[32] The pelvis may also be evaluated using the Trendelenburg patient position to help free abdominal fluid movement to the most dependent quadrants. Normal sonographic findings for this area include the absence of intraperitoneal fluid along with the normal echogenicity usually demonstrated in the abdomen and pelvis.

The anatomic region, common acoustic windows, and scanning planes for the FAST exam are presented for the abdomen and the pelvis. The examination includes the previously presented subxiphoid window to evaluate the pericardium and may also include the previously presented eFAST exam of the pleural spaces to evaluate the thorax.

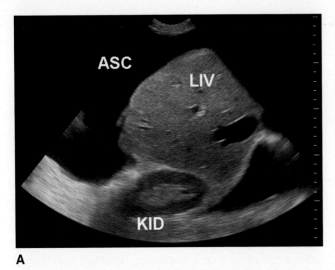

**A**

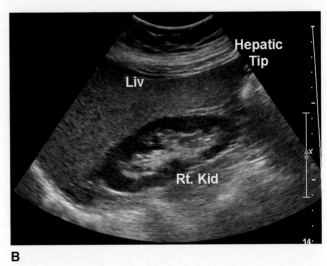

**B**

**Figure 25-4 A:** Coronal plane of right upper quadrant. The sonogram demonstrates free fluid (*ASC*, ascites). The liver (*LIV*) is noted anterior to the right kidney (*KID*). (Image courtesy of Zonare Medical Systems, Mountain View, CA.) **B:** Longitudinal image of right upper quadrant. The full extent of the liver is displayed. The hepatic tip annotates the inferior aspect of the liver. *Rt Kid*, right kidney.

## RIGHT UPPER QUADRANT

The probe is placed in the midaxillary line between the 8th and 12th rib space and uses the liver as an acoustic window to avoid air-filled bowel. A sagittal oblique and a coronal scanning plane are used with the notch of the probe placed toward the patient's head. This is an excellent scanning plane for visualizing the hepatorenal space (Morrison pouch) located between the liver capsule and the fatty fascia of the right kidney. Small superior probe angulations allow for evaluation of the right pleural space. With inferior probe angulations, the inferior pole of the right kidney and the right paracolic gutter can be surveyed. Both longitudinal oblique and coronal planes should be obtained to view the interface between the liver and right kidney (Fig. 25-4A). It is important to follow the lower edge of the liver caudally, until a sufficient view of the hepatic tip is obtained (Fig. 25-4B).

## LEFT UPPER QUADRANT

The scanning orientation is the same as for the right upper quadrant with the probe placed on the left side at the midaxillary line between the 8th and 12th rib space. This image plane will demonstrate the spleen and left kidney (Fig. 25-5). Both longitudinal oblique and coronal planes should be obtained to view the interface between the spleen and left kidney. With superior probe angulations, the left pleural space can be visualized. The probe should be rotated and angled to follow the renal anatomic plane to visualize fluid, if present, above the left kidney or in the left paracolic gutter.

## PELVIC CAVITY

With the patient in a supine position, the pelvis is the most dependent part of the peritoneal cavity. A fluid-filled urinary bladder, even if filling, is by way of a Foley catheter, provides a better acoustic window to investigate the presence of free fluid. A Trendelenburg patient position may be used if satisfactory images are not obtained in the supine patient position. The sonographer should evaluate the pelvic cavity using both longitudinal and transverse planes. For the longitudinal survey, the probe is placed in the midline, just superior to the pubic bone, with the probe notch placed toward the patient's head. A simple probe angling or rocking to the patient's right and then to the patient's left provides longitudinal sweeps through the cavity. After the longitudinal evaluation, turn the probe so the notch is pointing to the patient's right side and simply use probe angling or rocking superiorly and inferiorly to obtain transverse sweeps through the cavity. In both male and female patients, evaluate for free fluid in potential spaces. In the male patient,

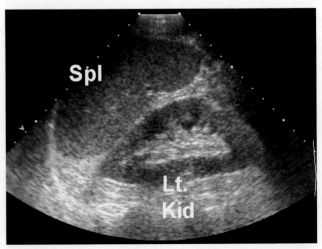

**Figure 25-5** Coronal image of the left upper quadrant. The sonogram demonstrates the relationship of the spleen (*Spl*) and the left kidney (*Lt. Kid*). There is no anechoic blood or fluid identified.

evaluate for fluid anterior to the bladder in the space of Retzius and between the bladder and rectum in the rectovesical pouch. In the female patient, the uterus should be noted midline, and one should evaluate both the vesicouterine and rectouterine pouches as well as the space of Retzius (Fig. 25-6A). If free fluid is present, it is most often located superior and posterior to the urinary bladder and the uterus.[8] Be aware of the possibility of a distended or overly distended urinary bladder being mistaken for free fluid in the pelvis (Fig. 25-6B).

## RIGHT AND LEFT PERICOLIC GUTTERS

To ascertain if there is free fluid in the pericolic gutters, sonography is performed in both longitudinal and transverse scanning planes through the peritoneal window inferior to the level of the ipsilateral kidney and next to the ipsilateral iliac crest.[8] A successful pericolic gutter evaluation is difficult if this acoustic window is not available due to the presence of a distended urinary bladder, a solid organ, or an air filled-bowel.

# DEEP VEIN THROMBOSIS

The clinical diagnosis of lower extremity deep venous thrombosis (DVT) is often hindered by its variable and unpredictable presentation, as well as the reality that many nonthrombotic conditions produce signs and symptoms suggestive of DVT.[33-35] The relatively superficial location and the lack of overlying skeletal structures or bowel gas allow for the seemingly simplistic evaluation of the peripheral veins.

A modification of the standard examination, which greatly abbreviates the traditional protocol, is typically utilized in the symptomatic, emergent patient.[36-40] The limited venous compression emergency protocol pursues areas in which turbulence poses the greatest risk

for developing thrombosis. This three-point evaluation includes the sonographic evaluation of the common femoral vein at the saphenous junction, the proximal deep and superficial femoral vein, and the popliteal vein. The superficial femoral vein is part of the deep venous system, but to avoid confusion, it may be referred to simply as the *femoral vein.*

The targeted evaluation of the deep venous system has two components: a primary and a secondary. The primary component uses gray scale imaging and a transverse plane to visualize the vein and to use the transducer to apply systematic, intermittent compression. Very little pressure is needed to collapse the vein because the wall is thin and venous pressure is low. Venous patency is confirmed with the release of the pressure. *Coaptation* refers to normal vein walls touching with compression. In the presence of a clot, the vein will not collapse.

The secondary component is the integration of Doppler techniques into the exam, assessing for flow characteristics and confirming venous patency in the setting of a suspected clot. In normal veins, color flow should fill the vessel lumen from wall to wall (Fig. 25-7A). In the presence of clot, areas of flow disturbances can be seen as blood flows around the obstruction, which does not allow the lumen of the vein to fill with color.

To begin the exam, place the lower extremities in a position of dependency. This can be done with the patient in a supine position and elevating the head of the bed approximately 15 to 40 degrees (reverse Trendelenburg). The leg in question should be abducted and rotated externally with slight flexion of the knee. A high-resolution linear array transducer with a frequency ranging between 5.0 and 9.0 MHz should be utilized. With the transducer perpendicular to the skin surface, at a level just inferior to the inguinal canal,

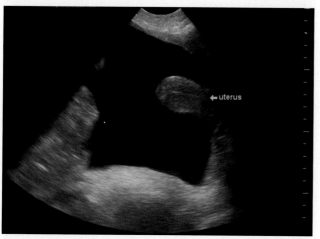

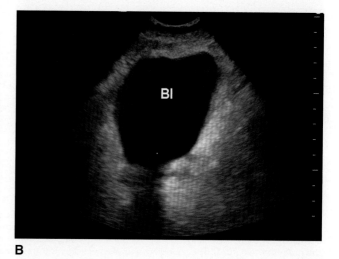

**A**                                                **B**

**Figure 25-6 A:** Longitudinal plane, midline pelvis. The uterus is noted to be surrounded by anechoic free fluid in the pelvis. **B:** Transverse plane, midpelvis. The urinary bladder *(Bl)* is distended. Care should be taken not to mistake the anatomy as a large free fluid collection. (Images courtesy of Zonare Medical Systems, Mountain View, CA.)

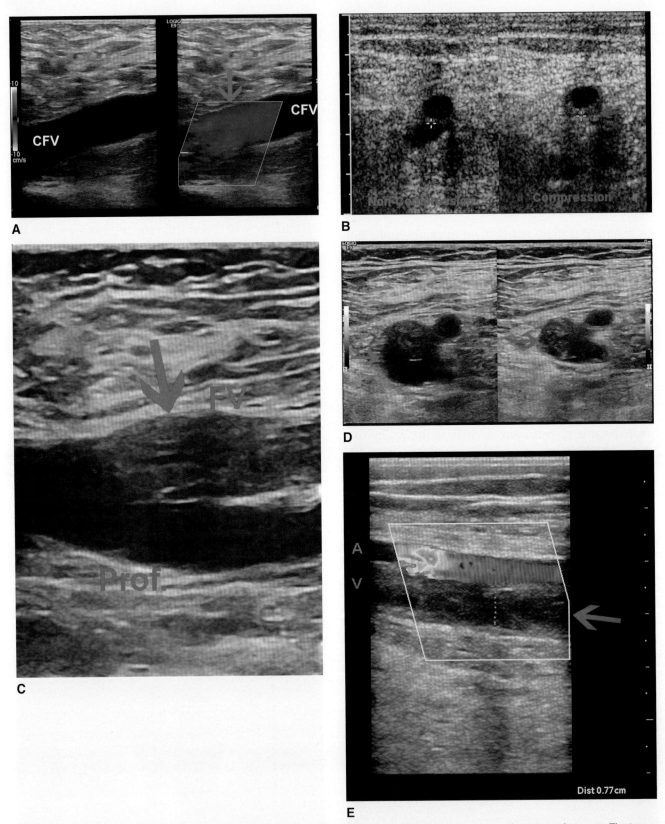

**Figure 25-7  A:** Longitudinal plane of the common femoral vein (*CFV*). The image on the left demonstrates the gray scale image. The image on the right displays normal intraluminal filling of the vein, with color Doppler (*arrow*). **B:** Transverse superior femoral artery (*A*) and vein (*v*). The image on the left shows the vessels without compression. The image on the right displays the position of the superior femoral vessels but with compression, there is a change in shape and the vein completely collapses (*arrow*). **C:** Longitudinal plane of the superior femoral vein (*FV*) and the profunda vein (*Prof*). The sonogram shows an echogenic intraluminal clot (*arrow*) seen in the femoral vein. **D:** Transverse mid femoral vein. The image on the left corresponds to a noncompressed vein with an echogenic clot in its lumen (*arrow*). The image on the right demonstrates the inability of the lumen walls to coapt with compression (*arrow*). **E:** Color Doppler imaging through the superior femoral vein (*V*) and artery (*A*). The artery displays good vascular flow (*blue color pixels*). In the femoral vein, there is no Doppler shift; thereby, it lacks color flow (*arrow*).

# Critical Thinking Questions

1. Following a motor vehicle accident, the FAST examination was performed on a 63-year-old woman who presented to the emergency department with acute thoracoabdominal trauma and hypotension. The subxiphoid scanning window was used to evaluate the four-chamber heart. The sonogram demonstrated a large anechoic stripe between the epicardium and the pericardium, a collapsed right ventricle, and paradoxical septal movement. Volume measurements of inferior vena cava during respiration demonstrated a loss of respiratory variation. Based on the clinical presentation and sonographic findings, what is the most likely diagnosis?

2. A 32-year-old man's right chest hit the handlebars as he was propelled off a motorcycle. The patient's vital signs were stable. The patient's pain and tenderness were located on the right side where he received the blunt thoracic trauma. His breath sounds were equal bilaterally. The sonography exam of the right and left hemithorax were performed using a 7-MHz linear probe. Lung sliding and comet tail artifacts were present throughout except on the longitudinal image obtain over the fifth right anterior intercostal space. Based on the clinical presentation and sonographic findings, what is the most likely

diagnosis? To complete the study, what should the sonographer try to document?

3. As a 4-year-old boy walks past a swing set, he gets hit in the abdomen, and is thrown several feet. Several hours later, the child is brought to the emergency department as his parents note his abdomen appears to be getting larger, appears more bruised, and he has abdominal tenderness. The FAST exam protocol is used on the patient. In the left upper quadrant, the splenic contour cannot be demonstrated, and it appears there is free fluid between the diaphragm and spleen interface and between the spleen and left kidney interface. Free fluid is also present in the rectovesical pouch. As the sonographer finishes the exam, the patient's condition progresses to hypovolemic shock. Based on the patient's condition and the sonographic findings, what is the preliminary interpretation of the sonography exam and what is the explanation for the diagnosis of hypovolemic shock?

4. On a patient being evaluated for deep vein thrombosis, what is a simple explanation for lack of compressibility in the vessel but spectral and color Doppler on the same vessel demonstrates laminar flow filling the vessel?

the common femoral vein and femoral artery should be noted in a transverse plane. With mild pressure applied to the transducer, on the surface of the leg, the normal venous lumen should completely collapse with immediate coaptation of its walls (Fig. 25-7B). The degree of pressure required varies and will depend on the depth and location of the vein. The artery often becomes misshaped but does not collapse.

Once the common femoral vein and artery are identified, transverse, systematic, and intermittent compression should be performed every 1 to 2 cm through the level of the superior femoral vein, past the junction of the common femoral, deep femoral, and superficial femoral vessels. Transverse compression should then be carried out in the popliteal fossa, at the level of the popliteal vein, and through the popliteal trifurcation.

In the presence of clot, an intraluminal hyperechogenicity is often seen, which leads one to suspect thrombus (Fig. 25-7C). Because an acute clot is often anechoic or hypoechoic and an older or chronic clot is more echogenic, the true hallmark diagnosis for DVT rests in the inability to completely compress the lumen of the vein with sonography (Fig. 25-7D). In the longitudinal plane, color Doppler should be applied to any venous segment in question of a successful compression or one containing internal echoes. If an obstructive process is located in the vein, color will not persistently fill the entire lumen (Fig. 25-7E).

## SUMMARY

- Bedside sonography in the emergency department holds a valued place in the traumatic patient workup.

- Emergency sonography is the ability to rapidly and accurately perform targeted emergent studies, which include FAST and eFAST examination protocols and compression and Doppler venous evaluation in the lower extremities.

- Emergency sonography allows for a more thorough and expedient care of critical patients and holds the potential of unveiling immediate data to manage emergent situations.

- Emergency sonography is an excellent imaging modality to evaluate for life-threatening injury and utilizing clinical expertise over time to evaluate patients for imaging triage or immediate surgical consultation.

- The emergency sonography examination relies on the skill, knowledge, and accuracy of the sonographer, knowing how to acquire focused examinations to benefit the care of the trauma patent.

### REFERENCES

1. Kortbeek JB, Al Turki SA, Ali J, et al. Advanced trauma life support, 8th edition, the evidence for change. *J Trauma.* 2008;64:1638–1650.

2. Hoffenberg S. The history and philosophy of emergency ultrasound. In: Cosby K, Kendall J, eds. *Practical Guide to Emergency Ultrasound*. Philadelphia, PA: Lippincott Williams & Wilkins; 2006;1–3.

3. American College of Emergency Physicians. Use of ultrasound by emergency physicians. *Acad Emerg Med*. 2001;38:469–470.

4. Rubin M. Cardiac ultrasonography. *Emerg Med Clin North Am*. 1997;15:745–762.

5. Heller M, Melanson SW. Applications for ultrasonography in the emergency department. *Emerg Med Clin North Am*. 1997;15:735–744.

6. Nelson BP, Melnick ER, Li J. Portable ultrasound for remote environments. part II: current indications. *J Emerg Med*. 2011;40(3):313–321.

7. American College of Emergency Physicians. Policy statement Emergency ultrasound guidelines. Available at: http://www.acep.org/workarea/downloadasset.aspx?id=32878. Accessed August 24, 2010.

8. American Institute of Ultrasound in Medicine. AIUM practice guideline for the performance of the focused assessment with sonography for trauma (FAST) examination. Available at: http://www.aium.org/publications/guidelines/fast.pdf. Accessed August 24, 2010.

9. American College of Radiology. ACR standard for the performance of an ultrasound examination of the abdomen and/or retroperitoneum. Available at: http://www.acr.org/SecondaryMainMenuCategories/quality_safety/guidelines/us/us_abdomen_retro.aspx. Accessed August 24, 2010.

10. Rugolotto M, Chang C, Hu B, et al. Clinical use of cardiac ultrasound performed with a hand-carried device in patients admitted for acute cardiac care. *Am J Cardiol*. 2002;90:1040–1042.

11. Hendrickson RG, Dean AJ, Costantino TG. A novel use of ultrasound in pulseless electrical activity: the diagnosis of an acute abdominal aortic aneurysm rupture. *J Emerg Med*. 2001;21:141–144.

12. Tang A, Euerle B. Emergency department ultrasound and echocardiography. *Emerg Med Clin North Am*. 2005;23:1179–1194.

13. Mandavia D, Joseph A. Bedside echocardiography in chest trauma. *Emerg Med Clin North Am*. 2004;22:601–619.

14. Tayal VS, Kline JA. Emergency echocardiography to detect pericardial effusion in patients in PEA and near-PEA states. *Resuscitation*. 2003;59:315–318.

15. Perera P, Mailhot T, Riley D, et al. The RUSH exam: rapid ultrasound in shock in the evaluation of the critically ill. *Emerg Med Clin North Am*. 2010;28:29–56.

16. Chan D. Echocardiography in thoracic trauma. *Emerg Med Clin North Am*. 1998;16:191–207.

17. Woo KC, Schneider JI. High-risk chief complaints I: chest pain—the big three. *Emerg Med Clin North Am*. 2009;27:685–712.

18. Volpicelli G. Usefulness of emergency ultrasound in nontraumatic cardiac arrest. *Am J Emerg Med*. 2011;29(2):216–223.

19. Dolich MO, McKenney MG, Varela JE, et al. 2,576 ultrasounds for blunt abdominal trauma. *J Trauma*. 2001;50:108–112.

20. Ma OJ, Mateer JR, Ogata M, et al. Prospective analysis of a rapid trauma ultrasound examination performed by emergency physicians. *J Trauma*. 1995;18:879–885.

21. Dulchavsky SA, Schwarz KL, Kirkpatrick AW, et al. Prospective evaluation of thoracic ultrasound in the detection of pneumothorax. *J Trauma*. 2001;50:201–205.

22. Kirkpatrick AW, Sirois M, Laupland KB, et al. Hand-held thoracic sonography for detecting post-traumatic pneumothoraces: the extended focused assessment with sonography for trauma (EFAST). *J Trauma*. 2004;57:288–295.

23. Abboud PC, Kendall J. Emergency department ultrasound for hemothorax after blunt traumatic injury. *J Emerg Med*. 2003;25:181–184.

24. Gilman LM, Ball CG, Panebianco N, et al. Clinical performed resuscitative ultrasonography for the initial evaluation and resuscitation of trauma. *Scand J Trauma Resusc Emerg Med*. 2009;17:34.

25. Stone MB. Ultrasound diagnosis of traumatic pneumothorax. *J Emerg Trauma Shock*. 2008;1:19–20.

26. Lichtenstein D, Meziere G, Biderman P, et al. The "lung point": an ultrasound sign specific to pneumothorax. *Intensive Care Med*. 2000;26:1434–1440.

27. Lichtenstein D, Meziere G, Lascols N, et al. Ultrasound diagnosis of occult pneumothorax. *Crit Care Med*. 2005;33:1231–1238.

28. Wherrett LJ, Boulanger BR, McLellan BA, et al. Hypotension after blunt abdominal trauma: the role of emergent abdominal sonography in surgical triage. *J Trauma*. 1996;41:815–820.

29. Reardon R, Moscati R. Beyond the FAST exam: additional applications of sonography in trauma. In: Jehle D, Heller M, eds. *Ultrasonography in Trauma: The FAST Exam*. Dallas, TX: American College of Emergency Physicians; 2003:107–126.

30. Moscati R, Reardon R. Clinical application of the FAST exam. In: Jehle D, Heller M, eds. *Ultrasonography in Trauma: The FAST Exam*. Dallas, TX: American College of Emergency Physicians; 2003:39–60.

31. Rothlin MA, Naf R, Amgwerd M, et al. Ultrasound in blunt abdominal and thoracic trauma. *J Trauma*. 1993;34:488–495.

32. Abrams BJ, Sukumvanich P, Seibel R, et al. Ultrasound for the detection of intraperitoneal fluid: the role of Trendelenburg positioning. *Am J Emerg Med*. 1999;17:117–120.

33. ACEP Clinical Policies Committee. Clinical policy: critical issues in the evaluation and management of adult patients presenting with suspected lower-extremity deep venous thrombosis. *Ann Emerg Med*. 2003;42:124–135.

34. Chopra A. DVT & pulmonary embolus. In: *The ABC's of Emergency Medicine*. 11th ed. Divisions of Emergency Medicine, Faculty of Medicine, University of Toronto; 2002. Available at: http://www.emergencymedicine.utoronto.ca/Assets/EmergeMed+Digital+Assets/education/ugrad/The+ABC$!27s+of+Emergency+Medicine.pdf. Accessed August 7, 2010.

35. Blaivas M, Lambert MJ, Harwood RA, et al. Lower-extremity Doppler for deep vein thrombosis—can emergency physicians be accurate and fast? *Acad Emerg Med*. 2000;7:120–126.

36. Kline JA, O'Malley PM, Tayal VS, et al. Emergency-clinician performed compression ultrasonography for deep venous thrombosis of the lower extremity. *Ann Emerg Med*. 2008;52:437–445.

37. Theodoro D, Blaivas M, Duggal S, et al. Real-time B-mode ultrasound in the ED saves time in the diagnosis of deep vein thrombosis (DVT). *Am J Emerg Med*. 2004;22: 197–200.

38. Fox J. Lower extremity venous studies. In: Cosby K, ed. *Practical Guide to Emergency Ultrasound*. Philadelphia, PA: Lippincott Williams & Wilkins; 2006: 255–266.

39. Jacoby J, Cesta M, Axelband J, et al. Can emergency medicine residents detect acute deep venous thrombosis with a limited, two-site ultrasound examination? *J Emerg Med*. 2007;32:197–200.

40. Jang T, Docherty M, Aubin C, et al. Resident-performed compression ultrasonography for the detection of proximal deep vein thrombosis: fast and accurate. *Acad Emerg Med*. 2004;11:319–322.

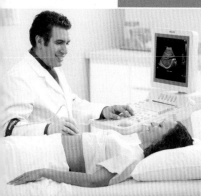

# 26 Foreign Bodies

Tim S. Gibbs

## OBJECTIVES

Identify and give examples of different types of soft tissue foreign bodies based on composition.

Explain sensitivity and specificity.

List the important information the sonographer should obtain from the patient interview and patient chart prior to providing a comprehensive sonography evaluation.

Differentiate the different sonographic appearances of soft tissue foreign bodies based on composition, location, age, and artifacts.

Describe the role of the sonographer prior to, during, and following sonography-guided foreign body removal.

Explain the limitations of sonography and the advantages of other imaging modalities used to image soft tissue foreign bodies.

## KEY TERMS

foreign bodies | granuloma | hypoechoic halo or rim | inorganic | organic | sensitivity | shadowing artifacts | soft tissue | specificity

## GLOSSARY

**granuloma** a tumor-like mass formation that usually contains macrophages and fibroblasts that forms as a result of chronic inflammation and isolation of the infected area

**hyperemia** an increase to the quantity of blood flow to a body part; increased blood blow as in the inflammatory response

**in vitro** when referring to a biologic process, it is made to occur in a laboratory vessel or in a controlled experimental environment but does not occur within a living organism or in a natural setting

**in vivo** when referring to a biologic process, it occurs or is made to occur within a living organism or natural setting

**occult** in reference to foreign bodies, the term refers to something hidden from view

**radiolucent** a tissue or material that allows transmission of X-rays and appears more dense (dark) on a radiograph; also known as nonradiopaque; for a foreign body, the material will often blend in and cannot be differentiated from the surrounding soft tissue

**radiopaque** a tissue, contrast, or material that attenuates or blocks radiation; the tissue, contrast, or material will appear bright on the radiograph

Conventional radiography, fluoroscopy, computed tomography (CT), magnetic resonance imaging (MRI), nuclear medicine, and sonography have been used to demonstrate the presence of foreign bodies. The purpose of this chapter is to present the sonographic scanning technique to recognize, locate, and assist in the removal of various types of soft tissue foreign bodies (STFBs) in superficial structures. Increasing sonographer and clinician awareness and confidence to choose sonography for STFB detection, localization, and removal may result in increased diagnostic accuracy and decreased diagnostic expense.

## COMPOSITION OF FOREIGN BODIES

Foreign bodies can be separated into three distinct categories based on their composition (Table 26-1). *Organic material* refers to biologic plant material and animal products. *Inorganic materials* are usually man-made products composed of minerals or

| TABLE 26-1 |  |
|---|---|
| **Composition of Foreign Bodies** |  |
| Organic | Plant material (thorn, wood, etc.) |
|  | Animal products (bee stinger, barb, etc.) |
| Inorganic | Glass, gravel, plastic (acrylic), pencil lead, graphite, and so forth. |
| Metallic | Wire, needle, fish hook, and so forth. |

made from minerals but are not animal or vegetable in origin. Metallic materials are those products with a metal alloy.

## SENSITIVITY AND SPECIFICITY

Radiographic imaging for foreign bodies has been used for many years with some degree of success. Because radiography relies on the density of the foreign body (FB), it has varied sensitivities for imaging the different types of FBs. Radiography detects 98% of radiopaque objects such as gravel, most glass, and metal[1]; however, radiography detects only 15% or less of radiolucent foreign bodies such as wood, plastic, some glass, and cactus spine.[2] Despite the poor sensitivity of radiography to demonstrate many organic objects and some inorganic objects, conventional radiography remains the most commonly used imaging study for the evaluation of FBs in the emergency department.[3] Consequently, many FBs are missed on initial evaluation. In fact, missed FBs are the second leading cause of malpractice lawsuits against emergency medicine physicians.[4,5] Wound care litigation constitutes 5% to 20% of lawsuit claims against

emergency medicine physicians and results in 3% to 11% of monetary rewards.[6,7]

Sonography performs well in demonstrating the FBs traditionally considered the most difficult to image on radiographic studies. In a retrospective studies where radiography failed to demonstrate a STFB, sonography had a sensitivity of 95% and a specificity of 89%.[8,9] In a prospective study using cadaver feet and wooden foreign bodies, Jacobson et al.[10] reported that sonography can reveal wooden FBs as small as 2.5 mm in length with 86.7% sensitivity and 96.7% specificity. At the time of this study, the resolution of the sonography equipment either makes visualizing FBs smaller than 2.5 mm more difficult or limits adequate visualization. Equipment today is capable of resolving objects within ±1 mm.

## SONOGRAPHY EQUIPMENT

Whenever possible, a 7- to 12-MHz high-resolution, linear array transducer should be used to obtain the images. A large footprint transducer is generally preferable for initial FB imaging and localization, but a small footprint transducer may be used when indicated. Maximizing image size by using a large, high-resolution monitor also facilitates FB identification. It may be difficult to identify small FBs on smaller monitors seen on some portable equipment. Visualization of superficial FBs may be facilitated by use of a water bath (Fig. 26-1). When it is necessary to increase the near field length for better visualization of the skin surface and to place a superficial FB in the focal zone, the sonographer can use a standoff gel pad[11–13] or something as simple as a thicker layer of scanning gel[10] (Fig. 26-2).

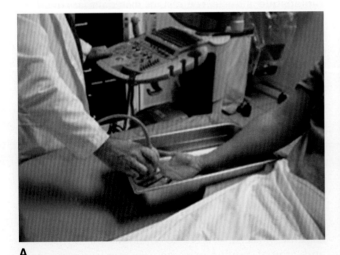

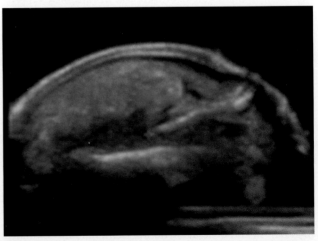

A

B

**Figure 26-1** Water bath. **A:** The photograph demonstrates using a water bath to scan the finger. **B:** The sonogram demonstrates a hyperechoic foreign body that was a broken toothpick located in the finger. (Photo and image courtesy and permission of Robert Tillotson DO, RDMS, FACEP, FAAEM, Stevens Point, WI.)

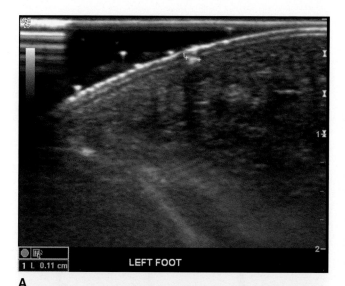

A    LEFT FOOT

B    LT PLANTAR TRANS

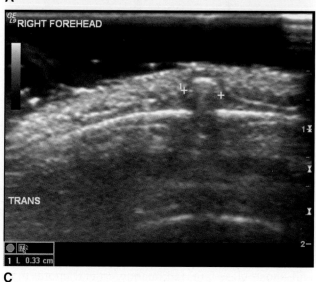

C    TRANS

**Figure 26-2** Increasing the near field length can be achieved by using a standoff gel pad or thicker layer of scanning gel, which can help to demonstrate superficial foreign bodies. **A:** On a sonogram of the foot, the punctate, hyperechoic material was diagnosed as gravel. **B:** The transverse sonogram of the left plantar image demonstrates glass as hyperechoic echoes in this foot of a 1-year-old infant. **C:** The transducer-to-skin surface distance of a standoff gel pad is seen on this transverse image, which demonstrates the hyperechoic glass located in the right forehead.

## IMAGING TECHNOLOGY

Shadowing and reverberation artifacts are helpful in both identifying and locating a FB. Newer technology does not provide any apparent improvement when imaging FBs and actually may make detection more difficult. Two of these instrumentation selections are tissue harmonics imaging (THI) and instrumentation that uses transmit beam-steering to create multiple imaging angles and then combines these microimages from different viewing angles into a single compounded image. The use of multiple imaging angles reduces shadow artifact, which is an important secondary sign in the detection of FBs (Fig. 26-3). The same is true for THI where shadowing is diminished or eliminated completely. Only the speckle reduction imaging (SRI) feature has helped improve image quality over normal imaging parameters (Fig. 26-4).

Color and power Doppler may further increase sensitivity as the normal inflammatory reaction materializes in a hypoechoic ring around the FB as a result of hyperemic flow.[14] Color Doppler parameters should be set to visualize slow flow (low velocity) to help determine if reactive hyperemia is present.[14] Varying the transducer angle in relation to the FB will assure the best color flow image will be obtained with the highest Doppler shift.

## EVALUATING THE COMPOSITION, LOCATION, AGE, AND APPEARANCE

Before beginning the imaging examination, conduct the patient interview and review the patient's chart. If a radiographic procedure has already been performed, review the radiographs. The information that is helpful prior to scanning includes ascertaining the type of

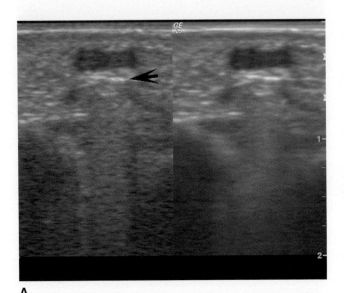

**A**

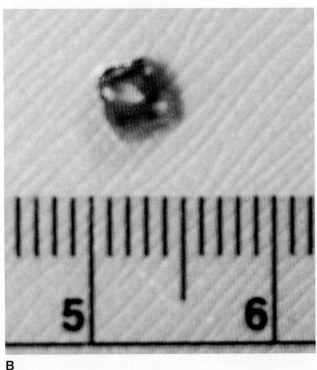

**B**

**Figure 26-3 A:** Compare the edge shadowing *(arrow)* and resolution of the glass foreign body of the image on the left made with normal instrumentation and the sonogram on the right made with crossbeam instrumentation. **B:** After removing the glass fragment, the foreign body is seen on the centimeter ruler.

material, the mechanism of injury to include the point of entry, and the duration of symptoms.

## COMPOSITION

The organic FB is the most difficult to locate and is rarely demonstrated on radiography; however, organic FBs are easier to locate and demonstrate on

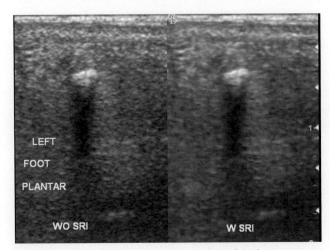

**Figure 26-4** A toothpick in the plantar surface of the foot is seen on these two images. Compare the foreign body image without speckle reduction *(WO SRI)* to the image with speckle reduction *(W SRI)*.

sonography. The echogenic pattern of an organic FB varies with its indwelling age. Some inorganic FBs can be difficult to image using radiography but present little challenge for sonography. The metallic FB can be seen on radiography and sonography. Metal and most glass are radiopaque (metal more than glass) and relatively easily seen with radiography (Fig. 26-5).

## LOCATION

When locating a FB, use radiographs if available to provide further information regarding location, depth, and composition of the FB. When used, radiographs should be obtained in two perpendicular projections (imaging planes) in order to triangulate the location. The FB will only be radiographically visualized if its density is greater than the surrounding soft tissue.

Radiographs may assist in targeting the location for initial insonation. This is especially helpful when external signs such as swelling or redness are not present. A working knowledge of the normal soft tissue structures can assist in separating normal structures from that of the FB (Fig. 26-6A). By documenting these anatomical structures and their relationship to the FB (veins, arteries, tendons, etc.), the physician can plan the best approach for its

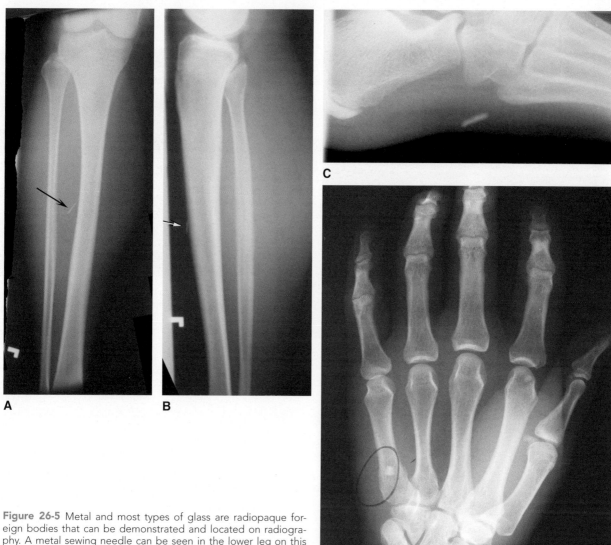

**Figure 26-5** Metal and most types of glass are radiopaque foreign bodies that can be demonstrated and located on radiography. A metal sewing needle can be seen in the lower leg on this **(A)** anterior to posterior projection and **(B)** the lateral projection of the tibia and fibula. **C:** A glass foreign body is seen on a lateral projection of the plantar surface of the foot. **D:** On a posterior to anterior projection of the hand, a glass foreign body is seen near the proximal end of the fifth metacarpal.

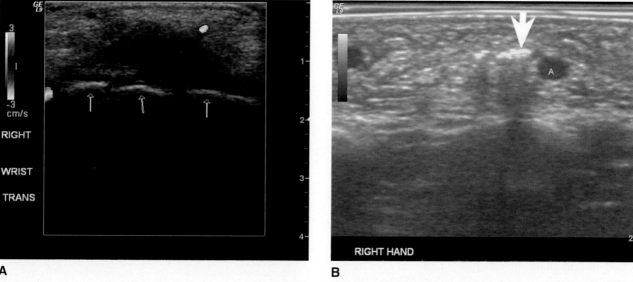

**Figure 26-6** Knowing soft tissue structures and anatomic relationships is important to enable differentiating anatomy from a foreign body and to identify the foreign body location. **A:** A transverse sonogram demonstrates three linear echogenic structures *(arrows)*. The structures are three right carpal bones but were mistaken for foreign bodies. **B:** A sonogram of the right hand shows the relationship of the foreign body *(arrow)* to an artery *(A)*.

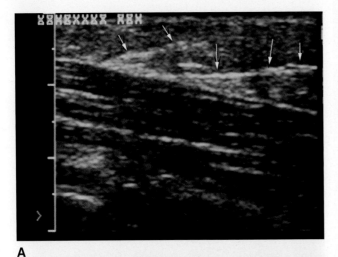

**A**

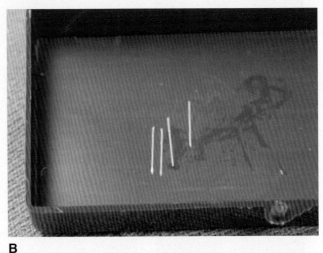

**B**

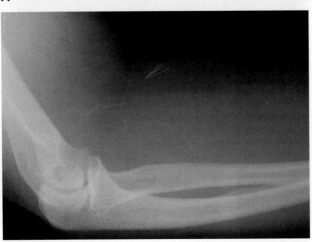

**C**

**Figure 26-7** This patient with 26-gauge hypodermic needles imbedded in her upper forearm presented a difficult challenge. **A:** Imaging perpendicular to the proximal forearm best demonstrated the needles *(arrows).* **B:** The superficial four needles were easily demonstrated and removed. **C:** The lateral view of the right elbows made with fluoroscopy during removal, demonstrates six radiopaque needles that were not seen sonographically.

removal to diminish postoperative complications[12] (Fig. 26-6B).

The smaller the FB, the more difficult it is to visualize.[15] The depth of the FB will determine the optimal frequency of the transducer. Ideally, the highest frequency possible that allows adequate depth of penetration should be utilized. Every attempt should be made to visualize the FB perpendicular to the transducer to minimize the potential errors in location and position within the soft tissue[12] (Fig. 26-7). When the FB is visualized, its location should be marked on the overlying skin for the physician to use during sonography-guided FB removal.

## AGE

Based on the duration of symptoms before imaging, the FB may be described in one of three age categories: acute, intermediate, or chronic[16] (Table 26-2). The sonographic appearance of a STFB will correlate with the type and with the age of the retained material.

In the acute phase, the FB will present as a bright echogenic structure with shadowing, which is due to the strong reflection of air in an organic FB, the material composition of an inorganic FB, or the alloy in a metallic FB. The term dirty shadowing is used when the reflection is due to the refracting properties of small gas bubbles and the high impedance of a gas.[3] The term clean shadowing is used when it is caused by attenuating properties (Fig. 26-8). A potential pitfall usually occurs with a projectile FB when there is air within the wound, which can obscure the visualization of the FB. This may be diminished or avoided by using multiple imaging angles after evaluating the FB with

| TABLE 26-2 |  |
|---|---|
| **Age of the Foreign Body** |  |
| Acute phase | Injury less than 3 days |
| Intermediate phase | Injury within 3–10 days |
| Chronic phase | Injury more than 10 days |

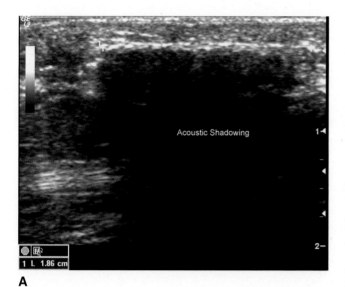

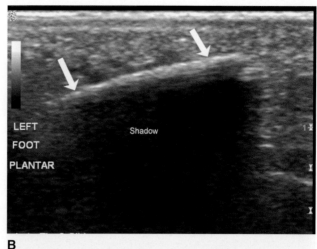

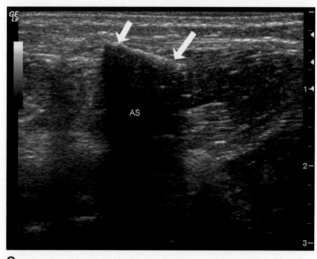

**Figure 26-8** Shadowing. **A:** The linear echogenic foreign body is seen with distal acoustic shadowing. **B:** The sonogram of an acute injury to the plantar surface demonstrates a linear echogenic toothpick *(arrows)* with distal shadowing. **C:** The sonogram of a slanted echogenic foreign body *(arrows)* shows distal clean shadowing *(AS)*.

perpendicular beam. After 24 hours from the beginning of the acute phase, a hypoechoic ring develops around the FB representing an inflammatory reaction to the FB.[17,18] The hypoechoic halo helps locate a FB as it highlights its location[14] (Fig. 26-9).

In the intermediate injury phase with an organic FB, air is slowly replaced with fluid. The sound penetrates through the FB without the shadowing artifact from the air that was present in the acute phase. At this point, the inflammatory response to the FB will appear with a more pronounced hypoechoic halo seen surrounding each type of FB. The hypoechoic ring can be used to improve both the sensitivity and specificity of the sonography examination.[17] Toward the end of this phase, the inflammatory response increases and the hypoechoic halo surrounding the FB becomes even more pronounced (Fig. 26-10). This inflammatory response may demonstrate an increased vascular perfusion on color or power Doppler.[14]

In the chronic phase, the appearance of the organic FB is similar to the acute phase in that air is replaced

by bodily fluid (Fig. 26-11). As the chronic stage progresses, a dense granular material develops encapsulating all three types of foreign bodies. This is the body's response to wall off the foreign material.[18] The inflammatory response can result in a clean shadow similar to that of bone (Fig. 26-12). If the granular material attenuates sound, the FB in this stage may be easier to locate and demonstrate with sonography. When located superficially, the FB and associated granuloma may easily be palpated aiding in the documenting its location.

## APPEARANCE

The changing sonographic appearance of retained FBs can assist in their detection and can be used to draw attention to the actual FB itself (Table 26-3). Most FBs are echogenic. Artifacts created by the FB may help identify their location. Comet tail artifacts can be seen with both metallic and glass foreign bodies[9,19] (Fig. 26-13). Clean or dirty posterior shadowing may also be seen with a FB or with fragments from a FB of varying thicknesses

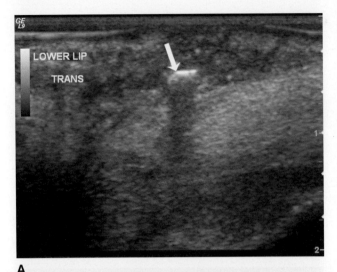

A

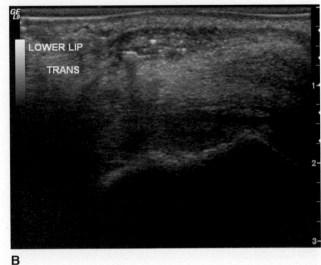

B

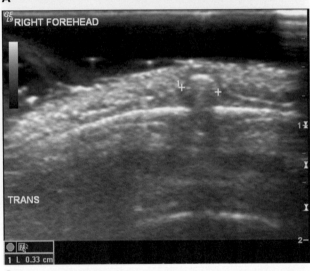

C

**Figure 26-9** Hypoechoic rim. **A:** The transverse sonogram shows a large broken tooth fragment imbedded in the lower lip with surrounding exudation. There is acoustic shadowing distal to the linear echogenic tooth fragment. **B:** On the same patient, a transverse sonogram shows multiple small tooth fragments, which appear echogenic and are located in the lower lip with a surrounding inflammatory process. **C:** On this patient, a transverse sonogram shows the glass foreign body in the forehead with the early formation of a hypoechoic rim.

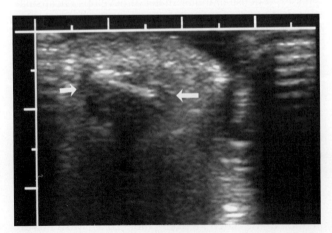

**Figure 26-10** This sonogram demonstrates a linear echogenic wood splinter in the finger with some distal acoustic shadowing. A hypoechoic halo (arrows) representing an inflammatory reaction to the foreign body is forming around the wooden foreign body.

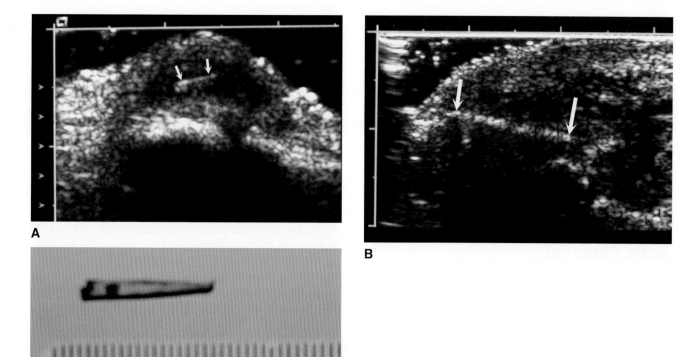

**Figure 26-11 A:** The longitudinal sonogram of the finger shows a linear echogenic wood foreign body *(arrows)*. The air normally seen in wood is replaced by fluid, which results in the loss of an acoustical shadow. **B:** On this patient, the sonogram was made on a wooden splinter *(arrows)* in the late intermediate early chronic stage. The splinter looses the acoustic shadow as air due to fluid replacement. **C:** The 2-cm splinter is seen after removal.

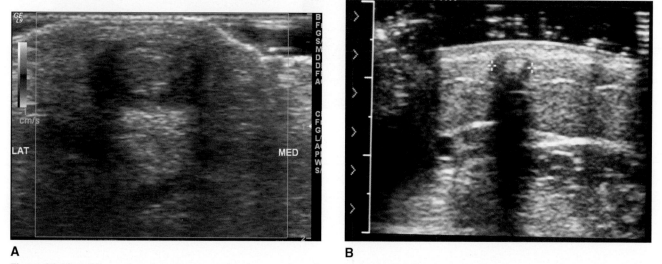

**Figure 26-12 A:** The transverse sonogram on the plantar surface shows the formation of a granuloma from a 3-month-old glass foreign body. **B:** This transverse sonogram shows a 5.6-mm granuloma from a retained bee stinger. In this patient, the attenuation by the granular material creates a clean shadow distal to the granuloma and foreign body.

**TABLE** **26-3**

Appearance of Retained Foreign Bodies

- Echogenic with clean shadowing
- Echogenic with dirty shadowing
- Echogenic with distal ring down
- Echogenic with hypoechoic ring surrounding it

and shapes. A potential pitfall of relying on shadowing is that air within the soft tissue can mimic the appearance of a FB (Fig. 26-14).

## SONOGRAPHY-GUIDED FOREIGN BODY REMOVAL

Once located, the depth, size, shape, and orientation or position of the FB should be determined and sonographically documented. A three-dimensional localization should be

made by scanning the area of interest in both the longitudinal and transverse orientations, with attention to detecting a FB and imaging any associated posterior acoustic shadowing or reverberation echoes.[11,17,18] It is important to mark the surface of the skin with an indelible marker directly over the FB. To facilitate this, a paperclip may be inserted between the patient and the transducer to create a shadow on the FB. The transducer is then removed and a mark is placed at the skin surface. If the FB is a small square or round BB sized object, a dot is sufficient to mark its location. If the FB is a linear object like a needle or toothpick, both ends of the FB should be marked and connected by a dotted line. This provides the physician with information regarding which direction to pull out the material (Fig. 26-15).

The location and distance of the FB from an acute entry wound can help the physician determine if removing the FB through the original track is feasible or whether a more direct approach is required. Trauma to

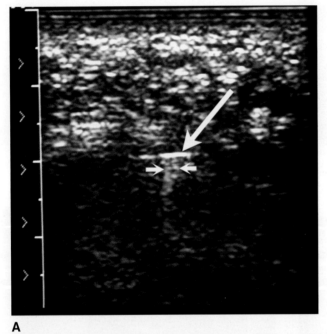

A

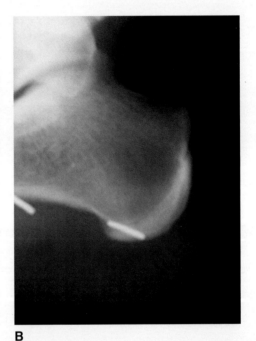

B

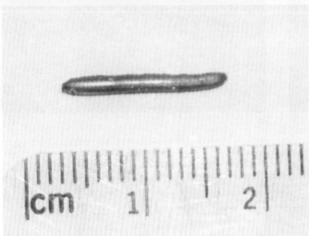

C

**Figure 26-13** This patient presented with a history of being injured with a wire. **A:** The sonogram shows the wire *(arrow)* located 2-cm deep, posterior, and lateral to the calcaneus. Distal to the wire, *short arrows* mark the comet tail artifact that are closely spaced reverberation echoes. **B:** The radiopaque wire can be seen on a lateral radiograph of the calcaneus. **C:** The 1.5-cm wire is measured after its removal.

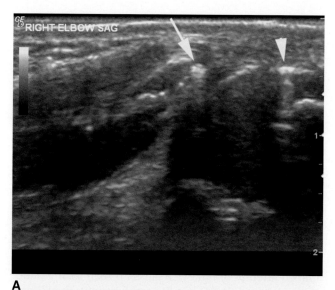

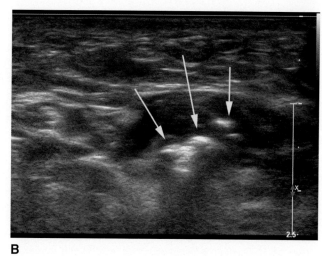

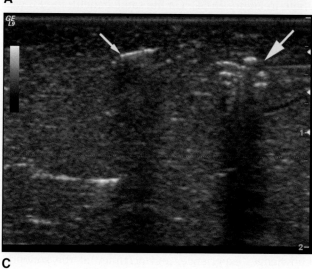

**Figure 26-14** **A:** The longitudinal sonogram of the right elbow demonstrates glass *(arrow)* embedded in soft tissue near air *(arrowhead)*, which can mimic a foreign body. **B:** The air *(arrows)* seen on this sonogram through soft tissue can mimic foreign bodies. **C:** On this sonogram, one can see shadowing from the foreign body *(small arrow)* and from the air *(large arrow)*, which was introduced with a lidocaine injection.

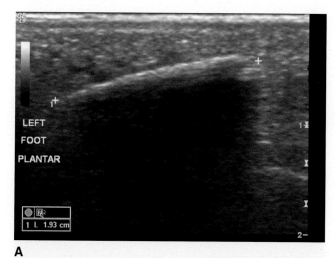

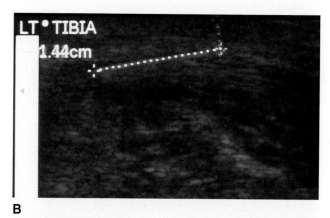

**Figure 26-15** Documenting foreign body location. **A:** The sonographer should annotate the image so the physician can see related anatomy and the angle of the foreign body in relationship to the skin surface. **B:** The annotation should include the length and depth of the foreign body in the soft tissue.

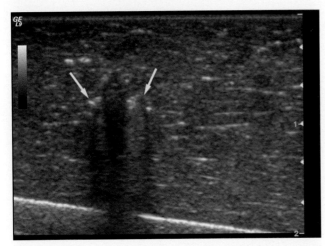

**Figure 26-16** During sonography-assisted removal, this sonogram shows the forceps *(arrows)* holding a glass fragment prior to removal.

the surrounding soft tissue is reduced whenever the FB can be removed through the original injury track. The physician may only need to enlarge the track slightly to provide access for the forceps. Using sonographic guidance for FB removal can result in reducing the size of incision with a less traumatic dissection to find and remove the material.[12] When using direct sonographic imaging to guide the forceps, it may be necessary to use a small footprint sector transducer in place of a linear transducer (Fig. 26-16).

When an open wound is present, the physician needs to determine if the FB may be removed through the tract it entered. In order to determine the best approach and minimize postoperative complications, the tract's angle and characteristics as well as the surrounding structures and their relationship to the FB should be ascertained. To further assist in removal of small foreign bodies, a needle or guide wire may be inserted with the tip placed at the FB. This provides a path of dissection through which the FB may be removed[12] (Fig. 26-17).

If the site is old and the original track has closed, determining the FB position can result in a smaller incision and decreased dissection for its removal. This results in decreased risk of complications as well as a faster recovery period. Untreated or retained foreign bodies can result in inflammation, infection, tendon or nerve injury, and allergic reaction[13,17,20] (Fig. 26-18). Infection is the most common complication with nerve injury a distant second.[2,17] If a patient presents with a history of recurrent localized infections, the patient should be asked about recent or remote trauma that may lead to a necessary search for a retained FB.[6]

Once the initial learning curve is overcome, sonographic guidance results in reduced time for FB localization and removal, smaller incisions, and less traumatic dissections.[12] A physician spent 20 minutes in a failed attempt to remove a glass FB seen on the radiograph in Figure 26-5D. On the same patient, the FB was removed in less than 1 minute using the sonography image seen in Figure 26-3A to reveal the FB location and the appropriate path of dissection.

After removal the site should be reimaged to evaluate if the removal was a complete success. A postremoval sonography evaluation precaution will help prevent retained FBs, which can result in inflammation, infection, tissue injury, and allergic reaction[13,17,20] (Fig. 26-19).

## LIMITATION OF SONOGRAPHY

Although sonography is effective in localizing FBs, there are limitations to its successful use. The major limitation is that the examination relies on the skill, knowledge, experience, and accuracy of the sonographer. While sonography has demonstrated superficial FBs less than 2 mm in size, sonography can be challenging for imaging objects that are smaller and/or not superficially located. FBs may also be obscured by

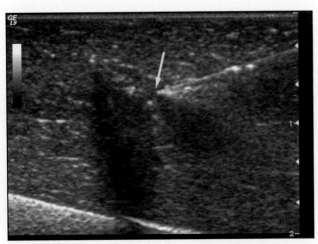

**Figure 26-17** The sonogram shows the placement of the needle tip *(arrow)* adjacent to a glass fragment.

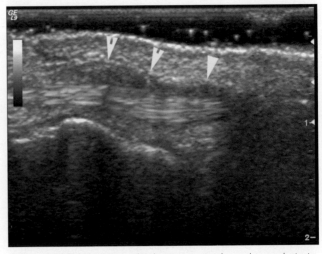

**Figure 26-18** The longitudinal sonograms shows hypoechoic inflammation *(arrows)*, surrounding the tendon.

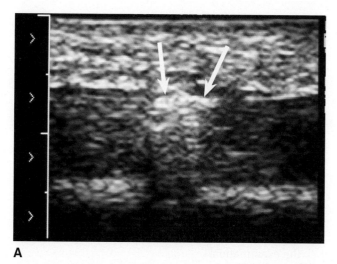

**A**

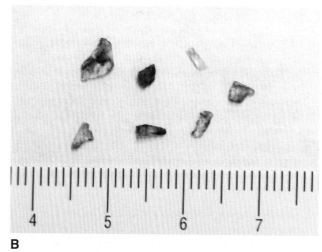

**B**

**Figure 26-19** Removing glass from the forearm. **A:** After sonography-guided removal of three small glass shards, the rescanning of the area showed foreign bodies *(arrows)* were still present. **B:** Seven more glass shards were eventually removed.

bony structures and air within the wound. Varying the imaging angles can decrease obscuration from bone. Imaging prior to wound exploration or irrigation may decrease introduction of air bubbles into the field of view. Air within the open cavity or removal site creates difficulty for sonographic imaging as it can mimic the appearance of a FB or obscure a FB. Air is introduced with the injection of a numbing anesthetic such as lidocaine and can result in almost total obliteration of a FB on the sonography image (Fig. 26-20).

False-positive findings can occur as a result from calcifications, scar tissue, fresh hematoma, or air trapped in the soft tissues.[17] Air within the tract created by the FB is seldom a problem for sonography if imaging is performed before any surgical intervention. Small glass fragments can mimic the appearance of air when the wound is still open. With a good understanding of normal anatomical structures, this potential risk with an open wound can be minimized (Fig. 26-20). Prior unsuccessful attempts at removing a FB can result in scar tissue that can distort the normal anatomical structures making a definitive identification problematic.

## COMPARING IMAGING MODALITIES

Conventional radiography is capable of visualizing metal, glass, and stone in bone, muscle, and air but is limited in demonstrating graphite only in muscle.[21] Most organic and inorganic foreign bodies are radiolucent and cannot be visualized on radiography in bone, muscle, or air.

On a CT image, wood is not seen in bone, is difficult to image in muscle, but may be seen in air.[21] CT imaging does detect metal, glass, stone, and graphite in bone and muscle. The greatest advantage of CT over conventional radiography or sonography is its capability of demonstrating foreign bodies in air.[21] CT scanning

is a more expensive imaging procedure, uses ionizing radiation, and may require sedation when used with pediatric patients.[17]

MRI is of limited use in the early detection of a FB as the modality is more expensive and its availability is more limited. For safety reasons, MRI should not be used for metallic foreign bodies and other unknown types of foreign bodies. The usefulness of MRI in FB evaluation is providing detailed information regarding tissue inflammatory reactions, osteoblastic or osteolytic changes, and secondary tissue reactions that can aid in determining the presence and location of an otherwise occult FB.[22]

Sonography has been proven more effective and less expensive than CT imaging eliminating the problem of radiation exposure.[9] The widespread availability and low cost of sonography make it the best choice for

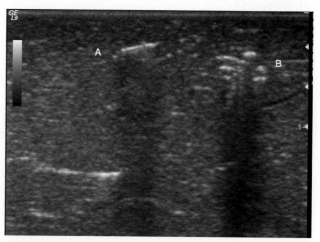

**Figure 26-20 A:** The sonogram on the left shows a glass foreign body as a linear echogenic structure in the tissue with some distal attenuation. **B:** Following injection with lidocaine, the sonogram on the right shows air bubbles interfering with visualizing the glass foreign body. Note the distal acoustic shadowing.

## Critical Thinking Questions

1. A 9-year-old boy has pain on the lateral border of the left foot. Radiography did not show any abnormality or explanation for a firm nodule with a purple tinge. The patient's mother wants this taken care of as soon as possible as the child will need to start wearing shoes again when he returns to school next week. When the patient was interviewed, the sonographer learns the child often played barefoot this summer in a heavily wooded area. What should the sonographer suspect and include in the imaging evaluation?

2. A fellow sonography student is looking for a research project and is interested in gaining a better understanding of the different foreign bodies. You explain to the student that much of the early research was performed using retrospective in vivo studies or prospective in vitro studies. Due to the limited time allocation for the research project and the limited number of studies which can be evaluated with a retrospective data collection, describe a prospective study to the student using turkey breasts. The student will be able to create a situation to evaluate the composition, location, and artifacts of the various foreign bodies embedded in the turkey breast. Why will it be difficult to evaluate the age of the foreign bodies?

3. During sonography evaluation of a foreign body, a hypoechoic rim or halo is detected and documented. Why does detecting and documenting a hypoechoic rim or halo improve the sensitivity and specificity of the examination?

4. During sonography evaluation for a foreign body, what conditions increase false-positive findings?

determining the presence of FB. A major reason sonographic utilization does not increase may be related to the lack of knowledge, experience, and confidence with sonographic findings, which prompt physicians to order other imaging procedures.[16] The American College of Emergency Physicians published guidelines recognizing foreign body detection and removal as a unique and evolving application of emergency sonography.[23] Sonography should become the main imaging tool used for the detection and localization of soft tissue FBs because of its sensitivity compared to the lack of sensitivity of other imaging modalities, it is noninvasive compared to ionizing radiation or magnet safety seen in other modalities, and it provides a high-resolution, real-time evaluation.[10,12,24]

## SUMMARY

- Sonographer and clinician awareness to use sonography for STFB recognition, localization, and removal may result in decreased diagnostic expense and increased diagnostic accuracy.

- When using high-frequency transducers to obtain high-resolution imaging, sonography is sensitive and specific for the detection of soft tissue foreign bodies, which has been demonstrated in vivo[11,12] and in vitro.[5,24]

- The sonography examination relies on the skill, knowledge, and accuracy of the sonographer who pays attention to the composition, location, age, and artifacts associated with foreign bodies.

- The experienced sonographer has an important role prior to, during, and following sonography-guided foreign body removal.

- Recognizing foreign body detection and removal is a unique and evolving application of emergency sonography.

- Sonography should become the main imaging tool used for the detection and localization of soft tissue foreign bodies because of its sensitivity, it is noninvasive, and it provides a high-resolution, real-time evaluation.

### REFERENCES

1. Manthey DE, Storrow AB, Milbourn JM, et al. Ultrasound versus radiography in the detection of soft-tissue foreign bodies. *Ann Emerg Med.* 1996;28:7–9.
2. Anderson MA, Newmeyer WL, Kilgore ES Jr. Diagnosis and treatment of retained foreign bodies in the hand. *Am J Surg.* 1982;144:63–67.
3. Lyon M, Brannam L, Johnson D, et al. Detection of soft tissue foreign bodies in the presence of soft tissue gas. *J Ultrasound Med.* 2004;23:677–681.
4. Dunn JD. Risk management in emergency medicine. *Emerg Med Clin North Am.* 1987;5:51–69.
5. Schlager D, Sanders AB, Wiggins D, et al. Ultrasound for the detection of foreign bodies. *Ann Emerg Med.* 1991;20:189–191.
6. Bass AM, Levis JT. Foreign body removal, wound. *Medscape: eMedicine.* January 2010. Available at: http://emedicine.medscape.com/article/1508207-overview. Accessed August 8, 2010.
7. Pfaff JA, Moore GP. Reducing risk in emergency department wound management. *Emerg Med Clin North Am.* 2007;25:189–201.
8. Bray PW, Mahoney JL, Campbell JP. Sensitivity and specificity of ultrasound in the diagnosis of foreign bodies in the hand. *J Hand Surg Am.* 1995;20:661–666.
9. Gilbert FJ, Campbell RS, Bayliss AP. The role of ultrasound in the detection of non-radiopaque foreign bodies. *Clin Radiol.* 1990;41:109–112.

10. Jacobson JA, Powell A, Craig JG, et al. Wooden foreign bodies in soft tissue: detection at US. *Radiology*. 1998;206:45–48.

11. Fornage BD, Schernberg FL. Sonographic diagnosis of foreign bodies of the distal extremities. *AJR Am J Roentgenol*. 1986;147:567–569.

12. Shiels WE II, Babcock DS, Wilson JL, et al. Localization and guided removal of soft-tissue foreign bodies with sonography. *AJR Am J Roentgenol*. 1990;155: 1277–1281.

13. Soudack M, Nachtigal A, Gaitini D. Clinically unsuspected foreign bodies: the importance of sonography. *J Ultrasound Med*. 2003;22:1381–1385.

14. Davae KC, Sofka CM, DiCarlo E, et al. Value of power Doppler imaging and hypoechoic halo in the sonographic detection of foreign bodies: correlation with histopathologic findings. *J Ultrasound Med*. 2003;22:1309–1313.

15. Tillotson R. Use of sonography in the evaluation of abscess, foreign bodies, and ocular evaluation. 2009 *SDMS* Annual Conference Proceedings, October 18, 2009, Society of Diagnostic Medical Sonography. Available at: http://www.sdms.org/members/AC2009Syllabi/syllabi/ SU-85.pdf. Accessed July 28, 2010.

16. Gibbs TS. The use of sonography in the identification and removal of soft tissue foreign bodies. *J Diagn Med Sonogr*. 2006;22:5–21.

17. Boyse TD, Fessell DP, Jacobson JA, et al. US of soft-tissue foreign bodies and associated complication with surgical correlation. *Radiographics*. 2001;21:1251–1256.

18. Saboo SS, Saboo SH, Soni SS, et al. High-resolution sonography is effective in detection of soft tissue foreign bodies: experience from a rural Indian center. *J Ultrasound Med*. 2009;28:1245–1249.

19. Ziskin MC, Thickman DI, Goldenberg NJ, et al. The comet tail artifact. *J Ultrasound Med*. 1982;1:1–7.

20. De La Torre C, Toribio J. Sea-urchin granuloma: histologic profile. A pathologic study of 50 biopsies. *J Cutan Pathol*. 2001;28:223–228.

21. Aras MH, Miloglu O, Barutcugil C, et al. Comparison of the sensitivity for detecting foreign bodies among conventional plain radiography, computed tomography, and ultrasonography. *Dentomaxillofac Radiol*. 2010;39: 72–78.

22. Bass AM, Levis JT. Foreign body removal, wound: treatment & medication. *Medscape: eMedicine*. January 2010. Available at: http://emedicine.medscape.com/article/1508207-treatment. Accessed August 8, 2010.

23. American College of Emergency Physicians. Emergency ultrasound guidelines. *Ann Emerg Med*. 2009;53:550–570.

24. Gooding GA, Hardiman T, Sumers M, et al. Sonography of the hand and foot in foreign body detection. *J Ultrasound Med*. 1987;6:441–447.

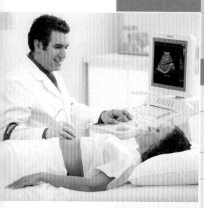

# 27 Sonography-Guided Interventional Procedures

Aubrey J. Rybyinski

## OBJECTIVES

Describe the benefits of sonography-guided interventional procedures.

Discuss the indications and contraindications for sonography-guided interventional procedures.

Explain the role of the sonographer during sonography-guided interventional procedures.

Discuss the difference between a fine-needle aspiration and a core biopsy and the benefits of each procedure.

List common sonography-guided interventional procedures and the potential complications involved in each.

## KEY TERMS

abscess drainage | adrenal biopsy | breast biopsy | liver biopsy | lung biopsy | lymph node biopsy | musculoskeletal biopsy | pancreatic biopsy | paracentesis | prostate biopsy | pseudoaneurysm repair | renal biopsy | sonography-guided procedure | thoracentesis | thyroid biopsy

## GLOSSARY

**coagulopathy** a defect in the body's mechanism for blood clotting

**core biopsy** a procedure that utilizes a hollow core biopsy needle to remove a sample of tissue frequently with a biopsy gun

**fine-needle aspiration** a procedure that utilizes a small needle attached to a syringe, a vacuum is created, and sample cells are aspirated for evaluation

**fresh frozen plasma (FFP)** a form of blood plasma that contains all of the clotting factors except platelets that is used to treat patients with a coagulopathy prior to interventional procedures

**international normalized ratio (INR)** a value used to standardize prothrombin time results between institutions as it adjusts for variations in processing and is expressed as a number

**partial thromboplastin time (PTT)** laboratory test used to evaluate for blood clotting abnormalities

**pneumothorax** a collection of air or gas in the pleural cavity of the chest between the lung and the chest wall that creates pressure on the lung

**prostate specific antigen (PSA)** a laboratory examination that measures the level of prostate specific antigen, a protein produced by the prostate gland, in the blood; an elevated level can indicate the presence of prostate conditions such as prostate cancer, benign prostatic hypertrophy, and prostatitis

**prothrombin time (PT)** laboratory test used to evaluate for blood clotting abnormalities; the time it takes the blood to clot after thromboplastin and calcium are added to the sample is recorded

**pseudoaneurysm** a complication that can occur after cardiac catheterization or angioplasty in which a hematoma is formed by a leakage of blood from a small hole in the femoral artery

The use of sonographic guidance has proven to be an invaluable asset to clinicians and patients for diagnostic and therapeutic procedures. Sonographic guidance techniques are continuing to improve with advances in transducer and equipment technology as well as increased operator experience. Sonographic guidance is frequently used for localizing organs, masses, and fluid collections in the abdomen, chest, neck, pelvis, and retroperitoneum. The most successful sonography-guided procedures have all personnel involved work together as a team and this includes the sonographer, physician, nurse, cytologist, and patient. This chapter focuses on those guidance procedures performed within the sonography department.

# SONOGRAPHY-GUIDED BIOPSY

Percutaneous biopsy has become the widely accepted technique for confirmation of suspected malignant masses and characterization of many benign lesions in various locations throughout the body. Many of these masses are in locations that once required computed tomography (CT) guidance or open surgery, but now the new equipment and procedures allow for successful sonography-guided biopsy. The popularity of sonography guidance has increased steadily because it is minimally invasive, accurate, and relatively safe. A minimally invasive procedure offers a cost benefit as it prevents the need to surgically remove tissue, it allows for a shortened hospital stay, and it enables a patient faster acclamation in resuming his or her usual activities. The ability to accurately characterize disease lowers the number of additional exams to confirm diagnosis potentially decreasing the amount of radiation exposure.

Unlike other imaging modalities, sonography is readily available, inexpensive, and reproducible and can provide guidance in multiple imaging planes allowing for multiple patient positions and approaches to be considered. The greatest advantage, however, is that it permits the real-time visualization of the needle tip as it passes through tissue planes into the target area. This allows for precise needle placement and avoidance of important structures. Studies have shown that an accurate diagnosis can be made in 95% of cases regardless of sample size. In addition, color flow Doppler imaging can help prevent complications by identifying and helping the clinician to avoid vascular structures that may be in the needle path.

Traditionally, the use of sonography for guided biopsy was for large, superficial, or cystic masses. With improvements in technology and biopsy techniques, small, deeply located, and solid masses can also undergo successful and accurate biopsy. Biopsy of deep masses and masses in obese patients can be difficult with sonography because of the difficulty in lesion visualization resulting from sound attenuation in the soft tissues. Similarly, not all lesions can be visualized by sonography, as they may be isoechoic to the surrounding tissues. Lesions located within or behind bone or gas-filled bowel cannot be visualized because of nearly complete reflection of sound from the bone or air interface. Frequently biopsies of the breast, liver, kidney, prostate, thyroid, parathyroid, and cervical nodes are easily performed. However, other sites within the body can undergo biopsy if the lesion is adequately visualized. A good rule of thumb is any mass that is well visualized on ultrasound should be amendable to a sonography-guided biopsy. A major factor in the success of sonography-guided biopsy lies in the experience and comfort level of the sonographer and radiologist.[1]

## INDICATIONS AND CONTRAINDICATIONS

A biopsy is performed to definitely diagnose the nature of a lesion. The major indication for biopsy is the suspicion of either primary malignancy or metastatic disease. As a diagnostic tool evaluating potentially malignant conditions, biopsy is indicated for initial evaluation before both surgical and nonsurgical interventions such as the administration of chemotherapy or radiation. For example, a biopsy could be performed to differentiate a metastatic mass from a second primary malignancy in a patient with a known primary malignancy. Frequently, biopsies are performed to evaluate the nature of an indeterminate lesion, such as a solitary solid hepatic mass in a patient with no history of malignancy. Infrequently, a biopsy is performed for confirmation of a mass that is suspected of being benign.[2]

The three contraindications to needle biopsy include uncorrectable coagulopathy, unsafe biopsy route, and an uncooperative patient. Although there are studies stating compromised coagulopathy is not a contraindication for fluid aspiration and superficial or low-risk biopsies, it is presented to provide general knowledge. If the patient's coagulopathy is unavailable within his or her medical record, the patient should get routine lab tests, known as a coagulation study. The three tests—prothrombin time (PT), partial thromboplastin time (PTT), and international normalized ratio (INR)—measure the time it takes for the blood to form a clot. These tests are simple and results are usually available within 2 to 3 hours. Due to the variability of the PT and PTT values between institutions, the World Health Organization (WHO) implemented the INR. This value standardizes results between institutions as it adjusts for variations in processing and is expressed as a number.

Mild coagulopathies may occur secondary to the use of blood thinners, such as aspirin and warfarin, and some antibiotics.[3] If a coagulopathy is present, the procedure may be delayed and the causative drug discontinued until the laboratory values return to normal. Patients that cannot wait for values to normalize can be administered fresh frozen plasma (FFP) or vitamin K. An important consideration is given to patients in whom the need for biopsy outweighs any risk.

The choice of biopsy route is crucial to success and a safe route must be obtained. A biopsy path going through major vessels or highly vascular structures increases the risk of hemorrhage. Bowel, the trachea, and other adjacent organs must also be avoided. An uncooperative patient also contraindicates needle biopsy. Patient cooperation is necessary for success as uncontrolled motion during the biopsy increases the potential for laceration and hemorrhage. It may be necessary to administer a form of sedation to a potentially uncooperative pediatric, senile demented, or mentally challenged patient.[4]

## TYPES OF SONOGRAPHY-GUIDED PROCEDURES

Sonography can be used for biopsies, core biopsies, needle placement for fluid drainage or mass localization, placement for a nephrostomy tube in an obstructed kidney, and collecting fluid from an abscess. Most often, the biopsies are used to confirm if a lesion is benign, malignant, or infected to help determine an appropriate treatment plan. These methods are less invasive than open and closed surgical procedures as the incisions of the latter are much larger and require some level of local or general anesthesia.

### Fine-Needle Aspiration

Fine-needle aspiration (FNA) with sonographic guidance is a widely accepted technique for the confirmation of suspected malignant masses and characterization of many benign lesions in various locations. For this type of biopsy, a "fine" or "thin" needle, most often 20- to 27-gauge are utilized and attached to a syringe (Fig. 27-1). These needles allow for multiple passes and are considered low risk because of the needle's relative thickness. As the name indicates, this technique uses aspiration to sample cells or fluid from a mass and is optimal for lesions lying superficially or at a moderate depth.[2] Specimens may also be obtained using a capillary action technique involving an up-and-down motion of the needle within the mass. This technique reduces trauma to the cells, which in turn decreases the amount of background blood on cytologic evaluation. FNA is a reliable and safe method of obtaining tissue samples allowing cellular evaluation for cytologic examination. The overall accuracy increases when a cytopathologist evaluates the specimens during the procedure to determine if additional tissue aspiration is required for diagnosis.[5]

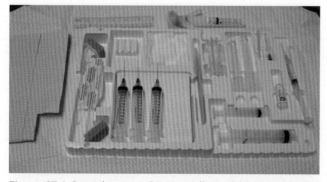

**Figure 27-1** Procedure tray. Commercially available prepackaged procedure trays contain antiseptic solution and needles attached to syringes. This procedure tray is set up for a thyroid fine-needle aspiration.

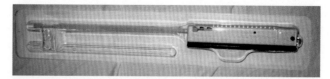

**Figure 27-2** Biopsy gun. Core samples throughout the body can be obtained using a commercially available biopsy gun. The sterile, prepackaged devices are available in a variety of gauges with different shaft and sample lengths.

### Core Biopsy

A core needle biopsy is a procedure that involves removing small samples of tissue using an automated hollow core needle commonly referred to as a "biopsy gun" (Fig. 27-2). The biopsy gun makes a loud noise when activated. It is important to make the patient aware of the noise to minimize patient alarm and patient motion during the procedure. As the name implies, the core biopsy needle facilitates the removal of a core sample of tissue and is a larger gauge than the needle used for FNA. Core biopsy needles are most often 14- to 19-gauge, offer various throw lengths, and have a tissue-cutting tip. The device is cocked and then inserted within the mass. A button is then pushed lunging the needle forward, which takes and stores a sample within a slot on the inner needle. In a core biopsy, the larger needle allows for a "core" tissue sample for analysis. The larger sample can be recut into smaller samples, which can be used for further analysis offering a more definitive histologic evaluation.[6] The larger sample can aid in the diagnosis of parenchymal disease, involving the breast, kidney, liver, prostate gland, and transplanted organs.

### Needle Selection

Each biopsy technique has its advantages and disadvantages, as does each needle type. There are a wide variety of needles commercially available, which vary in gauge, length, and tip configuration. An important consideration when choosing the appropriate needle is the amount of tissue required for accurate pathologic diagnosis.[7] The bore size of the needle is inversely related to its gauge. For example, a 16-gauge needle will offer a larger specimen than a 27-gauge needle. The choice of needle should be made with respect to the area being sampled and by knowing the risk of complications may increase from the use of a larger bore needle.

Although real-time visualization of the needle is one of the greatest strengths of sonography, it is often the most technically challenging. The sonographic appearance of a needle is either a hyperechoic line or dot depending on which imaging plane is used (Fig. 27-3). Larger caliber needles with a larger reflectivity surface are more readily visualized than the smaller gauge needles. If the needle is not visualized at first due to misalignment, usually maneuvering the transducer should

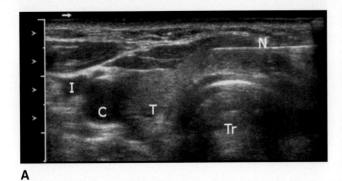

**A**

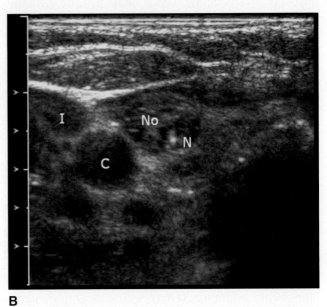

**B**

Figure 27-3 Needle visualization. **A:** The sonogram demonstrates the needle coursing through the thyroid isthmus perpendicular to the ultrasound beam. When the needle is visualized in the same plane as the transducer, the needle tip and shaft are visualized as an echogenic line. **B:** When the needle tip crosses out-of-plane to the sound beam as it does on this image, only the needle tip is represented as an echogenic dot within a thyroid nodule. *C,* carotid artery; *I,* internal jugular vein; *N,* needle; *No,* nodule; *T,* thyroid; *Tr,* trachea.

allow for visualization. The needle and transducer should be in the same plane to produce the best visualization. The ability to see the needle tip will improve the more perpendicular the needle is to the transducer. Needles are commercially available that are made specifically for sonography-guided procedures and are designed to aid in visualization, although any needle used for biopsy should be able to be visualized sonographically if aligned correctly. Experience results in improving both needle alignment and needle visualization.

# PROCEDURE

## ROLE OF THE SONOGRAPHER

The sonographer plays an important role in interventional procedures. It is important for him or her to locate the pathology of interest and offer his or her recommendation for the best and safest approach. Interventional sonographers not only possess basic sonographic knowledge but also must be able to optimize images for the detection of subtle masses and utilize features such as color Doppler to find a biopsy path that does not course through a blood vessel. The sonographer must also be familiar with instrumentation technologies to include harmonics, compound imaging, and consider transducer selection based on the area of interest, location, foot print size, and transmit frequency. During the procedure, the sonographer makes use of different patient positioning techniques that aid in the best approach and is aware of how breathing affects the movement of the mass. The sonographer is one of the first people the patient interacts with and can reassure the patient with a simple smile and an introduction to the procedure. Building a positive rapport from the beginning is invaluable. The sonographer can coach and

support the patient during the procedure to put them at ease and to make the procedure easier for all involved.

## PREPROCEDURE

After the patient's medical record is evaluated for appropriate history, lab values, and other imaging studies, informed consent must be obtained. Written informed consent has a detailed explanation of the major complications and should be discussed in the patient's native language. The patient should be apprised of the indications and alternatives, and should be able to understand and cooperate with instructions before and during the procedure.[8] After informed consent is obtained, everyone in the procedure room must pause for a time out. A time out allows the staff to verify the correct patient is present and confirm the procedure and procedure site. The sonographer may document the time out on an image (Fig. 27-4). Before, during, and

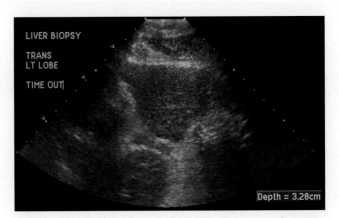

Figure 27-4 Time out. The procedure type, location, and time are documented when a "Time Out" is taken during the procedure.

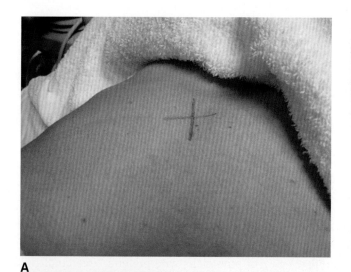

**A**

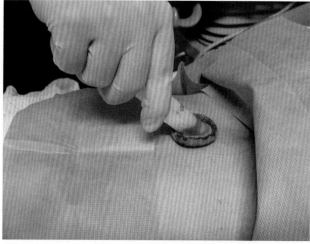

**B**

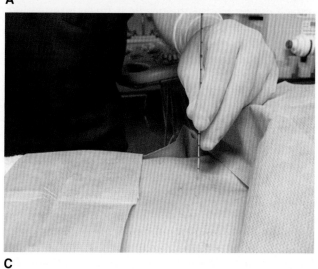

**C**

**Figure 27-5** Preprocedure. These images were obtained during the preprocedure setup for a left lobe liver biopsy. **A:** An "X" is placed over the best location for sampling. **B:** The area is then cleaned with an antiseptic solution and covered with sterile drapes. **C:** The biopsy gun is being lined up before being inserted for sampling.

after the procedure, a radiology nurse monitors vital signs by electrocardiogram (ECG) and pulse oximetry.

One of the pitfalls of biopsy is performing the procedure on the incorrect mass. The best way to avoid this is having the images from the prior exam in the procedure room for immediate and direct comparison. Next, a limited sonography examination must be performed to confirm the results of the prior exam and to determine the best biopsy approach. Possible approaches will be discussed with the performing physician and an "X" should be placed on the area where the needle will break the skin line (Fig. 27-5). Measuring the distance from the skin to the area of interest will help determine the length of the procedure needle needed (Fig. 27-6). During the procedure, it is preferable for the sonographer to stand on the opposite side of the stretcher than the physician but on the same side as the imaging equipment for ease of use. In the case requiring the sonographer to be positioned on the side opposite the sonography equipment or behind the physician, support staff can be directed to adjust instrumentation controls. It is always important to use optimal scanning ergonomics.

Most sonography-guided biopsies are performed on an outpatient basis and the patient can leave after completion or after a few hours of observation. There are generally no dietary restrictions before a biopsy; however, some institutions recommend nothing by mouth

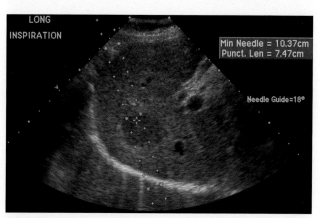

**Figure 27-6** Needle guide. By using the needle guide mode on the sonography equipment, the sonographer can determine the minimum needle and puncture lengths to the area of interest. Note the parallel white dots that offer a guide as to where the needle will travel during the probe-guided biopsy.

(NPO) or only having a light breakfast prior to a liver biopsy to contract the gallbladder. Patients may experience some level of anxiousness before the procedure and medication is prescribed and administered on a case-by-case basis. Many biopsies are performed using only 1% lidocaine as a local anesthetic to relieve pain. The injection of lidocaine can be described to the patient as a "bee sting." Increasing the pH of 1% lidocaine by adding one part of 1 mEq/mL of sodium bicarbonate to 9 or 10 parts lidocaine can reduce the discomfort and enhance anesthetic tissue dispersion. For deeper or painful lesions, conscious sedation with intravenous Versed (midazolam) or Valium (diazepam) and pain control with Dilaudid (hydromorphone hydrochloride) or Sublimaze (fentanyl) is used.[7] The level of sedation should be carefully monitored so that patients can still cooperate with inspiration and expiration requests. Intravenous access can be established to administer medications during or after the procedure.

## PROCEDURE

All patients are vulnerable to infection; therefore, aseptic or sterile technique must be maintained during the procedure. Sterile technique prevents contamination to the patient and to the specimen obtained by eliminating microorganisms. Those involved directly in the procedure will wear sterile gloves and the ultrasound transducer may be covered with a sterile plastic sheath (Fig. 27-7). The biopsy site will be cleaned with an antiseptic solution and draped. The transducer cover may degrade the quality of the ultrasound image and in such cases a povidone-iodine

(Betadine) solution can preserve sterility and act as an acoustic medium.

Because one of the greatest benefits is real-time visualization, the majority of sonography-guided interventional exams use the procedure. Biopsies are performed probe-guided or free hand. The probe-guided technique uses a needle guide fixed to the ultrasound transducer. The main advantage of this technique is that it keeps the needle within the plane of the sonographic image as it is advanced toward the biopsy target. The disadvantage is, however, the fixed relationship between the needle and probe reduces operator freedom in choosing the needle path.[9] When the transducer guide attachment is utilized, the needle guide mode on the sonography equipment can display the path the needle will travel (Fig. 27-8). For physicians who prefer a "freehand" approach during biopsy, the needle is freely inserted into the patient without the use of a needle guide. The freehand technique requires the operator to manipulate the sonography probe with one hand and the biopsy needle with the other (Fig. 27-9). The chief advantage is its versatility. The probe and needle can be positioned independently to achieve the best image of the lesion and a needle path free of intervening structures. To monitor the needle tip on its course to the target, the operator must maintain the needle within the plane of the ultrasound beam.[9]

## POSTPROCEDURE

Regardless of the method used for biopsy, representative images must be made during and after the procedure. Postprocedural images evaluate for

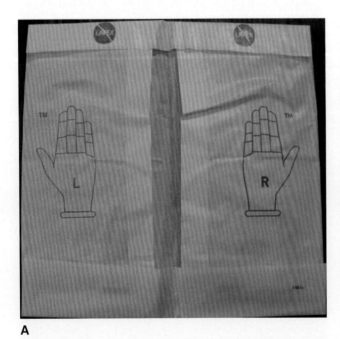

**A**

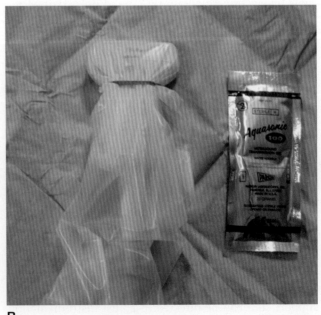

**B**

**Figure 27-7** Sterile technique. **A:** Sterile gloves and **(B)** a transducer covered by a sterile sheath help maintain an aseptic environment. The sterile gel is usually located within the transducer cover. The commercially available prepackaged sterile gloves and transducer covers help maintain sterile technique and reduce the risk of infection.

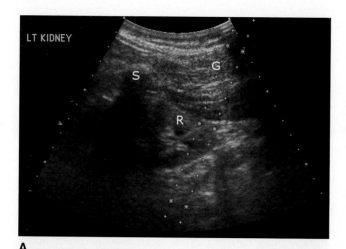

**A**

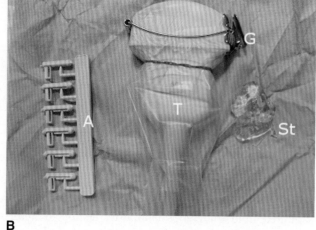

**B**

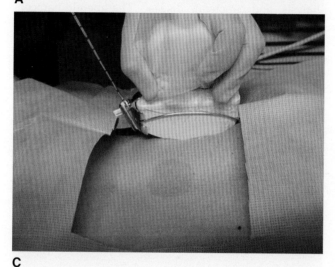

**C**

**Figure 27-8** Probe-guided procedure. **A:** The biopsy guide offers a representative pathway the needle will travel during the procedure. The image was right–left inverted for this renal biopsy. Inverting the image and transducer facilitates many biopsy procedures. *R,* kidney; *S,* rib shadow. **B:** The transducer *(T)* is prepared for the procedure. The reusable sterile biopsy bracket *(G)* is placed on the transducer over the sterile cover. The disposable sterile needle guides *(A)* are available in a variety of gauges and clip onto the biopsy bracket. Sterile gel *(St)* is placed on the sterile drape for use during the procedure. **C:** The needle is being inserted through the needle guide.

complications such as hematomas. After a superficial biopsy, the patient may be given an ice pack to hold over the incision site. Cold ice causes the capillaries to contract and facilitates clotting. The patient is typically monitored for 2 to 4 hours postliver biopsy. Vital signs will be taken after the procedure and before the patient is discharged.

## COMPLICATIONS AND RISKS

The complications of a sonography-guided biopsy are rare but those involved in the procedure as well as the patient undergoing the biopsy should be aware of them. The majority of these procedures are simple, safe, and performed as an outpatient procedure. Performing a minimally invasive biopsy can prevent the patient from undergoing unnecessary surgery. Localized pain, vasovagal reaction, and hematoma formation are the most commonly encountered complications, but the complications could become as serious as death. The incidence of hematoma is related to the number of passes and needle gauge necessary to obtain an adequate sample. Pain may be more common with lesions or masses that are situated deeply. Other complications include swelling, pancreatitis, biliary leakage, peritonitis, and pneumothorax. Anytime the skin is punctured, there is a risk of bleeding and infection, which diminishes by maintaining sterile technique. Infrequently, the needle may pass through a nonintended target such as a vessel, loop

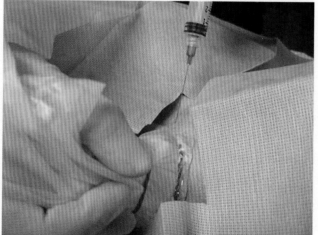

**Figure 27-9** Freehand technique. This left thyroid fine-needle aspiration is performed using the freehand technique. The needle is freely inserted into the patient without the use of a transducer guide using real-time visualization to guide positioning the needle.

of bowel, or an adjacent structure. The frequency of complications is often related to organ vascularity and location as well as needle gauge selected for the procedure.

## COMMON PROCEDURES

### ABSCESS DRAINAGE

The purpose of abscess drainage is to remove infected fluid, such as pus, from the body. An abscess can form after surgery or an infection such as appendicitis. Abscess drainages are usually performed if a patient has been on antibiotics with no change in symptoms. The aspirated fluid undergoes laboratory testing to determine what, if any, antibiotics could successfully treat the condition. An abscess can form anywhere in the body and the drainage may include the insertion of a tube or aspirating the fluid into a syringe (Fig. 27-10).

### ADRENAL BIOPSY

The adrenal glands biopsy on the organs located superior to each kidney may be performed if there is either a unilateral or a bilateral adrenal gland mass. Due to anatomic location, the right adrenal gland is more amendable to a sonography-guided biopsy through a transhepatic approach. Accurate patient positioning is crucial for success. The procedure may require an oblique, decubitus, or even a prone position.

### PARACENTESIS

A paracentesis procedure is used to remove ascites. The paracentesis can be performed for diagnostic or therapeutic reasons. Diagnostic indications include a new onset of ascites and ascites of unknown etiology. The collected fluid can be sent for laboratory examination to diagnose its cause and determine if it is infected. The most common causes of ascites are cirrhosis and malignancy. Other causes include heart failure, tuberculosis, dialysis, and pancreatic disease. Therapeutic paracentesis is performed when the cause is already known and the fluid is removed for patient comfort. The entire abdomen is evaluated before paracentesis to locate the largest or deepest pocket (Fig. 27-11). A left lower quadrant site is generally the best as the abdominal wall is relatively thinner and the depth of fluid is typically greater.[10] When evaluating the abdomen for the largest pocket of fluid, it is important not to apply excess probe pressure as it distorts and diminishes the actual volume of fluid (Fig. 27-12).

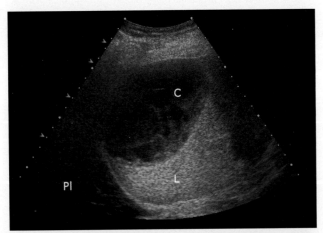

**A**

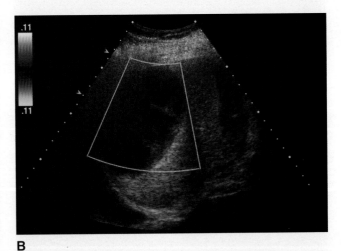

**B**

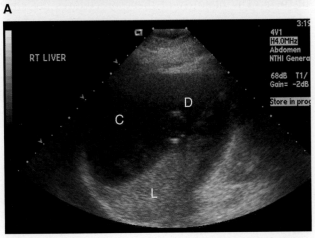

**C**

**Figure 27-10** Fluid drainage. The patient presents for a sonography-guided drainage procedure of the right liver. **A:** Longitudinal imaging of the right liver lobe shows a complex area in the liver and the patient also has a pleural effusion. **B:** The color Doppler demonstrates no flow within the complex area. **C:** The echogenic circle is the end of the drainage catheter. *C,* complex area; *L,* liver; *Pl,* pleural effusion; *D,* drainage catheter.

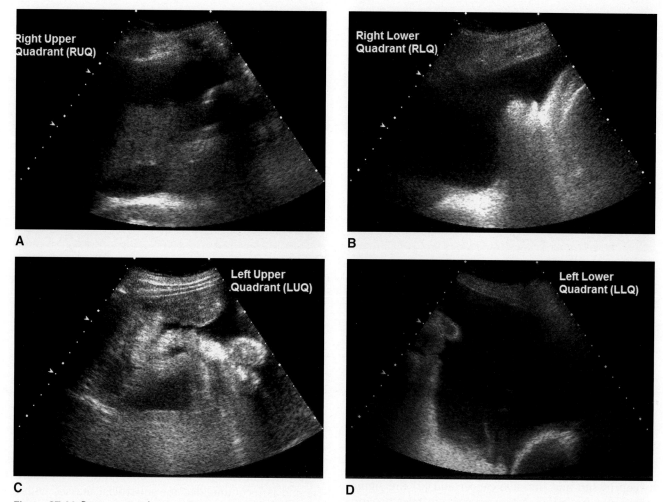

**Figure 27-11** Paracentesis planning. Prior to a paracentesis, images are made from all four abdominal quadrants. **A–D:** When comparing these longitudinal sections from the four anatomic locations in the same patient, ascites is demonstrated throughout the abdomen. For this patient, the best area for catheter placement is the left lower quadrant *(LLQ)*, which contains the most fluid.

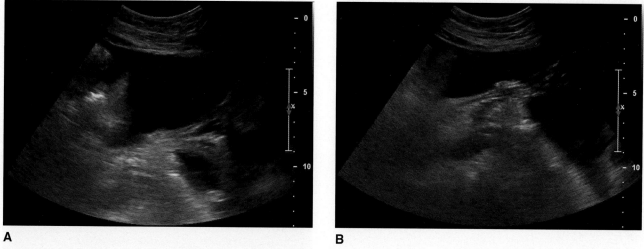

**Figure 27-12** Probe pressure. The two sonograms of the right upper quadrant show how probe pressure affects the amount of ascites visualized. **A:** Image made with light probe pressure. **B:** Image made with a moderate amount of probe pressure, which makes the amount of ascites appear less than in **(A)**.

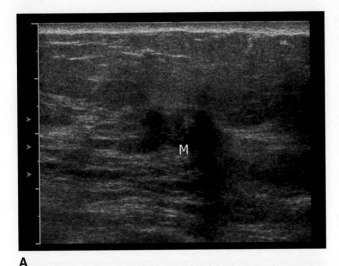

**A**

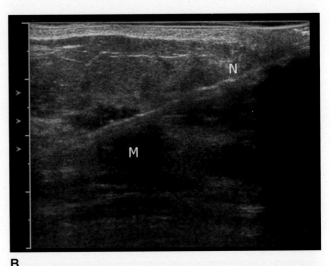

**B**

**Figure 27-13** Core biopsy. **A:** The sonogram made prior to the biopsy procedure demonstrates the location of a solid breast mass (M). **B:** During the core biopsy, the sonogram demonstrates both the solid breast mass (M) and the echogenic line of the needle (N) within the mass.

## BREAST BIOPSY

Patients presenting with suspicious breast findings are referred for core biopsy, FNA biopsy, or needle localization of a mass. The use of sonography is only advised if the suspected mass is well visualized. For palpable lesions, FNA is able to rapidly provide a diagnosis. A thin needle is used with FNA biopsy to obtain cells for cytologic evaluation. The main disadvantages of FNA breast biopsy are (1) the inability to distinguish between in situ and invasive cancer and (2) the significant rate of nondiagnostic samples and false-negative results primarily attributed to inexperience of the individual obtaining the biopsy.[11] A core needle biopsy offers a more definitive histologic diagnosis, avoids inadequate samples, and may permit the distinction between invasive versus in situ cancer (Fig. 27-13). For nonpalpable abnormalities, the core biopsy is replacing wire localization and excision.[11] A clip is placed in the area of a core sample to identify the region on follow-up examinations or subsequent wire localization and excision. Wire localization performed using ultrasound guidance is faster and better tolerated than the comparable mammographic localization (Fig. 27-14). In women with nonpalpable microcalcifications, the use of wire localization and excision is tailored to each case after collaboration between the radiologist and surgeon. Symptomatic cysts may undergo a sonography-guided aspiration (Fig. 27-15).

## LIVER BIOPSY

A liver biopsy is performed after a thorough clinical evaluation in patients with abnormal biochemical tests or liver lesions. Sonography-guided liver biopsy can be performed with either a fine needle (FNA) or by obtaining a core sample. Indications include the diagnosis, grading and staging of parenchymal liver diseases,

abnormal liver tests with unknown etiology, fever of unknown origin, diagnosis of a mass, and developing treatment plans based on histologic analysis.[12] Proper patient preparation is essential because it can reduce complications. Coagulation studies are obtained because some liver disorders elevate bleeding times. Patients are asked to remain NPO or have a light fatty meal to force gallbladder contraction so it is less likely to be injured. The success of sonography-guided focal liver lesions is highly dependent on obtaining enough tissue for analysis and is recommended for superficial masses with a diameter greater than 3 cm.[12] A liver FNA is used to sample suspected masses, whereas a core sample allows for parenchymal disease to be assessed (Fig. 27-16). The left lobe is easily biopsied using a subxiphoid approach. This approach is generally better tolerated by

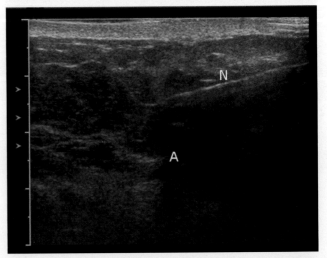

**Figure 27-14** Needle localization. The sonogram shows the echogenic line representing a needle (N), which was inserted near a suspicious breast lesion (A). The needle placement helps guide the surgeon to the area of interest. The patient did have the area removed and the specimen was evaluated for malignancy.

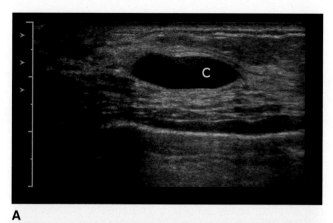

**A**

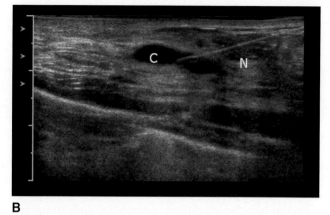

**B**

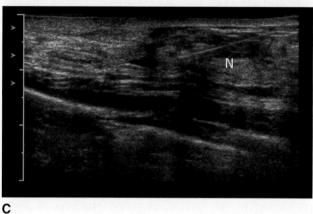

**C**

**Figure 27-15** Breast cyst aspiration. **A:** Prior to the aspiration procedure, a sonogram shows an anechoic cyst *(C)*. **B:** During the procedure, the needle *(N)* tip can be seen within the cyst *(C)*. **C:** As the procedure progresses, the sonogram shows the cyst was aspirated completely and the needle *(N)* is still seen in place.

patients and is more accurate than a blind right lobe biopsy.[13] Complications include bile leak, pneumothorax, and hematoma formation. After the biopsy samples are completed, postprocedural images should be obtained to evaluate for potential complications.

## LUNG BIOPSY

Sonography is becoming more widely accepted and offers a safer alternative to CT for biopsy of the pleural space, lung, and mediastinal masses. Indications

![Liver biopsy sonogram](Figure 27-16)

**Figure 27-16** Liver biopsy. The transverse sonogram made during a core biopsy of a hypoechoic liver mass *(M)* shows the needle *(N)* within the liver *(L)*. The pathology results on this patient confirmed the diagnosis of hepatocellular carcinoma. *I*, inferior vena cava. (Image courtesy of Maria Radke RDMS, RVT, Vineland, NJ.)

include evaluation of a previously found abnormality, mass, or pleural effusion. Sonography-guided lung biopsies are commonly performed on masses close to a rib or the diaphragm. Due to the variation of lung location during respiration, the procedure should be performed in a single breath to minimize complications. Depending on the location of the mass, different patient positions may be necessary in order to determine the safest approach. Complications include pneumothorax, bleeding in the lung, and infection.

## LYMPH NODE BIOPSY

Lymph nodes are part of the immune system and are found in the neck, behind the ears, in the axilla, and in the chest, abdomen, inguinal area, and groin. Normal lymph nodes are usually hard to feel and difficult to visualize sonographically. Lymph nodes can enlarge and become tender usually as a result of some type of infection. The swelling can also be caused by a cut, scratch, insect bite, tattoo, drug reaction, or malignancy. Most lymph nodes are superficial and amendable to a sonography-guided biopsy. The sonographer can use the curved or linear transducer and apply moderate pressure to reduce the distance the needle must travel and to move adjacent bowel out of the way. Color Doppler is used to avoid any blood vessels that course within the needle path. Lymph nodes can be sampled by FNA or core biopsy.

## MUSCULOSKELETAL BIOPSY

Sonography is used to localize masses found throughout the body for biopsy. Sonographic guidance can be used to efficiently acquire specimens from a variety of soft tissue tumors and disease processes. If biopsy of a soft tissue malignancy is performed, consultation with the surgeon is necessary to ensure that the biopsy tract is removed during the surgical procedure. Both fine-needle and core needle biopsy specimens can be obtained. Sonography can also be used to localize affected muscle groups and biopsy bone lesions when cortical destruction is present and to facilitate the passage of a needle into the medullary cavity.[7] Complications include bone fracture of the biopsy site, neurologic injury secondary to anesthetizing major motor nerves that may create paresis or paralysis, and bleeding or infection.

## PANCREATIC BIOPSY

Pancreatic biopsy is indicated whenever there is a pancreatic mass or pancreatitis of unknown etiology. Sonographically, the pancreas can be difficult to visualize due to its anatomic location and during biopsy bowel gas may obscure the image. During the procedure, moderate probe pressure can move and keep bowel loops away as well as shorten the needle path. Color Doppler is used to search for blood vessels and determine the safest biopsy route (Fig. 27-17). Despite its location and relational anatomy, complications during pancreatic biopsy are rare.

## THORACENTESIS

Thoracentesis is the removal of pleural fluid and the procedure can be performed for diagnostic or therapeutic purposes. Diagnostic indications include a unilateral effusion, bilateral effusions of different sizes, pleurisy, fever, an ECG and laboratory values inconsistent with heart failure, and an effusion that does not resolve with heart failure therapy. A sonogram to evaluate pleural fluid should be performed with the patient in the same position as during the thoracentesis, preferably upright leaning over a table. Sonography is used to localize fluid collections especially loculated effusions[14] (Fig. 27-18). The puncture site should be one to two rib spaces below the level at which breath sounds decrease or disappear on auscultation, above the ninth rib to avoid subdiaphragmatic puncture, and midway between the spine and posterior axillary line where the ribs are easily palpated. Therapeutic paracentesis is performed when the cause is already known and the fluid is removed for patient comfort. Complications include pain, bleeding, pneumothorax, infection, spleen or liver puncture, and vasovagal events.

## PROSTATE BIOPSY

The prostate is biopsied to confirm malignancy. Indications for biopsy include elevated prostate specific antigen (PSA), abnormal digital rectal examination, or palpable nodules. Before the procedure, the patient receives enema to clear the feces in the rectum that could obscure imaging. The patient is most commonly positioned in left lateral decubitus position. A high-frequency endocavitary transducer is inserted into the rectum to evaluate the prostate. The prostate should be surveyed in sagittal and coronal planes and a volume measurement should be recorded. Prostate cancer occurs most frequently in the peripheral zone; therefore, adequate sampling must be obtained from this region. Many techniques have been established but the most common uses the coronal plane and two representative samples are taken from the apex, base, and mid segments, from the right and left as well as a sample from the central zone. Additional samples should be obtained from suspicious or hypoechoic areas[15]

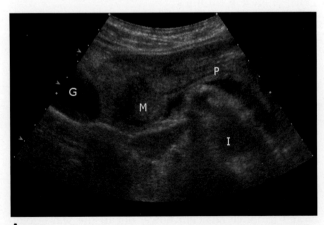

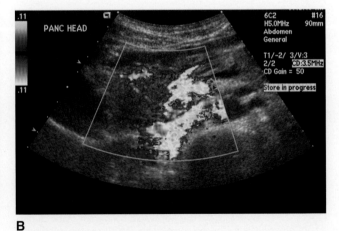

**A**     **B**

**Figure 27-17** Pancreatic mass. **A:** The gray scale transverse image of the pancreas (P) demonstrates a mass (M) in the pancreatic head. The gallbladder (G) is seen lateral to the pancreatic head. The inferior vena cava (I) is seen posterior to the pancreas. **B:** A color Doppler image demonstrates the surrounding vascularity. (Images courtesy of Maria Radke, RDMS, RVT, Vineland, NJ.)

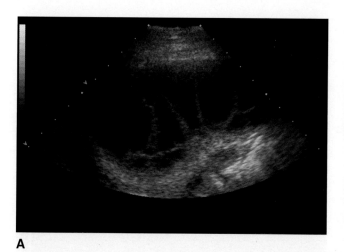
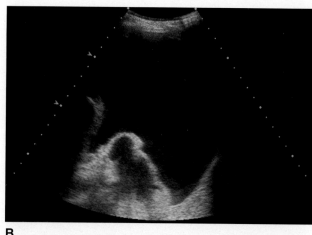

**A**                                                                      **B**

**Figure 27-18** Pleural effusion. **A:** The sonogram of the left pleural space prior to thoracentesis demonstrates loculations in the fluid. The loculations may limit the amount of fluid aspirated. **B:** This sonogram on a different patient demonstrates a large right pleural effusion.

(Fig. 27-19). When obtaining biopsy samples on the left side, puncturing the urethra is a complication that can be avoided by inverting the transducer right to left while rotating the transducer 180 degrees. Other complications include vasovagal episodes, rectal bleeding, and hematuria.

## PSEUDOANEURYSM REPAIR

A pseudoaneurysm forms when an arterial puncture site fails to seal, which allows arterial blood to spread into the surrounding tissues and form a pulsatile hematoma. They typically occur in the femoral artery and are iatrogenic. The number of pseudoaneurysms has increased significantly due to the exponential growth of interventional cardiology (Fig. 27-20). Several therapeutic strategies have been developed to treat this complication. They include sonography-guided compression repair, surgical repair, and minimally invasive percutaneous treatments such as thrombin injection.

It is important to note that sonography-guided compression repair has considerable drawbacks, including long procedure time, patient discomfort, and a relatively high-recurrence rate in patients receiving anticoagulant therapy. Compression repair has been shown to be less successful in patients with pseudoaneurysms larger than 3 to 4 cm in diameter and those who cannot tolerate the associated discomfort. Complications include acute pseudoaneurysmal enlargement, rupture, vasovagal reactions, deep vein thrombosis, atrial fibrillation, and angina. Moreover, sonography-guided compression repair requires the availability of an ultrasound device and the presence of skilled personnel during the procedure. The technique involves applying compression on the pseudoaneurysm neck with the ultrasound transducer until the flow within the neck is obliterated. Pressure is applied for a period of 1 minute, with the procedure repeated 10 times. At the end of each period, compression is released briefly to assess pseudoaneurysm patency and to reposition the transducer.

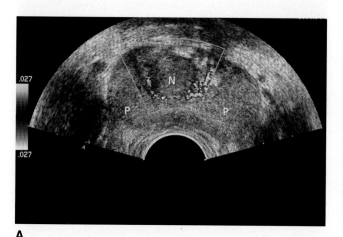
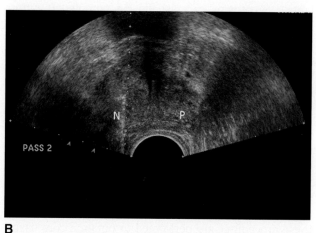

**A**                                                                      **B**

**Figure 27-19** Prostate biopsy. **A:** Before the biopsy, the prostate gland (P) is evaluated for nodules. This color flow image demonstrates a nodule (N) which will be sampled. **B:** During the biopsy, the prostate gland sonogram demonstrates the needle as an echogenic line (N) along the needle guide (dotted line).

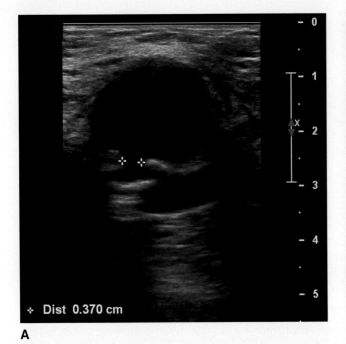

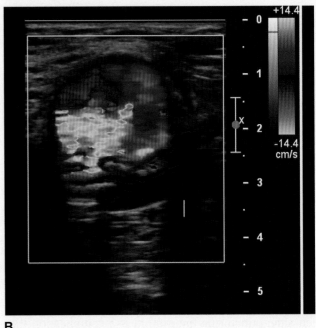

**A**                                                            **B**

**Figure 27-20** Pseudoaneurysm. **A:** A transverse sonogram on a patient following postcardiac catheterizations demonstrates pseudoaneurysm in the common femoral artery. The neck is marked by calipers and is small enough for a thrombin injection intervention. **B:** The color Doppler sonogram demonstrates turbulent flow within the pseudoaneurysm.

Care must be taken to avoid compromising flow within the underlying femoral artery. After successful thrombosis patients should be kept supine for a few hours, with the affected leg in the stretched position.

Percutaneous thrombin injection has gained popularity despite complications associated with the initial use of high-dose thrombin (average dose of 1,100 IU). The technique was refined when low-dose thrombin injections were studied and proven to have the same efficacy and consistently high-success rates. Compared with surgical repair, treatment of pseudoaneurysms with thrombin injection offers many advantages. The success rate of thrombin injection is 97%, even with patients treated with therapeutic levels of anticoagulants.[16] Treatment can usually be completed within several minutes. Complications of thrombin injection include distal migration of the thrombin. It is also possible that if the thrombin is injected in a diluted concentration, it may not remain in the cavity long enough to form a clot.

## RENAL BIOPSY

Renal biopsies are typically performed on the basis of clinical history or laboratory values. Indications include isolated glomerular hematuria, isolated nonnephrotic proteinuria, nephritic syndrome, acute nephritic syndrome, and unexplained acute renal failure. Generally, these procedures are performed to obtain a core tissue sample to evaluate parenchymal and glomeruli disease rather than sample a mass and as such, the kidney with

the least associated risk is biopsied.[17] Biopsy of a renal transplant can also be performed to evaluate for graft rejection. A lower pole biopsy site is optimal due to a decreased risk of major vessel puncture. Renal biopsies are performed probe-guided, not free hand to minimize risk and improve success. The kidney is sampled in the sagittal plane with the patient in the prone position. Inverting the image right to left and turning the transducer so that the notch points toward the patient's feet can aid in biopsy access (Fig. 27-21). Complications include

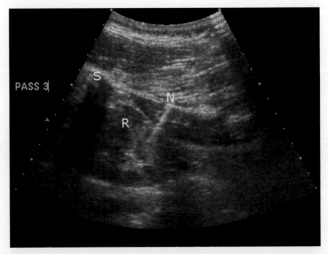

**Figure 27-21** Renal biopsy. The left kidney sonogram is inverted right-left, which facilitates both transducer and biopsy needle placement. The echogenic line represents the needle (N) as it obtains the sample. R, left renal tissue; S, rib shadow.

pain, infection, hematoma formation, and rarely, puncture of the adjacent organs.

## THYROID AND NECK BIOPSY

Thyroid, parathyroid, and other neck masses can be safely sampled by FNA. The success of FNA depends on the size of the lesion and the extent of cystic involvement.[18] Recent literature discourages FNA on nodules less than 10 mm because these microcarcinomas infrequently metastasize and carry a small risk of recurrence and mortality after surgical removal. Sonography offers real-time visualization; however, accurately aspirating cells from nodules smaller than 10 mm is difficult and may lead to false-negative results. The Society of Radiologists in Ultrasound (SRU) guidelines recommend FNA of nodules 10 mm or greater only when microcalcifications are present, 15 mm or greater if completely or predominantly solid or if coarse calcifications are present, and 20 mm or greater if predominantly cystic with a solid component[19] (Fig. 27-22). Cystic nodules offer a cytologic

diagnostic challenge because negative findings are not reliable but a finding of malignancy is reliable. For nodules that are complex, the cystic competent can be aspirated followed by sampling of the residual solid component.[20] If a large cystic mass is causing pain or discomfort, the cyst can be aspirated to alleviate symptoms (Fig. 27-23). Doppler ultrasound is used to evaluate any vessels that may lie in the needle path. Another technique used for obtaining cells is the fine-needle capillary (FNC) technique. Advantages of FNC include minimal trauma, tissue pressure, and capillary action. This method removes the syringe plunger and only uses the to-and-fro motion of the needle to obtain cells. The technique aspirates a smaller but more concentrated sample. FNC does not obtain as many cells as FNA and having a cytopathologist evaluate the specimens during the procedure drastically increases the overall accuracy as they can determine if additional tissues are required for diagnosis. For these procedures, the patient is supine and has both arms to the side. A rolled towel can be placed under the nape of the neck. This eases stress and makes the anterior neck

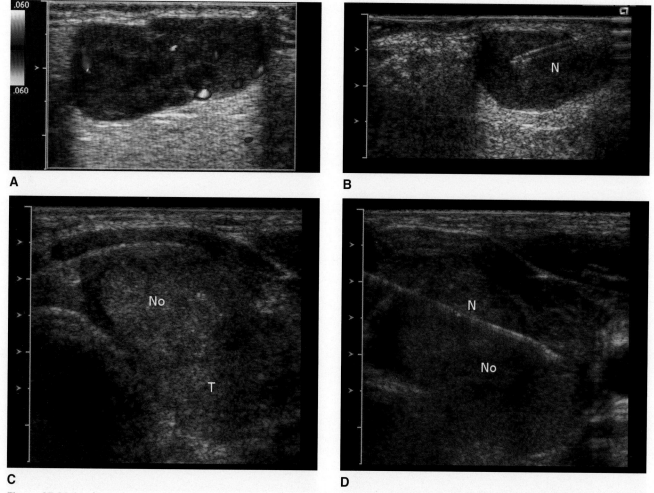

**Figure 27-22** Neck masses. **A:** A color Doppler image demonstrates a parotid mass. **B:** During fine-needle aspiration (FNA) biopsy of a parotid mass, the needle is clearly visible within the mass *(N)*. This mass was diagnosed as an early malignancy. **C,D.** The sonograms show a large thyroid nodule *(No)* that underwent successful FNA. The needle *(N)* can be seen within the nodule. *T,* thyroid. *(continued)*

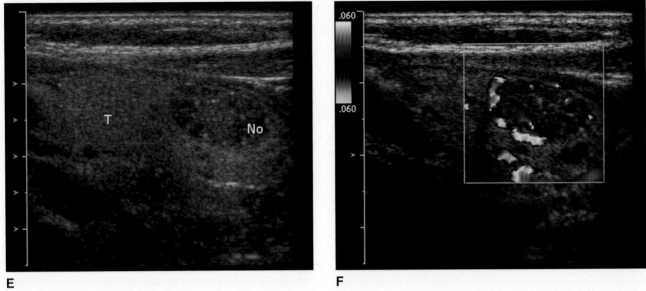

**E**

**F**

**Figure 27-22** *(continued)* **E,F:** The longitudinal sonograms of the thyroid gland *(T)* demonstrate vascular flow to a heterogeneous nodule *(No)* with microcalcifications in the lower pole of the gland. Microcalcifications increase the risk of malignancy.

more accessible. Complications include pain, bleeding, infection, and puncture of adjacent vessels such as the internal jugular vein or carotid artery.

## SUMMARY

- Sonography-guided interventional procedures include fluid drainages, tube placements, biopsies, fine-needle aspirations, and core biopsies.

- Benefits of sonography-guided interventional procedures include no ionizing radiation, less invasive than surgery, less expensive than alternative procedures,

can be performed with the patient in different positions, allows for real-time visualization of procedure, and color Doppler can aid in vessel visualization.

- Contraindications to sonography-guided procedures include coagulopathy, unsafe biopsy route, and an uncooperative patient.

- Fine-needle aspiration is performed with a thin needle, 20- to 27-gauge, attached to a syringe to remove cells for evaluation.

- Core biopsy is performed with a larger gauge, 14- to 19-gauge, biopsy gun and is used to remove a larger sample of tissue.

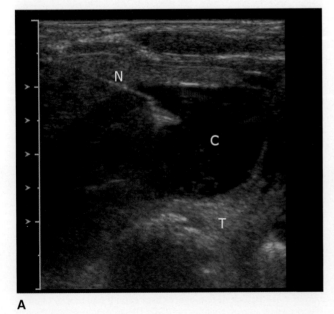

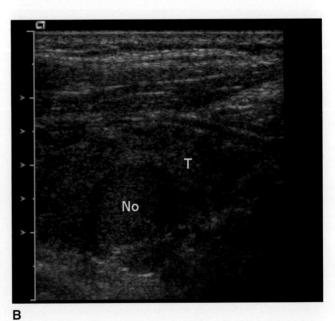

**A**

**B**

**Figure 27-23** Thyroid lesions. **A:** During an aspiration of a thyroid cyst *(C)* this sonogram was made and demonstrates the needle *(N)* within the cyst. *T,* thyroid. **B:** A subtle thyroid nodule *(No)* in the thyroid *(T)* parenchyma demonstrates the need to carefully survey the entire gland.

## Critical Thinking Questions

1. A patient presents for a fine-needle aspiration of a solid thyroid nodule. Explain the procedure to his or her including the potential risks.

2. A 58-year-old man presents with a palpable, pulsatile mass in his right groin 1 day postcardiac catheterization. What is the most likely diagnosis? Describe the options available to treat this condition.

3. What laboratory tests are indicated prior to an interventional procedure such as sonography-guided liver biopsy?

4. Which has a larger diameter, a 14-gauge needle or a 22-gauge needle?

5. What precautions are taken to limit the risk of infection during a sonography-guided interventional procedure?

• The size and type of needle chosen depends on the type of procedure, area of interest, amount of tissue needed for evaluation, and the risk involved. Needle gauge is inversely proportional to the diameter of the needle.

• A needle-guide keeps the needle in plane with the transducer for easier visualization but limits the path the needle can take; freehand procedures allow for more versatility, as the needle and transducer can be maneuvered independently, but needle visualization can be a challenge. The needle is best seen when the needle is in the same plane as the ultrasound beam and is more perpendicular to the transducer.

• Potential complications of interventional procedures include localized pain, vasovagal reaction, hematoma formation, and infection.

• Common sonography-guided interventional procedures include abscess drainage, adrenal biopsy, diagnostic and therapeutic paracentesis, breast biopsy, liver biopsy, lung biopsy, lymph node biopsy, musculoskeletal biopsy, pancreatic biopsy, diagnostic and therapeutic thoracentesis, prostate biopsy, pseudoaneurysm repair, renal biopsy, and thyroid biopsy.

### REFERENCES

1. DeJong R. Ultrasound-guided interventional techniques. In: Hagan-Ansert S, ed. *Textbook of Diagnostic Ultrasonography*. Vol 1. 6th ed. St. Louis, MO: Elsevier Mosby; 2006: 432–454.
2. Ultrasound-guided biopsy and drainage of the abdomen and pelvis. In: Rumack CM, Wilson SR, Charboneau JW, eds. *Diagnostic Ultrasound*. Vol 1. 3rd ed. St. Louis, MO: Elsevier Mosby; 2005:625–655.
3. Humes D. Kelley's *Textbook of Internal Medicine*. 3rd ed. Philadelphia, PA: Lippincott Williams & Wilkins; 2000.
4. Shin HJ, Amaral JG, Armstrong D, et al. Image-guided percutaneous biopsy of musculoskeletal lesions in children. *Pediatr Radiol*. 2007;37:362–369.
5. Afify AM, Al-Khafaji BM, Kim B, et al. Endoscopic ultrasound-guided fine needle aspiration of the pancreas: diagnostic utility and accuracy. *Acta Cytol*. 2003;47:341–348.
6. Shah VI, Raju U, Chitale D, et al. False-negative core needle biopsies of the breast: an analysis of clinical, radiologic, and pathologic findings in 27 consecutive cases of missed breast cancer. *Cancer*. 2003;97:1824–1831.
7. Hallet R. Musculoskeletal biopsy: percutaneous needle technique. Musculoskeletal procedures, 2009.*eMedicine: Medscape*. Available at http://emedicine.medscape.com/article/399094-overview. Accessed 24 May 2010.
8. Rockey DC, Caldwell SH, Goodman ZD, et al. Liver biopsy. *Hepatology*. 2009;49:1017–1044.
9. Pramit P, Brooks D, Wolfe R. Sonographically guided biopsy of focal lesions: a comparison of freehand and probe-guided techniques using a phantom. *AJR Am J Roentgenol*. 2005;184:1652–1656.
10. Thompson TW, Shaffer RW, White B, et al. Paracentesis. *N Engl J Med*. 2007;355:19–23.
11. Verkooijen HM. Diagnostic accuracy of stereotactic large-core needle biopsy for nonpalpable breast disease: results of a multicenter prospective study with 95% surgical confirmation. *Int J Cancer*. 2002;99:853–859.
12. Chhieng DC. Fine needle aspiration biopsy of liver: an update. *World J Surg Oncol*. 2004;2:1186–1194.
13. Plecha DM, Goodwin DW, Rowland DY, et al. Liver biopsy: effects of biopsy needle caliber on bleeding and tissue recovery. *Radiology*. 1997;204:101–104.
14. Koh DM, Burke S, Davies N, et al. Transthoracic ultrasound of the chest: clinical uses and applications. *Radiographics*. 2002;22:15–23.
15. Yang X. *Interpretation of Prostate Biopsy*. 3rd ed. Philadelphia, PA: Lippincott Williams & Wilkins; 2002.
16. Lenartova M, Tak T. Iatrogenic pseudoaneurysm of femoral artery: case report and literature review. *Clin Med Res*. 2003;1:243–247.
17. Campbell SC. In focus: renal cell carcinoma. *Clin Adv Hematol Oncol*. 2008;6:253–258.
18. Titton RL, Gervais DA, Boland GW, et al. Sonography and sonographically guided fine-needle aspiration biopsy of the thyroid gland: indications and techniques, pearls and pitfalls. *AJR Am J Roentgenol*. 2003;181:267–271.
19. McCartney CR, Stukenborg GJ. Decision analysis of discordant thyroid nodule biopsy guideline criteria. *J Clin Endocrinol Metab*. 2008;93:3037–3044.
20. Suen K. Fine-needle aspiration biopsy of the thyroid. *Can Med Assoc J*. 2002;5:167.

# Index